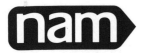

hiv & aids reference manual

edited by gus cairns

contributing editors Robert Fieldhouse (2000-2004)
Keith Alcorn (1995-1999)

August 2007

NAM, Lincoln House, 1 Brixton Road, London, SW9 6DE

In memory of
Martin Fright, Mike Rhodes, Simon Mansfield and Barry Jackson

HIV & AIDS Reference Manual
Twenty-eighth edition, August 2007

ISBN
978-0-9551678-5-0

Copyright ©
NAM 2007

Data conversion by
Thomas Paterson

Proofreading & typesetting by
Anu Liisanantti

Indexing by
Carolyn Partrick

Printed in the UK by
Lithosphere, London

NAM contact details:

email: info@nam.org.uk   tel: 020 7840 0050   fax: 020 7735 5351   website: www.aidsmap.com

NAM, Lincoln House, 1 Brixton Road, London, SW9 6DE   Registered charity number 1011220

NAM — For HIV information

This directory is one of five that makes up the NAM Manual. The Manual helps professionals in HIV sectors around the world with their work by providing the latest information on treatment and care, prevention, the social impact of the epidemic, and comprehensive listings of organisations in the UK, Europe and the world.

The Manual is dedicated to the memory of Martin Fright, Mike Rhodes, Simon Mansfield and Barry Jackson as a tribute to their inspirational contributions to NAM's development and to the broader community response to AIDS.

NAM was founded by Peter Scott in 1987. He was working at the heart of the community affected by HIV - at the London Lesbian and Gay Switchboard. At that time it was important to produce a clear, plain language resource in the face of extensive misinformation about HIV and AIDS, much of it confused and homophobic.

The Manual soon became the UK's primary source of high quality information on all aspects of the epidemic. As its users have grown and diversified within the UK and abroad, so it has been constantly revised, rewritten and adapted to take account of new needs.

NAM now also publishes a wide range of printed, audio and electronic materials for all communities of people with HIV and publishes on the internet at www.aidsmap.com. The work is rooted in the experiences of those most affected by the epidemic.

NAM believes information enables people to take control of their lives and healthcare, develop better dialogues with their healthcare staff and so live longer, healthier lives.

Table of contents

HIV testing

HIV prevention

Drug use and harm reduction

Hepatitis co-infection

TB and HIV

HIV and Black African Communities in the UK

Women and HIV

Children, adolescents and families

Haemophilia

HIV and prisoners

The law and HIV

Employment and HIV

Mental health and quality of life

HIV and AIDS

HIV

HIV stands for human immunodeficiency virus. It was originally isolated in Paris in May 1983 by Luc Montagnier. It belongs to a group of viruses called retroviruses.

Retroviruses copy their genetic material into the genetic material of human cells. This means that infected cells stay infected for the rest of their lives.

Through mechanisms which are still not fully understood, HIV prevents the immune system from working properly. Normally, the body's immune system would fight off infection. But HIV is able to infect key cells (called CD4 cells) which co-ordinate the immune system's fight against infection.

Many are destroyed during the first few weeks of infection. Subsequently CD4 cells, both infected and others which are not themselves infected, as well as other parts of the immune system, no longer work properly. This is thought to be because the presence of HIV keeps the immune system in a state of over-activation which eventually drains its resources.

AIDS

AIDS stands for acquired immune deficiency syndrome. AIDS is the result of the damage to the immune system caused by HIV.

A damaged immune system is unable to protect the body against certain specific 'opportunistic' infections and tumours. These are called opportunistic because they are caused by organisms which are normally controlled by the immune system but which 'take the opportunity' to cause disease if the immune system has been damaged.

The opportunistic infections which are considered to be 'AIDS-defining' are listed in the *HIV & AIDS Treatments Directory*. Unlike most other diseases, different people with AIDS may experience different clinical problems, depending on which specific opportunistic infections they develop. This is what a syndrome means - a collection of different signs and symptoms that are all part of the same underlying medical condition.

HIV and the causes of AIDS

It is generally accepted throughout the scientific community that infection with HIV is the necessary pre-condition for the development of AIDS.

It is evidently possible for an individual's immune system to be compromised in other ways, and in rare cases this can lead to the same kinds of infection as those seen in AIDS. This has been termed idiopathic CD4 lymphocytopenia or ICL. The immune suppression seen in ICL is not always the same as in AIDS however, often clearing up without treatment.

Opportunistic infections can also occur in patients whose immune systems have been suppressed by medical interventions, such as transplant patients and ones receiving cancer chemotherapy.

Although it is clear that HIV has a central role in the development of AIDS, other factors play an important role in the development of immune damage.

Some other diseases such as other sexually transmitted infections or malaria may play an additional role both in accelerating the course of AIDS and in making individuals more vulnerable to infection in the first place.

A person's general state of health is important; fatigue, poor nutrition and recreational drug use are among many other factors that may suppress the immune system. Some studies have found that people in certain developing countries develop AIDS faster, possibly for these reasons.

Lastly, so-called 'host factors' are very important. The individual's genetic makeup may make them more or less vulnerable to the damage caused by HIV.

See the *HIV & AIDS Treatments Directory* for a full discussion of these issues.

HIV transmission

HIV is present in the blood (including menstrual blood), semen and vaginal and rectal secretions of infected people, but can only be passed on to another person if those fluids get into his/her body. Although sophisticated laboratory techniques are able to isolate the virus from other body fluids of infected people, such as saliva, the level of virus in these fluids is far too low to be infectious.

Thus, the main ways in which HIV is transmitted are:

- Through unprotected anal or vaginal sex. HIV is unable to pass through good quality condoms, such as those bearing the CE mark, if they are used consistently and properly.

- It has been a subject of controversy for years as to whether HIV can be passed on during oral sex. It now does look as if a small proportion of infections - from 0.5% to 3% - get passed on this way. The risk is solely to the 'receptive' partner, i.e. the one 'doing it'.

- Through blood-to-blood contact. This mainly happens through the sharing of injecting equipment amongst injecting

drug users. In the past, before screening was introduced in the UK, this also occurred through blood transfusions or from infected blood products, such as the Factor VIII used to treat haemophilia. Occasionally it happens through occupational accidents amongst healthcare workers, such as needlestick injuries. Fortunately, follow-up studies have shown that fewer than 1% of individuals who receive injuries with HIV-contaminated needles become infected

- 'Vertically': this means from mother-to-baby during the course of pregnancy, birth or breastfeeding. The average risk of transmission during pregnancy is in the region of 25% if the mother is HIV-positive, although it may be higher if she has a higher viral load (the amount of HIV in her blood, which indicates the rate at which the virus is reproducing in the body) or has developed AIDS. Breastfeeding may add another 10-15% of infections, and should be avoided in countries where good alternatives to the mother's milk are available.

Detailed discussion of the modes of transmission of HIV can be found in *HIV transmission*.

The detection of HIV

Usually HIV infection is detected by an HIV antibody test. This detects proteins called antibodies which the body manufactures as part of its immune response to HIV.

The first test to be done, usually on blood, but possibly on saliva, is an ELISA (Enzyme Linked Immunosorbent Assay). Since this test can sometimes be positive even when someone is not infected - a 'false positive' result - a second test called the Western Blot is done. This can confirm an ELISA. Other kids of test are becoming available.

The amount of time between getting HIV infection and developing antibodies varies. The vast majority of people with HIV will produce detectable antibodies by six weeks after infection. However, in a small proportion it may take up to six months for antibodies to develop, and in a handful of people with HIV infection it has taken even longer or has not happened at all.

So a lack of HIV antibodies does not always mean freedom from infection, particularly if the person has been recently infected.

It is important to bear in mind that the HIV antibody test is not an 'AIDS test': there is no such thing. It is simply a test for one of the results of HIV infection and does not predict whether or not you will develop AIDS.

There are also a number of laboratory tests which can look for the virus or parts of the virus itself (antigen testing and viral load testing or PCR), or damage to the immune system, or other aspects of the body's response to the effects of the virus. These should not be confused with the HIV antibody test.

An antigen is a part of a virus that stimulates the production of antibodies. Someone who is antibody negative but antigen positive has the virus but has not yet produced antibodies.

For further information about HIV antibody testing see the chapter *HIV testing*.

Stages of HIV infection

Becoming HIV antibody positive

The earliest stage of HIV infection is called Primary HIV Infection (PHI). This stage lasts for three to six months after infection. Ordinarily, the body's immune system would fight off and clear viral infections during this stage, but, for reasons that are still not completely clear, the immune response that it develops to HIV cannot do this.

During primary infection, patients may have 10 to 100 times as much HIV in their body fluids as subsequently, which means they are very infectious.

The majority of people (about 50-80%) have a short illness soon after they become infected. This is called 'seroconversion illness' because it coincides with the time that blood ('serum') tests for antibodies to HIV become positive. The illness may take the form of a sore throat, a fever or a rash, or, rarely, more severe illness. However a large minority of people have no symptoms, and seroconversion illness may be mistaken for other illnesses such as flu.

Seroconversion illness

Around the time antibodies to HIV are appearing in the blood, some people may develop symptoms following exposure to HIV. This is known as seroconversion illness. The symptoms, which are caused by the body's immune response to the new infection, may include:

- Prolonged fever (4 - 14 days) and aching limbs

- Red blotchy rash over the trunk

- Sore throat (pharyngitis)

- Ulceration in the mouth or genitals

- Diarrhoea

- Severe headaches

- Aversion to light

Other symptoms, such as paralysis, meningitis and opportunistic infections as a consequence of severe immune suppression are much less common. Symptoms of seroconversion may occur in up to 80% of people infected, but the severity of the symptoms varies. Some people report only a mild flu-like illness two to six weeks after HIV exposure, but a few experience an illness severe enough to require hospitalisation. The longer the illness lasts, and the more severe it is, the more likely you would be to develop AIDS within five years, presuming you were not to use antiretroviral therapy.

Remember that these symptoms could be caused by other infections; flu, glandular fever, tonsillitis and a serious herpes attack have similar symptoms to those reported in seroconversion illness.

During recent years studies have been done to see if treating people during the early stages of HIV infection - before to shortly after seroconversion - would have the effect of slowing down or stopping the course of HIV infection and the eventual development of AIDS. Recent trials, some of which are still ongoing, have disappointed hopes that early treatment might alter for the better the subsequent course of illness. There are also disadvantages to taking anti-HIV therapy from the start such as experiencing drug side-effects, and possibly risking developing drug-resistant HIV, before it is necessary to do so. At present the British HIV Association (BHIVA) does not recommend that patients diagnosed during PHI routinely take anti-HIV therapy, but does say patients should be offered the choice to take part in one of the ongoing trials of early treatment.

Asymptomatic HIV infection

Initially any damage caused by HIV has no outward effect. This is called asymptomatic infection, which may last for many months or years.

Sometimes people with asymptomatic HIV infection may have swollen lymph nodes, which is called PGL, Persistent Generalised Lymphadenopathy. But this is not a sign of damage in itself.

People who have HIV and feel 100% well may nevertheless have signs of immune damage detectable by laboratory tests; for example, their CD4 count may be below normal levels. Viral load tests have also demonstrated that HIV is actively replicating inside the bodies of asymptomatic people from the moment of infection; at no time is the virus truly latent. The CD4 count and viral load are known as 'surrogate markers' and are discussed in the *HIV & AIDS Treatments Directory*.

Symptomatic HIV Infection

Statistical studies of people with HIV have shown that the more time passes, the more likely it is that the damage will become more severe and infections or tumours may develop. However, such statistics reflect population tendencies: individuals will have their own responses to HIV which may or may not lead to symptomatic disease.

The average time from HIV infection to the development of AIDS (in the absence of treatment) is usually quoted as 8-12 years. However this varies widely. Some people develop AIDS within a few years and a handful almost immediately. Equally, there are people who have had HIV for 20 years yet remain well and do not need to take treatment. Several different factors combine to influence the course of infection: the person's genetic makeup, their body's immune response to HIV, and the 'fitness' of their strain of HIV are all factors.

The infections that people with HIV develop are called opportunistic infections because they are infections with pathogens that are around us all the time - and which our immune systems can normally fight off with no problems. They only become a problem if the immune system is not working well, so that infections that were previously under control become reactivated.

Our bodies also contain cells that can start to divide uncontrollably at any given moment. Normally, these too are kept under control by our immune system. If, however, our immune system is damaged, these cells can cause opportunistic tumours or sometimes cancer.

In addition, HIV can have direct effects upon the body. For instance, the virus can also attack cells in the brain. These cells are involved in feeding the brain cells. If they are damaged, the brain, or some nerves, may not work as well as usual. This is called HIV-associated dementia.

When someone gets ill due to these infections or tumours, he or she is said to have symptomatic HIV infection.

It is important to understand that apart from the so-called 'wasting syndrome' and HIV-associated dementia, the symptoms of AIDS and of symptomatic HIV disease are the symptoms of particular conditions caused by opportunistic infections and tumours, and not directly by HIV itself. Therefore there is a wide range of possible symptoms, and it serves no particular function to answer the question: what are the symptoms of AIDS? Particular symptoms are associated with particular opportunistic infections.

An AIDS diagnosis

Before coming to a diagnosis of AIDS, doctors look at a variety of symptoms and tests. There is no single test for AIDS.

Doctors will look for one of the opportunistic infections or cancers in the presence of underlying immune deficiency. They might, for instance, do tests to try to seek a positive diagnosis of PCP, a type of pneumonia.

These tests are normally only available if you have already been diagnosed as HIV antibody positive, or sometimes if you are seriously ill.

The need for definitions

'AIDS' as the definition of a terminal illness has in some ways fallen out of date since combination therapy has enabled people to live in reasonably good health for many years, even if they have had a previous AIDS diagnosis. Some doctors these days prefer to talk about 'symptomatic HIV infection' as indicating a hopefully reversible effect of HIV.

However AIDS is still a useful definition in parts of the world where treatment is not so available, and as an indicator of the general health toll HIV is exacting on the population at a given time.

AIDS is also defined differently in different countries. In Europe it is still defined by the presence of one or more specific illnesses. In the USA, however, anyone with a CD4 count under 200 - about a fifth of the normal complement of CD4 cells - is deemed to have AIDS, even if they do not have current symptoms.

In reality, not all AIDS-defining disorders have the same prognosis, or outlook. For example, a gay man with a single lesion of Kaposi's sarcoma has AIDS, but has a much better outlook than a gay man with CMV disease or the brain infection PML. Age, race, gender and lifestyle factors can also mean that people who have the same defined HIV illnesses may have very different prospects.

Nevertheless, rigid definitions can be very useful in some circumstances. For example, in clinical and epidemiological studies, when large populations of people are being observed, it is essential to have well defined end points which mark the transition from one state of health to another. This is the only way that scientific principles can be observed and the studies can reach firm, reliable conclusions. It is also appropriate that these definitions change from time to time, as the epidemic evolves and we find out more.

However, definitions of HIV and AIDS as they have evolved have come to suggest that HIV infection is an inevitable, one-way process. In other words, they imply that everyone with HIV will initially be well, then they will get abnormal tests a little while before they get mild illness, and finally there will be a severe terminal illness.

This has been the pattern for many people, but others have had very different experiences. For example, people can get infections that would be diagnostic of AIDS and then become healthy again for a long while.

Improving treatments

The development of new and improved treatments both for the underlying HIV infection and the opportunistic infections has revolutionised the natural history of HIV and AIDS.

Early estimates of the proportion of people with HIV who will go on to develop AIDS were partly based on the experience of the epidemic in the years before such drugs became widely available. As new drugs against HIV and opportunistic infections have become available, these have had a dramatic impact on the prognosis for people with HIV.

Improving treatments for opportunistic infections mean that it is increasingly possible to develop an AIDS-defining illness, such as PCP, and have it successfully treated. Thereafter the individual may, to all intents and purposes, be just as healthy as they were before developing PCP, but nevertheless will now have been diagnosed as having AIDS. In practice, this means that very many people who meet rigid AIDS definitions can continue to lead healthy lives for long periods.

Prophylaxis, to prevent infections recurring or happening even a first time, has also changed the natural history of HIV disease. A number of studies in the early 1990s showed that, compared with the 1980s, people with HIV were experiencing a shorter survival time after they developed AIDS than previously. The reason for this was that prophylactic drugs have delayed the onset of AIDS, so that people are receiving their AIDS diagnosis when their CD4 cell count falls to, say, 75, when earlier in the epidemic they might have developed an AIDS-defining illness at a CD4 count of nearer 200. People with HIV who use prophylaxis are living with HIV without symptoms, and without an AIDS diagnosis, for longer.

The most dramatic developments in HIV treatment have occurred since 1995. Substantial reductions in death rates among HIV-positive people have been reported in many developed countries where infected people have access to the latest therapies. Early use of today's antiretroviral therapies, before HIV-related symptoms develop, may reduce an individual's risk of developing an AIDS-defining illness. Furthermore, many people with very advanced disease, including those with a prior AIDS diagnosis, have experienced remarkable recoveries in physical health, accompanied by rising CD4 counts and a reduction in viral load.

The exact degree to which deaths and illnesses caused by HIV have declined since the advent of good opportunistic infection treatment and HIV combination therapy varies from country to country according to factors such as whether the country offers universal treatment or excludes disadvantaged groups, and on the prevalence of co-infections like hepatitis B and C which may add to the disease burden in themselves, and make HIV more difficult to treat.

In the UK, AIDS diagnoses declined from a peak of 1800 a year in 1993-5 to about 800 a year today, and deaths due to AIDS from 1500 a year to 500 a year today. This is despite the number of people living with HIV in the UK nearly tripling during the same period. So the likelihood of an individual dying of AIDS in any given year has declined at least twenty-fold.

Surveys from countries like Denmark and the USA have revealed that while people with HIV who take appropriate treatment may now expect decades of life, life expectancy for people with HIV has in most cases still not reached that of the general public. However, treatments continue to improve.

The history of AIDS

The origin of AIDS

Understanding how the HIV epidemic emerged is necessary if future prevention work is to be directed towards useful goals.

The causes of epidemics are generally related to changes in human behaviours. Microbes frequently change their behaviour as a result of changes in the activities of their hosts. AIDS did not come from nowhere, but arose as a consequence of social changes which permitted the rapid dissemination of HIV.

Understanding how social changes assisted HIV's spread helps us anticipate the future course of the epidemic.

Where did HIV come from?

Through phylogenetic studies, we now have a reasonably clear picture of how SIV, the monkey and ape equivalent of HIV, crossed over into humans.

SIV stands for Simian Immunodeficiency Virus, but is a misnomer, as in its wild hosts it is tolerated at a high viral load without causing immune deficiency. It does, however, cause AIDS in non-African monkeys, such as Indian rhesus macaques, that have not seen the infection before.

There are many other conflicting theories (see below) as to the origin of HIV and AIDS but since 1999, studies by evolutionary biologists like Bill Hamilton of Oxford University, Paul Sharp of Nottingham University, Michael Worobey of the University of Arizona, Beatrice Hahn of the University of Birmingham, Alabama and other researchers from Montpellier, France, have - in a series of adventurous and sometimes dangerous trips to the jungles of west-central Africa - found SIV samples in chimpanzees, gorillas and (in the case of HIV-2) the sooty mangabey monkey that are so like the various types of HIV that there can be little doubt that they are the ancestral forms of the virus.

The story of the search for the origin of HIV is itself dramatic and ironically resulted in the death of Bill Hamilton, possibly the most celebrated evolutionary biologist of his generation. It is tragically ironic that a famous scientist essentially gave his life in the process of discovering the origins of the virus that has killed so many millions.

In 2000, Worobey, an assistant professor of ecology and evolutionary biology at the University of Arizona in Tucson, and Bill Hamilton went to the Democratic Republic of Congo to collect chimpanzee faeces. By collecting fresh samples they hoped to recover enough viral RNA to determine whether chimpanzees in the Kisangani region harboured the ancestor of HIV.

They worked with a team of hunters that tracked the chimps at night using their calls. The team carefully stored small samples of faeces in little screw-capped vials filled with a preservative.

The 2000 trip met with some calamities. Worobey contracted blood poisoning from a rattan palm spike that stabbed his hand. He hiked out of the forest to seek medical attention. His two companions, Jeffrey Joy and Bill Hamilton, came down with malaria. Hamilton later died from complications.

The faeces collected on that trip didn't yield any SIV genetic material, although tests of chimpanzee urine suggested that virus from the SIVcpz family was present in some of the chimps.

On his 2003 trip, Worobey was luckier. Although he hiked about 200 miles through the rainforest collecting samples, he did not fall ill.

Even so, out of 97 different samples collected, only one contained any SIV. But that was enough - the analysis revealed a brand-new strain, which Worobey and his colleagues named SIVcpzDRC1.

The sequence of the new SIV's genetic material definitively shows that HIV-1 didn't come from chimpanzees in that area, he said.

"This is one of only a handful of places in the world where SIVs are known to be circulating in chimpanzees. We know HIV-1 comes from chimpanzees, but we know little beyond this," he said. "I want to study this geographic area - get more samples, understand how the virus is maintained and transmitted in chimps, and understand why the virus is so pathogenic in humans but not chimpanzees."

Paul Sharp and colleagues such as Beatrice Hahn from the University of Birmingham, Alabama and others from the

University of Montpellier in France then took up the challenge, but concentrated their researches in Cameroon, the country which contains the widest variety of strains of HIV and which already appeared to be the place HIV-1 groups N and O came from.

Sharp presented his findings in a dramatic session at the 2006 Conference on Retroviruses and Opportunistic Infections, and his team later published their findings in Science Journal (Keele).

The two viruses that cause AIDS, HIV-1 and HIV-2, crossed over into the human population on at least 10 separate occasions during the 20th century, Sharp told the Retrovirus Conference..

But the vast majority of the world's HIV epidemic arose from a single transmission event between an unknown chimpanzee and an unknown human in a small corner of south-east Cameroon.

Sharp told the conference that he had narrowed down the chimpanzee equivalent of the virus that gave rise to most of the worldwide AIDS epidemic - the HIV-1 M group - to a small population of wild chimpanzees living in Cameroon close to the borders of the Republic of Congo and the Central African Republic.

Sharp explained that HIV comes in two varieties as different as cats and dogs - HIV-1 and HIV-2. HIV-2, which is less easy to catch and causes a milder version of AIDS, is restricted to west Africa and is pretty much the same as the simian or monkey immunodeficiency virus (SIV) found in the sooty mangabey monkey.

HIV-2 seems to have crossed into humans at least seven times, but four of these genetically distinct versions of HIV-2 have only ever been found in one human apiece, and one in two humans, showing that monkey-to-human virus transition may be a relatively common phenomenon but rarely gives rise to an epidemic (see Reeves and Dom). The variety of HIV-2 found in almost all human cases (it remains concentrated in west Africa and among west African immigrants in countries like Portugal) has been found in sooty mangabeys in the Tai National forest in the south-west corner of the Ivory Coast. These findings were presented at the 2004 CROI Conference by Beatrice Hahn's team (Santiago).

When it comes to HIV-1, which causes most of the world's AIDS, it was already known that it came from the SIV carried by chimpanzees (SIC_{cpz}), and that this SIV was itself a mixture of viruses carried by two other kinds of monkey, the greater spot-nosed monkey (*Cercopithecus petaurista*) and the red-capped mangabey (*Cercocebus torquatus*).

Previous research amongst captive chimpanzees had already found that SIV_{cps} is only carried by *Pan troglodytes troglodytes*, the subspecies that lives in central west Africa in countries like the Republic of Congo, Gabon, and southern Cameroon.

Sharp's team also knew that HIV-1 must have crossed into humans at least three times because it exists in three varieties called groups M, N and O - the latter two being rare.

Sharp's team went to west Africa and spent months collecting droppings from wild chimps and testing them for SIV. They found SIV of the type that crossed into humans only existed among chimps in southern Cameroon. They found SIV similar to HIV-1 group N in one site in the centre of the country. And they found SIV similar to HIV-1 group M - M for mainstream, which infects 40 million humans today - in two sites in the extreme south-east of the country. The scientist who actually obtained the sequences, Fran Van Heuverswyn, said that "two of the isolates more closely matched the HIV-1 causing the human epidemic than any found in the past". The viruses were 80% similar to HIV-1 group M.

This site where they found the type M-like virus is directly connected by river to Kinshasa, the capital of the Democratic Republic of Congo, where the first sample of blood containing human HIV was isolated in 1959 and where HIV in the human population continues to show the widest diversity today.

Sharp's findings have been disputed by writers such as Edward Hooper, champion of the oral polio vaccine theory of the origin of HIV, but previous research on the rate of genetic change of these viruses would seem to indicate that HIV-1 group M most likely crossed into humans around the 1930s - too early for initial infection, at least, to have taken place during the vaccine experiments of the 1950s.

This theory had already been called into question during 2000 with the release of data from researchers from Los Alamos National Laboratory in the USA which carefully examined the rate at which HIV sub-types diverged over the years.

This US study was presented by Dr Bette Korber of the Los Alamos National Laboratory in January 2000 at the Seventh Conference on Retroviruses and Opportunistic Infections. She suggested that the first case of HIV-1 infection of the M (main) strain, which gave rise to the global epidemic, occurred around 1930 in West Africa. The estimate of 1930 (which does have a 15 year margin of error) was based on a complicated computer model of HIV's evolution. If accurate, it means that HIV-1 strain M, at least, was in existence before many scenarios (such as the OPV and conspiracy theories) suggest.

Using the equivalent of 512 supercomputers for a whole day to perform their calculations, the researchers compared the genetic sequences of more than a hundred virus isolates, some dating from 1959 and the 1960s, to determine the average speed at which HIV sequences change over time. They used this information to back-calculate the amount of time it would have taken HIV to mutate from the genetic sequence of SIVcpz, its nearest relative.

The calculations established that HIV-1 group M, the root of virtually all the HIV-1 subtypes found in humans, is likely to have entered humans from chimpanzees in Africa between 1910 and 1940. The calculations found that sub-type D which is common in Africa began to evolve before 1950, and that sub-type B, which is common in USA and Europe began to emerge from sub-type D in the early 1960s.

Since then more research has filled in a missing piece of the jigsaw. Sharp's team found viruses that looked like HIV-1 types M and N, but not type O. He finally found an SIV that looked like type O - but in a completely expected source - gorillas.

Sharp told the Eighth Congress on Drug Therapy in HIV Infection in late 2006 that he had found the precursor of HIV-1 group O - but, to his surprise, in lowland gorillas, not chimps. He found it in two separate locations separated by 400 kilometres - one in central Cameroon and one on the coast, which may also indicate that group O crossed into humans earlier than group M. Six out of 213 (3%) of samples from gorillas carried group O virus almost indistinguishable from human group O.

It has been asked why, if HIV entered the human population as early as 1930, it was not noticed till 1981, and why no blood samples containing it were taken before 1959? Professor Sharp commented that HIV infection was probably a rare tropical infection caught from animals until modern urban living created the conditions where it could turn into an epidemic. He said that modelling the growth of epidemics showed that even in 1959 there might have been only 2000 people in the world with HIV, and we were lucky to find a sample that early. By 1980 300,000 people might have had it, and 40 million today.

Sharp's team is also narrowing in on the specific genetic mutation which, they believe, enables SIV viruses to change their nature so they can infect humans.

By comparing human and chimp viruses he found a single genetic change at a place called position 29 in HIV-1's matrix protein, which, produced by a viral gene called gag, forms part of its outer structure. At position 29 the amino acid methionine in chimps has been replaced by arginine in humans. This change is common to groups M, N and O.

When Sharp re-infected chimps with human HIV, the amino acid switched straight back to the chimp version.

He also found that - even though they are quite different species of virus - exactly the same mutation has happened in HIV-2, and speculates that this crucial change is what enables SIV viruses to infect humans.

Exactly what this part of the matrix protein does in HIV is as yet unclear, but it appears to interact with human proteins and subvert natural antiviral defences.

If Sharp's team can find out exactly what it does, they might find a defence against the cellular machinery that enabled SIV to invade humans and spark off a worldwide epidemic about 50-60 years ago.

Grounds zero: USA, Africa, Europe

HIV

The earliest stored blood sample which has tested unequivocally HIV-positive was taken from an unknown patient near what is now Kinshasa in the Democratic Republic of Congo in 1959.

AIDS was first identified as a distinct syndrome in 1981 as the consequence of a cluster of cases amongst gay men in US cities with established gay communities. A network of gay men has

been traced who came from Los Angeles, New York San Francisco, Florida and Texas US cities who all appear to have been connected sexually between 1978 and 1981 and who subsequently died of AIDS. One was Gaetan Dugas, the air steward who was identified by Randy Shilts in his book *And the Band Played On* as the 'patient zero' of the US epidemic. Dugas was displaying AIDS-related symptoms in 1979, but some of his contacts also became ill very shortly afterwards so it is impossible to tell who was in fact the US 'index case'.

Dugas had also travelled widely to Europe in his work, and apart from Arvid Noe, a Norwegian sailor who died in 1976 (see below), several other early cases of AIDS have been found in Europe, including two contrasting Germans - a soldier and an orchestral conductor - who both died in January 1979.

A presentation at the 2007 Retrovirus Conference suggested that HIV found its way to the USA via Haiti.

Michael Worobey told the conference that Haiti has the oldest HIV epidemic outside Africa and provided the source for the strain of HIV seen in North America and Europe.

Worobey's team of researchers found that the type of HIV most prevalent in Haiti, the United States and Europe - HIV-1 group M, subtype B - moved from Africa to Haiti in around 1966. HIV spread around Haiti before a single migration of the virus took it out of Haiti to the US and then worldwide between 1969 and 1972. The research also corroborates the idea that HIV-1 group M originated comparatively recently, probably no earlier than the early 20th century.

The exact circumstances surrounding the emergence of the strain of HIV in the United States and Europe have long been the subject of debate. Investigators from the US, Denmark and the United Kingdom recovered complete HIV-1 *env* gene sequences from samples obtained from five Haitian AIDS patients between 1982 and 1983 who were recent migrants to the United States. To test the hypothesis that subtype B has a Haitian origin, they conducted phylogenetic analysis of samples obtained from these patients and on a further 117 samples obtained from patients in 19 different countries.

A US or non-Haitian origin for subtype B was rejected by this analysis, strongly in favour of a Haitian origin. This was confirmed by analysis of the *gag* sequence of the viral samples.

According to the investigators' analysis, HIV-1 moved from Africa to Haiti in the mid-1960s - probably in or around 1966, a time when many Haitians professionals were returning home after working in the Congo.

Between 1969 and 1972, a single migration took subtype B out of Haiti. The investigators called this migration the "pandemic clade", representing "a key turning point in the history of the AIDS pandemic". HIV was probably transferred to the US by a single source early in the 1970s. This fits with subsequent epidemiology of HIV in the US. The first cases of AIDS were reported approximately ten years after HIV entered the US from Haiti - the interval between infection with HIV and progression to AIDS and death is in the region of ten years.

Interestingly, a single Haitian source was also identified for the subtype B epidemic in Trinidad and Tobago.

Haiti has had a long association with the origins of the AIDS epidemic. It was sometimes said - often disparagingly - that AIDS affected the three "H"'s - Haitians, homosexuals and haemophiliacs.

Dr Michael Worobey's presentation was greeted with an angry response by a Haitian delegate to the conference, who pointed to earlier studies that failed to find evidence of HIV infection in stored samples in the country. In response, Dr Worobey stressed that his study was not intended to "blame" any country or individuals for the origin of the HIV epidemic, but he again emphasised that phylogenetic analysis clearly showed a Haitian origin for the subtype B epidemic.

In terms of how HIV spread from its place or origin into the rest of Africa, to cause the 'hyperepidemic' that affects that continent today, retrospective analysis has also found large numbers of AIDS cases appearing in the Kagera and Rakai districts of Uganda in 1981-2. The theory is that HIV was brought to Uganda by Tanzanian soldiers who invaded in 1978 in order to overthrow Idi Amin. The circumstances of war, with violence, commercial sex and rape suddenly erupting in towns that were also key stopping points in a cross-Africa truck route, were what appear to have turned AIDS from a rare to a common disease in Africa.

In summary:

- HIV undoubtedly first appeared in western and central Africa.

- Two distinct, though related immunodeficiency viruses have crossed into human beings from two different species - the less virulent HIV-2 from the Sooty Mangabey, and HIV-1, the cause of the global epidemic, from the western subspecies of chimpanzee, *Pan troglodytes troglodytes* (more on this below).

- HIV-1 appears to have jumped the 'species barrier' not once but three times, as evidenced by three distinct subspecies circulating in humans - type M, the main type and cause of the global epidemic, and types O and N, which are rare and still largely restricted to central West Africa. HIV-2 also appears to have crossed over several times.

- Based on studies calculating the rate of genetic change, several events could have happened between 1910 and 1950, with the maximum likelihood around 1930. HIV-2 appears to be an older infection which may have crossed into humans at least seven times. HIV-1 crossed over three times and may yet do again; HIV-1 type N appears to be a more recent infection than types M and O.

- The important fact here is that HIV appears to be a very recent infection, unlike (say) tuberculosis, which has afflicted humanity for hundreds of thousands of years. Like SARS and H5N1 bird flu, HIV is an 'emergent virus', something new in nature (although SIV species could have crossed into humans in centuries before and never given rise to epidemics).

- It is its very novelty to the human immune system that gives HIV its lethal nature. It is not in the interest of microbes to kill their hosts too quickly, and viruses tend to attenuate (weaken) over time. Most monkeys live perfectly happily with their strains of SIV and do not develop illness despite having high viral loads.

- HIV may already possibly be getting less virulent: a Belgian study in 2005 (Arien) found that HIV from blood samples taken in 2002-3 was only 55% as fit as HIV taken from 1986-9 samples (though still fit enough to cause AIDS).

Early cases of AIDS

Subsequent review of the medical literature has revealed a plethora of inexplicable AIDS-like illnesses dating back to the late 1940s in the United States and Europe, although many of these scattered cases appear to be in people without classic HIV risk factors and could also be due to rare deficits in the immune system.

Pre-1981 cases fall into two categories: those for which stored blood samples have revealed HIV infection, and those for which no stored blood samples exist, but where the pattern of symptoms reported is highly suggestive of AIDS.

The oldest AIDS case for which an HIV diagnosis has been confirmed is that of Robert R, an American youth from St Louis who died in 1969. Robert's case is mysterious as he appears to have had no connection with Africa, and his sexual history is murky.

The case of David Carr, a Manchester sailor who is believed to have died of AIDS in 1959 has recently been called into doubt, following the discovery that the strain of HIV isolated from stored tissue samples was virtually identical to strains prevalent 30 years later. US researchers have argued that such a similarity is implausible unless the virus was a laboratory contaminant, because HIV would normally mutate considerably during a 30 year period.

Other than Robert R, the earliest proven AIDS case involved Arvid Noe, a Norwegian sailor who had travelled in Africa and then worked as a lorry driver in Europe. Not only he but also his wife and child died in 1976.

A Portuguese man who fell ill in 1978 has been retrospectively diagnosed as one of the earliest cases of AIDS caused by HIV-2.

The identified cases in which HIV was present are important because they challenge the belief that HIV is a virus which was introduced into the West in the 1970s. Although some of these cases indicate contact with Africa, the 1969 case of an American youth shows no evidence of an African connection.

Clinical records have also been used to identify pre-1981 cases. Historians have looked for unusual cases recorded in the medical literature which appear to fit the existing definition of AIDS. A surprising number of such reports exist, dating back to at least 1940 in North America and Europe. There are numerous reports of an AIDS-like syndrome which occurred in newborn children in Germany, Poland and Scandinavia, starting in 1939 and persisting until the late 1950s. The syndrome was characterised by *Pneumocystis* pneumonia (PCP), cytomegalovirus disease and hypergammaglobulinaemia (very high levels of antibodies), all characteristic of AIDS in newborn children today.

The Dutch researcher Jaap Goudsmit speculates that this eruption of an AIDS-like syndrome was connected to the re-use of needles in hospitals, a common practice before the development of disposable syringes in the 1960s. He also argues that it may have originated from a strain of HIV which was less harmful to adults than the forms of HIV now in circulation, and that it was introduced to Europe by German colonists returning from Cameroon prior to the outbreak of war. However, other researchers have long argued that these cases were due to malnutrition-induced immune deficiency, a point not addressed by Goudsmit. Edward Hooper's investigations suggest that all the outbreaks occurred in regions where uranium was being mined.

There have always been rare cases of immune system collapse in humans that aren't due to inherited immune deficiency, and cases still turn up in the literature of individuals with an AIDS-like picture of decimated T-cells but who lack risk factors and don't test positive for HIV antibodies. This syndrome has received the name ICL (idiopathic CD4+ lymphocytopenia), meaning 'deficit of CD4 cells of unknown origin', and while cases are extremely rare compared with cases of AIDS, many of these early reports could be ICL, singled out for report by doctors for case report precisely because they were unusual.

Similar detailed reports do not exist for Africa, except for data concerning Kaposi's sarcoma, which became epidemic in equatorial Africa in the late 1950s. This form of KS, which took the lethal form only in about 10% of cases, was not associated with HIV or with immune suppression, and affected Africans but not Westerners resident in Africa.

A dozen or so cases of AIDS-like illness have been identified by Edward Hooper in Kinshasa, Rwanda and parts of the Congo, the earliest properly documented case having been diagnosed in 1962. African doctors tend to agree that AIDS did not appear in Africa on a growing scale before the late 1970s, and that it became epidemic only in the early 1980s. In the early years of the epidemic the syndrome was known as 'Slim' in Uganda and other central African countries; it first appeared in Uganda on the north shores of Lake Victoria, in Burundi and Rwanda (states to the west of Lake Victoria), and in Kinshasa (the capital of Zaire), which lies at the crossroads of trade routes linking East Africa, West Africa, Angola and Zaire.

Isolated cases of AIDS-defining illnesses began to appear among gay men and injecting drug users from the early 1970s in New York and San Francisco. These were not linked by doctors until the beginning of 1981, when a cluster of orders for the drug pentamidine, used to treat PCP, sparked curiosity amongst officials at the Centers for Disease Control. Although the cluster of PCP cases was identified in 1981, it is possible that a low level of 'pneumonia' cases were treated with standard antibiotics and hence went undetected by the Centers for Disease Control

for some years before 1981. Some researchers argue that AIDS cases could have occurred at a low level in the population before the 1940s without exciting much suspicion, because of a greater frequency of infectious diseases. It was only when infectious disease became less common that immune deficiency became more remarkable and worthy of note. Prior to the introduction of antibiotics, tuberculosis and syphilis may have masked minor clusters of HIV disease, in the view of medical historian Mirko Grmek.

Alternative theories of origin

The polio vaccine link theory

Journalist Edward Hooper has spent years trying to prove that the most plausible explanation for the transfer of HIV into the human population is by the contamination of oral polio vaccine by SIV. The theory has been circulating since the early 1990s, although Hooper's book *The River* has renewed interest in this theory. Hooper suggested that chimp kidneys were used for the preparation of the attenuated virus used in the vaccine, and Hooper documents the potential for cross-species transfer of SIV between chimps in several camps used to collect primates for research purposes during the late 1950s.

Hooper also documents the locations in which oral polio vaccine potentially derived from chimp kidneys was administered. There is a close correlation between the sites of early vaccination drives (the Belgian Congo), the earliest reported cases of AIDS in Africa, and the highest seroprevalence in the early 1980s.

Hooper's theory is very logical and seductive. The oldest known case of AIDS in Africa occurred in a man from what was then Leopoldville and is now Kinshasa, capital of the Democratic Republic of Congo. Additionally, most of the early cases of HIV in Africa also occurred in Congo, Rwanda and Burundi, and most came from towns close to where the oral polio vaccine was tested.

In September 2000, scientists from around the world gathered at the Royal Society in London together with Edward Hooper to discuss the origins of the HIV epidemic.

Findings presented at this meeting showed no evidence of HIV or SIV infection in samples of the oral polio vaccine held by the Wistar Institute, developers of the vaccine alleged to have introduced HIV into humans in Africa in the 1950s.

The Wistar Institute deny that chimp kidneys were used in any vaccine preparation. Instead they say that the vaccine was cultivated in monkey kidneys. The question of which primate tissues were used is crucial because only chimpanzees have been shown to carry SIV.

Some of the earliest cases of HIV occurred in areas of the Congo where no-one was vaccinated. Conversely, some of the areas where vaccination was widespread did not report cases of HIV.

The contaminated needles theory

While Hooper may have been wrong in his specific assertion that HIV could have originated from the oral polio vaccine trials, he could still have unearthed a more general possibility; that the spread of what might have been a rare illness found only in people with close contact with chimpanzees may have initially been spread through the use of unsterilised needles. These could have been used not only in polio vaccine drives but in other vaccination programmes and in programmes to give people antibiotics for infectious diseases; many such programmes existed in west-central Africa around this time.

The WHO estimates that worldwide today, about five per cent of HIV infections come from the use of unsterilised needles.

In a series of papers published in 2002 and 2003, STI specialists David Gisselquist and John Potterat and psychologist Stuart Brody caused controversy by claiming that between 35% and 65% of HIV infections in Africa were caused by re-use of unsterilised needles rather than sex.

Gisselquist and colleagues based their theory on an analysis of early HIV infection reports received from countries in east and central Africa before 1990. They claimed to show that the number of medical injections reported by seroconverters was much better correlated with HIV infection than the number of sexual partners or STIs they had had.

Gisselquist also cited a South African study which found significant levels of HIV infection in children born to HIV-negative mothers, and evidence from Zimbabwe that falling STI rates were accompanied by rising HIV rates.

The work of Gisselquist and colleagues created enough controversy for the WHO to make an investigation of their theory. In an article published in the *Lancet* (Schmid) they reviewed Gisselquist and colleagues' arguments and refuted them:

- Transmission via unsterilised needles may possibly have contributed to the spread of HIV early on in the epidemic but Gisselquist had failed to review data since 1990, which showed an overwhelming *lack* of correlation between injections and HIV seropositivity (See, for instance, Lopman).

- Gisselquist was using 'reverse causality'; patients with HIV had had more injections because they had HIV-related illnesses, rather than acquiring HIV because they had injections.

- The South African study which found high rates of HIV infection in children of HIV-negative mothers was flawed, as the study authors admitted at the time; it had relied on oral HIV swabs self-administered by families and there was a lot of cross-contamination.

- More than twice as many injections with unsterilised needles are given in Asia (where the practice of getting vitamin shots from street-corner stalls is widespread) than in Africa. If HIV was largely spread by needles rather than sex, India would have the world's highest HIV prevalence.

- HIV has continued to increase in Zimbabwe and some other southern African countries as STIs have decreased because HIV prevalence is so high that most HIV infection is now occurring within marriage, where bacterial STIs are less likely to be commonly transmitted.

Has HIV become more dangerous?

Some scientists believe that HIV may have existed for many years as a relatively harmless virus in humans, but that changing conditions have made it more virulent. The simian immunodeficiency virus (SIV) has been observed to cause progressively more serious disease as it passes through a chain of chimpanzees, suggesting that adapting to a new host increases the virulence of an immunodeficiency virus. Conditions which encourage the repeated transmission of retroviruses will therefore encourage the development of progressively more dangerous strains of retroviruses.

When a retrovirus strain has few opportunities to encounter new hosts, natural selection will favour the persistence of strains of HIV which remain in a state of equilibrium with their host in order to continue reproducing itself. It is suicidal for the virus in such circumstances to kill the host. But if a strain of HIV begins to pass through a series of hosts, weaker hosts may allow the virus to grow unchecked and natural selection will tend to favour the multiplication of strains which are highly infectious and more likely to kill the host. In circumstances of frequent transmission to new hosts, virulent and pathogenic strains are just as likely to persist as quiescent, less pathogenic strains.

HIV-1 and HIV-2 serve as examples of divergent strains which may indicate the evolutionary path of HIV. HIV-2 causes disease less frequently than HIV-1, and seems to be more difficult to transmit through sexual intercourse. Until recently HIV-2 was confined largely to Western Africa, with its epicentre in the former Portuguese colony of Guinea-Bissau. HIV-1 may have diverged from HIV-2 a long time ago, and become more virulent as it became more widespread and more frequently transmitted.

However other more recent evidence suggests that HIV-1 may have become less, rather than more, virulent over time, at least since it became widespread in human beings - see the Arien study cited above.

Does HIV really originate in Africa?

The evidence points to an African source for HIV, not least the tight confinement of HIV-2 to Western Africa until the late 1980s. In addition, the presence of a larger number of genetic subtypes of HIV in Africa compared with anywhere else in the world suggests that the virus has been present for longer in the African population, and has diversified accordingly.

Another suggestive factor is that many early AIDS diagnoses (from 1959 to the early 1980s) occurred in individuals with connections with Africa, rather than in Europeans without African connections.

However, it is also important to note that there is virtually no reliable evidence from antibody testing to suggest that HIV was present on a significant scale in African cities before 1981, at least three years after HIV began to appear amongst gay men and drug users in North America. One study could find reliable evidence of HIV infection in only four out of 6,015 serum samples gathered between 1976 and 1984 in Africa, the period during which HIV was supposed to be spreading widely in Africa, and one of these samples came from a white European (Wendler). This finding is backed up by evidence from studies of blood gathered in Zambia and other Southern African countries, which failed to show conclusive evidence of HIV infection during the 1970s.

On the other hand, a study of blood samples in Zaire showed five out of 659 samples from 1976 to be positive and three of these samples came from individuals who later died of clinical syndromes suggestive of AIDS (Nzilambi). Furthermore, in 1984 Belgian doctors reported 18 AIDS cases, some dating from 1979, amongst Zairois attending hospitals in Belgium. This evidence suggests that the epicentre of the HIV-1 epidemic was somewhere in the Congo basin (Clumeck).

It was not until 1983 that AIDS was recognised by an Africa-based doctor, Dr Anne Bayley. From case reports it has been suggested that AIDS was occurring in Zambia from 1979 onwards. It is likely that the road and rail networks of Zambia contributed to the early spread of the virus (Hooper).

The Zambian epidemic is likely to have been predated by the epidemic in Rwanda by some five or six years. In his book *The River*, Edward Hooper documents the case of a Rwandese family consisting of three children and two parents. Within three months of the birth of the first child the mother presented with symptoms such as weight loss, diarrhoea, oral candidiasis. It is likely that these were the early symptoms of AIDS and this was in 1977 or 1978.

Could HIV have been genetically engineered or accidentally disseminated?

Claims that HIV was genetically engineered as a biological weapon are fanciful: until the advent of the epidemic, no scientist had the biotechnological tools necessary to create HIV from known lentiviruses. Conspiracy theories regarding the origins of the epidemic are invariably attempts to apportion blame for the social conditions which permitted HIV to become widespread.

It is also argued that HIV-2 was disseminated by polio vaccination. HIV-2 is related to a form of SIV found in sooty mangabeys, a species confined to West Africa. Edward Hooper suggests that a French vaccine used in this region by French and Portuguese researchers could have become contaminated if chimps were held in close proximity to sooty mangabeys, and chimp kidney was then used to produce the vaccine.

An alternate theory - HIV as a human virus

New research presented at the Eleventh International Congress on Virology in August 1999 has also challenged the dominant theory of the origins of HIV.

Professor Robert Garry's team from Tulane University, New Orleans, has confirmed that Robert R, a young man who was probably a sex worker died of HIV-related opportunistic illnesses in St Louis, USA, in 1969. The man's tissue was frozen at the time of his death and Professor Garry's team have since discovered that he was infected with a strain of HIV similar to HIV-1 subtype III/LAI.

This virus infects T-cells, rather than macrophages, and thus is less likely to be sexually transmitted, according to Professor Garry. He proposed that a more benign version of HIV has been infecting humans for hundreds or thousands of years, and that a recent mutation triggered the modern day pandemic.

The value of searching for origins

Scientific investigation of origins may help us to understand how to combat HIV most effectively. In terms of understanding the actual history of HIV, the virulence of the virus, and possible immunity to it, it is worth investigating populations who may have been exposed to HIV for many years, such as those in Africa. Furthermore, studying the immune response of primates infected with SIV may assist in vaccine development.

Further reading and references

Arien K et al. *Replicative fitness of historical and recent HIV-1 isolates suggests HIV-1 attenuation over time.* AIDS 19: 1555-1564, 2005.

Clumeck, Nathan et al *Acquired Immunodeficiency Syndrome in African Patients* NEJM 310(8): 492-497, 1984.

Gallo, Robert: *Virus Hunting Basic,* 1991.

Gao F et al. *Origin of HIV-1 in the chimpanzee pan troglodytes troglodytes,* Nature 397: 436-441, 1999.

Garrett, Laurie: *The Coming Plague.* Farrer, Strauss, Giroux, 1994.

Gisselquist D and Potterat J. *Heterosexual transmission of HIV in Africa: an empiric estimate.* International Journal of STD & AIDS 14: 162-173. 2003.

Goudsmit, Jaap: *Viral Sex: The Nature of AIDS,* Oxford University Press, 1997.

Grmek, Mirko: *History of AIDS: Emergence and Origin of a Modern Pandemic,* Princeton University Press, 1990.

Hooper Edward: *Sailors and starbursts, and the arrival of HIV* BMJ 7123, 1997.

Hooper Edward: *The River,* Penguin, 1999.

Keele BF et al. *Chimpanzee reservoirs of pandemic and nonpandemic HIV-1.* Science 313(5786):523-6. 2006.

Korber B et al. *Timing the Origin of the HIV-1 Pandemic.* Seventh Conference on Retroviruses and Opportunistic Infections, San Francisco, 2000.

Lopman BA et al. *Individual Level Injection History: A Lack of Association with HIV Incidence in Rural Zimbabwe.* PLoS Medicine 2(2): e37, 2005.

Nzilambi N et al: *The prevalence of infection with human immunodeficiency virus over a ten year period in rural Zaire* NEJM 318(5): 276-279, 1988.

Reeves JD and Dom RW. *Human immunodeficiency virus type 2.* Journal of General Virology 83: 1253-1265. 2002.

Santiago ML et al. *Endemic SIV$_{sm}$ Infection in Wild-living Sooty Mangabeys.* 11th Conference on Retroviruses and Opportunistic Infections, San Francisco. Abstract 380. 2004.

Schmid GP et al. *Transmission of HIV-1 infection in sub-Saharan Africa and effect of elimination of unsafe injections.* Lancet 363(9407): 482-488, 2004.

Sharp PM. *Where AIDS Came From.* 13th Conference on Retroviruses and Opportunistic Infections, Denver. Plenary lecture, abstract #70. 2006

Sharp PM. *Endemic Infection of Central Chimpanzee (Pan troglodytes troglodytes) by Simian Immunodeficiency Virus.* 13th Conference on Retroviruses and Opportunistic Infections, Denver. Oral presentation, abstract #35. 2006.

Sharp PM. *Where did it all Begin?* Eighth International Congress on Drug Therapy in HIV Infection, Glasgow. Keynote Lecture KL1. 2006.

Wendler I et al: *Seroepidemiology of human immunodeficiency virus in Africa* BMJ 293: 782-785, 1986.

Zhu T et al: *An African HIV-1 sequence from 1959 and implications for the origin of the epidemic.* Nature 391(6667): 594, 1998.

The spread of HIV

In the 40 years before HIV emerged, the world changed more rapidly than at any time since the European conquest of the Americas. Some of the changes were to facilitate the HIV epidemic, in the same way that social changes in the period following the discovery of the Americas encouraged the spread of syphilis in Europe and numerous infectious diseases in the Americas.

Population movements brought millions to big cities, and economic conditions frequently separated men and women from their partners. A growth in prostitution and polygamy occurred in African cities, and on trade routes between African countries. A dramatic growth in sexually transmitted diseases took place.

Medicine changed dramatically in Africa, with the increased use of injections and transfusions as part of treatment. Owing to lack of resources, needles were not always sterilised or disposed of between patients. Mass immunisation programmes took place without rigorous sterilisation of needles.

International travel made contacts between different countries and continents commonplace. For example, during the late 1970s, an increasing number of European gay men began to visit North America as airline travel became cheaper. Africans visited Europe more frequently, and large numbers of Europeans went to work in Africa. Sexual tourism to destinations such as Haiti and Thailand made a significant contribution to the local economies and attracted visitors from all over the developed world.

Taboos against homosexuality were vigorously challenged, especially in English-speaking countries and Northern Europe. Visible organised gay communities emerged in New York, San Francisco and Los Angeles during the 1970s which attracted gay men from all over the world to visit or settle. It is estimated that 50,000 gay men moved to San Francisco between 1969 and 1982.

Sexual freedom was a primary value and rallying point of these new communities, reflecting a wider sexual revolution in developed countries. Bathhouses and backrooms which allowed for multiple sexual contacts were also a key feature of these communities. Anther new feature of the emerging gay lifestyle was the versatility of sexual roles in an individual's behaviour. Until the 1970s much homosexual activity had been characterised by the maintenance of clear sexual roles of 'active' and 'passive' in anal intercourse, but as gay men became more open and liberated, this role separation was increasingly questioned and challenged. Fewer and fewer individuals were either exclusively active or passive.

Sexually transmitted infections, antibiotic use and recreational drug use amongst this population were all extremely high, and it was not at all uncommon for gay men in their thirties to have had over one thousand sexual partners in their lifetime. This was a very dramatic change from the limited numbers of sexual partners enjoyed by most gay men before the 1960s (Grmek; Root-Bernstein).

Blood transfusions became increasingly commonplace in medical practice, and an industry grew up dedicated to serving the requirement for both blood and blood products. In the United States paid donors were used - often, injecting drug users. This blood was sent around the world, and US blood donations were sold to Africa during the 1970s.

In the late 1960s haemophiliacs began to benefit from the discovery that Factor VIII could be synthesised from donated blood. Manufacturers were soon pooling Factor VIII from between 2,000 and 20,000 donors in order to produce Factor VIII concentrate for distribution all over the world. This increased the chance that haemophiliacs would be exposed to any new infections present in the blood donor population.

Intravenous drug use grew dramatically in the 1970s as heroin became increasingly available in the wake of the Vietnam war. The war introduced thousands of US troops to heroin, and the US government actively aided heroin smugglers in Laos who opposed the Communists, permitting huge quantities of heroin to flood to the West. Wars in Afghanistan and Lebanon also augmented the global supply of heroin, which was processed through Mediterranean ports such as Marseilles and Naples. Large drug dependent communities grew up in Southern European cities which acted as entry points for heroin. Large drug using populations emerged amongst minority populations in US cities, partially as a consequence of the exposure of servicemen to heroin in Vietnam (notably, a disproportionate number of US troops in Vietnam were black). Economic deprivation also led to depression and poverty which found outlets in drug use and drug dealing.

The growth in injecting drug use was also assisted by the arrival of disposable plastic syringes in the early 1970s, and drug-using institutions also developed in some large cities - shooting galleries - where addicts could go to score drugs and rent injecting equipment.

The growth of addict populations also led to an increase in prostitution to support drug habits, amongst both male and female drug users.

In Africa, civil and intra-regional wars may have provided the initial means of transfer of HIV from one country to another, as with the Tanzanian soldiers to Uganda. Similar spread occurs through migrant labour, as happened in the mass movement of male mine and other workers in South Africa in the 1970s-1990s from rural areas to work camps in urban parts of South Africa, and is happening now in China today. Finally, travel in the form of trucking has clearly been instrumental in the spread of HIV. Even today, HIV incidence concentrates around trucking routes and truckstops, not only across the African continent, but in other countries like India and Myanmar.

All these factors provided pathways for HIV to spread through more and more bodies, generating strains which perhaps became more virulent with each new host encountered.

Lessons to be learnt

A number of institutions played key roles in amplifying the epidemic: bathhouses, backrooms, shooting galleries and hospitals in some parts of Africa.

During the early 1980s there were bitter debates within the gay community over the wisdom of closing the bathhouses and policing sexual behaviour in backrooms on the grounds that these places were the sites in which unsafe sex was taking place. It is arguable that the worst epidemics of AIDS have occurred in those cities and countries where bathhouses existed, such as the United States and France, while it is arguable that Britain owes its relatively small epidemic by European standards to the fact that bathhouses and backrooms were illegal.

Closing the bathhouses was like attempting to put out a forest fire with a bucket of water (see *Early safer sex messages* below), although most histories of the epidemic consider their closure to have been an act of self-evident good sense (Fitzgerald: Shilts). In Holland, however, the bathhouses remained open throughout the epidemic, with one crucial difference from their North American counterparts: the provision of condoms and safer sex education. Today it is clear that educational efforts which target locations where HIV transmission may take place play an important role in limiting the spread of HIV during the early phase of an epidemic.

Shooting galleries also played a crucial role in the dissemination of HIV. Cities in which these institutions were a feature of drug using culture had earlier and larger epidemics of HIV and AIDS amongst injecting drug users (Joseph). Prevention efforts were never targeted at these locations or at other places where injecting drug use took place, largely for political reasons.

In Africa it is arguable that hospitals which did not sterilise needles between injections disseminated HIV to large numbers of patients. This may explain the parity of male to female seroprevalence figures for African cities, which have generally been interpreted as supporting the hypothesis that male-to-female transmission and mother-to-baby transmission are the key routes of HIV transmission. In fact, the African cultural preference for delivering medication by injection rather than pill or suppository may have influenced the development of the epidemic.

Another hypothesis suggests that these figures can also be interpreted as showing that the re-use of needles and blood transfusions are responsible for a sizeable proportion of infections in Africa (for further discussion of this view see Packard and Epstein in *AIDS: the Making of a Chronic Disease*).

A key form of prevention which could be targeted at hospitals is the provision of sufficient clean needles and/or sterilising equipment to ensure that transmission did not take place. Instead, prevention policies in Africa have focused almost exclusively on the 'social marketing' of condoms, in other words, encouraging people at risk to buy and use condoms. They have also emphasised monogamy, a message which may be counter-productive in a high prevalence population if monogamy means abandoning condoms. This message was promoted to gay men in the earliest years of the epidemic in advance of any firm knowledge about routes of transmission or prevalence of the infectious agent, and undoubtedly placed many individuals at greater risk.

Distance from the epicentre of the epidemic and travel also played a crucial role in determining the degree to which HIV had spread in the population by the time that the alarm began to be raised. In Britain for instance, this happened early in 1983, and one of the earliest informal methods of protection adopted by gay men was to avoid sex with Americans. This may have been an effective strategy at that time, since a high proportion of the early UK cases amongst gay men had US contacts. Another factor which may have minimised the harm of HIV was London's relative underdevelopment as a gay holiday resort compared with Paris or Amsterdam at this time. In this sense, London was culturally more distant from the epicentre of the epidemic than Amsterdam or Sydney.

In Africa the epidemic has spread along pathways which were already well-defined trade routes and highways. The development of prostitution to service truck drivers on transcontinental trade routes is one example of the way in which travel interacted with sexual activity to further the transmission of HIV. In the United States the epidemic spread outwards from the major gay communities and centres of drug use to regional nodes, which in turn served as centres for local epidemics, a phenomenon which should have allowed prevention efforts to be targeted not only at risk groups and risk behaviours but at risk regions.

These characteristics and institutions were of crucial importance in the early spread of HIV, and continue to be important factors in introducing HIV into new populations. However, other social factors tend to explain the continued spread of HIV once it has been identified in a population or region. These social factors are discussed in more detail in *Understanding the epidemic*.

Further reading

Elizabeth Fee and Daniel M.Fox (eds): AIDS: the making of a chronic disease, University of California Press, 1992.

Gould P. The Slow Plague, Blackwell, 1993.

Randy Shilts: And the band played on: politics, people and the AIDS epidemic, Penguin, 1997.

The epidemic since 1981

First case reports: 1981

The first identification of a pattern of illness related to immune suppression came in 1981. It was discovered that a rare cancer, Kaposi's sarcoma, was appearing amongst gay men in New York, Los Angeles and San Francisco and in June 1981 a short report was published in the weekly news bulletin of the Centers For Disease Control. The original report can be read at http://www.cdc.gov/hiv/pubs/mmwr/mmwr05jun81.pdf

A number of doctors had been aware of extraordinary levels of immunosuppression and sexually transmitted infections amongst sexually active gay men in New York and San Francisco for several years, and also of the widespread emergence of persistently swollen lymph glands (PGL-Persistent Generalised Lymphadenopathy) amongst gay men.

Many of these doctors were concerned that very high levels of sexual activity amongst urban gay men could eventually lead to chronic ill-health. During the late 1970s epidemic hepatitis B began to become a serious health problem amongst gay men, as did bowel infections such as giardiasis and amoebiasis. The first, mysterious cases of a rare skin cancer, later identified as Kaposi's sarcoma, began to appear amongst gay men in 1979 and 1980, but it was not until 1981 that a clear pattern emerged.

Reconstructing the first cases of HIV in North America has been hindered by genuine concerns about patient confidentiality. Much of the published literature provides nothing more than a general background. One paper that was published in 1984 entitled *AIDS Trends in the United States 1978-1982* by Curran, Haverkos and Selik divided the earliest cases of AIDS into four 'risk groups'. These were; gay and bisexual men (with the first cases appearing in the first quarter of 1978), intravenous drug users, Haitians (first cases appearing in the first quarter of 1980) and haemophiliacs (first cases appearing in the last quarter of 1981).

According to this paper, 4 cases of AIDS were diagnosed in the USA in 1978 and a further 8 in 1979. Eleven of the 12 cases were among gay men, 8 who lived in New York, 2 in California, 1 in Illinois and one whose place of residence was not specified.

Additional reports in the medical literature concerning the suspected AIDS cases in 1979 in the report above suggest that at least 5 of the 8 cases were genuine AIDS cases which resulted in death in 1979 or 1980. The four cases from 1978 may be more problematic in that it is likely that two of them may represent cases of classical KS.

The search for a cause

The disease was known at first as Gay Related Immune Deficiency, gay cancer or gay pneumonia. Within days of the first reports appearing in Morbidity and Mortality Weekly Report (MMWR), doctors from across the USA reported similar cases.

In 1981 cases of the inexplicable immune disorder appeared in injecting drug users in New York, but it was not until the summer of 1982 that the disorder was named the Acquired Immune Deficiency Syndrome. By this time cases had also been reported amongst Haitians living in the United States and amongst hæmophiliacs, but it was not until November 1983 that the first case of AIDS was reported in a recipient of an infected blood transfusion. All of these factors, and the first report of AIDS in a woman in August 1981, lent weight to a growing medical consensus that AIDS must be caused by a transmissible agent which could be passed on in blood and through sexual contact.

Pathology logs from 18 major US cities were analysed. These suggested that AIDS cases were not spread evenly throughout the USA, but rather were confined to the major centres of New York, Los Angeles, San Francisco and Atlanta.

A typical GRID patient was a gay man in his thirties, who frequented bars and saunas, and who used poppers as a sexual stimulant.

One of the first factors to be investigated as a cause was the use of poppers, or nitrite inhalants. Researchers found no link, but did notice that many of the earliest cases were linked: they had been one another's sexual partners. At this time researchers were working on the assumption that the disease had an incubation period of one year to eighteen months. With the benefit of hindsight, it is now reasonable to argue that this discovery was a case of drawing the correct conclusion from the wrong clues. Many of these early cases were unlikely to have been sources of infection for other cases in the early clusters; their linkage simply reflected the high turnover of partners amongst these men, and the very high level of seroprevalence of HIV in some sexual networks of gay men by 1981.

After the dismissal of poppers as a potential cause, opinion was divided between researchers on whether AIDS was caused by a single transmissible agent, in the same way as hepatitis B, or by a combination of immune suppressive factors. The latter theory, the immune overload theory, was developed as a result of the observation that all those who developed AIDS had immunosuppressive risks which might lead to the dramatic suppression of cell-mediated immunity seen in AIDS. In gay men, it was argued that repeated sexually transmitted infections combined with the use of antibiotics and the introduction of sperm into the rectum suppressed immunity. In hæmophiliacs, the repeated administration of blood products was blamed for suppressing immunity, whilst opiates and blood-borne infections were blamed for AIDS in injecting drug users. No explanation could be offered within this framework for the earliest cases of AIDS in women, except to insist that they must have been injecting drug users.

Subsequent research has shown that these factors alone cannot account for the immune suppression seen in the groups at risk of AIDS. For instance, gay men who report a high level of receptive anal intercourse but who remain uninfected with HIV do not develop AIDS. Hæmophiliacs who received Factor VIII not infected with HIV have not developed AIDS, although some studies have shown that Factor VIII is associated with a degree of immune suppression. Injecting drug users not infected with HIV do not develop AIDS either.

The search for a transmissible cause quickly became focused on the search for a retrovirus. Just months after the first cases of AIDS had been reported, virologists had already noted a similarity between the syndrome and the symptoms caused by feline leukemia virus, a retrovirus which affects cats. Research into viral causes for cancer was already well developed in the United States, and researchers in this field were quick to recognise that the hunt for an AIDS virus provided an exciting new area of research which could shed light on many of the problems they had been wrestling with for years.

HTLV-1 was the first cancer-causing retrovirus to have been identified, by Robert Gallo in 1980. His research team began looking for a virus in the same family. Meanwhile in Paris, researchers at the Pasteur Institute isolated a retrovirus from the lymph node of a gay man with early symptoms. Rather than causing lymphocytes (white blood cells) to divide, as the human leukemia virus (HTLV-1) did, this virus caused the cells to disappear. Luc Montagnier and colleagues called it lymphadenopathy associated virus (LAV). By mid-1983 Montagnier had isolated LAV from a gay man, a haemophiliac and a Haitian with AIDS, but in April 1984 the US Department of Health announced that the cause of AIDS had been discovered by Robert Gallo, in the shape of a virus named HTLV-3.

Gallo was subsequently accused of stealing Montagnier's discovery, sent as a sample to Gallo's laboratory, but Gallo claimed that LAV was a different virus. LAV and HTLV-3 have subsequently been shown to be identical. The French and US governments soon entered into a patent dispute over the discovery of the virus, because financial as well as public health interests were at stake in the discovery of HIV. Testing kits were to become a major source of revenue to those who had legal rights over the virus. Huge personal prestige was also at stake. It was subsequently established that LAV was indeed the virus described as HTLV-3, and that it had accidentally contaminated Gallo's cultures.

Further reading

Mirko Grmek: The History of AIDS: Emergence and Origin of a Modern Pandemic, Princeton University Press, 1991. All the research cited in this section is referenced in Grmek's History of AIDS, the best book available on the origins of the epidemic.

Edward Hooper: The River, Penguin, 1999.

Robert Root-Bernstein: Rethinking AIDS, Free Press, 1993.

The emergence of safer sex

Whilst scientists struggled to isolate a virus, the community most affected by AIDS was struggling to adjust to a new disease which appeared to be spreading rapidly. The responses of gay communities were to be instrumental in limiting the spread of AIDS and the harm caused by the epidemic. This section looks at those responses in some detail, in order that the roots of community-based responses to AIDS are not forgotten.

The earliest gay community response to AIDS came in the summer of 1981, with an article in the *New York Native*, a major gay newspaper. It drew attention to 'gay cancer', and called on gay men to donate money for research into the cause and for treatment research. A group of New York gay men also founded Gay Men's Health Crisis. At the same time the only national media attention to AIDS came in the form of a brief article in the New York Times with the headline 'Rare cancer seen in 41 homosexual men'.

The first safer sex guidelines, published in early 1983 (*How To Have Sex In An Epidemic* by Richard Berkowitz and Michael Callen), worked from the assumption that AIDS was caused by a repeated assault on the immune system by sexually transmitted diseases and other factors. They recommended 'no exchange of body fluids', and the use of condoms. Similar guidelines were evolved independently at the same time by an order of gay male nuns in San Francisco, the Sisters of Perpetual Indulgence, and the (then) San Francisco KS Foundation.

Early safer sex messages

It is important to understand the extraordinary shock which AIDS caused to a gay male culture organised around sex, and the speed with which that culture adjusted. The change in behaviour amongst gay men in large cities in North America and Europe can only be likened to the large-scale changes in human behaviour brought on by war. The first AIDS organisations were founded in 1982 by gay men in New York and other large cities in North America; in the UK the first AIDS organisation was founded in 1983.

The first information was disseminated in the gay press, by word of mouth and through sexual contacts, the most elementary forms of 'grass roots' peer education. It was also disseminated through doctors in GU medicine clinics, although advice from doctors may have been more cautious. In some cities the danger of infection through sexual activity was downplayed because the owners or major advertisers of the papers were also owners of the bathhouses, but the *New York Native*, Toronto's *Body Politic* and Boston's *Gay Community News* were especially important in conveying a number of messages to gay men:

- Cut down on your number of sexual partners.

- Don't exchange body fluids.

- Only have sex with people you know, who don't have AIDS.

Unfortunately, some of this advice provided no protection against the unknown agent, whilst for many, any advice was too late to prevent infection. It is estimated that new infections amongst gay men peaked in North American cities in 1983, and that more than half of all seroconversions occurred between 1978 and 1982, before any sort of warning had gone out to gay men.

Condom use was not part of the initial message which began to circulate amongst gay men. In the past, condoms had not been adopted to prevent other sexually transmitted diseases because most diseases were treatable and a pilot vaccine was becoming available against hepatitis B. Condoms were not part of the sexual culture of gay men, and their adoption took time.

What occurred between 1982 and 1985 was a drop in the number of sexual partners reported by gay men recruited to research studies, and an abandonment of anal intercourse. One survey showed a dramatic decline in cases of other STDs among gay men in New York from 2300 cases reported in 1981 to 500 in 1987.

Unfortunately, because HIV prevalence amongst gay men in large North American cities was already high by the time gay men started to adopt safer sex, the strategy of sticking to one partner failed to provide protection, though it may have helped to contain the epidemic during the 1990s.

The bathhouses debate

During 1983 and 1984 several North American gay communities were split over the question of whether bathhouses should be allowed to remain open in light of the widely accepted belief that many men were continuing to have unsafe sex in these places despite the warning that AIDS was caused by a sexually transmitted agent.

Some people argued that it was best to close the bathhouses in order to cut down on the potential for anonymous, unprotected sex. Others argued that the bathhouses should remain open, since they were ideal sites to educate sexually active men about the possible routes of HIV transmission. This argument was to happen in many countries, and was to rehearse a much broader political debate about the control of behaviour which was likely to put people at risk of HIV infection.

In both Europe and North America messages about the adoption of safer sex and risk reduction strategies seem to have been spread through a number of peer support networks: sexual partners, gay switchboards and support groups, alongside the gay press.

Further reading

Edward King: Safety In Numbers, Chps 1,2, Cassell, 1993.

Joseph Sonnabend: Acquired immunodeficiency syndrome: Opportunistic infections and malignancies in male homosexuals, JAMA 249: 2370.

AIDS in other population subgroups

Appearance of AIDS in hæmophiliacs

The first case of AIDS was recognised in a person with hæmophilia in the United States in January 1982, although it is now clear that a small number of cases had gone unrecognised as far back as 1979 in the United States. Despite this report, it took almost three years for public health authorities to act to safeguard the supply of clotting factor in some countries, resulting in thousands of infections which might have been avoided by the prompt introduction of heat treated Factor VIII, a process already recognised to reduce the hazard of hepatitis B infection. Even though the causative agent had not been isolated in 1983 and 1984, there were enough parallels between the incidence of hepatitis B and AIDS in different populations to make heat treatment a reasonable precaution.

For over a year and a half physicians debated whether Factor VIII was indeed the source of the agent which caused AIDS, and waited for action upon the blood banks which gathered the blood from which Factor VIII is isolated. Most seroconversions among haemophiliacs occurred in 1983 and 1984 in the United States and Europe, and infected blood products continued to be distributed until the end of 1985 in France. As a result, half of all hæmophiliacs in France were infected, whilst in the UK one quarter of hæmophiliacs were infected. In general, those with the most serious hæmophilia were most likely to have been infected, owing to their greater intake of Factor VIII; those who received greater quantities of imported blood were also at greater risk (see *HIV transmission through blood transfusions and blood products* and *Haemophilia* for further details of these findings).

Appearance of AIDS in blood transfusion recipients

The first case of AIDS in a person with no other risk except for blood transfusion was diagnosed in a New York hospital in the summer of 1982. Amazingly, the report of this case was rejected for publication by several medical journals, and it was not until December 1982 that the first case of AIDS due to blood transfusion was officially recognised by the US Centers for Disease Control.

During this period the blood banks refused to accept that a clear public health risk existed in the United States, although the British Blood Transfusion Service began to ask individuals from high-risk groups (gay men and drug users) to refrain from giving blood in August 1983. As one historian has commented, the CDC 'moved with great consideration for the institutions in question'. The blood banks objected to demands for screening on the grounds that there was still no proof that AIDS had a transmissible cause, whilst gay groups objected on civil rights grounds to calls for gay men to refrain from donating blood. When the CDC proposed that the antibody test for hepatitis B be used as a surrogate test for those at risk for AIDS (88% of those diagnosed with AIDS at the beginning of 1983 had antibodies to hepatitis B) the blood banks objected on the grounds of cost. They estimated that it would cost around $100 million a year to test for hepatitis B, and this outlay was for a route of transmission that remained unproven, they argued.

The key problem in the US was the for-profit nature of blood donation. In contrast to the voluntary, unpaid donation system run largely by non-profit organisations in Europe, the United States had a system of paid donors, and blood banks in turn sold the blood to hospitals. The paid donor system was particularly abused by injecting drug users who donated blood frequently in order to obtain money.

It was not until March 1984 that an antibody test for HIV became available for commercial use in the United States. In the UK all blood donated since November 1985 has been screened for antibodies to HIV.

AIDS in children

The first case of AIDS in a child was identified in late 1981 at Albert Einstein Hospital in New York; several more were to follow in the next year. All were children of mothers who injected drugs. In May 1983 a report of AIDS in children in the *Journal of the American Medical Association* sparked mass panic after one of the reporting physicians speculated that AIDS had developed as a result of casual household contact. His views were echoed by Dr Anthony Fauci of the National Institutes of Health, who said 'If routine close contacts can spread the disease, AIDS takes on an entirely new dimension'.

In fact, the claim that the cases were a consequence of casual household contact was strongly disputed by other doctors reporting cases of AIDS in children in the same issue of the journal. For neither the first nor the last time, accuracy in AIDS reporting was sacrificed for sensationalism.

There had been little evidence of panic over casual transmission of AIDS before this report. It triggered a panic which is still

being dealt with by health educators. Although it is often argued that fears of contagion accompany any new disease, it is also arguable that clear guidance by public health authorities can allay such fears. The unwarranted speculation of public health officials and their exaggeration by the media was to prove a huge obstacle to future education efforts.

Further reading

Randy Shilts: And the band played on: Politics, people and the AIDS epidemic, Penguin, 1987.

The AIDS panic begins

The speculation about casual household transmission was reported by US news agencies with the headline 'AIDS Disease Could Endanger the General Population' in May 1983. Within days firefighters and policemen in San Francisco had been issued with rubber gloves and face masks, fanning fears that AIDS was contagious. In the months to come hundreds of incidents stoked public fears that the 'gay plague' might be airborne or passed through food handling, touch, clothing and bedding. Television crews in several cities refused to work in studios in which people with AIDS were being interviewed, and jurors in a San Francisco court case demanded to be released from jury service when it emerged that one of their number had AIDS, lest they be infected by sitting with him. Nurses refused to care for AIDS patients and funeral directors refused to handle the bodies of people who had died of AIDS. In June 1983 a quarter of Americans questioned for a Gallup poll feared they could get AIDS by casual contact with an infected individual.

This hysteria was to have several important consequences. It posed a major problem for health education, since huge numbers of people were ill-informed about the disease and its routes of transmission as a result of media coverage. The hysteria also made the issue of the identification and surveillance of people with AIDS hugely controversial.

Demands quickly emerged for the quarantine of people with AIDS in order to protect the general population, and it was the fear of misuse of information about people with HIV and AIDS which led to opposition to HIV testing and proper surveillance of HIV diagnoses in the United States. As a consequence, it is still impossible to track accurately the spread of HIV in the United States owing to completely anonymised testing.

In contrast, the UK established a system of confidential reporting which protected the identity of people with HIV whilst allowing public health authorities to track the development of the epidemic. The hysteria also amplified prejudice against people with AIDS, who were already shunned in many cases because of their sexuality.

The 'gay plague'

As AIDS moved from being represented as a minor problem affecting homosexuals to being a major threat to the general population, anti-gay prejudice became vehement. Media coverage gave the impression that the gay lifestyle and the gay movement in themselves were responsible for AIDS, rather than the presence of a virus amongst the gay population. In the UK, *The Sun* described AIDS as 'the gay plague', whilst in the USA syndicated newspaper columnist Patrick Buchanan pronounced that 'the homosexuals have exacted a terrible price for their lifestyle'.

Those who expressed the view that AIDS represented the wages of sin were given prominent coverage in news media throughout the developed world, whilst any sense that an extraordinary natural disaster was befalling gay men was entirely missing from news coverage. Hæmophiliacs and those infected through blood transfusions began to be represented as 'innocent' victims, rather than as victims of institutional neglect and corporate greed.

It is sometimes easy to forget the depth of prejudice which was vented in the media and by the general public during the first few years of the AIDS epidemic. From 1983 onwards the tabloid press in the UK gave increasing attention to homosexuality in a way which was bound to inflame prejudice. Up until 1981 opinion polls had shown that a growing proportion of British voters supported equal rights for lesbians and gay men; after 1981 support diminished dramatically at the very time when an organised lesbian and gay movement was beginning to emerge at both national and local level.

In 1986 Geoffrey Dickens MP called for the re-criminalisation of homosexuality, and Sir Alfred Sherman, a close friend of Margaret Thatcher, wrote in *The Times* that AIDS was a problem of 'undesirable minorities ... mainly sodomites and drug abusers, together with numbers of women who voluntarily associate with this sexual underworld'. There is little doubt amongst observers that Margaret Thatcher regarded homosexuality with distaste, even though apologists for her regime have claimed she counted homosexuals amongst her best friends. Like Ronald Reagan, she regarded homosexuality as an unfit subject for public discussion and a political embarrassment to a government whose core constituency was more likely than most to have strong prejudices against homosexuals and drug users.

This view was most clearly articulated by the Conservative Family Campaign (CFC), which called for the re-criminalisation of homosexuality and the isolation of the infected. As representatives of public opinion favoured by a number of journalists and newspaper proprietors, the CFC was able to win great prominence for its views, and played a key role in whipping up anti-gay prejudice. Today the CFC wins little public attention and has dwindled to a handful of members, its dreams of power dashed after repeated failures to influence public policy.

During the early 1980s lesbian and gay concerns began to be addressed in local government in London in the fields of education, policing and discrimination; by 1986 homosexuality was a major political issue in the UK and in 1987 the Conservative Party characterised the Labour Party's education policy as one of 'gay lessons' provided against the wishes of parents. The negative publicity was undoubtedly damaging to the Labour Party and had a serious effect on the political acceptability of prevention work targeted at gay men.

In late 1987 the Conservative government drafted Section 28 of the Local Government Act, intended to prevent the promotion with taxpayers' money of homosexuality as an acceptable alternative lifestyle. This legislation dissuaded many local authorities and health authorities from carrying out HIV prevention work with gay men despite the fact that HIV prevention was specifically exempted. Section 28 was finally abolished on 17th November 2003.

Moral panic and stigmatisation

In the developed world AIDS was widely characterised as having brought about the end of an era. In 1983 the American author Andrew Holleran wrote that AIDS 'had subverted the pleasures of promiscuous sex as abruptly as OPEC had ended the era of cheap energy', whilst in England Martin Amis described AIDS as 'the closure of the sexual revolution'. Even in 1994 such metaphors were still alive and kicking; a new history of the UK epidemic was entitled *The End of Innocence*.

Whilst it is clear that major changes in behaviour took place in the years following the emergence of AIDS, the role of AIDS in motivating those changes except amongst the high-risk groups is questionable.

'While it seems fairly clear to us that the sexual revolution is no longer careering along on its carefree course, what we have actually seen in the broad population is a levelling off in the rate of sexual experimentation rather than a reversion to the values of earlier days' wrote Masters and Johnson in their 1987 call to arms *Crisis: Heterosexual Behaviour in the Age of AIDS*. This levelling off had already begun amongst heterosexuals before the mid-1980s AIDS panic hit the heterosexual population, and appears to have been related in part to the massive increase in herpes infections amongst heterosexual men and women and misgivings about the safety of some forms of contraception. It

was also due to an increasingly conservative social and economic climate in which pleasure became secondary to work. Business became a lifestyle in the 1980s, but many social commentators were quicker to seize upon the media hype that surrounded AIDS than to recognise how AIDS fitted into the political economy of the 1980s.

In the UK some Marxist commentators saw the AIDS panic as a plot by right-wing governments to scare the working class into embracing 'family values', yet what is remarkable about public information campaigns in the developed world is the extent to which they eschewed moralising and concentrated on giving 'the facts'. In fact the shift to family values in the rhetoric of some right-wing politicians was an appeal to the confusion created by rapid social change and inflation, and events such as AIDS were merely a fleeting motif in a wider defensive action intended to create an illusion of social stability by reinforcing the centrality of the family in political discourse.

Subsequent surveys have shown that the fear of AIDS has tended to reinforce cautious sexual behaviour amongst those who have fewer sexual partners, but that in the UK at least, it has had little effect on the behaviour of young people who have more than two sexual partners per year (Johnson).

References

Simon Garfield: The End of Innocence: Britain in the time of AIDS, Faber & Faber, 1994.

Anne Johnson et al: Sexual Attitudes and Lifestyles, Blackwell, 1994.

William Masters et al: Crisis: Heterosexual Behaviour In The Age of AIDS, Weidenfield and Nicolson, 1988.

Simon Watney: Policing Desire, Routledge, 1987.

Simon Watney: Practices of Freedom, Rivers Oram, 1994.

State neglect of the epidemic

While gay communities in large cities began to treat AIDS as an emergency, governments in the United States and other countries responded slowly to the threat of AIDS. It was not until 1985 that governments in the US or the UK took serious steps to inform the population, and it was not until the late 1980s that information was targeted at those most at risk. When Health Minister John Patten first suggested an education campaign in early 1985, the need to educate gay men was dismissed by his Cabinet colleagues. Even when the British Government launched a national educational campaign in the mainstream press in 1985, it was criticised by Tony Whitehead of the Terrence Higgins Trust for failing to target gay men and injecting drug users as a matter of urgency. The first pamphlet on AIDS issued by the Health Education Council (as it was called at the time) in January 1985 did not mention anal intercourse, and it was not until 1989 that the Health Education Authority (as it was called then) produced any advertising aimed specifically at gay men.

In the United States some city governments were more responsive than others to calls for action. In San Francisco the city's Department of Public Health was quick to seek out community organisations through which to build a consensus about the need for behaviour change (including closure of public sex facilities), and the city quickly moved to fund health education and care services. In New York by contrast it took more than a year for the city's administration to acknowledge the epidemic. The city's health commissioner opposed attempts to establish a programme of co-ordinated care between the city's social services, hospitals and voluntary organisations. At the end of 1983 Mathilde Krim of the American Foundation for AIDS Research said no one in city government 'gave a damn' about the need for AIDS services in the US city worst affected by AIDS.

It was the same with injecting drug users. Vigorous opposition to a policy of needle exchange, to the distribution of bleach to addicts or any prevention activity which appeared to condone drug use made it extremely difficult to prevent infection. There was also widespread denial amongst drug users and drugs workers that a problem existed, and it was not until 1985-86 that widespread education work began (Des Jarlais). The city of

New York began a needle exchange programme in 1988, but this was terminated in 1990 for political reasons.

In the UK education aimed at drug users didn't begin until 1986, when it became evident that injecting drug users in the Edinburgh area had a high prevalence of HIV infection. Needless to say voluntary organisations such as the Terrence Higgins Trust, Standing Conference on Drug Abuse (SCODA) and Scottish AIDS Monitor had to carry out such work.

The core reason for neglect was an unwillingness to allocate money to socially unpopular groups, particularly those which did not have concentrated voting power capable of determining elections. In the United States the apportionment of public money is strongly influenced by the activities of pressure groups representing political constituencies, and the political weakness of AIDS-affected communities makes neglect of their needs a politically viable decision for legislators at national and local level in the US (see Kayal for a discussion of funding allocation).

AIDS organisations initially lacked proper lobbying skills and were unable to influence Congress by a mass mobilisation of public opinion in the same way as the Christian right consistently manages to do. Recently US AIDS activists have begun to discuss what can be done to improve this situation, but much political attention has been diverted away from AIDS issues by the involvement of gay activists in the campaign to elect President Clinton and subsequent demands to legalise lesbian and gay military service.

In the UK it is less easy to claim that the Government has neglected the epidemic as a whole, but it is certainly accurate to say that the Government has consistently ignored the most affected community - gay and bisexual men. There has been little pressure until recently from AIDS organisations to rectify this imbalance, and none from gay campaigning organisations such as the Stonewall Group.

Further reading

Dennis Altman: AIDS and The New Puritanism, Pluto, 1986.

Don Des Jarlais: The First City: HIV among intravenous drug users in New York, in AIDS: The making of a chronic disease, eds Elizabeth Fee and Daniel M. Fox, University of California Press, 1992.

Philip Kayal: Bearing Witness: Gay Men's Health Crisis and The Politics of AIDS, Westview, 1993.

Larry Kramer: The Normal Heart (1985); Reports from the Holocaust, Penguin, 1993.

Randy Shilts: And The Band Played On, Penguin, 1987.

Injecting drug use

The 1980s in Britain was an era in which the recorded prevalence and spread of drug use increased among most sectors of the population. In the last five years of the decade, the Home Office Notifications of new drug users (Misuse of Drugs Act, Class 1) increased by 46% and the number of renotifications has also continued to increase. However, these statistics perhaps represent as little as 10% of the overall number of long-term users.

In 1982 in their Treatment and Rehabilitation Report, the Advisory Council on the Misuse of Drugs (ACMD) recommended the development of Drug Advisory Committees to co-ordinate local services both within the voluntary and statutory sectors. Since the NHS and Community Care Act Drug Advisory Committees may have a role in advising purchasing authorities.

In its first report, Aids and Drug Misuse (1989), the ACMD stated that 'the spread of HIV is a greater danger to individuals and the public than drug misuse'. This promoted a shift towards harm reduction policies.

It became a priority to draw as many drug users as possible into services, in order to prevent the spread of HIV infection and minimise drug related harm.

By the end of 1986 MPs were debating whether or not to fund needle and syringe exchange programmes; Scottish Office

Minister John Mackay told the Commons, 'AIDS is a totally self-inflicted illness', but in 1987 the Department of Health set up a pilot programme to monitor the effectiveness of needle exchanges and mounted the first education programme for injecting drug users in the autumn of 1987. From 1988 onwards an increasing number of drugs projects set up needle exchanges, and the availability of clean needles together with a relatively well developed network of drugs projects and treatment services has played a key role in preventing the spread of HIV in the UK. Policies on drug use and HIV have been far more pragmatic in the UK than many other countries, and are widely regarded as a model for other European countries.

The emergence of voluntary organisations

In the United States the first voluntary organisations to be established were Gay Men's Health Crisis in New York and the Kaposi's Sarcoma Research and Education Foundation in San Francisco (later the San Francisco AIDS Foundation). Initially these organisations were established to raise money for research into the new disease, and to disseminate information to gay men, and it was to be several years before these organisations began to develop the much broader roles of service provision and policy advocacy. The organisations also established helplines, and had close links with the leading doctors treating people with AIDS.

In the UK the first organisation to emerge was the Terrence Higgins Trust, which was founded in 1982 in memory of one of the first British gay men to die of AIDS. The Trust was re-launched in May 1983 with the object of providing education and support by volunteers from London Gay Switchboard, which organised a conference in May 1983 to discuss the new disease.

These UK initiatives followed the broadcast of a BBC2 Horizon documentary Killer In The Village, arguably the single most important programme on AIDS to be broadcast in Britain. It alerted thousands of gay men to the new disease. By the end of 1983 the Terrence Higgins Trust had published its first information leaflet on AIDS and opened a helpline in early 1984. The first safer sex leaflet was launched in late 1984, and it was at this point that the gay press and most gay men in the UK began to realise that safer sex precautions required more than just the avoidance of Americans (Berridge; Garfield; Scott).

Trust volunteers met with the Chief Medical Officer to lobby for public education, and used the gay press to promote the adoption of safer sex. For several years the gay press, and Capital Gay in particular, remained the only regular source of information on AIDS in the UK.

The Terrence Higgins Trust grew during the 1980s from an organisation with a very small staff to the largest employer in the HIV voluntary sector and the biggest provider of services to people with HIV. The Trust's early work concentrated on plugging the gaps left by government neglect, which meant that the organisation was amongst the first to work not only with gay men but with drug users, prisoners, women, young people, faith communities, families and children. The organisation's great strength is its basis in volunteers' direct experience of the epidemic. One of the first services to be developed was an idea copied from the American model, buddying, intended to counter the isolation and shock felt by people diagnosed with AIDS.

Scottish AIDS Monitor (SAM) was also founded in 1983, but was forced to close in 1995.

A support group for people diagnosed HIV-positive was founded soon after the HIV antibody test became available in the UK in late 1984. People with HIV identified the need for peer support as crucial. Body Positive started out as a support group within the Terrence Higgins Trust, but swiftly became a separate organisation from February 1985, and during 1985 founded a helpline, a hospital visiting service and a newsletter. The Body Positive drop-in centre opened in June 1989 and the group held its first annual conference in 1989.

A national network of Body Positive groups formed from 1986 onwards as people diagnosed HIV-positive outside London sought the support of self-help groups. The Body Positive movement was a reflection of the large asymptomatic population of HIV-infected people in the UK and the relatively small number of people with AIDS. In contrast, American activism was concentrated on PWA (people with AIDS) groups from very early on in the epidemic, leading to very different models of advocacy and support.

Frontliners was founded in 1986, once again within the Terrence Higgins Trust, but also grew into a separate organisation with its own premises and branches outside London. Frontliners provided support, advice and information as well as monitoring services provided to people with HIV and AIDS. The organisation opened its own premises in 1990, but was forced to close for financial reasons in 1991.

In 1993 a new organisation for people living with HIV and AIDS was founded. The UK Coalition of People Living with HIV and AIDS also provides advocacy, support and information.

Positively Women was started in 1987 by a group of HIV-positive women who found that existing services were unable to meet the needs of women diagnosed with HIV.

The National AIDS Trust (NAT) was founded in May 1987 with finance from the government. Its role would be to co-ordinate the activities of the voluntary sector, and fundraising chairman Robert Maxwell promised that the Trust would raise £50 million. Unsurprisingly, virtually none of this money materialised, and it was to be left to trusts such as CRUSAID and the Red Hot AIDS Charitable Trust together with trust funds set up by two pop stars, Elton John and Freddie Mercury (posthumously) to perform the bulk of independent fundraising in the UK. As a co-ordinator of voluntary sector activity the National AIDS Trust's record has been mixed; whilst the organisation has done much to provide 'seed' funding for new organisations and has been quick to recognise new needs, critics of NAT say that the organisation had failed until recently to grasp the extent to which the political climate was changing or the needs of gay men were being ignored.

Further reading

Dennis Altman: Power and Community: Organizational and Cultural Responses to AIDS, Taylor and Francis, 1994.

Simon Garfield: The End of Innocence: Britain in the time of AIDS, Faber & Faber, 1994.

Philip Kayal: Bearing Witness: Gay Men's Health Crisis and the Politics of AIDS, Westview, 1993.

Edward King: Safety In Numbers (Chapter Five), Cassell, 1993. Peter Scott: White Noise: How gay men's activism gets written out of AIDS prevention, in: Acting on AIDS, Eds Josh Oppenheim and Helena Reckitt, Serpents Tail, 1997.

AIDS becomes a public emergency: 1985-89

The death of Rock Hudson

It was the death of movie star Rock Hudson in August 1985 which paradoxically began to change public perceptions of who was at risk for AIDS and how much of a public health priority AIDS ought to be.

Rock Hudson's death triggered huge media interest in AIDS, presaging the extent to which future coverage of AIDS would hinge upon its impact on celebrities. AIDS ceased to be regarded as a minority issue after Hudson's death, as speculation increased about the extent of the epidemic likely to occur amongst heterosexuals. This was highly ironic, given that Hudson was the victim of the epidemic occurring amongst gay and bisexual men, but his heterosexual image continued to deflect attention away from his sexuality even in death.

The emerging heterosexual epidemic 1985-87

In the second half of 1985 several factors combined to create a renewed AIDS panic, this time focused on fears that HIV was breaking out into the heterosexual population via 'bridging groups' - injecting drug users and bisexual men. In the United States HIV was beginning to be diagnosed amongst the female partners of injecting drug users with increasing frequency, leading to speculation that a chain of transmission could develop amongst heterosexuals who did not inject drugs, and that AIDS would 'break out' of the high risk groups by this route.

Public health officials also looked to Africa with growing concern, where available evidence suggested that an HIV and AIDS epidemic was occurring amongst heterosexuals. In September 1986 the British ambassador to Zaire warned in a dispatch to the Foreign Office of the frightening possibility that HIV might behave in the same way amongst heterosexuals in the developed world.

Armed with this limited knowledge, public health officials and journalists began to speak in terms of tens of thousands of AIDS cases amongst heterosexuals unless sexual behaviour changed. In October 1986 the US Surgeon-General Everett Koop published a report on the US AIDS epidemic which predicted that AIDS would increasingly become a heterosexual problem in the United States. A major public education campaign was launched, to be followed a few months later by a similar initiative in the United Kingdom. British efforts were characterised by an extraordinary degree of co-operation between government and broadcasters as television networks planned a week of programmes for February 1987 in collaboration with the Department of Health. AIDS was treated in practice as the greatest national emergency since the Second World War, the first occasion on which broadcasters had sought to co-ordinate their programmes to ensure that all viewers would be exposed to the message 'Everyone Is At Risk'.

One of the key effects of this campaign was to create widespread anxiety amongst heterosexuals over minimal HIV risks and to create a new category of those in need of services, the 'worried well'. This panic did not exist before the Government advertising campaigns, yet the massive increase in the number of people needlessly seeking tests has been interpreted as an indicator of the success of public education! Any rational public health analysis would see this as a grotesque misallocation of resources, and any rational public health policy would not have continued to panic people unnecessarily, long after the point at which it became evident that the risk to the general population was relatively minimal.

The formation of AIDS policy in the UK

The Public Health Laboratory Service (as it was then called) began to monitor AIDS in the UK in August 1982 and by 1983 it was clear that public health measures would be necessary in order to respond to the disease. The first area in which public policy was developed was with regard to blood transfusions and blood products. In August 1983 the Blood Transfusion Service issued an appeal for donors from high-risk groups to refrain from giving blood, and in late 1983 the Chief Medical Officer Donald Acheson first met with representatives of the Terrence Higgins Trust to put on record his concern over the spread of AIDS.

Acheson was to be the key figure in the British government response to AIDS during the 1980s. It was he who convinced Government ministers of the importance and urgency of AIDS as a public health issue, and it was he who steered the Government away from panic measures through the recruitment of an Expert Advisory Group on AIDS (EAGA), composed of specialists already working in the field.

EAGA was convened in early 1985 to guide the Department of Health in the formulation of policy and the development of health education messages. EAGA recommended that no special measures were required to control people with HIV and AIDS, and that existing VD and infectious disease legislation was adequate to monitor and control the disease. In years to come this decision was to be condemned by right-wing writers as a capitulation to the gay lobby, but in truth the Terrence Higgins

Trust had little influence on this decision. It was taken by medical professionals and civil servants, who saw not only the danger of driving underground those suffering from the disease, but also how anomalous this would be in the history of post-war public health.

Coercive public health measures had declined during the 20th century after a lively history of implementation during the early years of the public health movement. Legislation which could be used to quarantine people with infectious diseases had developed during the 19th century, but as democracy developed during the 20th century and infectious disease declined in incidence, coercive public health measures were less likely to be used. During the 1970s public health had become more politicised as a political analysis began to develop of the relationship between inequality and health and of the power of the medical profession.

Whilst the Government took the advice of EAGA on matters of public health policy, it was reluctant to accept the advice of EAGA and the associated Advisory Group on Health Education and AIDS when it came to setting the tone of health education. One member of the Health Education group reported that the unanimous suggestions of the group were invariably rejected by politicians, resulting in delays and obscure advertising which did more to confuse than inform the public (see Garfield). 'There will always be limits to what can be said in national advertisements' the Chief Medical Officer told EAGA members in July 1986, but the coyness of early advertising was laughable. Department of Health officials devised the phrase 'rectal sex' to describe the most high-risk activity. 'Why not use words like bumfucking?' asked Tony Whitehead of the Terrence Higgins Trust when the first adverts were published.

In October 1986 the Government's view of the severity of the problem was transformed with the publication of the Surgeon-General's Report in the United States, and civil servants and ministers moved swiftly from foot-dragging to crisis mode. Cabinet Secretary Robert Armstrong is reported to have remarked that nothing had caused him greater loss of sleep during his career as a public servant than the threat of AIDS, and in late 1986 he could be forgiven for sleepless nights. Predictions of the likely spread of AIDS based on extrapolations from Africa and New York were terrifying; the disease could engulf Western societies within a decade, decimating the most productive generations, claimed newspaper reports.

Within weeks civil servants had agreed with broadcasters that unprecedented steps would be taken to put across the message to the general public that AIDS was potentially a risk for everyone, and at the beginning of 1987 an advertising campaign together with a leaflet drop to every home in Britain took place. 'Don't Die of Ignorance' was the message, the iceberg its metaphor for the invisible threat of AIDS. The leaflet stressed that AIDS was 'not just a homosexual disease', a line supposed to quell prejudices that AIDS was a gay disease. Donald Acheson was concerned that unless correctly handled, one of the major effects of the campaign would be to increase prejudice against gay men. But given the degree of prejudice that had already been unleashed by media coverage of AIDS, it is hard to see how things could have got any worse - unless the Government were to give in to demands for punitive action against the gay community and people with HIV, who were blamed for visiting this scourge upon society. Were fears of the imminence of open repression amongst the gay community well founded, and was the Chief Medical Officer already alert to sympathy with such views amongst Government ministers?

In March 1987 TV channels co-operated to broadcast a week of programmes on AIDS, an unprecedented move in peacetime. Virtually none of these programmes were able to speak frankly to gay men; it was easier to speak frankly about injecting drug use than to approach the taboo subject of anal intercourse on the air.

Government policy was to continue to be formed by an alliance of experts and civil servants throughout the late 1980s and early 1990s. Yet there was never any coherent national plan for fighting AIDS, or a sense of long-term planning. This was to become painfully evident in the early 1990s.

Further reading

Keith Alcorn: The Public Sphere of AIDS in Taking Liberties, Serpents Tail, 1989.

Virginia Berridge: The early years of AIDS in the United Kingdom 1981-6: historical perspectives in Epidemics and ideas: essays on the historical perception of pestilence, Cambridge University Press, 1992.

Michael Fumento: The Myth of Heterosexual AIDS, Basic, 1990.

Simon Garfield: The End of Innocence (Chapter Six), Faber and Faber, 1994.

Edward King: Safety In Numbers (Chapter Five), Cassell, 1993.

The HIV test

It took just over a year from the announcement that the virus which caused AIDS had been isolated to the introduction of antibody testing kits which could be used to screen blood donations and test individuals who wanted to know whether they were infected. In most developed countries the test became available during 1985, and screening of blood donations began by the end of 1985. There was considerable demand amongst those in high risk groups for AIDS to know whether they were infected with HIV, but there was also considerable anxiety amongst the affected communities and especially amongst gay men over the ways in which the HIV antibody test could be used to discriminate against people with HIV.

The availability of a diagnostic test for HIV stimulated demands for the introduction of a number of traditional coercive and semi-coercive public health measures to control the spread of HIV. The availability of the test provided the technological means for the organisation of a conventional public health response to disease: the identification of carriers. In the United States the medical profession widely argued that AIDS and HIV infection should be treated the same as other sexually transmitted diseases, and that existing VD legislation was adequate to deal with the problems. This included:

- The power of physicians to test without consent.

- Mandatory testing of all persons seeking wedding licences or joining the armed forces.

- The requirement to notify partners of the infected and compel them to attend for treatment.

- The power to quarantine those who wilfully spread the disease.

- The routine testing of pregnant women to protect the unborn.

- The named reporting of carriers to allow full clinical follow-up (to prevent further spread of the disease).

All of these measures have been partially adopted with the exception of testing without consent. Mandatory testing of all persons requiring wedding licenses has been abandoned as too expensive by most American states which adopted the policy in the mid-1980s. Voluntary testing was quickly accepted as the only practical way to ensure that the civil liberties concerns of the gay community and people identified as HIV-positive were adequately addressed. Compulsory testing has been declared to be contrary to the European Convention on Human Rights.

In the United States antibody testing was seen as a key instrument of HIV prevention; there was a widespread faith amongst public health officials that simply knowing one's antibody status would result in behaviour changes. Yet amongst the gay community there were strong misgivings about the value of the test and its civil liberties implications. From late 1984 onwards the gay press in both Britain and America covered debates about testing in ways which sought to highlight the drawbacks of testing - the potential for discrimination as a result of the test, the lack of diagnostic information which the test provided and the chance of false positive results. But as the epidemic developed outside the gay community the civil libertarian opposition to testing diminished.

The protection of the 'innocent' through the introduction of ante-natal HIV screening in the United States was the first move towards more routine testing, but it was the developing notion of 'early intervention' - antiretroviral drug treatment and prophylaxis against PCP - which tipped the balance towards testing amongst gay men. Organisations such as the San Francisco AIDS Foundation and Gay Men's Health Crisis urged testing in order to gain access to treatment, especially early treatment with AZT, on the assumption that the drug delayed the development of AIDS. In 1993, however, the results of the Concorde trial of AZT showed no additional benefit if AZT was taken whilst asymptomatic compared with AZT taken at the onset of symptoms.

From 1987 onwards HIV antibody testing in the UK became more commonplace amongst heterosexuals, with demand driven largely by media campaigns.

These arguments ignore the social discrimination which has characterised the AIDS epidemic, the way in which discrimination has encouraged the spread of HIV amongst certain social groups and the way in which this discrimination structures the experience of HIV testing, diagnosis and disclosure. Fears that information about HIV status would be misused were well-founded in the mid-1980s. At that time there was no guarantee that people with HIV would be treated well; in the political climate of the period many feared that the ascendancy of the moral right could lead to more punitive measures against the infected.

In 1990 the Chief Medical Officer suggested that the medical benefits of testing now outweighed the disadvantages, whilst still acknowledging that the insurance industry's questions regarding HIV testing remained a disincentive to testing. In 1994 the Association of British Insurers announced that insurers would henceforth abandon questions about negative test results, and in October 2004 that it would stop asking applicants about their sexuality or refuse applications on the basis of assumptions about their sexuality.

Even if gay and bisexual men test HIV-negative, they will still be required to provide information on their medical history because they have been designated 'high-risk' by the insurance industry.

Chris Morgan of Compass Independent Financial Advisors, who advised the ABI on the change, forecast several more years' wait before movement on HIV infection itself, and said, "Even with the better life expectancy of HIV-positive people, it's still going to be a difficult issue."

In the U.S. a company called Impaired Risk Specialists, part of the Guarantee Trust group, has offered life insurance for people with HIV since 1997. But it sets quite strict conditions: Applicants must be 21 to 49, be working, lead an "active life" and have a low viral load.

In November 2004, African Life, a South Africa-based insurance company, has announced that it is lifting HIV/AIDS exclusions on its life insurance policies.

And in March 2005, the six largest members of the Dutch Union of Insurers, who represent more than 80% of the Dutch market, announced that they had decided to offer policies to some people with HIV, based on a finding that mortality in people with HIV had fallen to less than 0.5% a year - considerably lower than that due to insulin-dependent diabetes.

A positive effect of the availability of testing has been access to treatment and the encouragement of safer sex, but the overwhelming negative effect of testing has been the bestowal of uncertainty on many seropositive individuals, which has been psychologically damaging for many.

Further reading

Ronald Bayer: Private Acts, Social Consequences: AIDS and the politics of public health, Rutgers University Press, 1991.

Cindy Patton: Inventing AIDS (Chapter Two) Routledge, 1990.

The degaying of AIDS

In the developed world, the most significant event which took place during the second half of the 1980s was the overestimation of risk to the heterosexual population. This was to determine the subsequent course of policy, just as the appearance of AIDS in the gay population had determined policy in the first half of the decade.

Predictions were based on limited and incomplete information, and thus led to the construction of imprecise epidemiological models. Such computerised models require information about the average number of sexual partners, the turnover of sexual partners (or rate of partner change), variations between different groups within the population in terms of rates of partner change and average number of sexual partners, and mixing between those groups. The models also require information about the likelihood that HIV will be transmitted on each occasion of sexual intercourse with an infected person, the incubation period before the development of symptoms and the existing prevalence of HIV in the population. All of these items of data were missing or incomplete in 1985-86 when the first predictions were made on the basis of extrapolation from the gay population and the African epidemic. Unsurprisingly they were wrong, and it was not until the late 1980s that enough data were available with which to make accurate predictions.

The first predictions were seized upon and highlighted by the media and by those who worked in the field in order to alert the general public and those responsible for policy decisions to the danger of a rapid spread of HIV into the heterosexual population. It is often argued that gay organisations deliberately used the tactic of over-inflating the potential risk of a heterosexual epidemic to win funding, yet gay organisations only had access to the same data as everyone else and did not have magical access to a true picture of the unfolding of the epidemic which they withheld from the public health authorities.

Ironically, since 2000 the same situation has operated in the reverse direction in the UK: forecasts that the number of gay men living with HIV would continue to outstrip the number of heterosexuals were almost immediately proved wrong as a new wave of HIV diagnoses in people coming form the world's highest-prevalence countries finally achieved a 'heterosexualisation' of the epidemic that would not have occurred if cases had been restricted to UK nationals.

The campaign to re-gay AIDS

In 1991 a number of reports to medical journals provided evidence that the practice of unprotected anal intercourse was increasing amongst gay men, and that HIV infection was spreading more rapidly as a consequence. These findings were reinforced by reports from the United States where psychologists had adopted the label 'relapse' to describe the phenomenon of unsafe sex amongst men who had previously practised safer sex. These indicators confirmed what a number of educators, NAM amongst them, had been stressing for some years, namely the need for sustenance in safer sex education for gay men.

In May 1992 a survey published jointly by the National AIDS Manual (as NAM was then called), The Terrence Higgins Trust, NW Thames HIV Project and a newly formed group, Gay Men Fighting AIDS (now called GMFA), highlighted the extent to which HIV prevention work for gay men was being neglected in the UK. The survey found that only 4% of organisations conducting HIV prevention work in the UK had carried out any substantial efforts to educate gay men.

At the same time Gay Men Fighting AIDS was launched to lobby for a re-direction of resources towards safer sex education for gay men, arguing that gay men had been neglected despite the clear epidemiological evidence that they continued to be at far greater risk than heterosexuals, owing to the vastly greater prevalence of HIV amongst the gay population than amongst the general population.

Gay Men Fighting AIDS also sought to pioneer innovative forms of safer sex education, including the use of sexually explicit imagery, which had been shied away from by other organisations dependent on direct funding from the Department of Health. Interestingly, by 1994 the Terrence Higgins Trust felt able to publish posters which were just as sexually explicit as those published by GMFA in 1992, despite continuing to receive Government funding.

The report and other accumulating evidence led to significant changes in the field of HIV prevention over the next two years as the Department of Health emphasised the need for health authorities to target gay and bisexual men. By 1994 many organisations had begun to target HIV prevention messages specifically towards gay men.

A survey published by the Health Education Authority (as it was then called) in 1994 showed that there had indeed been a rethink by HIV prevention agencies throughout the country: overall, 86% of health purchasing agencies had funded targeted HIV prevention work at gay men or bisexual men in the preceding year (1993/4).

A similar survey commissioned by the Local Authority Association's Officer Working Group on AIDS into local government response to HIV and AIDS showed that though there had been considerable improvement in targeting gay men and bisexual men, still only half of the authorities in the country with social services departments did so.

In both cases an increased recognition of the importance of targeting gay men and bisexual men had not necessarily led to substantial commitments of resources to this target group.

References

Edward King, Michael Rooney, Peter Scott: HIV Prevention for Gay Men: A Survey of Initiatives in the UK, North West Thames Regional Health Authority, 1992.

Will Anderson, Ford Hickson, Clive Stevens: Health Purchasing, HIV prevention and gay men. Results of a survey into the purchasing of HIV prevention work for gay and bisexual men by health authorities in England, NAM/Health Education Authority, 1994.

Will Anderson, Ford Hickson: Local government, AIDS and Gay men. Results of a survey into the HIV and AIDS services of local government in England and Wales, with a particular emphasis on work with gay men and bisexual men, NAM/ Local Authority Association's Officer Working Group on AIDS, 1994.

The early heterosexual epidemic challenged

In November 1989 Lord Kilbracken suggested to the House of Lords that the Government had been exaggerating the risk of AIDS to the heterosexual population, and that funds would be better targeted at the high-risk groups. The risk of heterosexual transmission was 'statistically invisible', he claimed. His statement sparked a media campaign which was to end the national consensus on the risk of AIDS to heterosexuals.

Kilbracken's views were taken up by a number of right-wing newspapers including The Sun and The Daily Mail. Whilst Kilbracken's arguments were true in essence, they became the vehicle for a campaign which proclaimed to readers of the tabloid press that 'Straight Sex is safe'. Journalists confused the chances of meeting an HIV-infected heterosexual partner in the UK with the chance of infection through vaginal intercourse if a partner was infected. Sir Reginald Murley, former head of the Royal College of Surgeons, was widely quoted on his view that the young woman being featured at the time in HEA AIDS advertising was only at risk if she injected drugs or 'allowed herself to be buggered'.

The complete disavowal of any risk attached to heterosexual vaginal intercourse was to be a theme repeated for several years to come, and posed an important dilemma for HIV prevention work. Whilst the statistical chance of meeting an HIV-infected heterosexual partner was low, vaginal intercourse with an HIV-infected partner was certainly high risk. Unfortunately, rather than devoting more attention to the identification of

particular risk groups within the heterosexual population, many health educators thought it better to continue to emphasise the risk to everyone. It was to be a strategy which gradually undermined the credibility of all AIDS education targeted at heterosexuals as the predicted epidemic did not materialise.

Policy makers were understandably reluctant to commit themselves to any predictions about the spread of HIV in advance of the Day Report in 1990, which made epidemiological predictions on the basis of far more comprehensive data than any reports which had gone before. When the Day report reduced the estimates made by the 1988 Cox report, some media commentators took this as a sign that earlier predictions had been exaggerations. In fact, the estimates were reduced because of the uptake of safer sex amongst gay men.

The questioning of the risk to heterosexuals gathered force in 1990 with prominent reporting by The Sunday Times of The Myth of Heterosexual AIDS, an investigation of debates about the potential for a heterosexual epidemic in the developed world by US author Michael Fumento. His analysis was one of the most thorough critiques of existing prevention messages and their basis in epidemiological fact, but his agenda in reporting on AIDS was not to re-direct resources and education towards the most affected communities, but to re-direct resources away from AIDS entirely on the grounds that the threat had been exaggerated by the gay lobby and moral conservatives for political ends (Fumento).

In 1992 a major media scare erupted around an HIV-positive Birmingham hæmophiliac alleged to have infected women after becoming aware of his HIV status. The case was used to demand new controls on HIV-positive people, including the criminalisation of HIV transmission in circumstances where an individual knows his or her status. Some newspapers published reports claiming that the man had engaged in anal intercourse with some of his partners, evidence that was used to support the view that HIV could not be transmitted through 'normal' vaginal intercourse, but only through 'unnatural' anal intercourse.

Current predictions about the spread of HIV and who is at most risk of HIV infection are discussed in more detail in Epidemiology.

Further reading

Michael Fumento: The Myth of Heterosexual AIDS, Basic Books, 1990.

Simon Garfield: The End of Innocence: Britain in the time of AIDS, Faber & Faber, 1994.

Initiatives in other countries

There are few examples from the early days of the epidemic of countries that initiated successful prevention measures. One often quoted is Uganda, the first country in Africa to be seriously affected.

In 1986 President Yoweri Museveni responded to the emerging HIV crisis in Uganda by embarking on a nationwide tour to tell people that avoiding AIDS was a patriotic duty, and that they should abstain from sex before marriage and then go on to remain faithful to their partners and to use condoms. Uganda's Health Minister announced to the World Health Assembly that there was HIV in Uganda, and the first AIDS control program in Uganda was established. It focused on providing safe blood products, and educating people about risks.

Museveni's campaign gave rise to two famous slogans which have come to be used throughout Africa: 'ABC' (Abstinence, Be faithful, use a Condom) and "Zero grazing", meaning not to have sex with casual partners.

HIV prevalence fell in Uganda from 21% in pregnant women and 15% in the general population in 1990/1 to around 4% in 2004, though there is much argument as to whether this is due to the HIV prevention programme or to natural attrition through people dying of AIDS - see *Epidemiology* for more details - and the national figures have been disputed by independent activist bodies like the National Guidance and Empowerment Network.

In **Thailand** the "100 per cent condom campaign" in 1990-92 is often seen as one of the most successful HIV prevention programmes of all time. It slashed HIV incidence among young men from 2.5% a year to 0.5%, reduced prevalence among army recruits from 10% to 2.5%, and it is estimated that HIV prevalence in Thailand today is still - a decade after the campaign ended - 50% lower than it would have been if it had not happened.

Its success was partly due to good timing and an accurate perception that a widespread culture of commercial sex was responsible for the rapid growth of HIV at the time. It was also partly due to it being an easily enforceable target. The campaign put pressure on brothel owners to enforce 100 % condom use in their establishments and ensured that ones not conforming to this rule were closed by the police.

Other countries like **Brazil**and **Senegal**, who have managed to contain HIV prevalence to less than 1%, are perhaps less celebrated because they never allowed HIV to get out of hand and become a generalised epidemic. An example of how a country has to take radical steps to contain HIV comes from Senegal, where in the 1990s a number of HIV cases were traced to transmission within all-male Islamic seminaries. Though obviously this was due to male-male sex, the subject of homosexuality was never specifically addressed, but HIV education posters and classes were introduced into a setting that would in some other Islamic countries be completely inadmissible.

It is perhaps more instructive to look at countries that failed to institute timely prevention programmes to see what can happen. One example is South Africa, where an epidemic mainly concentrated among the country's gay population turned into one of the worst generalised epidemics in the world. This was partly due to the anti-apartheid struggle and the institution of democracy reaching their peak and distracting attention at the time HIV was taking hold, and an ambiguous and lukewarm government attitude towards prevention and especially treatment since.

A current example may be Russia, were HIV prevalence increased sevenfold between 2002 and 2004. Another may be the USA, where the failure to take HIV messages to new populations at-risk has led to a hugely disproportionate HIV prevalence among the US black population.

See **Epidemiology** and **Prevention** for more data on developing countries.

Scientific advances

During the early 1980s scientific researchers anxious to track the course of the new disease had recruited large groups of those at risk, principally gay men, in order to collect data on the prevalence of the disease and possible routes of transmission. As the decade went on, these cohorts and others subsequently recruited were to provide hugely valuable information which continues to provide our most reliable guide to the effects of HIV.

These cohorts were able to provide information on three major concerns: the routes of transmission; how long HIV might take to cause AIDS; and whether other factors (or 'co-factors' might be involved in the disease).

Although routes by which HIV could not be transmitted were fairly clear by 1985, it was still unclear at this time how likely it was that HIV could be transmitted by routes such as oral sex, from a woman to a man during vaginal intercourse or through needlestick injuries. As new cohorts and case reports updated

our knowledge on these issues, some media commentators took changes in advice as signalling that scientific opinion was, and is, deeply uncertain over the routes of HIV transmission. 'Do scientists know everything there is to know about the transmission of HIV?' was the angle of such stories, and they sought to grab attention by proposing new and improbable routes of transmission, often based on questionable laboratory evidence rather than epidemiological observation in the real world. Transmission by mosquitoes and through kissing have been two of the most persistent examples.

Another cause of confusion is the length of the incubation period between infection and the appearance of symptoms (the asymptomatic period). Confusing evidence on this subject has lent fire to the arguments of those who question the role of HIV in AIDS, and has caused much anxiety amongst HIV-positive people.

In the first years of the epidemic doctors assumed that the incubation period was no more than a year, on the erroneous assumption that individuals who reported sexual contact with those diagnosed with AIDS tended to develop AIDS within a year of sexual contact. It is more likely that these individuals had been infected for considerably longer, and that their contact with earlier AIDS cases was merely the consequence of the high prevalence of HIV within the gay population.

The predicted incubation period gradually lengthened as cohort observations were able to show that people infected in the early 1980s were taking longer than previously assumed to develop symptoms. Current cohort data suggests that this period is, on average, around 10 years (with considerable variation). However, while some will develop AIDS quickly, perhaps within one to two years of infection, others may still be healthy twenty-five years after infection.

Cohorts have also been able to answer the question of whether other factors apart from HIV might be responsible for immune deficiency in those at risk of AIDS. Cohorts have shown conclusively that HIV is the primary factor associated with immune deficiency in all groups at high risk of AIDS, that AIDS-defining illnesses occur very rarely in the absence of HIV infection, and that factors such as drug use do not cause immune deficiency. However, cohorts have also shown that a number of co-factors appear to increase the likelihood that AIDS will develop in HIV-positive people. The clearest influences on disease progression are age, income and access to care; older people and the very young develop AIDS much more quickly than those in their 20s and 30s. Those with incomes at or below the poverty line have been shown to progress to AIDS far more quickly than those with high incomes.

Treatment before the advent of combination therapy

In the first few years of the epidemic, treatments failed to have a great effect on the life expectancy of people with AIDS. Despite optimistic claims that the discovery of HIV promised a swift breakthrough in the search for vaccines and treatments, the progress in the search for effective antiretroviral drugs was slow in coming.

The first major antiretroviral drug to be licensed for use in people with AIDS was AZT, which became available in 1986. It is now clear that the Phase 2 trials which led to the licensing of AZT were conducted with insufficient rigour, and there have been allegations of fraud made against the investigators in this trial. It is important to bear in mind that investigators and drug regulators were under huge pressure to make available a drug which might offer hope to thousands. Consequently they cut corners in ways which compromised the value of data gathered in this study. AIDS activists demanded that regulatory authorities abandon 'business as usual' procedures intended to safeguard the public, and regulators were persuaded that emergency circumstances justified less stringent precautions. It took nearly eight years for the limited nature of AZT's benefits to become fully apparent, a process which is argued by some to have seriously impeded the search for other more effective treatments (Harrington).

Treatments against opportunistic infections have been developed more successfully, the most important being prophylaxis against pneumocystis pneumonia (PCP). A number of studies have now shown that PCP prophylaxis is the factor responsible for extending the lifespans of people diagnosed with AIDS (See *Opportunistic Infections* in the *HIV & AIDS Treatments Directory* for further details of this research). PCP prophylaxis was introduced as a standard measure only after vigorous campaigning led by People with AIDS groups in the United States.

Political pressure to release AIDS drugs has played a major role in expanding the treatment options of people with HIV through lobbying of drug companies and drug regulators. Until the AIDS epidemic began it was extremely rare for drug companies to release promising drugs on a compassionate, one-off basis to people in urgent need before they had been licensed. In the case of experimental tuberculosis drugs, it was decided that the most ethical approach was to use all available drugs to conduct research in order to benefit as many patients as possible in the long term. In the case of HIV infection, companies have learnt that compassionate release of experimental drugs is a shrewd form of publicity and marketing.

The early release of AIDS drugs has also been brought about by a shift in the underlying drug regulation philosophy in the United States. From the early 1960s the US Food and Drug Administration strictly regulated the release of new drugs onto the market in order to prevent disasters such as the birth defects caused by thalidomide. Drugs companies were required to put compounds through years of tests in order to prove their safety. In the 1980s the FDA began to face pressure from free market advocates for a speeded-up process, one which would reduce the costs of industry and increase the choice of consumers. AIDS was one of the first areas in which drug approval was speeded up, after ferocious criticism from AIDS activists who charged that people were dying for want of effective drugs whilst the FDA deliberated on safety regulations not designed with a public health emergency in mind.

Many people with HIV and AIDS have become experts on the treatments available to them, a development which substantially altered the balance of power between doctors and patients. Following on from the developing awareness of the importance of informed consent amongst feminist health activists and cancer patients, AIDS activists have promoted the principles of fully informing people about the risks and benefits of treatments and of allowing individuals more control over access to experimental treatments.

In the field of complementary therapies there have been few major breakthroughs which demonstrate that complementary treatments are clearly effective, but an increasing number of people with HIV have turned to complementary therapies and report benefits from those therapies. The use of complementary therapies has in turn stimulated a greater interest amongst doctors in the benefits of such treatments and the ways in which they can be combined with orthodox treatments.

References

Mark Harrington: The Crisis In Clinical AIDS Research, Treatment Action Group, New York, 1993.

PWA self-organising and AIDS activism

Almost as soon as AIDS organisations were started, support groups for people diagnosed with AIDS emerged on the model of self-help groups for other diseases. These groups quickly became more than support groups however; they provided welfare advice, information on treatments and advocacy for the needs and rights of people with AIDS.

PWA support groups also spawned buyers' clubs and treatment newsletters as people with HIV sought to obtain experimental treatments. In the mid-1980s several drugs not licensed in the US, including isoprinosine, were smuggled into the US from Mexico by what became known as the AIDS underground, hence the label 'underground' treatments. Treatment newsletters such as *AIDS Treatment News* in San Francisco were founded to provide information on the underground and experimental treatments being used by people with AIDS.

In 1987 a new organisation emerged as a voice for people affected by AIDS. The AIDS Coalition to Unleash Power (ACT UP) was founded in New York in 1987 as a radical protest group intended to draw attention to the lack of progress in research and discrimination against people with AIDS. Its targets were Federal drug regulators, researchers and the media, and it drew attention to issues by a mixture of media-friendly street protests and well-informed lobbying. Amongst the group's targets were the Food and Drug Administration (the US authority responsible for licensing new drugs), the National Institutes of Health (the body responsible for running AIDS drug trials) and *The New York Times* (for failing to report the impact of the epidemic in New York).

ACT UP groups soon sprang up in other US cities and in other countries, the most successful and largest outside the USA being in Paris.

In retrospect, some of the group's campaigns are questionable. For instance, in 1989 ACT UP targeted New York City Health Commissioner Stephen Joseph after he revised downwards estimates of AIDS cases for sound epidemiological reasons. His rationale for doing so was widely misrepresented by ACT UP and the gay press as homophobic, but the estimates which Joseph chose to use as a basis for service planning turned out to be accurate. Campaigns promoting safer sex to lesbians were another example of misguided priorities; whilst ACT UP did virtually nothing to promote safer sex amongst gay and bisexual men, significant amounts of energy were devoted to highlighting virtually non-existent risks to lesbians. This was paradoxical given the organisation's commitment to correcting misinformation about modes of transmission in the mainstream media, and reflected the extent to which ACT UP became driven by the agendas of caucuses within the organisation rather than attention to the realities of the epidemic.

Even in 2004, ACT-UP Paris's involvement in stopping trials of pre-exposure prophylaxis to see if oral HIV drugs could be used in high-risk negative people to prevent infection has been criticised by other activists, though others saw their protests against the trials as leading to advances in the development of guidelines for the ethical conduct of prevention trials in resource-poor settings.

Further reading

Bruce Nussbaum: Good Intentions, Atlantic Monthly Press, 1991.

Peter Arno & Karen Feiden: Against The Odds: The Story of AIDS Drug Development, Harper Collins, 1992.

John S. James (Ed.): AIDS Treatment News Vols 1-2, Celestial Arts 1989, 1991; Vol 3 (Alyson),1994.

AIDS dissidents/denialists

During the early 1990s the media began to give considerable prominence to the views of Prof. Peter Duesberg, the prominent retrovirologist, who questions whether HIV is the cause of AIDS. Prof. Duesberg has provided the focus for a wide assortment of people who question various aspects of orthodox opinion on HIV infection and AIDS.

In the UK a number of television documentaries broadcast on Channel Four between 1989 and 1993 questioned the scientific basis for the belief that HIV causes AIDS, attacked the use of AZT in the treatment of HIV and AIDS as misconceived and possibly dangerous, and questioned whether an epidemic of AIDS caused by HIV was really taking place in Africa. All three programmes contained serious scientific inaccuracies.

For a while *The Sunday Times* gave increasingly prominent coverage to the views of Peter Duesberg, and was strongly identified as a promoter of dissident theories about AIDS. Unfortunately the paper's coverage of those dissident theories has been highly selective and sensationalised, and has served to polarise debate rather than opening it up.

Several studies have shown an overwhelming association between testing positive for HIV antibodies and the subsequent development of AIDS. A review of deaths amongst haemophiliacs in the UK showed a tenfold greater chance of death amongst HIV-positive haemophiliacs in the UK when compared with their HIV-negative counterparts over the period 1978-92, and deaths related to AIDS-defining illnesses occurred exclusively in the HIV-positive group (Darby).

A study in Uganda showed a 64-fold higher chance of death over a two-year period amongst HIV-positive individuals in Rakai province compared with HIV-negative individuals.

A study of babies born to HIV-positive mothers showed 21 AIDS-related deaths in HIV-positive children over 26 months of follow-up, compared with just one death (due to child abuse) in the HIV-negative children. Mothers of HIV-negative and HIV-positive children were equally likely to have a history of drug use and to have used similar levels of drugs.

A study in haemophiliacs showed that development of AIDS in haemophiliacs is not a function of the volume of Factor VIII to which an individual has been exposed, but of infection with HIV. Seventeen HIV-positive haemophiliacs were matched with HIV-negative haemophiliacs who had received similar quantities of clotting factor; there were 16 AIDS-related events in the HIV-positive group over a ten-year period, compared with none in the HIV-negative group (Phillips).

Arguments about the causes of AIDS are discussed in more detail in the *HIV & AIDS Treatments Directory*. The US National Institute of Allergies and Infectious Diseases publishes a useful factsheet summarising the arguments - see below.

References

Darby S et al: Mortality in the complete population of UK haemophiliacs before and after HIV infection. Nature 377: 79-82, 1995.

NIAID (National Institute of Allergies and Infectious Diseases). The Evidence That HIV Causes AIDS. Last updated February 27, 2003. Can be viewed at http://www.niaid.nih.gov/factsheets/evidhiv.htm

Compensation for people with haemophilia

In November 1987 the Hæmophilia Society lobbied parliament for recognition of infection due to medical and administrative negligence, and for compensation. Lobbying was rewarded with a £10 million one-off payment. This was administered by the newly set up charity, the MacFarlane Trust, to give individuals and families a bonus of £35 per week. The DHSS made it clear that this was not compensation. The money was provided for the relief of need. This meant that no HIV-positive people with hæmophilia had an absolute right to payment.

Kenneth Clarke took over the new Department of Health in summer 1988 and found writs from 20 people with hæmophilia sitting on his desk. By then, people with hæmophilia in West Germany had received £50,000 each in government compensation; the New Zealand, Danish and Norwegian governments responded similarly to their liability.

The Hæmophilia Society advised their members to continue pursuing their law suits and recommended a government payment of £100 million. This resulted in the much publicised release of £24 million to be administered by the MacFarlane Trust as lump sums of £20,000 to people with hæmophilia and HIV or their bereaved families. Again, the message was that there was 'no concession to the principle of fault' and that litigation would have to continue if people with hæmophilia wanted more money.

The Hæmophilia Society continued to press for an out of court settlement. By February 1990 the overwhelming majority of all people with hæmophilia infected with HIV, or the families of those who had died, had issued a writ against the Department of Health.

The Hæmophilia Society persuaded the 1922 Committee of Tory backbenchers to support their campaign, but Margaret Thatcher continued to refuse to settle the issue (increasing her unpopularity). It was only after she had resigned and John Major's government was established that a settlement was reached in December 1990.

Amounts made available varied according to marital status, age, and whether children were involved. The figures concerned were between £20,000 and £60,000. This was on top of the assigned £20,000 awarded in 1988. The MacFarlane Trust is also now making weekly payments. The 1990 settlement was made on the condition that individuals dropped their court action. People with hæmophilia and HIV accepted the award, although a limited number have continued their actions, on legal advice, where negligence could be proved.

In August 2001 Lord Owen, the former UK Health Secretary under the Callaghan Labour government, accused the Health Department of failing to implement instructions issued whilst he was Health Secretary in the 1970s which should have ensured that the UK became self-sufficient in blood products. This would have eliminated the risk of people with hæmophilia becoming infected with HIV or other viruses like hepatitis C.

Imports of blood products, especially from the US, continued to be received in the UK, without the knowledge of Lord Owen. Lord Owen made a call for compensation for people who have contracted viruses from contaminated blood. A Haemophilia Society spokesman said that although the Government had set up a compensation scheme for people who had contracted HIV, it had done nothing for those infected with hepatitis C.

The Department of Health said they found it difficult to respond to events that occurred so long ago, but that, as Secretary of State for Health, it was Lord Owen's job to ensure that his policy was carried out.

After sustained pressure from haemophiliacs and their advocates in the UK, on 19 February 2007 - in the case of HIV, some 23 years after the event - Lord Morris of Manchester announced the Archer Independent Public Enquiry into how a generation of people with haemophilia were infected with HIV and/or hepatitis C and its consequences.

The Haemophilia Society Chairman, Roddy Morrison, said: "The Archer Enquiry's importance to the haemophilia community cannot be overstated. All across the United Kingdom those infected and their families will rejoice that all the facts are finally to be brought out into the open.

"It is particularly important that the inquiry will be examining the consequences of the disaster for the haemophilia community for those living with infection/s. Many have suffered unduly with financial hardship; some have even had to give up their homes. Many more have found themselves to be uninsurable, unemployable and unable to make adequate provision for their dependants.

Women as an affected group

In early 1987, a couple of HIV-positive women began to meet in each other's homes. They were extremely isolated and felt that the existing AIDS service providers were not responsive to their needs. Desperate to meet other women, they distributed simple posters and placed advertisements in the press. As their numbers slowly grew they were offered a meeting place by an established agency - SCODA, the Standing Conference on Drug Abuse. Soon after that, THT provided them with a small office and Positively Women (PW) was officially founded as an organisation. PW has grown significantly since then, and now boasts a small team of workers, and offices near central London, where women can drop in for support groups, complementary therapies and advice. Support groups are also run in the premises of other agencies throughout London.

PW is a fine example of peer-led support responding to a major gap in appropriate service provision. The need for services for women living with HIV and AIDS is now recognised as an important component in AIDS support, and many agencies are finding ways to integrate this as a part of their services. In general, services tailored to the needs of African women remain underdeveloped, although some service providers in London are beginning to address the specific needs these women encounter.

Women carers

The response to AIDS for women is more than responding to the needs of women who know themselves to be living with HIV or AIDS. Women who are the informal and formal carers of people with HIV, relatives, lovers and workers in the AIDS sector or the caring professions all need appropriate and focused services. Women are disproportionately represented in the caring professions (e.g. nursing, social work), and are frequently most called upon as informal carers (mothers, sisters, friends). Yet women are also notoriously resistant to accepting support and care for themselves. Of course, there is also a vital need for HIV prevention to be targeted at women. The number of women being diagnosed as HIV-positive grew rapidly throughout the 1990s, with women, the majority of black African origin, now accounting for around 35% of new diagnoses each year.

Responses to the diversity of needs women encounter in respect of HIV began at the end of 1990, when World AIDS Day focused on 'Women'. Around that time, many groups described the range of ways in which women can be affected by AIDS. For example, the Women Health and Screening Delegation joined forces with the National AIDS Trust and developed a series of seminars entitled 'Women, AIDS and the Future'. These seminars sought to raise awareness among mainstream women's groups, for example the Women's Institute. These types of initiatives have, however, been criticised for trying to cover every way in which AIDS affects women, so that little is addressed in depth, especially the principal risks to women of acquiring HIV.

HIV prevention for women

It could be said that women have been targeted by HIV prevention messages since 1987. The government's notorious 'Don't Die of Ignorance' campaign ran with a strap line that included the words: 'Gay or straight, male or female, anyone can get AIDS from sexual intercourse.' This type of Equal Opportunities discourse became commonplace in the general AIDS awareness campaigns of the late 1980s, and was supported by numerous media messages about an imminent 'Heterosexual AIDS Epidemic'. In these responses the particular needs of women were obscured in a generalist appeal to 100% safer sex 100% of the time.

The other mainstream form of HIV prevention work incorporating women shows women as a danger to men. In late 1988 the Health Education Authority (as it was then called) ran a series of newspaper advertisements showing a head and shoulders photograph of an attractive, vampish woman with a strap line asking how she would look in a few years time if she

had HIV. The next photograph was the same, and concluded, 'Worrying, Isn't It'. The advert was targeting men who would want to have sex with her, rather than targeting women themselves. This is only the most notorious of many initiatives which have used women in this way. Many discussions about women who work in the sex industry are fuelled by the perceived need to avoid transmission from women workers to their male clients. Fortunately, some grassroots initiatives (for example, ScotPEP in Edinburgh) developed peer education projects which sought to empower women to avoid acquiring HIV, not simply to reduce transmission.

The other focus of HIV prevention and women concerns maternity. Since 1992 there have been a range of guidelines to encourage pregnant women in 'high prevalence areas' to test for HIV during their pregnancy. This follows anonymous seroprevalence testing showing that as many as one in 125 pregnant women in central London is HIV-infected, but only one in five of these women is known by health carers to be HIV-positive. The encouragement to test is sometimes couched in terms of women's need to know in order to access services.

In 1999 the guidelines regarding antenatal HIV testing in high prevalence areas in the UK were extended to cover the whole of the UK. At the time of writing, (May 2003) Government targets to have 80% of women in the UK take up the offer of an HIV test in pregnancy. For further discussion of this issue, see **Women and HIV.**

Public attitudes to AIDS

Diana, Princess of Wales and red ribbons

Bigoted responses to people with HIV and AIDS have persisted throughout the epidemic, fanned by the tabloid press. Raising public awareness by using celebrities and members of the royal family began around the time that public education began to stress the risk to the heterosexual population. Until this time celebrities had been reluctant to publicly associate themselves with AIDS for fear that it would be taken as a public admission of homosexuality.

In 1987 the TV AIDS Awareness Week used celebrities such as singer Ian Dury to deliver messages about safer sex to young people; it was felt that celebrity endorsement of condom use would be more credible than the advice of doctors.

Celebrities were also used in other ways: to raise money and to project a message of compassion towards people with AIDS. In 1987 Princess Diana opened the Broderip Ward at London's Middlesex Hospital, the first of many supportive public appearances designed to show the Princess's concern for people with AIDS. Of particular note to the press was her decision not to wear protective clothing or gloves, presumed by many to be a prerequisite for contact with the infected. It was to be the first of many gestures which did a great deal to change public attitudes, and the Princess was to show an impressive commitment to AIDS whilst facing severe public criticism for her association with AIDS 'victims'; 'Does she really want to go down in history as the patron saint of sodomy?' asked John Junor in The Sunday Express. Princess Diana's commitment also served to make the issue respectable; when celebrities and the wealthy saw the Princess prepared to commit her time and public profile to such a controversial issue, it is likely many others felt it safe to do so as well.

The death of pop star Freddie Mercury was another transforming moment. Mercury's death of AIDS at the end of 1991 was the occasion for equal outpourings of grief and homophobic venom, and the single 'Bohemian Rhapsody' was re-released to raise money for the Terrence Higgins Trust. Subsequent royalties from a string of Mercury posthumous releases were given to the Mercury Phoenix Trust, and in May 1992 a major concert pulling together many of the world's major rock stars was held at Wembley. Its aims were AIDS awareness and fundraising, and it was the event which launched the red ribbon into the national consciousness.

The red ribbon had been adopted as a symbol of AIDS awareness in the United States during the 1991 Gulf War as an activist protest against the amount of money being poured into the war at a time when the Bush administration was cutting AIDS funding in real terms. Activists chose the red ribbon symbol as a contrast to yellow ribbons being worn to remember US service personnel in the Gulf. The ribbon outlived the Gulf war however, and began to achieve an international currency as a symbol of concern about AIDS. The ribbons were publicised as a symbol through a series of 'product placements' which linked them with celebrities and with one of the communities most affected by AIDS, the entertainment industry. The red ribbon appeared at the US Emmys in 1991, the Oscars, the Freddie Mercury AIDS awareness concert in 1992, World AIDS Day in 1992 and President Clinton's inauguration in 1993.

AIDS becomes a global pandemic

The recognition of AIDS in Africa and Haiti soon after its emergence in the United States was just the first stirrings of an epidemic that was raging on every continent within ten years. Unlike well established infectious diseases, AIDS has been dubbed 'the slow plague' by some commentators because of the way in which the disease spreads invisibly for many years before the first signs of its arrival in a region or population group. This has made governments in impoverished regions reluctant to adopt prevention policies until they see signs of AIDS; by then it is often too late to prevent a major epidemic.

The first region outside Africa and North America in which AIDS emerged was Europe, because of the continent's connections with both epidemics. South America was the next region to be affected, with Brazil suffering most. Caribbean states such as Haiti, the Dominican Republic and Trinidad also became affected at this time. But until the late 1980s most cases in these regions were probably a result of sex between men or transfusion with infected blood products. It was only in the late 1980s that the first evidence emerged of the spread of HIV through vaginal intercourse.

In 1987 the World Health Organisation began to characterise the spread of HIV according to different patterns. Pattern 1 countries were those in which the spread of HIV had occurred predominantly through sex between men, injecting drug use and blood products. Pattern 2 countries were those in which transmission had occurred primarily between men and women and through blood products and unsterilised needles. Pattern 3 countries were those in which the spread of HIV was very limited and in which cases of AIDS could be attributed to contact with Pattern 1 or 2 countries or the import of infected blood products. This classification is now questionable given the development of Pattern 2 and Pattern 1 type epidemics simultaneously in countries such as Thailand. The spread of HIV in Asia and Eastern Europe has challenged earlier assumptions about which societies would be vulnerable. In the 1980s Lee Kuan Yew, the Prime Minister of Singapore, expressed the view that the superior morals and sexual restraint of Asian people would minimise the threat of AIDS in South East Asia.

It was not until the mid-1980s that HIV began to spread in Asia and Eastern Europe, at first as a consequence of injecting drug use. In Thailand for instance, HIV prevalence amongst injecting drug users in Bangkok increased from virtually nil to 30% in less than six months following a prison amnesty which released HIV-positive drug users into the community in the autumn of 1987. Subsequently however, sexual transmission of HIV has taken place on a large scale.

HIV has continued to spread rapidly in Africa, India, south-east Asia and the Caribbean. Since 2000, new epidemics have taken

hold in the former Soviet countries of eastern Europe and central Asia, individual countries like Papua New Guinea (though unprotected sex) and Iran (though injecting drug use) that had previously been largely AIDS-free developed epidemics of their own, and the HIV virus continues to surprise us with its tendency not only to erupt in places where it is not expected but also to unexpectedly become less widespread in others. For further discussion see **An Overview of the Global Epidemic** in **The Epidemiology of HIV**.

Further reading

Jonathan Mann, Daniel Tarantola and Thomas Netter: AIDS In The World: A Global Report, Harvard University Press, 1993.

1996: the year of treatment breakthroughs

1996 must rank as the year of greatest optimism in the treatment of HIV and AIDS since the epidemic first began. By the beginning of 1997 it was clear that treatment advances implemented during 1996 had had dramatic effects on rates of death and illness amongst people with HIV.

These advances included:

- A much improved understanding of the progression of HIV infection due to viral load testing

- The validation of changes in viral load in response to drug therapy as an accurate predictor of the clinical benefits of a drug

- The discovery that the development of drug resistance could be delayed indefinitely if viral activity could be reduced to minimal levels

- The identification of treatment regimens which could reduce virus activity to minimal levels in 8-12 weeks

- The discovery that immune reconstitution can take place after viral activity is shut down, leading to reduced levels of opportunistic infections

- The licensing of a new class of drugs (protease inhibitors) of great antiretroviral power, especially when used in combinations

- The commercial availability of viral load testing for use in clinical practice.

All these developments took place between September 1995 and September 1996, and completely transformed the clinical outlook for people with HIV. Prior to this point, clinicians in the UK had been very cautious about the prospects of controlling HIV infection with antiretroviral therapy. This caution was encouraged by the results of the Concorde trial, which had shown only a very short-term advantage to AZT treatment prior to the development of symptoms, and an agreement that AZT delayed disease progression by an average of one year, no matter when it was initiated. Such results made doctors and patients cautious about antiretroviral treatment, and AIDS organisations showed little enthusiasm for treatment education. NAM was the only AIDS organisation to provide regular treatment information prior to 1995.

In September 1995 the results of the Delta trial encouraged a new sense of optimism about the potential of antiretroviral treatment. The Delta trial of combination antiretroviral therapy showed that combining AZT with ddI or ddC may significantly improve survival in people with HIV. The trial found a 38% reduced incidence of death over two years in people who received combination therapy compared with those who received AZT alone.

However, the Delta study also showed that people with previous exposure to AZT did less well than those who were AZT-naive, with no greater clinical benefit visible after two years when they were compared to the AZT-only group.

The results of Delta were backed up by another US trial ACTG 175, which confirmed the superiority of combination therapy in delaying disease progression. Dual combination therapy was adopted as the standard of care by larger treatment centres in the UK within months of these results, but research by *Positive Nation* magazine in October 1996 showed that some treatment centres were still prescribing AZT monotherapy over one year later.

The arrival of viral load testing

The development of a test which could detect HIV more accurately than the p24 antigen test came with the refinement of polymerase chain reaction (PCR) testing. This technique amplifies strands of genetic material in such a way that levels of a minute gene fragment can be measured. It is no longer necessary to isolate organisms or to culture them in the laboratory, provided that their genetic make-up is well mapped. The latest PCR test can detect as little as 5 genetic sequences in a millilitre of blood (compared with 10,000 in 1995), making the test a highly sensitive instrument for observing HIV.

The viral load test has given scientists a tool for detecting HIV during the asymptomatic phase of infection. The p24 antigen test and direct virus culture techniques were the only means of detecting HIV previously, and both these techniques were insensitive to the presence of low levels of HIV.

However, viral load measurements of the blood of asymptomatic people yielded startling information. Refuting the previously established view that HIV is latent until just before the development of symptoms, researchers such as David Ho discovered that high levels of viral activity were going on throughout the asymptomatic period.

Viral load testing of stored blood samples also demonstrated that individuals with high viral load had a much greater risk of disease progression. Analysis of changes in viral load after eight or twelve weeks of drug treatment in several clinical trials, most notably ACTG 175, revealed that the greater the fall in viral load after the first few weeks of treatment, the greater the long-term clinical benefit. The viral load test made it possible to detect within months whether a treatment regimen was likely to offer long-term clinical benefit to a patient, and transformed the way in which therapy was conceptualised by most doctors.

Viral load testing made possible the beginning of an era of 'individualised therapy', in which patients would no longer be prescribed drugs according to the results of a clinical trial, with one combination routinely prescribed to thousands of patients. In future, HIV therapy would be tailored to the individual viral load of a patient, and to their previous treatment history.

The licensing of protease inhibitors

Viral load testing also made it possible to assess the impact of new class of drugs much more quickly than has been the case in previous AIDS research. Protease inhibitors went from initial trials in humans to widespread prescription in less than four years, and offered new hope to many patients who had exhausted all other options.

Protease inhibitors attack HIV at a different point in its life cycle from drugs such as AZT or d4T (nucleoside analogues). They prevent the production of new HIV particles by blocking the action of an enzyme called HIV protease. Unlike other anti-HIV drugs, they were designed specifically to do this job after careful study of the exact structure of the protease enzyme. They are one of the first major examples of drug design aided by 3D computer techniques, and drugs to inhibit protease enzymes in many other viruses are now being developed as a result of the work that was done on HIV protease inhibitors.

However, protease inhibitors are very expensive in comparison with many other drugs, and one of the major problems facing people with HIV is the unwillingness of governments to pay for the drugs despite accumulating evidence that these drugs are a highly cost-effective addition to existing treatments. One year's treatment with a protease inhibitor currently costs around £3300 - £4000 per year compared with £2000-£3000 for the nucleoside and non-nucleoside reverse transcriptase inhibitors, or, to put it in the context of combination therapy, a first-line regimen of AZT/3TC/efavirenz costs about £6800 a year compared with around £9000 if the second-line regimen is tenofovir/FTC/lopinavir/ritonavir.

The new understanding of HIV disease

By the middle of 1996 it was clear that old understandings of how HIV infection should be treated were being swept away. First casualty of the paradigm shift was the idea of monotherapy (treatment with one drug), discredited by the results of the Delta trial. Next to go was the assumption that HIV is latent during the asymptomatic phase. Perhaps the biggest shift was the realisation that drug resistance lay at the root of treatment failure.

Drug resistance was identified as crucial by following a number of leads. The first was the discovery that patients who suffered rebounds in viral load after a period of successful drug treatment always showed evidence of drug resistance. Secondly, patients whose viral load stayed low didn't have the same levels of resistance as those who had rebounded. Even more significantly, the lower a patient's viral load went under the pressure of drug therapy, the less chance there would be of the development of drug resistance.

Hence, drug resistance was the motor behind the resurgence of the virus, and if it could be prevented, HIV could be suppressed indefinitely. If drug resistance occurred, patients could be switched to other drugs, and viral load would fall again, in theory.

Research presented at the Vancouver International AIDS Conference in July 1996 showed clearly that three drugs were much more likely than two drugs to maintain suppression of the virus and prevent the development of resistance.

The adoption of triple therapy as a new standard of care

Following the Vancouver conference a consensus emerged amongst clinicians that triple drug therapy was the optimum form of treatment for HIV disease. It presented the best available option for shutting down HIV replication and halting or significantly delaying disease progression.

Some countries were quicker to adopt this standard of care than others. Some doctors in the US had begun to switch to triple therapy in early 1996, as soon as protease inhibitors became available, and in France funds were made available to allow doctors to prescribe triple therapy in the summer of 1996. In the UK however, the implementation of triple therapy even for patients with advanced disease was a slow process. Due to the devolution of responsibility for spending decisions to local health authorities, there were no nationally agreed standards for prescribing, or any guaranteed rights regarding access to treatment. Standards of care were determined by the willingness of local health authorities to fund improvements in care out of existing funds. Unlike in France, where funds were allocated specifically to prevent regional inequalities in access to treatment, no new funds were made available by the Department of Health to pay for improved HIV treatment during 1996. It was not until April 1997 that new funds became available to fund improved treatment, and even then the funding increase was not adequate to cover the increased uptake of treatment or the introduction of viral load testing.

The great unknowns: duration, tolerability and cure

Whilst the future of HIV treatment looks much brighter than it did pre-1996, there are still several unknown factors which could darken this picture.

The first is the durability of the effects now being seen with triple combination treatment. Whilst the majority of patients randomised to receive triple therapy in clinical trials continue to show no signs of rebounds in viral load, it is important to note that people who take part in clinical trials tend to respond better to therapy than those who receive treatment as part of routine clinical care. It is not yet known what proportion of patients will cease to benefit from this treatment after five or more years. Professor Andrew Phillips, a statistician at the Royal Free Hospital Medical School in London, has concluded that so long as complete adherence to Highly Active Antiretroviral Therapy (HAART) can be maintained over the long-term, today's therapies appear able to suppress viral replication for more than ten years.

With the use of a triple combination therapy based on non-nucleosides (NNRTIs) as a first-line regimen, one based on boosted protease inhibitors as a second-line, and in 2006-8 the emergence of new- easy-to-take drugs of other classes such as integrase inhibitors and CCR5 inhibitors, not to mention improved PIs such as darunavir, the potential now exists for drug-naïve patients without primary drug resistance to have as many as four effective regimens, giving them the chance of having their HIV controlled over decades. Cohort studies in the USA, France and Denmark have shown that the life expectancy of people with HIV, particularly those that manage to maintain reasonably high CD4 counts, is still not a match for the general public but is approaching normality.

Reports of the longer-term **side-effects** of protease inhibitors (and, as it later became clear, the thymidine analogue nucleoside drugs too) began to emerge during 1998. Though rates of prevalence vary greatly from study to study, a proportion of patients have experienced body fat changes and lipid abnormalities after being treated with protease inhibitors and thymidine analogues. Other studies have linked long term side-effects to the NNRTI efavirenz (psychological) and to tenofovir (bone and renal).

The major reason why patients cease to benefit from triple therapy is because they develop drug resistance, and the major determinant of drug resistance is a lack of adherence to treatment. If blood levels of a drug fall too low, drug resistance can develop. Resistance to some HIV drugs can develop very rapidly; patients who missed less than 5% of their doses during one six month trial developed resistance, and doctors are currently advising patients to take every dose at the appointed time to be certain of continued benefit.

However, treatment adherence is a major drawback of the new treatment regimens. Many patients complain that they find it very difficult to take all the drugs, and mechanisms to assist people with adherence have taken on increasing importance. In recent years regimens have become simpler as drugs are co-formulated to be taken in one pill and as new drug formulations deliver more active ingredient in smaller pills.

Resistance to one drug may also lead to resistance to other drugs (cross-resistance). Cross-resistance is currently universal between the NNRTI drugs; it causes major problems in sequencing the nucleoside drugs, as high-level resistance to some may cause low-level resistance in others; and slowly gathering resistance, much f it cross-resistance happens even with the boosted protease inhibitors, which are designed to have a high barrier to resistance.

All current HIV drugs are virustatic rather than virucidal drugs: the stop the virus reproducing as long as they are taken but they do not eliminate it form the body. **Eradication** of HIV is conceptually difficult because, as a retrovirus, it stitches its genes (and therefore the instructions for making new viruses) into many long-lasting cells in the immune system. Eradication with the current therapies is now widely regarded as impossible, though strategies to achieve this are still being researched; the latest was the use of valproic acid to stimulate dormant HIV-infected cells to reproduce HIV again and therefore become targets for antiretrovirals.

Immunogenic drugs that work on the immune system rather than on blocking HIV have been studied for years but have failed to find a permanent place in the HIV treatment repertoire. This is for several reasons. Firstly, HIV exerts hugely complex effects on the immune system, and a drug that simply boosts the number of immune cells may be counter-productive as it could simply provide more opportunities for HIV to replicate. Secondly, the immune attrition of AIDS is thought to be caused at least as much by overstimulation and burnout of the immune system as it is by the direct cytotoxic effects of HIV itself. People with AIDS actually might benefit from having some parts of their immune systems suppressed rather than enhanced. Thirdly, some on the immunogenic drugs that have been tried so far, like interleukin-2, are difficult to take and produce unpleasant side-effects. Nonetheless in theory there is no reason why a drug that subtly stimulates the right parts of the immune system or even, as a therapeutic vaccine, 'primes' the immune system to fight back better against HIV, cannot be developed. Studies of the cytokine interleukin-7 are the latest in a long line of immune-booster trials. **Long-lasting formulations** of HIV drugs are probably a more practical way forward. There are already drugs in trials like the monoclonal antibody TNX-355 which is taken as an intravenous infusion (drip) every two weeks. If this period could be stretched further and alternative delivery systems for other HIV drugs like implants or patches be developed, it might make adherence a lot easier.

A vaccine for HIV?

When the discovery of HIV was announced in 1984, Margaret Heckler, the then US Secretary of Health and Human Services, predicted that a vaccine against it would be available in two years. Even at the time scientists listening blanched at her over-confidence. It took 47 years from the discovery of the polio virus to the development of a vaccine, and even hepatitis B took 16 years.

There are particular reasons why the development of a vaccine against HIV is an especially daunting task. All most vaccines have to do is to stimulate the body into mounting the immune response against the vaccine that it would do to the disease anyway. But in the case of HIV, a vaccine would have to do 'better than nature' because the immune response the body mounts against HIV is insufficient to contain it - and indeed even contributes to the development of AIDS.

At the 2004 World AIDS Conference in Bangkok, the WHO's José Esparza, in contrast, predicted that given the current state of HIV vaccine development, a workable one would not be found before 2017 at the earliest. Only two years previously at Barcelona he had predicted there would be one by 2009.

The apparently receding prospects for an HIV vaccine are due to the fact that the first and simplest strategy tried - a vaccine that induced antibodies against HIV - failed in early 2003 when the VaxGen AIDSVAX vaccine, the first and only one so far to complete a phase III clinical trial, failed to offer protection.

There are worrying signs that the second strategy tried - vaccines that generate cellular immunity in the shape of anti-HIV CD8 cells - is likely to fail too, because in some experiments HIV has found a way to develop resistance to them.

The third generation relies on a mixture of CD8 cell response and the generation of special, so-called 'broadly neutralising' antibodies, but development is still at a very early stage.

Some scientists think that a preventative vaccine against HIV will prove impossible to make and that the best option for long-term control involves the development of some kind of therapeutic vaccine or immune modulator that slows progression to AIDS in those already infected.

However much excitement may have been generated by advances in HIV treatment over the past few years, the impact of these improvements will represent a mere drop in the ocean unless an effective vaccine against HIV can be developed soon.

Although it is unrealistic to expect that the first generation of HIV vaccines will provide 100% protection to 100% of those vaccinated, finding a vaccine which is even 50% effective raises a host of difficult logistical and ethical issues, not least, who will pay for it and who will it be tested on?

Preventing the global spread of HIV requires two things apart from a vaccine, one probably more feasible than the other. One is a vaginal microbicide, a chemical which can be used by women during sex to kill HIV. The other is a huge reduction in the supply of heroin and the use of injectable drugs. But underlying these requirements, say prevention experts, are much greater changes in the structure of societies and the global distribution of wealth. The vulnerability of women and the global trade in heroin are just symptoms.

However, a microbicide could be closer than a vaccine. Experts are agreed that a prevention method which could be controlled by women rather than men would have a significant impact on infection rates in developing countries. Several products are now entering large-scale clinical trials, but even if an effective, convenient and safe microbicide is developed in the next few years, it is unclear how women in developing countries will be able to afford how to use it.

The British microbicide and vaccine researcher Robin Shattock has suggested that a practical HIV vaccine would in fact look more like a microbicide. Shattock points out that because an HIV vaccine needs to help the body develop mucosal as well as or instead of systemic protection, it might best be delivered in the form of a microbicide-vaccine which, applied as a gel, would stimulate the Langerhans cells that cover the mucosa, and which are the first to be infected with HIV or transport that infection to other cells, to mount a long-lasting anti-HIV response. However a microbicide-vaccine would not protect against parenteral transmission, i.e. through needle-sharing and needlestick injury.

Further discussion of vaccines and microbicides can be found in **Developing prevention technologies.**

The slow normalisation of HIV

Getting to the point where HIV infection is a manageable chronic condition rather than a dramatic and terminal disease has had its negative consequences, too. The huge amount of interest and public concern that was poured into HIV and AIDS between 1985 and the late 1990s has ebbed away even as the number of people with HIV grown - both in the UK and in other countries. The upshot has been that, while the medical picture for people with HIV continues to get brighter, facilities for peer support, social care and voluntary organisations have got ever more stretched and AIDS has lost a lot of its 'special' status. HIV voluntary organisations continue to close and merge - even while writing this paragraph in 2007, there are rumours that two more UK voluntary organisations may be about to close - and even making the case for HIV-specific services other than medical ones becomes more difficult.

Changing services
During the early 1990s a major re-structuring of public health services began (and continues) which was to transform dramatically the way in which AIDS services were funded and

provided. Two reforms - the introduction of an internal market into the health service and the introduction of community care legislation designed to establish a market in social services - have transformed the relationship between the voluntary sector and funders.

The internal market in the health service has given district health authorities and trusts the task of purchasing services from providers, often agencies which previously formed part of the health service. Purchasers also increasingly buy services from voluntary organisations. For instance, regional health authorities in London have contracts with a range of voluntary organisations in London which provide services to people with HIV or which do prevention work. The introduction of this system has required voluntary organisations to introduce careful monitoring procedures in order to provide purchasers with information on the users of their services, and to engage in consultation with service users and potential service users to ensure that their needs are being met.

In 1993 the Department of Health announced that funding to a number of organisations which had been receiving Section 64 (new charity development) money was to be cut. The move was interpreted as a sign that AIDS was being downgraded as a Government priority, especially in the light of the fact that the Department would make no commitment to the continuation of ring-fenced AIDS funding (money designated for AIDS funding only) or current levels of funding after 1995. The Health Secretary told the press that AIDS would henceforth have to compete for funding with other health problems, and that the Department would be looking at ways of targeting funding more effectively in the future.

Another factor which has seriously affected the coordination of AIDS services is the abolition of regional health authorities and the transfer of health services commissioning to district health authorities. This shift has made life even more difficult for service providers, especially in London, by forcing them to seek funding from many different sources.

Rationalisation of the UK HIV sector
In 1999 and 2000 several major mergers and closures in the UK HIV sector signalled that the proliferation of voluntary sector organisations had halted, and that the sector has grasped the need for a rationalisation of services to meet the new financial realities. In 1997 and 1998 Health Service Commissioners in London signalled that significant cuts in voluntary sector grants would be forthcoming as the cost of combination therapy increased.

In 1999 the Terrence Higgins Trust merged with a number of regional service providers to form a national organisation for England, and in 2000 Body Positive closed after serious financial problems (despite high demand for its services). The London Lighthouse and Terrence Higgins Trust joined together and the AIDS Treatment Project's phoneline was absorbed by the Trust following ATP's financial collapse.

Changes were not confined to the social care arena, which has been the subject of much scrutiny. Changes in the HIV prevention sector also occurred. In London, Rubberstuffers lost the contract to provide free condoms for gay men in a price competition, whilst Healthy Gay Manchester merged with the city's Lesbian and Gay Switchboard to form a new gay health organisation.

In August 2002 Blackliners, the national organisation for black and ethnic minority people with HIV, also collapsed after funding contracts were not renewed. Much of its work has now been taken over by the African HIV Policy Network, by a number of smaller African organisations, and by non-HIV organisations such as the Citizen's Advice Bureau.

The end of ring fenced funding for HIV prevention
In April 2002 the protected status of HIV prevention funding, known as 'ring-fenced' monies was terminated. HIV prevention

funding became mainstreamed. This occurred at the same time as some of the most substantial organisational changes in the NHS in its history.

The mainstreaming places HIV firmly within a sexual health policy agenda. In England, from the old Health Authorities, Primary Care Trusts (PCTs) were created. Since April 2002, PCTs have been responsible for commissioning local services. In Wales, Local Health Groups will begin commissioning services this year (2003).

Over the past year there has been anxiety within the HIV sector that these changes could facilitate widespread disinvestment in local HIV prevention services since HIV will be forced to compete with a range of other health areas for the same funding.

Some anxieties have not been borne out in most areas. After an initial period of confusion PCTs in urban areas like London and Manchester formed consortia to purchase and allocate HIV services regionally, though inequalities of service still exist elsewhere.

Of greater concern is the relentless increase in HIV prevalence in the UK. This has led to a soaring HIV treatment budget with increases in HIV prevention, community care and funding for other STIs not keeping pace.

Of even more importance is the decision by the government to exclude HIV and sexual health from the system of National Service Frameworks (NSFs) which were devised at the time of the PCT reorganisation. NSFs bind PCTs to achieve tight targets in dealing with cancer, coronary heart disease, diabetes, mental health and several other areas. Some organisations like the Terrence Higgins Trust have attributed the lack of an NSF for sexual health for the increase in HIV among gay men and the considerable increases in STIs among both gay men and young people in general. A target to provide a consultation for every person seeking care at a GUM clinic within 48 hours has failed to be achieved for the fourth year in a row, with no discernible progress being made towards the target.

A sexual health and HIV commissioning toolkit, designed to support the implementation and development of PCT plans from April 2003 was published in January 2003. It advises on partnership models; how to undertake local needs assessments; include examples of good practice in providing information to the public, and to people with HIV specifically, on sexual health and HIV.

The National Strategy for Sexual Health and HIV

Background to the strategy

The Government's commitment to developing a national sexual health strategy was announced by Tessa Jowell, Minister for Public Health. This strategy aimed to set a programme of action on sexual and reproductive health for England. In May 2000 it was announced that the Government planned to join up the Social Exclusion Report into Teenage Pregnancy and the developing HIV/AIDS strategy into an overarching strategy. The need to address sexual health had been highlighted in the Government's White Paper *Saving Lives*. Professor Michael Adler, Professor of Genitourinary Medicine/Sexually Transmitted Diseases at University College London Medical School was seconded to the Department of Health for a year in the first instance to lead on this work which he had begun back in September 1999 and alongside Dr Sheila Adam, Deputy Chief Medical Officer became the lead for the development of the strategy.

The first national strategy on sexual health and HIV services was published in July 2001. It was backed by an investment of £47.5 million to support the range of initiatives set out in the strategy.

The strategy aims to modernise and restructure services to meet patients' needs, aiming to prevent the spread of sexually transmitted infections (STIs) and HIV and improve care and treatment for those who need it.

The key elements of the strategy include:

- The first ever national information campaign aimed at the general public to span prevention of sexually transmitted infections, HIV and unintended pregnancy, to safeguard sexual health.

- New targets to reduce the numbers of newly acquired HIV infections and gonorrhoea infections.

- Targeted screening for chlamydia.

- A model for sexual health services that can be delivered by every Primary Care Trust, increasing access and bringing a broader role for nurses and other staff working in primary care.

- Routine HIV testing will be offered in all sexual health clinics to reduce the number of undiagnosed cases.

- More people will be offered hepatitis B vaccine in sexual health clinics to protect them against sexually transmitted infection.

- New one-stop sexual health services will be piloted and evaluated.

- Local stakeholders will review sexual health and HIV services in each area and ensure that sexual health services are delivered in each PCT. The Strategy requires a ten-year commitment to deliver what it proposes.

Aims of the strategy

- to reduce the transmission of HIV and STIs, with a national goal of achieving a 25% reduction in the number of newly acquired HIV and gonorrhoea infections by 2007.

- to reduce the prevalence of undiagnosed HIV and STIs - in particular, by setting a national standard that all GUM services should offer an HIV test to clinic attendees on their first screening for STIs, and working towards shorter waiting times for urgent appointments in GUM services.

- to begin a programme of screening for Chlamydia for targeted groups during 2002.

- to stress the importance of open access to GUM services and, over time, improving access for urgent appointments.

- to increasing the uptake of hepatitis B vaccine.

- to reduce unintended pregnancy rates - including setting a national standard.

- to improve health and social care for people living with HIV.

- to reduce the stigma associated with HIV and STIs.

The sexual health and HIV strategy implementation action plan was published on the Department of Health's website on Monday 24 June 2002.

The action plan set aside the first £14 million of the strategy to pay for a range of sexual health services, including a £1.5 million roll-out of chlamydia screening, which will offer a urine test to women attending GUM clinics or having their first smear or pregnancy.

A £2 million Department of Health information campaign, directed at young adults, was launched in the autumn of 2002 to warn of the risks of unprotected sex. Sexual health telephone helplines were improved to offer more information and to refer people to specialists, where required. Additionally, the help on sexual health through NHS Direct, the national telephone advice service was also stepped up.

A total of £276.3 million was allocated to primary care trusts in England for HIV/Aids treatment and care in 2001-2. This included £52.3 million for GUM services. This represented an increase of £41 million to the previous year's budget.

From 2003 extra Department of Health funding meant that all visitors to a GUM clinic will be offered an HIV test at their first sexually transmitted infection check.

The first public information campaign

The first public information campaign to increase awareness of the risk of sexually transmitted infections (STIs) among 18 - 30 year olds and to highlight the importance of practising safe sex in preventing STIs was announced by the Health Minister Hazel Blears on November 28th 2002. It used radio, web-based advertising and 'ambient' media such as beer mats, scratch cards and washroom posters. The £4 million campaign is anticipated to run initially for two years. A new website - http://www.playingsafely.co.uk/ - and a telephone information line - 0800 567 123 - support the headline messages with more in-depth information.

The campaign strapline was "Don't play the Sex Lottery. Use a condom"

What has happened since 2001: the transformation of the UK epidemic

In a sense, the National Sexual Health and HIV Strategy was out of date before it was even issued. It was certainly overtaken by events. Its appearance took place during the most rapid period of transformation the UK HIV epidemic has ever been through.

HIV prevalence in the UK doubled in the five years between 1999 and 2004. From infecting one in 1,000 people living in the UK, it now infects one in 500. In 1999, 3,000 people were diagnosed with HIV; in 2005, 7,700 were diagnosed.

In 1999 diagnoses of HIV among heterosexuals overtook those among gay men; in 2001 diagnoses among heterosexual *women* overtook those among gay men; and in 2004, for the first time, more heterosexuals than gay men were being seen for HIV treatment and care in the UK.

This increase is largely accounted for by heterosexual Africans who caught HIV in high-prevalence countries and have come to the UK as asylum seekers, workers or students. Other European countries have seen a similar transformation in the makeup of their HIV-positive population, but none as dramatic a change as the UK. The *Eurosurveillance* website comments that, of the European countries that have comprehensive HIV reporting: "Trends.are largely driven by the United Kingdom, which accounts for 28% of the population but for 53% of all reported HIV infections in recent years."

This is not because diagnoses among gay men have gone down. In fact the yearly total of diagnoses among gay men has increased by 60%, from 1400 to 2200, during that time. Most of this is accounted for by more gay men coming forward for testing and there being fewer undiagnosed; about 25% of UK gay men who have HIV were undiagnosed in 2004 as opposed to 33% in 1999. However this also adds to the strain on services. There is certainly no evidence that the infection rate among UK gay men is slowing down (see **Epidemiology**).

In addition to HIV, the last ten years have seen big increases in sexually transmitted diseases. Between 1996 and 2004, gonorrhoea diagnoses doubled, chlamydia diagnoses more than

tripled, and syphilis diagnoses went up 17-fold in men, 8-fold in women, and 29-fold in gay men. Taking the long view, these are increases from a historically low point in the early 1990s, and do not come near the STI rates of the 1970s, but the Government appears to have failed to anticipate any increases at all.

The author of the Sexual Health and HIV Strategy himself, Professor Michael Adler, told the BBC in 2003 that the $47.5 million allocated for the entire Strategy in 2000 would not even pay for one part of it, the chlamydia screening programme. And in 2004 he told the British HIV Association Conference in Cardiff that part of an extra £15 million allocated on top of the Strategy money to modernise GUM services had not got to the clinics but had been diverted to finance other areas by PCTs.

There has been almost no progress towards achieving the target of getting everyone seen within 48 hours at STI clinics. Figures released in June 2005 showed that only 38% of GUM clinic patients in England were seen within 48 hours, and that another 29% were not seen within two weeks. Even eight per cent of cases classed as 'emergencies' had to wait more than two weeks. The figures from 2006 showed a slight improvement.

The chlamydia testing programme has gone ahead, as has the 'Sex Lottery' campaign - only to receive criticism from activists, including NAM, that it gave the impression that white teenagers were a risk group for HIV and that it was not targeting prevention campaigns at those who needed them most (see "Where it's Really Hurting", *The Guardian,* 10 September 2005).

The upsurge in cases among Africans led to stories in the media in 2004 that "health tourists" posed both a public health and an economic problem to the UK. The government responded by:

- imposing visa restrictions on Zimbabweans, who had been the largest single group of immigrants from a high-prevalence country.

- increasing deportations and turning down asylum appeals on the basis that HIV treatment was now available in countries of origin.

- in April 2004, rescinding a concession that allowed visitors to the UK without residency status to receive HIV treatment if they had managed to stay in the UK for more than a year.

This resulted in an HIV 'underclass' of anything from 1,000 to 4,000 people with HIV who are able to receive emergency treatment for TB and other AIDS-related conditions, but who cannot access antiretrovirals on the NHS. In addition a large proportion of people with HIV in the UK are now unemployed, not because they are too ill to work, but because they are not allowed to.

The geographical spread of people with HIV in the UK has also changed, partly owing to the dispersal of HIV-positive immigrants away from London. Sixty per cent of new HIV diagnoses were made within London in 2000; in 2004 the proportion was 41%.

HIV organisations in the UK have had to respond fast to a quickly-changing client group. The Terrence Higgins Trust has established itself as the main HIV service provider in parts of the UK such as the West Midlands, Yorkshire and the west of England, but elsewhere and in Scotland independent organisations such as George House Trust and Waverley Care have had to change the services they provide very quickly.

In London mergers between local organisations continue to occur, with the latest being the 2005 merger between the London East AIDS Network and the Globe Centre to form Positive East. The THT continues to be the biggest service provider in London, but the UKC (UK Coalition of People Living with HIV and AIDS) expanded from its original remit as an advocacy and information organisation to provide a range of training and re-employment services as the lead organisation for Ensuring Positive Futures, a partnership of six HIV organisations.

The closure of Blackliners in March 2003 left a gap in HIV service provision for Africans and Caribbeans, and small African organisations originally only serving people from certain parts of the continent, or certain parts of London, such as HAAZ (the HIV/AIDS Association of Zambia) UAAF (the Ugandan AIDS Action Fund) and ACIA (the African Community Involvement Association) have had to scale up rapidly to provide services to a standard funders expect. In the regions, there has not been the same growth in African-specific organisations apart from the consolidation of the already-existing Black Health Agency and its associated AIDS Helpline in Manchester. Rather, already-existing organisations face having to cater for two widely-different groups of people with HIV within their existing structures.

With more NHS restructuring on the horizon (there are plans to take back commissioning of services to the 28 Strategic Health Authorities that have previously only had a monitoring and guidance function), voluntary organisations continue to face an uncertain financial and organisational future in a country with an increasingly large, diverse and marginalised population with HIV.

Will the UK continue to reach out to marginalised groups and protect them from HIV as it dared to do for Edinburgh heroin users in 1985? Will it continue to provide universal free treatment? Or will it become an increasingly American-style society where the groups most likely to get HIV are the very ones who are left untargeted by prevention messages and who cannot get NHS treatment?

The global picture since 2000: treatment comes to the developing world

Several pivotal events and developments have changed the response to the global AIDS epidemic enormously since this Manual was last fully rewritten.

The Geneva World AIDS Conference in 1998 had as its slogan "Bridging the Gap" (presumably between rich and poor countries) but was marked largely by an appreciation of how big that gap was, with activists from the developed world finally facing the possibility of years of healthy living as their developed-world counterparts still battled with the devastation of AIDS.

AIDS activism moves south

In contrast the Durban World AIDS Conference in 2000 felt like a genuinely pivotal event. The first to be held in a developing country, its opening and demonstrations that took place around that opening introduced many developed-world AIDS workers for the first time to a new breed of AIDS Activist and a new set of demands.

South Africa's Treatment Action Campaign, prominent at the conference in purple T-shirts bearing the words HIV-positive, were only the most prominent of a new generation of developing-world equivalents of ACT-UP who shifted the debate on to the possibility of something previously regarded as impossible - the provision of antiretrovirals for people with HIV in poor countries. Other organisations like Thailand's Thai Drug Users' Network, the National Guidance and Empowerment Network in Uganda and some of the local branches of GNP+, the Global Network of People Living with HIV and AIDS, are only the most prominent of a plethora of local organisations representing people with HIV that do everything from provide basic services to serve as lobbyists to international bodies.

These combined with multilateral organisations like the United Nations, private philanthropic trusts like the Bill and Melinda Gates Foundation and the Open Society Foundation, international NGOs like Médecins Sans Frontières and ActionAid, and existing

anti-globalisation lobbyists to force through huge cuts in the price of HIV drugs to the developing world, so that a typical first-line regimen such as AZT/3TC/efavirenz, which costs $10,000 a year in the USA, can be provided for $200-350 a year in developing countries.

HIV drugs cost so much because of the financial structure of the pharmaceutical industry, which enables companies to recoup their enormous development costs by having a monopoly on selling their new drug while it is still under patent protection. A pivotal event was the forcing through of an agreement at the World Trade Organisation talks in Doha in 2001. Normally patent protection rules under TRIPS, the Trade-Related aspects of Intellectual Property Rights agreement, would make it illegal to sell any drug that was still under a patent. However, following the Doha conference, ministers agreed that TRIPS should not prevent members from taking measures to protect the public health of its citizens. It therefore agreed that countries should be able to manufacture generic drugs made before the 1995 introduction of TRIPS and could produce newer drugs under a system called compulsory licensing.

What this meant was that the large pharmaceutical companies had an incentive to cut prices for drugs intended for the developing world because otherwise their business in those regions would be undercut by generics companies that, in the case of countries like India and Brazil, has already been making generic antiretrovirals (and flouting the WTO rules in the process).

In the meantime parallel developments were happening which brought new money and new funding mechanisms onstream to pay for the huge scale-up of HIV treatment provision.

Indeed, it was not just treatment that was scaled up. One finding of the drive towards universal treatment is that spending money on treatment also means providing better HIV prevention too. This is partly because, given hope at last that something can be done about HIV, far more people come forward for testing. Evidence is emerging that ART availability leads to an upsurge in demand for HIV testing and counselling and other prevention services. In one district in Uganda, introduction of ART led to a 27-fold increase in demand for HIV testing and counselling.

Another is that in areas like Africa public health systems had been so starved of investment for so long that they were barely extant, let alone capable of delivering complex drug regimens on a regular band continuing basis to thousands of people. Indeed the numbers that would have to be treated to meet the need of all people with AIDS in the developing world would put rich countries' health systems under strain.

In terms of institutional change, several pivotal events made the development of a global AIDS initiative possible.

The millennium goals and UNGASS

In 2000 the United Nations announced its Millennium Development Goals. These are a set of targets to alleviate world poverty, ignorance and disease by 2015, which the United Nations acknowledges will be impossible to achieve unless the impact of HIV/AIDS is mitigated.

The Declaration of Commitment on HIV/AIDS was adopted by the world's governments at the Special Session of the United Nations General Assembly on HIV/AIDS in June 2001.

For the first time ever, time-bound targets to which governments and the United Nations may be held accountable were established.

These are part of the wider targets of the UN's Millennium Development Goals, a set of targets to be achieved by 2015. It is acknowledged that majority of them will be impossible to meet unless the impact of HIV/AIDS is mitigated.

The Millennium Development Goals are:

- **Hunger and poverty:** To a) reduce by half the proportion of people living on less than a dollar a day and b) to reduce by half the proportion of people who suffer from hunger.

- **Education:** To ensure that all boys and girls complete a full course of primary schooling.

- **Gender equality:** To eliminate gender disparity in primary and secondary education preferably by 2005, and at all levels by 2015.

- **Child mortality:** To reduce by two thirds the mortality rate among children under five.

- **Maternal mortality:** To reduce by three quarters the maternal mortality ratio.

- **HIV/AIDS and other diseases:** To halt and begin to reverse the spread of HIV/AIDS, and the incidence of malaria and other major diseases.

- **Environment:** To a) Integrate the principles of sustainable development into country policies and programmes and reverse loss of environmental resources, b) to reduce by half the proportion of people without sustainable access to safe drinking water and c) to achieve significant improvement in lives of at least 100 million slum dwellers, by 2020.

- **Global trade and development** A set of seven goals to enhance free and fair trade and new technologies and to reduce debt.

- Drug access subgoal: One subgoal of the last goal is **"In cooperation with pharmaceutical companies, to provide access to affordable essential drugs in developing countries."**

UNAIDS and its co-sponsors have established a set of yardsticks for tracking movement towards The HIV targets. Work on the first report measuring progress against these indicators will begin in 2003, and will be based on progress reports provided in March 2003 by the 189 countries that adopted the Declaration.

Already there is substantial evidence of progress. More countries are recognising the value of pooling resources, experiences and commitment by forging regional initiatives to combat the epidemic. For example:

The Asia Pacific Leadership Forum, which is tasked with improving key decision-makers' knowledge and understanding of HIV/AIDS and its impact on different sectors of society.

Members of the Commonwealth of Independent States have developed a regional Programme of Urgent Response to the HIV/AIDS epidemic, which government leaders endorsed in May 2002.

In mid-2002, the Pan-Caribbean Partnership against HIV/AIDS signed an agreement with six pharmaceutical companies as part of wider-ranging efforts to improve access to cheaper antiretroviral drugs.

In sub-Saharan Africa, 40 countries had developed national strategies to fight HIV/AIDS by 2002 (almost three times as many as two years previously), and 19 countries now have National AIDS Councils (a sixfold increase since 2000).

However, fewer than 4% of people in need of antiretroviral therapy in low- and middle-income countries had access to those medications at the end of 2001, and fewer than 10% of people with HIV/AIDS had access to palliative care or treatment for opportunistic infections.

Aside from the prohibitory cost of many medications, insufficient capacity of health sectors, including infrastructure and shortage of trained personnel, are major barriers to health service delivery in many countries.

Then, in June 2001, the United Nations convened a General Assembly Special Session on AIDS and HIV (UNGASS), the first ever such session to be convened on an issue not directly to do with war or security.

This session ended up with the signing of a Declaration of Commitment on HIV/AIDS. This 103-paragraph document contained resolutions countries bound themselves to deliver in order to mitigate the impact of HIV and AIDS ranging from political leadership and institutional restructuring to research into vaccines and microbicides.

The Declaration pledged to spend $10 billion on the global epidemic by 2005 (an amount in fact comfortably exceeded), and the very last paragraph, number 103, pledged to "Explore, with a view to improving equity in access to essential drugs, the feasibility of developing and implementing, in collaboration with non-governmental organizations and other concerned partners, systems for voluntary monitoring and reporting of global drug prices." ·

The Global Fund

The next event was the development of **The Global Fund to Fight AIDS, TB and Malaria ('The Fund').**

There were already international AIDS programmed being run by bodies such as the World Bank and the UK's Department for International Development, but this initiative, suggested by UN Secretary-General Kofi Annan at UNGASS in 2001 and started in 2002, is an attempt to develop a completely new and multilateral funding mechanism for AIDS and HIV. The Fund currently finances 300 programmes in 174 countries. At present about 61% of the money goes to African nations, 23% goes to Asia, the Middle East and North Africa, and 16% goes to Latin America, the Caribbean and Europe.

A grand total of $9.8 billion has been pledged to January 2007. The Fund has approved a total of US$ 7 billion to over 450 grants in 136 countries, including the latest grants to receive approval for Phase 2 funding (years three to five of the grant lifespan). Of the US$ 7 billion approved, US$ 3.3 billion has now been disbursed to public and private recipients in 130 countries. And to date, 83% of approved grantees have signed grant agreements.

The Fund does not dictate how much donor countries should give nor does it either run the programmes countries spend money on nor seek out programmes to finance; it is purely a funding mechanism. Its recipient countries (who in some cases are also donor countries; Uganda, for instance, has pledged $2m to The Fund), decide on what AIDS, TB and malaria projects need funding and make bids for them through committees called **Country Co-ordinating Mechanisms.** These include representatives from government, NGOs and in some cases organisations of people with HIV.

The Fund has been criticised for being over-elaborate in structure, and has struggled to match the level of funds it has to disburse with the levels of demand. It is also been unable to enforce efficient usage of funding once it actually gets to the country concerned. In several countries there have been financial scandals. In some, funds have been received but have taken an inordinate time to get used. In India, for instance, owing to government inertia not one dollar of $112m available for HIV treatment was used for over a year. In August 2005 The Fund announced that it had devised 'EARS' (Early Warning and Response System) in order to alert it when programmes were running into trouble at the country end.

In other cases, funds have also apparently disappeared into the pockets of corrupt officials (or, at the very least, into Byzantine accounting practices) in, for instance, Uganda. And countries with totalitarian regimes, such as Myanmar, have placed such restrictions on international aid workers that they have been unable to carry out Fund-financed programmes. The Fund finally showed its 'teeth' in 2005 when it refused to pay out any more money to Uganda (or Myanmar until, in the case of Uganda, the apparent corruption was investigated, or, in the case of Myanmar, restrictions on aid workers were lifted.

Part of the Fund's problem is that the USA developed its own international HIV treatment and prevention programme, the **President's Emergency Plan for AIDS Relief (PEPFAR)**.

PEPFAR

This programme was announced by George W Bush in January 2003, when he asked the US Congress "To commit $15 billion over the next five years, to turn the tide against AIDS in the most afflicted nations of Africa and the Caribbean".

PEPFAR is in many ways a mirror-image of The Global Fund. It is completely unilateral, and seeks out programmes to fund. Where The Global Fund has an explicit 'No Strings' policy which has no guidelines that restrict what kind of programmes it is prepared to finance, PEPFAR only funds programmes of its own choosing - which explicitly exclude programmes for groups that provide abortion, needle exchange to drug users and groups that don not specifically sign a declaration opposing sex work (a reason why Brazil turned down a $40 million grant in 2005). It also largely concentrates on funding programmes in 15 'focus countries" (Botswana, Côte d'Ivoire, Ethiopia, Guyana, Haiti, Kenya, Mozambique, Namibia, Nigeria, Rwanda, South Africa, Tanzania, Uganda and Zambia, with Vietnam being added in 2004), although in fact PEPFAR can finance programmes in any country that has already received AIDS relief from the USA, and has done so (for instance) in India.

Congress mandated that PEPFAR money be divided up so that 55% was spent on the treatment of people with HIV/AIDS (of which 75% must be spent specifically on antiretroviral drugs); 15% on palliative care for people with AIDS; 20% on HIV prevention (of which at least 33% is to be spent on abstinence until marriage programs), and 10% for helping orphans and vulnerable children.

PEPFAR has critics not just because of its 'strings attached' funding policies but also because it has been accused of fiddling its statistics and overstating the amount of money it has spent and the number of people it has placed on treatment. For instance, PEPFAR claims that it has put 33,000 people in treatment in Botswana because it makes a small contribution to clinics that are in fact largely financed by The Global Fund. It has also, if anything, been almost too treatment-focused and has actually spent less than the mandated 20% on prevention, probably because it is a more politically controversial area.

However it has also been praised for being more speedy and efficient in getting antiretroviral drugs to where people need them and not being vulnerable to local political inefficiency, unlike The Fund. It devised a phased programme of introducing funding by 'tracks' so that organisations already providing treatment programmes were initially financed and newer programmes were allowed to get 'up to speed' and be funded by later tracks. It also confronted one of the most difficult aspect of providing ARV treatment, which even the USA cannot always get right for its own citizens; ensuring a constant supply of a commodity where gaps in supply would be quickly lethal. It has awarded a contract to organise a foolproof Supply Chain Management System to the international NGO John Snow International.

PEPFAR and The Global Fund are by no means the only international HIV funding mechanisms to arise in the first half of the 'noughties' (the decade from 2000 to 2010). Ex-President Bill Clinton has developed his own Clinton Foundation which both runs its own treatment and prevention programmes and has also helped run aspects of The Fund's work (it stepped in to sort out the India mess, for instance). The Bill and Melinda Gates foundation has made a speciality of funding innovative prevention programmes such as IAVI, the International Partnership for Microbicides and pre-exposure prophylaxis trials. George Soros's

Open Society Foundation has concentrated on parts of the world and groups ignored by other programmes such as sex workers and drug users in the former Soviet states. And existing programmes such as the UK's DfID and the World Bank continue to fund their own programmes.

The 3 by 5 Campaign

Access to Treatment - The 3 by 5 Campaign

As a result of UNGASS and the drug-access activism that had preceded it at the Durban World AIDS Conference in 2000, the World Health Organisation (WHO) announced in 2003 a campaign to get three million people treated with antiretroviral drugs by the end of 2005 (half the number thought to be in life-or-death need).

The WHO announced in June 2005 that nearly one million people were now on antiretrovirals (ARVs). This was 600,000 fewer than their target for that month and they admitted that the three million goal would not be met.

However '3 by 5' does seem to have served as a catalyst for accelerated drug access during the two years of its existence. In sub-Saharan Africa, half a million people -11% of those in need - are now thought to be on ARVs (up from 310,000 six months earlier). In south and south-east Asia the number on ARVs increased threefold from 55,000 to 155,000 in the year from June 2004 to June 2005. In Latin America 63% of people in need of ARVs are now taking them. And in Eastern Europe the number on ARVs has nearly doubled, from 11,000 to 20,000.

'3 by 5' has been the first set of HIV treatment goals specifically linked to a programme of action and it has involved countries and international agencies finally tackling the huge barriers to the treatment of disease previously thought so expensive, complex and life-long that scaling-up treatment was impossible. In order to do this the WHO included the following basic recommendations if scale-up or ARV treatment was to become a reality:

- *Political commitment:* Of 49 WHO/UNAIDS "focus countries", 40 have established national targets for treatment access, and 34 are developing or have completed implementation plans. These plans are a first step toward rapidly scaling up ART access. The WHO/UNAIDS report calls for countries that do not have concrete plans to put them in place quickly.

- *Standardized approaches and increased capacity:* The countries making the most significant progress in providing quality ART to the greatest number of people are those that have adopted standardised drug regimens and clinical monitoring procedures. These countries are also addressing bottlenecks in procurement and supply chain management and in human resources capacity - by training non-physician health workers to safely and effectively administer ART. More countries should follow these leads.

- *Technical support:* WHO and other UN agencies are in the process of increasing technical assistance to countries in scaling up their ART programmes and strengthening their health sectors overall. A key WHO initiative employs new mapping software to help countries pinpoint the greatest unmet needs for a range of health services, in order to best target available resources. Overall, there is a need for technical assistance agencies to better coordinate with each other and with donors. The new UNAIDS Global Task Team is one forum for promoting this kind of improved cooperation.

- *Sustainable financing:* Donors have committed a total of US$27 billion over the next three years for HIV/AIDS treatment, care, and prevention efforts. However, not all of these commitments have been delivered, and the total amount pledged leaves a projected shortfall of at least US$18 billion for the period 2005-2007. Donors should accelerate funding disbursements to countries, increase their commitments, and pledge long-term, predictable funding. Developing countries should continue to invest their own resources. The new G-8 debt relief proposal provides an opportunity for several countries to reallocate significant resources to HIV/AIDS.

- *Linking treatment and prevention:* Evidence is emerging that ART availability leads to an upsurge in demand for HIV testing and counselling and other prevention services. In one district in Uganda, introduction of ART led to a 27-fold increase in demand for HIV testing and counselling. The WHO/UNAIDS report recommends steps for countries to integrate HIV treatment with testing and prevention, including using the same health clinics to offer both treatment and testing, and training health workers who administer ART to also offer prevention.

Of these, the biggest barrier to scale-up is technical and human capacity. Universal ARV treatment will involve an extraordinary expansion and in some cases re-creation of healthcare systems reduced to skeleton services by years of neglect, underfinancing and the 'brain drain' or qualified medical personnel to developed countries.

ARV scale-up can be a challenge even to middle-income countries. In South Africa the 3 by 5 campaign estimates that 10-14% of the population in need of ARVs currently gets them, with wide disparities between different provinces. The South African Health Department plans to get ARVs to one million people by 2009 - pretty much the total of people who need them now, in September 2005. But the research organisation Health Systems Trust calculated that this would cost the country US$1 billion - 20 times what was being currently spent. An additional 3,200 doctors, 2,400 nurses, 765 social workers and 765 dietitians would be required to distribute and monitor ARV treatment.

Faced with this, one of the most exciting developments in some countries has been the recruitment of people with HIV themselves as peer treatment support workers.

Other barriers to access include:

- **HIV stigma.** Although studies have found that HIV stigma generally reduces when people realise that treatment works and is available, there have been reports from countries like Ghana and Nigeria that reluctance to come forward for voluntary counselling and testing was restricting the number of people treated. In Botswana President Festus Mogae announced in 2004 a controversial policy of routine opt-out HIV testing for people having medical checkups to increase the proportion of people who, in a country with 35% prevalence, know their HIV status from 8% to 100%.

- **Resistance.** In 2004 a study (Kamya) found that one-third of a group of 137 patients at Mulago Hospital in Kampala, Uganda had failed antiretroviral therapy after an average follow-up period of 38 weeks, with 22% acquiring resistance to NNRTIs.

- **Second-line treatment.** The proportion of people who respond virologically to first-line regimes is 50% to 80% - similar to the proportion in developed countries, confounding predictions of poor adherence, but dependent on the potency and purity of drug regimens. Second-line treatments generally involve the more expensive protease inhibitors. During the summer of 2005 Brazil, which has pioneered universal HIV treatment in non-rich countries, was involved in a protracted negotiation with major Pharmaceutical company Abbott to reduce the price of its PI *Kaletra* (lopinavir/r). In September 2005 a group of Ugandan doctors criticised the country's national HIV programme for only supplying drugs to drug-naïve people, saying that people who had been able to pay for first-line regimens were being discriminated against if they found they could not afford second-line ones (Colebunders).

- **Drug prices.** Although huge reductions in the prices of drugs have been negotiated, many countries still require patients to make co-payments on their ARVs. In the Uganda study cited above the main reason for treatment failure and the acquisition of resistance was poor adherence. In a cross-sectional questionnaire, eleven per cent of patients had missed a dose in the previous four days and 18% in the previous two weeks. The main reason cited by patients for poor adherence was the fact that some patients had to pay a contribution to the cost of therapy. Researchers reporting to the Bangkok World AIDS Conference in 2004 found that in Haiti a programme of completely free access had resulted in 80% virological success, but a similar programme in Malawi where patients had to pay a contribution to medication was only 50% effective. As a result a group of health economists led by the South African Professor Alan Whiteside launched a campaign called 'Free by 5' in 2005 demanding free provision of ARVs to the developing world.

- **Side-effects.** ARV programmes in the developing world use fixed-dose generic combinations such as *Triomune* (d4T/3TC/nevirapine). D4T has largely stopped being used in the developed world due to its association with lipoatrophy (fat loss). One study in India (Pujari) found that lipoatrophy was detected in 26% of patients receiving d4T/3TC/nevirapine and 10% of those receiving AZT/3TC (p=0.08). Another study from Nigeria (Imarhiagbe) found that three out of eleven people given *Triomune* developed progressively higher triglyceride levels in their blood.

Universal Treatment Access

In July 2005 the G8 summit at Gleneagles announced the goal of universal HIV treatment access by 2010.

Funding will be crucially important to meet this goal

With UNAIDS calculating that the current cost of universal treatment, prevention and care for HIV being in the region of $27bn a year, but with the two largest funding mechanisms, the US Presidential Emergency Fund for AIDS Relief (PEPFAR) and The Global Fund for AIDS TB and Malaria, between then providing no more than $6bn a year, the international money to fight HIV/AIDS needs to be drastically upscaled if the epidemic is not to outrun the resources available to deal with it.

Access to Treatment - 2007 update

The WHO released another report on 17 April 2007 giving a new update on treatment access.

Significant progress has been made towards the goal of universal access to HIV drugs, the WHO said.

But the report found that the *rate* of increase had slowed down and that there needed to be significant improvements if the majority of people with HIV treatment needs were to get antiretrovirals by 2010, as promised by the 2005 G8 summit.

The WHO highlighted Africa, the world's hardest-hit continent, as the place where treatment had improved most dramatically. In fact Africa's HIV-positive people in 2007 were now more likely to have access to treatment than people in most of Asia, Russia or the middle east.

However the agency said that significant gaps remain.

Treatment for children was lagging behind treatment for adults; the provision of drugs to pregnant women to stop children getting HIV in the first place remained scandalously patchy; TB programmes are missing the chance to detect HIV in their patients and co-treat them; and some groups such as intravenous drug users were missing out treatment, especially in Russia, the country with the biggest needle-driven outbreak.

HIV testing needs to be improved, too, says the report; at present in Africa's hardest-hit countries fewer than one in four HIV-positive men, and fewer than one in six women, know their HIV status and only one in nine adults have taken a test.

The report contains a couple of surprises too. More women than men were getting HIV drugs in the majority of countries. And although the average price of the cheapest drug regimens had continued to decrease in the last year, in had done so only by 10% to 20%, and in the case of the regimen with the fewest side-effects, the average price had actually increased.

The report said that In December 2006 over two million people in the developing world were on HIV treatment plus another 600,000 in the developed world, and 700,000 got the drugs for the first time in 2006.

In Africa 28% of people who need HIV pills were now getting them, a 65% increase in a year and a 13-fold increase since 2003. In Botswana over 90% of Botswana nationals who needed the drugs was getting them and in Rwanda and Namibia over 70%.

Coverage remained poor, however, in Nigeria, Africa's most populous country, with only 10% who needed treatment getting it.

In Latin America 72% of people who needed treatment were now getting it; although there was substantial variation between countries, the WHO commented that "the overall coverage appears to be approaching universal access".

However in south and south-east Asia fewer than one in five(19%) of people who needed treatment was getting it; this was largely driven by the situation in India where at most nine per cent and possibly as few as four per cent of HIV patients were getting the drugs they needed. In contrast Thailand and Cambodia now had over 80% coverage.

In eastern Europe and central Asia the position was even worse, with only 15% coverage in the region as a whole and, scandalously in what is now a rich country, only 3% in Russia.

The Russian situation is largely driven by stigma against drug users, who form 87% of people with HIV but only 8% of the 3% who get antiretroviral therapy - this means only one in 400 drug users with HIV is on treatment.

The poorest-served area was north Africa and the middle east, where only 6% of those who needed treatment were getting it. Although this part of the world is a low prevalence area for HIV, there are growing epidemics amongst drug users in Libya and Bahrain and the beginnings of one amongst gay men.

Although in most cases equal proportions of men and women were getting treatment, where they weren't, the situation tended to be biased against men. Worldwide 48% of people with HIV are women but they represented 57% of those getting treatment.

In South Africa while 58% of people with HIV are women, 70% of those who were getting treatment are women, while in China, women formed 28% of the positive population but 45% of those

on treatment. This may be because women get the opportunity to be tested and treated in antenatal care.

Dr Charlie Gilks, the head of WHO's HIV treatment department, told reporters in Geneva that "The encouraging progress that was made . . . has been sustained." He said that one of the main reasons for the success was the significant drop in the cost of drugs.

However there were ominous signs that prices might not drop much further. Prices of the four cheapest combinations only fell between 10% and 20% in 2005-6, and the cheapest combinations also tended to be the ones that caused the worst side-effects, as they contain d4T (stavudine), a drug that has fallen out of favour in the rich world because it causes fat loss.

The average price of the WHO-approved combination that causes the fewest side-effects, AZT/3TC/efavirenz, had actually increased by nearly 40% in 2004-6.

Treatment when it was accessed was generally as successful as it was in the rich world, the report found. Surveys had shown that 80% of people were still on their first drug combination after a year and 75% after two years, with slightly higher failure rates than in the west, largely driven by the fact that people were often more ill when they started treatment.

However the price of second-line therapy was still considerably beyond the pockets of most countries. While the average price of the cheapest combination, 4T/3TC/nevirapine, cost $123 a year in the poorest countries and $145 in middle-income ones, the most frequently-used second-line therapy, ddI/abacavir/Kaletra, cost $1,698 in poor countries and $4,735 in middle-income ones.

The dispute between the Thai government and drug company Abbott over the price of *Kaletra* in early 2007 showed that intense negotiations over the price of the second-line protease inhibitor drugs would be necessary if treatment success was to be sustained.

It needs to be, because the bottom line is that access to antiretrovirals is starting to work. In Botswana, where 30% of the population has HIV and 90% of those who need treatment get it, mortality peaked in 2003 with one in 166 citizens dying every year compared with one in 500 in 1994.

In 2006 this had declined to one in 220 and the trend towards increased upward life expectancy seemed to be accelerating.

Global HIV treatment, long thought to be impossible, may now be a realistic hope, and with it may come the first real reductions in the global toll of AIDS.

Progress towards HIV treatment - selected countries - January 2007

Country	Adults in need	Adults on ARVs reported	Percentage treated
Argentina	40,000	19,812	50%
Botswana	77,000	60,741	79%
Brazil	210,000	174,000	83%
Cambodia	21,500	16,685	78%
Cameroon	92,000	23,114	25%
China	110,000	30,118	27%

Country	Adults in need	Adults on ARVs reported	Percentage treated
Côte d'Ivoire	95,000	19,739	21%
Dem Rep Congo	160,000	17,509	11%
Estonia	1,900	242	12.5%
Ethiopia	150,000	38,446	35%
Ghana	55,000	4,635	9%
Haiti	19,000	7,597	39%
Honduras	9,600	3,856	40%
India	1,055,000(?)	52,383	c. 6.5%
Jamaica	4,400	2,122	49%
Kenya	240,000	80,803	33%
Malawi	160,000	53,853	33%
Mozambique	250,000	31,076	12%
Nigeria	460,000	46,810	10%
Papua New Guinea	8,500	371	4%
Peru	18,000	7,822	44%
Russia	140,000	4,520	3%
Rwanda	41,000	27,550	68%
Somalia	7,100	49	1%
South Africa	910,000	163,433	18%
Swaziland	39,000	15,731	40%
Tanzania	240,000	41,920	18%
Thailand	120,000	73,363	60%
Uganda	190,000	45,946	24%
Vietnam	40,000	3,196	8%
Zambia	190,000	65,383	34%
Zimbabwe	310,000	26,327	9%

The future global burden of HIV

So we are well on the way towards universal treatment access and HIV will become worldwide what it is in the developed world, a chronic manageable condition, yes?

It may well become more chronic and more manageable, but a 2006 forecast by Colin D Mathers and Dejan Loncar of the WHO and published in the Public Library of Science predicts that AIDS, even if 80% ARV coverage is reached by 2012, will continue to exact a huge burden on global health.

The WHO report predicts that AIDS will be the number one cause of sickness and disability in the world by 2030. HIV-related sickness will disable more than twice as many people as the next-worst chronic illness, depression. The WHO also finds that AIDS will be the third-biggest killer after heart attacks and strokes which, because they generally kill suddenly, do not exact the same price in terms of chronic illness.

There will however, be one worse killer than AIDS, the WHO warned: tobacco. Because it's a cause of disease rather than a disease itself, cigarettes are not on the list, but they will cause eight million deaths a year by 2030, while AIDS will kill 6.3 million.

The WHO report is the first attempt to forecast life expectancy and cause of death for the next 25 years since a similar report in 1990. The old report and the new one come to the same overall, optimistic conclusion: although the number of deaths per year will rise, this is due to increased population, and the overall death rate will fall. Fewer people will die young, and more people from diseases of old age.

Life expectancy will increase in all areas and in high-income countries will reach 85 for women and nearly 80 for men. The average life expectancy will be over 65 for men and women in every part of the world except in Africa, where, because of AIDS, people will still only look forward to an average 55 years of life, though that is ten more than today.

The biggest improvement in health will be due to the control of infectious disease other than AIDS, and in particular infant mortality. With better medicines for childhood killers like diarrhoea and malaria, twice as many children will live to become adults.

The death rate due to most other conditions will fall or remain neutral, though only modestly in some cases. The two biggest exceptions other than AIDS will be caused by increasing affluence, WHO predict.

Diabetes, a disease overwhelmingly caused by obesity, will cancel out gains in controlling heart attacks and strokes as the human race becomes, on average, fatter. And more people will die of road traffic accidents as the world's cities clog up with cars.

But the death rate due to these two factors will only increase by just over one per cent a year. HIV-relayed deaths will increase at twice this rate in women and three times this rate in men, WHO predicts.

If it was not for HIV, the proportion of the world's deaths caused by infectious diseases would almost halve from over 15 million deaths a year in 2002 to eight million by 2030. But add on AIDS, and you get only a modest decline from 18 million today to 15 million in 2030. AIDS, by then, will cause 42% of all deaths due to infectious disease, compared with 15% today.

Then, as now, the biggest killer of all will still be cardiovascular disease; but AIDS will have overtaken all other causes, including cancer.

That is if things carry on as they are - and "as they are" includes the relatively optimistic prediction that 80% of the world's HIV sufferers will have access to antiretroviral drugs as needed by 2012. If only 60% get them, the toll will be worse.

What can we do about HIV? The WHO model predicts that for the next few years antiretroviral drugs will save lives. But from about 2012, because more people will be living longer with HIV, and more will be catching it, the death rate will rise - unless comprehensive HIV prevention programmes are put in place.

If a comprehensive prevention package for HIV is put into place for everyone in poor countries and for high-risk groups in rich ones, including increased testing, universal access to condoms, and comprehensive safer-sex advice, then AIDS deaths will stabilise at around 3.5 million a year - half the figure they will otherwise be, and lower than cardiovascular disease ((7 million), cancer (5.5 million) and infant mortality (4.8 million).

The health gap between the rich world and the rest is starkly underlined in the report, and its biggest effect is the difference in the burden of AIDS. While AIDS will be the biggest killer in poor countries and the fourth-biggest in middle-income ones, it appears nowhere on the list of top 10 killers in the rich world. There, apart from diseases of old age like Alzheimer's, all the top ten slots are filled by diseases at least partly caused by smoking (lung cancer, emphysema, pneumonia), poor diet (diabetes, stomach cancer, colon cancer) or both (heart disease and strokes).

The WHO report doesn't take account of the unexpected - such as a medical breakthrough (like an HIV vaccine) or a dramatic shift in behaviour (we all stop smoking or driving cars). In general, its predictions set three conditions for people who want to live a long life: eat sensibly, don't smoke - and have safer sex.

References

Blackstock O. Curing Stigma - The Limits of Antiretroviral Access. NEJM 353(8): 752, 2005.

Colebunders R et al. Free antiretrovirals must not be restricted only to treatment-naïve patients. PloS Medicine 2 (10): e276, 2005.

Health Systems Trust: South African Health Review 2005. See http://www.hst.org.za/publications/682

Imarhiagbe FA et al. Hypertriglyceridemia in Antiretroviral Therapy. Medscape General Medicine 7(3), 2005.

Kamya M.R. et al. Treatment outcomes for antiretroviral therapy in a routine clinical setting in Kampala, Uganda. Seventh International Congress on Drug Therapy in HIV Infection, Glasgow, abstract PL4.4, 2004.

Mathers CD and Loncar D. Projections of Global Mortality and Burden of Disease from 2002 to 2030. PLoS Medicine, 3(11): 2011-2030. 2006.

Millennium Development Goals: see http://www.un.org/millenniumgoals/

Pujari SN et al. Lipodystrophy and dyslipidemia among patients taking first-line, World Health Organization-recommended highly active antiretroviral therapy regimens in western India. JAIDS 39: 199-202, 2005.

'3 by 5' campaign: see http://www.who.int/3by5/en/

Crystal ball gazing: the future of the HIV epidemic

HIV has continually wrong-footed 'experts' who predicted what it would do next or how the epidemic would develop. It has just as often failed to fulfil terrifying predictions (for instance, in not starting a generalised heterosexual epidemic in developing countries) as it has erupted with terrifying speed into new populations (as for instance, as we write, into Papua New Guinea). It is perhaps better to look at 'themes' and see how these may work themselves out as humanity and its most recent plague adapt to each other over the next decade.

- **More women.** There is no indication that the continued 'feminisation' of HIV will slow down; the epidemic shows a consistent pattern in being predominantly male in the areas where is has most recently appeared, and predominantly female in the areas where it has been around longest, in the absence of prevention programmes that protect women. The absence of those prevention programmes may hopefully start up a new wave of women-directed HIV prevention - which won't always go in directions men like (as, for instance, the recent campaign among HIV-positive women in France *for* the jailing of men who transmit HIV).

- **The next crisis in treatment provision.** The above paragraphs witness an extraordinary global treatment initiative that no one could have predicted coming to fruition only five years ago. However what the world as yet appears to be unprepared for is what to do when first-line treatments fail. It is not just that second-line drugs like protease inhibitors are more expensive (hence the recent stand-offs between the Brazilian and Thailand governments and Abbott Laboratories over the price of *Kaletra*). Who will pay for and administer the viral load and resistance tests that will be necessary to keep people's HIV treatment working? If we do not pay for these diagnostic tests and use 'clinical monitoring', which basically means waiting till people get sick before switching, will be see a global epidemic of drug-resistant HIV?

- **More treatment, more people, more HIV.** As we have seen in the developed world, the immediate result of successful HIV treatment is a great many more people living with HIV. And more people living with HIV means more sexually-active people to spread it. Global treatment provision is not an alternative to prevention; on the contrary, it will compel new, more complex and possibly politically difficult approaches towards prevention.

- **More travel, more internet, more gay men - more sex!** HIV isn't just affecting the poorest of the poor, it is affecting people in 'tiger economies' like India and China. Even in Africa, there are predictions that some countries may bounce back from the development rut AIDS seemed to have condemned them to. What this means is that, short of there being a global fuel crisis and resultant recession, or swingeing financial penalties on carbon-wasting activities, more people will travel; the use of the internet and other new communication technologies will continue to expand exponentially; and people will use these technologies to find who they want sexually. There is already evidence that the internet is not just being used by gay men to find each other but is encouraging men to try gay sex who wouldn't have done so before. This particularly applies to the developing world where the internet often offers the only possibility of contact. However the internet also offers a radical new space in which to do HIV prevention.

- **The coming plague of stigma.** Universal HIV treatment in some ways removes stigma because people with HIV are not feared any more as vectors and embodiments of death and disease. However people with HIV in developed countries have found it replaced by other forms of stigma. Will a rise in the number of sexually active people with HIV give rise to more criminal prosecutions for transmission? Will re-emergence into the workforce mean more discrimination at work? And will immigration become an even hotter political potato as more and more countries worry about the cost of treating migrants with HIV? Above all, will HIV turn from the scary to the scuzzy - from a terrifying, tragic but at least interesting disease into just the most serious, chronic and expensive of the list of embarrassing sexually transmitted infections?

- **A new emphasis on sexual responsibility.** One development that almost certainly *will* happen is an increasing number of prosecutions of people with HIV for infecting others. In recent months the number of UK convictions for reckless infection has increased to 13. A high-profile case in Australia has led to calls for a ban on HIV-positive travellers and for phylogenetic testing to trace contacts. There have been calls for the death penalty for men who infect women with HIV through rape in Uganda and Zimbabwe. While HIV campaigners will continue the question the value and public health consequences of prosecuting 'bedroom GBH', and while better expert defence may secure a larger number of acquittals in future, prosecutions for HIV and possibly other STDs will almost certainly continue. HIV prevention organisations, caught on the hop, may need to teach people with HIV a new balance between rights and responsibilities.

- **Will the world get bored?** HIV had slipped off the media agenda in the countries where people no longer die from it. The result of this 'ignoral' is usually that it is prevention programmes that get neglected, rather than treatment. The result of taking the eye off the ball in prevention is that HIV then finds its way into populations that have no culture of HIV prevention, and regains a foothold. An example seems to be young African-Americans. There HIV prevalence has reached a scarcely believable 48% in young gay men and incidence in one city, Baltimore, 8% a year.

- **HIV slips to the margins** A linked phenomenon is that as groups who are easily reached by prevention and treatment programmes (such as white, educated gay men) are reached, so the virus can only go in one direction - towards people who are ever more marginalised, poor and hard to reach such as prisoners, drug users, homeless people, the mentally ill, MSM and sex workers in the developing world, and so on.

- **The pipeline dries up.** So far drug companies have shown a remarkable ability to stay ahead of HIV's ability to mutate around their products. However as treatments get more successful so the financial rewards for developing new ones get less, as there are a smaller and smaller group of failing patients who desperately need them. In addition, the easy targets are the ones first developed, and as HIV drugs get more sophisticated they get pricier. The list of new drugs pulled out of development in the last two years is a long one, and includes T-1249, two CCR5 inhibitors, a CXCR4 inhibitor, an integrase inhibitor, a CD4 inhibitor, and several members of existing classes such as capravirine. Will we get stuck with the drugs we have now? Will drug companies ever consider it profitable to develop therapeutic vaccines people could take once a year? And will 'narrowcast' medicines specifically tailored to particular people's genetic makeup ever be financially realistic?

- **New prevention technologies - miracle - or impossibility?** We have already detailed above why trying to find a vaccine for HIV is so difficult. Prevention campaigners are now placing their faith in microbicides, pre-exposure prophylaxis, circumcision and other biological methods of HIV prevention to work where persuasion, education and behaviour change don't. However the current generation of microbicides may only be 60% effective at best and the phase III trials are on the knife-edge of not being powered to produce a meaningful result; PREP appears to be almost impossibly controversial; and widespread circumcision, if attempted, won't protect women, injecting drug users and gay men.

- **HIV will continue to transform societies.** Universal treatment is a very long way off and may never be a possibility; there will still be a lot for vulnerable people to get angry about; societies will still have to face up to and dialogue with their most stigmatised members in order to prevent HIV, or pay the penalty. We will not see the end of the epidemic, or even its 'normalisation', over the next decade.

The epidemiology of HIV

Epidemiology is the study of the way diseases spread through populations. It monitors the spread of diseases and tries to predict how epidemics will grow and who is likely to be affected by them.

Epidemiologists monitor patterns of illness, and sometimes identify new diseases as a result of this work. AIDS is a notable example. The possibility that a new illness characterised by immune suppression might be emerging was first suggested when the Centers for Disease Control (CDC, now known as the Centers for Disease Control and Prevention) in the United States noticed an unusual number of requests for drugs to treat *Pneumocystis* pneumonia (PCP, fomerly known as *Pneumocystis carinii* pneumonia), which at that time was a very rare condition.

Epidemiology tells us:

■ How an epidemic has developed.

■ Where the epidemic is now.

■ How the epidemic is likely to develop.

A proper understanding of the current nature of the HIV epidemic and its likely development over the medium and long-term is crucial if services - including both care provision and HIV prevention activities - are to be properly planned, accurately targeted and effectively delivered.

The collection of data

Epidemiology provides information on two distinct but closely related issues:

- How HIV is transmitted

- Who the epidemic affects (in the past, present and future).

In Britain information about individuals who test HIV antibody-positive or who are diagnosed with AIDS is reported in an anonymised form to either the Health Protection Agency (HPA) in London, or the Scottish Centre for Infection and Environmental Health (SCIEH). GPs, NHS hospitals and clinics as well as private hospitals and clinics all take part in this scheme.

Since the beginning of 2000 clinicians in England and Wales and Northern Ireland have been asked to report all first UK diagnoses of HIV infection in those aged 14 and over to the HPA.

Previous to this time, reports were made by the laboratories that actually performed the HIV tests on samples. Clinician reporting has greatly enhanced the quality of information available about the epidemic in the UK. For example, details of ethnicity were given on ninety-nine per cent of clinician reports. This compared to 48% of laboratory reports.

Surveillance programmes have to reach a compromise between completely anonymised reports, which may be inaccurate because there could be numerous duplicates of the same individual if they attend different clinics, and names-based reporting, which has been opposed because it was thought that both doctors and patients would object to the breach of confidentiality.

When AIDS monitoring was first set up in 1984 it was decided that reports of AIDS and (when HIV antibody testing became available in 1985) HIV should be sent to what was then the Public Health Laboratory Service (PHLS) in an anonymised form. The patient's name and identifying details such as date of birth and address are stripped from the report, leaving the following demographic details:

- Age

- Gender

- Region of Residence

- Probable mode of HIV transmission

- Probable country where HIV was acquired

- Probable mode of transmission and country of acquisition of the infecting partner

- Ethnic origin (since 1995)

Individual diagnosis reports are identified by a code number which is issued by the HIV or GUM clinic or GP practice where the diagnosis is made. The code is a Soundex code, a method of transforming surnames into a simple numerical code that was first used in the US census of 1880.

Some surnames have unique Soundex codes but the majority of codes are shared between different surnames (the point of developing the code in the first place was to be able to trace people who spelt their surname inconsistently). It is based on the pattern of consonants in the surname. For instance the Soundex code for this writer's name (Cairns) is C652 and is shared by the surnames Carmichael, Carrington, and Cornish, among others.

In theory the HPA could ask the clinic to identify the person behind a particular diagnosis report but in practice this is never done. The point of using the Soundex code as opposed to complete anonymity is to weed out probable duplicate reports. By the end of 1994 over 93% of the 20,407 reports on the HPA database had been Soundex coded, and 22% of the reports of

HIV infection were recognised as duplicating earlier reports of infection. It also enabled 70% of AIDS reports to be linked to independent reports of HIV infection.

The collected data allow the HPA to assemble profiles both of the cumulative epidemic, and any changes in its form over time.

The HPA uses a number of exposure categories in order to identify the routes of infection amongst heterosexual men and women and to monitor whether HIV is spreading from particular subgroups amongst heterosexuals. This system is very useful, because it monitors for the spread of infection from groups recognised as being at higher risk of infection ('second generation' transmission).

Estimates of the total number of HIV-infected people in different exposure categories are important for public health planning. It is also useful to know the prevalence of undiagnosed infection in the community, and the future number of people with severe HIV infection.

The 'direct' method of estimating the total number of both diagnosed and undiagnosed prevalent HIV infections among adults in the United Kingdom (UK) uses a combination of data from different sources.

The total number of prevalent diagnosed HIV infections in England and Wales was derived by adjusting the number of reported infections from the National Survey of Prevalent Diagnosed Infections (SOPHID) for both under-reporting and failure to access services annually.

The total number of prevalent undiagnosed HIV infections was calculated by applying undiagnosed HIV prevalence estimates, obtained from the Unlinked Anonymous Prevalence Monitoring Programme (UAPMP), to different categories of the population at different levels of risk of HIV infection. These categories included 'sex between men', 'sex between men and women', and 'injecting drug users'. Estimates of the total population within these categories were produced by combining the proportion of the population with particular behavioural characteristics, based on the results of the second National Survey of Sexual Attitudes and Lifestyles (Natsal 2000), with mid-year population estimates from the Office for National Statistics (ONS). Each population denominator was then multiplied by the relevant HIV prevalence estimate to derive the number of undiagnosed HIV-infected persons within that category.

The direct method protocol has been developed to include evidence-based adjustments that take account of differences in prevalence between subgroups within the population categories. The behavioural characteristics of the population have been updated using data from Natsal 2000.

In addition to the collection of HIV and AIDS diagnoses, the HPA also compile two other ongoing sets of data.

Unlinked Anonymous Prevalence Monitoring Programme (UAPMP)

This provides similar information without the biases involved in voluntary, 'elective' testing. In anonymised seroprevalence studies, samples of blood taken for other medical purposes at hospitals, clinics, casualty departments and maternity units are tested for HIV. Any information which could identify the individual is removed, leaving only the basic demographic information.

At present the HPA has three anonymised seroprevalence studies in its Unlinked Anonymous Prevalence Monitoring Programme (UAPMP). These are:

- Attendees at GUM clinics: samples provided for syphilis serology are tested.

- Injecting drug users: unlinked anonymous saliva samples are collected from drug users in contact with over 50 specialist agencies in England, Wales and Northern Ireland.

- Pregnant women and their newborn babies: samples collected from women attending antenatal clinics and from newborn infants.

Survey of Prevalent HIV Infections Diagnosed (SOPHID)

This provides data on those patients diagnosed with HIV and attending HIV-related care in clinics throughout the UK. As well as the data collected in initial diagnosis reports, information on the stage of disease reached and the level of antiretroviral therapy used is collected too.

After all the information has been compiled and analysed, the statistics are released in the form of monthly updated bulletins from the HPA. The Department of Health also issues these as press releases. Standard monthly statistical updates include only AIDS statistics; quarterly tables also include HIV figures. More detailed breakdowns are made widely available to such people as senior medical figures and health authority managers. More complex surveys such as the anonymised seroprevalence surveys are published in journals such as HPA's *Communicable Disease Report Weekly*.

Limitations to the available statistics

Firstly, the interpretation of the data related to diagnosed infections must take account of who comes forward for testing. By definition, reported positive HIV antibody test results include only those individuals who have taken the test. Those who choose to get tested may not be representative of the total population of HIV-infected people.

Secondly, people who visit sexually transmitted infection clinics are likely to be among the more sexually active members of the population. HIV infection rates among them may therefore be higher than among the population as a whole. However, they are also more likely to test for HIV.

In 2003 the HPA estimated that based on figures from the UAPMP, the proportion of gay men attending GUM clinics who were HIV-positive but did not know it was 25%. However, in 2005 they revised their estimate of the total proportion of gay men who were undiagnosed upwards to 34%, after anonymised surveys in London, Manchester and Brighton suggested a higher figure (see the Dodds survey under **Will we observe increases in HIV infection amongst gay men?** below).

They also estimated that 28% of women and 39% of men (including gay men) with HIV were undiagnosed. It is clear that only a proportion of those who are HIV-positive come forward for testing, and this proportion may well be different in the various risk groups and in different parts of the country. Furthermore, reporting of identified infections and AIDS cases may be incomplete or delayed.

Conversely, despite the weeding out of duplicate reports by Soundex code, it is clear that a proportion of patients still get 'double counted' because they have presented for care at several clinics. HIV diagnoses may also overestimate the overall prevalence on HIV in the country (once the likely proportion of undiagnosed people has been estimated) because many people with HIV come from highly mobile populations and may leave the UK after diagnosis.

The same applies to intravenous drug users. A recent study in which saliva samples were collected by street agencies in touch with drug users that did not use traditional drug agencies[1] found that HIV prevalence was higher among these largely younger users, especially in London.

Having said this, the UK probably has one of the best HIV surveillance programmes in the world. In the USA, for instance, each state has its own surveillance programme for HIV diagnoses. Some use a system of codes based on names, as in the

UK; others first collect epidemiological data by name before coding them and sending them to the federal Centers for Disease Control; others keep the patients' names linked to their data and rely on agreements to maintain patient confidentiality. As a result, the CDC is still unable to issue reliable figures for HIV infection that cover all 50 US states because it is not confident that each state collates statistics to the same standard of accuracy. It has recently announced that federal funding will from 2006 be withheld from states that do not adopt confidential names-based reporting, which they regard as the only safe method of weeding out duplicate records.

AIDS diagnoses, on the other hand, have by federal law to be reported on a name-by-name basis so, whatever concerns there may be about patient confidentiality, at least state-by-state comparisons are possible and the CDC can issue reliable national figures.

In Europe surveillance systems range from the completely anonymous, as in France and Germany, to Iceland, which has a fully named-patient system. Other countries add a measure of traceability to patient records by retaining initials and/or part of the patient's social security number. No other country uses the Soundex code. Some countries like Italy and Ireland do not have a mandatory national surveillance system but rely on extrapolations from a sample of lab reports. France only recently instituted a national system in 2003, though because this was done so late; its national patient database is now probably the most sophisticated in the world.

Nonetheless HIV statistics are usually more reliable than those for other diseases, since most developed countries at least instituted some kind of systematised reporting of HIV and AIDS. Compare, for instance, the situation with hepatitis C. The UAPMP figures suggest that about one-third of the people with HIV in the UK are undiagnosed. The HPA can therefore make an estimate of the number of new infections (incidence) and the number living with HIV (prevalence) which has a statistical uncertainty of about 18% either way: that is, UK prevalence is in the order of 45,000 to 65,000.

In contrast there could be anything between 250,000 and 500,000 people living with hepatitis C in the UK, an uncertainty factor of 50% either way. Because reporting is not mandatory, there were only just over 8,000 new hepatitis C diagnoses notified to the HPA last year, scarcely more than the 7,500 or so HIV diagnoses.

How statistics are presented

The month-on-month developments in the HIV and AIDS statistics provide an indication of the evolving dynamics of the epidemic. However, unless viewed with caution and an awareness of their limitations they can be more confusing than enlightening.

The fact that HIV infection usually remains asymptomatic for years means that new positive HIV antibody tests in a given month or year do not necessarily reflect transmission patterns as they are taking place at that time. A person may choose to take the HIV antibody test one month after becoming infected, only many years later or when they already have symptoms suggestive of AIDS. Thus HIV statistics can only reveal the cumulative shape of the epidemic, rather than provide a snapshot of trends at any given moment.

This problem is all the more significant with AIDS statistics. Although it is likely that AIDS statistics are more fully documented than positive HIV antibody test results, simply because a person who develops AIDS is likely to seek medical attention, the long average period between the contracting of HIV infection and the development of symptomatic disease means that AIDS statistics are unlikely to be representative of current patterns of HIV transmission.

Incidence and prevalence

Epidemiologists use two different measures of the severity and burden of diseases and it is important to understand the distinction between the two.

Incidence is the number of new cases of the disease diagnosed within a specific time period. It measures the **spread** of the disease. It is usually expressed as the number of cases per patient-years. Incidence in vulnerable groups may be very much higher: for instance gay men in the UK are probably between 50 and 100 times as likely to get HIV as a member of the general population.

Incidence depends critically on case reports and tests and can't be retrospectively determined from anonymous prevalence surveys, nor, in the case of a long-term chronic disease like HIV, is it the same as the number of new diagnoses (though it would be for an acute disease like flu or SARS).. Therefore **the rate of new diagnoses of HIV is not indicative of current incidence**.

For instance the number of gay men diagnosed with HIV each year in the UK has increased by 75% since 1998. But the number of gay men who take an HIV test when they go to a GUM clinic has during the same period increased by 60%. So most of the increase in diagnosis is due to more testing and only perhaps 15% of the increase is due to an actual increase in the rate of new infections.

Given the 'time lag' in diagnoses, how can true incidence be estimated? There are a couple of clever ways to estimate incidence within given populations who do not all come forward for testing. At present these are only used as research tools but some, for instance, a **detuned assay** (see HIV testing) which detects which HIV diagnoses are of recent infections (usually ones contracted in the last six months) can determine the proportion of people testing HIV-positive who have recent infections and therefore the overall recent incidence in the population.

It was by using anonymous HIV testing coupled to a detuned assay that, for instance, a survey in Baltimore in the USA this year2 found an annual HIV incidence of 8% among gay men, four times larger than the proportion of men reporting HIV diagnoses.

Conversely the incidence in San Francisco was only half of the new diagnosis rate, and previously estimated incidence, of 2.2%, indicating a possible move among gay men in the city towards behaviours less likely to result in IV infection.

Prevalence is the total number of people who have the disease at any one time. For instance in the UK about 60,000 people or one in 1,000 of the general population are currently living with HIV. Prevalence measures the overall **burden** of disease in a society rather than its spread. It depends crucially not only on the incidence but also on mortality from the disease (and from other causes) or on spontaneous recovery or cure rates if the disease is not lifelong like HIV.

Only by mapping both incidence and prevalence is it possible to predict whether an epidemic is getting more severe or waning.

While in general the fewer people suffer from a serious infection like HIV the better, there are situations in which increasing prevalence may be a form of good news; and in which declining prevalence may be bad news.

For instance: there are currently about ten times as many people living with HIV in the UK as catch it every year. But because the death rate among people with HIV is now only 6% of the annual incidence, it can easily be seen that this figure will continue to grow for the foreseeable future. The increasing prevalence of HIV in the developed world is primarily a sign of success in reducing the death toll from AIDS rather than failure to contain HIV.

Conversely where the mortality from a disease is particularly high, prevalence may fall even though incidence remains stable. This was the case in Uganda in the 1990s. HIV prevalence among people in the Rakai district fell from 17.6 to 11.4% from 1990 to 2002, even though the annual incidence remained unchanged. This was largely because more people were dying from AIDS at the time than were catching HIV; the wave of deaths was reflecting the extremely high incidence of the previous decade.

The fact that this declining prevalence was seen as evidence for the success of the HIV prevention programmes of the preceding few years shows how the significance of prevalence and incidence figures can get very confused in people's minds. The undoubted success of the Ugandan 'zero grazing' campaigns of the late 80s-early 90s were reflected in declining HIV incidence at the time But in terms of any reversal in the reduced life expectancy exacted by AIDS, we have only seen an improvement since 2000, as in the graph below.

The epidemiologist Roy Anderson sums up the situation with regard to HIV thus:

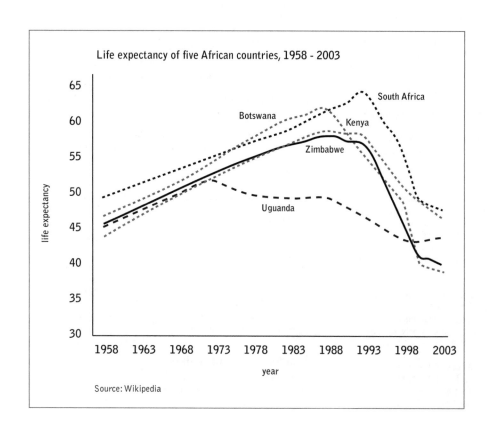

"*The prevalence of HIV in a particular population will not grow indefinitely, it will saturate at some level. Following the initial spread of HIV there is likely to be a fall in the incidence of infection followed in turn by a resultant reduction in prevalence. A fall in incidence is likely to precede the fall in prevalence, as the time scale over which the epidemic saturates is likely to be more rapid than the time scale on which HIV associated mortality increases.*"

Thus, even in a situation where there is no HIV treatment, and mortality runs unchecked, there may be a considerable time lag between a fall in incidence and one in prevalence. This is likely to be prolonged by decades in a country that has universal HIV treatment, and if incidence remains unchecked, prevalence will not decline until the number of 'at risk' people in the population is saturated (see chart below).

This means that prevention campaigns have to be extremely successful to have a short-term effect on prevalence. This does appear to have happened in Thailand, where the institution of near-universal condom use among men visiting sex workers in the early 1990s brought the HIV incidence in young men down from 2.5% in 1991 to 0.5% in 1993. This rapid fall in HIV incidence was followed equally rapidly by a fall in prevalence (see second chart below).

HIV-1 prevalence in Thai military conscripts

This may be one of the few occasions in which an HIV prevention campaign has had such an immediate effect, apart from very early in the history of the epidemic, where rapid behavioural changes accompanied by high mortality achieved permanent declines in prevalence rates in groups like intravenous drug users in the UK.

Incidence and prevalence figures will tend to run 'neck and neck' in an acute infection such as influenza, and indeed prevalence is rather a meaningless term in a situation where prevalence during one week is a 'snapshot' of recent infection with virtually the same meaning as incidence, and by the end of the year may be zero.

In non-infectious conditions like cancer, changes in incidence are the most useful tool to map both factors giving rise to the disease and the effect of treatment. If incidence changes quickly, an unusual influence like an environmental agent may be suspected.

In a chronic, slowly-accumulating infectious disease like HIV, incidence therefore is the best measure of whether behavioural change or prevention interventions are having an effect on the epidemic, and can also be used to make predictions as to future prevalence. Prevalence (current and projected) is the best indicator of the burden of the epidemic and is the figure to use in planning services.

Difficulties in using statistics to plan services

At a local level, primary care trusts often experience

Prevalence/Incidence

$R_t > 1$ $R_t < 1$ $R_t = 1$

- - - HIV prevalenceNRTI
- - - Incidence of HIV-associated mortality
—— HIV incidence

$R_0 > 1$ time (years)

Source: WHO

HIV-1 prevalence in Thai military conscripts

North

National

Source: Jugsudee et al. 1996

problems in obtaining up-to-date and comprehensive data on the numbers of people testing positive in their district (and demographic breakdowns of potential service users) due to a lack of provision for the exchange of data between services, lack of resources to collate and analyse such data, and insistences that all data must remain confidential.

Even when data have been obtained from clinics, for instance, it may still not relate to actual service needs in particular districts because people may take HIV antibody tests at clinics outside their district of residence.

There is even a phrase - 'perverse incentives' - that refers to the fact that area-based health services like PCTs have a disincentive to improve open-access services like GUM clinics, as they will attract more patients and increase running costs.

The lack of data sharing between districts may perpetuate the phenomenon of local residents going outside the district for HIV/AIDS services. If health authorities and local authorities perceive an apparently low demand for services within the district, they will not consider it necessary to provide them. For instance, districts in south London may not be aware of the extent of their HIV-positive populations because people are using hospitals north of the river, or Welsh PCTs because of patients using English clinics.

Despite the need for reliable data for use as a basis for planning, many hospitals and local authorities have not had the resources to devote time to data collection, analysis or publication. The quality of epidemiological data is strongly related to the financial incentives available to district health authorities. Thus, if funds are allocated on the basis of HIV reporting, districts will have an incentive to invest in improved reporting and analysis, which in turn will yield more cost effective targeting of services.

More detail on how UK statistics are compiled can be obtained from the Health Protection Agency's website at www.hpa.org.uk. Links to this site and other useful sources of statistical information on HIV can be found at **aidsmap.com**.

High-risk groups and high-risk behaviours

Epidemiologists use the phrase 'risk groups' to refer to people who may be vulnerable to a particular medical or social condition. For example, smokers are a risk group for lung cancer and need specially targeted health education. Or, for example, an outbreak of meningitis in Gloucestershire means that people who live there constitute a risk group with special needs. So the idea of risk groups is useful for identifying the need for particular resources and services.

While everyone is biologically susceptible to infection with HIV if exposed to the virus, this does not mean that everyone is equally at risk from the virus. For example, a gay man having unsafe sex is at much greater risk of becoming infected with HIV than a heterosexual man having unsafe sex. This is for the simple reason that in Britain to date, HIV has disproportionately affected certain definable groups within the population, namely gay men and injecting drug users. In some parts of the country up to one in five gay men may be HIV-positive. Gay men are thus far more likely to encounter sexual partners who have HIV than are most heterosexuals.

To this extent, definable groups within the population may be accurately described as high-risk groups, because they are at the greatest statistical risk of being or becoming HIV-positive through unsafe sex. This recognition should be seen as benign, rather than stigmatising or hostile, since it allows priorities in HIV education and care service provision to be established. In a world of limited resources, it makes sense that resources are targeted to the areas of greatest need.

Unfortunately, this benign concept has been misused throughout the epidemic. The identification of gay men and injecting drug users as high-risk groups in the early 1980s did not result in education and care services being targeted to them; indeed, it was left largely to underfunded voluntary groups to 'look after their own'. Instead, members of the high-risk groups were falsely believed to be a risk to others, rather than to be at increased risk themselves. Gay men and drug users were consequently targeted with hysterical blame, prejudice and discrimination.

The misunderstanding of 'high-risk groups' also contributed to the idea of bridging groups, and the related idea that HIV spreads from gay men through bisexual men and hence to women and thus the general public.

Because of these phenomena, AIDS educators in the 1980s went to considerable lengths to discourage the use of the high risk group terminology. But now, with the advantage of hindsight, it is clear that the rejection of the concept may have done more harm than good.

AIDS education which stressed that everyone was potentially at risk from HIV has been widely misunderstood as meaning that everyone is equally at risk. Consequently, HIV prevention work in the 1980s was generally characterised by vague and untargeted campaigns for the 'general population', and initiatives focusing on those most at risk were almost entirely neglected.

The harmful consequences have been twofold. First, non-drug-using heterosexuals have realised that they are not at such great risk of HIV infection as many campaigns indicated, and appear now to distrust any AIDS education that is directed to them. Secondly, safer sex campaigns for gay men have been neglected. This is likely to be one of the reasons why increases in unsafe sex and in new HIV infections have been reported among gay men since the late 1980s.

In the UK, the bridge communities of bisexual men and injection drug users have failed to have a great impact on the spread of HIV into the general population through heterosexual sex.

In 1990 2.6% of the total diagnosed with HIV in the UK, 12.3% of diagnosed heterosexuals, and approximately 40% of heterosexuals who had acquired their HIV in the UK, were heterosexuals who had acquired HIV from an injecting drug user or (known) bisexual man. By 2004 that proportion had gone down to 0.5% of total infections, 0.9% of heterosexual infections, and no more than 7% of infections acquired by heterosexuals within the UK.

While 'bridges' between risk groups may be important in other situations (for instance, between married men who have sex with men and their wives in certain developing countries), in the UK it appears that there are discrete epidemics within each risk group.

Reference

Anderson R. Trends in HIV incidence and prevalence: natural course of the epidemic or results of behavioural change? UNAIDS, 1999. See
http://www.emro.who.int/asd/backgrounddocuments/uae03/surv/trends%20in%20HIV%20incidence%20and%20prevalence.pdf

An overview of the UK epidemic

UK AIDS and HIV current figures

The most up-to-date figures are made available in the quarterly AIDS reports of the Health Protection Agency (HPA - 020 8200 6868). To view the latest statistics, visit the *Links* section on our website aidsmap.com and select *Statistics*.

Where not otherwise referenced, all the data in this section have come from the HPA website at http://www.hpa.org.uk/.

Since the beginning of AIDS reporting in 1982 to the end of December 2006, 84,730 reports of HIV infection have been recorded in the UK. This represents a 16% increase since the figures were last summarised by the AIDS Reference Manual in June 2005.

Of these, 22,745 (27%) were diagnosed with AIDS (at the time of testing or subsequently). 17,329 of those diagnosed with HIV have died - of any cause - so it can immediately be seen that there are far more people living with HIV in the UK today than have died from it.

This would imply a maximum figure of about 67,000 people diagnosed with HIV currently living in the UK, though this is likely to be an overestimate as included in the total there will be some reports of individuals who have left the country, and unrecognisable multiple reports of others.

The SOPHID data (see below) report that up to the end of December *2005* - a year earlier -47,025 individuals accessed HIV-related care in the UK. Add in 5505 so far notified in 2006 - and figures will rise as late reports come in - and the total will reach about 54,000. It is estimated that approximately one-third of people living with HIV in the UK remain undiagnosed, implying that the true total of the HIV-positive population is probably at least 75,000, giving a national prevalence of 0.12%. On other words about one in every 475 Britons has HIV - though for some age groups this proportion is far higher. The prevalence for people in their 40s is about 0.4%, or one in 250.

As we said above, so far for 2006, 5,505 new HIV diagnoses have been made. This is expected to rise further once late reports have been received. For instance, when the AIDS Reference Manual reported in December 2002, the total stood at 4,204, but another 2,024 cases have now been added to the total for this year as late reports came in.

The annual total of new diagnoses has risen each year from 1994 to 2005, with the annual figure trebling over that time from over 2,500 to over 7,500. It looks possible that for the first time in over a decade the total for 2006 may be slightly lower. Even if it isn't, since 2003 the steep rate of increase in diagnoses seen in the early 2000s has slowed considerably, despite more people coming forward for tests. This appears to be accounted for by a fall in heterosexual infections, driven largely by lower immigration figures from sub-Saharan Africa.

Infections in gay men remained flat during the 1990s at around 1400-1500 infections a year, but since a low point in 1998 have increased slowly and so far for 2005 have totalled 2,404, with more expected to be added as late reports come in.

This 75% increase in the annual total of diagnoses for gay men since 1998 appears largely to be driven by increased rates of testing. Incidence in this group (which comprises 75% of all people who acquire HIV within the UK) has varied between about 3% and 4% a year since 1995 with little sign either of increase or decline.

The interval between HIV infection, AIDS being diagnosed or death occurring, and the event concerned being reported to the surveillance system can be considerable. This means that all totals based on the year of an event are subject to revision as

further reports are received, and that numbers, particularly for recent years, are likely to rise as further reports are received.

In the year 2006 there had so far been:

- 1685 new diagnoses reported as a result of sex between men (38% of those with a known source).

- 2492 new diagnoses reported as a result of sex between men and women (58%), of which 63% were in women.

- 108 new diagnoses reported as a result of injecting drug use (2.5%).

- 81 (1.8%) new diagnoses reported as a result of mother-to-child transmission.

- 25 (0.57%) new diagnoses reported as a result of blood/tissue products.

- And another 1114 infections whose source remained undetermined. These undetermined diagnoses are not expected to change the percentages of infections attributable to different risks by much, as there is no evidence that infections from one group get reported any later than others.

Although more heterosexuals than gay men are being diagnosed, the relative proportions are changing. The last time this chapter was updated, figures to the end of December 2004 indicated that 31% of diagnoses had been in gay men and 65% had been in heterosexuals.

The UK: a unique epidemic?

The UK remains a low-prevalence country for HIV, with about one in 500 of the adult population infected compared with (for example) one in about 160 in the USA. However the *growth* in HIV diagnoses in the early 2000s was almost uniquely steep. HIV incidence doubled in the four years between 1998 and 2002, and incidence in heterosexuals trebled during the same period. For comparison, it was thought newsworthy when it was announced recently that HIV prevalence in Japan had doubled in the eleven years between 1991 and 2002.

The growth in the UK epidemic has been fuelled largely, though not entirely, by HIV diagnoses among immigrants from sub-Saharan Africa. Although 56% of HIV diagnoses were among heterosexuals in 2004, only 16% of these heterosexuals acquired HIV within the UK. The rest were acquired abroad, overwhelmingly (87%) in Africa. The position in gay men is exactly the reverse: the HPA estimate that 16% of gay men acquired their HIV infection *outside* the UK.

Furthermore, of the 16% of home-grown heterosexual infections, in about 75% of cases the infecting partner acquired their infection outside the EU. However the proportion of heterosexual cases that were acquired in the UK has increased from 11% to 16% in the last two years. As relatively fewer HIV-positive immigrants arrive from high-prevalence countries, and as those who stay here develop relationships here, we may see a continued growth of heterosexual transmission in the UK - though there are epidemiological reasons why it is unlikely ever to reach the level of ongoing transmission seen amongst gay men.

Nearly half - 47% - of all new HIV cases in the UK in 2004 were among people of Black African ethnicity (to use the HPA's term), which would include some African gay men and Africans who acquired HIV within the UK.

The transformation of the UK's epidemic can be seen in the following two graphs. The first includes all risk groups (with heterosexuals divided into men and women) and the total of infections. The second compares the three major risk groups (heterosexuals, gay men and Africans). Africans, as pointed out above, would include Africans from all risk groups, but it can be seen how the growth in African infections echoes the heterosexual curve. (see below)

drug users have declined as a proportion of newly-diagnosed HIV-positive individuals in Scotland from 77% prior to 1986 to 3% in 2002.

However here are early signs that HIV infections might be increasing amongst drug users, as 1.7% of new diagnoses in 2004 were among this group but 2.5% in 2006.

Injecting drug users make up 37% of all diagnosed HIV-positive individuals in Scotland, compared with 6% across the rest of the UK.

Two epidemics

What we see above is not one HIV epidemic, but two: one a long-standing epidemic concentrated almost entirely among gay men and largely acquired in the UK; the other a fringe or penumbra of the HIV pandemic in sub-Saharan Africa, consisting of HIV cases caught in the most high-prevalence countries of the world but diagnosed here.

Is this a unique situation? There are historical reasons why the UK should be particularly affected by HIV in Africa: it is estimated that 54% of the world's people with HIV live in African countries within the British Commonwealth and the eight highest-prevalence counties in the world happen to be ex-British colonies (in order of prevalence, Swaziland, Botswana, Lesotho, Zimbabwe, South Africa, Namibia, Zambia and Malawi). But other countries have colonial ties with Africa too.

In Belgium HIV diagnoses went up by 42% between 1997 and 2002 and it is estimated that 60% of cases in 2002 were among people from sub-Saharan Africa. In Switzerland diagnoses rose by 25% between 2001 and 2003, and of the 42% of diagnoses that were among heterosexuals, 65% were in people from sub-Saharan Africa. Other western European countries have seen similar increases.

However it is only Ireland and the Scandinavian countries that have seen heterosexual cases from Africa come to dominate in the same way they have done in the UK. Ireland saw HIV diagnoses jump 33% in once year between 2002 and 2003; 63% of cases in 2002 were among heterosexuals and of those 77% were acquired in Africa, figures very similar to the UK. And in Sweden it is estimated that two-thirds of cases in the last two years have come from people infected in the global epidemic (to quote the *UNAIDS* fact sheet on the country), with only 21% of cases among gay Swedes. However the Scandinavian countries continue to have very low prevalence, about half that of the UK.

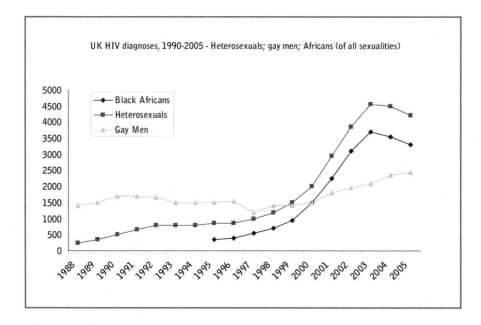

Source: HPA

To the end of December 2006, 4,582 injecting drug users have been reported to be HIV-positive in the UK. 70% are men (3,185 men, 1,397 women). This represents around 5.4% of the total reported HIV infections in the UK.

The majority (40%) of all HIV diagnoses among injecting drug users have been in London, and the overwhelming majority of the remainder have been diagnosed in Scotland (32%). Injecting

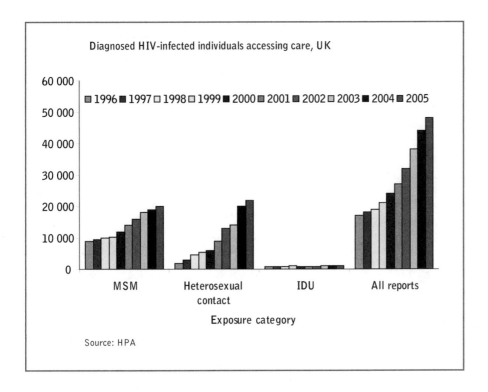

Diagnosed HIV-infected individuals accessing care, UK

■ 1996 ■ 1997 □ 1998 □ 1999 ■ 2000 ■ 2001 ■ 2002 □ 2003 ■ 2004 ■ 2005

Exposure category

Source: HPA

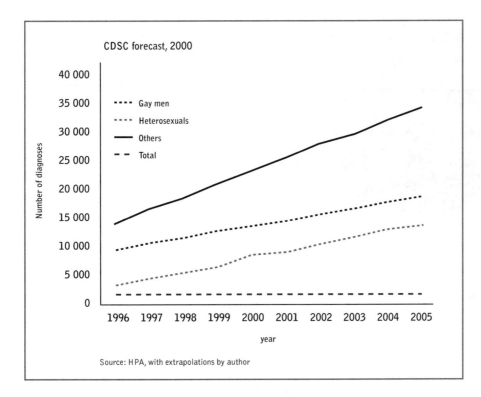

CDSC forecast, 2000

- - - - Gay men

- - - - Heterosexuals

——— Others

– – Total

Number of diagnoses

year

Source: HPA, with extrapolations by author

Multiply this figure by the estimated HIV prevalence in gay men and you get a figure substantially in excess of those seeking HIV care.

However NATSAL's figures are usually regarded as conservative because people do not tend to tell the whole truth to sex researchers and it may also underestimate the HIV incidence and prevalence among gay men who frequent the commercial gay scene but do not attend GUM clinics.

Whatever the exact figures, it is clear that the upward curve in prevalence was not foreseen. In 2000, the CDSC (forerunner to the HPA) issued its own figures for prevalence up to 2000 and the estimated increase up to 2005, and this forecast makes an interesting contrast with what actually happened. The estimated totals seen for care were simple linear extrapolations of what had already been happening. The 'actual total' line comprises the actual SOPHID data from 1996-2005. The sudden rate of increase in diagnoses from 2001 onwards is obvious (see CDSC forecast 2000, left).

The way that heterosexual infections were about to outstrip gay ones was completely unforeseen, and shows how, even in the developed world, political and economic turmoil can suddenly transform the shape of epidemics. In 2003, for instance, the biggest single nationality among newly-diagnosed people (larger than UK nationals) was Zimbabweans, many seeking asylum from the Mugabe regime.

This tripling of prevalence since highly active antiretroviral treatment (HAART) became available has in turn had a knock-on effect on HIV services and created considerable political turmoil and policy changes, such as the withdrawal, from April 2004, of entitlement to NHS HIV treatment to anyone who could show they had been in the UK more than twelve months. These changes are documented elsewhere in this Manual, under **African communities in the UK.**

This also led to a situation where, in 2003, gay men became for the first time less than half the total of those living with HIV in the UK they were 51% of the total in 2002 and 45% in 2003.

The overlap of gay men and ethnicity

Of course, we are not seeing two *completely* separate infections. Gay men exist in Africa and the rest of the developing world too.

The UK's sudden increase in HIV diagnoses has led to a doubling of prevalence since 2000. The first chart above is based upon the SOPHID data and includes only those diagnosed and seeking care in the relevant year. It may therefore miss some people that get diagnosed and then do not see a clinic for more than a year. But it also excludes the estimated 34% of people with HIV who don't know they have it.

The HPA's estimate for the number of undiagnosed people is based in part on an estimate of the number of sexually active gay men culled from the 2000 National Survey of Sexual Attitudes and Lifestyles (NATSAL). This found that 2.8% of UK men had had sexual experience with another man in the last five years.

They may both be a source of HIV infections and be vulnerable to infection by UK gay men.

The HPA has hitherto only collected the likely country of infection data for heterosexuals, though it plans from next year to collect these figures for gay men too. In gay men, country of possible infection, country of birth, and STD clinic attendance have only been collected through clinician reporting, and so are not available for diagnoses.

What we do know about the country of infection and ethnicity of gay men is presented here:

- The UK was the country of probable infection for 83% of newly-diagnosed gay men, with 7% from the rest of Europe, and between 3% and 1% from other continents.

- Nine per cent of HIV-infected black and ethic minority people seen for care in 2005 were gay men/MSM.

- Seventy-two per cent of newly diagnosed gay and bisexual men were born in the UK, 14% in other parts of Europe, and between 5 and 2% born in other continents.

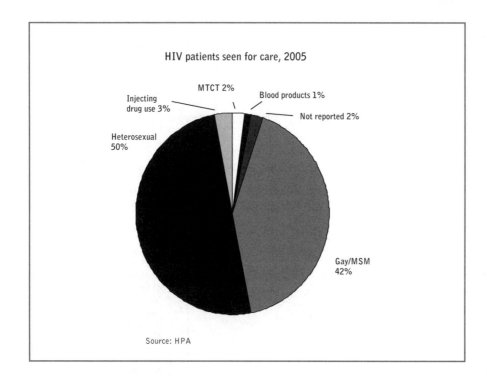

HIV patients seen for care, 2005

Source: HPA

- We can see from this that when it comes to gay men the UK is more likely to be the place where gay men catch HIV than where they are born: when gay men come to the UK they are usually coming from a lower-risk environment to a higher-risk one, the opposite of the situation for most heterosexuals.

- The majority of men (87%) were white, 6% 'other' or mixed, 3% blackCaribbean, 2% black African, 1% black 'other', and 1% Asian.

Prevalent diagnosed HIV infections

Information on prevalent diagnosed HIV infections is provided by the survey of prevalent diagnosed HIV infections (SOPHID) in England, Wales, and Northern Ireland, and CD4 monitoring in Scotland.

In 2005, the latest year with full figures available, 47,025 individuals were receiving care of which at least 31,082 (66%) were receiving antiretroviral therapy.

The proportion of newly diagnosed infections attributed to heterosexual contact has increased to 65% of the total reported in 2004, and heterosexuals accounted for the majority of the prevalent diagnosed caseload for the first time in 2003 (see chart, opposite).

The decline of AIDS

There has been a marked fall in the number of new AIDS diagnoses amongst people who have been aware of their HIV status for some time, suggesting that anti-HIV therapy is having an impact on disease progression. An increasing proportion of new AIDS diagnoses are occurring in people who had never been tested or had only been diagnosed with HIV less than three months before the onset of an AIDS-related illness. For them, their HIV diagnosis probably comes too late for anti-HIV therapy to delay the onset of AIDS (see chart next page).

In the UK, AIDS diagnoses have fallen from a high of 1,851 in 1994 to 777 cases diagnosed in 2004. In the period 1994-2001 new AIDS diagnoses fell in all regions of the UK. Deaths due to AIDS fell from 1531 in 1994 to 231 in 1999, and have since then stayed at more or less this level, while death from other causes has increased slightly, from 169 in 1994 to 242 in 2004. This was the first year that more deaths in people diagnosed with AIDS were due to non-AIDS-defining illnesses than AIDS itself.

The SOPHID survey says that in 2005 44% of those seen for HIV care in the UK were asymptomatic, 29% had 'pre-AIDS' symptoms and 23% has AIDS-defining symptoms, though this tells us nothing about how long people remained ill. There were 270 AIDS-related deaths amongst the patient population in 2005; this represent 0.6% or one in 166 of those seen for care.

Although there is no evidence that Africans in the UK have a shorter life expectancy once they have been diagnosed with AIDS (compared with other groups of people with AIDS), the rate of new AIDS diagnoses amongst African people has hardly fallen at all. Every year Africans diagnosed with AIDS form a larger proportion of UK AIDS cases, and whilst new AIDS diagnoses fell 35% amongst gay men in 1997, they fell by only 6% amongst Africans.

London loses some of its dominance

Since the beginning of the HIV epidemic London has been the epicentre of HIV in the UK, with 56% of all diagnoses made in the Greater London area and another 9% in the south-east. However, though London and the south-east remain dominant, they are much less so than previously. In 2004 41% of HIV diagnoses were made in London and an additional 12% in the south-east (see second chart opposite).

The proportion of all new HIV diagnoses that were made in London has declined steadily: from 64% in 1990 and 60% in 2000 to 53% in 2002 and 41% in 2004. In the same time period the proportion of all new HIV diagnoses made in the south-east has risen from 7.5% to 12% and in the Eastern region the proportion has increased from 2% to 8%. The North West region has the third largest number of HIV diagnoses in the UK after London and the south-east, accounting for 8.5% of all new diagnoses in 2004.

When it comes to patients seen for care, the graphic overleaf from HPA eloquently illustrates the extent to which HIV has spread from two epicentres in London and Edinburgh. The area with the second-highest number of patients after London remains the north-west of England. However the areas that have seen the steepest *increases* in the number of patients are the north-east, and the east and west Midlands.

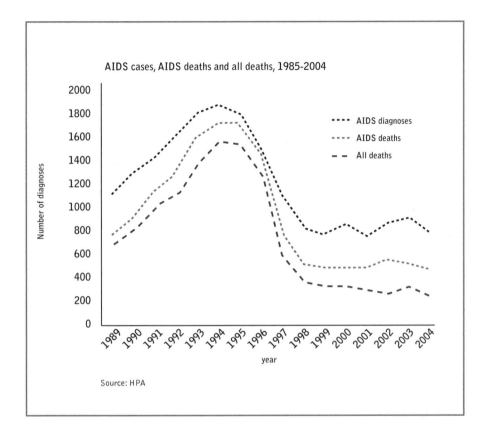

AIDS cases, AIDS deaths and all deaths, 1985-2004

····· AIDS diagnoses
····· AIDS deaths
— — All deaths

Number of diagnoses

year

Source: HPA

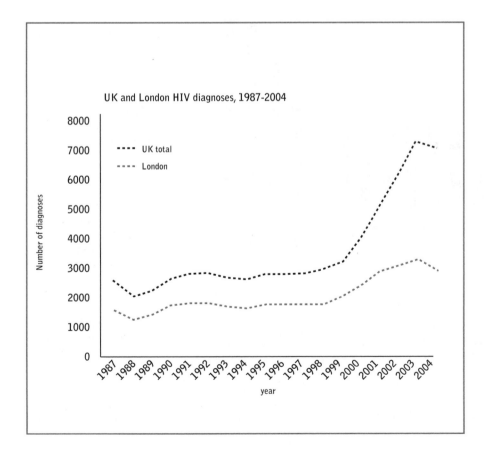

UK and London HIV diagnoses, 1987-2004

····· UK total
····· London

Number of diagnoses

year

The north-west, south-west and Kent and Sussex areas have the highest proportion of patients who are gay men (66-70%): this is largely accounted for by the large gay communities in Manchester, Bournemouth and Brighton. The east and west midlands, east Anglia and Yorkshire all have a much lower proportion of their patient population as gay men (about 40%); conversely about 55% are Africans. Much of this increase in the population of Africans with HIV outside London is attributed to the Home Office's policy of dispersal of asylum seekers outside London, though it is also partly due to African immigrants choosing to move to areas where house prices and rents are cheaper.

Scotland has seen an increase in its HIV diagnoses over the same period, with the large rise that started in the rest of the UK in 2000 starting in 2002 and so far showing no signs of stopping, with the largest year-on-year increase recorded so far between 2003 and 2004. So far there have been 28% more cases of HIV recorded in 2004 than the previous year, and late reports will probably take this increase up to 35% or more. There were already twice as many new cases of HIV recorded in 2004 as in 2001.
(see charts next page)

The perils of late diagnosis

The British HIV Association recommends that anti-HIV treatment should start before the CD4 count has fallen below 200, if the patient is ready for the commitment of treatment.

Around 33% of people who test positive every year in the UK already have CD4 counts below 200, the level at which immediate prophylaxis against *Pneumocystis* pneumonia is recommended, and the AIDS-defining limit in the USA.

Among gay men, the average CD4 count when diagnosed HIV-positive has remained

Rates of adults accessing HIV care by residence

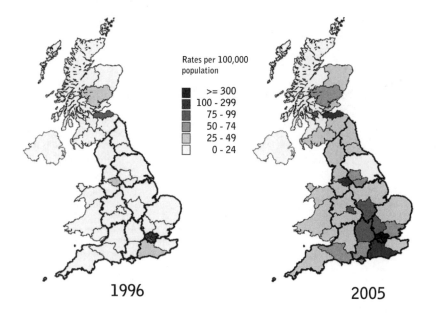

Rates per 100,000 population

■	>= 300
■	100 - 299
■	75 - 99
■	50 - 74
■	25 - 49
□	0 - 24

1996

2005

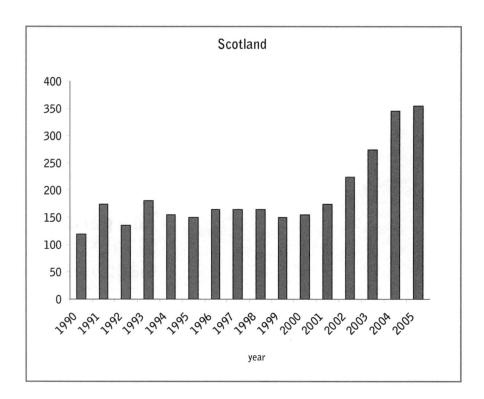

Scotland

year

Amongst those who have contracted HIV through injecting drug use, the average CD4 count at diagnosis is 315 cells. The proportion with CD4 counts under 200 at diagnosis was 37% in 2002.

In contrast, heterosexuals (the majority of whom are African) are being diagnosed with HIV at much lower median CD4 counts (around 200 to 260), with African men being diagnosed at an extremely late stage of infection (200 cells). Forty per cent of female heterosexuals and 49% of male heterosexuals (70% of whom are African) were diagnosed when their immune systems were already severely immunosuppressed.

Amongst Africans in the UK, fewer than 25% know their HIV status at least two months before developing an AIDS-defining illness. An increasing proportion of these 'short interval' AIDS diagnoses amongst heterosexuals are cases of tuberculosis, which may occur at higher CD4 counts than other opportunistic infections (in other words, earlier in the course of HIV infection).

A survey from north London's Royal Free Hospital HIV clinic found that half of all cases of AIDS diagnoses at the clinic occurred in the 15% of patients who did not come for an HIV test till their CD4 count was dangerously low (under 50).

Altogether 110 patients out of the 719 treated at the Royal Free between January 1996 (when combination therapy became available) and December 2002 were in this group of late testers.

Late diagnosis among those at low risk of infection

While most late HIV diagnoses in England, Wales and Northern Ireland are currently seen in black African heterosexuals, late diagnosis is also a problem for a smaller number of

almost constant since 1990, at around 350, but the proportion whose CD4 count was below 200 at diagnosis declined steadily, from 38% in 1993 to 25.4% in 2002. However the average CD4 count in those testing late was a life-threatening 60, compared with an average figure of 450 in the early testers, and the proportion of all deaths in gay men with HIV that happened in the year after diagnosis went up, from 8% of all deaths in 1996 to 27.5% in 2001.

mainly UK nationals who may have low risk for HIV, may not be aware of their partners' risks or may not acknowledge their own high risk of infection.

Newly-diagnosed and reported HIV infections in the UK are followed up if their exposure route requires clarification. In-depth confidential interviews are conducted if both the clinician and patient agree. In many cases HIV diagnosis is only made after frequent attendances with a range of symptoms to primary care physicians (GPs).

During 2001, the Communicable Disease Surveillance Centre (now the HPA) interviewed 265 people (155 men and 110 women) who had been diagnosed with HIV despite fitting into none of the known risk groups.

More than half of these individuals had not been diagnosed till the appearance of AIDS-related symptoms, and 60% had been infected in the UK or a low-prevalence country.

Of these 84 had been reported with an undetermined risk for acquiring HIV infection, 134 with a heterosexual risk, but without additional information and 47 were believed to have acquired their infection in the UK from partners not known to have a risk factor for HIV infection. After interview, 20% of the group turned out to have had high-risk sex abroad, but in low-prevalence countries, and 16% had had sex with a 'high risk' partner, generally a bisexual man.

Just under one quarter (23% or 62 individuals) were diagnosed because of the identification of an HIV-positive child or partner. In total 14% (37) were diagnosed because they were screened as a blood donor, at an antenatal or STI clinic, for insurance or for a visa. 8% (21) were tested of their own volition.

The majority of individuals reported frequent visits to their GP with a range of health concerns prior to diagnosis. For 213 of those interviewed, no risk factors for HIV were identified other than heterosexual contact, the majority of which occurred in the UK with partners believed not to be at any risk of HIV infection. Of the individuals diagnosed late (after the appearance of HIV-related symptoms, which were often misdiagnosed), 71% were men, compared with 42% of individuals diagnosed before symptoms appeared.

Almost all did not perceive themselves to be at risk of HIV infection and over half claimed little knowledge of HIV. A large proportion had been in a relationship for five years or more and this may have reinforced their sense that HIV was not of concern to them.

All those diagnosed late due to illness stated that no partners had contacted them to inform them of their possible HIV risk. In response to their own diagnosis, almost one third (of the 49 individuals asked) chose not to inform any of their partners. It is likely that some of the partners of those diagnosed late will also themselves be diagnosed late, as they will not perceive themselves to be at risk of HIV infection.

Primary care physicians should be encouraged to consider HIV testing as a possibility when patients "without risk" for HIV infection present with symptoms not responding to established treatments. The fact that these individuals presented to their GP on multiple occasions is particularly worrisome in light of Government plans to devolve some responsibility for HIV testing to primary care.

Undiagnosed HIV infections

About one-third of people in the UK with HIV are thought to be unaware of their infection. This undiagnosed proportion varies both between and within risk groups.

The HPA estimates that about 32% of people with HIV in the UK are undiagnosed: this figure was revised upwards from 26% in 2005 when it was realised that the methodology the HPA had used led to unreliable estimates.

Of the undiagnosed adults about 45% were gay men/MSM, about 27% were heterosexual women, about 25% were heterosexual men and about 2.4% were IDUs. Heterosexual women are less likely to be undiagnosed than either gay or straight men: this is largely due to antenatal screening.

The proportion of undiagnosed infections also varies within risk groups. The annual HIV Prevalence and Sexual Behaviour Survey of gay men on the commercial scene in London, Manchester and

Brighton, which gave anonymous saliva HIV tests to participants, found in 2003 that 33% of those with HIV were unaware of their infection and no less than 44% in London.

In contrast, the HPA found that in 2005 3.2% of gay men nationally and 3.8% in London attending GUM clinics had undiagnosed HIV infection - suggesting that it may be people without STI symptoms, who think they have not been at risk, or who simply are scared to be tested that form the majority of the undiagnosed.

References

Gilbart VL. Late diagnosis of HIV infection amongst individuals with low, unrecognised or unacknowledged risks in England, Wales and Northern Ireland. abstract WePeC6078 Fourteenth World AIDS conference.

Gupta SW et al. CD4 cell counts in adults with newly diagnosed HIV infection: results of surveillance in England and Wales, 1990-1998. AIDS 14: 853-861, 2000.

More on specific risk groups: gay men

Although HIV *diagnoses* in gay men have increased every year since 1999, it is impossible to say as yet whether HIV *incidence* - the rate of new infection - is increasing. All we can say is that incidence appears not to be decreasing. The majority of the increase in diagnoses is accounted for by an increase in the number of gay men coming forward for testing and the frequency with which they test. In short, the increase in diagnosis may be as much good news (more infections detected) as it may be bad news (more infections per se).

However testing rates amongst gay men have not increased as fast as testing rates amongst heterosexuals and in the last two years there is some evidence of a levelling-off of testing. The HPA graphics on the right depict the proportion of people attending GUM clinics that accepted the offer of an HIV test, and the proportion of those who went away with their HIV infection undiagnosed. It appears that there may be a 'hard core' of 20% or so of gay men (and possibly heterosexuals) who do not wish to test, and that about 40% of the 3.2% of gay male GUM clinic attendees who had previously undiagnosed HIV infection go away from GUM checkups with their HIV still undiagnosed, or about 1.4% of all gay men who have STD checkups.

However this figure may be misleading. While there may be a hard core of 'won't testers', anecdotally not all gay men who are already aware of their HIV infection choose to declare it when they have an STD checkup, and some choose to go to a different GUM clinic for their STD checkups than for their HIV care. This may be to avoid disclosing that they have had unprotected sex.

So has the rate of new infections increased? Incidence is quite difficult to measure because of the difficulty of establishing the exact date of infection. Incidence was worked out by taking the number of infections in GUM clinic attendees recorded by the UAPMP and then performing a second 'detuned' assay on a random selection of them. A detuned assay has a deliberately lower sensitivity to antibodies, and so fails to pick up on infections less than six months old (because these have lower antibody titres). It is important to emphasise that this is a relatively small sample and the results of the chart below do not reach statistical significance. However if they reflect the population of gay GUM clinic attendees at large, then during the last two years about 3-4% of gay men in London and about 2% outside London became infected with HIV. For comparison, this represents a considerably greater incidence than the estimated 1.2% a year among gay men in San Francisco discovered by similar means but less than half of the 8% incidence found in Baltimore.

So large increases in sexually transmitted infections among gay men in recent years have only so far appeared to translate into a steady state, or at most, a modest increase in HIV infections. It

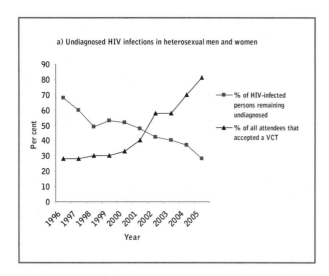

a) Undiagnosed HIV infections in heterosexual men and women

- % of HIV-infected persons remaining undiagnosed
- % of all attendees that accepted a VCT

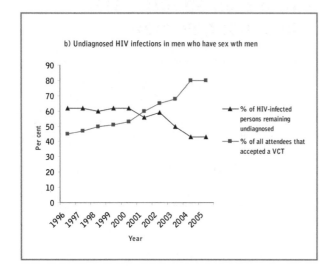

b) Undiagnosed HIV infections in men who have sex wth men

- % of HIV-infected persons remaining undiagnosed
- % of all attendees that accepted a VCT

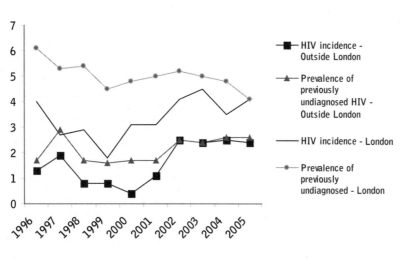

Prevalence of previously undiagnosed HIV infection and estimated HIV incidence among MSM attending GUM clinics

- HIV incidence - Outside London
- Prevalence of previously undiagnosed HIV - Outside London
- HIV incidence - London
- Prevalence of previously undiagnosed - London

Source: HPA

is also worth pointing out that this relatively slow increase occurs against the background of a constantly increasing proportion of gay men in the population who have HIV. This may be indicative that gay men in the UK are increasingly adopting behaviours like serosorting (see **HIV prevention: D is for disclosure, serosorting and negotiated safety**).

Rates of prevalent diagnosed HIV infection acquired through sex between men have been calculated using the numbers of males aged from 15 to 49 years for each region/country of the UK, with the highest rates seen in the London Region (351 per 100,000), followed by the South East Region (65 per 100,000) and the North West Region (64 per 100,000).

The annual London Gay Men's Sexual Health Survey (LGMSHS), which asks over 8,000 gay men in community venues about their sexual behaviour and asks them to provide an anonymous saliva sample to test for HIV prevalence, found an overall HIV prevalence in London of 10.9% when its findings were last published in a journal (in 2004, from a series of surveys ending in 2000).

The London Gay Men's Sexual Health Survey has now been expanded to include Brighton and Manchester. In March 2005 the lead researcher Julie Dodds told the 2005 8th CHAPS gay men's prevention conference in Bristol that the most recent survey for which figures had been compiled (2002) found HIV prevalence among gay men in Brighton of 14%, London of 12.5%, and in Manchester of about 8%. The lower prevalence in Manchester was largely due to the fact that this group was, on average, younger. Results of the 2005 survey, reported in 2007, showed little difference in self-reported HIV status.

HIV prevalence is heavily skewed by age in the gay population, with the 2000 survey finding that only 1.6% of under-25s had HIV. This rose to a peak of 19.7% among men aged 35-40 and was lower in men above 40. This almost certainly reflects the peak incidence of HIV in gay men around 1990; peak prevalence in 2005 would probably be in the 40-45 age range. However it also attests to the fact that the more sex you have had, the more likely you are to have HIV, and older men are more likely to have it simply through the accumulation of sexual exposures.

It also found that HIV prevalence was skewed by ethnicity (with non-whites 50% more likely to have HIV) and education (men who left school at 16 had an 18% prevalence).

Cohort studies

It is very important to realise that the UAPMP programme only tracks the testing behaviour and results of gay men who attend GUM clinics. It is completely unable to do so for gay men who don't have STD checkups - perhaps because they feel at less risk. As for the The London Gay Men's Sexual Health Survey, this also tracks a subset of gay men, namely those who frequent the commercial gay scene in three cities, and who therefore might be expected to have higher-than-average rates of HIV.

The only UK study which has been able to track a cohort of gay and bisexual men is *The National Gay Men's Sex Survey*, carried out by Sigma Research.

This also cannot be an objective survey of the gay male population of the UK, as like virtually any imaginable gay survey it depends on respondents who self-select as gay. However its respondents are probably more diverse than GUM clinic attendees or gay venue patrons.

Sigma recruit their respondents in three ways: 1) Via a booklet questionnaire picked up at community venues 2) via an online survey accessed via a number of gay websites and 3) up until 2004, via clipboard questionnaires at gay festivals.

Reports from this cohort may be able to offer a useful counterbalance to trends in voluntary HIV test reporting as a way of demonstrating trends in the incidence of HIV infections amongst gay and bisexual men, but neither can claim to capture an objective sample of gay men adjusted for confounding factors like age and sexual activity.

Both HIV prevalence and HIV testing history among the SIGMA cohort have remained remarkably similar in the nice years from 1997 to 2005, with absolutely no apparent increase in the number of testing and very little in the number with HIV (see chart below).

How do we reconcile an increase in the annual number of diagnoses (according to the HPA) with no significant increase in the proportion of testers who report they are positive (according to Sigma)? There has been a decrease in the number of men who have tested who refused to disclose their status to the Gay Men's Sex Survey over this time, so this cannot be the explanation.

In their 2005 survey Sigma quote a paper (Dougan et al.) which hazards four explanations:

- the rate at which men become infected (HIV incidence) has increased;

- an increase in the number of men with HIV moving to the UK from abroad;

- fewer diagnoses are going unreported (ie. improved reporting);

- changes in the uptake of HIV testing are reducing the number of men with undiagnosed infection and reducing the average length of time between infection and diagnosis.

The second possibility seems not to be the case, in fact the proportion who report their infection was acquired abroad has declined during this time, from 25% to 16%.

However the composition of the Sigma cohort has changed over time. In recent years a higher proportion of respondents have come from the online part of the survey, relatively fewer from booklet questionnaires picked up at community venues, and the 'festival' section of the survey was dropped altogether for 2005 because it was labour-intensive. Online respondents have consistently tended to be younger and to have tested less often for HIV than respondents via booklets and festival questionnaires, and it is at least possible that the apparent lack of change in HIV prevalence Sigma found may be confounded by a change in the demographics of the respondents, due to the lower prevalence identified in younger men and higher prevalence in older men; the average age at diagnosis has also increased during this time, though amongst gay men not very significantly, from 32 to 34 (greater increases in the median age at diagnosis were seen for heterosexuals, especially women, and IDUs).

During this period, according to the UAPMP, incidence among gay men over 35 did appear to increase, however. For older men it was under 2% a year between 1997 and 2001 but then increased to 4-5% between 2002 and 2004.

Conversely the one group amongst whom diagnoses did not increase was younger gay men in London (under 35) - even though more got tested for HIV, and rates of STIs went up amongst them.

Probably the best we can say at present, then, is that HIV incidence amongst gay men in the UK is holding steady at present at a rate of about 3% a year, but that the average age at which gay men acquire HIV has somewhat increased.

Reference

Dodds JP. *Increasing risk behaviour and high levels of undiagnosed HIV infection in a community sample of homosexual men.* Sex Transm Infect 80: 236-240, 2004.

Dougan S, Elford J, Chadborn T et al. *Does the recent increase in HIV diagnoses among men who have sex with men in the United Kingdom reflect a rise in HIV incidence or increased uptake of HIV testing?* Sexually Transmitted Infections, online publication, sti.2006.021428v2. November 2006.

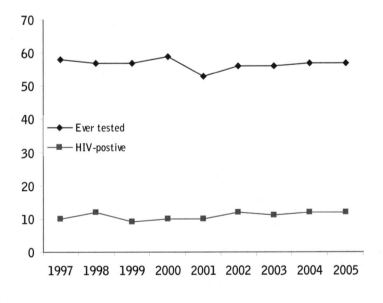

Gay Men's sex Surveys 1997-2005: proportion testing for HIV and proportion of testers HIV-positive

- Ever tested
- HIV-postive

Source: Sigma Research

HIV infection acquired through sex between men and women

Since 1999 the number of reports of new diagnoses of infections attributed to heterosexual sex has outnumbered other routes of infection and is now the major source of new infections. By the end of June 2005 there had been a total of 68,712 infected individuals reported in the UK. 36,671 (53%) of these were infected heterosexually.

The majority of the heterosexual HIV infections diagnosed in the UK are acquired abroad by people HIV-infected before moving to the UK, though HIV infection is also contracted heterosexually by individuals from the UK working or travelling abroad.

Of all diagnoses of heterosexually acquired infections made during 2004, 70% were attributed to infection in Africa. However, the numbers of UK diagnoses of infections heterosexually acquired in Asia and in Latin America/Caribbean has risen in the latter part of the 1990s, while those from North America, Europe, and Australasia have increased more slowly, and decreased relative to the total of infections (see chart below).

Reports received to the end of June 2002 showed that 52% (305) of the total of 590 infections reported as acquired in Asia

risk' (see chart on next page). In 2006 the HPA started breaking down these 'high risk' partners: about two-thirds appear to be partners who acquired HIV through intravenous drug use and about one-third are bisexual men who have sex with men.

HIV transmission within UK

In addition to the sharp rise in HIV diagnoses in people who have acquired their HIV heterosexually outside the UK, there has also been a rise in the number of new diagnoses of HIV infections acquired heterosexually in the UK, from a partner also presumed to have been infected heterosexually.

Most of the rise in diagnoses is attributable to infections acquired through heterosexual contact in the UK, with individuals themselves infected heterosexually outside Europe. Altogether 5.8% of heterosexual infections come into this category, though 6.4% of heterosexual infections in 2004 were of people infected in the UK by partners infected abroad. For 79% of this group (576/731) the partner's infection was attributed to heterosexual contact in sub-Saharan Africa.

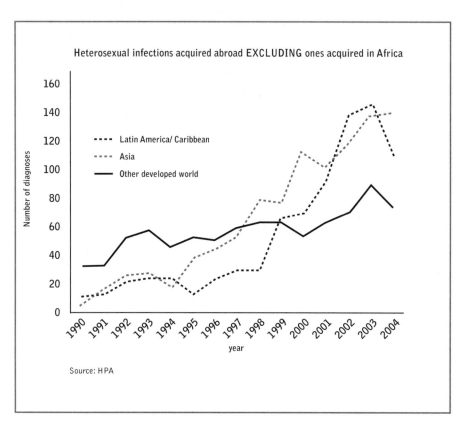

Heterosexual infections acquired abroad EXCLUDING ones acquired in Africa

- - - - Latin America/ Caribbean
- - - - Asia
——— Other developed world

Number of diagnoses

year

Source: HPA

The number of infections recorded where *both* partners acquired their HIV in the UK has increased only slightly and has decreased as a proportion of those infected. It stood at about 70 infections in 2004, or just 1.7% of the heterosexual total for that year, and totals 798 out of 27,902 heterosexual infections recorded, or under 2.9% of the total.

The HPA calculate that of all heterosexual cases of HIV ever recorded where infection appears to have happened within the UK, 50% of infections were acquired from partners who were infected in Africa and 24% were acquired from partners who acquired HIV within the EU (mainly in the UK). The other 26% of partners either acquired their HIV in other parts of the world or their infection source could not be traced.

More women diagnosed than men

More heterosexually acquired infections have been diagnosed in women than in men. By the end of December 2006 the number of heterosexually infected women diagnosed was 21,111 and the number of men was 13,450 (61% women). In 2006, of reports received so far, 926 men and 1566 women (63% women) have been diagnosed.

were associated with Thailand, often affecting individuals visiting that country from the UK for business or tourism. Diagnoses of infections acquired in Latin America/Caribbean increased overall from a cumulative total of 320 at the end of March 2001 to 480 by the end of December 2002.

Bridging communities

During the early years of the epidemic it was thought that groups recognised as being at high risk of HIV infection, such as bisexual men and injecting drug users, would provide a 'bridge' for the virus to cross into the general population through heterosexual sex. In the UK this route does not seem to have had a great impact on the spread of HIV. Annually there have been fewer than 90 new diagnoses of infections acquired in this way throughout the last decade, and the number has been going down, not only as a proportion of the total, but in absolute terms. Overall 4.4% (1229/27,902) of heterosexually infected individuals diagnosed by the end of June 2005 were categorised as infected through contact with a partner classified as 'high

In those infected through contact with members of high-risk groups the number of diagnoses in women is much higher than men. This is because those in the high-risk groups are predominantly male. There are also more females than males among those recorded as heterosexually infected in Africa, and among those infected heterosexually in the UK by a partner infected heterosexually outside Europe. The female predominance overall has been contributed to by an increased uptake of testing as a result of initiatives to improve the rates of maternal antenatal diagnosis. It may also reflect the differing attitudes to healthcare between men and women.

Increase in heterosexuals receiving care

The annual survey of prevalent diagnosed HIV infections (SOPHID) collects information for every patient seen for

HIV-related treatment and care in the previous year. It therefore reflects current prevalence whereas the cumulative reports referred to above also include people who have died and people who may later have left the country. Largely as a result of the increasing numbers of diagnoses of heterosexually acquired HIV, for England and Wales reports to the SOPHID survey of individuals with heterosexually acquired HIV infection receiving care rose from 5,357 in 1999 to 22,320 in 2005 - a fourfold increase.

The focus of the epidemic in the UK is in London and the south-east of England, but the heterosexual epidemic is less concentrated on London than the gay one, possible due to dispersal of asylum seekers. All areas of England and Wales except for London, the north-west and the south-west have more heterosexuals receiving care than gay men (see chart below).

Of those heterosexually infected, 10,289 (47%) lived in the London region - compared with 10,286 (56%) gay men.

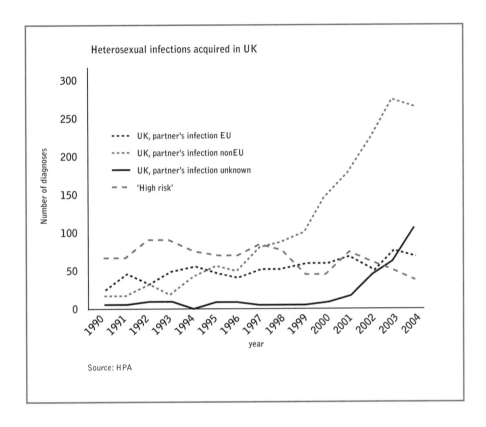

Source: HPA

Seventy per cent of heterosexuals receiving care in 2005 were black African in ethnicity and 18% were white (not necessarily UK white). The other heterosexuals feed into the ethnic categories used by the HPA thus: Caribbean (3.8%), 'Black-other' (2.1%), Indian/Pakistani/Bangladeshi (1.5%), other Asian/oriental (1.5%) and other/mixed (2.5%).

Since 1996 the proportion of heterosexuals seen for care who are black African has increased from 52% to 70% and the proportion that are white has decreased from 37% to 18%, with other ethnic categories essentially remaining unchanged as a proportion of the total, though not in number.

Results from the UAPMP survey of genitourinary clinic attendees in 2003 found that the prevalence of HIV infection among heterosexual GUM clinic attendees was 1.01% in London, compared with 20.7% among gay men and 0.38% outside London (excluding Scotland), and compared with 5.6% in gay men.

Since the UAPMP does not record the ethnicity of the people whose anonymous samples are surveyed, this reflects HIV prevalence in the sexually-active heterosexual population generally. Prevalence among vulnerable groups like African is higher. A survey in 2001 found that among heterosexuals born in sub-Saharan Africa and attending London GUM clinics in 2000/2001, one in 21 men (4.75%) and one in 13 women (7.7%) was HIV-positive, compared to one in 428 men (0.23%) and one in 573 women (0.17%) born in the UK.

Of the heterosexuals with HIV infection, 50% had not had their infection diagnosed previously, with a slightly higher proportion of women than men undiagnosed. This is more than double the proportion of gay men turning up with undiagnosed infections.

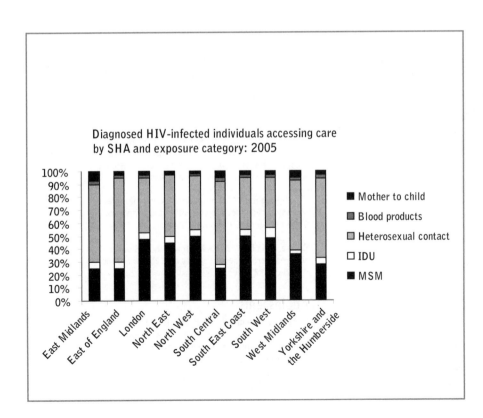

Of these previously undiagnosed GUM clinic attendees, 41% went away from their STI checkup without their HIV infection being diagnosed, compared with 27.5% of gay men.

Thus while gay male GUM clinic attendees are 15 times more likely to have HIV than heterosexual attendees, they are 'only' 7.5 times more likely to have undiagnosed infections, and 'only' five times more likely to have infections that remain undiagnosed after a GUM clinic visit.

Subtype B gets less common
The HPA reports of where infection was acquired are subject to some uncertainty since it is often the patient or clinician's best guess as to where they were infected that gets recorded on the monitoring form.

One independent indicator that heterosexuals in the UK are acquiring HIV that at least originated in Africa lies in the proportion infected with HIV subtype B, the most common in the developed world. This proportion has fallen significantly in recent years, according to data presented to the HPA's annual scientific conference in 2002.

Gary Murphy told delegates that between 1997 and 1999, the proportion of subtype B new HIV infections amongst heterosexuals fell to less than 5% of the total, while the number of heterosexuals found to be recently infected with non-B subtypes increased, in particular HIV subtype A (found, more than anywhere else, in Kenya), subtype C (found throughout eastern and southern Africa) and subtype AG (a 'cross' between A and a virus found in central west Africa).

Dr Murphy said it was not possible to determine if the infections had happened in the UK, but researchers suspected that the overwhelming majority of heterosexual infections were acquired outside the UK, particularly in sub-Saharan Africa.

Whilst the number of new subtype B infections fell overall amongst heterosexuals regardless of sex, they remained disproportionately concentrated amongst men.

Some researchers believe that the fact that heterosexual men are somewhat more likely than women to be infected with subtype B is evidence of covert homosexual behaviour or injecting drug use not admitted at the time of HIV testing.

Pregnant women
The UAPMP of pregnant women found that in 2003 0.44% of all pregnant women in London had HIV (one in 228), compared with only a tenth as many outside London (0.39% or one in 2570).

It was estimated that nearly all pregnant women now have their HIV infections diagnosed prior to giving birth - a huge improvement from the last time this was reported in this manual, in the year 2000, when 82% in inner London, 65% in outer London, and 56% in the rest of England and Wales had had their infection diagnosed prior to giving birth. The Government set a target of 90% uptake of HIV testing by the end of 2002.

In 2003, the prevalence of HIV was highest in inner London with 0.56% (one in 179 women) who gave birth to live-born infants in this area being infected with HIV. In the same time period in outer London, 0.36% (one in 277 women) gave birth to live-born infants. This was a substantial rise since 2000. Within London, the prevalence varied considerably according to maternal health authority of residence and was highest in Lambeth Southwark and Lewisham.

Outside London, the prevalence of HIV infection among women giving birth to live-born infants has remained lower than the rate for the population as a whole.

Estimates of the prevalence of HIV in pregnant women have also been made for health authorities in the UK not covered by the UA programme. These estimates have been derived using available data from the dried blood spot programme and the survey of prevalent HIV infections diagnosed (SOPHID).

In 2004, of the 600 women known to be HIV-positive during pregnancy, 552 were already diagnosed before the current pregnancy, and 48 diagnosed during antenatal care.

Children
Since the beginning of the epidemic up till June 2005, 4828 children have been reported to have been born in the UK to HIV-infected mothers, of whom 1390 (29%) became infected with HIV before or during birth, or as infants. Another 1374 have yet to have their HIV serostatus determined, but as these are all children born recently, most will prove to be uninfected.

By March 2006, 1846 HIV-infected children had been reported to the National Study of HIV in Pregnancy and Childhood (data available upon request from nshpc@ich.ucl.ac.uk, tel. 020 7829 8686 or 020 7905 2692). About 19% of all infected children ever reported in the UK & Ireland are known to have died, and about 10% have left the country or are otherwise lost to follow up. Around 95% of those currently living with HIV had acquired infection from their mothers perinatally.

The transmission rate has improved over time. In 2003, assuming the same transmission rate, of 819 babies born to mothers with HIV, about 170 babies would have acquired HIV in the absence of prevention methods. In fact, only 35 (4.2%) did. It is estimated that HIV infection could have been prevented in half of these 35 infected babies if every pregnant women with HIV had her infection detected before delivery, and in fact for the latest year we have figures, 2005, only about 2.3% of children born to HIV-positive mothers became infected. Of the HIV-positive women giving birth in England in 2001, 70% lived in London and 77% were born in sub-Saharan Africa.

The proportion of diagnoses of HIV that are due to mother-to-child transmission has stayed remarkably constant over time, varying from 1.8% to 3.7% of the total since 1992, despite the proportion of HIV diagnoses that are among women increasing during that time from 18% of the total to 42%. This reflects both increased detection of HIV infection in pregnant women before delivery, and improvements in the use of antiretroviral therapy and delivery methods to prevent mother-to-child infection.

Of infected children, 833 (61%) were born in London whereas of those known to be uninfected, only 56% did. Of the 1362 children with HIV, 255 (19%) are known to have died.

About 10% of children in the UK and Ireland born to HIV-infected women were born abroad, so the sum total of children reported was 6604, of whom 1387 (21%) were known to have HIV, with another 21% undetermined. Of these, 55% were reported from London, 28% from the rest of England and 11% from the Republic of Ireland.

Not all children with HIV acquire their infection from their mother. As well as the 1387 children above, another 267 acquired their HIV through blood product treatment and another 54 through blood transfusion or tissue transplant, while in 60 the source of infection could not be ascertained.

By 2002, about 70% of children were taking antiretrovirals. Mortality rates declined by 80% and progression to AIDS by 50% between 1997 and 2002.

By the end of 2003 it was known that about 150 of these children were under five years old, 280 were aged 5-8, 250 aged 9-12, and 130 were 13-15.

Adolescents
Another 75 teenagers aged 16-19 had acquired HIV when they were born, so altogether there are 205 young people who have reached the age of adolescence, having lived with HIV throughout their childhood.

Another 360 teenagers aged 15-19 have acquired HIV through sexual transmission or injecting drug use.

The SOPHID survey for 2005 found that 362 teenagers aged 16-129 were accessing HIV care through adult clinics. Of these 86 had acquired HIV from their mother, 195 through heterosexual contact, 46 through gay sex and the others through other routes or undetermined.

References

Ades AE, Walker J, Botting B, Parker S, Cubitt D, Jones R. Effect of the worldwide epidemic on HIV prevalence in the United Kingdom: record linkage in anonymous neonatal seroprevalence surveys. AIDS 13: 2437-2443, 1999.

HPA. AIDS and HIV infection in the United Kingdom: monthly report. HIV infection in women giving birth in the UK - trends in prevalence and proportions diagnosed to the end of June 2000. Commun Dis Rep CDR Wkly [serial online] 2001 [cited 11 April 2002]; 11 (8): HIV/STI. Available from http://www.phls.org.uk/publications/cdr/archive/hivarchive.html

Duong T, Ades AE, Gibb D, Tookey P, Masters J. Vertical transmission for HIV in the British Isles: estimates based on surveillance data. BMJ 319: 1227-1229, 1999.

Expert Group on Antenatal HIV Targets. Targets aimed at reducing the number of children born with HIV: report from an Expert Group. London: Department of Health, July 1999.

Tookey P. Obstetric and paediatric HIV surveillance data from the UK and Ireland: Data to the end of June 2005. Institute of Child Health, July 2005. Powepoint presentation at: http://hpa.org.uk/infections/topics_az/hiv_and_sti/hiv/epidemiology/files/NSHPC_slide_set_July_2005.ppt

Ethnicity and HIV

Information on ethnicity has been requested on the AIDS reporting forms, which are completed by clinicians, since the start of surveillance in the early 1980s. The reporting of diagnoses of HIV infection from microbiology laboratories began in the mid-1980s when tests for HIV antibody were developed. Information on ethnicity was first requested on this report form in 1993 when the ethnic categorisation was aligned with that used in the 1991 UK national census. The proportion of new HIV diagnoses where ethnicity was reported has increased from 44% (1150/2636) in 1995 to 83% in 2003 and 2004.

Ethnicity and AIDS

Information on ethnicity has been collected since the early 1980s when surveillance of AIDS began. By the end of March 2002, data on ethnicity were available for almost 94% of cumulative reported AIDS cases. This has risen from 92% completeness at the end of 1997. A table of cumulative AIDS cases by exposure category and ethnic group can be viewed in the HIV/AIDS quarterly surveillance tables, available on the PHLS website at: http://www.phls.org.uk/topics_az/hiv_and_sti/hiv/epidemiology/quarterly.htm

Of the 57,250 individuals diagnosed with HIV whose ethnicity has been recorded since 1995, 19,451 (34%) are white, of which 14% are women. 22,341 (39%) are black African, of which 64% are women.

The annual survey of prevalent HIV infections diagnosed (SOPHID) records the ethnicity of patients seen for HIV-related care in England, Wales, and Northern Ireland during the preceding year. In 2003, the survey recorded 35,428 individuals seen for HIV-related care. Information on ethnicity was available for 34,345 (97%) individuals. Of these 53.2% were white, 37.1% black African, 3.2% black Caribbean, 2.7% other or mixed, 1.4% black other, 1.3% SE Asian and oriental, and 1.1% Indian/Pakistani/Bangladeshi.

Injecting drug users

To the end of June 2005, 4,582 injecting drug users have been reported to be HIV-positive in the UK, 70% of them men.

There is relatively little ongoing transmission of HIV among injecting drug users (IDUs) in the UK. In 2006 the proportion of HIV diagnoses attributable to intravenous drug use was 2.5% of the total.

The fact that only about 3.5% of the HIV-positive population got HIV through injecting drug use in probably the UK's biggest prevention success. Not only the proportion, but the absolute number, of HIV infections in IDUs consistently declined between the late 1980s and 2000, at the time infections in other groups have increased. Since then there have been slight signs of an increase, especially amongst drug users in London and those who are not seen by agencies. In 2002, for instance, the proportion of HIV diagnoses attributable to intravenous drug use was only 1.7% of the total (see chart).

Nonetheless, in comparison 22% of people with HIV in France acquired it through injecting drugs, 28% in the USA, 34% in Ireland and 49% in Portugal, while in the countries of Eastern Europe injecting drug use is (as yet) the predominant mode of acquisition (76% of cases in Russia).

The majority (40%) of all HIV diagnoses among injecting drug users have been in London, and the overwhelming majority of the remainder have been diagnosed in Scotland (29%). Injecting drug users have declined as a proportion of newly diagnosed HIV-positive individuals in Scotland from 77% prior to 1986 to 4% in 2004.

Injecting drug users make up 30% of all diagnosed HIV-positive individuals in Scotland, compared with 3.5% across the rest of the UK.

Twenty-nine per cent of IDUs have been reported as having AIDS. This is the same proportion of AIDS cases and among all people with HIV. But 36% are known to have died as opposed to just 23% of all people with HIV. A large proportion (42%) died without AIDS being reported. This is to be expected, since liver disease due to hepatitis B and hepatitis C and drug overdoses are common among injecting drug users.

Data are available on country of infection for around 30% of all HIV diagnosed injecting drug users; 817 reported a probable country of infection. Thirty two per cent (262/817) gave the UK as their probable country of infection. This was

Rate of infections among injecting drug users

infections/year

Source: HPA

followed by Italy (20%, 162), Spain (13%, 108), Portugal and the Azores (8%, 66) and Ireland (4%, 34). This would indicate that infections acquired abroad, particularly in Southern Europe, are making a significant contribution to HIV infections reported in the UK.

It is difficult to be sure how widely HIV has spread amongst injecting drug users owing to the difficulty in estimating how many people have injected drugs and shared injecting equipment at some time in the past. The issue is further complicated by the fact that UK estimates have tended to be based on surveys of the current UK population, and do not take into account the extent of migration amongst injecting drug users. The likelihood of having injected drugs in the past is greater for migrants from southern European countries.

Nevertheless a number of strong clues exist regarding prevalence. 2.5% of both male and female IV drug users who seek an HIV test have been HIV-positive (see Public Health Laboratory Service Quarterly Tables). Unlinked anonymised seroprevalence studies suggested a prevalence of 4.7% in drug users attending syringe exchanges or drugs agencies in London in 1995 (less than 2% in men under 25, but up to 8% amongst those between 30-34, suggesting that those who were more likely to have been injecting in the mid-1980s were most likely to be infected. The same wasn't true for women; under 24s were the most likely to be infected).

By 1997 the HIV prevalence among male injecting drug users in London had fallen very slightly, to 4% in men and 1.5% in women. Prevalence declined more significantly outside London, to 0.3%. In 1999 prevalence of HIV infection among those who had begun injecting in the UK in the previous 3 years was estimated at 0.1%. This had fallen from 0.3% in the mid 1990s.

HIV has spread much less widely amongst injecting drug users in the UK than in southern European countries. For the large part this is due to the widespread introduction of needle/syringe exchange schemes before HIV had become widely disseminated amongst the drug using population in the UK. The number of cases of HIV infection and AIDS amongst injecting drug users may also be lower than other European countries because less injecting drug use has taken place in the UK and because less needle sharing took place. A Public Health Laboratory study in 1995 estimated that between 50,000 and 77,000 people in England and Wales were currently injecting drugs, with a subset of between 10,000 and 15,000 who risked blood-borne infection by sharing injecting equipment (Heptonstall).

Although prevalence surveys amongst drug users in several British cities have shown stable or even declining prevalence in the past few years, new infections may still be occurring at a significant rate. Apparently declining or stable prevalence could be explained by:

- Seropositive drug users entering methadone treatment and hence no longer being recruited to prevalence studies through syringe exchanges.

- Migration of HIV-positive drug users to other cities, and their replacement in prevalence studies by HIV-negative users.

- Lack of contact between drug users who continue to share and drugs services which are offering treatment, from which prevalence studies have been recruited.

Apparently stable prevalence may also be explained by increasing levels of HIV testing amongst injecting drug users, which leads them to access drugs services and hence be more likely to be recruited to prevalence studies. This would cancel out the effect of injectors moving to other locations or dropping out of the drug using population.

However, the 1997 Anonymised Seroprevalence report noted that of 292 injecting drug users who had reported starting to inject in the past three years, only one had HIV infection. In comparison, almost 10% were already infected with hepatitis B.

The Unlinked Anonymous Prevalence Monitoring Programme survey of injecting drug users provides prevalence data for hepatitis B and C as well as HIV. Prevalence data are available for those injecting drug users who began injecting in the three years before the date of the survey which they were included in. Many of those who have been injecting for less than three years (so called new injectors) will have been aged under 25 at the time of the survey, however, many young injectors will have been injecting for more than three years and other individuals started injecting later in life.

HIV-positivity amongst injecting drug users is highest in London, Edinburgh and Dundee. Outside these cities very low levels of infection have been found.

In Edinburgh, prevalence amongst current injecting drug users was around 20% in a 1992 survey, although a 1989 study amongst current injectors attending a general practitioner in the worst affected district of Edinburgh showed seroprevalence of 64%. The rate of new infections is thought to be very low due to a decline in syringe and needle sharing and the decline in injecting amongst HIV-positive drug users, many of whom are now receiving methadone treatment or have ceased drug use altogether.

In 1995 the Communicable Disease Surveillance Centre reported that nearly one in five people injecting drugs and attending specialist agencies in London and the South-East reported recent sharing of injecting equipment, and that sharing was more common amongst younger drugs users and amongst women. A similar rate was found in 1997, and when the definition of sharing was expanded to include the sharing of spoons, filters and water, the proportion increased to 57%. These findings have particular relevance for hepatitis C prevention, which is much more easily transmitted by these practices than HIV.

Injecting drug use has been raised as a particular problem in prisons, but preliminary UK studies suggest that there has been little spread of HIV through needle-sharing in prison in comparison with other European countries. Nevertheless, research in the UK indicates that around a third of drug users inject whilst in prison, that a majority of injectors report sharing needles in prison and that between half and three quarters of injectors report have been in custody whilst dependent on drugs or shortly after ceasing drug use.

Twenty-five per cent of injecting drug users in a 1992 anonymised study of a Scottish jail were HIV-positive, although only 4.5% of all prisoners in the jail were infected. A screening exercise at Glenochil prison identified at least 13 inmates who are believed to have been infected from the same source through sharing needles whilst imprisoned, and it is estimated that between 22 and 43 inmates had been infected altogether.

Two recent surveys suggested that in London undocumented HIV infection among drug users could be on the increase. A survey of 27,932 drug users given unlinked anonymous HIV saliva tests found that HIV prevalence specifically in London was 5%, four times the national average and 13 times the prevalence outside London.

Annual incidence among new drug users was estimated to be 2.5% - comparable with that in gay men - though this fell to 0.8% after the first year as people became more informed about HIV risks and better at cleaning 'works'. Drug users recruited in community settings (streets, needle exchanges etc) had six times the HIV prevalence of drug users using established agencies, suggesting a population of newer users underserved by standard programmes.

Another survey of 428 drug users mainly in London found an HIV prevalence of 4%, a hepatitis C prevalence of 44%, and found that 24% of individuals at baseline saying that they had shared needles and syringes and 54% reporting the sharing of drug use paraphernalia.

References

Donoghoe M et al: HIV testing and unreported positivity among injecting drug users with no treatment experience, AIDS 7: 1105-1111, 1993.

Heptonstall J et al: How many people in England and Wales risk infection from injecting drug use? Communicable Disease Report 5: 40-44, 1995

HIV and AIDS in injecting drug users in the United Kingdom. Communicable Disease Report 9: 35, 1999.

HIV and AIDS in injecting drug users in the United Kingdom. CDR Weekly 10: 34, 2000.

Hope V et al. HIV prevalence among injecting drug users in England and Wales 1990 to 2003: evidence for increased transmission in recent years. AIDS 19(11): 1207-1214. 2005.

Judd A et al. Incidence of hepatitis C virus and HIV among new injecting drug users in London: prospective cohort study. BMJ, November 13th, 2004.

Scottish Affairs Committee (1994): Drug Abuse In Scotland, First Report: Volume 1, HMSO, 1994.

Turnbull P et al: Drug Use In Prison, AVERT, 1994.

Antiretroviral therapy usage in the UK in 2001

Of the 47,025 people receiving care in England, Wales and Northern Ireland in 2005, 31,082 (66%) were using some form of antiretroviral therapy (mono-, dual, triple or quadruple therapy).

In total 24,344 patients were taking triple combination therapy. This represents 52% of all people being seen for HIV-related care. As expected, a much smaller proportion (1,462 individuals or 3% of all people being seen for care) were taking mono or dual therapy. Some of these would be pregnant women with high CD4 counts taking mono or dual therapy to prevent transmission, while others would be multi-drug-resistant patients kept on one or two drugs to maintain immune function as best as possible till new options became available. A total of 5,754 individuals were taking four or more anti-HIV drugs, 12% of all patients receiving HIV-related care.

In 2004, outside of London and the South East, where 15,398 individuals or 66% of all people on treatment reside, the regions with the biggest number of people on therapy were, in descending order, the North West (1,892 individuals), the Eastern region (1,250 individuals), the West Midlands (1,033 individuals), the South West (902 individuals), Yorkshire and Humberside (890 individuals) and the East Midlands (844).

The reliability of epidemiological projections

One of the key problems faced by epidemiologists when making projections about the future spread of HIV is the lack of information about some of the factors which may influence the speed at which HIV spreads amongst different risk groups within the population. Nevertheless it is possible to be fairly confident about some of the key factors which will continue to determine the development of the epidemic simply by looking at past patterns.

In the mid-1980s a series of projections were made from the limited data available at that stage which greatly overestimated the spread of HIV amongst the UK population. These projections created expectations about the development of the epidemic which did not materialise, and have led to claims that the scale of the epidemic was exaggerated in order to win funding.

What do epidemiologists need to know to make projections?

In order to make accurate projections, epidemiologists need to take into account the following variables. They are closely interrelated and it is not possible to single out one as more important than the others.

Virulence of HIV and infectivity of HIV-infected persons

It is likely that individuals are most infectious in the six to eight weeks after infection until antibodies are produced to suppress HIV in the blood, semen and vaginal and cervical fluid. Thereafter very low levels of HIV are present in these body fluids for much of the time that individuals are asymptomatic. Virtually all the viral burden is confined to the lymph tissue (the lymph nodes, the spleen etc.). Increasing viral load tends to correspond with the development of symptoms, and individuals are once again highly infectious. For example, one study has shown that semen is most likely to contain HIV in individuals with CD4

counts below 100, and it was very difficult to find HIV in the semen of men with CD4 counts above 200 (for further discussion of factors which influence infectivity see *HIV transmission*).

These fluctuations of infectivity may help to explain the shape of the epidemic. For instance, reductions in viral load in infected gay men, together with the effectiveness of community-based safer sex education, probably account for the apparent fall-off in new infections amongst gay men in the mid-1980s in Europe and North America.

Because the periods of high infectivity are relatively short, the levels of unprotected sex or needle sharing with different partners (and the choice and location of those partners) during those periods are very important in determining how many people become infected and where the virus spreads. This explains why gay men and injecting drug users have been seriously affected; members of these groups with large numbers of contacts are more likely to come into contact with people who are going through a period of high infectiousness.

This is not to say that HIV is not passed on at other times by HIV-positive people. But the current distribution of HIV infection in the UK and other countries in the developed world does suggest that much HIV infection can be accounted for by contacts which take place during those periods of high infectivity. If HIV-positive people were very infectious much of the time, the virus would have spread even more widely in the core groups, far more frequently to contacts of the core groups, and far more frequently to their other partners in turn.

The frequency of partner change amongst different groups in the population:

As noted above, the more contacts take place when an individual is infectious, the more infections will result. If there is a low level of partner change this will tend to minimise the spread of HIV. Levels of partner change amongst heterosexuals have been overestimated in the past.

Extent of mixing between different groups

If there is little mixing between bisexual men and female partners, there will be little spread of HIV by this route. But if many bisexual men have large numbers of female partners whilst highly infectious, HIV will be widely disseminated amongst women. The same is true with injecting drug users, and with people from high prevalence locations.

One interesting explanation for why HIV rates are so much higher in African-American men than in other ethnic groups in the USA, despite the fact that rates of unsafe sex are if anything lower, was put forward by a paper presented to the Toronto World AIDS Conference in 2006 (Berry). The researchers found that African-American men were more likely to exclusively have sex with men of their own ethnicity than other groups, so they were more likely to encounter an HIV-positive man than other gay men. Conversely, they tended to have sex with a wider age range than gay men of other ethnicities, who tended to stick to partners within five years either side of their own age.

Age-mixing is an important factor in the shockingly high rates of HIV incidence on young women in Africa, and it may be part of the explanation in black gay America too.

Extent of risk-taking behaviour amongst different groups

Even if many injecting drug users in a locality are infected with HIV, there will be little HIV transmission unless needle-sharing takes place. HIV will not spread if a large proportion of individuals have adopted behaviour which minimises the risk of infection, or if they don't engage in risk behaviour in the first place.

Prevalence of HIV in different groups and locations

Glasgow is a good example of a city which has been insulated from an HIV epidemic amongst injecting drug users by a low initial prevalence of HIV amongst injecting drug users and the adoption of behaviour which minimises the risk of HIV infection.

The levels of HIV infection amongst migrants to the UK from Africa and the European Union

This has turned out to be the biggest single influence on HIV diagnoses in the last five years. The largest proportion of AIDS and HIV cases amongst the heterosexual population is found in people who are migrants to the UK. If increasing numbers of people entering the UK are HIV-positive, this will affect the size of the UK epidemic.

The effect of treatment more alive, but less infectious

Improvements in treatment mean that people with HIV will live longer without symptoms, and that people will live longer with AIDS. Antiretroviral treatment which reduces viral load will play an especially significant role in limiting transmission, rather than increasing the potential 'pool' of infectious persons by keeping people alive.

Underestimates of the size of the key risk groups

Predictions are partly based on estimates of the frequency of homosexual and drug injecting behaviour, yet no one really knows how frequently these things happen. Epidemiologists have to use indirect indicators such as the incidence of hepatitis B infection amongst injecting drug users, the incidence of rectal gonorrhoea amongst gay and bisexual men and the size of the population of GUM clinic attenders as surrogates for measuring the level of risk-taking behaviour.

The emergence of increasingly virulent strains of HIV

Although this variable is unlikely, we cannot predict with any certainty how HIV will evolve. It may become more infectious or more deadly, or less so.

Understanding of the UK HIV epidemic relies on being able to establish how the individuals reported to the data set probably acquired infection, and if the route is heterosexual, how or where they or their partners are likely to have become infected. All reports of new diagnoses of HIV infection that are received with insufficient information to ascertain the probable route of infection are subject to follow-up. Where necessary this follow-up may include interview by a research nurse, subject to the agreement of the diagnosing clinician and patient. The time taken to complete this process means that the proportion of reports for which infection route is unresolved is higher for recent time periods than for the data set overall.

Reference

Berry M et al. *Sexual networks and risk behaviors among racial/ethnic groups of men who have sex with men*. XVI International AIDS Conference, Toronto. Abstract no. TUPE0617. 2006

What may happen in the next five years?

As we have said above, few people writing about the epidemiology of HIV in the UK at the turn of the millennium could have predicted that the rate of new diagnoses would more than double over the next five years, that twice as many heterosexuals as gay men would be diagnosed by 2003, and that more heterosexuals than gay men would be living with HIV in the UK by 2004.

What happens over the next five years depends to some degree on issues that HIV prevention programmes can affect, such as reversing the upward trend in gay male infections and in heterosexual infections acquired in the UK.

We quite suddenly have a large group of heterosexuals with HIV in the UK and it is difficult to predict to what degree a 'home grown' heterosexual epidemic will take off. So far the number of UK-acquired infections is relatively small, but they have risen proportionately in line with heterosexual infections in general, though ones where both partners acquired HIV in the UK have so far not increased. It is difficult to tell whether this is due to lack of partner mixing between HIV- positive heterosexuals and others, or between the most affected community (Africans) and others, or whether we are just seeing the beginning of the much shallower bell-curve typical of a heterosexual epidemic.

Although surveys have consistently documented rises in both unprotected sex among gay men, and serodiscordant unprotected sex, the upward trend in gay diagnoses is due primarily to two factors: a larger population of gay men living with HIV, and increased uptake of HIV testing as a result of the routine offer of the test by GUM clinics. Although evidence from the USA suggests that once diagnosed people with HIV take steps to limit their chances of infecting others, these do not outweigh the fact that in (for example) London, a gay man with HIV, in the absence of disclosure of status, is going to meet seven times as many partners who are HIV-negative as HIV-positive, so has many more potential opportunities to transmit HIV than an individual HIV-negative person has to contract it. This imbalance is one reason why some HIV organisations have suggested that prevention campaigns need to be increasingly directed at people with HIV.

However the greatest influence on HIV in the UK in the last five years has been immigration. Owing to restrictions by the Home Office, including the institution of visas for Zimbabweans; an increasing rate of deportations; faster processing of asylum claims and legal judgments that lack of antiretroviral treatment in the home country is not a reason to uphold an asylum claim, the number of immigrants from sub-Saharan Africa has started to drop. This will probably lead (and may already be leading) to a considerable slackening off in the rate of increase in new infections, and possibly a decline.

Two parts of the world that may exert an unknown degree of influence are India and Eastern Europe. Indians form the second-largest ethnic minority in the UK, and India has a rapidly-expanding HIV epidemic, with a highly-disputed figure for HIV prevalence that may be approaching 1%. Relatively few Indians are new immigrants - most are second- or third-generation settlers - but the proportion and number of heterosexual infections caught in South Asia has climbed in recent years and the effect of travel to and from home countries, and bringing husbands and wives from India, has an unknown effect at present.

There are no immigration restrictions at all on the recent new member states of the EU, the ex-Iron Curtain states of Poland, the Czech Republic, Slovakia, Hungary and Slovenia, and the Baltic states of Lithuania, Latvia and Estonia.

Most of these countries have low HIV prevalence themselves, considerably lower than the UK, with the exception of the small states of Latvia (0.6%) and Estonia (1.1%). For Poles, Czechs and Bulgarians, therefore, coming to the UK may represent coming to a higher-risk environment for HIV.

Next door, however, and separated only by porous borders, are the huge countries of Ukraine (HIV prevalence 1.4%) and Russia (1.1%), home of the world's fastest-growing HIV epidemics. The main affected community in the former Soviet states is drug users, who may be too poor, too stigmatised and (in the absence of treatment) to ill to form a sizeable proportion of the large increase in Eastern Europeans working in the UK and other EU countries, but as the relatively recent Eastern European epidemic matures we may begin to see more cases among heterosexual people from this part of the world in the UK. So far, however, rumours of high levels of HIV in Eastern European sex workers have proved false, though there was a syphilis outbreak in this group in East London in 2004.

Impact of immigration and international travel on HIV in UK

Worldwide travel has increased in the past decade due, in part, to its increasing accessibility and affordability. Affluent, widely-travelled gay men were among the first to be affected by HIV back in the early 1980s. After the establishment of the HIV epidemic in the UK, most transmission occurred within gay male communities in the UK. But in recent years the epidemiology of HIV in the UK has changed completely, as we saw above.

The number of migrants to the UK including refugees and asylum seekers increased from the mid-1990s.

The 2005 BBC 'Born Abroad' survey found that 7.5% of people living in Britain were born abroad (4.3 million out of 57.1 million), and that between 1991 and 2001, half of Britain's population and peaked in 2002. London had by far the biggest number of non-nationals and has also experienced the biggest rise in immigrants, with a 45% increase in Londoners born abroad between 1991 and 2001. However areas that had previously had very few immigrants like the north-east also had big increases.

Immigrants come for a wide variety of reasons and have a number of different legal statuses ranging from full naturalisation through work permits and student visas to refugees and asylum seekers - both documented and

undocumented. An illustration of this variety is the fact that some of London's richest (Hyde Park, Chelsea) and poorest (East Ham, Tottenham) districts are among those with the highest immigrant populations. So is the list of countries with the biggest migrant populations in the UK. Excluding the Republic of Ireland, the top five are India, Pakistan, Germany, the Caribbean nations and the USA, with two countries with high HIV prevalence - South Africa and Kenya - coming in at numbers seven and eight.

The countries that have contributed the biggest net increases of migrants during the 1990s are also a varied list, showing how immigration is equally a phenomenon of skilled workers travelling to the UK for jobs and people fleeing the world's trouble spots. The nationalities with the biggest net population increase during the 1990s were Afghanistan, Albania, China, former Yugoslavia, Finland, Greece, Sierra Leone, South Africa, Sweden and Zimbabwe.

In terms of people 'pushed' by persecution rather than 'pulled' by economic advantage, applications for asylum peaked in 2002 at 84,130 but have since fallen dramatically and in 2004 stood at 33,930. In terms of applicants per head of population, the UK is about midway down the list of EU countries, with Austria getting 3.9 times as many applicants per capita and Italy getting a fifth as many.

The country of origin of asylum seekers varies rapidly according to the war and human rights conditions in different parts of the world. The 'top five' countries for applicants over the last five years are as follows:

2001	2002	2003	2004
Afghanistan	Iraq	Somalia	Iran
Iraq	Zimbabwe	Iraq	Somalia
Somalia	Afghanistan	China	China
Sri Lanka	Somalia	Zimbabwe	Zimbabwe
Iran	China	Iran	Iraq

Obviously some countries, like China, are on the list because of their high populations. In terms of asylum seekers per head of population, 2004's 'top five' looks like this:

Asylum seekers per 10,000 population in originating country:

- Somalia 3.1

- Zimbabwe 1.6

- Iraq 0.7

- Iran 0.5

- China 0.018

Other small African countries like Eritrea (2.5 asylum seekers per 10,000) are also over-represented.

Equally, asylum seekers come from countries with widely varying HIV prevalence. Zimbabwe has nearly the highest HIV prevalence in the world at 24.6% of the adult population, according to UNAIDS. In 2002 there were more Zimbabweans diagnosed with HIV in the UK than British citizens. The number of Zimbabwean entrants has since declined to less than a third of the 2002 since the introduction of via requirements for Zimbabweans in 2003.

Somalia's HIV prevalence is unknown, as the country's civil disorder has prevented adequate surveillance, but appeared to be about 1% in surveys done in 2003-4; Iran, China and Iraq all have prevalence under 0.1%, though the first two are experiences rapid HIV increases in vulnerable populations.

Equally many migrants come from other countries that have high prevalence but are not in a state of war or problems with human rights violations, like South Africa.

These migrants are predominantly young people aged less than 35 years and are likely to be a sexually-active population. However the majority of migrants from South Africa are white, and HIV prevalence has been found to be low on this portion of the South African population.

Additionally, worldwide travel has increased in recent years, including both UK residents travelling abroad and nationals from other countries visiting the UK.

Recent studies have shown evidence of population-wide changes in sexual behaviour in the past decade, including the acquisition of new partners abroad. Taken together, these factors contribute to the increased probability of encountering STIs and HIV.

Between 2000 and 2001, following the introduction of new HIV diagnosis reporting by clinicians, country of infection was recorded for 84% of newly diagnosed HIV infections. The UK was the likely country of infection for 28% (1,042 of 3,727) of those diagnosed, while for 47% (1,755) it was an African country, 3% (105) Europe, and 3% (112) Asia. Stark differences can be observed by exposure category; 85% (758 of 892) of HIV infections attributed to sex between men acquired in the UK, compared to 13% (284 of 2,243) of heterosexual infections.

Between 2000 and 2001, 83% of heterosexuals diagnosed with HIV in the UK were born abroad. Of the heterosexuals born in the UK (358) 10% (37) were probably infected in Thailand, while 47% were infected in the UK. For male heterosexuals born in the UK, where country of infection was known, 18%

(35 of 196) were probably infected in Thailand compared to 30% in the UK.

Who is at risk: a summary

What these figures show is the extent to which HIV and AIDS remain highly concentrated within some population groups. They also show the extent to which newspaper reporting and commentary on these figures distorts the risk to the least vulnerable and draws attention away from the highest risks.

Whilst it may be correct to say that everyone is potentially at risk, the chances of the majority of heterosexual people meeting an HIV-positive sexual partner are very low. Similarly the claim 'each time you sleep with someone you sleep with all their previous partners' may be scary, but there's little evidence that HIV is currently being transmitted in the UK through lengthy chains of heterosexual partnerships as some health educators have claimed. If this was the case there would probably be much larger numbers of HIV-positive heterosexual men and women identified as HIV-positive. A PHLS investigation of 15 cases of second-generation transmission could find only one suspected case in which a chain of transmission could be demonstrated (Gilbart). It is unlikely that a radically different pattern holds true amongst the untested.

Whilst it is also true to say that knowing your partner may not protect heterosexual men and women from being infected, it will go some way to providing protection. In particular, knowing that your partner is likely to have had unprotected sex abroad, injected drugs or had sex with another man would be a useful indication of potential risk.

References

BBC 'Born Abroad' Database, 2005. See http://news.bbc.co.uk/1/shared/spl/hi/uk/05/born_abroad/html/overview.stm

Gilbart V et al: Second generation heterosexual transmission of HIV-1 infection. CDR 2(5), 1992.

Home Office: Asylum statistics, fourth quarter, 2004. See http://www.homeoffice.gov.uk/rds/pdfs05/asylumq404.pdf

Using epidemiology to plan services

The importance of targeting

An editorial in the *New England Journal of Medicine* summarised current thinking amongst epidemiologists and public health planners on the value of targeting.

The argument for targeting HIV prevention is based on the marked difference in rates of HIV infection and AIDS amongst those engaging in various types of high-risk behaviour, living in various areas, and belonging to various demographic groups.

Publicly emphasising that large numbers of people are at low, but not at zero risk, has potentially serious political consequences. People are not very good at processing information about low-probability events in which there could be a highly negative outcome. They tend to greatly over-estimate or under-estimate the likelihood of such events, and their estimates can be unduly influenced by small amounts of new information.

Public emphasis on the low but not quite zero risk of HIV infection may thus lead many people to overestimate their chances of becoming infected. If later information, including personal experience, contradicts these exaggerated fears, people are likely to revert to their previous underestimation of risk.

In addition, they may conclude that their fear of HIV infection was deliberately manipulated by health officials, AIDS activists and researchers to advance other agendas.

An effective programme to prevent HIV infection must have both universal and targeted components. The universal component includes reducing HIV-related discrimination, removing commercial restrictions on the materials necessary for safer behaviour, and providing information about the risk of HIV transmission. The targeted component involves focusing the limited resources for intensive programmes of behavioral change on situations in which the risk of HIV transmission is highest.

Such a strategy would follow the dictum of 'Warn widely and spend wisely' (Des Jarlais).

'Targeting' is a term loosely used in HIV prevention, often without a clear understanding of what it implies. In fact, 'targeting' refers to a chain of decisions made in HIV prevention work. It refers to:

- The assessment of local need (ideally with reference to national and local epidemiological data).

- The recognition of particular risk groups/needs.

- The decision to allocate resources to meet particular needs (prioritisation).

- The development of strategies to address the target group.

- The evaluation of the impact of targeted work.

- The adjustment of strategy to take into account the results of evaluation and the impact of targeted work on epidemiological trends.

See also: *HIV prevention: which methods work?*.

Who should be targeted for HIV prevention?

The data discussed above show that HIV infection remains highly concentrated amongst certain groups in the UK which are reasonably easy to target with services intended to minimise HIV transmission.

- Targeting of gay men will address the group in which the chances of HIV infection continue to be highest. A UK gay man in London has about 200 times as much chance of coming across a sexual partner with HIV as a British-born heterosexual outside London, and gay men still account for four out of five HIV infections caught within the UK.

- Despite this, funding for gay-specific HIV prevention campaigns has been disproportionately low. The CHAPS gay men's HIV prevention partnership had funding of about £1.7 million in 2004 (lower than its budget in 1998). Adding other gay men's initiatives brings the sum spent on gay men to about £3.5 million, or about 15% of the total HIV prevention budget.

- In a report for the England and Wales AIDS Funders Forum in March 2007, Sigma Research (see Weatherburn et al), found that:

Of 70 new information, advice and advocacy interventions gained by voluntary organisations in the past three years, only four were for gay men, and the survey did not establish how many of the 22 lost were for gay men

Whereas there were net gains in the provision of information and advice, social support, mental health and even written info, there was hardly any gain in prevention interventions

And yet gay men as a group were seen by providers and commissioners as better served than many other groups and therefore less prioritised for new services.

The two areas that received most new services by the voluntary sector were financial and social support for immigrants, especially undocumented ones, and employment/retraining/living well schemes, even though these are seen as the areas least well provided for.

One unnamed respondent said that "Gay men with HIV, indigenous to Britain, are invisible to most funders."

- Targeting of injecting drug users will continue to be necessary despite apparently declining prevalence amongst this group (see *Injecting drug users* above). This is because the number of new drug users and registered addicts continues to increase. Whilst the situation amongst injecting drug users in the UK remains relatively stable, this is highly dependent on the continued provision of needle/syringe exchange schemes and ongoing education in prisons.

- Strategies which promote condom use amongst injecting drug users and their partners will have a significant impact on new infections through sexual intercourse.

- African communities in the UK will continue to experience a high incidence of AIDS; educational methods appropriate to these communities need to be stepped up. This group has been particularly neglected by HIV prevention initiatives in the UK despite widespread awareness that a terrible epidemic is going on in sub-Saharan Africa.

- Other ethnic groups in the UK will be vulnerable to HIV according to the degree that HIV and AIDS are affecting an ethnic group's country of origin and the extent to which members of that group travel back and forth between the UK and the country of origin.

- Female sex workers are at high risk of HIV infection, but seem to have remained remarkably unaffected by HIV compared with other European countries. This is probably due in large part to low levels of infection amongst injecting drug users in the UK, but sex workers will only continue to remain unaffected provided that current educational efforts continue.

- Infection while travelling abroad accounts for a growing proportion of cases amongst heterosexual men and women; travellers and workers abroad can be targeted by a variety of methods depending on their destination. For instance, it is reasonable to assume that anyone who requires vaccination against tropical infections will also be in particular need of education about the risks of HIV infection abroad. Similarly, seafarers are likely to be at risk.

- Women are more vulnerable to infection than heterosexual men in the UK because they are more likely than heterosexual men to have partners who are bisexual or who are injecting drug users. Many women report that they were unaware of being at risk until they learnt of their HIV status either through ante-natal testing or through diagnosis as a consequence of illness.

- Partner notification programmes may be one of the most appropriate mechanisms by which new infections amongst heterosexual women can be prevented.

These are the core groups at risk for HIV infection in the UK. Targeting also needs to address the discrimination experienced by these groups and by people with HIV and AIDS generally.

Reference

Weatherburn P et al. *The Growing Challenge: A strategic review of HIV social care, support and information services across the UK*. Sigma Research, ISBN 1 872956 88 2. 2007.

An overview of the global epidemic

(In this section on the global epidemic, all references unless otherwise indicated come from the UNAIDS AIDS Epidemic Update for December 2004 see http://www.unaids.org/en/HIV_data/epi2006/default.asp - and the individual-country UN Epidemiological Fact Sheets on HIV and Sexually Transmitted Infections.)

As of December 2006, the United National Global AIDS Programme, UNAIDS, estimated that 39.5 million people were living with HIV worldwide. These included 2.3 million children under fifteen years of age and 17.7 million women. Women accounted for 48% of all adults living with HIV worldwide, and for 59% in sub-Saharan Africa.

UNAIDS' figures are never exact, for reasons explored below, so the possibly range of uncertainty was from 34.1 million to 47.1 million. Similar ranges of uncertainty are to be understood for many of the figures below; we will only cite the possible range when it is particularly relevant, but it is wise to remember that these are estimates, arrived at by using a combination of sentinel and population surveys and epidemiological modelling. In some countries the uncertainty is much greater than in others.A total of 4.3 million people are thought to have been newly infected with HIV during 2006, 530,000 of whom were children aged under 15 years. This represents a significant decrease of 12% in adults and 17% in children on the estimated number of new infections in the year 2004, last time this section was updated.

The total number of AIDS deaths in 2004 was 2.9 million, also a decrease. In 2002 and 2004 this figure was 3.1 million, though this 6% decrease is within the boundaries of uncertainty. However the decline in the estimated number of deaths of children is significant - in 2004 UNIDS estimated that 640,000 children had died of AIDS that year, but in 2006 this figure was

40% lower at 380,000. Twenty-five million people have died of AIDS since the epidemic began in 1981.

About 11,800 new HIV infections occurred every day in 2004: one every 7.3 seconds, with an AIDS death every eleven seconds. Ninety-five per cent of them were in the developing world. Of the 10,400 new infections occurring each day in adults, 50% are in women and 50% are in young people under 25.The global prevalence of HIV is still increasing, but at present the rate of increase has slowed (see chart)

Although UNAIDS' estimate of the total number of people living with HIV and acquiring it every year has been revised downwards in recent years, this is a real slowdown. At present, the epidemic in the most severely affected parts of the world has got to the mature point where as many people are dying of HIV as are catching it. Prevalence in southern Africa may be beginning to stabilise and in east Africa has already fallen.

It is important to remember that much of reason for the decline in the rate of increase of prevalence is because mass dying is taking place. Prevalence may rise again if universal treatment access becomes a reality, as it has in the developed world (contrast this chart with the UK charts in the previous sections), unless it goes hand-in-hand with effective prevention measures.

However, some epidemiologists are more optimistic. In an article in *The Lancet* in March 2006, epidemiologists James T Shelton, Daniel Halperin and David Wilson said that the global epidemic of HIV may have started to decline. Lancet readers, they say, "may be surprised.that HIV incidence has peaked overall in Africa."

An accompanying study (Kumar) showed that in southern India, long forecast to be the next global hotspot for HIV, HIV prevalence had fallen in young women from 1.7% in 2000 to 1.1% in 2004.

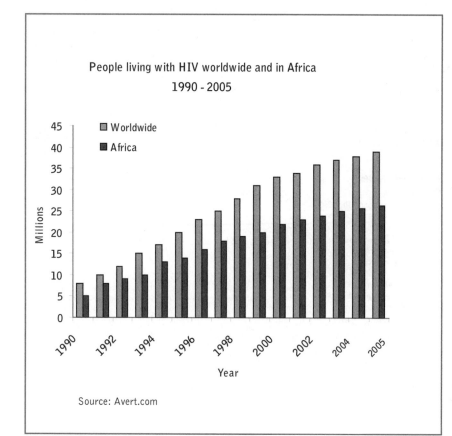

People living with HIV worldwide and in Africa
1990 - 2005

- ■ Worldwide
- ■ Africa

Source: Avert.com

HIV incidence in Uganda peaked in 1987, when 4% of Ugandans could expect to catch HIV every year. Now that rate is less than 0.5%. In neighbouring Kenya, incidence peaked in 1992 at 2% - now incidence is 0.2%, or only one new case in 500 Kenyans a year. In one of the world's worst-hit countries, Botswana, incidence peaked at over 10% in 1995, although it is still running at 6%, a rate twice that seen in US and UK urban gay men. Only in Mozambique, amongst African countries surveyed, did incidence still appear to be increasing. Even in much-criticised South Africa, incidence appears to have peaked in 1997. Only in Mozambique, amongst countries surveyed, did the rate of new HIV infections still seem to be increasing (see chart on next page).

Prevalence, the total proportion of the population with the disease, lags behind incidence, because HIV is a chronic infection and the peak death rate happens years after the peak infection rate. But even so, in Kenya, prevalence peaked in 1997 when 10% of Kenyans had HIV. Now 6% do. In Uganda, 'first in

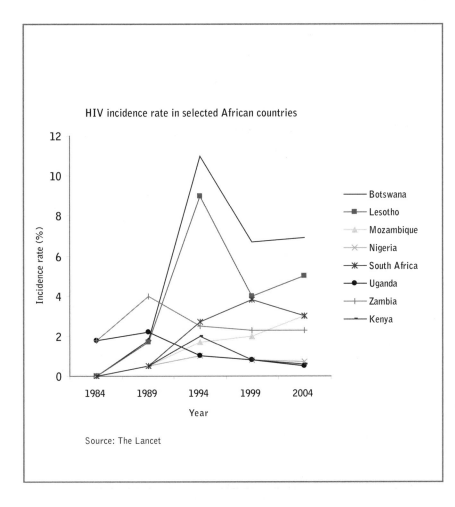

HIV incidence rate in selected African countries

Source: The Lancet

Legend:
- Botswana
- Lesotho
- Mozambique
- Nigeria
- South Africa
- Uganda
- Zambia
- Kenya

of HIV seen in some southern African countries will probably never be seen again:

"Their genesis probably reflects a 'perfect storm' of factors, including limited male circumcision and significant networks of concurrent sexual partnerships involving both men and women, which fuelled a chain reaction of rapid transmission from one highly infectious, newly-infected person to another."

What has caused the decline in incidence? Partly, it's a natural phenomenon where HIV spreads among the most susceptible people first and kills them off, as happened to a whole generation of gay men in the early 1990s in the USA and Western countries. The US peak of incidence among gay men was way back in the early 1980s, before there was even a name for HIV.

However in some countries - notably Kenya, Uganda, Thailand and Cambodia - HIV prevalence has fallen further and for longer than would have been expected due to these effects alone. All these countries have featured comprehensive, hard-hitting, country-wide HIV prevention programmes - at least among heterosexuals - and appear to have reaped the benefit.

and first out' of African countries, a quarter of the population had HIV in 1990 - now less than 5% do.

More recent declines in prevalence have been reported from Zimbabwe, Ethiopia, and Malawi and across the Caribbean, in Haiti. In Botswana, sentinel surveillance of pregnant women revealed an HIV prevalence of 37.4% in 2003; in 2005 this had declined by over 10% to 33.4%.

The ultimate goal of the world community's fight against HIV is, of course, to reduce the death toll from AIDS and there are signs that this is beginning to happen even in the most grievously affected countries. In Botswana, for instance, the death toll from AIDS meant that general mortality amongst the population peaked in 2003 with one in 166 citizens dying every year compared with one in 500 in 1994. In 2006 this had declined to one in 220 and the trend towards increased upward life expectancy seemed to be accelerating.

In countries with universal treatment, however, the time delay between a decrease in incidence and the overall HIV rate is much longer, because people are not dying and so reducing the pool of infected people, and in countries like the UK and USA the number of people with HIV continues to increase -- as it does in countries slower to catch on to HIV prevention in Africa, like South Africa.

One incidence peak may follow another, as HIV infection 'saturates' one population but then spreads into new, susceptible populations. In the graph above it can be seen that incidence is starting to rise again in Botswana and Lesotho, possibly due to infections in older people. The clearest example of this may be Russia, where incidence appeared to peak in IDUs in 2000-02 (though this may be an artefact of fewer tests being carried out subsequently), and has since then declined, while continuing to spread from IDUs into the heterosexual population. However, Shelton and colleagues say that the generalised 'hyper epidemics'

But, *The Lancet* warns, we cannot be complacent: "Incidence is still unacceptably high, especially in southern Africa, and can reverse course if gains from behavioural changes slacken."

A reminder that HIV can suddenly break out anew in populations that haven't had safer-sex advice and help was seen recently in Thailand, where there was a tripling of the HIV rate in young gay men in the last two years in a country normally seen as an HIV success story. And some other countries are only just starting to experience the initial phase of the epidemic, characterised by the rapid expansion of the epidemic in very high-risk populations such as injecting drug users and/or sex workers: these notoriously include Russia and many of the other former Soviet republics (though even here, incidence seems to have peaked) but also several previously very low-prevalence Arab countries including Libya and Bahrain.

Sentinel versus population surveillance

HIV and AIDS surveillance is a far less precise science in many countries than it is in the UK. Even the USA is unable to release accurate estimates of how many of its inhabitants have HIV, due to different reporting systems in different states, though all states in the USA will finally move to names-based HIV reporting (which has always existed for AIDS reporting) in 2007.

Some European countries like Italy and Spain still do not compile HIV figures from every region. And when it comes to poor countries with inadequate health infrastructure, UNAIDS has to rely on 'sentinel' HIV surveillance among groups likely to come into contact with health workers and epidemiologists - such as pregnant women, sex workers, STI clinic attendees and tuberculosis patients. They are also more likely to be city-dwellers, who in most (though not all) countries have higher HIV prevalence than the rural population. UNAIDS has come to realise that these groups may tend to have higher HIV prevalence than the general population. If HIV surveillance in the UK relied on attendees at London GUM and antenatal clinics, for example, it would overestimate UK prevalence anything up to six-fold. Sampling pregnant women may in other cases underestimate HIV if the epidemic is concentrated among gay men and injecting drug users.

The other method is to use random population sampling to determine HIV prevalence. This risks bias in the opposite direction to sentinel surveillance. It will tend not to sample enough members of vulnerable communities such as sex workers and men who have sex with men, and are of little use in countries with tightly-focused epidemics. Voluntary sampling is likely to underestimate prevalence due to HIV stigma. A study comparing the two methods in Africa found that population-based sampling, compared with sentinel surveillance, tended to underestimate HIV prevalence in men and overestimate it in women - possibly because women are more often at home to be surveyed (Boerma 2003).

As a result, even in Uganda, for example, one of the most-researched and documented of African countries, UNAIDS estimates that about 530,000 people or 4.1% of the adult population is living with HIV, but gives high and low estimates of 350,000 and 880,000 (2.8% and 6.6%) as representing the spread of uncertainty. In neighbouring Kenya, a survey in January 2004 found a national prevalence of 6.7% (4.5% in men and nearly 9% in women); previous estimates had been as high as 15%.

In some countries - and in particular the two countries thought to have the highest numbers of people living with HIV, South Africa and India - the true number of people living with HIV has caused huge political controversy. Prominent anti-apartheid journalist Rian Malan questioned South Africa's HIV figures in 2001. However he based his claim that prevalence was a great deal lower than the official figures on death certificates and other documented causes of death by AIDS. Subsequent investigation found that families were very reluctant to have HIV recorded on death certificates and in fact previous estimates had been up to 40% too low (Groenewald).

India bases its HIV figures on sentinel surveillance in publicly-funded antenatal clinics. As has previously been noted, surveillance among pregnant women may over- or underestimate HIV prevalence considerably, and India has the additional problem that 80% of its healthcare takes place in privately-run clinics. In addition India has an extremely variable HIV epidemic, with sentinel surveillance prevalence ranging from zero in Haryana state (which didn't mean it was zero, it meant no HIV infections were found at antenatal clinics) to 2.25% in Andhra Pradesh.

As a result the Indian government was able to make the nonsensical claim in May 2005 that HIV incidence countrywide had fallen by 95% in a single year, from 520,000 in 2003 to 28,000 in 2004.

In fact the figures previous to 2004 were inflated; in 2003, a change in data collection methods included an increase in sentinel surveillance sites and an expansion of testing from mostly high-risk populations to include low-risk populations. Previously, the prevalence among the high-risk populations was reported as if it was the general prevalence in the population. New HIV infection figures for 2003 also included many cases that erroneously had not been recorded in previous years, making the number of new HIV infections between 2002 and 2003 appear larger than they were.

The controversy in India continues: see under that country for more information.

References

Boerma JT et al. *Estimates of HIV-1 prevalence from national population-based surveys as a new gold standard?* Lancet 362: 1929-1931, 2003.

Groenewald, Pet al. *Identifying deaths from AIDS in South Africa.* AIDS 19(2): 193-201, 2005.

Kumar R et al. *Trends in HIV-1 in young adults in south India from 2000 to 2004: a prevalence study.* Lancet 367: 1164-1172. 2006.

Malan, Rian. *AIDS in Africa: in Search of the Truth.* Rolling Stone Magazine, November 22, 2001

Misra, Neelesh, *HIV Cases Show Huge Drop in India, but It's a Glitch in the Statistics.* Associated Press, 31 May 2005.

Shelton JD et al. *Has global HIV incidence peaked?* The Lancet 367:1120-1122. 2006.

UNAIDS: AIDS Epidemic Update, December 2006.

UNAIDS estimates for the next twenty years

Even if global HIV prevalence is nearing its peak, the HIV epidemic is far from burnt out, background prevalence and there could be 68 million HIV-related deaths between 2000 and 2020 unless prevention and treatment programmes to combat the disease are expanded drastically. Such a level of AIDS related mortality would represent a three-fold increase on the 21 million deaths attributed to AIDS in the 20 years before 2000.

As suggested earlier, prevalence rates in some countries with very high rates are beginning to stabilise. In the worst-affected region of all, southern Africa, prevalence appears to be still going up in South Africa itself, but it has remained static in Zimbabwe since 1997 and appears to be stabilising in Zambia, Malawi and Mozambique. Meanwhile there have been real falls in prevalence not only in Uganda - where this happened in the early 1990s - but more recently in Kenya, Burundi and Ethiopia.

Even in Uganda, this appears largely due to the fact that the death rate has reached saturation point. UNAIDS is also projecting that 50% of South African new mothers could die because of HIV, and that mortality amongst 15 to 34 year-olds will be 17 times higher because of AIDS.

HIV spreading in new areas

However if the prevalence and death curves start going up again, they will probably do so due to the spread of HIV to other parts of the world, notably India, the Far East and Eastern Europe. This has prompted UNAIDS to warn that even though 40 million people are currently infected with HIV worldwide, the HIV epidemic is potentially still in an early phase unless the newly-affected countries can adopt effective prevention measures fast. The number of people living with HIV in East Asia (China and its neighbours) increased by 50% between 2002 and 2004, and in Eastern Europe and Central Asia (largely Ukraine and Russia) by 40% during the same period and by another 21% from 2004 to 2006. There was a 70% increase in new infections in the region between 2004 and 2006.

In South and South-East Asia, the number of new HIV infections rose by 15% in 2004-2006, while in the Middle East and North Africa it grew by 12%.

Countries with previously low prevalence can experience sudden upsurges of HIV for the same reason as Scotland did in 1984 - due to HIV suddenly arriving among injecting drug users. This happened in Indonesia and 1999-2000 and appears to be happening right now in the formerly low-prevalence countries of central Asia such as Uzbekistan.

Young people are bearing the brunt of infections, with approximately 50% of all new cases of HIV in people aged 15 to 24. Almost 12 million young people under 25 are thought to be infected with HIV, and 14 million children have lost one or both parents due to AIDS. UNAIDS are predicting that "this number will continue to grow rapidly, as the numbers of adults dying of AIDS rises over the coming years."

"The face of HIV is now the face of a young woman"

Even more than young people, women are now disproportionately affected. Nearly half - 48% - of the world's positive people are women, but in Africa, 59% are now female. The proportion of people with HIV who are women ranges from 26% to 59% in different regions but there is no part of the world where that proportion that are women has not grown. Other parts of the world where the majority or almost the majority of the epidemic is female include the Caribbean, north Africa and the middle east, and the Pacific.

In the parts of the world where the epidemic is 'mature' it follows a remorseless spread from vulnerable groups like sex workers, gay men and drug users into bisexual men, drug users' partners and sex workers clients, and from there into a group of people formerly at low risk - namely, married or monogamous women.

In some parts of the world marriage is actually a risk factor for HIV. "Focusing programmes on persuading girls to abstain from sex until marriage is of little help to many young women," is UNAIDS' comment.

Among sexually active girls in the cities of Ndola in Zambia and Kisumu in Kenya, HIV infection rates were 10% higher in married women under 25 than in single women. Ninety per cent of women testing HIV-positive in Indian antenatal clinics say they are in a long-term monogamous relationship, 90% of HIV-positive women in Lima, Peru, say they have had no more than two sex partners in their life, and in Uganda 88% of girls with HIV under 19 are married. In Thailand in 1992, 90% of HIV transmission was occurring between sex workers and their clients. By 2002, 50% of HIV infections occurred within marriage, as former sex-worker clients infected their wives.

In South Africa, Zambia and Zimbabwe young women aged 15-24 are three to six times as likely to have HIV as young men - in Ghana nine times more likely - and more than three-quarters of people living with HIV under 25 in Africa are female. Half the people with HIV in the Caribbean are also female.

There is an urgent need for more prevention options that women can use other than attempting to persuade men to use condoms.

Female condoms have not taken off in the developed world, but have become popular in parts of Africa and Asia. In Senegal, the condoms are sold with noisy "bine bine" beads; an erotic accessory that women wear around their hips. The rustle of the polyurethane during sex is now associated with the clicking of the beads. In Zimbabwe a new word - kaytec-yenza - has entered the vernacular to describe the "tickle" created by the inner ring rubbing against the penis. And in India sex workers allow clients to insert the condom themselves - a huge thrill, in a culture where touching the vagina or viewing it closely is taboo.

However the female condom is expensive and is not an option for married women, which is why increasing amounts of money are being put into the development of microbicides. One study estimates that if a 60%-efficacious microbicide was used by only 20% of women in 73 low-income countries, 2.5 million infections could be averted over three years among men, women and children.

At the moment the world waits to see if any of the first generation of candidate microbicides will prove to be effective - even in the context of a clinical trial. The closure in December 2006 of the CONRAD-sponsored trial of the microbicide cellulose sulphate when significantly more HIV infections were found amongst women using the microbicide at one trial site than amongst women using a placebo was a reminder that there may be no 'magic bullet' prevention method that will make women less vulnerable to HIV.

Surveys that ask questions about how women are culturally and institutionally vulnerable to HIV tend to reveal that they are for the same reasons they lack control over reproduction, and that the ultimate answer to reducing women's vulnerability to the virus will be to enable to world's women to achieve a decent standard of education and of financial independence.

Sex workers

One way women have, over the centuries, attempted to become financially independent, or simply to survive, increases their vulnerability to HIV - to become **sex workers**. In most developing

countries of the world apart from in sub-Saharan Africa, sex workers and their clients have been the second group of people into whom HIV has spread after establishing a foothold in injecting drug users. This was the case in Thailand and Cambodia in the early 1990s and appears to be happening right now in China, Russia and parts of the Middle East.

A huge and polarised ideological debate has arisen as to whether sex work is a mark of the exploitation and degradation of women, and the way to reduce women's vulnerability to HIV is to suppress it, or whether it will always happen, is at least potentially a route out of dependence on men, and the way to reduce women' vulnerability in the trade is to educate them and support sex workers' moves towards self-organisation.

Both may be true according to context. The trafficking and effective slavery of poor Nepali girls into India (see Human Rights Watch) and east European women into London (Dickson) are just the best-researched examples of what is acknowledged to be a worldwide phenomenon that exposes women to disease, violence and exploitation and not only them, but their clients, to HIV. Since many of those clients are outwardly 'respectable' married men, sex work then becomes a means by which HIV spreads into the general heterosexual population.

In May 2005 Brazil became the first country to turn down financial assistance from the US PEPFAR (President's Executive Programme for AIDS Relief) programme because its conditions included a requirement that grant recipients should not support programmes that in any way supported sex workers (Boseley and Goldenberg).

On the other hand, sex workers have shown a remarkable ability in disparate countries to self-organise and self-educate themselves about HIV. Examples such as Calcutta's Sonagachi project (Biswas) and Cambodia's Women's Network for Unity are a reminder that HIV and its associated stigma have in some cases forced previously marginalised and powerless communities to band together and claim a voice on the global stage. This has not always been a smooth process, even within the AIDS activist community, with campaigners against sex work and trafficking co-existing alongside self-help projects in places like Cambodia, each claiming to represent the interests of "the community". It is this kind of political tension that contributed to the closure of the tenofovir pre-exposure prophylaxis trial in that country - see **HIV Prevention** for more.

References

Biswas R. *The Red Lights of Sonagachi*. Positive Nation, issue 85/6, December 2002.

Boseley S and Goldenberg S. Brazil spurns US terms for AIDS help. The Guardian, 4 May 2005. For the PATHWAY Act which established PEPFAR see www.pepfarwatch.org/pubs/WomenandAIDSLeeBill.pdf

Burt K. *Whatever happened to the Femidom?* The Guardian, 23 August 2005.

Dickson S. *Sex in the City: Mapping Commercial Sex across London.* Poppy Project report, 2004. See www.endviolenceagainstwomen.org.uk/documents/Sex%20in%20the%20City.pdf

Human Rights Watch. *Rape for Profit: Trafficking of Nepali Girls and Women to India's Brothels.* HRW reports 12(5), October 1995. See www.hrw.org/reports/1995/India.htm.

Women's Network for Unity: see www.womynsagenda.org/programs/sexworker/SW/swnu.html

The invisible men

There is some evidence that many of the husbands of women who infect them with HIV are not picking up the virus from female sex workers, but from other men. In the developed world, gay men are often the most visible and best-informed group of people with HIV. In the developing world, the opposite is usually the case, with men who have sex with men (MSM) often the most marginalised, least researched and least visible at-risk group. In the Caribbean, UNAIDS comments: "Sex between men, which is heavily stigmatised and in some places illegal, remains a significant - but still neglected - aspect of the epidemics." In Chennai, India, six per cent of men reported sex with other men, and 57% of them also reported that they were married to women. A study from Galle in Sri Lanka (Perera) found that 12.5% of male teenagers aged 18-19 reported having had anal sex - and only 0.8% of female teenagers.

In the parts of the world where there actually is surveillance of HIV among men who have sex with men, high rates of HIV are found. HIV prevalence among gay men in Bangkok was 17% in 2004; in 2006 this had increased to 28.4%, and this appears to be the tip of an iceberg of increasing HIV infection amongst MSM in cities widely spaced around south-east Asia. The same has long been the case in Latin America, where MSM have always been the most-affected population. In Lima, Peru, HIV prevalence in MSM in 2004 was 22%, and 87% of Peruvian men who had sex with men also reported sex with women; in Guayaquil, Ecuador, prevalence was 27% in 2005 compared with only 7% in the rest of the country outside the capital Quito, reminding us that gay epidemics as often highly localised. And in one survey of gay men in five cities in the USA, the infection rate among black men who have sex with men has now reached a scarcely believable 48%.

Sex between men remains a virtually unresearched area in Africa. One poster (Zulu) at the International AIDS Society Conference in Rio in 2005 sought out men who have sex with men in Zambia. It found complete ignorance of homosexual HIV risks. One in five men said they had had a sexually transmitted infection, but thought you could only catch STIs from women, and three-quarters of them believed having anal sex with a man was safer than having sex with a woman.

Since then a few more studies of MSM in Africa have been conducted. At the 2006 International AIDS Conference, Frits van Griensven of the US CDC, who conducted the prevalence surveys amongst gay men in Bangkok, cited studies that had found HIV prevalence amongst MSM in Africa of 38% in Kilifi, Kenya (compared with 6.1% in the general population); 21.5% in Dakar, Senegal (general prevalence: 0.9%); and 9.3% in Khartoum, Sudan (general prevalence: 1.6%).

Given estimates of the proportion of men in the different locations who were MSM, this meant that 10% of the adult HIV prevalence in Kenya might be due to sex between men; 17% in Sudan; and 36% in Senegal.

In contrast, in Ukraine, of the 62,365 people officially reported as having HIV since 1987, only 44 cases have been attributed to sex between men - an equally unbelievable figure. Gay men are only found where they are looked for, and UNAIDS' comment is that this is "a curiously low figure which lends credence to concerns that HIV might be spreading largely undetected among men who have sex with men."

It is not just in the developing world that marginalised communities of gay men are significant drivers of HIV. In the USA the epidemic has shifted from being on largely concentrated in gay men and intravenous drug users, largely white, to being a black epidemic with heterogeneous risk factors and with ten times the infection rate in black Americans as in white. A high proportion of these infections are in young black men who may or may not identify as gay.

Centers for Disease Control researchers examined trends in new HIV diagnoses (with or without AIDS) among persons 13 to 24 years of age between 1994 and 2003 in 25 US states with longstanding, name-based HIV reporting.

Results indicate that new diagnoses declined significantly among young women, but rose among young men. Among 13 to 24 year-old females, new HIV diagnoses fell 20% over the 10-year period. HIV diagnoses also declined among young men for the first few years of the period (by 30% from 1994 to 1998); but the decline was offset by a 41% increase from 1999 to 2003. The increase among young men was driven by a 47% rise in diagnoses among MSM ages 20-24, 60% of whom were black, and 67% of whom were unaware of their HIV status.

References

Perera PB. *Unprotected anal sex: an important risk factor for HIV in a resource-limited population in Asia*. Third IAS Conference on HIV Pathogenesis and Treatment, Rio de Janeiro, abstract MoPe11.10C10, 2005.

Thebody.com. *Data From 2005 National HIV Prevention Conference Give Clearer Picture of U.S. HIV Epidemic and Improved Strategies to Confront It*. 13 June 2005 - see http://www.thebody.com/cdc/prevention_conference.html

Van Griensven S. *What's Driving the Global MSM Epidemic?* 14th Conference on Retroviruses and Opportunistic Infections, Los Angeles, 2007. Abstract 55.

Zulu KP. *Anal sex and HIV - an ignored tragedy, a case of Zambia*. Third IAS Conference, Rio de Janeiro, abstract MoPe10.7P03, 2005.

Who's at most risk?

Despite the image of HIV as predominantly affecting certain groups of people, the global epidemic in fact affects very different proportions of the primary at-risk groups depending on which part of the world they live in.

The following chart is adapted from UNAIDS, CDC and HPA data and shows the proportion of adults living with HIV who were infected through sex between men, injecting drug use, and heterosexual sex and other exposures in five different parts of the world: the USA, the UK, Latin America, Eastern Europe and Central Asia, and South and South-East Asia (excluding India, where the majority of exposures appear to come from non-commercial heterosexual contact, and where the sheer population size drowns out the signal from other countries in the region.

It is of course no indication of the relative numbers infected in the different regions, only the relative contribution different avenues of infection make to the epidemic in the five areas. It is also subject to caveats such as the above-cited invisibility of homosexual sex, and the sometimes blurred definition of what constitutes 'commercial' sex. In the USA the small number 94%) of gay men who were also injecting drug users has been divided evenly between the categories.

UNAIDS goes one step further and in Latin America, Eastern Europe and Central Asia subdivides heterosexual infections into ones acquired between commercial sex workers and their clients, and ones acquired in through non-commercial heterosexual sex.

It can immediately be seen that the virus is 'targeting' very different groups of people and because of this resources spent on treatment and care and above all prevention must be allocated differently. In the USA we see a steady or slightly increasing number of gay infections, a declining number of ones acquired through injecting drug use, and an increasing number of heterosexual ones. In the UK a predominantly gay epidemic has been transformed into a 50/50 gay/heterosexual epidemic, but one where the predominant mode if infection within the country is still sex between men. In Latin America there is and always has been a much more varied epidemic, partly due to bisexual behaviour amongst men. In Eastern Europe and Central Asia the epidemic is still overwhelmingly led by injecting drug users, but there are worrying signs that heterosexual infections are starting to increase. And in most countries of south and south-east Asia there is still a chance to direct prevention messages towards commercial sex workers and their clients in an effort to stem a rising epidemic amongst heterosexuals.

These regional charts of course generalise badly and don't take account of between-country differences; but they do serve as a reminder that one size does not fit all when it comes to targeting prevention messages.

More than one in four has access to HIV treatment

In the 2002 edition of this manual, about 4% of people in the developing world who were in need of antiretrovirals to treat AIDS had access to them. By 2004, this had increased fourfold to about 16%. By 2006 this had near-doubled again to 28%, though access is very uneven. It ranges from nearly 90% in countries like Brazil and Botswana, to 35-40% in Uganda, Kenya and Rwanda, but still only 5% in some other African countries such as Tanzania, and less than that in some countries of eastern Europe - including Russia, a country which 'on paper' is rich enough to afford ARVs..

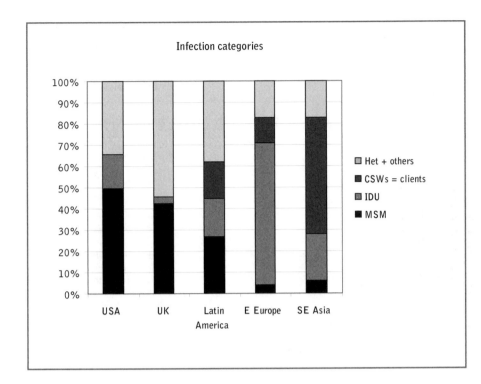

Infection categories

Ugandamade against AIDS in the 1990s, and HIV prevalence has again been rising in some rural areas.

See under Uganda for more.

Africa

Sub-Saharan Africa has just over 10% of the world's population, but is home to nearly two-thirds (62.5%) of all people living with HIV. The overall prevalence of HIV in Africa is 5.9%. In no other part of the world is it more than a fifth of this figure. Current estimates from UNAIDS are that 24.7 million people are living with HIV or AIDS in sub-Saharan Africa, of whom 13.3 million (59%) are adult women, nine million are young people (aged 15-24) and almost three million are children under 15. An estimated 2.8 million Africans became infected with HIV in 2006, and 2.1 million died of AIDS, representing nearly three-quarters (72%) of global AIDS deaths.

This expansion in treatment, with an estimated one million people worldwide on ARVs by July 2005, was in part due to the '3 by 5' campaign to get three million people on treatment by the end of 2005. See **The History of AIDS** for details.

Successful prevention efforts

UNAIDS report highlights the successful slowing of the spread of HIV in some countries, suggesting that "the world is finally waking up to what it takes to bring [HIV] under control" and that "political commitment has grown hugely in the past two years.grounded in the increasing involvement of community and religious organisations, businesses, individuals and activists."

Highlighted for praise are Zambia which has managed to reduce HIV prevalence amongst women in both urban and rural areas, and Poland, which, unlike much of Eastern Europe, succeeded in curtailing the HIV epidemic amongst injecting drug users and preventing it from spreading to the sexually active population.

In June 2005, it was suggested that HIV prevalence amongst pregnant women in South Africa may have levelled off at 25%, with statisticians noting a slight fall in new cases of HIV detected in under 25s. The 2006 UNAIDS report found evidence of increased safer sex behaviours (increased age at sexual debut and/or reduction in average number of partners and/or increased condom use) amongst young people aged 15-24 in at least nine Africa countries (Ivory Coast, Cameroon, Kenya, Malawi, South Africa, Uganda, Tanzania, Zambia and Zimbabwe) and also in Haiti.

In other cases, however, there are worrying signs that successful HIV prevention efforts are being reversed. Thailand's achievement in cutting HIV prevalence in the early 1990s is now under threat because of 50% prevalence among the one group of people who were excluded from this strategy - injecting drug users. India stands poised on the edge of a generalised HIV epidemic, at least in certain states, as does Russia.

Uganda, praised as "Africa's greatest success story in the fight against AIDS," is a complex case, with both successes and failures. At the end of 2001 adult HIV prevalence had fallen from 8.3% in 1999 to 5%. The South African government's HIV awareness campaigns with young people are also singled out for praise, the 2004 UNAIDS report noting increased rates of safer sex amongst the young. However the 2006 report notes that "new research indicates a possible erosion of the gains

In the early 1990s, no-one really saw quite how massive a problem HIV could become in sub-Saharan Africa. Some countries have seen rises to levels that were previously thought extremely unlikely. There are ten countries in which more than one-tenth of the adult population aged 15-49 is HIV-positive. In four, more than one adult in five now has HIV.

However one cannot really talk about one HIV epidemic in Africa. Although the situation may again change, there are about four different patterns of infection in Africa, though there are individual countries which are exceptions to the rule even in their regions.

The world's epicentre of HIV lies in nine countries in southern Africa. In this so-called 'hyper epidemic', HIV affects more than one in 10 of the population. Amongst these countries, only in Zimbabwe has a scientifically-reliable decline in prevalence been demonstrated since 2004, though there are early signs that prevalence may be starting to decrease in South Africa and Botswana. In other countries like Mozambique HIV has not yet reached its peak.

There is then a fringe of countries round this in eastern and west-central Africa - plus a few outliers like Cote d'Ivoire - where HIV prevalence in many is still higher than it is in any other continent, but to nothing like the level seen in southern Africa. In some east-African countries like Kenya and Uganda, former hyper epidemics of HIV appear to have burned themselves out, at least for now, as the first generation to get HIV have mainly died. The potential for increased incidence and prevalence remains, however.

In other west African countries like Nigeria and Cote d'Ivoire there are signs of a slowly-increasing epidemic or one that has stabilised at a relatively high level. West Africa started to experience high HIV incidence rates later than other parts of the continent and unless treatment and prevention efforts are stepped up, some more of these countries my developed high-prevalence generalised epidemics.

Finally it's important to remember that there are a number of countries in Africa where HIV has been kept within relatively modest limits - lower, for instance than the rate in Haiti (3.8%),

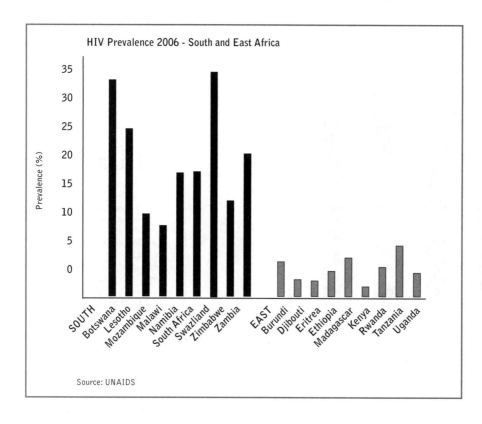

HIV Prevalence 2006 - South and East Africa

Source: UNAIDS

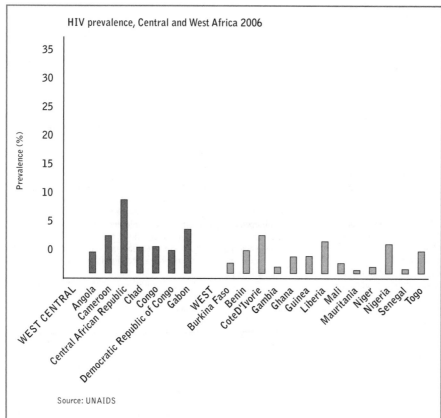

HIV prevalence, Central and West Africa 2006

Source: UNAIDS

hyper epidemic such civil war, a long HIV history, large numbers of displaced persons and extreme poverty, seem to be doing a better-than-expected job of containing HIV.

This is all relative, of course. There is not a single country in mainland Africa that has a lower HIV prevalence than the developed country with the *highest* prevalence, namely the USA.

East Africa

In East Africa, the countries that first bore the brunt of African HIV infection in the 1980s have either successfully made progress in controlling their epidemic during the 1990s or appear to be doing so now.

Even in **Ethiopia**, a populous and poor country tipped to be one of the next to see a large generalised epidemic, HIV prevalence among pregnant women usually seen as the best indicator in the absence of population surveys dropped from 14% in 1997-98 to 11.8% in 1999-2000 and has remained there since, while in Addis Ababa specifically prevalence fell much more sharply form 24% in 1997 to 11% in 2003. Countrywide, surveillance has been unusually inadequate and UNAIDS at present is saying cautiously that the true HIV prevalence in the country could be anything between 0.9% and 3.5% - but this is considerably lower than its 2004 estimate of 4.4%.

Somalia is slowly recovering from a decade or more of civil wars but at present is split into unilaterally-independent areas. A 2004 survey determined prevalence to be 0.9% but noted "zonal variations." In the self-declared autonomous regions of Somaliland and Puntland, prevalence was 1.4% and 1.0%, respectively. Antenatal prevalence in Somaliland rose from 0.9% in 1999 to 1.4% in 2004, while prevalence was 3.5% among STD patients and 5.6% among TB patients (Reference: Agence-France Presse).

the world's highest-prevalence country outside Africa, or Belize (2.5%), the continental country with the highest rate. These include countries in west Africa and the Horn of Africa that have so far remained - at least by African standards - relatively untouched by HIV, often through adopting prevention programmes in time. However there are promising signs that some central African countries like Rwanda and the Democratic Republic of Congo, despite having numerous risk factors for a

Eritrea next door is also recovering from decades of war; its first comprehensive surveillance programme in 2003 found HIV prevalence of 2.4%.

In **Kenya** HIV appears to be continuing to decline. There data from antenatal clinics show HIV prevalence in pregnant women falling from 13.6% in 1997-8 to 9.4% in 2002-03. Figures from **Rwanda**and **Burundi** also show some signs of a decline.

Tanzania up till 2004 was the one exception to this east African success story. Its overall prevalence has now fallen. In parts of the country where there have been intensive prevention programmes, prevalence has fallen from 20.5% to 14.6% in pregnant women between 1994 and 2000, whereas in areas that have not seen programmes, it rose from 22.5% to the very high figure of 30.2%. However both intensified prevention efforts and the beginnings of treatment access appeared to be paying off in 2005/6 and the latest estimate for the country's HIV prevalence put it at slightly lower than Uganda's.

For **Sudan,** see North Africa and the Middle East.

The case of Uganda

Uganda has long been lauded as a success story of HIV prevention. Although much of the decline in prevalence is due to the fact that, as the first country in the world with a generalised epidemic, much of the first high-prevalence generation has now died. But without the prevention campaigns of the late 1980s, its current prevalence of 5-6% would look a lot more like the 24% prevalence back in 1990.

In a late breaker presented at the Twelfth Annual Retrovirus Conference in early 2005, it was suggested that mortality, not behavioural change, had been the main cause of the decline in HIV prevalence seen in Uganda during the 1990s. Maria Wawer of Columbia University in New York said that increased deaths due to AIDS contributed 5% of the 6% decline in prevalence seen in the Rakai district between 1993 and 2004.

Annual incidence had not declined during the same period, and prevalence among young people under 19 had also not changed.

She also found that while condom use has increased sharply over the last ten years, this has been counterbalanced by increases in other sexual risk behaviour and that Ugandans, at least in Rakai, appear to be less abstinent and less faithful than they were. The implication is that if HIV treatment starts to reduce mortality in the area, HIV prevalence may actually increase, following a pattern seen in parts of the developed world.

Wawer was presenting findings from the Ugandan Open and Positive Programme, which has conducted continuous surveillance of HIV incidence and prevalence (via blood tests) and sexual behaviour (via questionnaires) of 44 communities in the Rakai district since 1993.

Wawer said HIV prevalence during that time had declined from about 20 to 13% in women and from 15 to 9% in men. However the incidence of new cases had not changed. It was 1.3% a year in 1993 / 4 and 1.7% in 2003 / 4, a non-significant difference.

Condom use had increased among men and women significantly during that time. For instance, in male teenagers (15 - 19) with casual partners it had doubled from 19 to 38%. Women reported using condoms 28% of the time among non-married partners but only 1% of the time with husbands.

However other sexual risk-taking behaviour had increased. Forty per cent of 15 to 19 year-old males were sexually active in 1993 / 4. This had increased to 50% by 2003 / 4. The number of men (aged 15 - 49) reporting two or more sexual partners in a year increased from 22 to 27% in the decade. Of particular concern was that 48% of men diagnosed with HIV during 1993 / 4 reported two or more sexual partners. This had increased to 69% in 2002 / 3. Wawer commented that there was no way of telling if extramarital sexual activity was a cause of, or subsequent to, their HIV infection.

Given a flat incidence rate, the main cause of the decrease in prevalence was death. The mortality rate due to AIDS increased in Rakai from 12% in 1990 to 14% in 2002. In 2001 to 2003 there were 125 new cases of HIV among the study population,

and 200 deaths. Death therefore contributed to more than 80% of the decline in prevalence.

There is considerable concern that in other parts of the country prevalence appears to be on the rise again.

In a second study in 2006 (Baryarama), a team of Ugandan researchers sifted through the positive diagnoses amongst no fewer than 203,000 people who came forward for HIV testing between 1992 and 2003. They calculated what proportion of the previously HIV-negative became positive during the course of each year.

They found that, based on figures from people coming forward for testing, annual incidence increased from 0.9% a year in 1993 to 2.3% in 2003. In other words, whereas about one in every 110 Ugandans caught HIV in 1993, one in every 44 caught it in 2003.

The researchers also found that, in line with national surveys, though not as dramatically, HIV prevalence amongst the population decreased from 23% in 1999 to 13% in 2000. Since than, however, it has started going up again and now stands at 15%, though this is not as yet a statistically significant trend.

This rate is higher than those calculated for the whole population since this is the rate amongst people coming forward for testing. The age at which people catch HIV has also increased over time, with the most at-risk age period shifting from people in their mid-20s in the early 90s to people in their early 30s today.

This survey's results may well be disputed as they depend on extrapolating from diagnosis figures, and they also make assumptions about the death rate from AIDS. However they certainly don't support the widespread idea that, since 1993 at least, Uganda has been an HIV success story.

"Our analysis reveals a new phase of the HIV epidemic in Uganda," say the researchers. "These findings support the need for intensified prevention interventions among middle-aged persons."

So, is Uganda a success story or a failure? The answer is probably that, although the majority of the decline in prevalence in Uganda in the 1990s was due to AIDS mortality, early and comprehensive prevention efforts also helped ensure that the eventual, ongoing HIV prevalence in the country was lower than it otherwise would have been.

Southern Africa

Southern Africa is now by a long way the most affected part of the world. In all nine countries in the region more than one adult in ten has HIV and four countries more than one in five. A third (32%) of people with HIV globally lives in these countries and a third of AIDS deaths occur there.

South Africa itself continues to have the most people with HIV of any country in the world, and the epidemic here does not appear to have reached saturation point, with prevalence among pregnant women continuing to rise in all states except Free State and Gauteng. Overall it was 27.9% in 2003 compared with 26.5% in 2002, and was at the hyper epidemic level of 37.5% in KwaZulu Natal. In 2006 the latest data showed a continuing, rising trend nationally in HIV infection levels among pregnant women attending public antenatal clinics to 30.2% in 2005

However, HIV prevalence among young people may be stabilising. Antenatal surveillance suggests that HIV prevalence among 15- 24- year-old pregnant women has remained relatively stable since 2000 at 14%-16% among 15-19- year-olds and 28%-31% among 20-24-year-olds.

The most tragic consequence is that, having started later, South Africa's epidemic has now reached the stage where increasing numbers of people are dying of AIDS. The latest official mortality data show total deaths (from all causes) in South Africa increased by 79% from 1997 to 2004. Death rates from natural causes for women aged 25-34 years increased fivefold between 1997 and 2004, and for males aged 30-44 they more than doubled.

Nine countries in Africa, all in the south with the exception of the Central African Republic now have life expectancies at birth of less than 40 years. In Namibia, adult female mortality was 3.5 times the level in 2000 than it was in 1993. In **Zimbabwe**, life expectancy at birth was 34 in 2003, compared with 52 in 1990. And in the South African province of KwaZulu Natal, half of all adults were dying of AIDS or HIV-associated TB by 2000. In southern Africa, the Great Dying has begun, with incalculable effects on the fabric of society.

There are some signs of hope. Up till 2004 there was early evidence that the epidemic in **Zambia** might be following a similar course to Kenya and Uganda; HIV rates among pregnant 15-19 year olds in the capital Lusaka almost halved from around 28% to near 14% between 1996 and 2002. However the country's HIV prevalence now seems to have stabilised at 17%, with little change between 2004 and 2006.

The only 'success story' in terms of prevalence, if it can be called that, is **Zimbabwe.** Here antenatal clinic data show HIV infection levels in pregnant women, which were hovering at 30%-32% in the early 2000s before declining to 24% in 2004. In the capital, Harare, prevalence among pregnant women peaked at over 36% in 1996 before falling to approximately 21% in mid-2004. The observed declines in prevalence appear to be related to a combination of factors, especially reductions in casual sex relations with non-regular partners, along with increases in condom use and later sexual debuts.

Whereas in the early 2000s it Zimbabwe was on track to overtake Swaziland and Botswana as the world's worst-affected country, a combination of factors, including despite chronic economic mismanagement, a relatively intact health infrastructure, seems to have helped it avoid this distinction. Nonetheless, Zimbabwe still has one of the worst HIV epidemics in the world, with one in five of its citizens living with HIV.

Tiny **Swaziland** now has this dubious distinction, though even here mass-media HIV prevention campaigns and more recently an increasing interest in male circumcision may help to reverse the course of the epidemic.

In the middle of all this devastation is **Botswana**, a small-population country with a quarter of its population HIV-positive, relative prosperity by African standards and, uniquely not only for Africa but for most of the developing world, 90% of its citizens who need them on antiretrovirals and a programme to get every adult to test for HIV. Botswana is in many ways a fascinating experiment into what might be possible and the limits of HIV treatment. No one has ever tried putting a large proportion of the population of a country on HIV treatment before. It will be interesting to see what happens to its life expectancy and if the huge cost of its programme can be maintained.

So far the signs seem to be good: the proportion of people with HIV in Botswana has fallen from one in three to one in four in two years, a third of the country's adult population has taken an HIV test, and AIDS mortality apparently peaked in 2003. In this year, one in every 166 Batswana died compared with one in 500 in 1994, but by 2006 this had declined to one in 220 and the trend towards increased upward life expectancy seemed to be accelerating.

However, astonishingly, comprehensive knowledge of HIV remains low: only about one in three young people aged 15-24 both correctly identified ways of preventing the sexual transmission of HIV and rejected major misconceptions about HIV transmission.

West Africa

In West Africa, HIV prevalence exceeds 5% in five countries in west and central Africa, namely Cameroon (5.4%), the Central African Republic (10.7%), Côte d'Ivoire (7.1%), the Congo Republic (5.3%) and Gabon (7.9.

In west-central Africa, the sharp rise in HIV prevalence among pregnant women in **Cameroon** (more than doubling to over 11% among those aged 2024 between 1998 and 2000), shows how suddenly the epidemic can surge, but in this country and the neighbouring **Central African Republic** prevalence in pregnant women now seems to have stabilised, albeit at the high level of 10%.

Encouragingly, prevalence in the **Democratic Republic of the Congo** continues to decline slowly, from 5% in 2002 to 4.2% in 2004 and to 3.2% in 2006. Cô´¥|#160;dIvoire remains the worst-affected country in West Africa, but even here prevalence has fallen from 13% in 1999 to 6.4% in 2003. West Africa also contains success stories like **Senegal**, which has kept its prevalence below 1% throughout the epidemic, with imaginative and bold HIV prevention campaigns taking place in Islamic schools and elsewhere, though prevalence among female sex workers in the capital Dakar was recently reported to be around 15% and higher in other towns.

But the big epidemic in West Africa is in **Nigeria**. Because of its large population (137 million), its 3.9% prevalence means that is has 2.9 million people living with HIV - the third-largest number after South Africa and India. In this diverse and large country, prevalence ranges from a low of 2.2% in the south west, to 7% in the conservative Muslim north and10% in centre of the country.

In 2002 the Nigerian government started an ambitious treatment programme to get 15,000 people on to ARVs within 1 year. In 2004 the programme suffered a major setback when it was hit by a shortage of drugs- some people received no treatment for up to three months, a stark warning about the importance of capacity. The programme eventually resumed but has not yet achieved the 2002 goal because of poor infrastructure and management.

Nigeria is also a country that has seen many people afraid to come forward for testing and treatment due to stigma against people living with HIV. HIV-positive people often lose their jobs or are denied healthcare services because of the ignorance and fear about HIV and AIDS. One recent survey found that 60% of healthcare workers thought HIV-positive patients should be isolated from other patients.

Nineteen African countries have set up national HIV councils or commissions at senior levels of government even Somaliland, an autonomous region of Somalia, set up one in 2005 - and local responses are growing in number. Across the region, 40 countries have completed national strategic AIDS plans evidence of their determination to reach the targets outlined in the UN Declaration of Commitment on HIV. Also encouraging is the active involvement of regional bodies, such as the Economic Commission for Africa, the Africa Union, and the Southern African Development Community, in tackling HIV as a development issue.

AIDS orphans

When one considers that half of all people who become HIV-positive do so before they reach their 25th birthday and progress to AIDS and death by the time that they reach 35, it is hardly surprising that a generation of children are left parentless, to be brought up by their grandparents or often among child-headed households.

Current estimates suggest that the cumulative number of children who have lost their mother or both parents to AIDS before the age of 15 since the epidemic began stands at 12,100 000 for sub-Saharan Africa alone. By 1997, in many African countries, the proportion of children who had lost one or both parents to AIDS had reached between 7 and 11%. Pre-AIDS estimates of orphans in developing nations pitched the rate at 2%.

Across Africa, many governments have rallied support in order to set up mechanisms to care for the children left behind. As early as 1986, Janet Museveni, wife of the Ugandan President Yoweri Museveni set up UWESO, the Uganda Women's Effort to Save Orphans. It was intended to assist orphans in the resettlement camps used after the civil war and eventually return the children to their extended families. The organisation now has 35 branches nationwide and funds education and training for the children as well as helping the guardians of the children -usually female relatives of the children- to set up small businesses.

The impact on education

It has been suggested that children finish school when their parents die, regardless of their age. Large household surveys are beginning to validate these claims. Certainly, it would appear that when both parents die the likelihood of a child continuing in education diminishes even further.

It is not uncommon for dying parents to marry their daughters off, partly to ensure that she is cared for after their death. In one study of orphans in Kenya, 41% of girls left school to get married and 28% because they became pregnant.

HIV has been shown to take up precious resources, and even when a child has two parents who are alive, the cost of care for them should they become sick, can have a direct effect upon the amount of money that is available for education.

In the Central African Republic, a recent study has shown that as many as 107 schools have closed due to staff shortage, and only 66 remain open. Over 85% of deaths among teachers between 1996 and 1998 were due to AIDS. As many teachers died between 1996 and 1998 as retired.

In Zambia, around 2000 new teachers are trained each year. During the first ten months of 1998, the country lost 1300 teachers to AIDS. It has been suggested that HIV has further exacerbated the gap between educational achievement in rural areas and the cities. Many teachers are disinclined to work in rural areas, largely because of a desire to be close to some kind of health care.

The impact on the economy

HIV has the potential to restrict economic growth through:

- reducing the number of workers available and increasing production costs which, in turn, could reduce international competitiveness.

- decreasing personal, corporate and public sector savings as a result of HIV-related expenses.

- reducing the amount any government can invest in infrastructure, as spending on HIV increases.

Food insecurity

HIV devastates the agricultural sector. It causes farm labour losses and depletes family income that would normally purchase food, with a resultant impact on the health of the entire population. A recent famine in Zimbabwe - a country formerly known as 'the breadbasket of Africa' - was in part caused by HIV reducing adults' capacity to work on the land.

AIDS is intensifying chronic food shortages. In Zambia, research shows the poorest economically active households rely heavily on cash income for food. When the price of food increases, poor families are hit hardest.

In high-prevalence countries, a vicious cycle exists between food shortages, malnutrition and AIDS. In Zimbabwe, by 2000, AIDS had robbed the country of between 5 and 10% of its agricultural workforce. By 2020, farm labour losses will approach 25%. In Malawi, households that lost females under age 60 were twice as likely to experience a food deficit as households in which men in the same age bracket had died. In Uganda, 1990s research demonstrated food insecurity and malnutrition were the most serious problems for many female-headed AIDS-affected households.

Food insecurity is especially damaging for people living with HIV because they need more calories than uninfected individuals.

Furthermore, malnourished HIV-infected people progress more quickly to AIDS. HIV prevention, nutritional care, and AIDS mitigation measures need to be incorporated into general food security and nutrition programmes.

A security issue

Development in countries badly affected by HIV has clearly been undermined. HIV in sub-Saharan Africa is now deadlier than war itself. To put this in context, during 1998 200,000 people died as a result of war in sub-Saharan Africa. The number lost to AIDS in the same year was already ten times higher, at 2 million.

AIDS is rapidly becoming the major issue for human security in sub-Saharan Africa. On the 10 January 2000 the United Nations Security Council held a meeting on AIDS in Africa. This was the very first time that the Security Council had discussed any health issue.

The prevalence of HIV among military personnel is often higher than in the population as a whole, following the long-established pattern of other sexually transmitted infections. This has serious implications for the role of the military within societies as well as internationally, in peacekeeping operations.

An even deeper concern raised by HIV and AIDS is that large numbers of orphans, lacking in education and adult guidance, may be recruited into militias and armies that then destabilise the continent. The breakdown of government and society in Sierra Leone and Liberia is seen as an awful warning of what could happen elsewhere.

This concern can be overdone: some have suggested that the current regimes in Uganda and Rwanda, which are credited with having restored order and improved government to deeply traumatised countries, were both installed by "armies of orphans".

References (Uganda):

Baryarama F et al. *Estimating HIV incidence in voluntary counseling and testing clients in Uganda (1992-2003)*. JAIDS 44(1):99-105. 2007.

Wawer MJ et al. *Declines in HIV prevalence in Uganda: not as simple as ABC*. Twelfth Conference on Retroviruses and Opportunistic Infections, Boston, abstract 27LB, 2005.

Asia (From Iran to Japan)

There were an estimated 8.6 million people living with HIV in south, south-east and east Asia, 2.4 million of them women, in December 2006. Unlike in Africa, where the figures were revised slightly downward between 2002 and 2004, this represented an increase of 23% between 2002 and 2006 and a 33% increase among women. Approximately 630,000 people are estimated to have died of AIDS in the past year, a 16% increase in the AIDS death toll since 2004.

Over the whole of this vast area HIV prevalence about 0.5% - one in 200 people - but because Asia contains 55% of the world's population this means a lot of people with HIV. There is considerable variation between countries, both in terms of prevalence per head of population and because Asian's countries range from the world's two most populous countries to some of its smallest, in terms of absolute numbers.

In China, Bangladesh, Pakistan, the Philippines and Sri Lanka, HIV prevalence is still lower than it is in the UK, and in far-flung Mongolia it is virtually zero. But Thailand has ten times as many people living with HIV as the UK in a country with comparable population, Cambodia's 1.6% approaches west African levels, and India, because of its vast population, may already have taken over from South Africa as the country with the most HIV-positive people in the world (but beware: India's HIV figures are unusually uncertain - see below for more details)..

The apparent low prevalence in Asia may be misleading - rates of HIV infection among specific populations, such as sex workers or

Top twelve Asian countries in order of prevalence and absolute numbers with HIV

Country	HIV prevalence	Country	Number with HIV
1. Cambodia	1.6%	1. India	5,700,000
2. Thailand	1.4%	2. China	650,000
3. Myanmar	1.3%	3. Thailand	580,000
4. India	0.9%	4. Myanmar	360,000
5. Malaysia	0.5%	5. Vietnam	260,000
5. Nepal	0.5%	6. Indonesia	170,000
5. Vietnam	0.5%	7. Cambodia	130,000
8. Singapore	0.3%	8. Pakistan	85,000
9. Iran	0.2%	9. Nepal	75,000
10. China	0.1%	10. Malaysia	69,000
10. Pakistan	0.1%	11. Iran	66,000
10. Laos	0.1%	12. Japan	17,000

All other countries have less than 0.1% prevalence, i.e. less than half of UK prevalence

intravenous drug users (IDUs) within each of these countries may be much higher. HIV rates among drug injectors in China range from 18% to 56%; prevalence in Thai drug users approaches 50% and in gay men, 15-30%; and India is a patchwork of localised epidemics, with prevalence ranging (as far as can be told from its inadequate surveillance system) from very low in some states to over 3% in others.

Within the largest Asian nations, some regions may have a greater number of inhabitants than most African countries as well as having HIV prevalence rates much higher than the national average.

In Asia, there is immense social pressure on men to marry and have children. A well-established gay identity is non-existent, and men who have sex with men tend to be married too. Men who engage in male-male sex as well as heterosexual sex with their wives, or female partners, are more likely to be HIV-positive than their exclusively heterosexual counterparts.

Throughout the region, injecting drug use offers the epidemic huge scope for growth. Upwards of 50% of injecting drug users already have acquired the virus in parts of Malaysia, Myanmar, Nepal, Thailand and in Manipur in India.

In Japan, prevalence is still low with about 17,000 people (most of them males) with HIV, but this number slowly increased between 1994 and 2004 and then jumped by 5,000 (42%) in two years. Here, the virus is spreading increasingly among young people. A reportedly growing trend of casual sex with multiple partners (known as sukusutomo or 'sex friends'), along with falling condom sales, suggests that new patterns of HIV spread could widen significantly.

Nearly 40% of new HIV infections in 2001 were among people in their teens and twenties-a development that seems to match reports of increased rates of sexually transmitted infection among Japanese men (up 21% between 1998 and 2000) and women (up 14%) under 24.

India : the world's largest HIV epidemic - or just the most complex?

The exact number of people living in the world's second-largest and probably most varied country is a highly contentious subject. UNAIDS gives wider margins of uncertainty than it does for nearly any other country, estimating that though the best guess is something near 5.7 million people, it could be as low as 3.4 million or as high as 9.4 million (even at the low end, it is nearly an order of magnitude larger than any other Asian HIV epidemic in terms of numbers). We have explained above why India's patchy surveillance system and largely private health care makes assessing accurate figures particularly difficult.

In parts of north-east India, widespread injecting drug use helped establish an early entry-point for HIV. In Manipur in 1988 the prevalence of HIV was hardly detectable. Just four years later, HIV prevalence had risen to over 70% among injecting drug users and has stayed at this level ever since, and prevalence in pregnant women has risen from 1% to 5% in the cities, though prevalence in the state as a whole is only around 1.5%, not as high as in Maharashtra and Andhra Pradesh (2.5-3.0%). Typically, the majority of injecting drug users are men who will eventually pass HIV to their wives, girlfriends or other sexual partners through unprotected sex.

UNAIDS comments that "there are signs that injecting drug use is playing a bigger role in India's epidemics than previously thought." In Chennai in the high-prevalence state of Tamil Nadu, for instance, 64% of injecting drug users had HIV by 2003. Nearly half of them lived with a wife or regular sex partner.

A different pattern has been seen in southern and western states. By the mid- 1990s, a quarter or more of sex workers in cities such as New Delhi, Hyderabad, Madurai, Pune, Tirupati, and Vellore tested positive for HIV. By 1997 the prevalence of HIV among sex workers in Mumbai had reached 71%, despite long-established HIV prevention programmes. In 1996, 14% of truck drivers in Tamil Nadu reported recent unprotected sex with a sex worker.

In the central belt of India, running from Mumbai and Goa in the west to Hyderabad and Pondicherry in the east, there is a generalised HIV epidemic which has spreads into the general heterosexual population. Consequently, women account for a growing proportion of people living with HIV (some 38% in 2005), especially in rural areas. In the higher-prevalence states of the south, most HIV transmission appears to be occurring between sex workers and their clients, and their other sex partners. In Karnataka, for example, almost one quarter (23%) of 1100 female sex workers taking part in a recent study were HIV-infected.

We have already mentioned that a considerable number of men appear to have sex with men in India and though this taboo area is little researched, a few studies do give a glimpse into the gay element to India's epidemics. A study of 6,661 MSMs contacted through parks and cruising areas in Andhra Pradesh in central India showed that the vast majority of them (87%) had had unprotected anal sex, nearly half had had it in the last two weeks, and 20% in their last sexual encounter. Although 85% had heard of AIDS and 70% knew condoms could prevent it, nearly a quarter of them had never even heard of condoms. Forty-one per cent of the men were currently married (though, intriguingly, 2.3% said 'to a man'), and that half of them had had sex with a woman in the last three months, most of it without condoms.

In the two states where such data have been collected, HIV prevalence of 6.8% and 9.6% were found among men who have sex with men in Chennai and Mumbai, respectively. In more recent surveys, HIV prevalence of 12% was found among men who have sex with men seeking voluntary counselling and testing services in Mumbai, and 18% prevalence was found at 10 clinics in Andhra Pradesh

Countrywide, awareness of HIV is high, with roughly three-quarters of adult Indians (aged 15-49) aware that correct and consistent condom use can prevent sexual transmission of HIV. But, in general, awareness and knowledge of HIV remain low in rural areas and particularly among women.

Behavioural studies in India suggest that prevention efforts directed at specific populations (such as female sex workers and injecting drug users) are paying dividends in some states, in the form of higher HIV knowledge levels and condom use. However, HIV prevalence among these key groups continues to increase in some states, underlining the need for well-planned and sustained interventions on a large scale.

At the beginning of this section, under **Sentinel versus population surveillance**, we said that there had been huge controversy about the true burden of HIV in India. This controversy continues.

According to a late-breaker presentation at the Sixteenth International Conference in Toronto in August 2006, population-based HIV prevalence estimates in Andhra Pradesh, the south Indian state thought to have the highest prevalence of HIV, were found to be two-and-half times lower than estimates based on sentinel screening at antenatal and sexual health clinics.

At the end of 2005, India's National AIDS Control Organisation (NACO) estimated that there were 5.21 million people living with HIV, although this figure had been criticised by some as an underestimate.

NACO extrapolates data from the public health system - primarily women testing for HIV during antenatal care, as well as anonymous surveillance from sexual health clinics - in order to estimate HIV prevalence in India, and until now no population-based study had systematically examined the validity of this extrapolation.

Investigators from the Administrative Staff College of India and the Institute of Medical Sciences in Hyderabad sampled 13,838 adults aged 15-49 from 66 rural and urban clusters that represented the 4.5 million adults in the Guntur district of south India's Andhra Pradesh state, which is thought to have the highest HIV prevalence in India. Demographic data were obtained from a total of 12,617 individuals (91.2% of those sampled), and dried blood spots obtained at the same time were tested for HIV antibodies, p24 antigen and HIV RNA. The results were then compared with the HIV estimates from NACO's sentinel surveillance data.

The investigators found that the adjusted HIV rate in adults was 1.72%, with a slightly higher prevalence in men than women. Prevalence was also slightly higher in urban than rural settings, and twice as high in people who were in the lower half of the Standard of Living Index(i.e. poorer), compared with those in the upper half (2.58% vs. 1.20% respectively).

Around 23% of pregnant pregnant women had accessed antenatal care through the public health system in the previous two years. Significantly, they discovered that very poor women were over-represented, which resulted in an unusually high HIV prevalence rate (3.61% versus 1.08% of pregnant women who did not use the public health system). This would have skewed the surveillance-based data which found antenatal clinic HIV prevalence to be 3%.

The investigators calculated that their population-based estimate for the Guntur district is 45,925 adults after adjusting for underrepresented high-risk groups. In contrast, NACO's surveillance-based estimate was 112,635 adults. In other words, population-based HIV prevalence was two-and-a-half times lower than the sentinel surveillance data.

By applying the investigator's population-based estimates to the entire state of Andhra Pradesh, this results in a reduction from 1.44 million adults living with HIV to just over half a million -

and if extended to the whole country would reduce UNAIDS' estimate from 5.7 million to under 2.5 million.

Reference

Dandona L et al. *A population-based study suggests that the HIV estimate for India needs major revision.* Sixteenth International AIDS Conference, Toronto, abstract ThLB0107, 2006.

Thailand

Around 580,000 people were believed to be living with HIV at the end of 2006 in Thailand, or 1.4% of the adult population, though as in India there is a considerable margin of uncertainty as to the actual figures, with low and high limits of 310,000 and one million. This is due concentrated epidemics occurring among two of the most marginalised groups in Thai society - injecting drug users and migrant workers, largely from Myanmar. However in general HIV prevalence continues to edge lower.

The main route of transmission is heterosexual sex. It is currently thought that more than half of all new cases are occurring through transmission within marriage. Thailand, with its '100% condom campaign' in 1992, is one of the few countries to have made a real and demonstrable difference to its HIV epidemic with a comprehensive campaign. But sexual mores in Thailand are changing, and a campaign targeting sex workers and their clients is of less relevance in a society adopting more 'westernised' sexual behaviour, including sex before marriage between teenagers. One study released in advance of the Bangkok World AIDS Conference in 2004 found only 25% of Thai teenagers used condoms. HIV rates among pregnant women are about 2%, particularly in the southern provinces.

About 20% of infections continue to occur through injecting drug use, which was very important in the early establishment of HIV in Thailand, compared with about 5% a decade ago. Median HIV prevalence among IDUs varies from 31% to 51% and despite a strong activist movement among drug users which sprang up in the wake of a rash of extra-judicial killings in 2002/3, needle exchange is still illegal. Methadone maintenance therapy is allowed, but this is of limited use as many of Thailand's more recent IDU HIV infections have been in people injecting 'ya baa' - methamphetamine. Whereas in 1996 70% of Thailand's IDUs were injecting heroin, in 2001 70% were injecting the same drug known to western gay men as 'crystal' or 'Tina'.

In contrast to the pattern seen with blood-borne infections in North America and Western Europe, where sexual transmission and injecting drug use transmission seem to be remarkably separate, there has been a shift in Thailand from a dominance of subtype B virus among IDUs to a dominance of 'subtype E', matching the strain that is most commonly transmitted through sex.

Recent reports suggest that the main modes of transmission may be changing. Whereas most HIV transmission in the 1990s occurred through commercial sex, half the new HIV infections now appear to be occurring among the wives and sexual partners of men who were infected several years ago. There are also indications that unsafe sexual behaviour is on the increase among young people in Thailand.

Finally, as we have already said above, there are alarming signs of extremely high rates of infection amongst young gay men and other MSM in Thailand - and indeed in urban centres in neighbouring countries.

The same survey that found an HIV rate of 17% amongst MSM in Bangkok in 2003 found a rate of 28.3% in 2005. The increase was across the board, in all ages and in gay men recruited at a variety of venues. In 2005 the same survey was extended to Thailand's second city, Chiang Mai, and its largest resort, Phuket. It found prevalence amongst MSM of 15.3% in Chiang Mai and 5.5% in Phuket. Gay men seemed to be catching HIV very young, too - the average prevalence in Bangkok men aged 21 and under was 22.3%.

It is difficult to generalise to other countries in the area as different study methodologies were used, but in Thailand there is hard evidence that there is a rapidly increasing HIV epidemic underway in gay men. Thailand's reputation for relative sexual liberalism only extends to the Thailand tourists see, and non-commercial male-male sex between Thais is still very much a hidden activity. Thai MSM, therefore, missed out on the messages from the '100% condom campaign' in the early 90s. At the start of 2006, in response to the alarming HIV prevalence in gay men, the Thai Ministry of Public Health in conjunction with the charity Family Health International developed a western-style HIV prevention campaign for gay men called "Sex Alert" that will disseminate information through magazine and radio adverts, phone text messages, the internet and on 'mobile media' such as taxis.

Myanmar (previously Burma)

In the previous edition of the AIDS Reference Manual we said that "this oppressed and impoverished country has become the latest candidate for the development of a severe generalised epidemic of HIV in Asia."

Luckily, this appears not to be happening, with HIV remaining concentrated amongst high-risk groups such as IDUs and MSM. The latest figures indicate that the epidemic might be diminishing. HIV infection levels have declined among pregnant women (1.3% in 2005, down from 2.2% in 2000) and among men seeking treatment for other sexually transmitted infections (from 8% in 2001 to 4% in 2005).

Nevertheless, the country is experiencing a serious epidemic, with an estimated 360 000 people living with HIV at the end of 2005, and national adult HIV prevalence of approximately 1.3%. "HIV prevalence of 2.2% among young people aged 15-24 in 2005 is a cause for serious concern," says UNAIDS.

Myanmar's former status as the world's number one producer of opiates (Afghanistan has now taken over) meant that there was an early epidemic among injecting drug users, and 45 to 80 of IDUs have tested positive for HIV in sentinel surveillance every year between 1992 and 2003.

Genetic typing of HIV shows that with the exception of one outbreak in China, virtually all the strains of HIV now circulating in Asia -- from Manipur, India, all the way to Vietnam, from mid-China all the way down to Indonesia, come from Myanmar, with research teams showing that these various HIV strains can be tracked along four major routes, all originating in the country.

Myanmar has not been helped by its oppressive military government: in August 2005 The Global Fund withdrew $35.7 million worth of funding from the country because severe travel restrictions imposed on aid workers meant that, in the Fund's view, they could not mount an effective programme.

Cambodia

Cambodia has about 130,000 people living with HIV, and this 1.6% prevalence rate is the highest in Asia, but the country can count itself in recent years as an HIV success story - estimated prevalence has gone down at least 25% in the last two years. Cambodia has followed Thailand in a very active programme of HIV prevention which has had some success despite the lack of resources available within the country.

It has been the norm in Cambodia for men to engage in premarital and extramarital sex, particularly with women who are paid. There is some evidence that condom use among men using sex workers has increased dramatically in recent years and there are encouraging signs of a decline in HIV rates among pregnant women - from 3.2% in 1997 to 2.3% at the end of 2000. The proportion of men under 24 visiting sex workers in 2003 was 8% - three years previously it had been 19% - and male teenagers are about nine times more likely to use condoms than older men, suggesting prevention programmes are on target.

It has been reported that consistent condom use among direct female sex workers has increased from 43% in 1997 to 96% in 1999. Among non-brothel-based indirect sex workers, consistent condom use increased from 9.6% to 84% over the same period.

HIV prevalence among men who have sex with men in Cambodia was estimated at 15% in a 2000 survey. More recently a survey found a prevalence of 8.9% in the capital Phnom Penh but only 0.8% outside the capital.

Cambodia has reported stabilising levels of infection, along with decreasing levels of high-risk behaviour. HIV prevalence among pregnant women in major urban areas declined slightly from 3.2% in 1996 to 2.8% in 2002. Prevalence among brothel-based sex workers declined from 43% in 1995 to 21% in 2003, according to the latest data we have, with the decline most pronounced among sex workers under 20.

China

China still has a low HIV prevalence of about 0.1% and UNAIDS estimates that there are about 650,000 people with HIV in this, the world's most populous country. China has had an unusual HIV history in that HIV spread from the country to the towns and not the other way round. HIV was originally concentrated among injecting drug users in peripheral provinces such as Yunnan and Xinjiang and 44% of HIV infections are still caused by injecting drug use. The epidemic amongst IDUs is still increasing, and spreading to other provinces. HIV prevalence has exceeded 50% among injecting drug users in parts of Xinjiang, Yunnan and Sichuan provinces. China has now instituted needle exchange, with 92 sites in the affected areas, with the result that the use of non-sterile needles ranged from 27%-79% when the projects began, but had fallen to 12%-56% by end-2005

HIV later erupted into Henan province in mid-China via the selling of infected blood. It has now spread to all 31 provinces. HIV prevalence among Yunnan drug injectors is 21%.

There are also signs of heterosexually transmitted HIV epidemics spreading in at least three provinces (Yunnan, Guangxi and Guangdong) where HIV prevalence in 2000 was as high as 11% among sentinel sex worker populations. Many sex workers inject drugs and in Sichuan province only 40% reported using condoms with clients.

The onward sexual transmission of HIV by people who became infected when they sold their blood to collecting centres that ignored basic blood-donation safety procedures poses a massive challenge, as does the need to provide them with treatment and care.

As in much of the rest of Asia the contribution of men who have sex with men is unknown. A 2005 survey in Beijing found prevalence of 4.6% among gay men in Beijing but only 1.5% in Shanghai.

Unlike India, there are still very low rates of HIV awareness in parts of China. However there are signs that China's strong centralised government is now waking up to its potential HIV problem. Condom distribution schemes have taken off in cities like Guandong.

Vietnam

Vietnam is now in the grip of an increasing HIV epidemic. The number of people living with HIV has doubled since 2000, and reached an estimated 260 000 [150 000-430 000] in 2005. Some 40 000 people are being infected with HIV each year. Rates in IDUs have risen from 9% in 1996 to 30% in 2003 and a 2005 survey in Haiphong and Hanoi found that two-thirds of drug injectors had HIV. Haiphong, the country's largest fort, has an HIV prevalence in female sex workers of 30% in 2005 compared with 12% in Ho Chi Minh City at the other end of the country.

Japan

There are an estimated 17,000 people living with HIV/ AIDS, or 0.03% of the adult population. However annual incidence appears to be accelerating. It doubled between 1992 and 2004 and rose by 2,000 from 2002-4 then by 5,000 between 2004 and 2006. There has been a marked shift in the proportion of transmission due to homosexual sex, which has risen to more than double the proportion due to heterosexual sex; until 1999 the proportions were equal.

Indonesia

Another vast and varied country, Indonesia is still a low-prevalence area for HIV but in the last few years has seen an explosive epidemic happening among injecting drug users. Rates among IDUs in the capital, Jakarta, rose from 8% in 1998 to 48% in 2001 and have stayed at that level, but even in far-flung areas like Kalimantan (Borneo) some surveys have shown that the majority of IDUs are now infected.

Low-prevalence countries

Several highly populous countries in Asia still have low HIV prevalence and, as UNAIDS comments, have the opportunity to keep it that way with imaginative HIV prevention projects. An example is **Bangladesh** where needle-exchange programmes in cities like Dhaka have not only shown a decrease in needle reuse among participants but a 'spin-off' in the form of lower rates of unprotected sex too. As a result for such a [populous and poor country Bangladesh has maintained an extraordinarily low HIV prevalence - only one in 12,000 Bangladeshis appear to have HIV compared with, for instance, one in 500 people in the UK.

Malaysia has just inaugurated needle-exchange - despite protests from conservative Islamists - and as its epidemic is still largely restricted to IDUs it stands a chance of staying a low-prevalence country, though a recent survey found that 17% of HIV transmission was due to unprotected sex. **Pakistan** and the **Philippines** face regular predictions of the eruption of HIV but so far have shown little sign of encroaching HIV prevalence even in high-risk groups like sex workers. In the Philippines the official number of cases of HIV stands at 2,200. UNAIDS estimates that 10,000 HIV-positive people lived in the country in 2003, but even so this is only just over 0.1% of the population. Risk behaviour points to a potential for an epidemic in some of these countries, but so far outreach campaigns seem to have contained HIV with, for instance, the rate of condom use among freelance sex workers in the Philippines increasing from 65 % in 1997 to 72% in 2000 and 80% in 2002.

Pakistan saw its first outbreak of HIV among IDUs in 2004 but so far this does not seem to have spread to the rest of the population, though a 2005 study amongst male sex workers and *hijras* (eunuchs) in Karachi found that 7% of the male sex workers and 2% of the *hijras* were HIV infected, indicating that HIV is starting to spread amongst MSM.

The Caribbean

The Caribbean is the second-most affected area in the world after sub-Saharan Africa, with a regional prevalence of 1.2% or one in 83 adults living with the virus, largely concentrated in five countries with prevalence above 2% - the Bahamas, Belize, Guyana, Haiti and Trinidad and Tobago, though the Dominican Republic and Jamaica, because of their population, have the largest number of people with HIV after Haiti. Nearly three quarters of the 250,000 people living with HIV in the Caribbean are in the two countries of the island of Hispaniola.

UNAIDS estimates that 27,000 people became infected with HIV in the area in 2006 - an eight per cent increase on 2004. Over the past decade, the ratio of men with HIV to women with HIV has narrowed considerably and now nearly as many women as men are infected - about 49% of the total.

By and large the epidemic in the Caribbean is concentrated among heterosexuals, with sex between men and women being the main route of transmission. UNAIDS comments that infections "are being fuelled by a thriving sex industry, which services both local and foreign clients."

Not all of this is heterosexual, though figures are very hard to come by for sex between men as homosexuality is highly stigmatised throughout the area. INAIDS estimates that about 10% of infections come from sex between men. Rates of seroprevalence among men who have sex with men in Jamaica rose from around 10% in 1985 to 15% in 1986, then doubled to 30% over the next decade, but there have been no sentinel surveys among gay men since 1996, and present prevalence among gay men in a country where homosexuality is violently stigmatised is unknown.

There is also evidence of a high rate of HIV infection among injecting drug users in Puerto Rico, where 43% of all HIV cases were among injecting drug users.

Among heterosexuals, a similar disparity is opening up between men and women in infection rates as in Africa. In the Dominican Republic, women under 24 were twice as likely to be infected as their male peers and in Jamaica teenage girls (10-19) are 2.5 times as likely to have HIV as boys. The heterosexual epidemic of the Caribbean has two major driving forces; the early initiation of sexual relationships and the high turnover of sexual partners, common among young people. As is the case in Africa, girls are placed at risk of infection because of the fact that there is much sexual mixing, with young girls frequently becoming the partners of older men.

Twelve countries in this region, including the Dominican Republic and Haiti, several Central American countries (such as Belize and Honduras), and Guyana and Suriname, have an estimated HIV prevalence of 1% or more among pregnant women.

Haiti

Around 190,000 people or 3.8% of the adult population are estimated to be living with HIV. Haiti has by far the worst epidemic of all the countries in the Caribbean, and it is a long-standing epidemic: Haiti appears to be the first country in the western hemisphere to experience AIDS (see **the History of AIDS**). By the end of 1999, it has been estimated that almost 75,000 children had become orphaned by the epidemic. Data from 2004 suggested a decline in HIV prevalence, with rates among women attending antenatal clinics falling from 4.5% in 1996 to 2.8% in 2003/4. However the most recent data, says UNAIDS, suggests that "Haiti's epidemic could take a turn for the worse." There is evidence of ongoing high rates of infection in young women - always a sign that a new generation is becoming infected. New data show that 4.2% of young women in the West, Nippes and North departments of Haiti were HIV-infected in 2005, more than double the 2% prevalence among young men. The one bight spot is that despite being the poorest county in the Americas, Haiti has made slow but steady progress in developing access to antiretrovirals, though still only 12% of the population in need is covered.

Dominican Republic

In this country, sharing the island of Hispaniola with Haiti, about 66,000 people are living with HIV/AIDS, or 1.1% of the adult population.

Sentinel surveillance data from 1991 to 2001 suggest that HIV prevalence among pregnant women has stabilised or perhaps begun to decline in the Dominican Republic (where estimated adult HIV prevalence was 2.5% in 2001). These findings appear to correlate with evidence of increased condom use among female sex workers (from 75% to 94% in 12 months in the capital, Santo Domingo, in 12 months), due to a campaign to promote safer commercial sex in the city. There has also been a reduction in the number of sexual partners among men. Nonetheless, ongoing transmission continues through commercial sex both with tourists and local men, and HIV prevalence amongst female sex workers has been found to range from 2.5% to over 12%, depending on the locale.

Jamaica

Jamaica has about 25,000 people with HIV, or 1.5% of the adult population. It was thought in 2004 that nearly half of infections were amongst young women, but the latest data suggests that about 7,000 women over 15 are infected of 28% of the total, giving rise to suspicions that sex between men, in one of the most homophobic countries of the world, is a hidden driver of the epidemic. The island has a long-established epidemic which means that it has the highest number of AIDS cases in the region after Haiti, with about 1300 deaths due to AIDS reported in 2004, twice as many as the 640 reported from 2002. However the most recent round of surveillance suggests no slackening off in the epidemic, with rates of 8% in men and 5% in women attending STI clinics and prevalence among pregnant women consistently at about 1.4%.

Guyana

This country is on the South American mainland but is generally counted as a Caribbean country because of its ethnic makeup and historical ties to the UK. It is the worst-affected country in South America, with 12,000 people affected or 2.4% of the population.

Recent statistics reveal that the country is faced with a generalised HIV/AIDS epidemic affecting both males and females, and also children as a result of the predominantly heterosexual transmission of the epidemic. However sex between men is also a significant factor with one survey finding that 21% of men who have sex with men in its Demerara-Mahaica region (in the northeast) were infected with HIV. Meanwhile a third of female sex workers in the capital, Georgetown, were found to have HIV too.

AIDS is currently the leading cause of death among persons in the 25-44 year age group, and the second leading cause of death overall. A cumulative total of 2588 deaths has been officially recorded.

One bright spot, however, is that **Guyana**'s antiretroviral therapy programme had, as of mid-2006, reached more than half of the persons in need of treatment.

Other countries

Trinidad and Tobagois seeing a steadily rising epidemic, with around 2.5% of the population infected. Life expectancy on the two islands is projected to be nine years lower than it would have been without AIDS in 2010. In contrast **The Bahamas** and **Barbados**seem to have had some prevention success. In the Bahamas HIV prevalence among pregnant women fell from 4.8% in 1993 to 3% in 2002 and in Barbados from 0.7% in 1999 to 0.3% in 2003. New HIV cases fell in the Bahamas from 734 in 1994 to 396 in 1999 and have remained at that level. **Belize** is another mainland country that is counted as ethnically and historically Caribbean. Its small population means that its 2.1% prevalence translates into 3700 people with HIV, and innovative youth awareness project, Youth for the Future, appears to have had some success in reducing HIV transmission amongst young people.

Cuba is the exception among Caribbean nations, with 3,300 people infected or considerably under 0.1% of the adult population. This is partly due to Fidel Castro's highly controversial policy of quarantining people with HIV in the 1980s - a policy now abandoned. Cuba also provides comprehensive antiretroviral treatment with locally-made generics. However there has been a fivefold increase in new cases between 1995 and 2000, largely among men who have sex with men.

Latin America

There are an estimated 1.7 million people living with HIV/AIDS in Latin America (0.6% of the adult population), of whom 610,000 (36%) are women. UNAIDS estimates that 240,000 people were newly infected with HIV in 2004 and 95,000 people died due to AIDS in that year.

Two thirds of the 1.7 million live in the four largest countries: Argentina, Brazil, Colombia, and Mexico. However, estimated HIV prevalence is highest in the smaller countries of Central America where it was just under 1% in El Salvador, Guatemala and Panama, 1.5% in Hondurasand 2.5% in Belize(which is dealt with under the Caribbean).

Only Guatemala and Honduras have HIV prevalence above 1% but there are much higher rates of HIV in vulnerable communities. In Central America (except for the relatively more prosperous Costa Rica) and the countries that line the Caribbean coast the majority of HIV infection is occurring through sex between men and women.

Brazil, which because of its large population contains one in three Latin Americans with HIV, is also experiencing a significant heterosexual epidemic, but there are also high seroprevalence rates among men who have sex with men and injecting drug users.

By comparison, the HIV epidemic is largely confined to men who have sex with men and injecting drug users in Argentina, Mexico and Colombia. In Costa Rica, the epidemic almost entirely centres on men who have sex with men. Studies among men who have sex with men in Costa Rica suggest that seroprevalence rates were as high as 10-16% as long ago as 1993.

Many countries in Latin America have begun to provide antiretroviral drugs to their inhabitants, and Brazil has been able to make treatment available to everyone who needs it. Local production and bulk purchasing of imported antiretrovirals has led to significant decreases in the programme's drug costs.

As of 2006, 72% of people in Latin America had access to antiretroviral drugs, though the proportion per country varied from 86% on Brazil to 39% in Ecuador.

Brazil

There are an estimated 620,000 people living with HIV/AIDS or 0.6% of the adult population. The Brazilian government has embarked upon HIV prevention campaigns which have been credited with a fall in prevalence of HIV among injecting drug users in particular. This has been pursued with a strong commitment to health care and protecting the rights of people living with HIV. The government is committed to provide free antiretroviral therapy to all those who need it; an estimated 157,000 Brazilians were receiving antiretroviral treatment by the end of 2004. Since the introduction of this policy in 1996, AIDS deaths have almost halved. Opportunistic infections declined by between 60-80% between 1996 and 1999.

Condom use among men who have sex with men increased dramatically between 1989 and 1995, rising from 34% to 69%. At the same time the proportion of men reporting anal sex in the past 6 months rose from 67% to 76%.

Amongst heterosexuals, while the percentage of young people who are sexually active changed little between 1998 and 2005, condom use rates increased dramatically-by more than one third among 15-24-year-old men and women. Among Brazilians of all ages, condom use increased by almost 50% during the same period.

However in the more impoverished parts of Brazil, particularly the north-eastern region, it is claimed there are very few prevention activities and unprotected sex remains highly prevalent.

In Sao Paolo, the rate of new HIV infections among men who have sex with men was a steady 2% between 1994 and 1997 and among sex workers 7% A study among pregnant women in the southern state of Rio Grande do Sul found HIV prevalence of 3% to 6% in pregnant women.

Prevention programmes among injecting drug users have contributed to a substantial decline in HIV prevalence in this population in several large metropolitan areas. The HIV prevalence among injecting drug users in Salvador fell from 50% in 1996 to 7% in 2001.

In addition, a national survey in Brazil has shown increasing condom use among injecting drug users (from 42% in 1999 to 65% in 2000)-a sign that sustained education and prevention efforts are bearing fruit.

Mexico

There are an estimated 180,000 people living with HIV/AIDS, or 0.3% of the adult population, concentrated in Mexico City, Baja California, Yucatan and Quintana Roo states. The epidemic is still largely concentrated among men who have sex with men (where prevalence has been measured as up to 15%) and injecting drug users (7%). However, seroprevalence rates among female sex workers are estimated to be below 1% and data from a programme to reduce the transmission of HIV from mother to infants suggest that less than 1 in 1000 women of childbearing age is infected.

Argentina

There are an estimated 130,000 people living with HIV/AIDS, or 0.7% of the adult population, with 65% of infections occurring in Buenos Aires city and province. Injecting drug use was formerly the principal means of transmission in Argentina as also in Chile and Uruguay, but sexual transmission of HIV to male and female partners of drug users is now more common, and the male-to-female ratio among people living with HIV narrowed from 15:1 in 1988 to 3:1 in 2002. There are very few prevention efforts directed at men who have sex with men despite prevalence of 14% being found among them in Buenos Aires, with only one in seven aware of their status. In neighbouring **Uruguay** the prevalence among MSM was 21%.

Honduras

Honduras is the worst-affected country in Latin America (not counting Belize or Guyana), with 63,000 people living with HIV or 2% of the population. HIV prevalence among MSM was measured as 13% in 2001 and among prisoners, 7%.

Guatemala

There are an estimated 73,000 people living with HIV/AIDS, or 1.38% of the adult population. Seroprevalence rates among pregnant women and sex workers are higher in the coastal cities and the capital than in more rural cities.

Eastern Europe and Central Asia

There are an estimated 1.7 million people living with HIV/AIDS in Eastern Europe and Central Asia, as of December 2004. This is 0.9% of the adult population - a 21% increase within the last two years, a 54% increase in the last four, and a twenty-fold increase in less than a decade.

UNAIDS considers this to be the fastest-growing series of epidemics in the world, mainly driven by increasing rates of injecting drug use. In 2006 there were an estimated 270,000 new infections, representing a 70% increase over then umber of new diagnoses in 2004. AIDS claimed the lives of 84,000 people in this region during 2006 - nearly twice the number in 2004, and a sign that the epidemics are maturing. The majority of

people with HIV live in two countries: the Russian Federation and Ukraine,which together account for approximately 90% of all people living with HIV in this region.

While the number of cases reported in people infected heterosexually has risen, largely due to sexual contact with injecting drug users, rates of HIV among gay and bisexual men in this region have remained very low - or appear to be low, though little surveillance among men who have sex with men has happened.

Newly diagnosed people tend to be much younger in Eastern Europe. Eighty per cent of new infections reported in adults/adolescents in 1997-1999 occurred in people less than 30 years old, compared with 30% in this age group in western Europe. It is estimated that up to 1% of the population in these regions is injecting drugs. Those injecting drugs can be very young. One study among Moscow secondary-school students revealed that 4% had injected drugs.

Urgent measures are needed to limit transmission among injecting drug users and prevent the further diffusion of HIV into the sexually active population, though this is to some extent already happening. In 2006 37% of HIV infections in the region occurred through sex and the proportion of people with HIV who are women has risen to 41%.

In the Russian Federation, and in many of the Central Asian Republics, the wave of injecting drug use is closely correlated with socioeconomic upheavals that have sent the living standards of tens of millions of people plummeting, amid rising unemployment and poverty levels. Another factor has been the fourfold increase in world production of heroin in the past decade, along with the opening of new trafficking routes across Central Asia.

High rates of sexually transmitted infections continue to be found in Eastern Europe and Central Asia, suggesting widespread unsafe sex and increased risk of HIV infection. In the Russian Federation between 200,000 and 400,000 cases of syphilis are reported annually.

Another casualty of the socioeconomic upheavals and structural chaos has been access to treatment. Progress in expanding access to antiretroviral therapy has been slow. As of mid-2006, fewer than 24 000 people were receiving antiretroviral treatment, 13% of the estimated 190 000 people who need the drugs, with an even lower proportion in Russia. This is despite the fact that Russia now has the per capita income of a developed country. Injecting drug users fare particularly badly: although the make up two-thirds of people with HIV throughout the region, they only represent one quarter of those receiving antiretrovirals.

Russian Federation

Russia has the fastest-growing HIV epidemic of any large country. In 2002 the UNAIDS estimate for the number of people living with HIV in Russia was 130,000, or 0.18% of the adult population. The 2006 estimate is 940,000 people or 1.1% of the adult population - a sevenfold increase in four years. Of these 350,000 have been registered.

HIV prevalence among pregnant women countrywide rose more than elevenfold in five years, from 0.01% in 1998 to 0.11% in 2003. But even this doesn't reflect the more-than-exponential growth in HIV in certain areas. The epidemic in Russia is concentrated into just ten of the country's 89 oblasts (provinces), all but one of them on the European side of the Urals. This means that other areas still have the chance to stem HIV. But in the most affected large city, St Petersburg, HIV prevalence increased one-hundredfold in four years, from 0.013% (one in 7700) in 1998 to 1.3% (one in 77) in 2002.

In the Russian Federation, there are an estimated 2.5 million drug users. With such a large pool of potential candidates for infection, it is likely that infection rates among injecting drug users will continue to rise, and may also begin to infiltrate other parts of the population. Injecting drug use is still the main route of transmission in the countries that make up the former Soviet

Union. Rates of infection remain low, but the speed of transmission has been astounding. New infections in Russia during the first half of 2000 increased by 305% compared to 1999, with a total of 22,068 cases being reported during the first six months of the year. HIV epidemics have been discovered in more than 30 cities and 86 or the country's 89 regions. Up to 90% of the registered infections have been attributed to injecting drug use.

The drug users with HIV are tragically young, even more so than in Ukraine. In Irkutsk, Siberia, HIV prevalence among drug users in 2004 was 65% and 90% of those were still in their teens.

There are also a significant number of babies being born with HIV in Russia - the total has now risen to more than 9,000.

In terms of actual diagnoses, The annual number of new reported HIV cases in the Russian Federation rose rapidly in the late 1990s, peaked at more than 87 000 in 2001, then declined steeply before stabilizing at 33 000-36 000 in 2003-2005. This was partly due to a reduction in testing: there were 50% fewer tests done in 2000-04 than there were in 1996-2000. However it also appears to reflect a real decline in incidence in injecting drug users. This is due to three factors. The overall number of drug users appears to have decreased; there were 17% fewer newly registered drug users in 2003 compared with 2002, for example. Secondly, HIV infection may have reached saturation point in certain populations. But thirdly, the epidemic is changing: the proportion of new HIV cases likely to have been linked to non-sterile injecting drug use equipment has also shrunk, from more than 90% in 2000 to 66% in 2005.

We may be seeing a similar pattern to Ukraine where an initial outbreak of cases in IDUs falls away only to be replaced by a slower epidemic through sexual transmission. One piece of evidence suggesting that this may be happening is that the proportion of people infected with HIV who were women went up from 24% in 2001 to 38% in 2003. Relatively few surveys have been done in Russian sex workers, but one found HIV prevalence of 14% among female sex workers in Moscow. In St Petersburg one survey found - not unexpectedly - that female sex workers and IDUs were often the same people. Four out of five sex workers said they infected drugs; when tested, 48% of them had HIV, rising to 64% among 20-24 year olds. The fact that 8% of injecting drug users in Moscow and 20% in Volgograd have been found to have syphilis indicates that unprotected sex is common among many injecting drug users.

Prisons have been another hothouse for HIV in Russia, with prevalence among prisoners estimated at 2 to 4% and with HIV and TB (much of it multi-drug-resistant) reinforcing each other's incidence and severity. The epidemics amongst IDUs and prisoners are, of course, linked, with IDUs (and sex workers) subject to often arbitrary arrest and imprisonment.

As in Ukraine, reported rates among men who have sex with men remain low, but UNAIDS comments that Russia's surveillance system captures so little information about gay men that it's impossible to say what their contribution is to the epidemic. In one study, carried out in Tomsk and Ekaterinburg in 2003, 0% and 4.8% HIV prevalence, respectively, was found in men who have sex with men. What little countrywide evidence we have suggests comparatively low, but increasing rates of infection in this group, from 0.2% amongst men coming forward for testing who reported sex with other men, to 0.5% in 2004.

The situation in Russia can potentially be contained. HIV prevalence remains very low (from 0.0001% to 0.15%) in 66 of Russia's provinces and ten provinces contain over half the reported cases. Some HIV prevention activities are taking place in prisons, such as distribution of bleach to clean needles.

Treatment levels for people with HIV in Russia dismal, considering this is a country with an increasingly developed economy: the 2006 WHO report into ARV access estimated that no more than 5% and probably only 3% of those who are in need of HIV treatment are getting it, and even as they are in Ukraine, with fewer than 4,500 people accessing ARVs - and only about 120 of those are drug users. The former Soviet

countries have failed to drive the bargains with drug companies that other developing and middle-income countries have, so HIV treatment in Russia is currently as expensive as it is in the UK, with a year's course of drugs costing more than the average annual income; because of the country's high per capita income, it also is not eligible for grants from the Global Fund and many other treatment funders. Substitution treatment for heroin addiction is also not available, with methadone and buprenorphine still being listed as illegal drugs.

Ukraine

With an estimated adult prevalence rate of 1.5% - a 50% increase since 2002 - Ukraine is the most affected country in the region and in the whole of Europe, with an estimated 377,000 people living with HIV. Ukraine has an exceptionally young HIV epidemic, with up to 60% of women with the virus under 25. Annual HIV diagnoses have more than doubled since 2000, reaching 13 786 in 2005 and bringing to over 97 000 the total number of officially recorded HIV infections.

Although the epidemic started in drug users, and 45% of new diagnoses are still in this group, new diagnoses of HIV in persons infected through heterosexual intercourse accounted for 30% of all new cases reported in 2003 - up from 15% in 1998. An initial sharp rise in HIV cases took place between 1995 (1499 cases, with only 399 reported before that from the start of the epidemic) to 8934 in 1997. Cases then seemed to slacken off, with 5830 reported in 1999. However yearly cases have increased ever since.

"Ukraine," says UNAIDS, "presents a vivid example of how swiftly an HIV epidemic can move beyond the most at-risk populations and into the general population." The proportion of persons infected through heterosexual transmission of HIV has increased from 14% of new cases during 1999-2003 to over 35% of new cases in the first six months of 2006.

HIV prevalence among pregnant women in Ukraine is now among the highest in all of Europe: 0.31% in mid-2006. However one Ukrainian success story has been the provision of antiretrovirals to mothers to prevent mother-to-child transmission, with more than 90% of diagnosed HIV-positive mothers now receiving ARVs. This has brought the mother-to-child infection rate down from 28% to 8% and this continues to decline. The fact that it is not lower is because a high number of mothers - especially ones who are IDUs or partners of IDUs, fear reporting to antenatal clinics for HIV screening.

Provision of ARVs to the general population is less impressive; currently about 25% of those who are in urgent need of antiretroviral drugs get them. This is however an enormous improvement on 2004, when only 1.1% of the population in need was getting treatment. Although this is at least better than Russia, injecting drug users, similarly, miss out disproportionately on ARV provision.

The deadly combination of tuberculosis and HIV is a serious problem in Ukraine, which has the world's highest proportion of TB cases that are multi-drug resistant - 10-15%.

Up to 2004 only 44 cases of the 62,365 people officially reported by that time as having HIV since 1987 were attributed to sex between men. This unbelievably low figure may say more about the stigma against homosexuality in the region than it does about the true prevalence among gay men. Limited HIV sentinel surveillance in this population group has revealed HIV prevalence of 28% and 9%, respectively, in the cities of Odessa and Mykolayiv.

There are a few signs of hope. Drug users appear to increasingly be adopting safer-sex behaviour and the Health ministry has at least provided treatment to stop babies getting HIV from their mothers; the proportion of babies born with HIV from infected mothers decreased from 27% in 2001 to 12% in 2003.

Other countries

Although the HIV epidemic in the other former soviet states are dwarfed by those in Russia and Ukraine, the rate of new HIV diagnoses in **Georgia** and **Moldova** has doubled since 2001 and has quadrupled in Uzbekistan - see below.

In **Belarus**very approximately 26,000 or 0.5% of the adult population are infected, though surveillance is so inadequate the true figure could be anything between 12,000 and 40,000. The epidemic continues to expand with a constant annual increase of around 700 new cases per year. Transmission by injecting drug use represented 71% of reported cases. There is a clear trend towards increasing number of persons infected by sexual mode of transmission (from 27.16% in 2001, 34.9% in 2002, to 50.4% in the first 11 months of 2004) and a generalisation of the epidemic. In 2006, a grand total of 87 adults and 32 children received antiretroviral treatment - 54 more than in 2004.

Central Asia

HIV prevalence remains very low in most of the central Asian and Caucasian republics. However one stark warning comes from **Uzbekistan**which now has the dubious distinction of having the youngest and fastest-growing HIV outbreak in the world. All but 9% of the cases of HIV ever diagnosed in the country have occurred since 2000, and have risen 14-fold in five years from 153 cases reported in 2000 to 2198 cases in 2005. UNAIDS estimated that 11,000 people in the country now have HIV. Infections have almost entirely occurred amongst injecting drug users: the country straddles the trade route between Afghanistan, now the world's largest opium-growing economy, and Russia and Europe.

Neighbouring **Kazakhstan** has the same prevalence, though cases have risen more slowly. The small, poor and mountainous republics of **Kyrgyzstan** and **Tajikistan**currently have low prevalence but are seen as very vulnerable owing to their position between the world's top opium growing country, Afghanistan, and one of its main markets, Russia. However the Kyrgyz Republic has become a model for other former Soviet countries and beyond in its methadone-maintenance and syringe-exchange programmes in its two main cities of Bishkek and Osh. In the Caucasus **Azerbaijan**shows some signs of a developing epidemic, with HIV rates of 25% among drug injectors and 11% among street sex workers in the capital, Baku, and as noted above, HIV prevalence in **Georgia** has doubled since 2001. Only **Armenia**, of all the former Soviet republics, remains a low-prevalence country and one where infection rates are not even especially high in IDUs.

The Baltic States

These states, Lithuania, Latvia and Estonia, as EU members, are now under **Western Europe.**

North America and Western Europe

There are an estimated 2.14 million people living with HIV in the developed-world countries of North America and Western Europe, as of the end of 2004, 1.3 million in north America (all but 60,000 of them in the USA) and 740,000 in western and central Europe. The adult HIV prevalence rate in north America is 0.8% and in Europe is 0.3%, though with considerable variation between countries. Women constitute 26% of the total infected adult population. In 2002, 65,000 people were newly infected in this region and 30,000 deaths due to AIDS were recorded.

Western and Central Europe

Reference: The figures used for Western Europe here come from the latest HIV/AIDS Surveillance in Europe report from the European Centre for the Epidemiological Monitoring of AIDS. See http://www.eurohiv.org

In 2005 about 25,000 new cases of HIV were diagnosed in the countries of western and central Europe, the vast majority (22,700) from western Europe. The

It is surprisingly difficult to get accurate HIV figures for the whole of Europe and to compare rates between countries. This is because three of the highest-prevalence countries, the Netherlands, France and Spain, only ever reported AIDS cases and do not systematically collect data on HIV diagnoses: France and the Netherlands finally started doing this in 2003. Italy has collected data since 1999 from six out of its 20 regions which are then extrapolated to form an estimated total. Several other countries only started collecting HIV (as opposed to AIDS) data relatively recently. Portugal, which has the highest HIV prevalence in Western Europe, started in 2000, and Austria in 1998.

In the 16 out of 23 countries for which reporting data is available at least since 1998, HIV cases, which had been rising slowly since 1998, increased markedly from 9,657 in 2001 to 12,135 in 2002 (a 28% increase) and again by a further 9% to 13,184 cases in 2003.

As a result while we have a pretty accurate figure for HIV prevalence in countries such as the UK that have always had good HIV surveillance, we are extremely uncertain about the true HIV prevalence in others; this is partly due to undiagnosed infections but much more to do with diagnosed infections not being centrally reported. For instance, the

WHO estimates that HIV prevalence in the UK is between 0.19% and 0.22% of the general population. But for France, Italy and Spain, respectively, the high and low prevalence estimates are 0.20-0.68% (France); 0.24-0.77% (Italy); and 0.29-0.92% (Spain).

The following table has been compiled from the EuroHIV list above, from UNAIDS country profiles, and also from data provided by Dr Srdan Matic of the WHO.

Just over one third (35%) of HIV infections diagnosed in 2005 in western and central Europe occurred during sex between men, while more than half (56%) were acquired during heterosexual intercourse.

Heterosexual sex accounted for just 43% of reported risk factors in 1998 but 56% in 2005, and is now the predominant mode of transmission in newly diagnosed people in every country in Western Europe except for Germany and the Netherlands, where gay men still make up the largest proportion of new diagnoses. In line with this the proportion of people diagnosed who were women increased from 27% in 1998 to 36% in 2003.

However after slow declines up to 2001, cases in gay men also rose by 22% in 2002 and remained at the 2002 level in 2003. Some of this may be due to an increased uptake in testing - half of the gay men diagnosed in the UK in 2002 had been infected for more than six years - but, as UNAIDS comments, "HIV infection is now the fastest-growing serious health condition in England." In Germany testing campaigns had already boosted uptake in the late 1990s so an increase in diagnoses from 642 in 2000 to 742 in 2001 probably reflects a real increase.

In contrast, and unlike the situation in Eastern Europe, cases due to injecting drug use have declined across the region since 1998, even in countries such as France, Portugal, Switzerland and Spain where it contributed to what was for Europe very high prevalence. In countries where aggressive HIV prevention efforts targeted at injecting drug users have been implemented, the HIV prevalence rate among injecting drug users has been contained at below 5-7%.

Selected European Countries, HIV prevalence
(WHO estimates)

Country	No living with HIV	Country	Prevalence
1. Italy	150,000	1. Estonia	1.3%
2. Spain	140,000	2. Latvia	0.8%
3. France	130,000	3. Spain	0.6%
4. United Kingdom	68,000	4. Italy	0.5%
5. Germany	49,000	5. France	0.4%
6. Portugal	32,000	5. Switzerland	0.4%
7. Poland	25,000	5. Portugal	0.4%
8. Netherelands	18,000	8. Belgium	0.3%
9. Switzerland	17,000	8. Austria	0.3%

In all other European countries the prevalence of HIV in the general population is 0.2% or lower.

To a certain extent if diagnoses in people who acquired HIV outside Europe are excluded, the historical difference in HIV prevalence in Europe is very largely to do with how quickly each country moved to tackle HIV infections in injecting drug users.

Spain recorded 16,000 new HIV cases a year in the mid-80s but levels have declined considerably since due to a comprehensive harm-reduction programme, though up to a third of IDUs in Catalonia are HIV-positive. In Portugal, which has only begun to tackle its HIV and drug problem, over 50% of new HIV infections were still due to injecting drug use in 2002, 40% were among heterosexuals, and only 10% among gay men.

In the 11 countries that give source of infection, an increasing proportion of these cases were in people who caught their HIV in countries with generalised epidemics, from 30% of heterosexual infections in 1998 to 58% of them in 2003, over 90% of whom were migrants from sub-Saharan Africa.

The number of heterosexual diagnoses in Europe would in fact be less than half of those reported in gay men were it not for immigration into Europe from the world's high-prevalence countries, primarily sub-Saharan Africa. About three quarters of heterosexually acquired HIV infections in Europe were among immigrants and migrants, and most of the difference in prevalence between European countries that is not explained by needle exchange policy is explained by the proportion of black African immigrants in their population. Amongst these two variables is one constant; HIV diagnoses amongst gay men have been rising slowly but steadily in virtually every western European country of the 'old EU' since the late 1990s.

The United Kingdom's position in Europe

The HIV/AIDS Surveillance in Europe Report comments that:
"Trends in the West are largely driven by the United Kingdom,

which accounts for 28% of the population but for 53% of all reported HIV infections in recent years."

And in its latest AIDS Epidemic Update, UNAIDS says: "The largest increases in HIV diagnoses in western Europe have been reported in the United Kingdom, where HIV remains one of the principal communicable disease threats."

These statements are not quite so startling as they look, as without longstanding figures from France, Spain, Portugal and the Netherlands in the Eurosurveillance list, the UK's contribution to the figures is disproportionate. But it does underline the fact that the UK's HIV epidemic has been one of the faster-growing ones.

Furthermore this is not entirely due to heterosexual cases among immigrants. In 2003 the United Kingdom had:

- The second-highest rate of new HIV infections (117 new cases per million) behind Portugal (228 cases per million) - Italy and Spain excluded (the tiny country of San Marino also had a higher rate of cases). This compares with a figure of 81 cases per million population throughout western Europe (excluding France)

- The highest rate of new diagnoses in gay men in the whole of Europe (33 cases per million) after San Marino - Italy, Spain and Austria excluded

- The second-highest rate of heterosexual cases after Portugal (65 cases per million - higher than the official figure in Ukraine) - Spain, Italy and Austria again excluded.

The 'home grown' epidemic in the Northern European countries such as the United Kingdom, the Netherlands, Germany and Scandinavia has therefore continued to be primarily concentrated among gay and bisexual men, and although most countries have reported an increase in the number of heterosexually acquired infections over time, much of this is among migrant populations from Africa and other regions where heterosexual transmission is dominant, rather than heterosexual transmission in-country. In the UK 48% of all infections in 2004 and 88% of heterosexual infections were acquired abroad. In Sweden in 2003, more than 80% of all infections were heterosexual ones acquired abroad.

AIDS cases as a guide to HIV prevalence

As we say above, HIV diagnoses and prevalence are very hard to compare between countries in Europe, due to differing levels of reporting. However AIDS cases are reported by all countries in western Europe, and most countries now have comparable treatment coverage too, so some degree of cross-country comparison is possible. The relative frequency of AIDS cases therefore reflects relative HIV prevalence with reasonable accuracy.

Cases of AIDS in western Europe have declined every year from 1996, when 21,786 cases were reported, to 2005, when 7065 cases were reported.

In 1996 the countries with the highest AIDS burden were (in order of new AIDS diagnoses per million population) Portugal (101 cases per million), Spain, (91) Italy (42) Switzerland (38) and France (32), with the UK sixth on the list at 13.6 cases per million population

In 2006 that order remained little changed but had declined or remained steady everywhere - with the exceptions of the UK and Ireland. The list now reads Portugal (77 per million), Spain (48), Switzerland (38), Italy (28) and France (22) with the UK still on the list in sixth place but with the case burden increased to 15 per million.

The increase in the UK and Ireland (and no decrease in Sweden and Belgium) is not, of course, an increase in the death rate due to AIDS amongst people with HIV, but rather underlines the fact that these countries during this decade have had the fastest-growing HIV epidemics in the region - largely driven by immigration. Sweden, Belgium and Ireland are the three countries in Europe where more than 60% of HIV diagnoses in 2005 were amongst people coming from high-prevalence countries, and in the UK 55% of diagnoses were amongst this group. This compares with only 16% in Portugal.

Other significant epidemics

France

In FranceIt is estimated that 130,000 people are living with HIV/AIDS, or 0.4% of the adult population. To date, 55,000 AIDS cases have been reported. Accurate figures are unavailable for France because testing is anonymised. In September 1999 French doctors recommended to the Health Ministry that anonymised reporting of HIV diagnoses should become mandatory in order to improve surveillance, and this came into force in 2003. In France, HIV prevalence among injecting drug users rates ranged between 10% and 23% in 2000.

Spain

Spain and Italy have the largest number of people living with HIV of any western European country - exactly which has the largest HIV-positive population is very difficult to say as both countries continue to have inadequate HIV surveillance.

Spain has the higher prevalence because of its lower population, at 0.6% of the adult population or the same as the USA. It is estimated that between 115 000 and 155 000 Spaniards are living with HIV/AIDS, and that about 75% of them are aware of their serostatus.

Although injecting drug use remains the main mode of transmission in Spain, about one-quarter of all HIV infections have been heterosexually transmitted.

Data from the regions that do report HIV cases show that during the 1980s, HIV spread widely among IDUs and, to a much lesser extent, MSM. The large number of sexually active young adults among HIV-positive IDUs led to the infection of non-injecting sexual partners and, through vertical transmission, children. By the start of the 1990s, more than 100 000 people had already been infected with HIV, and HIV-related mortality ranked first in 1994 among the major causes of adult death and potential years of life lost.

As of December 2005, most of Spain's reported AIDS cases (66%) were IDUs. A further 16% had been infected heterosexually, and 14% were MSM. Spain has the largest cumulative total of AIDS cases, and of IDUs with AIDS, of any European country.

The Spanish AIDS epidemic appears to have peaked in 1994, followed thereafter by a rapid decline in the number of annually reported cases: from 7428 new cases in 1994 to 1549 in 2005. The number of AIDS deaths peaked in the mid-1990s with more than 5000 deaths annually. Since then, there has been a rapid decline in the number of deaths, reflecting the impact of HAART since its introduction in 1996.

During 2005, approximately 100 000 PLWHA were seen for care for their condition, and estimated 75 000 Spaniards (39 000 IDUs, 53 000 males) were receiving HAART.

Reported HIV prevalence among injecting drug users in Spain in 2000 was 20-30% nationwide. HIV prevalence among injecting drug users declined by half in Barcelona (44% to 21% between 1995 and 2001-2003) and Sevilla (44% to 22%), both cities with long-standing harm reduction programmes. In contrast, in Madrid, where such programmes were introduced only in the late 1990s, HIV prevalence among injecting drug users remained stable (37% in 1995 and 35% in 2001-2003).

Italy

There is probably less data on HIV in Italy than from any other European country, and indeed than many other world countries. HIV incidence for 2004 was estimated to be between 3500 and 4000 new infections, with 65% males and 20% people born outside the country.

Early on in the epidemic, the main route of transmission was through injecting drug use. However, in recent years transmission has predominantly been due to sexual contact. In 2005, around 47% of new AIDS cases were among cases infected through heterosexual sex, 22% among men having sex with men and 30% among injecting drug users. In 1994, just fewer than 2% of AIDS cases were found in foreigners, whereas in 2005, 21% were among non-Italians.

AIDS incidence in Italy varies greatly by region. The cities of Rome and Milan have the highest annual AIDS incidence rates (4.9 and 4.8 AIDS cases per 100 000, respectively), followed by Genoa (4.1/100 000) and Bologna (3.7/100 000). In 2005, 100 000 people were seen for care, and 75 000 were receiving HAART as of December 2005.

Portugal

Portugal had the highest HIV prevalence in western Europe in 2002, but since then prevalence has decreased, largely due to the belated introduction of harm reduction]programmes for IDUs. Prevalence was estimated as 0.7% in 2002 but is now estimated to be about 0.4%. HIV diagnoses among injecting drug users were almost one third (31%) lower in 2005, compared with 2001 (857 versus 1247).

Portugal still has the highest AIDS incidence in Europe (88 cases per million population in 1999). To the end of 1999 there had been 6,558 cases of AIDS reported.

Portugal's serious epidemic among injecting drug users still accounts for half of newly diagnosed HIV infections, though the number of reported HIV infections among injecting drug users has declined significantly since 2001.

Portugal is the only country in Europe to report a significant number of cases of HIV-2 infection.

Further information on AIDS in Europe can be obtained from the European Centre for the Epidemiological Monitoring of AIDS, Hôpital National de Saint-Maurice, 14 rue du val d'Osne, F-94410, France. Quarterly European HIV & AIDS statistics are also available online at http://www.eurohiv.org

This site and other statistical sources are included in the *Statistics* links selection at NAM's website aidsmap.com

Central Europe

There may be cause for moderate optimism in Central Europe, where countries continue to hold the epidemic at bay; the overall HIV incidence remained exceptionally low in 2001 (7-10 reported infections per million persons). Prevalence remains low in countries such as the Czech Republic, Hungary, Poland and Slovenia, where well-designed national HIV/AIDS programmes are also in operation.

Overall the countries of central Europe - the former 'Iron curtain' states - remain remarkably free of high levels of HIV, partly due to imaginative HIV prevention and outreach programmes being instituted early. Since 1996 21,000 cases of HIV have been reported, a tenth of the number reported in West Europe, and incidence and prevalence similarly runs at about a tenth of Western European rates, though some of this may be due to fewer people coming forward for testing.

Poland, the most populous country in the area, reported 652 new cases of HIV in 2005. This represents a new infection rate of 16.9 per million population compared with the United Kingdom's 117 cases per million. Poland has an HIV prevalence among injecting drug users of around 9%, far higher than in any other country in Central Europe, but this has fallen from a peak of 13% in 2000 thanks to needle exchange and harm reduction programmes. All other countries in the region reported lower new infection rates than Poland except for tiny Slovenia (18.3 cases per million)

In **Romania**, cases in children who were infected around 1990 through blood transfusion and multiple injections with improperly sterilised needles account for around 70% of all infections (5,000 of an estimated 7,000).

The Baltic States

Geographically these are part of eastern Europe, but are now EU members. They include the two highest-prevalence countries in the European Union.

Reported infections in **Estonia,** a small country of 1.4 million people, soared from 12 in 1999 to 1474 in 2001 and 7700 in 2004, with 621 new infections in 2005, a rate of 467 per million population, or some 86% higher than the country with the next-highest new-diagnosis rate, Portugal. Its adult prevalence rate of 1.2% makes it the highest-prevalence country in the European Union. However the rate of new diagnoses has gone down since 2002 when 899 new diagnoses were made.

The same applies to **Latvia**; here new reported infections rose from 25 in 1997 to 807 in 2001, and where a further 308 new HIV cases had been registered by the end of June 2002. However the sudden increase in the number of HIV infections diagnosed around the turn of the century appears to have abated and the HIV epidemics are now growing at a slower pace. There has been a steady decrease in the number of new HIV diagnoses in Latviasince 2001 and in 2005 only 299 were reported.

UNAIDS estimates about 7500 people with HIV in the country, or about 0.6%. **Lithuania** has got off more lightly so far with 1300 people with HIV or 0.2%, though there was a major outbreak in one of its prisons in 2002, when 284 inmates (15% of the total) were diagnosed HIV-positive.

North America

The USA

In the USA and Canada there were an estimated 1.3 million people living with HIV at the end of 2004, 58,000 in Canada and all the rest in the USA.

In the USA an estimated 0.6% of the population is living with HIV, making it one of the highest-prevalence countries in the developed world. There are only seven countries in the world estimated to have more people living with HIV in their population than the USA.

38,133 people were newly diagnosed with HIV in 2003 in the 33 states that used names-based reporting. The other 18 states (and the District of Columbia) currently use code-based anonymised reports which the Centers for Disease Control regard as unreliable. If they were included the estimated number of people newly infected during 2003 was about 60,000 in that year 17,000 deaths occurred due to AIDS. The availability of antiretroviral treatment has brought a decline in death rates.

However there is continuing transmission of HIV and it is increasingly concentrated among ethnic minority populations in the USA.

African-Americans, for example, form 13% of the population of the USA. But they constituted 40% of all people living with HIV in 2005; 60% of all women living with HIV; 48% of new HIV diagnoses; and 50% of all AIDS cases.

Hispanics are also disproportionately affected, though not to quite the same extent as African-Americans. Forming 14% of the population, in 2005 they formed 20% of AIDS cases.

The US epidemic is still primarily concentrated among gay men with large minorities of intravenous drug users and

heterosexuals. Amongst the 33 states that report HIV diagnoses, 49% are amongst men who acquired HIV through sex with men and another 4% were gay men who injected drugs, so could have caught HIV through either route. Another 14% cited injecting drug use as their main risk factor and 32% appear to have caught HIV heterosexually. (It is important to note that for AIDS surveillance purposes the USA now uses a different definition of AIDS from the one employed in Europe. Since 1993 anyone with a CD4 count below 200 is considered to have AIDS. In Europe a diagnosis of AIDS can only occur after the diagnosis of specified opportunistic infections).

African American women account for 72% of all new HIV diagnoses in women, meaning they are 21 times as likely to get HIV as their white counterparts. In the 33 states, the bulk of HIV infections among 13-19-year-olds reported in July 2000-June 2001 were among females (56%), a disproportionate percentage of them African-American. Most young women had acquired the virus through heterosexual intercourse.

Furthermore the gay epidemic had become far more a black gay epidemic. In the 33 states 42% of new diagnoses of HIV in 2005 were amongst white non-Hispanic gay men, 36% amongst African American men and 19% amongst Hispanic men. In one study HIV prevalence in black gay men in five urban centres was nearly 50%, five to ten times what it was in white men. In the 33 areas with names-based reporting 46% of new cases of HIV in 2003 were in whites, 35% in blacks and 17% in Hispanics (with the other two per cent is Asians, Pacific Islanders and Native Americans), but the 18 areas excluded from these figures include urban areas with high black populations.

The ethnicity of people with AIDS has changed so that in 1985 60% of PWAs where white, 25% black and about 15% Hispanic. By 1994 AIDS cases in blacks equalled those in whites, and in 2002 about 30% of AIDS cases were in whites, over 50% in blacks and about 20% in Hispanics. ~In 2002 the death rate due to AIDS was twice as high in blacks as in whites.

In a sense the USA is seeing a whole new epidemic of HIV superimposed on top of the old one; not an imported epidemic from high-prevalence countries as in the UK and other European countries, but an epidemic among the 'third world in the first' of impoverished black US citizens, many with multiple HIV risk factors and with limited access to adequate healthcare. One recent study has suggested that the high rates of incarceration of African-American men (approximately one in 12 of whom have been in jail or prison) could be associated with the disproportionate HIV infection rates among African-American men and women.

HIV reporting in the United States is not universal (though AIDS reporting is); 18 states have anonymised testing systems which prevent reporting, and in none of these states does HIV reporting extend back as far as 1985. Data on HIV infection are thus highly incomplete. However most states are now moving towards names-based reporting.

1996 was the first year in which the US reported a fall in the incidence of AIDS since the epidemic first appeared. The fall is attributed to improvements in treatment. The number of deaths declined 12% from 24,900 in the first six months of 1995 to 22,000 in the first half of 1996. During the first half of 1997 AIDS diagnoses fell by a further 15% compared with the first half of 1996.

However, there are significant variations between racial groups and between genders. Whilst deaths declined by 21% amongst whites in 1996, they declined only 2% amongst African/ Americans, and deaths have increased by 3% amongst women. In part these variations can be explained by the differing rates at which HIV spread amongst these population groups during the 1980s, but they are also a reflection of access to, and uptake of, treatment.

Death rates in the major cities declined further than the national average. New York, San Francisco, Los Angeles, and Miami all reported a decline of 20% in the death rate in the first half of 1996 compared to 1995.

According to a 2002 CDC report, AIDS-related illnesses remained the leading cause of death for African-American men aged 25-44 and the third-leading cause of death for Hispanic men in the same age group.

HIV prevalence levels are exceptionally high among African-American men who have sex with men in the USA-up to 48% among 23-29-year-olds, according to one six-city survey. About 64% of the women diagnosed with HIV in 2001 in the United States were African-American. A significant number of these women acquired the virus from men who also have sex with men.

Surveys regularly conducted among several thousand gay men in San Francisco have identified a continuing increase in the proportion of men who are reporting multiple partners and unprotected sex over the past six months. The San Francisco survey reveals that risk behaviour has increased most rapidly among men under 25. The survey identified an increase in the percentage of men reporting unprotected sex and multiple partners from 22% in 1994 to 32% in 1997. The prevalence of HIV among men presenting for voluntary counselling and testing almost tripled from 1.3% in 1997 to 3.7% in 1999.

Since then unprotected sex levels have stabilised, but at a much higher rate, with around a third of HIV-negative men reporting unprotected sex and about 50% of HIV-positive men. Despite this, HIV incidence has actually fallen in some areas such as San Francisco (halving from 2.4% to 1.2% a year) despite continuing high levels of STIs. This appears to be because gay men, when they have unprotected sex, are increasingly finding ways of doing it solely with men of their own HIV status, the amount of *serodiscordant* (different-status) unprotected sex has decreased since 2001 from 30% to 20% in HIV-positive men and from 20% to 5% in HIV-negative men.

Nonetheless, unprotected sex will still expose men to STIs, and rectal gonorrhoea among gay men had been declining until 1993, but since that time has been steadily increasing, in line with the reported increase in unprotected anal sex. In New York, it is estimated that nine out of ten cases of HIV acquired through sex between men and women are related to sex with a drug user.

Canada

In Canada, meanwhile, there are an estimated 58,000 people living with HIV/AIDS, or 0.3% of the adult population. The makeup of the HIV-positive population is the same as the USA, with 46% of infections coming from sex between men, 14% from injecting drug use, and 37% form heterosexual sex. Aboriginal persons accounted for 9% of new HIV infections in 1999, although they constituted only 3.3% of the general population. Injecting drug use accounted for 53% of new infections among Aboriginal Canadians and sex between men only 10%.

Australasia and the Pacific

In the whole of the Australasia and the Pacific region it was estimated that 81,000 people were living with HIV in 2005 and that 7100 people became newly infected. Three-quarters of those people are in Papua New Guinea, where the epidemic is serious and growing.

In Australia and New Zealand there were an estimated 17,400 people living with HIV/AIDS in 2002, 16,000 of them in Australia, or 0.1% of the adult population, and fewer than 1,000 of them women - the lowest female to male sex ratio in the world. Fewer than 200 deaths occurred due to AIDS in 2002.

However, the annual number of new HIV diagnoses in **Australia** has gradually increased from 650 in 1998 to 899 in 2005 and 954 in 2006. A resurgence of unsafe sex between men appears to be the major risk factor for these new infections.

The epidemic tends to be confined largely to gay men with 85% of new HIV diagnoses accounted for by gay sex, 8.5% by heterosexual sex and 4% by injecting drug use. A study in the Australian cities of Sydney and Melbourne in 1998 found that a third of gay men were less concerned about HIV infection since the introduction of antiretroviral treatments. These men were found to be 40% more likely to have had recent unprotected anal sex than men whose fear of infection was unchanged by the introduction of new therapies.

The per capita rates of HIV diagnoses among Australia's indigenous peoples has been similar but there is a higher proportion of diagnosis among women (36% of the total) and injecting drug users (20%) and much lower in gay men (42%).

In **New Zealand**, though prevalence is still low, new HIV diagnoses reached a high of 218 in 2005, the highest number since testing began in 1985. Just over half of cases were amongst gay men and 37% amongst heterosexuals, 90% of whom acquired their infection abroad.

Papua New Guinea

Just across the Torres Strait from Australia is the nation with the highest HIV rate in the Pacific region and one with an accelerating HIV epidemic, which UNAIDS fears is the best candidate for an African-style generalised epidemic outside Africa. In 2002 there were an estimated 5,400 people living with HIV/AIDS in Papua New Guinea (PNG), or 0.22% of the adult population. By 2004 this was 16,000 people (4,800 of them women), or 0.6% of the population. And by 2006 it was estimated that 57,000 people in the country were living with HIV or 1.8% of the population. The epidemic has therefore expanded more then tenfold in four years. There were 2120 new diagnoses recorded in 2003 and for the first time the majority of them were in women, and new diagnoses have ben running at 2000+ a year since.

The annual number of new infections has been increasing steadily since they first started being detected in any significant amount in 1995. In 2003 1.4% of pregnant women in the capital, Port Moresby, tested HIV-positive and 2.5% in the northern town of Lae. More than twice as many young women under 24 have been diagnosed as men of that age. Available data suggests that the epidemic is centred on commercial and causal sex, most of it heterosexual. One study in rural and peri-urban areas found that 55% of interviewed women had exchanged sex for money and/or goods and 36% of men had paid for sex. In addition, up to 12% of men living in rural and peri-urban areas reported occasionally having sex with other men.

Recent surveys in **Irian Jaya** (West Papua) in the Indonesian half of New Guinea found that unmarried young women were almost ten times and young men five times more likely to be sexually active compared with other Indonesians and that 29% of young sexually active Papuan women reported having sex with a man more than ten years older than themselves.

North Africa and the Middle East

There were an estimated 460,000 people living with HIV/AIDS in North Africa and the Middle East at the end of 2004, about 0.2% of the population, according to UNAIDS, although it considers surveillance systems to be inadequate to be very confident about such estimates. An estimated 36,000 people died from AIDS in 2004 and 68,000 people were newly infected. Women constitute 46% of the infected adult population.

HIV/AIDS arrived late in these regions and infection rates remain at very low levels in most countries, however, in several places HIV infection rates are increasing and denial of the problem among social and political leaders in some countries may provide the epidemic with an ideal environment for continued growth.

In some countries such as Libya, Bahrain and Iran (see **Asia**) the epidemic is largely being driven by injecting drug use while in others such as Algeria, Morocco and Saudi Arabia unprotected sex seems to be the main risk factor. At some antenatal clinics in the south of Algeria, more than 1% of pregnant women have tested HIV-positive

Systematic surveillance remains inadequate, making it very difficult to deduce accurate trends in many countries. It is possible that hidden epidemics could be spreading in this region. Better surveillance systems (such as those introduced in Iran, Jordan, Lebanon and Syria) will enable more countries to accurately track the development of the epidemic and mount more effective responses.

Sudan

Sudan straddles the divide between North Africa and sub-Saharan Africa, and this is reflected in its mixture of peoples, in its war-torn history and its HIV prevalence. Latest estimates show that about 350,000 Sudanese or 1.6% of the adult population were living with HIV at the end of 2003. Although the true number could be anything between 120,000 and 1.3 million, even the lower estimate means that more than 80% of people in the Middle East and North Africa are living in Sudan. HIV prevalence is up to eight times higher in the south of the country than in the capital, Khartoum, though HIV is present in the capital; surveys have shown infection rates of 1% in police officers and 9.3% amongst men who have sex with men. Sudan's slow emergence from decades of civil war could unfortunately accelerate the spread of HIV as people resume normal patterns of travel and trade.

Libya

Libya has three times the HIV prevalence of its immediate neighbours, at 0.3%. This is due to a rapidly-growing epidemic among injecting drug users. Almost 90% of the officially-reported 5160 HIV infections among Libyans (as of December 2002) had occurred in 2000-02 alone. Over 90% of cases were attributed to injecting drug use and about 50% of drug users receiving treatment in the capital Tripoli were HIV-positive in 2003.

Saudi Arabia

Saudi Arabia's HIV prevalence is low (about 8,000 people) and the majority of HIV cases (54%) are in migrant workers rather than in Saudi Nationals, concentrated in the port city of Jeddah. Saudi Arabia was recently criticised for its treatment of migrant workers with HIV following news reports that they were being locked in secure wards without access to ARVs till deported.

Israel

Israel is a low-prevalence country for HIV, with 4,300 people living with HIV. However there have been signs of a rapid increase recently, and a shifting of transmission patterns towards heterosexual sex. In 2004, Israel reported a rise of 9% in new HIV cases and the proportion of women rose from 20% to 30%. In 1998 the average age of women newly infected with HIV was 30 years but in 2004 was reported to be 19 years.

The epidemiology of HIV-2

HIV-2 in the UK

HIV-2 is extremely rare in the UK. By the end of September 2006, 109 diagnoses of HIV-2 infection in individuals without HIV-1 infection had been reported in the UK. A further 20 diagnoses of HIV-1 and HIV-2 dual infections were also reported. Most of the cases have been identified by anonymous testing, so it has been impossible to identify their origin.

In terms of actual clinic diagnoses, between 1985 and 2003 inclusive, 1324 individuals diagnosed and reported with HIV in the UK had probably been infected in West Africa, where HIV-2 originates. Of these 917 (69%) were HIV-1 infected and 52 (6%) HIV-2 or HIV-1/HIV-2 co-infected. For 355 (27%) the HIV type was not reported.

The proportion of HIV-2 and HIV-1/HIV-2infections varied by country of infection (p<0.001): ranging from the Gambia (11.7%-15.2%) to Nigeria (0.7%-1.0%). A further 130 individuals of west African origin were probably infected through heterosexual intercourse within the United Kingdom by a heterosexual partner infected in West Africa. 89 (68%) were HIV-1 infected and three (2%) HIV-2 infected or HIV-1/HIV-2 co-infected. For 38 (29%) HIV type was not reported.

Five children born to HIV-2 infected mothers have been reported: two children have been shown to be uninfected, two are still HIV-2 indeterminate, and one has been lost to follow-up.

Three of the five surveys in the unlinked anonymous (UA) testing programme identified HIV-2 positive specimens. From 1990 to 2000, the programme identified 36 specimens positive for HIV-2 alone, and a further 17 positive for both HIV-1 and HIV-2, out of 1,730,573 specimens tested. There were 11,131 specimens positive for HIV-1 infection only.

In some cases the same individual may have been included more than once, and if they have had a diagnostic test they may also be included among the 83 cases described in the first paragraph of this section. The UA programme has shown, however, that HIV-2 is making a very small contribution to the numbers of HIV-infected individuals in the UK: the ratio of HIV-1 infections to HIV-2 is over 250:1.

Reference

Dougan S. Diagnoses of HIV-1 and HIV-2 in England, Wales, and Northern Ireland associated with west Africa. Sexually Transmitted Infections 81: 338-341, 2005.

HPA. AIDS and HIV infection in the United Kingdom: monthly report. HIV-2 infections identified in the UK. Commun Dis Rep CDR Wkly 11 (21): 15, 2001. Available online at www.hpa.org.uk/publications/Cdr/PDffiles/2001/cdr2101.pdf

HIV-2 globally

HIV-2 is highly concentrated in West African countries such as Senegal, Ivory Coast, Cape Verde, Gambia, Guinea-Bissau, Liberia, Ghana and Nigeria. It has tended to spread only to countries with strong links to these West African countries - France, Portugal, Angola and Mozambique. Very few cases have been reported outside these countries.

A number of factors suggest that HIV-2 is unlikely to spread in the same way as HIV-1:

- A number of strains of HIV-2 have been identified, classified into four clades (A, B, C, D) which are no more closely related to each other than they are to different strains of an SIV (simian immunodeficiency virus) found in wild sooty mangabey monkeys in West Africa. It therefore appears that the different clades represent separate transmissions of the virus at some time in the past from sooty mangabeys to people.

- HIV-2 infection appears to be less pathogenic than HIV-1. It is much more difficult to isolate HIV-2 from the blood of infected individuals than in cases of HIV-1 infection.

- Immunodeficiency caused by HIV-2 infection takes much longer to develop. Individuals infected with HIV-2 are asymptomatic for much longer, and may not develop high levels of virus in their blood for fifteen to twenty years after infection, by which time they may be much less sexually active or past child-bearing age.

- HIV-2 is not easily transmitted during the lengthy asymptomatic phase of infection due to the very low levels of virus found during this time, which may explain why the virus is less widespread. Studying sex workers in Senegal, researchers found that whilst HIV-1 spread very rapidly (the number of new cases of HIV-1 was greater during each year of the study than the preceding year), HIV-2 spread much

more slowly (the number of new cases each year was almost identical). Researchers estimated that it would take 5 years for the number of HIV-1 cases to double, but 31 years for the number of HIV-2 cases to double (Kanki).

- HIV-2 is less easily transmitted from mother to baby, perhaps because of much lower viral load in HIV-2 infected mothers (Gayle).

References

HPA. AIDS and HIV infection in the United Kingdom: monthly report. HIV-2 infections identified in the UK. Commun Dis Rep CDR Wkly 11(21): 15, 2001.Available online at www.phls.org.uk/publications/Cdr/PDffiles/2001/cdr2101.pdf

de Cock K et al: Epidemiology and transmission of HIV-2: why there is no HIV-2 pandemic. JAMA 270(17): 2083-2086, 1993.

Gayle HD et al: HIV-1 and HIV-2 infection in children in Abidjan, Côte d'Ivoire. JAIDS 2(5): 513-517, 1992.

Hishida O et al: Clinically diagnosed AIDS cases without evident association with HIV type 1 and 2 infections in Ghana. Lancet 8825: 971-972, 1992.

Kanki P et al: Slower heterosexual spread of HIV-2 than HIV-1. Lancet 343: 943-946, 1994.

HIV type O and viral diversity

In 1994 researchers in Cameroon reported that they had identified a new variant of HIV, named type O, which was not picked up by standard antibody tests for HIV-1. This was seen as representing a distinct branch of HIV-1 from the main "M" group of viruses, as a result of a separate transmission of the virus to people from its original host, the common chimpanzee. However later investigations found that, unexpectedly, type O may have come from a different host - the gorilla.

A further group of isolates from the same area have been described as an "N" group, which is more closely related to known chimpanzee viruses than either O or M, and is therefore likely to represent a more recent inter-species transmission event.

Type O accounts for only a minority of infections even in Cameroon and Gabon (10% in Cameroon) and are extremely rare elsewhere, while type N has only ever been found in 12 patients.

Antibody testing kits for use in initial screening, including rapid tests, have increasingly been adapted to include antigens from type O viruses as well as type M and from HIV-2.

Other variants of HIV-1 are less divergent, and are already detectable by standard antibody testing kits. References to these variants, or subtypes, are becoming more frequent in scientific literature. The subtypes each predominate in different parts of the world, and the occurrence of the same subtype in countries far apart provides clues about the global dissemination of HIV.

- Subtype A is found in Central Africa, especially in Kenya.

- Subtype B is the predominant strain found in the developed world amongst injecting drug users and gay men. It is common in the Americas, Europe, Australia and Thailand (predominantly amongst injecting drug users and their sexual partners, although subtype E is now increasingly dominant among both groups).

- Subtype C is found in India, Brazil, Ethiopia, Tanzania, China and southern Africa and is now the most widespread virus on a global scale.

- Subtype D is found in Central Africa.

- Subtype E is not found as a separate subtype in itself but is only ever found in a recombinant form, as half of a 'spliced' virus where its genes are mixed with subtype A virus. It is found in the Central African Republic and in Thailand. It has been given the alternative name of 'CRF 01-AE'.

- Subtype F is found in Brazil, Romania and the Democratic Republic of the Congo.

- Subtype G is found in the Democratic Republic of the Congo, Gabon and Taiwan.

- Subtype H is found in the Democratic Republic of the Congo and Gabon.

Recombinant forms of the virus, between different subtypes, are increasingly important in some parts of the world, especially West Africa, where most people with HIV have viruses described as 'AG' recombinants - though these often include sections of other subtypes too.

The large number of variants in Africa strongly suggests that HIV has been present in humans in Africa for longer than in other parts of the world.

It has been suggested that some variants of HIV may be transmitted more easily by vaginal intercourse, whilst some may be better adapted to transmission through blood, but research is still going on to answer this question. Recent work in Kinshasa has identified a number of viruses in the M group that cannot be classified in existing subtypes. This suggests that the whole sub-type phenomenon is nothing more than a sampling effect from the human population in which the virus was first established on a large scale, and in which it then diversified at random.

Reference

HIV-2 infections identified in the UK. CDR Weekly 11: 21, 2001.

HIV transmission

The established modes

The bottom line

HIV can be transmitted through unprotected sexual intercourse, sharing injecting equipment or receiving blood transfusions and other blood-related products from an infected person. It can also be transmitted from an HIV-positive mother to her baby.

Unprotected sex

Established and common routes:

- Unprotected anal penetration

- Unprotected vaginal penetration.

Possible but less common routes:

- Oral transmission: it is now thought that between less than 1% to 3% of all HIV cases in the UK may be due to oral transmission. Most cases suggest that oral transmission depends on either damaged tissue in the mouth or throat, the presence of an untreated STI in the throat, or an ulceration on the penis. It may also need an exceptionally high viral load in the transmitting partner.

- Any sexual activities where significant amounts of blood may be shared (e.g. fisting, piercing, etc). Small amounts of blood are unlikely to transmit HIV.

- Through blood in otherwise uncontaminated body fluids: in the mouth or the rectum, during menstruation.

- Through shared sex toys etc.

Needles and sharps (non-medical)

Established and common route:

- Sharing injecting equipment.

Possible but less common route:

- Needle-stick and sharps injuries.

Possible but very uncommon route:

- Tattooing, acupuncture, electrolysis, shaving equipment. In these cases it is assumed that infection is possible but extremely unlikely. A case of infection through unsterilised acupuncture needles has been reported.

Medical (iatrogenic) transmission

Possible but less common routes:

- Unsterilised needles used for injection. This risk should be non-existent in the UK, but worldwide the World Health Organization (WHO) estimates that five per cent of HIV infections in developing countries are spread by this route.

- Blood transfusions, blood products and donations (organs, skin). Since 1985 blood donations in the UK have been screened, and screening began at roughly the same time in most other countries which could afford such programmes. Organs and tissues for donation have also been screened since that time, whilst blood products such as Factor VIII have been heat- treated since 1984.

- Surgical and other invasive procedures: fortunately very uncommon and the risk needs to be seen in the light of the far greater risks involved routinely in these invasive health care procedures.

- Occupationally through blood splashes onto broken skin and needle stick injuries.

- Donations of blood, organs, tissues, semen, breast milk and bone marrow - in each of these instances a very small number of cases have been reported.

The mechanisms of HIV transmission

First principles

It has now been proved that for HIV transmission to happen, three conditions need to apply:

- Live virus has to be present either in the body of an infected person or in a contaminated body fluid or body tissue (Presence).

- There has to be a sufficient amount of the virus present (often called technically 'tissue culture infectious dose') (Quantity).

- It has to get into the body of the uninfected person through an effective route for transmission to occur. In this respect HIV is no different from any other virus: it can only be transmitted through certain now well-understood routes. There must be susceptible receptor cells at the site of entry and inadequate host defences (Route and Susceptibility).

Additionally, there are two sets of co-factors which may be said to encourage transmission or make it more likely:

- Physical co-factors.

- Social co-factors.

These principles can be used to determine the following:

- Clear guidelines on the established and predominant modes of transmission.

- Clear guidelines on biologically possible but unlikely modes of transmission.

- Clear guidelines on 'impossible' modes of transmission and reassurance against unfounded concerns about HIV and AIDS.

All of these factors are now discussed in more detail immediately below.

The grounds for confidence in this knowledge are discussed in *The evidence for HIV Transmission*, later in this chapter.

Comparing risks

There are problems in establishing the comparative degrees of risk of particular activities. This is because:

- They vary with the co-factors described immediately below.

- Different studies have shown some conflicting results in different populations.

- The size of statistical samples has not been large enough to do away with statistical possibilities of error.

However, it is possible to suggest orders of magnitude of risk.

Beyond distinguishing such orders of magnitude, however, any greater precision can rarely form a safe basis for making individual judgements about preventing HIV transmission in particular circumstances.

For example, although it is probably true that unprotected anal sex is more likely to transmit HIV infection than unprotected vaginal sex, any reliance upon protection through switching from one to the other would fail to reduce the risk sufficiently for it to be an acceptable mode of protection. Thus advice to

heterosexuals to refrain from anal intercourse in order to be safe is not good advice. People often 'mix' risks, too; but any change in behaviour (a good example is changing from breastfeeding to bottle-feeding your baby) has to be complete.

Conversely, we know that the correct use of a condom of an appropriate quality will reduce the order of magnitude of risk quite substantially.

The use of the categories 'high risk', 'medium risk', 'low risk' can become confusing, particularly where different agencies or countries classify the same activity at different levels of risk.

However, it is becoming increasingly clear from epidemiological evidence that the activities classified as 'high risk' in the earliest years of the epidemic remain the preponderant routes of transmission, whilst those classified in the past as 'medium risk' have in fact been discovered to be very low risks.

The very highest-risk activities

- Unprotected receptive or insertive anal sex.

- Unprotected receptive vaginal sex.

- Sharing unsterilised injecting equipment.

- Being born to or breastfed by an untreated HIV-positive mother.

High-risk activities

- Unprotected vaginal sex.

- Receiving donated blood or organs or injections with unsterilised needles in countries with inadequate screening procedures.

Less risky activities

- Penetrative sex with appropriate barrier (condom or female condom), when used correctly: there is a (not insignificant) residual risk because incorrect use may lead the condom to fail.

- Oral sex receptively.

- Sharing injection equipment if improperly sterilised.

- Occupational risks in invasive surgical and medical contexts.

- Laboratory work with superconcentrates of HIV.

- Being born to or breastfed by an HIV-positive mother receiving antiretroviral treatment.

Very low risk activities

- Sharing penetrative sex toys.

- Sharing razors, toothbrushes, etc.

- Rimming if blood present in stool.

'Never mind the facts, just give me the figures'

Medical and helping professionals are time and again asked by people afraid they have put themselves at risk of HIV to give precise estimates for the likelihood of infection.

For reasons specified above and below, precise estimates of the risk level of individual activities are hard to come by and vary enormously according to many different criteria:

- Whether the source was known to be HIV-positive.

- If not, the prevalence of HIV in the population or among the specific risk group the person belonged to.

- The stage of infection and viral load of the positive person.

- Whether they were on HIV medication.

- The general state of health of both partners.

- The presence of sexually transmitted infections, including the presence of any ulcers or lesions in either partner.

- The quantity of infectious body fluid transferred.

- The virulence of the particular strain of HIV.

- Whether the recipient has some degree of natural or acquired immunity to HIV.

- .and many other reasons.

However, HIV advisors and recipients of advice have often complained that repeatedly telling someone their activity has been 'low risk' is no help unless some degree of quantification is attempted. Therefore, and with all the above caveats in mind, we will here list the best estimates (or guesstimates) of the likelihood of infection per exposure for specific activities and incidents.

Per Exposure means the risk of infection **for each individual incident HIV transfer could have occurred.** This is a more precise measure of risk than 'per sexual partner' (because sexual partners may or may not have HIV) or 'per head of population' (because people's risk behaviour varies so much).

The problem with this measure of risk is that it makes things look not very risky. What it does not take into account is that people do certain things (e.g. have sex) a lot more often than they do other things (e.g. prick themselves with an infected needle.) Health advisors have been reluctant to give figures like this before, because they felt that if they told someone who had done the sexually most risky possible thing (had receptive unprotected anal sex with someone recently infected) that they had a one in 33 chance of infection, the person would think, "Only one in 33. Well, that's worth risking."

What this one in 33 figure means is that the person would only have to have sex with the source partner 17 times - easily done within, say, a month in a new relationship - for it to become **more likely than not** that they will catch HIV.

However, figures can also exaggerate perceived risk, too. The figures below are all on the basis that the source partner is known to be HIV-positive.

Where the serostatus of the source partner is unknown, the prevalence of HIV in the source partner's risk group has to be taken into account. This makes certain activities very much less risky than they otherwise would have been if the partner was known to be positive. In other cases it makes relatively little difference.

For instance, about one in eight gay men in London has HIV whereas about one in 500 UK adults in general has it (unless they are in another higher-risk group).

So where the source partner's serostatus is unknown this would mean that the chance of contracting HIV from a single act of unprotected receptive anal sex with a gay man in London is at most one in 33 times eight = one in 264.

However, the chance of getting HIV from a similar act of unprotected vaginal sex if you are a woman having sex with a man who is not from a high-prevalence community would be at most 0.00164%, or about one chance in 61,000.

Having said this, 'from a high prevalence community' is not something that can be easily judged and is susceptible to stereotyping.

Once you have read this table, continue to the 'now read on.' section

Table: Estimated HIV risk per exposure for specific activities and events

Activity	Risk per exposure	Notes
Vaginal sex less than five months after infection of source partner	0.82% (1:123)	Because viral load likely to be higher: See 'now read on...' below
Vaginal sex less than six weeks after infection of source partner	less than 2% (1:50)	High-end estimate
Vaginal sex, partner in chronic infection (but not with AIDS)	0.08% (1:1250)	
Vaginal sex, chronic infection, with condom	0.0012% (1:8333)	Assuming condom failure rate of 15%
Vaginal sex, partner with AIDS and not on treatment	0.45% (1:222)	From study in Africa: sex woth partner 5-15 months before their death
Insertive vaginal sex (overall)	0.06% (1:1666)	Ten to 25 times more risky if partner recently infected
Receptive anal sex amongst gay men, partner unknown status	0.27% (1:370)	

Activity	Risk per exposure	Notes
Vaginal sex, partner with AIDS and not on treatment	0.45% (1:222)	From study in Africa: sex woth partner 5-15 months before their death
Insertive vaginal sex (overall)	0.06% (1:1666)	Ten to 25 times more risky if partner recently infected
Receptive anal sex amongst gay men, partner unknown status	0.27% (1:370)	
Receptive anal sex amongst gay men, partner HIV-positive	0.82% (1:123)	
Receptive anal sex less than five months after partner's infection	3% (1:33)	Because viral load likely to be higher. See 'now read on...' below
Receptive anal sex less than six weeks after partner's infection	less than 11% (1:9)	High-end estimate
Receptive anal sex with condom, gay men, partner's HIV status unknown	0.18% (1:555)	
Receptive anal sex less than five months after partner's infection, with condom	0.45% (1:222)	Condom failure rate 15%
Insertive anal sex, gay men, partner unknown status	0.06% (1:1666)	Ten to 25 times more risky if partner recently infected
Insertive anal sex, gay men, partner HIV-positive	0.18% (1:549)	
Insertive anal sex with positive partner less than six weeks after infection	4.5% (1:22)	High-end estimate
Insertive anal sex with condom, gay men, partner unknown status	0.04% (1:2500)	
Receptive oral sex	0.04% (1:2500)	Maximum estimated figure
Sharing injecting equipment	1.4% (1:71)	Estimated range: 1:48 to 1:150

Table references

Vaginal sex: Wawer M J et al. HIV-1 Transmission per coital act, by stage of HIV infection in the HIV+ index partner, in discordant couples, Rakai, Uganda. Tenth Conference on Retroviruses and Opportunistic Infections, Boston, abstract 40, 2003.

Vaginal sex: Gray R H et al. Probability of HIV-1 transmission per coital act in monogamous, heterosexual, HIV-1-discordant couples in Rakai, Uganda. Lancet 357(9263): 1149-1153, 2001.

Vaginal sex: Galvin SR and Cohen MS. The role of sexually transmitted diseases in HIV infection. Nature Reviews Microbiology (2-1), 2004.

Anal sex between men: Vittinghoff E. Per-contact risk of human immunodeficiency virus transmission between male sexual partners. American Journal of Epidemiology 150(3): 306-311, 1999.

Oral sex: Vittinghoff, above.

Oral sex: Page-Shafer K et al. Risk of HIV infection attributable to oral sex among men who have sex with men and in the population of men who have sex with men. AIDS 16(17): 2350-2352, 2002.

Sharing injecting equipment and needlestick injury: Gaughwin MD et al. Bloody needles: the volume of blood transferred in simulations of needlestick injuries AIDS 5(8): 1025-1027, 1991.

Needlestick injury: Becker C et al: Occupational infection with HIV, AIM, 110(8): 653-656, 1989.

Needlestick and mucous membrane exposure: Ippolito G et al,, Italian Study Group on Occupational Risk of HIV Infection. The risk of occupational human immunodeficiency virus in health care workers. Arch Int Med 153: 1451-1458, 1993.

Blood Transfusion: Ward JW: The natural history of transfusion-associated infection with human immunodeficiency virus: factors influencing the rate of progression to disease, NEJM 321(14): 947-952, 1989.

Now read on: two big exceptions

1. Acute HIV infection

Immediately after infection and before the body starts trying to defend itself against HIV by making antibodies, people often have dramatically higher levels of HIV in their blood and other body fluids than thereafter, during chronic infection. During the period of HIV infection before and during seroconversion (see *HIV Testing*) people can quite often have viral loads 100 or more times greater than the ones they have during chronic infection.

This means they could be up to 100 times more infectious with HIV. One mathematical model (Fraser) estimated that people are at least 24 times more infectious.

This has led epidemiologists to suspect that a great deal of HIV is spread by people who have recently become infected themselves. Mathematical models have estimated that anything between 14% (from the Fraser study above) and 50% (Cates) of HIV is transmitted by people in acute HIV infection.

If so, this represents a considerable problem when it comes to HIV prevention. It is also attested from studies that people who know their HIV status reduce their risk behaviour by anything between 40% and 85%. People in acute infection are unlikely to know or even suspect they have HIV, especially if they do not have (or do not yet have) obvious seroconversion symptoms.

It also means that - in theory at least, though this has never been researched - that the HIV risk of some activities could be very considerably higher if they are done with a partner in acute HIV infection. In short, what may be low or medium risk at other times may be medium to high risk at these times. This might explain some cases of transmission through routes like oral sex.

Up till 2007, all of the estimates of the proportion of infections due to primary infection had been produced by mathematical models: but mathematical models are only as good as the data put into them. The low-rate estimate (14%) above was mainly influenced by the consideration that the period of very high viral load is in fact very short. Most people may only have viral loads in the millions for a week to a month - or, at most, six weeks - after infection. Thus, it was reasoned, no matter how infectious people are during this period, they simply haven't the time in which to contribute to more than a minority of infections.

The first direct evidence of the amount of HIV spread in acute HIV infection came from a study presented at the 2007 CROI Conference (Brenner) - and it came in at the high end: it estimated that nearly 50% of all HIV infections are transmitted by people in acute infection. Although the evidence is still indirect, and based upon phylogenetic analysis of the different viruses people carry and the way they 'cluster' into closely related groups suggestive of chains of infection, it is much firmer evidence than that provided by modelling.

Blum and Brenner and colleagues from the McGill AIDS Centre in Montréal found that just under 50% of HIV infections in a group of 593 people who'd been diagnosed less than six months after infection clustered into closely-related groups, suggesting chains of infection between newly-infected people.

These clusters featured HIV viruses so genetically similar that they were almost certainly connected; on average only 0.015% of their genetic make-up was different from other viruses in the cluster (one part's difference in 7500). About half these groups were small, consisting of duos, threesomes or foursomes of newly-infected people. But the other half of these clusters of infection had an average of nine connected infections. Nine out of ten infections in these clusters took place within two years of each other, suggesting an average time between acquiring HIV and passing it on of about three months.

Brenner also looked at a comparable group of 795 patients either diagnosed in chronic infection (135 people) or who had been diagnosed for some time and who had been on treatment (660 people). She found that only 3.2% of these infections fell into clusters, and that that only 5.4% of patients who'd been infected with HIV for less than six months had infections that clustered with the HIV belonging people in long-term infection. When they did, the long-term infected person was only one-third of a duo of infections, not a member of a big group. This suggests that when a long-term-infected person transmits HIV it's usually a one-off event, caused maybe by pure bad luck or maybe for other medical reasons such as acquiring an STD or failing therapy.

Altogether Brenner found 75 clusters of connected infection in the Quebec study, and the largest connected group featured 17 people infected over a three-year period. Brenner calculated that recently-infected people were responsible for a minimum of 49.4% of transmissions, and chronically-infected people for 27.5% of transmissions, evenly split into people who'd never taken antiretroviral drugs and ones who had but had a detectable viral load.

This doesn't add up to 100% because these are minimal estimates and express the degree of uncertainly of the figures.

In an accompanying editorial UK HIV specialists Martin Fisher and Deenan Pillay commented that if 50% of HIV is transmitted

by people who've recently caught it and if (as they suspect) at least 50% of these don't know it, this presents prevention strategists with a problem as many prevention strategies depend on someone knowing they have HIV or at least not assuming they're negative.

They urge an expansion of testing and the use of add-ons to traditional HIV antibody testing such as antigen testing and pooled viral load testing, which can pick up recent infections earlier and increase the number of positive tests by 10%.

"Strategies to improve recognition of recent infection, in addition to identifying undiagnosed chronic infection, are crucial to effective implementation of prevention strategies," they write.

References

Brenner BG et al. High rates of forward transmission events after acute/early HIV-1 infection. J Infect Dis 195: 951-959, 2007.

Pillay D and Fisher M. Primary HIV infection, phylogenetics, and antiretroviral prevention. J Infect Dis 195: 924-926, 2007.

Cates W et al. Primary HIV infection--a public health opportunity. Am J Public Health. 87(12): 1928-1930, 1997.

Fraser C et al. Quantifying the Impact of Primary Infection on HIV Transmission and Control. 13th Conference on Retroviruses and Opportunistic Infections, Denver, abstract 162, 2006.

2. Acquired immunity

The other consideration operates in the opposite direction, by reducing the amount of HIV transmission that might be expected rather than increasing it; but it may have had similarly distorting effects on our estimates of the relative and absolute risks of transmission for different acts.

This is the phenomenon of acquired immunity. An HIV-negative partner exposed to their HIV-positive partner's virus may in the end build up a degree of immunity to it sufficient to make transmission much less likely.

This possibility had been known about since the early 1990s and studies of people such as the well-known group of Kenyan sex workers that appeared to have antibody-mediated immunity to HIV infection despite (or, indeed because of) frequent HIV exposure lent credence to the idea that it might be a common phenomenon.

In 2004 Dr Barry Peters and colleagues from St Thomas's Hospital in London studied 29 monogamous heterosexual serodiscordant couples who had had frequent unprotected intercourse for more than six months. They compared the anti-HIV immune responses in the negative partner to those in a control group of 15 HIV-negative women and 10 HIV-negative men who had had no sex, or only protected sex, for at least the previous six months.

They took CD4 cells from all the subjects and attempted to infect them with various different strains of HIV in the test tube.

It was found that CD4 cells in women who had had unprotected sex with HIV-positive men were only 10% as likely to be infected with HIV (of the type that is more often transmitted) as CD4 cells from women who'd had protected or no sex.

The HIV-negative men who'd had unprotected sex with positive women had half that degree of protection: their CD4 cells were 20% as likely to be infected with HIV as cells from men who'd had protected or no sex.

So the mucosal immunity generated by frequent sexual exposure to HIV - meaning the immunity generated by cells lining the genital membranes - can be as high as 90% immunity in women and 80% in men, though the degree of 'in vivo' i.e. real life protection will probably be less.

In an accompanying editorial, *The Lancet* cautioned against jumping to the wrong conclusions from this study:

"*Most epidemiological evidence indicates that unprotected intercourse dangerously exposes most individuals to HIV infection...Peters' observations must never, of course be interpreted as a suggestion for individuals to have unprotected intercourse for the purposes of immunisation."*

In a study presented at the Bangkok World AIDS Conference the same year, Dr Tuofu Zhu found evidence of he same phenomenon amongst long-term gay male couples.

Zhu was studying "long-term exposed seronegative" partners of HIV-positive gay men. The group consisted of the HIV-negative partners of HIV-positive men who had been diagnosed between 1994 and 1998.

Out of 94 HIV-negative regular partners of positive men, he found 14 who had in fact become HIV-positive -- a rate of only 15%, despite regular unprotected sex with their partners over a period of years.

Two of the partners appeared to have caught HIV from their partners early on in their relationship, but to have mounted a successful immune response to it, becoming so-called "exposed seronegatives". This meant that they had no antibodies to HIV and did not test HIV antibody positive. The fact that they had HIV at all could only be detected by hypersensitive viral-load testing, which picked up HIV in their blood at a count of 0.05 copies - one thousandth of the amount usually called "undetectable" by standard "ultrasensitive" tests.

The other 12 of the 14, however, had recognisable HIV infections with positive antibody tests. Some maintained low viral loads in the 500-2,000 range and showed some evidence of an immune response to HIV; others had "standard" viral loads in the tens of thousands. But all 12 had clearly not caught HIV from their regular partners. Genetic analysis of the virus they carried showed that not only was it completely different in each case from the virus their partner carried, but that on average it was more different than any randomly selected North American strain would have been.

When they had a strong immune response to HIV, their virus tended to change in a completely different way to their partner's and become more unlike it as time went on. When people only had a weak response to their partner's HIV, their viruses became more similar.

Although no one is recommending that long-term negative partners of positive men have unsafe sex, this study does add to the evidence that a degree of immunity to "familiar" HIV can be built up, but that these immune responses are narrow and do not protect you against "stranger" virus.

More evidence for acquired immunity comes form the finding that HIV superinfection - the acquisition of a second strain of HIV from a positive partner - is common in the first year of contact with a new partner but becomes less so as time goes on. Studies have found evidence of superinfection in 2 to 5% of persons in the first year of infection (Smith) but found no evidence of superinfection in long-term relationships (Gonzales). In fact 95% of all cases of superinfection so far documented have occurred through contact with a partner less than three years intro a relationship. Interestingly, superinfection is also more common in people with recent HIV infection anyway and much less common in people with long-term infection - possibly because viral mutation and diversification in the person 'auto-immunises' them against a wider range of other types of HIV.

What does this mean for our estimates of HIV transmission? The estimates for the risk during vaginal intercourse above were taken from a longitudinal study of long-term monogamous heterosexual discordant couple - exactly the kind of people where the negative partner may have acquired immunity to HIV. Since the majority of sexually-acquired HIV is spread in casual sex situations or between new partners, this may mean that estimated for the per-exposure risk for certain activities maybe anything up to 10 times too low when applied to casual sex situations.

References

Gonzales MJ, Delwart E, Rhee SY, et al. Lack of detectable human immunodeficiency virus type 1 superinfection during 1072 person-years of observation . Journal of Infectious Diseases. 188: 397-405, 2003.

Peters B et al. Effect of heterosexual intercourse on mucosal alloimmunisation and resistance to HIV-1 infection. Lancet 363: 518-524, 2004.

Smith DM et al. Incidence of HIV superinfection following primary infection. JAMA 292(10): 1177-1178, 2004.

Zhu T et al. Breakthrough HIV-1 infection in long-term exposed seronegative individuals. XV International AIDS Conference, Bangkok, abstract TuOrA1141, 2004.

More on transmission risks

The prevalence of HIV

HIV will inevitably be more prevalent in some groups of people than others because of the history of the epidemic.

This will mean that the same act will carry different levels of risk in different groups of the population and different places:

The prevalence in different core groups varies from place to place and over time, e.g. between gay and bisexual men in the USA and the UK. For instance, prevalence in both gay men and heterosexual women in at least twice as high in London as it is in the rest of the UK. However this is for different reasons; while prevalence in London gay men as a whole is higher, it is only so in women because more African women live in London. So it would be misleading to say that prevalence in women in general as a population group is higher in London.

- Statistical scientific knowledge about prevalence rates in groups of the population cannot always be safely translated into practical knowledge of individuals' risk factors in particular cases.

- Groups defined by a common sense of identity are not functionally the same as groups defined by their actual behaviour. Thus, many people have mistakenly believed themselves not to be at risk because they saw themselves as heterosexual even though they were also engaging in unsafe homosexual activity in practice.

Identification and avoidance of people with HIV is not an effective or desirable line of defence against HIV for individuals who engage in activities which can transmit the virus. This is because, at any time the majority of people with HIV cannot be identified by external physical signs. Moreover, any attempt to fit individuals into broad and blunt risk categories (although useful in the planning of public health services) is likely to fail on an individual level most of the time. It is not always possible to detect the sexual or drug using history of partners with sufficient accuracy for this to offer sufficient protection.

The presence and concentration of HIV

HIV may be present in many body fluids, but it does not follow that its presence will constitute a risk for infection. This is because it may be present in many body fluids only in very low concentrations. Research shows that levels of HIV vary hugely across time in the same individual, with the highest levels detectable just after infection and at the development of symptomatic HIV disease. It was estimated by Galvin, for instance, that the risk of HIV infection to a woman from a single instance of unprotected vaginal intercourse varied from one in 25 to one in 1,000 if the man is in the first three weeks of HIV infection, but that this falls to one in 1,000 to one in 10,000 if he is chronically infected.

It is important to note that it is almost impossible to isolate HIV from some body fluids, such as urine.

Reference

Galvin SR and Cohen MS. The role of sexually transmitted diseases in HIV infection. Nature Reviews Microbiology (2-1), 2004.

In what form is HIV infectious?

HIV's genetic material may be passed from one individual to another in several different forms.

It may be passed as free virus particles (HIV RNA), which are able to bind onto cells with CD4 markers.

It may be passed within HIV-infected lymphocytes as proviral DNA. In this case the virus is transcribed into the genetic material of the host cell and will begin to replicate when that immune system cell is activated.

In semen, for instance, it exists in both forms; as virus particles in the nutrient carrier fluid; and as proviral DNA within lymphocytes. It is not present in sperm cells themselves.

The difference between viral load and infectious particles

Throughout this chapter you will see the terms 'viral load' and 'infectious particles' used. These terms refer to different measurements:

- 'Infectious particles' refers to the number of viruses present in millilitre of a body fluid. This is assessed by a test which detects whole viruses. It is slow and laborious to conduct, and if there are very low levels of HIV present in a body fluid the test will not detect the HIV particles.

- 'Viral load' refers to the results of a test designed to amplify any genetic material of the virus in a sample of a body fluid. This test uses a template which corresponds to a genetic sequence of HIV which does not tend to vary between individuals. The test detects the genetic sequence and amplifies it by attaching a marker chemical to make the genetic sequence visible. The test will go through several rounds of amplification to increase the chance that HIV's genetic sequence can be detected. The final result is described as the number of HIV RNA copies per millilitre. The number is usually at least tenfold greater than the number of infectious HIV particles.

Repeat viral load tests of the same blood sample can give results that vary by a factor of 3. This means that a meaningful change would be a drop to **less than 1/3** or an increase to **more than three times** the previous test result. For example, a change from 200,000 to 600,000 is within the normal variability of the test. A drop from 50,000 to 10,000 would be significant.

It is important to note than no more than 2% of the HIV in a person's body is in the blood at any one time; the viral load test does not measure how much HIV is in body tissues like the lymph nodes, spleen, or brain. HIV levels in lymph tissue and semen go down when blood levels go down, but not at the same time or the same rate.

The viral load test, also known as the polymerase chain reaction test, is a technology devised to detect very small genetic fragments. It cannot judge whether these fragments are infectious.

The viral load tests currently available all have lower limits of detection which vary between 500 and 5 copies per millilitre.

Log changes in viral load

Throughout this chapter reference will be made to 'log' changes in viral load. The log scale is the measurement used by researchers to describe the changes in viral load in an infected individual, and in this case refers to changes to the power of 10. The scale is used because the magnitude of changes in viral load during antiretroviral therapy is immense, and can only be captured on graphs or diagrams by using a logarithmic scale.

A 1 log change refers to a tenfold change, a 2 log change to a hundredfold change and a 3 log change to a thousand-fold change.

Viral load below 10,000 copies is considered to be low viral load, whilst viral load in the range of 10,000 to 50,000 copies is considered to be moderately high, and above 50,000 copies is considered to be high.

Blood

HIV has been isolated from blood at levels of up to 5,000 infectious particles per ml, but some researchers have found it much more difficult to isolate HIV from the blood of HIV-positive individuals.

Although levels of free infectious virus may be very low in the blood of asymptomatic individuals (below 200 HIV RNA copies per ml), asymptomatic individuals may have viral load above 1,000,000 HIV RNA copies per ml.

Antiretroviral therapy using a combination of drugs usually reduces viral load by at least 90% within a few weeks of initiating treatment. Blood from individuals receiving antiretroviral therapy may be less infectious, although many cases have been reported of viral burden rebounding to extremely high levels when resistance to antiretroviral drugs emerges, or when treatment is discontinued.

References

Ho DD et al: Quantitation of human immunodeficiency virus type 1 in the blood of infected persons. NEJM 321: 1621-1625, 1989.

Levy JA: Pathogenesis of human immunodeficiency virus infection. Microbiological Reviews 57: 185-289, 1993.

Semen

Between 10 and 30% of seminal fluid samples studied have been shown to contain either free infectious virus or cell-associated virus (infected lymphocytes). However, levels of cell-associated virus are much higher; there are up to one million lymphocytes in each millilitre of semen; even if only one per cent of these lymphocytes are infected with HIV, this means that each millilitre of semen may contain up to 1,000 infected lymphocytes. The average male ejaculation is 5ml of semen, although this varies considerably.

Lymphocytes and cell-associated virus are most likely to be present in individuals suffering from infections which cause inflammation in the urethra and other regions of the genital tract. Untreated sexually transmitted infections, even those which cause no detectable symptoms, are likely to increase the viral load in semen.

The relationship between viral load in blood, immune status and viral load in semen is full of uncertainties. Recent studies have produced very contradictory results.

Viral load in semen is usually greater in those with lower CD4 counts. Several studies have shown that HIV is more frequently isolated from the semen of men with CD4 counts below 200, especially if they are symptomatic. A 1994 study found HIV in the semen of 87% of men with CD4 count below 100, but in only 40% of men with CD4 counts between 100 and 200. Only in men with CD4 counts below 100 was it possible to find more virulent forms of HIV (the SI phenotype), which are believed to be more easily transmitted during vaginal intercourse (Vernazza). A 1996 study found that HIV RNA levels were at least tenfold (1 log) higher in men with CD4 counts below 200 compared to men with CD4 counts above 500 (Dyer).

A 1991 study found that whilst HIV was most commonly isolated from the semen of men with CD4 counts below 200, it could also be isolated from the semen of 43% of a group of asymptomatic men on at least one occasion out of six monthly

tests, suggesting fluctuating levels of HIV in the semen of infected men.

Although most studies show that the majority of men treated with antiretroviral drugs demonstrated parallel declines in plasma and seminal viral load, all studies have shown considerable individual variation in responses.

The following patterns have been observed:

- Viral load becomes undetectable in plasma weeks or months before doing so in semen.

- Viral load becomes undetectable in semen but not in plasma.

- Plasma viral load rebounds after a period of undetectability but seminal viral load remains undetectable.

Studies of gay men (Taylor) suggest that at any one time about 12% of HIV-positive men on ARV treatment may have detectable HIV in their semen even if they do not have it in their blood; this has been linked to the presence of (often asymptomatic) urethritis.

Seminal and plasma viral loads were obtained from 72 HIV-positive men who were not taking HIV therapy in a research project involving investigators from London and Birmingham. Earlier research from these investigators established that in men taking antiretroviral therapy, a detectable seminal viral load was associated with untreated gonorrhoea.

Although none of the men in the study had a blood plasma viral load below the limit of detection (400 copies/ml), 22 men (30% of the sample) did have undetectable seminal viral loads. These men were classified as "non-shedders". Low levels of HIV, on average 4,000 copies/ml, were detected in the semen of 58% of men, who were classified as "seminal shedders". Their blood plasma viral load was significantly higher than non-shedders at 100,000 copies/ml versus 10,000 copies/ml.

12% (n=9) of men had extremely high seminal levels of HIV, on average 398,000 copies/ml, and these nine men were classified as "seminal super- shedders" and were considered particularly likely to pass on HIV during unprotected sex.

Blood plasma viral loads, CD4 cell counts and stage of HIV disease did not differ significantly between super-shedders and seminal shedders. However, the investigators did find that super-shedders were generally older, with an average age of 48 years compared to 35 for the sample as a whole, and were more likely to have an STI (33% of super-shedders compared to 3% of total sample).

The investigators conclude that men shedding viral load in their semen were likely to have higher blood plasma viral loads than non-shedders. In addition, a small number of men are super-shedders, and although they have comparable blood levels of HIV to normal shedders, super-shedders tend to be older and have an STI which may assist local reproduction of HIV in the genital tract.

A comprehensive discussion of research findings in this area can be found in the "HIV & AIDS Treatments Directory", or at aidsmap.com. See *Anti-HIV Therapy: Choosing your treatment strategy*.

References

Dyer JR et al: Effects of disease stage and CD4 lymphocyte count on shedding of HIV-1 in semen, Eleventh International Conference on AIDS, abstract WeC.335, 1996.

Ilaria G et al: Detection of HIV-1 DNA sequences in pre-ejaculatory fluid, Lancet 340: 1469, 1992.

Levy JA: Pathogenesis of human immunodeficiency virus infection, Microbiological Reviews 57: 185-289, 1993.

O'Brien TR: Inverse association between zidovudine therapy and the isolation of HIV in the semen of HIV-positive men, Seventh International Conf on AIDS, abstract MC 3092, 1991.

Pudney J et al: Pre-ejaculatory fluid as potential vector for sexual transmission of HIV-1, Lancet 340: 1470, 1992.

Taylor S, Sadiq T, Sabin C, et al. Seminal super shedding of HIV: implications for sexual transmission. Tenth Conference on Retroviruses and Opportunistic Infections; Boston, Massachusetts, abstract 454, 2003.

Vernazza PL: Detection and biologic characterization of infectious HIV-1 in semen of seropositive men, AIDS 8(9): 1325-1329, 1994.

Vaginal and cervical secretions

Levels of HIV in the vagina increase at the time of menstruation because of the presence of blood and other cell-associated virus. Levels of macrophages which could harbour HIV also increase in the vaginal fluid at the time of menstruation. It is believed that sexually transmitted infections and inflammation in the vagina will boost the level of lymphocytes. The hormone progesterone, a component of some oral contraceptives, has also been associated with increased HIV RNA levels (Mostad).

Levels of HIV RNA in plasma and vaginal fluid have been shown to correlate very closely, but nearly 35% of women tested in one study had no detectable HIV RNA in their vaginal fluids despite detectable HIV in their plasma once the single occasion sampling took place (Hart).

HIV RNA levels in vaginal fluid have been shown to decline after the initiation of antiretroviral therapy. Antiretroviral therapy was associated with a median 1.4 log decline (approx 95%) in viral burden in vaginal fluid after three weeks of therapy. Antiretroviral therapy consisted of one or two nucleoside analogues (Lennox).

References

Hart C et al: Correlation of cell-free and cell-associated HIV RNA levels in plasma and vaginal secretions, Fourth Human Retroviruses Conference, abstract 347, 1997.

Lennox J et al: Effect of antiretroviral therapy on vaginal HIV RNA level, abstract 498, Fourth Human Retroviruses Conference, 1997.

Mostad S et al: Cervical and vaginal HIV-1 DNA shedding in female STD clinic attenders, Eleventh International AIDS Conference, abstract We.C.333, 1996.

Vogt MW et al: Isolation patterns of the human immunodeficiency virus from secretions during the menstrual cycle of women at risk for the acquired immunodeficiency syndrome, AIM 106(3): 380-382, 1987.

Rectal secretions

A 2004 study of gay men found that levels of HIV RNA in rectal mucosal secretions were higher than those in blood or semen - by about 500% in the case of blood and 2,500% in the case of semen.

The study found that viral loads in swabs taken from the rectum were 25 times higher than semen viral loads in the 58% of the men not taking HIV treatment, and four times higher in the 37% of men on treatment who had detectable viral loads.

The average rectal viral loads were 316,000 and 4,000 respectively.

There was also a much less strong relationship between the use of treatment and reduction of viral load in the rectal swabs than there was with blood or semen.

During anal intercourse, the rectum secretes a protective, lubricating mucus to accommodate penetration. Although the mucus eases penetration and repeated thrusting, it by no means protects either partner from cuts and abrasions that can lead to the passage of HIV infection, which is why proper lubrication and condom use is necessary. In fact, the mucus may be far more dangerous than any other fluids either partner might be exposed to.

The study suggests that gay or bisexual men who have insertive unprotected anal sex and encounter this mucus are at far higher risk of HIV infection than previously thought. Formerly, most literature on HIV protection named blood or semen as the main culprit in HIV transmission.

Reference

Zuckerman, Richard et al. HIV-1 RNA in rectal mucosa secretions and seminal plasma; considerations for microbicide efficacy. First Microbicides conference, London, abstract 02679, 2004.

Brain tissue and cerebrospinal fluid

HIV was cultured from the cerebrospinal fluid of 13 out of 14 people suffering from AIDS-associated neurological disorders, in much higher quantities than any other body fluid apart from blood (Levy). Another study was able to isolate HIV from brain tissue and cerebrospinal fluid in 24 out of 33 people suffering from AIDS-associated neurological disorders (Ho).

References

Ellis RJ et al. Progression of neuropsychological impairment in human immunodeficiency virus infection predicted by elevated cerebrospinal fluid levels of human immunodeficiency virus RNA. Archives of Neurology 59(6): 923-928, 2002.

Ho DD et al: Isolation of HTLV-III from cerebrospinal fluid and neural tissues of patients with neurological syndromes related to the acquired immunodeficiency syndrome, NEJM 313(24): 1493-1497, 1985.

Levy JA et al: Isolation of AIDS-associated retroviruses from cerebrospinal fluid and brain of patients with neurological symptoms, Lancet (ii): 586-588 (Sep 14), 1985.

Bronchoalveolar fluid

Faeces

HIV has never been isolated from faeces in an infectious form. Genetic material from HIV has been detected, but it has never been possible to culture the virus in the laboratory from faeces.

Saliva

HIV has been successfully isolated from saliva on only a handful of occasions despite many attempts, and even then only in tiny quantities compared with blood, semen and vaginal fluid. This low recovery rate is probably explained by the presence in saliva of substances that prevent hIV from infecting new cells.

Tears

Researchers have found it difficult to isolate HIV from the tears of HIV-positive people. In one experiment it was possible to find HIV in the tears of only one person with AIDS out of seven tested, and impossible in five HIV-positive people with no symptoms (Fujikawa). Another experiment using highly sensitive techniques looked at 50 HIV-positive people and failed to find HIV in the tears of any of them (Mueller).

Urine

Although HIV antibodies are detectable in urine, HIV capable of infecting cells has not been isolated from urine; in one study HIV could not be isolated from the urine of any of the 48 people studied.

References

Fujikawa LS et al: Isolation of human lymphotropic virus type III from the tears of a patient with the Acquired Immunodeficiency Syndrome, Lancet (ii): 529-530 (Sep 7), 1985.

The effects of antiretroviral therapy on infectivity

Drug activity in the genital tract of men

Although most studies show that the majority of men treated with antiretroviral drugs demonstrated parallel declines in plasma and seminal viral load, all studies have shown considerable individual variation in responses.

The following patterns have been observed:

- Viral load becomes undetectable in plasma weeks or months before doing so in semen.

- Viral load becomes undetectable in semen but not in plasma.

- Plasma viral load rebounds after a period of undetectability but seminal viral load remains undetectable.

- Discrepancies between the emergence of resistance in the blood and semen.

In the first case, prolonged HIV production in the genital tract may be explained by the fact that long-lived cells which have been infected by HIV continue to pump out virus copies because anti-HIV drugs cannot adequately penetrate these particular cells. Another explanation might be that virus production continues because latently infected cells are triggered into virus production by the presence of infections or inflammation.

One particular infection that has synergy with HIV infectivity is genital herpes (HSV2). The presence of (often asymptomatic) herpes infection in the genital tract both increases the amount of HIV produced by infected cells in the HIV-positive person and makes cells in the genital and anal tracts of the HIV-negative person more susceptible to infection. It does this both by directly affecting the genetic turnover of HIV and by stimulating the release of inflammatory cytokines like IL-4 which make cells both more expressive of, and more receptive to, HIV. In vivo studies report that aciclovir treatment can produce a survival benefit in HIV-1-infected patients and that recurrent genital herpes appears to be linked to HIV-1 transmission by both boosting plasma retroviral load and providing a portal of entry and exit for HIV-1 (reviewed in Palu 2001).

However, even when HIV is 'undetectable' by bDNA testing in semen, this does not mean that it has disappeared. The viral load test cannot detect viral load below 1,000 copies in semen, and more sensitive tests must be used to establish whether semen still contains infectious HIV. These tests look for HIV's DNA. The presence of HIV DNA suggests the presence of actively replicating infectious HIV.

One small study found that three out of eleven patients on antiretroviral therapy with undetectable viral load in semen still had detectable HIV DNA when more sensitive tests were conducted.

A larger study of over 100 men on treatment examined blood and semen samples for HIV RNA and DNA. Only two treated men (2%) had HIV RNA in their semen in comparison to 67% of untreated controls. Of the 53 treated men tested for cell-associated HIV DNA, nine had detectable HIV DNA in contrast to 21 of 55 untreated controls. These statistically significant differences suggest that antiretroviral therapy does reduce the amount of HIV in semen. However, some HIV may remain in semen and HIV transmission through the exchange of sexual fluids remains a possibility despite treatment (Vernazza 1998).

Another study of 52 HIV-infected men has found a substantial minority do not have a correlation between seminal and blood plasma viral load. Twenty men had seminal viral load equivalent or higher than their blood plasma viral load (Tachet 1999).

Whilst some doctors have argued that reducing viral load in semen will have a beneficial effect on transmission rates, others caution that this is not yet proven (Vernazza, Albrecht).

A 58-week study of eleven men taking antiretroviral therapy found that different viral variants emerged in plasma and semen in seven out of eight men in whom drug resistance mutations could be identified. These findings suggest that different forms of drug pressure are operating in the plasma and the male genital tract, and lends some support to the view that protease inhibitors do not penetrate the male genital tract in high enough concentrations to prevent the development of resistance (Eron). Analysis of mutations in HIV taken from semen and blood has led some researchers to propose that a separate seminal HIV reservoir exists in some men.

The largest study to date, in 85 Brazilian men who had been followed for at least six months after starting antiretroviral therapy, found that 74% of individuals had detectable HIV in their semen at baseline. All had undetectable viral load within four months of starting therapy, but by month 6, 44% had experienced viral load rebound in plasma, compared to only 25% in semen (Barroso).

Poor penetration of protease inhibitors into the genital tract has also been reported. A study of drug levels in eight patients receiving ritonavir, saquinavir and stavudine (d4T) showed undetectable levels of saquinavir in semen despite high plasma levels in some patients, and sub-therapeutic levels of ritonavir (Taylor). Protease levels in the semen were generally less than 5% of the levels attained in the blood. Despite the poor penetration, viral load was reduced to undetectable levels in the semen and blood plasma after six months of treatment.

Sub-therapeutic levels might encourage the development and transmission of drug-resistant virus. Poor penetration of PIs is probably due to the protein binding of protease inhibitors and the high protein content of semen, or to the low levels of polyglycoprotein (Pgp), a substance which pumps protease inhibitor molecules out of cells. Pgp is present at very low levels in cells of the brain and testes.

Other conditions such as urethritis (inflammation of the urethra) may be associated with detectable HIV RNA in semen. One study of seven HIV-positive men found that seven had asymptomatic urethritis, four of whom had detectable virus in their semen, despite anti-HIV treatment (Winter).

A recent study found that in the majority of gay men the presence of chlamydia or NSU did not result in seminal viral load becoming detectable. However four men in the study had gonorrhoea and all had detectable viral loads, possibly because gonorrhoea is particularly inflammatory. It may also be worth noting that the study found that although the majority of men with no sexually transmitted infections and an undetectable plasma viral load also had an undetectable seminal viral load, this was not always the case (Sadiq).

Drug activity in the genital tract in women

Several large studies (52, 55 and 112 women tested) have found a strong association between the level of viral load in blood and the level of viral load in cervicovaginal fluid (Hart, Hoesley, Cuuvin). The initiation of antiretroviral therapy significantly reduced HIV RNA in vaginal fluid in one study.

However, there is some evidence that antiretroviral therapy may have discrepant effects on blood and on cervicovaginal fluid, especially when a genital infection is present. An American study of eleven women on antiretroviral therapy showed that viral load in vaginal fluid was significantly higher. The presence of genital tract infections such as thrush or inflammatory lesions of the vulva or cervix was predictive a discrepant response to anti-HIV treatment. The authors of the study have noted that their results should be treated with caution due to the small sample size and the fact that none of the women were receiving protease inhibitor treatment (Stephens).

Another small study has found that HIV in blood and in cervicovaginal fluid (CVF) is genetically distinct, suggesting that HIV in CVF is being produced by activation of local immune cells (Subbarao).

The presence of herpes infection is also associated with a greater risk of transmission by HIV-positive women and acquisition of HIV by negative women, and using the drug aiclovir has resulted in modest reductions in viral load amongst HIV-positive women and significant reductions in HIV acquisition amongst HIV-negative women - see **Using antiretrovirals for HIV prevention.**

References

Albrecht H et al. Seminal viral load. AIDS 12(3): 333, 1998.

Barroso PF et al. Effect of antiretroviral therapy on HIV shedding in semen. Annals of Internal Medicine 133 (4): 280-284, 2000.

Cuuvin S et al. HIV-1 RNA levels in the genital tract of women on anti-retroviral therapy. Fifth Conference on Retroviruses and Opportunistic Infections, Chicago, abstract 713, 1998.

Eron J et al. Penetration of HIV protease inhibitors into seminal compartment may be limited. AIDS 12: 7397-7405, 1998.

Eyre RC et al. Evidence for a distinct reservoir of HIV in semen. 94th Annual Meeting of the American Urological Association, Dallas, 1999.

Hart CE et al. Correlation of HIV type 1 RNA levels in blood and the female genital tract. Journal of Infectious Diseases 179 (4): 871-882, 1999.

Hoesley C et al. Quantification of cervicovaginal lavage and plasma HIV-1 RNA in HIV-1 seropositive women. Fifth Conference on Retroviruses and Opportunistic Infections, Chicago, abstract 712, 1998.

Palu G et al. Molecular basis of the interactions between herpes simplex viruses and HIV-1. Herpes. 8(2): 50-55, 2001

Sadiq ST et al. The effects of antiretroviral therapy on HIV-1 RNA loads in HIV-positive patients with and without urethritis. AIDS 16: 219-225, 2002.

Stephens P et al. HIV viral load in cervical, vaginal and menstrual fluids as compared to peripheral blood levels in women with HIV/AIDS. Twelfth World AIDS Conference, abstract 23477, 1998

Subbarao S et al. Genotypic evidence of local HIV expression in the female genital tract. Fifth Conference on Retroviruses and Opportunistic Infections, Chicago, abstract 708, 1998.

Tachet A et al. Detection and quantification of HIV-1 in semen: identificaiton of a subpopulation of men at high potential risk of viral sexual transmission. AIDS 13(7): 823-831, 1999.

Taylor S et al. The impact of ritonavir/saquinavir/stavudine on viral load in seminal fluid and plasma compartments. Twelfth World AIDS Conference, abstract 23397, 1998.

Taylor S et al. Poor penetration of the male genital tract by HIV-1 protease inhibitors. AIDS 13(6): 859-860, 1999.

Vernazza P. Quantification of HIV in semen: correlation with antiviral treatment and immune status. AIDS 11: 987-993, 1997

Vernazza P. Effect of antiviral treatment on the shedding of HIV-1 in semen. AIDS 11: 1249-1254, 1997.

Vernazza PL et al. Potent antiretroviral treatment results in marked suppression of seminal HIV-RNA and -DNA shedding. Fourth Congress on Drug Therapy in HIV Infection, Glasgow, abstract OP 6.3, 1998.

Winter AJ et al. Asymptomatic urethritis and detection of HIV-1 RNA in seminal plasma. Fifth Annual Meeting of the British HIV Association, abstract 01, 1999.

Summary

HIV is not present in:

- Urine, faeces, vomit, sweat.

HIV is present in negligible quantities in:

- Saliva (only ever detected in very small quantities in the saliva of a very small number of people)

- Tears

- Blister fluid.

HIV is present in infectious quantities in:

- Blood and blood-derived products

- Semen and possibly pre-ejaculatory fluid

- Vaginal and cervical secretions or juices

- Rectal secretions

- Breast milk (this raises special issues which are discussed in *Mother-to-baby transmission*, below).

These are, for all intents and purposes, the key body fluids and materials to take precautions against.

In addition, HIV has also been detected in sufficient quantities in:

- Amniotic fluid

- Cerebrospinal fluid

- Tissue and organ donations

- Skin transplants

- Bone marrow transplants.

All of these are only a potential risk in invasive surgical procedures and may be covered by the same precautions and guidelines.

The route of transmission

HIV can only be transmitted and cause infection if it gets into the body via a route where vulnerable cells are plentiful.

On a cellular level, HIV can infect CD4 cells and CD8 cells in the blood as well as cells in the lungs, the brain, the gastrointestinal tract and the kidneys. But to reach these cells, HIV must pass through cells in the mucous membranes called dendritic cells and Langerhans cells.

Dendritic cells are in fact designed precisely to 'ferry' infectious particles to the lymph nodes where they act as antigens that stimulate the immune response; it is exactly this otherwise protective activity that HIV exploits in order to achieve infection.

Dendritic cells do not become infected with HIV themselves but the virus's gp120 envelope protein attaches itself to a 'sticky' molecule called DC-SIGN which coats the cells (see Geijtenbeek 2000).

Therefore, blood splashed onto the skin will not come into contact with the Langerhans cells beneath the skin because these are not exposed. The skin must be damaged, lacerated or deeply wounded for this to happen. In the rectum and vagina by contrast, infected blood or semen will reach the Langerhans cells far more easily because they are close to the surface and lack the covering of the thick dead epithelial layer which is the dry surface of the skin.

The effective routes for transmission to occur are:

- Directly into the blood (parenterally) through a wound; through a cut or sore or damaged skin; an injection using contaminated and unsterilised injection equipment; an invasive surgical procedure such as an organ transplant or blood transfusion

- Through particular 'interior' sections of skin called mucous membranes in the rectum, the vagina and cervix; the urethra (which is in front of the vagina in women and the tube of the penis in men); mucous membranes in the eyes and mouth in rare circumstances.

It should be noted that in these cases, trauma or damage to the tissue is not always necessary for infection to occur. These mucous membranes will allow HIV to be absorbed into cells which facilitate infection. In the early years of the epidemic it was thought that damage to these tissues might be the precondition of infection. We now know that infection occurs without such damage, although damage will certainly increase the chances of infection.

There are only four proven, substantial routes of transmission:

- Unprotected intercourse with someone who is infected.

- Sharing unsterilised injection equipment which has been previously used by someone who is infected.

- Injection or transfusion of contaminated blood or blood products, and donations of semen (artificial insemination), skin grafts and organ transplants taken from someone who is infected.

- From a mother who is infected to her baby (this may be during the course of pregnancy, at birth and through breastfeeding).

Physical cofactors that encourage transmission

Factors that may increase the risk of infection if exposed to HIV include:

Sexually transmitted infections

Having other sexually transmitted infections at the time, such as herpes or syphilis, especially, but not only, if they cause genital ulceration, may increase the risk of HIV transmission. Genital ulceration provides an enhanced route of infection. In Thai women with HIV-positive partners, a history of syphilis, herpes, gonorrhoea or chlamydia all increased the risk of infection, and women were twice as likely to be HIV-positive if their partners had a history of sexually transmitted infections since seroconversion (Nelson).

Sexually transmitted infections also increase the quantity of HIV-bearing cells present in the vaginal fluid or semen, although some infections appear to increase levels of viral shedding more than others. A study amongst commercial sex workers in Kenya found that active gonorrhoeal infection was much more strongly associated with viral shedding than chlamydial infection (Mostad). A study amongst female sex workers in Cote d'Ivoire found that the presence of cervical or vaginal ulcers, gonorrhoea or chlamydia were most strongly associated with HIV-1 shedding in cervicovaginal fluid (Ghys). Similarly, gay men studied in the US had a threefold greater likelihood of viral shedding in their semen if they also had detectable cytomegalovirus infection in their semen (Dyer).

The genital shedding of herpes simplex virus (HSV) and HIV is closely correlated, meaning that a person shedding HSV is more infectious for HIV.

Investigators screened women for HIV who were receiving hormonal contraceptives at the Coast Provincial General Hospital in Mombassa, Kenya between May 1996 and September 1999. In total 210 women tested HIV-positive and were eligible for the study, which involved baseline tests including taking blood samples, plasma viral load, and CD4 cell counts, and the taking of cervical swabs to detect the shedding of HSV and HIV. Follow-up was one and two months later.

The lower limit of detection for the plasma HIV viral load tests was 50 cells/ml and 125 cells ml for the cervical swabs. Detectable cervical HIV was present in 66.7% of women (28/42) with detectable cervical HSV and in 65.8% of women (98/149) without, leading the investigators to comment that "the detection of cervical HSV DNA was not significantly associated with HIV-1 levels greater than 125 copies/swab or with the detection of HIV-1 infected cells."

However, the investigators add that although there was no relationship between detection of the two viruses, there was a significant relationship between the quantities of HSV and HIV found in cervical secretions of HSV shedding women. A 10-fold (one log) increase in the amount of cervical HSV was associated with a 1.36-fold increase in cervical levels of HIV. This relationship remained unchanged when differences in CD4 count and plasma viral load were adjusted for. No significant relationship was found between the shedding of cervical HSV and plasma HIV viral load.

The investigators speculate that "local interactions between HSV and HIV-1 may provide a plausible explanation for the association between the genital shedding of the two viruses". They conclude that "HSV suppression could be an important means of decreasing" the spread of HIV, and given the high levels of HSV infection in their study population call for "additional prospective studies of the relationship between HSV and HIV-shedding."

The relationship between HSV and HIV infectivity and disease progression is the subject of intensive investigation. A study conducted in the US before the introduction of HAART found that treatment for HSV resulted in a modest reduction in HIV viral load, and a recent South African study found that recent HSV infection was associated with HIV seroconversion.

The health status or disease progression of the infected partner

It has been theorised that individuals are most infectious at two points during HIV infection: during primary infection (the period before antibodies appear) and the symptomatic phase (after symptoms appear). However, research to test this theory has produced contradictory results. As discussed above, levels of HIV in semen and vaginal fluid are unpredictable and not always closely associated with virus levels in blood (see *The presence and concentration of HIV* above). For example, one study found no difference in seminal viral load between individuals tested during primary infection and others who had more advanced HIV infection (Dyer). But these results need to be treated with caution because they refer to 3 individuals from a study of 101 men.

A large study in Thailand which investigated HIV transmission in 467 couples where the male partner had been identified as HIV-positive found that even when the man's CD4 count was above 500, 39% of women were already infected. These findings suggest that viral load is high even during early disease, although it was not possible in this study to distinguish between infection in primary infection and infection after an immune response had reduced viral load (Nelson).

Another study in Thailand could find no difference in infection rates between women exposed to partners during their primary infection phase and women who began sexual relationships with men after their partners had become infected (Duerr).

An unequivocal link between recent HIV-infection and high risk of HIV transmission was reported at the tenth Conference on Retroviruses and Opportunistic Infections in Boston in February 2003.

The researchers calculated the incidence of HIV transmission per monogamous, vaginal heterosexual act as thus: in the five months immediately following seroconversion, rate of transmission was ten times greater than during chronic infection at 8.2 per 1000. In late stage infection (five to 15 months before death) it was 4.5 per 1000. During chronic infection, once the viral load set point had been reached - after 5 months and before late stage HIV disease - the transmission rate was 0.8 per 1000.

Although it has been understood for some time that there was an association between the very high viral loads seen during the primary infection and a greater likelihood of infecting others, this report from the Johns Hopkins University Rakai Project Team suggests that much HIV prevention work would benefit greatly by focusing on those currently untested or very recently infected.

The strain of virus

There have been recent claims by some scientists that different strains of HIV have differing infectivity, and that strains which are predominant in developing countries could be more easily transmitted through vaginal intercourse and from mother-to-baby.

The evidence that HIV subtypes have differing levels of infectiousness is conflicting. The main evidence comes from test tube experiments which tested the ability of different HIV subtypes to replicate in immune cells called Langerhans cells, which are plentiful in the wall of the vagina. Researchers found that subtype E, which is more common in Asia and Africa, could replicate faster in these cells than subtype B. They suggested that this showed subtype E was likely to be transmitted more easily through vaginal intercourse than subtype B (Soto-Ramirez).

Thai researchers found that when all other factors were controlled for, female partners of men infected with subtype E were 3.1 times more likely to be infected with the same strain than female partners of men carrying subtype B (Kunanusont).

These findings have raised the fear that subtypes such as E may spread rapidly in Europe and North America. However, these subtypes have been transmitted in European countries such as Belgium and the UK without showing a more pronounced transmission rate (although this may be a function of sexual mixing patterns and lower levels of STDs in those countries).

A review by the US Centers for Disease Control and Prevention found little epidemiological evidence that some subtypes are more infectious (Mastro). They made a number of observations:

- Transmission rates of different subtypes are similar from mother to baby in countries such as Thailand where several different subtypes are present in the population.

- Different transmission rates of subtypes amongst the adult population can be explained by the fact that subtypes which first appear in injecting drug users are likely to spread faster because a greater number of high risk contacts take place in this group.

- Where HIV subtypes appear to be confined to particular population groups, this may be a consequence of the route by which HIV entered that population group, not a consequence of its ease of transmission by a particular route. For example, although subtype B HIV is predominant amongst drug injectors in Thailand, whilst subtype E is predominant amongst those who acquired HIV through sexual intercourse, this is almost certainly a consequence of the fact that HIV was introduced into the drug injecting population by drug injectors from the US or Europe, where subtype B predominates.

The question of varying infectiousness remains unanswered, and will require close surveillance in years to come.

Damaged tissue

Damage to tissue in the throat or mouth may facilitate infection; in reported cases of infection through oral sex, inflammation of the throat because of allergy and frequently bleeding gums have been cited along with pharyngeal gonorrhoea as co-factors for infection. In women, oral contraception can sometimes cause cervical ectopy, in which cells in the cervix are exposed on the surface where they can easily be broken, allowing for easier HIV transmission.

Immune system activation

Generalised immune system activation may play some role, as yet unclear, in facilitating HIV infection, in the view of some researchers. They point to increases in viral load when other active infections, such as tuberculosis, are present. However, a study in Tanzania failed to find any evidence that people with a previous history of tuberculosis were more likely to acquire HIV during a five-year follow up period (Borgdorff).

However a 1996 study (Goletti) found that levels of HIV in the bloodstream increased from five- to 160-fold in HIV-infected people who develop active tuberculosis. The findings may help explain why HIV-infected people with active TB have a poorer prognosis than HIV-infected people without TB.

References

Borgdorff MW et al: Tuberculosis infection and HIV incidence in Africa, Lancet 348: 1743, 1996.

Druett A et al: Heterosexual transmission during the seroconversion versus the post-seroconversion period, Eleventh International AIDS Conference, abstract Mo.C.571, 1996.

Geijtenbeek, T.B.H. and others. DC-SIGN, a dendritic cell-specific HIV-1-binding protein that enhances trans-infection of T cells. Cell 100(5): 587-597. March 3, 2000.

Ghys A. HIV shedding, STD and immunosuppression. AIDS 11(12): F85-F93, 1997.

Goletti D, et al. Effect of Mycobacterium tuberculosis on HIV replication: role of immune activation. Journal of Immunology 157: 1271-1278, 1996.

Mastro TD et al: Why do HIV-1 subtypes segregate amongst persons with different risk behaviours in South Africa and Thailand? AIDS 11(1): 1997.

McCutchan, F: HIV Genetic Diversity, Eleventh International AIDS Conference, Abstract No. M02, 1996.

McClelland RS et al. Association between cervical shedding of herpes simplex virus and HIV-1. AIDS 16: 2425-2430, 2002.

Mostad S. Shedding of HIV-1 in the female genital tract. AIDS 10: 1305-1315, 1996.

Nelson K et al. High rates of transmission of subtype E human immunodeficiency virus type 1 among heterosexual couples in northern Thailand: role of sexually transmitted diseases and immune compromise. Journal of Infectious Diseases 180: 337-343, 1999.

Wawer M J et al. HIV-1 Transmission per coital act, by stage of HIV infection in the HIV+ index partner, in discordant couples, Rakai, Uganda. Tenth Conference on Retroviruses and Opportunistic Infections, Boston, abstract 40, 2003.

Gray R H et al. Probability of HIV-1 transmission per coital act in monogamous, heterosexual, HIV-1-discordant couples in Rakai, Uganda. Lancet 2 Apr 14; 357(9263): 1149-1153, 2001.

Social cofactors which encourage transmission

While it has been important to focus down on the specific details of how transmission occurs at a cellular and bodily level, it is important for the purposes of prevention and reassurance in the real world to be aware that all transmission is by definition always interpersonal i.e. it involves two or more people. As such, it needs to be understood as a social phenomenon as much as a biological one.

Resistance to infection

Research in Kenya has identified a particular genetic tissue type which is associated with a low risk of HIV infection despite repeated exposure to HIV. Women with the HLA-28 genetic marker were much more likely to be seronegative in the Nairobi sex workers study.

Some of the genetic patterns seen in persistently seronegative women in Nairobi have not been seen in North Americans or Europeans. These patterns are rare in the Nairobi cohort; however, they have also been seen amongst men persistently seronegative despite repeated exposure to HIV-positive partners.

The more dissimilar the mother and baby's MHC 1 profile, the lower the chance of transmission from mother to baby. The closer the fit, the greater the likelihood of transmission.

More recently a number of studies in Africa have found that different MHC 1 profiles vary in their reactivity to HIV by as much as eleven-fold (Frahm 2004; Kiepiela 2004), and that there was a strong correlation between subject's reactivity to HIV and their viral load, which varied from 200,000 and above in those with the least reactive MHC types to a few hundred with the most reactive. These surveys are the most comprehensive yet that map out a huge degree of genetic variability in susceptibility ti HIV infection and progression to AIDS.

Cytotoxic T-cell protection against HIV

In Gambia, British researchers have found female prostitutes with immune responses to HIV yet no evidence of infection. The researchers took samples of CD8 lymphocytes (cytotoxic lymphocytes or CTL) from women persistently seronegative despite a high risk of exposure. These lymphocytes were then exposed to genetic material from HIV to determine whether they recognised this material. If the CD8 lymphocytes had encountered these genetic sequences in the past, they would show a response. In three out of six women they observed immune responses to HIV despite no evidence of infection.

In Nairobi, British vaccine researchers have identified a similar group of women, and have also made a disturbing discovery about the mechanisms which maintain this form of immune response. The group found that 6 persistently seronegative women with cytotoxic T-lymphocyte responses to HIV seroconverted after they stopped commercial sex work for a period (and therefore reduced the amount of unprotected sex they engaged in). This finding implies that repeated exposure to HIV might be necessary in order to maintain the cytotoxic response (Kaul).

Investigations are now going on to determine what degree of overlap exists between the two forms of resistance. For example, does a strong immune response to HIV depend on possessing a particular genetic type? Or is a CTL response to HIV a function of exposure to very small amounts of HIV which 'prime' the immune system to recognise HIV in the future?

Another interesting observation is the finding that nearly 50% of seronegative Ethiopians tested in Israel have specific immunity to HIV, but no evidence of HIV infection or HIV antibodies. Furthermore, specific cellular immunity was found to increase over the course of one year in these individuals, although 5 of the 21 had evidence of HIV RNA after one year of follow-up. It is possible that all 21 have undetectable HIV infection which is extremely well controlled, to the extent that viral expression has been halted (hence the lack of antibody response), rather than resistance to HIV.

The authors speculate that a high burden of parasitic infections in these individuals could have enhanced their ability to mount an immune response to HIV, but if this were the case one would expect to see this degree of HIV-specific immunity on a far larger scale in Africa. It is more plausible that this group of individuals were exposed to a geographically confined, defective strain of HIV, resulting in either immunity or very easily controllable infection (Bar-Yehuda).

In 2003 a UK team published findings showing that the negative partner in serodiscordant couples in long-term relationships who had unprotected sex acquired a degree of immunity to their partner's HIV (Peters 2003).

Dr Peters' team studied 29 monogamous heterosexual serodiscordant couples who had had frequent unprotected intercourse for more than six months. They compared the anti-HIV immune responses in the negative partner to those in a control group of 15 HIV-negative women and 10 HIV-negative men who had had no sex, or only protected sex, for at least the previous six months.

They took CD4 cells from all the subjects and attempted to infect them with various different strains of HIV in the test tube.

It was found that CD4 cells in women who had had unprotected sex with HIV-positive men were only 10% as likely to be infected with CCR5-tropic HIV as CD4 cells from women who had had protected or no sex.

The HIV-negative men who had had unprotected sex with positive women had half that degree of protection: their CD4 cells were 20% as likely to be infected with HIV as cells from men who'd had protected or no sex.

A study, presented by Dr Tuofu Zhu (see reference) at the 2004 Bangkok World AIDS Conference found evidence of the same immunity in gay men.

Zhu was studying "long-term exposed seronegative" partners of HIV-positive gay men. The group consisted of the HIV-negative partners of HIV-positive men who had been diagnosed between 1994 and 1998.

Out of 94 HIV-negative regular partners of positive men, he found 14 who had become HIV-positive.

Two of the partners appeared to have caught HIV from their partners early on in their relationship, but to have mounted a successful immune response to it. They had no antibodies to HIV - in other words, they did not test HIV-positive by conventional tests. The fact that they had HIV at all could only be detected by hypersensitive viral-load testing, which picked up HIV in their blood at a count of 0.05 copies - one thousandth of the amount usually called "undetectable" by standard tests. There were no infections from regular partners more than 18 months after the start of the relationship.

The other 12 of the 14, however, had recognizable HIV infections with positive antibody responses. Some maintained low viral loads in the 500-2,000 range and showed some evidence of an immune response to HIV; others had standard viral loads in the tens of thousands. But all 12 had clearly not caught HIV from

their regular partners. Genetic analysis of the virus they carried showed that not only was it completely different in each case from the virus their partner carried, but that on average it was more different than any randomly selected North American strain would have been.

When they had a strong immune response to HIV, their virus tended to change in a completely different way to their partner's and become more unlike it as time went on. When people only had a weak response to their partner's HIV, their viruses became more similar.

Chemokine receptor mutations and resistance to infection

Viruses have a particular host cell in the host animal or plant and HIV is no exception. Hepatitis viruses have host cells in the liver and herpes simplex virus (causing cold sores) live in peripheral nerve cells. The host cells for HIV are those carrying CD4 molecules - macrophages and CD4 T lymphocytes (CD4 cells). HIV uses proteins on its surface called gp120 and gp41 to attach to the CD4 molecule on cells. Specific antibodies to gp120 can block the attachment to CD4 molecules.

In 1996 it was discovered that HIV also binds to a second protein on the surface of human cells, called chemokine receptor 5 or CCR5, as part of the process of infecting a cell. The genetic instructions for producing this protein are contained in a gene called the CCR5 gene. Everyone has two copies of this gene, but a significant proportion of the population (about one in seven US whites, and one in 59 US blacks) have a mutation in one or both of these genes which interferes in the production of the protein.

People who have two mutant CCR5 genes may be partially protected against infection with NSI strains of HIV. However, they are not completely protected against HIV infection, since they remain susceptible to SI strains of HIV. There have now been four separate papers describing cases in which people with two mutant CCR5 genes have become infected with HIV.

Studies have found that among HIV-positive people who were infected sexually, those who have one mutant CCR5 gene experience slightly slower HIV disease progression (characterised by one researcher as 'only a couple of years'). No reduction in disease progression was seen among people infected by other routes, such as blood products or drug injecting, perhaps because they were probably exposed to larger amounts of HIV when they became infected.

The CCR5 protein is believed normally to act as a receptor for three chemokines (immune system chemicals) known as RANTES, MIP-1 alpha and MIP-1beta. Studies have shown that HIV-positive people who do not progress, and HIV-negative people who have been repeatedly exposed to the virus through unprotected sex yet do not become infected, often have unusually high levels of these chemokines. They are thought to inhibit HIV either because they bind to the CCR5 protein on CD4 cells and 'block' it, or because their presence causes the shape of the CCR5 protein to change, or because they cause the cell to display fewer CCR5 proteins on its surface. In any event, this prevents HIV from using the receptor and so reduces the chance that the cells will be infected. It is speculated that levels of these chemokines may fall with age, which might explain why older people tend to experience faster HIV disease progression than younger people.

The level of CCR5 expression per CD4 cell appears to be increased in an environment of high immune activation, which may explain why HIV infection is more frequent in Africa and Asia. A research team in Israel compared levels of CCR5 expression in HIV-negative Ethiopians and an HIV-negative Israeli control group and found significantly higher levels of CCR5 expression. However, they also found higher levels of CCR5 expression in Ethiopian immigrants resident in Israel for more than five years, despite no differences in immune activation levels when compared to an Israeli control group. This finding suggests that there may be a genetic predisposition to increased CCR5 expression in some African populations that could also account for higher prevalence (Kalinkovich).

These discoveries about co-receptors have now enabled the development of a new class of drugs - the chemokine receptor inhibitors. By the end of 2007, the first of these, the CCR5 inhibitor maraviroc, will probably be licensed for prescription in both the US and the EU. Others are likely to follow. See the Treatments directort for details.

References

Dean M et al. Genetic restriction of HIV-1 infection and progression to AIDS by a deletion allele of the CCR5 structural gene. Science 273: 1856-1862, 1996.

Deng HK et al. Identification of a major co-receptor for primary isolates of HIV-1. Nature 381: 661-666.

Frahm N et al. Consistent CTL targeting of immunodominant regions in HIV across different ethnicities. J. Virol. 78(5), 2004.

Kalinkovich A et al. Increased CCR5 expression in Ethiopians: Relevance to the rapid spread of HIV infection in Africa? XIII International AIDS Conference, Durban, abstract MoPeA2016, 2000.

Kaul R et al. Late seroconversion in HIV 'resistant' Nairobi prostitutes is associated with a preceding decrease in HIV exposure. Seventh Conference on Retroviruses, San Francisco, abstract 489, 2000.

Kiepiela P et al. Dominant influence of HLA-B in mediating the potential co-evolution of HIV and HLA. Nature, 432(7018): 769-775. 2004.

Peters B et al. Study of Allo-immunization in Humans During Sexual Intercourse and Effects on HIV Infectivity. Tenth CROI, Boston, abstract 424, 2003.

Zhu T. Breakthrough HIV-1 infection in long-term exposed seronegative individuals. 15th International AIDS Conference, Bangkok, abstract TuOrA1141, 1994.

Superinfection

There is an increasing scientific consensus that individuals infected with HIV may be at risk of acquiring other strains of HIV. As discussed in *The Origins of AIDS*, at least eight major subtypes of HIV-1 have already been identified, and one major subtype of HIV-2 has also been identified. It has recently been established that:

- Individuals can be infected with two different subtypes at once.

- Individuals can be infected with wild-type virus after initially being infected with drug-resistant virus.

- Chimpanzees can be infected with one subtype of HIV after having already seroconverted in response to another sub-type. This suggests that an immune response to one sub-type may not be protective against another sub-type, and that re-infection is a theoretical possibility.

- Subtypes of HIV can re-combine to form new subtypes. For example, subtype E is believed to have been a product, or 'mosaic', of co-infection with subtypes B and F at some point in the history of the epidemic. Subtypes G and I are also recombinants related to subtype A. It is unknown whether different subtypes have different biological properties such as greater infectiousness or speedier disase progression (although see *The strain of virus* above for discussion of this issue).

At the XIII International AIDS Conference in Durban, Dr Francine McCutcheon presented evidence that the number of recombinant viruses is growing, and that these viruses are particularly common in West and Central Africa. Some recombinants appear to contain genetic information from up to six different viruses, she reported, indicating a far rate of re-infection than hitherto imagined. However, high levels of recombinant viruses in the population appears to be associated with a lower HIV prevalence, suggesting that these viruses may not be transmitted as efficiently as 'purer' viruses.

- Re-infection with the same subtype may also be cause for concern even in populations where one subtype predominates, especially if it is possible for drug resistant viruses to pass to hosts already infected with HIV. This

raises the prospect of drug-resistant HIV being transmitted within the HIV-positive population.

- Transmission of drug-resistant HIV could also lead to the recombination of HIV variants resistant to several different drugs, leading to the faster emergence of multiple drug resistant HIV.

Persuasive evidence which seems to support these theories was presented to the XIV International AIDS Conference in Barcelona. Two cases of documented superinfection with different strains of HIV were reported. In one case a man presented to doctors with an acute retroviral syndrome (the flu-like illness which develops when a person first develops antibodies to HIV after infection with the virus) following a number of unprotected sexual contacts. The man was already known to be HIV-positive and had been on HAART for over two years. Tests after a viral rebound indicated that the man had originally been infected with subtype AE, but was also infected with subtype B. The possibility that he was infected with subtype B before the rebound was eliminated by performing a polymerase chain reaction (PCR) test, which confirmed the absence of subtype B before the viral rebound. In addition, the type of subtype B the man was infected with closely related to subtypes found in Brazil, where the man had had recent unprotected sexual contacts.

In a second similar case, a man was found to be superinfected despite having a strong and effective immune response to his existing HIV infection. The case involved a man who had been enrolled on a treatment interruption study, and after three cycles of treatment and interruption had mounted an effective immune response to HIV. When a viral rebound occurred, detailed analysis of the man's viral profile revealed that he had been superinfected with a new strain of subtype B. Despite having a strong immune response to the original strain of subtype B, the man's immune system was less able to recognise the new strain leading to uncontrolled viral replication.

The May 2nd edition of the journal *AIDS* carried a case report of a man who has been superinfected with wild-type (drug-sensitive) HIV after initial infection with drug-resistant virus.

The patient was enrolled in a cohort of people who were initially infected with drug-resistant HIV. Four months later, however, a separate and distinct wild-type viral population was detected.

At enrollment the man had a CD4 cell count of 711 cells/mm^3 and viral load of 2,413 copies/ml. Plasma and peripheral blood mononuclear cell samples were taken in order to identify resistance mutations. Resistance mutations in reverse transcriptase codons 181 and 184 were identified.

However, the presence of a second, distinct viral population was confirmed four months later by the sequencing of the 1302 bp fragment of the gag-pol region. It showed that, unlike the initial strain of HIV detected in the man, the second strain was drug-sensitive at codons 181 and 184 of HIV reverse transcriptase where drug resistance was initially detected.

Both strains of HIV were from the type B subtype, which is prevalent in the US. Further tests were conducted to rule out the possibility that the man had been initially infected with both a drug-sensitive and drug-resistant strain of HIV. These included clonal sequencing and genetic reconstruction of viral populations. These tests failed to detect a mixed population of HIV before or after the point at month four when the man was superinfected. Coinfection was further ruled out by analysis of the length polymorphism of the V4-V5 region of HIV gp120 which showed that the man was initially infected with a single strain of HIV.

Superinfection with the wild-type HIV had a negative impact on the man's viral load and CD4 cell count. Coinciding with detection of the second strain of HIV the man's viral load increased from a stable level of between 2,400 copies/ml and 7,000 copies/ml to a little over 34,000 copies/ml at month four, almost 200,000 copies/ml at month six and 170,000 copies at month nine. At the same time, the man's CD4 cell count fell from almost 800 cells/mm^3 to a low point of 283 cells/mm^3 at eleven months.

"These data indicate that four months after infection by drug-resistant HIV this patient was infected by a second, drug-sensitive virus", note the investigators.

The potential health implications of infection with two different viral populations, which are not equally susceptible to the patient's immune system, are emphasised by the investigators, with the fitter wild-type virus causing "an abrupt increase in plasma viremia" in this patient.

Superinfection could also impact on the effectiveness of HAART. Standard tests to detect drug resistance would not reveal a drug resistant strain of HIV after superinfection with a second, fitter, wild-type strain. "Nevertheless, if the patient were to initiate therapy, it seems likely that drug-resistant virus would quickly re-emerge."

At the Eleventh Retrovirus Conference in 2004 (Smith 2004) a group of investigators from Los Angeles and San Diego provided long-awaited information on the incidence of sexually-acquired superinfection, concluding that, amongst their cohort of 78 recently infected individuals not on therapy, the annual rate of superinfection was 5%.

Smith and colleagues retrospectively analysed blood plasma samples from 78 individuals - the majority of whom (90%) were gay men - who were enrolled in the San Diego and Los Angeles Acute HIV Infection and Early Disease Research Programmes between December 1997 and June 2003, and looked for independent clusters of the *pol* gene. When superinfection was suspected, they rigourously tested the samples using four different lines of molecular investigation: clonal (V3) and dye-primer (*pol*) sequencing, and length polymorphism analysis (V1-2 and V4-5).

Three cases of superinfection were identified in the cohort. In each case, superinfection occurred between five to 13 months after the estimated date of initial infection. Each superinfecting HIV strain was associated with a change in susceptibility to antiretrovirals, even though none of the men were on therapy. Two were initially infected with drug-resistant HIV and then became superinfected with a wild-type strain, while the other was initially infected with a wild-type strain and then was superinfected with a drug-resistant strain. Within six months of acquiring the superinfecting strain, their viral loads increased by an average of 1.6 logs and their CD4 counts decreased by an average of 132 cells/mm3 (p< .05).

All three of the cases were gay men who had multiple sexual partners, making identification of the person who superinfected them (the index case) impossible. Without the index cases, the possibility of co-infection - that is, infection with two different viruses at the same time - cannot be completely ruled out. However, since the method they used to identify superinfection is considered to be somewhat conservative, Smith noted that their 5% annual rate may actually be an underestimate, although previous studies in chimpanzees and injection drug users found a similar 5% incidence rate.

However other doctors disagree as to the frequency of superinfection. At the Seventh International Congress on Drug Therapy in HIV Infection Dr Mark Wainberg talked about instances of superinfection he had detected in a cohort of patients followed since primary HIV infection.

One patient out of the 31 in the PHI cohort was not only initially infected with a multi-drug-resistant virus but later acquired a second MDR virus some 30-40 weeks after his first infection. The superinfection was detected because the patient's viral load, which had been very low (in the region of 200-1,000 copies) suddenly increased tenfold to several thousand copies/ml.

Genotyping showed that a different pattern of resistance mutations had taken over; while the first virus had thymidine analogue mutations, the second one lacked these, while still having the M184V mutation and the V108I NNRTI mutation.

The clinical consequences of infection with MDR virus were unpredictable, Wainberg said.

The physician actually responsible for the care of the superinfected patient was in the audience, and in response to a question added that his patient had failed several regimens and was now on a treatment break with a CD4 count of under 200.

Wainberg added that he personally thought superinfection, at least with resistant viruses, was a relatively rare event, being observed in only one out of 31 patients in six years' observation of this closely-followed cohort.

Since then instances of superinfection continue to be reported, but it is still unclear how common it is as a phenomenon. Most of the cases reported have only come to light because of adverse clinical consequences such as the sudden appearance of HIV drug resistance. It may be that superinfection is quite common but does not often have adverse effects; equally it may be that some resistance attributed to poor adherence is in fact due to superinfection.

There is evidence that superinfection is common in the first year of contact with a new partner but, due to acquired immunity, becomes less so as time goes on. Studies have found evidence of superinfection in 2 to 5% of persons in the first year of infection (Smith) but found no evidence of superinfection in long-term relationships (Gonzales). In fact 95% of all cases of superinfection so far documented have occurred through contact with a partner less than three years into a relationship. Interestingly, superinfection is also more common in people with recent HIV infection anyway and much less common in people with long-term infection - possibly because viral mutation and diversification in the person 'auto-immunises' them against a wider range of other types of HIV.

References

Gonzales MJ, Delwart E, Rhee SY, et al. Lack of detectable human immunodeficiency virus type 1 superinfection during 1072 person-years of observation . Journal of Infectious Diseases. 188: 397-405, 2003.

Smith D et al. Incidence of HIV Superinfection Following Primary Infection. 11th CROI, San Francisco, abstract 21, 2004.

Wainberg M. Evolution of transmited wild-type and drug-resistant virus in primary HIV infection. Seventh International Conference on Drug Therapy in HIV Infection, Glasgow. Plenary PL2.3, 2004.

Sources of evidence about HIV transmission

Introduction

One of the features that has undermined much HIV/AIDS education so far has been the tendency to provide disempowering rather than enabling information. Information which over-emphasises very small risks at the expense of concentrating on the demonstrably greater risks of penetrative intercourse and sharing injecting equipment is likely to undermine the success of HIV prevention strategies which concentrate on risk reduction rather than risk elimination (See *HIV prevention: which methods work?* for a discussion of risk reduction and risk elimination approaches).

This section looks at how information about HIV transmission has been gathered, and at cases which appear to suggest new routes of transmission in addition to the well-established routes of sexual intercourse, sharing injecting equipment, mother-to-baby and blood transfusion/blood products. We provide a detailed account of some of these anomalies because they have bred so much uncertainty.

We also offer a critical method for looking at any new proposed routes of transmission, since one of the key tasks facing anyone giving advice on AIDS and HIV is responding to the seemingly endless flow of new possible risks and old misinformation.

Sources of evidence

Our picture of how HIV transmission can or cannot take place is based upon evidence and arguments drawn from many different sources. The overall picture is made up of many different forms of information collected in many research studies over a number of years.

Broadly, the key methods that have been used to come to our understanding of HIV transmission can be summarised under the following categories (which are dealt with immediately below in the rest of this section):

- Epidemiological evidence, or information drawn from observation of patterns of illness, infection and behaviour.

- Virological evidence, or information drawn from the study of HIV and knowledge of other viral infections and the human immune system.

- Risk analysis, or the likelihood of certain events happening given a specific combination of factors e.g. infection of patients by surgeons compared with other risks.

However, it is important to be aware that the complete picture of risk assessment depends upon using all these methods together in combination.

On its own, evidence drawn from any one discipline can lead to the wrong conclusions. This is especially the case because not all pieces of evidence are of equal weight, of equally valid methodology, or of equal accuracy.

For example, if one were to take virological evidence alone, kissing would seem to be a plausible route of transmission because of the occasional isolation of HIV in saliva. Yet epidemiological evidence consistently fails to show kissing to be a risk for HIV infection.

Epidemiological evidence

The epidemiological evidence that confirms our knowledge of the modes of transmission of HIV is drawn from

- Case reports (morbidity and mortality reports).

- Cohort studies and case control studies.

- Seroprevalence surveillance of whole populations, i.e. surveys of incidence and prevalence.

- Correlation analysis.

Case reports

Case reports were crucial in establishing new trends and risks. Clusters of cases of Kaposi's sarcoma and immune suppression amongst gay men in North America led to the recognition of a new epidemic syndrome. This is how the epidemic first began to be detected, some time after it was underway, because of the lag between HIV infection and symptomatic HIV disease. The possible sexual link between these cases was gradually narrowed down by detailed interviewing which asked questions about many lifestyle factors presumed to be common to all those affected by AIDS. These included the use of poppers and recreational drugs, and sexual practices such as fisting, rimming, watersports and anal intercourse. It was eventually discovered that the only common link was anal intercourse, either insertive or receptive.

Case reports may also be useful for detecting particular modes of transmission, e.g. transplants and transfusions, where accurate follow-up is possible.

However, case reports are a crude instrument which tell us very little information with accuracy. They cannot, on their own, be used to establish transmission risks - only to indicate areas of

possible risk which can then be investigated by using more sensitive epidemiological methods.

It was only when more sophisticated epidemiological instruments were employed that the specific modes of transmission, as opposed to undefined sexual contact, were discovered.

Cohort studies and case control studies

A cohort study refers to a study that follows up a group of people, asks questions about their possible risk activities, compares this with their developing status in respect of HIV infection and as a result draws conclusions about which of these possible risk factors is or is not a real risk factor in transmission.

Essentially there are two sorts of cohort study from which information about HIV transmission has been drawn:

- Particular dedicated cohort studies (gay men, family settings, people with haemophilia, etc.)

- Cohort studies established for other reasons (e.g. hepatitis B) plus retrospective analysis of epidemiological data.

Cohort studies are one of the most powerful epidemiological instruments and provide us with our most scientifically reliable information. They do, however, have the drawback that time and resources are required to achieve statistical power. Thus cohort studies have been extremely important in showing:

- That unprotected penetrative anal sex is by far and away the greatest risk factor for gay men and other men who have sex with men.

- That safer sex practices are extremely effective in substantially reducing HIV transmission.

- That the risk from oral sex is low.

However, because cohort studies look at a group made up of individuals who are as randomly chosen as possible from within that group of the population, it can be very difficult for them to distinguish small differences in very low possible risks. For instance, it has been shown that although most cohort studies have shown no detectable statistical risk in oral sex between men, this would still be the case if there were a very small risk of, say, 1%. This is because it is not easy to find a large enough number of gay men who only suck and don't engage in other possible risk activities to provide sufficient statistical power to detect such a low order of risk. One way of doing this might be to recruit a cohort of men through an international multi-centre cohort study (for further discussion of the risks of oral transmission see *Oral transmission*, below).

Seroprevalence surveillance of whole populations

This may be undertaken in various ways:

- Pooling of case reports (by CDC, HPA and equivalent bodies).

- Annual STI reports from GUM clinics.

- Epidemiological distribution in the population as a whole through anonymised seroprevalence surveillance.

- Screening of blood donations.

- Anonymised seroprevalence surveys of GUM clinic attenders and other groups.

This will reveal for instance that, with the exception of those babies born to mothers who are HIV-positive, pre-pubertal children in general are not being infected with HIV. This provides firm evidence to link HIV transmission to certain activities (sexual and drug using) which sexually mature adults undertake but children on the whole do not. It also helps demonstrate that a whole range of messy, 'unhygienic' social contact activities which children engage in more than other sectors of the population are not in themselves a risk factor for HIV transmission between children.

Correlation analysis

This is a way of checking the accuracy or otherwise of our predictions and may be regarded as the nearest thing to a true experiment that can be achieved in epidemiology.

The correlation of predictions may work through comparison of a group with itself at a later date or through comparing different groups of the population.

A correlation between groups of people affected by AIDS and people affected by hepatitis B was noted even before HIV was discovered, leading to the assumption that the agent which caused AIDS must be transmitted through blood and sexual contact.

Risk analysis

It is often suggested that contracting HIV by some routes is less likely than being struck by lightning or being knocked over by a bus. Whether or not these are accurate comparisons, it is well understood that these risks can be quantified on a statistical basis (e.g. a one in a million chance of being struck by lightning during a storm). Actuarial calculations of life expectancy can quantify the risk of death based on whether or not one smokes or drives a car by referring to statistics on deaths attributed to these activities and the frequency of such 'acts of god'

It is less easy to quantify some risks of HIV transmission, such as the risk of transmission during any one occasion of sexual intercourse with an infected person.

On the other hand, it is easy to analyse the likelihood of certain risks of HIV transmission based on epidemiological and biological evidence, along with some common sense. Thus we can say with some confidence that the likelihood that someone will be infected through being bitten by a dog which has just bitten an infected person is so remote as not to be worth discussing. This is both because the conditions needed for transmission to occur are unlikely to be fulfilled (see *The mechanisms of HIV transmission*), and because dogs bite two people in succession very rarely. Furthermore, the chances that one will be standing next to someone with HIV when this unfortunate event occurs are remote, to say the least.

The limitations of the evidence

One drawback of much scientific 'evidence' is the extent to which it relies, at some level, on self-reporting by subjects under study. Thus in the case of illness doctors will use laboratory measurements in addition to the subjective reports of symptoms given by a patient in order to produce accurate information about the course of an illness. This is more difficult in the case of an illness which is the consequence of stigmatised behaviour. It's important to have a realistic scepticism about the likely shortcomings of any non-statistical or anecdotal data produced about risks for HIV transmission. This is because people may have good reason not to tell the truth at a particular time or place.

Unfortunately, common sense often goes out of the window when dealing with anything to do with AIDS. A healthy scepticism about anomalous individual case reports which cannot be substantiated by other methods is often absent, and information which is highly provisional is accepted as a well-established scientific fact.

Some examples of the need for such scepticism are discussed below.

Healthcare workers

A reappraisal of the figures for healthcare workers infected occupationally, which took into account the greater risk from

their sexual or drug-using practice, made it clear that occupational transmission was even more of a rarity than previously thought. In the USA it has been shown that the fear of losing occupational compensation can be an important factor deterring people from mentioning any non-occupational risks they have run.

Oral sex

A 1992 Dutch study found that five out of nine gay male seroconverters who had at first denied anal intercourse later reported that it had taken place in the twelve months prior to seroconversion (Keet). Of the 20 men who denied having had receptive anal intercourse in their questionnaire, 11 later contradicted this statement. Of the 82 men who did report having had receptive anal intercourse, only one later contradicted this statement. Researchers concluded that strong reasons may exist for 'forgetting' or failing to report anal intercourse. These might be:

- Shame at failure to practise safer sex

- 'Forgetting' in order to blot out the memory of risky sexual activity

- Desire to please researchers by demonstrating an adherence to safer sex guidelines

- Refusal to acknowledge taboo sexual practices i.e. anal intercourse.

It is worth noting that much epidemiological evidence is dependent to some degree upon interviews with people who have been infected in order to find out what they have or have not been doing. Because sex and drug use are activities which people are not used to telling the truth about (especially to officialdom), any scientific method must be prepared to take into account not only the answers to questions but how sensitively the questions were asked in the first place.

At the Retroviruses conference held in San Francisco in 2000, researchers from UCSF presented data which suggested that 8 cases or 6.6% of the study sample (total 122) had contracted HIV through oral sex. No other route of transmission could be identified. Whilst concluding that oral sex represented a lower transmission risk, the authors felt that it may be an important mode of HIV transmission due to the relative frequency with which it occurs. Each of the men who had contracted HIV through oral sex believed it to represent no or minimal risk.

The authors did not present any data on the co-factors that influence the risk of transmission through oral sex such as the role of ejaculation, and the presence of sores in the mouth or bleeding gums. It was subsequently revealed that ejaculation occurred in six of the eight cases and around half of seroconverters also had significant gum disease or ulcers.

Additionally, the study could provide no insight into the role viral load played in transmission.

For more information on oral sex risks, see page 119 later in this chapter.

How information on risk is received

Just as important as using scientific methods to gather the information is a critical awareness of how different ways of presenting the same information will lead to differing popular perceptions of what that knowledge means. For instance, the way in which a case report in a scientific journal is presented is likely to lead to very different conclusions than if it is reported in the popular press.

The use of tentative scientific language is intended only to lead to tentative and provisional conclusions. Most scientists will be reluctant to rule out events like HIV transmission by insects until a process of hypothesis, investigation and disproval has been undergone, because this is the tried and trusted scientific method. This is time consuming, and meanwhile it leaves areas of uncertainty. Unfortunately, this process of scientific dialogue is open to radical misinterpretation through other media which deal in fast and easy answers.

For example, medical journal discussion on the possibility of transmission through kissing was subject to widely differing interpretations. In 1989 Italian doctors reported on the results of experiments in which they had measured the amount of blood present in saliva after eating, deep passionate kissing and tooth brushing (Piazza). Whilst small quantities of blood were measured in saliva after kissing or eating, considerably larger quantities were detected in saliva after tooth brushing. The authors of the letter argued that this suggested some risk of HIV transmission through kissing.

This statement was highlighted by the media as suggesting that HIV transmission could be transmitted through kissing after all. The authors of the report did not appear to have grasped the extent to which their findings would be misinterpreted, or the inadequacy of their method for providing information on which to base a major reassessment of safer sex guidelines.

Those reporting the evidence as 'news' failed to make a common-sense judgement about the scale of the epidemic if kissing were a mode of transmission.

Dealing with new evidence

Sometimes a 'theoretical' method will be proposed for how blood to blood or body fluid to blood contact may occur through a hitherto unmentioned route. This is what happened at one stage with the suggestion of transmission of HIV by an insect vector. This 'theoretical' method has been found to be impossible for all practical purposes in two ways. Virological evidence has shown that there would be insufficient virus in such a method of transmission to be able to transmit effectively; and epidemiological evidence has shown that the patterns of HIV infection in populations all over the world show no correlation whatsoever with patterns of the population that are most bitten by insects. One method without the other may not provide convincing evidence. Together they show why certain 'theoretical' modes of transmission are impossible.

Another example is the way in which researchers have employed both epidemiological and biomedical knowledge to explain why oral transmission seems so uncommon.

Occasionally a doctor will write a letter to, say, *The Lancet* or the *British Medical Journal* in which a new mode of transmission is proposed on the basis of their cross-examination (or 'history') of one of their patients who has developed HIV infection.

If, however, this contradicts what we know from epidemiological studies it will generally be the case that closer scrutiny of the methodology used to take the history shows that it is invalid: either because of certain assumptions that were made or because

of other questions that were not asked. Some of these examples are discussed in *Low and theoretical risks*.

The more precise the epidemiological evidence needed, the longer it takes to gather. Therefore epidemiological evidence on its own may not be any more precise than to suggest that a range of activities together are implicated in HIV transmission. It then requires virological knowledge and sociological knowledge to differentiate activities implicated in this way into those that are functionally linked and those that are only coincidentally linked.

However, it is important to understand the logical sequence: epidemiology establishes the risk and virology refines it, and not vice versa. We should always be sceptical of theoretical virological routes, therefore, which have no basis in epidemiological evidence.

Anticipating future anxieties

In analysing any report which seems to propose a new route of transmission, there are a number of questions worth asking:

- Where has this been reported? What is the track record of that publication?

- Is there some 'line' the article is trying to push which requires it to overstate e.g. a distraction from the established and predominant risks?

- Is there actual new evidence being reported? Or is this opportunistic reviewing of old evidence?

- If this is a letter or opinion expressing concern about a 'possible' new mode of transmission, is it really one that isn't already in fact accounted for by our existing knowledge?

- How big a sample of people is it? If only one, or ones and twos, how rigorous is the methodology?

- Does the article reveal the methods used? If not, why not?

- What steps were taken to guard against simply taking someone's fallible memory or opinion as scientific fact?

- Does the article state what conditions have had to be disproved in order to establish the authenticity of this point of view?

- Is this in fact anything new in principle as opposed to in manifestation?

References

Keet I et al: Orogenital sex and the transmission of HIV amongst homosexual men, AIDS 6(2): 223-226, 1992.

Piazza Et al: Passionate kissing and microlesions of the oral mucosa: possible role in AIDS transmission; JAMA 26: 245-246, 1989.

Anal and vaginal transmission

Introduction

This section provides a summary of what is currently known about the transmission of HIV through sexual intercourse. References are summarised for each section rather than for the chapter.

The basis for our knowledge

Sexual intercourse was identified as a key route of transmission of the agent assumed to be causing AIDS even before HIV was discovered. Information about the sexual transmission of HIV has been gathered from a large number of epidemiological studies in Africa, North America and Europe. These have been conducted with several different groups of people:

- Couples in which one partner is HIV-positive and one partner is HIV-negative at the beginning of the study ('discordant couple' studies). The European Study Group on Heterosexual Transmission of HIV is an example of this sort

- Gay men recruited to cohort studies specifically for the purpose of studying sexual risk factors for HIV infection, or gay men previously recruited to hepatitis B vaccine studies

- Female sex workers in African cities.

Information has also been gathered from laboratory studies of body fluids and tissues, providing information about infectivity and mechanisms of infection and possible immunity from infection.

In addition the viability of vaginal transmission has been established through reports of HIV infection through artificial insemination by donor. These are discussed in more detail below.

Anal intercourse between men

Unprotected anal intercourse (having intercourse with) between men is a highly efficient means of transmitting HIV because of the delicacy of the tissue in the rectum, and because cells are present in the tissue of the rectum which are vulnerable to infection by HIV.

It also allows HIV in blood to come into contact with the delicate tissue on the head of the penis and in the urethra.

Studies of gay and bisexual men show a number of factors increase the likelihood of HIV infection through anal intercourse even further:

Rectal bleeding

This could be caused by piles, warts, herpes lesions, by the prior use of sex toys, or by fingering and fisting. But even if none of these occur, anal intercourse can still cause bleeding and tiny abrasions in the lining of the rectum. The failure to use some form of lubrication is likely to increase the chance of bleeding.

Sexually transmitted infections

See *Transmission through vaginal intercourse*

Viral load in semen

This topic is covered in more detail in *Transmission through vaginal intercourse* later in this section.

In terms of studies specifically of gay men, a study presented in 2003 (Taylor) found that a small number of "seminal super-shedders" who have disproportionately high HIV viral loads in their semen may be particularly likely to transmit HIV during unprotected sex.

The Taylor study found that while a large minority were exceptions to the rule, there was at least a correlation between viral load in plasma and in semen. But a 2001 study (Kalichman) of gay men with multiple partners found no correlation at all; the subjects were as likely to have a higher viral load in semen than in blood as the other way round.

Kalichman took blood and semen samples from 35 sexually active gay men and found that seven on the 35 had undetectable HIV in their blood but high levels of HIV in their semen - from 10,000 to a million copies.

An equal number of men had HIV in their blood but not in their semen, while the rest had virus in both body fluids, but there was no correlation at all between the viral load in blood and that in semen.

Altogether more than half of the men had detectable HIV in their semen.

He said that studies found that although there was no link between how much unprotected sex men with HIV had and whether they were optimistic about their HIV treatment, there was a link if they believed the HIV drugs made them less infectious.

It was clear that a lot of the men with an undetectable viral load in their blood thought they were not infectious, because the men who were 'undetectable' in their blood recorded an average of four instances of insertive anal sex over the previous month whereas the average for men with detectable plasma viral loads was only 0.3 instances.

In a subsequent study, Kalichman found that out of 20 gay men, 10 switched their behaviour from always using condoms to sometimes not using them when they were told they were 'undetectable'.

Kalichman acknowledged his study conflicted with others. He suggested that the high semen viral loads seen in his gay men were due to high levels of sexual activity and resultant high levels of subclinical urethritis.

These studies are of concern because there is more evidence that some gay men are using viral load in a positive partner to guide decisions about unprotected sex.

In one study (Guzman), the San Francisco Department of Public Health and the US Centers for Disease Control and Prevention questioned 507 men who have sex with men (MSM) recruited from social venues, street locations and community agencies.

Seventy-eight per cent of those questioned were familiar with the term 'viral load' and one third (111 of the total sample) had discussed viral load with a partner of a different HIV status during the previous year in order to make decisions about which sexual practices to engage in. Of those who had discussed viral load, more than half estimated that they used viral load disclosure to guide sexual decision-making in at least 70% of their sexual encounters.

Among study participants, HIV-positive individuals were more likely than HIV-negative men to use viral load information to make sexual decisions, and African Americans were more likely than whites to base sexual risk behaviour on such information. Significantly, among HIV-negative men with serodiscordant partners, those who discussed viral load reported a greater willingness to engage in unprotected sex with a partner whose viral load was undetectable.

Study authors note that while they surveyed a limited number of men in a single metropolitan area, these findings suggest that many MSM are using viral load disclosure to make sexual risk decisions, contrary to guidance from public health officials. Researchers recommend that HIV prevention programmes targeting gay and bisexual men underscore the limitations of using viral load as an individual indicator of infectivity.

Use of poppers (nitrite inhalants)

In the early years of the epidemic there was speculation that poppers contributed to the development of AIDS by suppressing the immune system. This was because use of poppers was a practice common to all the earliest AIDS cases. Scientific debate has continued on the role of poppers in the epidemic, and some continue to argue that poppers are in themselves sufficient to cause the immune suppression characteristic of AIDS. Whilst poppers may cause a degree of immune suppression (although not of CD4 and CD8 cells) in healthy individuals, a recent analysis comparing seropositive and seronegative men over ten years showed that seronegative men retained stable CD4 counts despite long-term poppers use, whilst seropositive men who used poppers and other recreational drugs suffered declining CD4 counts (Dax; Schechter). The view that poppers and other toxic drugs cause AIDS is discussed further in the *HIV & AIDS Treatments Directory*.

The relationship between poppers and HIV infection is more suggestive. Seage reported in 1992 that a cohort of gay men who almost always used poppers during receptive anal intercourse were twice as likely to be HIV-infected as those who did not use poppers during receptive anal intercourse. It is speculated that nitrite inhalants dilate the blood vessels in the rectum, making them more vulnerable to infection and to bleeding. As yet there has been little investigation of the role poppers might play in altering immune function and thereby diminishing a protective immune response to HIV infection.

These factors place both partners at risk of HIV infection. The receptive or passive partner) is at greater risk from receiving semen in the rectum, but the insertive or active partner is also at risk of infection, due to the presence of blood in the rectum. Abrasions to the delicate tissue on the head of the penis and underneath the foreskin put the active partner at risk from blood in the rectum if he is not using a condom.

The risks to active and passive partners

A dangerous myth of the AIDS epidemic is the belief amongst some gay men that the insertive/active partner) will not get infected. It is difficult to establish the relative risks of receptive and insertive anal intercourse because many of those infected will have taken both roles in anal sex. Evidence from a number of cohort studies (especially Keet 1992) demonstrates that the insertive partner in anal intercourse can become infected.

However, when examining evidence from the same cohort study, it is also clear that HIV infection is most common amongst those who engage in both roles, or only practice receptive anal intercourse, whilst those who confine themselves only to the insertive role are much less likely to have been infected (Van Druten).

A review of serconverters from three US cities calculated that the risk of infection through unprotected receptive anal intercourse was approximately ten times greater than the risk of infection through insertive anal intercourse.

The per-contact risk of acquiring HIV infection during unprotected receptive anal intercourse with a man known to be HIV-positive was 0.82% (eight in one thousand), whilst the per contact risk of acquiring HIV from unprotected insertive anal

intercourse with any partner was more than ten times lower (0.6 in one thousand). Receptive oral sex that involved ejaculation carried a per-contact risk of 0.4 in one thousand (Vittinghoff).

A study (Zuckerman - see **Rectal secretions** above) suggests that gay or bisexual men who have insertive unprotected anal sex and encounter this mucus are at far higher risk of HIV infection than previously thought. Formerly, most literature on HIV protection named blood or semen as the main culprit in HIV transmission.

The risk from precum in anal intercourse

It is sometimes assumed that if the active/insertive partner does not ejaculate inside his partner, then the risk is significantly reduced. Although the chances of infection from pre-cum are probably lower than if ejaculation occurs, it is not possible to be certain about this, because levels of HIV in pre-cum vary. A person in very early or symptomatic stages of infection may have higher levels of HIV in pre-cum than someone who is asymptomatic (Ilaria). See also *Oral transmission: What is the risk of infection from pre-cum?* below. It is therefore hard to be confident that withdrawal before ejaculation will protect the receptive partner from being infected. Nevertheless, withdrawal before ejaculation is likely to constitute less of a risk.

References

Dax EM: Amyl nitrite alters in vitro human immune function, Immunopharm and Immunotox 13(4): 577-587, 1991.

Guzman R et al. Communication of HIV viral load to make sexual risk decisions with serodiscordant partners among a diverse sample of men who have sex with men. National HIV Prevention Conference, Atlanta, USA, presentation TP-113, 2005.

Kalichman SC et al. Human immunodeficiency virus in semen and plasma: investigation of sexual transmission risk behavioral correlates. AIDS Res Hum Retroviruses 10: 17(18): 1695-1703. 2001.

Keet I et al: Orogenital sex and the transmission of HIV among homosexual men, AIDS 6(2) 223-226, 1992.

Seage GR et al: The Relation between Nitrite Inhalants, Unprotected Receptive Anal Intercourse, and the Risk of Human Immunodeficiency Virus Infection, Am J of Epidem 135(1): 1-11, 1992.

Schechter MT et al: HIV-1 and the aetiology of AIDS, Lancet March 13: 658-659, 1993.

Schechter MT et al: HIV and the aetiology of AIDS (Letter), Lancet May 8: 1222-1224 1993 (See also letters from Ascher and Dalgleish in the same issue, and from P Duesburg in The Lancet April 8 and June 12 1993).

Taylor S, Sadiq T, Sabin C, et al. Seminal super shedding of HIV: implications for sexual transmission. Program and abstracts of the tenth Conference on Retroviruses and Opportunistic Infections, Boston, Massachusetts, abstract 454, 2003.

Van Druten HAM et al: Homosexual role separation and the spread of HIV. Eighth International Conference On AIDS, Amsterdam, abstract ThC 1518, 1992.

Vittinghoff E et al. Per-contact risk of human immunodeficiency virus transmission between male sexual partners. American Journal of Epidemiology 150: 306-311, 1999.

Zuckerman, Richard et al. HIV-1 RNA in rectal mucosa secretions and seminal plasma; considerations for microbicide efficacy. First Microbicides conference, London, abstract 02679, 2004.

Anal intercourse between men and women

The same physical factors which increase the chance of infection in anal intercourse between men also apply to anal intercourse between men and women. These are:

- Sexually transmitted infections.

- Bleeding.

- Use of poppers.

Anal intercourse has been downplayed as a route of transmission between men and women, yet there is now evidence that it plays an important role in HIV transmission amongst heterosexuals. In 1992 the European Study on Heterosexual Transmission of HIV highlighted anal intercourse as one of the factors which increased the likelihood of transmission amongst the couples in the study, and showed that amongst couples where the infected partner was still asymptomatic (and not likely to be highly infectious), the chance that infection was likely to have taken place through anal intercourse was five times greater than through vaginal intercourse. Caution should be exercised when drawing conclusions from these findings, because of the small numbers involved.

In 1987 Padian reported that the risk of infection for a woman from one act of anal intercourse was 2.3 times greater than from vaginal intercourse. This study did not distinguish between partners at different stages of disease progression (and therefore, potential infectivity).

It has also been suggested that anal intercourse will not be a significant route of transmission amongst heterosexuals because it is not practised by significant numbers of heterosexuals. This is not the case. Ten per cent of heterosexual women in the United States report having anal intercourse regularly, and a quarter engage in it occasionally. A 2004 telephone survey of heterosexuals under 35 conducted by the US Association for Social Health found that 47% of respondents 'sometimes or never' used condoms for vaginal sex. It also found that of the approximately seven per cent of heterosexuals that said they had anal sex, an even higher proportion did not use condoms - some 65%.

In the UK, 12.3% of male respondents and 11.3% of women who responded to the National Survey of Sexual Attitudes and Lifestyles (2000) reported anal intercourse with a partner of the opposite sex in the previous year. It is not a practice which is confined to particular ethnic groups, nor one which takes place predominantly between prostitutes and their clients. It is practised by large numbers of sexually active adults on a regular basis for pleasure, and should be considered as one of the key issues in the prevention of HIV transmission amongst heterosexuals.

References

American Social Health Association Press Release: SURVEY SUGGESTS LACK OF AWARENESS HEIGHTENS RISK FOR SEXUALLY TRANSMITTED DISEASES. See http://www.planetout.com/health/hiv/?sernum=2778 6 April 2004.

European Study Group on Heterosexual Transmission of HIV: Comparison of female to male and male to female transmission of HIV in 563 stable couples, BMJ 304: 809-813, 1992.

European Study Group: Risk factors for male to female transmission of HIV, BMJ 298: 411-415, 1989.

Padian N et al: Female to male transmission of Human Immunodeficiency Virus, JAMA 266(12): 1664 -1667, 1987.

Transmission through vaginal intercourse

Numerous studies have now shown the ease with which HIV infection can be transmitted during unprotected vaginal intercourse. A number of factors unrelated to condom use seem to increase the chance of infection through vaginal intercourse. These are the following:

The level of HIV in semen or vaginal fluid

Levels of HIV vary in both semen and vaginal fluid, partly as a result of disease progression, with higher viral load observed later in HIV infection; in a 1992 study only 4% of those with CD4 counts over 200 produced semen from which it was possible to culture HIV, compared with 24% of those with CD4 counts under 200. In a 1994 study HIV isolation was most frequent from the semen of men whose CD4 count was below 100 (87% vs. 40% of men with CD4 count of 101-200) (Anderson; Vernazza).

However, virus levels in semen appear to be unpredictable, and some studies have reported no correlation between virus levels in blood and virus levels in semen (see under *Viral load in semen* above).

This may be partially explained by the presence of undiagnosed or asymptomatic genitourinary infections in individuals with high viral load in semen but low plasma viral load (see *The mechanisms of HIV transmission* in this section).

The European Study Group on Heterosexual Transmission of HIV noted in 1994 that partners of men or women who had a CD4 count below 200 at the beginning of the study were much more likely to have seroconverted after 20 months than partners of HIV-positive men or women who remained asymptomatic throughout the 20 month follow-up period (De Vincenzi 1994).

A study in Uganda has confirmed that viral load is the most important factor in determining whether HIV is transmitted. But it is unclear how these findings can be translated into a Western setting where people are using antiretroviral drugs, experts warn.

415 couples in whom one partner was HIV-positive were identified in the Rakai district of Uganda. The couples were identified by confidential HIV testing. All couples were offered counselling in condom use and the opportunity to learn their HIV status at the beginning of the study, and access to free condoms throughout the study. People diagnosed HIV-positive were left to decide whether or not to inform their partners, a decision criticised in an accompanying editorial in the *New England Journal of Medicine* (Quinn).

Sexually transmitted infection treatment was offered at regular intervals as part of another study to half the participants. The other half were required to seek free treatment if they experienced any symptoms. HIV antibody status and exposure to sexually transmitted infections was tested every ten months.

Viral load prior to transmission was determined by measuring the viral load of the HIV-positive partner at the check-up prior to seroconversion of his or her partner. To estimate the relative risk, this viral load result was matched with one from another individual of similar age and sex who had not seroconverted.

In this study, every year of follow-up for an individual counts as a person year. In this study 415 couples were enrolled and followed for a median of just under two years. This means that the study followed people for approximately 800 person years.

The key findings of the study were:

- 22% of all partners seroconverted during the follow-up period.

- Men were just as likely to become infected as women at any given level of viral load.

- Circumcision appeared to be protective: none of the circumcised male partners of HIV-positive women became infected, whereas 40 out of 197 uncircumcised men became infected.

- Symptomatic sexually transmitted infections did not affect an individual's likelihood of catching HIV, but a history of genital discharge in the HIV-positive partner was associated with an increased risk of HIV infection ($p < 0.05$).

- Viral load above 50,000 copies in the HIV-positive partner was most strongly associated with the risk of transmission, at a rate of 23 infections per 100 person years.

- 5.6% of all transmission occurred in couples where the HIV-positive partner had a viral load between 400 and 3,499 copies, indicating that transmission can take place even from individuals considered to be at very low risk of disease progression. This translates into 2.2 cases per 100 person years, a tenfold lower risk than seen in couples where the HIV-positive partner had viral load greater than 50,000 copies.

- No infections occurred in couples where the HIV-positive partner had viral load below 1500 copies.

In an editorial accompanying the publication of the study, Dr Myron Cohen of the University of North Carolina noted that the findings did not necessarily support the view that lowering viral load with antiretroviral treatment would reduce HIV transmission rates:

HIV-1 can still be cultured from the genital secretions of some patients who are receiving antiretroviral therapy and who have undetectable levels of HIV-1 RNA in blood, a finding that means that one cannot reassure patients that they are not contagious. Indeed, if the use of such therapy increased the likelihood that HIV-1-infected patients would practice unsafe sex in the mistaken belief they were unable to transmit the virus, it could offset the benefit of viral suppression, he wrote.

The levels of HIV in vaginal fluid tend to vary too. Levels of HIV are likely to be highest around the time of menstruation when HIV-bearing cells shed from the cervix are most likely to be found in the vaginal fluid, along with blood (Mostad).

However, avoiding sexual intercourse during menstruation is likely to provide little protection to male partners of HIV-positive women: the 1992 report of the European Study Group showed that almost half the men infected by female partners in the study were men who avoided intercourse during menstruation.

One study (Lennox) has found that subclinical inflammation within the female genital tract might also increase cervicovaginal shedding of HIV.

Putting these studies together, the clinical relevance becomes clear: High blood plasma viral load means that genital tract viral load is also likely to be high, as the two appear to be reasonably correlated in most studies.

However, clinical or asymptomatic genital inflammation will further increase genital HIV shedding, and there appears to be a small number of patients with no apparent genital tract infections who still may have exceptionally high genital tract viral loads and only moderately elevated plasma viral loads.

The evidence concerning the effects of anti-HIV treatment on the levels of HIV in semen and vaginal fluid is discussed in detail in *Treating HIV in genital fluids* in *Anti-HIV-therapy: Choosing your treatment strategy* in the *HIV & AIDS Treatments Directory* or at aidsmap.com.

Sexually transmitted infections

Ulcers caused by sexually transmitted infections may provide a route of infection for HIV. This is due to damage to the mucous membranes and the increased presence of the white blood cells which HIV infects. Bleeding from these ulcers may also increase the chance of infection (Padian). Non-ulcerative sexually transmitted infections such as gonorrhoea, chlamydia, bacterial vaginosis and trichomoniasis also appear to assist HIV infection according to epidemiological evidence, although the precise mechanism is unclear. It is impossible to say at present whether genital warts play any role in assisting HIV infection (Laga).

In 1994 the European Study Group on Heterosexual Transmission of HIV reported that those with sexually transmitted infections were three or four times as likely to be infected after 20 months of follow-up than those who reported no sexually transmitted infections (De Vincenzi 1994).

In 1999 a study of Thai women with HIV-positive partners showed that women whose partners had a history of sexually transmitted infections were twice as likely to be HIV-positive as women whose partners did not. In this study women with other possible exposure routes were excluded, and CD4 counts were also measured. Women almost always had higher CD4 counts than male partners, suggesting later exposure to HIV (Nelson).

Studies in Malawi and Cote d'Ivoire amongst men and women respectively (Cohen; Ghys) have demonstrated that HIV levels in sexual fluids are reduced by treatment of urethritis and gonorrhoea.

If an HIV-infected person is also concurrently suffering a sexually transmissible infection, this is likely to increase the infectivity of his semen or her vaginal fluid. HIV infection is also likely to lead to an increased incidence of ulcerative sexually transmitted diseases, such as herpes and cancroid. Sexually transmitted diseases play a key role in HIV infections amongst heterosexuals. Thrush (candida infection) also makes women more vulnerable to HIV infection, for the same reason, and women with a history of thrush infection who are HIV-positive seem more likely to pass HIV to their male partners.

One study estimates that the presence of an ulcerative genital infection on a man's penis increases the per-sex act transmission risk from a woman to a man 50-300 fold (Hayes).

In 1995 a study conducted in the Mwanza district of Tanzania showed that at a population level a reduction in the prevalence of sexually transmitted infections and a syndromic treatment programme for STIs were associated with a reduction in the incidence of new HIV infections. These findings suggest that the control of sexually transmitted infections can play a major part in HIV prevention (Grosskurth). (Syndromic treatment is a simplified, rule-based approach for settings where diagnostic facilities are limited.)

However, in 1999 another group working in the Rakai district of Uganda reported that in a region with higher HIV prevalence (15.9% vs 4%), a randomised study of mass STI treatment did not find any difference in HIV incidence between those who received STI treatment and those who did not. The authors suggested that in a more mature epidemic, STIs may not play the same role as in an early epidemic, where they might be amplifying transmission opportunities amongst individuals recently infected with HIV and their partners. In the early stages of an epidemic, these individuals are likely to be those with the largest number of sexual contacts with other individuals who also have a high number of sexual contacts. In a more mature epidemic, other host factors (such as degree of natural immunity) and the number of sex acts with each partner will play a more important role. An initial core group of HIV-infected individuals might just as easily infect 100 people if they have repeated sex with those individuals as if they had single sexual contacts with thousands of people, irrespective of STD incidence (Hitchcock; Wawer).

In a 2004 study of gay men (Buchacz), syphilis infection in HIV-positive men was associated with an increase in viral load and reduction in CD4 cell count. The study investigators believed that their findings indicate that HIV-positive men with syphilis were potentially more infectious and called for integrated public health campaigns to prevent the spread of both HIV and syphilis.

There has been considerable debate about the role of STI treatment programmes within HIV prevention programmes. One of the key points to remember is that the two studies discussed above are not entirely comparable, not only because the epidemic may have been more mature in the latter study, but also because the nature of the treatment programmes differed. In the latter study a one-off programme of treatment took place, but experts point out that single dose antimicrobial treatment of the kind used in the Rakai study would have no impact on conditions such as herpes, syphilis and bacterial vaginosis, all of which may be implicated in HIV transmission (Grosskurth 2000). Herpes simplex in particular was a much more common condition in the Rakai district; 43% of diagnosed genital ulcers were caused by HSV-2, compared with less than 10% in the Mwanza district.

The role of genital herpes in HIV transmission is receiving attention. Herpes simplex virus II (HSV-2) is the most common cause of genital ulcers worldwide and it has long been suggested that by disruption of the epithelial barrier and general inflammation, it may increase the chances of infection with HIV.

In a South African study 400 female sex workers at truck stops between Durban and Johannesburg were screened for HIV. Only 198 were found to be HIV-negative and they were monitored monthly over three years. Of the women who seroconverted during the study, all but six became HSV-2 positive before they became HIV-positive, suggesting to the investigators that "immediately after infection with HSV-2, the risk of contracting HIV-1 increases significantly."

However, investigators also found that women who were already HSV-2-positive at the start of the study had a lower risk of HIV seroconversion than those who were HSV-2-negative at the start of the study. The investigators speculate that the women already infected with HSV-2 were protected from reinfection with HSV-2, thus reducing the chance of acquiring HSV-2 ulcerative lesions which are a risk factor for HIV.

HIV subtype

Research from Thailand shows that HIV-1 subtype E is more frequently transmitted through vaginal intercourse than HIV-1 subtype B (the subtype predominant amongst drug injectors and gay men in the West). When all other factors were controlled for, female partners of men infected with HIV-1 subtype E were 3.1 times more likely to be infected with the same strain than female partners of men carrying HIV-1 subtype B (Kunanusont). This finding may explain why epidemiologists have calculated that the risk of heterosexual transmission per episode of sexual intercourse in the Thai population was 31-fold to 56-fold higher than estimates for the US population (Mastro). Subtype E has also been shown to reproduce more efficiently than subtype B in immune cells called Langerhans cells, which are numerous in the vaginal wall.

However, many researchers are still sceptical about differences in transmission rates between HIV subtypes (see *Physical co-factors which encourage transmission* earlier in this chapter). A Thai/American group found that viral load was significantly lower (approximately 0.5 log) in the semen of 87 Thai men infected with subtype compared to 70 men infected with subtype B (Coombs).

Individual cases studies also suggest that HIV-1 is a great deal more easily transmitted than HIV-2. Austrian doctors reported in 1994 that a woman infected with HIV-1 by a partner co-infected with HIV-1 and HIV-2 did not seroconvert for HIV-2 despite nearly 14 months of follow-up (Most).

Damage to the tissue of the genitals

More violent sexual penetration of the type often associated with rape may lead to vaginal or penile abrasions which may increase the chances of HIV infection. This is most likely to be caused by rough sex and/or dryness in the vagina, and will create small abrasions which make it more easy for the virus to get into the bloodstream.

Bleeding from damaged tissue on the penis may also facilitate infection to the female partner.

A number of studies have also suggested a possibly increased risk of HIV infection when the hymen is broken on the first occasion of sexual intercourse.

Reduction of vaginal lubrication becomes more common with age, and some researchers say that this is one reason why some studies show higher rates of HIV infection amongst post-menopausal women. Younger women in early puberty may also produce less vaginal and cervical secretions, perhaps increasing their vulnerability to HIV infection and contributing to the disproportionate prevalence of HIV amongst adolescent women. Hysterectomy in older women has also been reported as a factor which may pre-dispose to the risks of HIV infection in older women (Holmberg).

Vulnerability of the cervix

Cells particularly vulnerable to HIV infection are located beneath the surface of the cervix (Pomerantz). These cells are more vulnerable to infection in adolescence and during a woman's first pregnancy, perhaps accounting for the higher prevalence of HIV amongst women under 30 than amongst men under 30 in Africa.

These cervical cells may also become vulnerable as a consequence of changes in the cervix caused by human papilloma virus and chlamydia. Sexual health programmes which seek to reduce the incidence of unprotected sex amongst adolescent women may therefore be particularly important.

Circumcision

For further discussion of the effects of circumcision on HIV transmission see *C is for circumcision* in the chapter *HIV prevention*.

Female genital mutilation (female circumcision)

In women, the practice of female genital mutilation, the cutting of the genitals, is speculated to assist HIV infection, but a comparison of areas of high HIV prevalence in Africa with areas in which female genital mutilation is commonly practised has shown no clear correspondence.

A study from Tanzania presented at the 3rd IAS conference found that female genital mutilation actually had a negative effect on HIV transmission (Stallings).

Number of exposures

One sexual contact is enough for a man to be infected: 8.2% of 73 men followed for an average of 13 weeks seroconverted after one sexual contact with a woman (all had genital ulcer disease, five were uncircumcised) (Johnson).

One exposure to infected semen is enough for a woman to be infected; this is demonstrated by the 1990 report of HIV infection following artificial insemination (MMWR). A 1995 review of 199 women at five US fertility clinics exposed to HIV-infected semen from a single donor found that seven women were infected from a single exposure (Araneta).

Seroconversion is dependent on sexual intercourse with an infectious partner; 100 sexual contacts with a partner who has a very low level of infectivity is probably far less risky than sexual contacts with 100 different HIV-positive partners. This is because there is a high probability that at least one of these partners is highly infectious.

There is no evidence that seroconversion occurs after a cumulative process of infection - in other words, the more times one has sex with an infected person, the more virus one becomes infected with, until a critical mass is achieved and seroconversion occurs. This belief has arisen in part because of lay beliefs about health and illness, but also from the observation that many partners of HIV infected people have gone for long periods without being infected. This is due to the fact that conditions which permit infection may not exist all the time.

Immune function

Although there is some evidence that despite repeated exposure to HIV, some people do not become infected, the significance of these observations is not fully understood. We do not know if this means that some people can resist HIV infection, and what the factors might be which confer some kind of resistance to infection.

There are several possible explanations for this phenomenon:

Genetic susceptibility to HIV is a hypothesis supported by a number of observations, notably the identification of a common genetic marker on the immune cells of some people who appear to have resisted infection, correlated with the identification of a number of genetic markers on the immune cells of people who have developed AIDS.

Resistance to infection within a population develops through generations of interactions between the host immune system and infectious organisms, and develops by a process of natural selection; those with the best resistance will survive the infection and pass their genetically conferred resistance onto some of their descendants. This is the way in which populations adapt to some conditions; an example of this is the adaptation of Europeans to various forms of pox virus (e.g. smallpox), and the lack of resistance shown by inhabitants of the Americas when Europeans first introduced these viruses. Resistance to HIV infection is discussed in *Resistance to infection* earlier in this chapter.

Stronger cellular immunity: Some people have been observed to have consistently higher CD4 counts, higher levels of CD8 cells and lymphocytes throughout periods of study than comparable individuals who seroconvert during the course of the study (Visscher). It may be that the overall state of the immune system plays an important role in preventing or allowing infection, but the mechanism is still unknown. Some research has suggested that exposure to very small amounts of HIV may have an immunising effect by stimulating cell-mediated rather than antibody responses to HIV, but this view remains to be proven.

Defective form of HIV: An alternative suggestion is that individuals who have apparently resisted HIV infection may simply have encountered a defective or less virulent form of HIV. In 1995 considerable publicity was given to the case of a child who had cleared HIV infection after perinatal infection. Researchers subsequently demonstrated that the child had been infected with a defective strain of HIV and had been able to clear the virus and revert to HIV-negative by twelve months of age (Bryson).

For more on immune function and HIV, see **Cytotoxic T cell protection against HIV** above.

Nutritional deficiency

Deficiency in blood levels of the mineral selenium has been associated with increased rates of vaginal HIV shedding in a study conducted among women in Kenya. HIV-positive women with selenium deficiency were almost three times more likely to have evidence of HIV DNA in their vaginal fluids when sampled (once only) (Baeten).

Although the authors of this study have suggested a potential role for selenium supplementation in reducing transmission, the confounding effect of viral load was not taken into account in this study. While the authors controlled for the effects of CD4 count, they did not test for plasma viral load, and it is possible that an independent association might exist between plasma viral load levels and selenium deficiency.

References

Anderson DJ et al: Effects of disease stage and zidovudine therapy on the detection of human immunodeficiency virus type 1 in semen, JAMA 267: 2769-2774, 1992.

Araneta MRG et al: HIV transmission through donor artificial insemination, JAMA 273(11): 854-858, 1995.

Baeten J et al. Selenium deficiency is associated with shedding of HIV-1 infected cells in the female genital tract. XIII International AIDS Conference, Durban, abstract MoOrA226, 2000.

Bryson YJ et al: Clearance of HIV infection in a perinatally infected infant, NEJM 332(13): 833-838, 1995.

Buchacz K et al. Syphilis increases HIV viral load and decreases CD4 cell counts in HIV-infected patients with new syphilis infections. AIDS 18: 2075-2079, 2004.

Cohen M. Reduction of concentration of HIV-1 in semen after treatment of urethritis: implications for prevention of sexual transmission of HIV-1. Lancet 349: 1868-1873, 1997.

Coombs RW et al. Does viral sub-type determine HIV-1 shedding in semen? Annual Meeting of the American Urological Association, abstract 1111, 1999.

De Vincenzi I et al: A longitudinal study of human immunodeficiency virus transmission by heterosexual partners, NEJM 331(6): 341-346, 1994.

Ghys A. HIV shedding, STD and immunosuppression. AIDS 11(12): F85-F93, 1997.

Gray R et al. HIV incidence associated with male circumcision in a population-based cohort, and HIV acquisition/transmission associated with circumcision and viral load in discordant couples: Rakai, Uganda. XIII International AIDS Conference, Durban, abstract MoOrC193, 2000.

Grosskurth H et al: Impact of improved treatment of sexually transmitted diseases on HIV infection in rural Tanzania: randomised controlled trial, Lancet 436: 530-536, 1995.

Grosskurth H et al. Control of sexually transmitted diseases for HIV-1 prevention: understanding the implications of the Mwanza and Rakai trials. The Lancet 355: 1981-1987, 2000.

Hayes RJ et al: The cofactor effect of genital ulcers on the per-exposure risk of HIV transmission in sub-Saharan Africa, J Trop Med Hyg 98: 1-8, 1995.

Hitchcock P, Fransen L. Preventing HIV infection: lessons from Mwanza and Rakai. The Lancet 353: 9152, 1999.

Holmberg SD, Horsburgh CR: Biologic factors in the sexual transmission of human immunodeficiency virus, J Inf Dis 160(1): 116-125.

Ilaria G et al: Detection of HIV-1 DNA sequences in pre-ejaculatory fluid, Lancet 340(8833): 1469, 1992.

Johnson AM et al: Heterosexual transmission of HIV, AIDS(S1): 549-556, 1988.

Kunanusont C et al: HIV-1 subtypes and male to female transmission in Thailand, Lancet 345: 1079-1083, 1995.

Laga M: Interactions between STDs and HIV infection, Transcript 28, Aug 1992.

Lennox J et al. Subclinical inflammation in the female genital tract is strongly associated with vaginal viral shedding independent of plasma viral load. Program and abstracts of the tenth Conference on Retroviruses and Opportunistic Infections, Boston, Massachusetts, abstract 101, 2003.

Mastro TD et al: Probability of female-to-male transmission of HIV-1 in Thailand, Lancet 343: 204-207, 1994.

Most J: Differences in heterosexual transmission of HIV-1 and HIV-2, Lancet 344: 1572-1573, 1994.

Mostad S: Shedding of HIV-1 in the genital tract, AIDS 10: 1305-1315, 1996.

Nelson KE et al. High rates of transmission of subtype E human immunodeficiency virus type 1 among heterosexual couples in Northern Thailand. Journal of Infectious Diseases 180: 337-343, 1999.

Padian N et al: Female to male transmission of Human Immunodeficiency Virus, JAMA 266(12): 664 -667, 1987.

Pomerantz RJ et al: Human immunodeficiency virus infection of the uterine cervix, Ann Int Med 108(3): 321-327, 1988.

Ponce de Leon, S et al: Gossypol suppresses p24 antigen in semen, Eighth International Conference on AIDS, PoC 4538, 1992.

Quinn CT et al. Viral load and heterosexual transmission of human immunodeficiency virus type 1. New England Journal of Medicine 342(12): 921-929, 2000.

Ramjee G et al. Herpes simplex virus type II infection is a risk factor for HIV seroconversion. South African MRC policy brief 3, August 2002.

Stallings RY. Female circumcision and HIV infection in Tanzania: for better or for worse? Third IAS Conference, Rio de Janeiro, abstract TuOa0401, 2005.

Vernazza PL et al: Detection and biologic characterization of infectious HIV-1 in semen of seropositive men, AIDS 8(9): 1325-1329, 1994.

Visscher B et al: Levels of immune cells in HIV-resistant men. Eighth International Conference On AIDS, abstract WeA 1048, 1992.

Wawer MJ et al. Control of sexually transmitted diseases for AIDS prevention in Uganda: a randomised community trial. The Lancet 353: 9152, 1999.

Male-to-female transmission

A number of large studies have now shown that a woman is usually at greater risk of HIV infection from vaginal intercourse with an HIV-positive man than vice versa. Several factors may explain this:

Ejaculation

The chances of infection occurring if ejaculation does not take place may be very low. The European Study Group on Heterosexual Transmission of HIV noted that after 20 months, none of the couples who had consistently practised withdrawal experienced the seroconversion of the HIV-negative partner. This suggests that the risk of infection from pre-ejaculate is small (De Vincenzi 1994).

Quantity of infectious fluid taken into the body

A woman may often take large quantities of semen into her vagina, which quickly comes into contact with the more vulnerable tissue of the cervix.

Presence of sexually transmitted infections

See *HIV transmission*

The acidity of the vagina

HIV may be vulnerable to a more acidic environment. 'Healthy' vaginal secretions are acidic, thus providing some protection against the virus. Vaginal secretions become more alkaline on contact with blood or semen, in the presence of vaginal infections, or during oral contraceptive use.

Damage to the vaginal wall and cervix

This may occur as a result of infections or abrasions, or erosion because of oral contraceptive use.

In summary, taking sperm/semen into the vagina appears to suppress local mucosal immune defences, making HIV infection more likely. Attention is now being focused on microbicides which boost the natural immune defences of the vaginal and cervical regions. These may provide protection in circumstances where condom use is either impossible or inconsistent.

References

De Vincenzi I et al: A longitudinal study of human immunodeficiency virus transmission by heterosexual partners, NEJM 331(6): 341-346, 1994.

Gresenguet G et al: HIV infection and vaginal douching in Central Africa, AIDS 11: 101-106, 1997.

Female-to-male transmission

The key determinants of whether HIV transmission is likely to occur from a woman to a man are:

Infectivity

Sex with a partner who has a high level of virus in their blood, either just after infection or as symptoms develop, significantly increases the risk of female-to-male infection.

Sexually transmitted infections

These increase the vulnerability of a man to HIV infection in two ways. They may increase the infectiousness of the female partner (see *Sexually transmitted infections* above), whilst an ulcer on the penis (such as those caused by syphilis or herpes) increases the vulnerability of the male partner.

Circumcision

Men who are uncircumcised appear to stand a greater chance of HIV infection than men who are circumcised. This may be due to the delicacy of the tissue of the foreskin, and the frequency with which it may be torn during intercourse, particularly when there is a lack of vaginal lubrication. It may also be to do with the fact that vaginal fluid containing HIV may be held under the foreskin after intercourse, increasing the period during which HIV infection may occur. For more see **C is also for Circumcision.**

References

European Study Group on Heterosexual Transmission of HIV: Comparison of female to male and male to female transmission of HIV in 563 stable couples, BMJ 304: 809-813, 1992.

Padian N et al: Female to male transmission of Human Immunodeficiency Virus, JAMA 266(12): 1664 -1667, 1987.

Vogt MW et al: Isolation patterns of the human immunodeficiency virus from cervical and vaginal secretions, AIM 106(3): 380-382, 1987.

Transmission through artificial insemination

A number of cases of HIV infection through donor insemination have been reported dating from prior to the introduction of the HIV antibody test. In one case the partner of an HIV-positive haemophiliac was infected by artificial insemination from her partner, despite the fact that the semen had been processed to reduce the chance of HIV infection (MMWR 1990).

The most detailed study of the risks involved in donor insemination comes from Los Angeles, where public health officials investigated a number of cases in which women with no known risks developed AIDS or tested HIV-positive. They found that some of these women had undergone artificial insemination prior to 1986, and traced back the semen to find out whether it had come from donors who subsequently developed AIDS. Seven women were identified as HIV-positive in the course of this investigation; all had received artificial insemination before 1986 (Araneta).

However, the study also found that the vast majority of women who received semen from HIV-positive donors did not seroconvert. In one case 29 out of 30 recipients of semen from one HIV-positive donor tested HIV-negative on follow-up, and it was calculated that the risk of infection per insemination exposure in this study was 0.50%.

'Sperm washing' is a method of reducing the risk of partner insemination from a known HIV-positive partner, pioneered by Augusto Semprini in Milan Italy, and also available at the Chelsea and Westminster hospital in London and some other European centres. As of 2001, 300 healthy children had been born after more than 3000 cycles of sperm washing and intrauterine insemination treatment or in vitro fertilisation, with no reported seroconversions in either partner or children.

For more on sperm washing, see *Women and HIV.*

References

Anderson DJ et al: Effects of disease stage and zidovudine therapy on the detection of human immunodeficiency virus type 1 in semen, JAMA 267: 2769-2774, 1992.

Araneta MRG et al: HIV transmission through donor artificial insemination, JAMA 273(11): 854-858, 1995.

Baeten J et al. Selenium deficiency is associated with shedding of HIV-1 infected cells in the female genital tract. XIII International AIDS Conference, Durban, abstract MoOrA226, 2000.

Bryson YJ et al: Clearance of HIV infection in a perinatally infected infant, NEJM 332(13): 833-838, 1995.

Cohen M. Reduction of concentration of HIV-1 in semen after treatment of urethritis: implications for prevention of sexual transmission of HIV-1. Lancet 349: 1868-1873, 1997.

Coombs RW et al. Does viral sub-type determine HIV-1 shedding in semen? Annual Meeting of the American Urological Association, abstract 1111, 1999.

Dax EM: Amyl nitrite alters in vitro human immune function, Immunopharm and Immunotox 13(4): 577-587, 1991.

De Vincenzi I et al: A longitudinal study of human immunodeficiency virus transmission by heterosexual partners, NEJM 331(6): 341-346, 1994.

European Study Group on Heterosexual Transmission of HIV: Comparison of female to male and male to female transmission of HIV in 563 stable couples, BMJ 304: 809-813, 1992.

European Study Group: Risk factors for male to female transmission of HIV, BMJ 298: 411-415, 1989.

Ghys A. HIV shedding, STD and immunosuppression. AIDS 11(12), F85-F93, 1997.

Gilling-Smith C. HIV and infertility: time to treat - Editorial. BMJ 322: 566-567, 2001.

Gray R et al. HIV incidence associated with male circumcision in a population-based cohort, and HIV acquisition/transmission associated with circumcision and viral load in discordant couples: Rakai, Uganda. XIII International AIDS Conference, Durban, abstract MoOrC193, 2000.

Gresenguet G et al: HIV infection and vaginal douching in Central Africa, AIDS 11: 101-106, 1997.

Grosskurth H et al: Impact of improved treatment of sexually transmitted diseases on HIV infection in rural Tanzania: randomised controlled trial, Lancet 436: 530-536, 1995.

Grosskurth H et al. Control of sexually transmitted diseases for HIV-1 prevention: understanding the implications of the Mwanza and Rakai trials. The Lancet 355: 1981-1987, 2000.

Hayes RJ et al: The cofactor effect of genital ulcers on the per-exposure risk of HIV transmission in sub-Saharan Africa, J Trop Med Hyg 98: 1-8, 1995.

Hitchcock P, Fransen L. Preventing HIV infection: lessons from Mwanza and Rakai. The Lancet 353: 9152, 1999.

Holmberg SD, Horsburgh CR: Biologic factors in the sexual transmission of human immunodeficiency virus, J Inf Dis 160(1): 116-125.

Ilaria G et al: Detection of HIV-1 DNA sequences in pre-ejaculatory fluid, Lancet 340(8833): 1469, 1992.

Johnson AM et al: Heterosexual transmission of HIV, AIDS(S1): 549-556, 1988.

Keet I et al: Orogenital sex and the transmission of HIV among homosexual men, AIDS 6(2): 223-226, 1992.

Kelly R et al. Age of male circumcision and risk of prevalent HIV infection in rural Uganda. AIDS 13: 399-405, 1999.

Kunanusont C et al: HIV-1 subtypes and male to female transmission in Thailand, Lancet 345: 1079-1083, 1995.

Laga M: Interactions between STDs and HIV infection, Transcript 28, Aug 1992.

Lavreys L et al. Effect of circumcision on incidence of human immundeficiency virus type 1 and other sexually transmitted diseases: a prospective cohort study of trucking company employees in Kenya. Journal of Infectious Diseases 180: 300-336, 1999.

Levy JA: Pathogenesis of Human Immunodeficiency Virus Infection, Microbiological Reviews: 183-289, March 1993.

MMWR: HIV-1 infection and artificial insemination with processed semen, MMWR 39 (15) 249: 255-256 1990.

Mastro TD et al: Probability of female-to-male transmission of HIV-1 in Thailand, Lancet 343: 204-207, 1994.

Moses S et al: Male circumcision and risk for HIV infection: A review of epidemiological studies conducted to date, Ninth International Conference on AIDS Po C11-2838 1993.

Most J: Differences in heterosexual transmission of HIV-1 and HIV-2, Lancet 344: 1572-1573, 1994.

Mostad S: Shedding of HIV-1 in the genital tract, AIDS 10: 1305-1315, 1996.

Nelson KE et al. High rates of transmission of subtype E human immunodeficiency virus type 1 among heterosexual couples in Northern Thailand. Journal of Infectious Diseases 180: 337-343, 1999.

O'Farrell N et al. Circumcision in men and the prevention of HIV infection: a meta analysis re-visited. Int J STD AIDS 11(3): 137-142, 2000.

Padian N et al: Female to male transmission of Human Immunodeficiency Virus, JAMA 266(12): 1664 -1667, 1987.

Pomerantz RJ et al: Human immunodeficiency virus infection of the uterine cervix, Ann Int Med 108(3): 321-327, 1988.

Ponce de Leon, S et al: Gossypol suppresses p24 antigen in semen, Eighth International Conference on AIDS, PoC 4538, 1992.

Quinn CT et al. Viral load and heterosexual transmission of human immunodeficiency virus type 1. New England Journal of Medicine 342 (12): 921-929, 2000.

Seage GR et al: The Relation between Nitrite Inhalants, Unprotected Receptive Anal Intercourse, and the Risk of Human Immunodeficiency Virus Infection, Am J of Epidem 135(1): 1-11, 1992.

Schechter MT et al: HIV-1 and the aetiology of AIDS, Lancet March 13: 658-659, 1993.

Schechter MT et al: HIV and the aetiology of AIDS (Letter), Lancet May 8: 1222-1224 1993 (See also letters from Ascher, Dalgleish in the same issue, and from P Duesburg in The Lancet April 8 and June 12 1993).

Van Druten HAM et al: Homosexual role separation and the spread of HIV. Eighth International Conference On AIDS, Amsterdam, abstract ThC 1518, 1992.

Vernazza PL et al: Detection and biologic characterization of infectious HIV-1 in semen of seropositive men, AIDS 8(9): 1325-1329, 1994.

Visscher B et al: Levels of immune cells in HIV-resistant men, Abstract WeA 1048 Eighth International Conference On AIDS 1992.

Vittinghoff E et al. Per-contact risk of human immunodeficiency virus transmission between male sexual partners. American Journal of Epidemiology 150: 306-311, 1999.

Vogt MW et al: Isolation patterns of the human immunodeficiency virus from cervical and vaginal secretions, AIM 106(3): 380-382, 1987.

Wawer MJ et al. Control of sexually transmitted diseases for AIDS prevention in Uganda: a randomised community trial. The Lancet 353: 9152, 1999.

Oral transmission

Summary

- The risk of getting HIV through oral sex is low, but not non-existent. Infection via *receptive* oral sex ('doing it') is biologically plausible and almost certainly happens occasionally. However the difficulty of gathering evidence means that scientists do not agree on the proportion of sexually-transmitted HIV infections that come from oral sex.

- The most plausible minimum and maximum figures are 0.1% (one infection per 1000 HIV infections) and 5% (one infection per 20).

- The UK's Health Protection Agency estimates that between 1% and 3% of HIV cases result from oral transmission of the virus.

- Infection is thought to be much less likely if ejaculation into the mouth does not happen; and some evidence suggests that mouth lesions may need to be present.

- There are a couple of case reports of HIV infection from a woman to a man via cunnilingus.

- Infection via *insertive* oral sex ('having it done to you') is probably exceedingly low risk and may be impossible.

- It is not possible to contract HIV infection through kissing.

The difficulty of getting proof

The risk of HIV transmission through the mouth is certainly smaller than through vaginal or anal intercourse or through sharing injecting equipment. No cases have been reported of HIV transmission through kissing. Very few cases of transmission through oral sex have been reported amongst gay men despite the continued practice of oral sex (often with ejaculation into the mouth) by large numbers of men participating in cohort studies over the past decade.

Although two cases have been reported in which transmission has been attributed to performing cunnilingus on an HIV-positive woman, significant doubts have been raised about the reliability of the evidence in these cases.

Most of the reports of oral transmission lack even the basic safeguards of cohort studies (see *The evidence for HIV transmission* earlier in this chapter). Anecdotal and self-reported evidence is largely presented in the form of letters to medical journals rather than peer review journal articles, and depends upon close questioning of individuals by doctors in order to follow through all possible avenues.

It is important to note that only a handful of reported cases of oral transmission come from cohort studies (in other words, people questioned about their sexual practices on a regular basis and tested for HIV antibodies) or from studies in which there has been a rigorous follow-up of patients.

Even the most reliable cohort studies report wildly different figures for the proportion of HIV caught through oral sex.

The lower limit: zero to 0.7%

A long-standing study (1990-2002) of heterosexual serodiscordant couples where the positive partner attends an HIV clinic in Madrid paid specific attention to oral sex. It found that out of 135 couples who reported oral sex, with 19,316 individual acts of exposure over 210 person-years of study, not one HIV seroconversion happened. This would set a lower limit of zero and an upper limit of 0.74% for the proportion of HIV infections due to oral sex - at least, that is, in heterosexuals.

The upper limit: 21 per cent

In Sweden, a three year study of men attending Stockholm's Gay Men's Health Clinic between 1990 and 1992 identified six men out of 28 seroconversions (21%) who are believed to have seroconverted as a consequence of oral transmission (Grutzmeier). There are several reasons to consider these findings more reliable than some other case reports:

- The serostatus of the individual's sexual partners and confirmatory accounts of the sexual acts which took place has been obtained for each case through the Swedish compulsory partner notification scheme.

- The serostatus of the presenting patient was matched to his previous test result, obtained through clinics in Stockholm. Almost all cases had tested negative within the previous year. Repeat testing by seronegative gay men is the norm in Sweden.

The Swedish researchers suggested that as the rate of new infections through anal intercourse decreases, very small numbers of cases of oral transmission will become more visible in cohort studies. However, it is important to be cautious about such an assumption, as a recent Dutch study shows.

The study found that five out of nine gay male seroconverters who had at first denied anal intercourse later reported that it had taken place in the twelve months prior to seroconversion (Keet). Of the 20 men who denied having had receptive anal intercourse in their questionnaire, 11 later contradicted this statement. Of the 82 men who did report having had receptive anal intercourse, only one later contradicted this statement. Researchers concluded that strong reasons may exist for 'forgetting' or failing to report anal intercourse. These might be:

- Shame at failure to practice safer sex.

- 'Forgetting' in order to blot out the memory of risky sexual activity.

- Desire to please researchers by demonstrating an adherence to safer sex guidelines.

- Refusal to acknowledge taboo sexual practices, i.e. anal intercourse.

- Believing that vaginal or anal sex with a condom is zero risk, when in fact condoms only reduce the risk of HIV transmission by 85 to 90%.

Nevertheless, the same study concludes that four out of 102 seroconverters in the cohort may have been infected through oral sex between 1985 and 1990.

Other studies

A study presented at the Seventh Retroviruses Conference in San Francisco in January 2000 postulated that 6.6% of new infections were due to oral sex. The study examined 122 infections identified in San Francisco between 1996 and 1999. Eight men had no other potential risk factors, and all said that they viewed oral sex as carrying little or no risk for HIV infection.

However, the finding of this study have been called into question as some of the men who had reported oral sex as their only risk activity subsequently reported unprotected anal intercourse.

However, the partner of one of the eight people corroborated that they had only had oral sex, and genetic sequencing confirmed that he was indeed the source partner. Unless both partners were lying, what can be said from this study is that it appears to indicate that something between one and eight per cent of sexual HIV infections might come from oral sex.

Analyses presented at the conference did not focus on the co-factors that may influence the risk of HIV transmission. It is known that around half of the seroconverters also had significant gum disease or ulcers and that ejaculation in the mouth occurred in six of the eight men thought to have been exposed to HIV through oral sex. The researchers concluded that oral sex may be an important mode of transmission due to the relative frequency with which it occurs.

In San Francisco (Page-Shafer 2002), 239 gay men seeking HIV testing between 1999 and 2001 who reported exclusively having oral sex were identified. None tested HIV-positive. Taking into account the number of partners and HIV-positive partners the men reported, the authors calculated that the maximum "population attributable risk" of getting HIV from one oral sex partner (i.e. the proportion of HIV infections that would be attributable to oral sex, per partner) was 0.1% of all infections. Page-Shafer's study is probably one of the more reliable ones as the subjects were asked about their sexual behaviour in advance of testing, and were therefore less likely to be trying to explain away a perceived lapse from safer sex.

However risk per-partner is not a very useful measure of risk, as most gay men and many heterosexuals have more than one oral sex partner. The per-contact risk is a better measure.

On 14 March, 2003, HIV InSite convened a panel of experts, including Kimberly Page-Shafer, who works at the University of California-San Francisco's Center for AIDS Prevention Studies, to try to come to some consensus on the risk of HIV transmission via oral sex (HIV InSite). By this time Page-Shafer's dataset from the same study had expanded to 363 HIV testees reporting oral sex only, and she had still not uncovered one seroconversion. This enabled her to calculate the upper bound of the per-contact risk as 0.04% - that is, HIV might be passed on in one in 2,500 acts of oral sex between serodiscordant people.

This might not sound like much - but you only need 100 different partners, or 100 contacts with one HIV-positive partner, for that risk to become one in 25, which is not negligible.

A risk of one in 2,500 exposures is approximately 20 times lower than the estimated risk for receptive anal sex, but is only half the risk estimated for receptive vaginal sex with a partner during chronic infection. However it is the upper bound of a mathematical model calculation - in other words, using only the evidence from the Page-Shafer study, the risk could be anywhere between zero and one in 2500 per exposure.

In contrast, for instance, a Spanish study (Castilla) of monogamous heterosexual couples from the same cohort as the del Romero study above found a general seroconversion rate via vaginal and anal intercourse, from man to woman and vice versa, of only 0.049% or one transmission in 2040 exposures. However this was the documented seroconversion rate in a closely-followed cohort and therefore likely to be a median rather than a maximum.

The HIV InSite panel ultimately could not come to a consensus on the proportion of infections due to oral sex. While Kimberly Page-Shafer suggested from one in 100 to one in 1,000, Susan Buchbinder of the San Francisco Department of Public Health thought one in 100 a minimum figure, with a maximum of one in 20 (5%). Ultimately it appears to come down to whether researchers believe people are telling the truth when they say that oral sex has been their only risk factor.

When is oral sex risky?

Much speculation about the risks of oral sex has concentrated on the likelihood of infection through cuts in the mouth, but it is equally plausible to argue that the key factor in determining infection through oral sex is viral load in semen or vaginal fluids. The quantity of infectious fluid which enters the mouth may also play a role. If this is the case, it would suggest that fellatio is more risky than cunnilingus.

American epidemiologist James Koopman has calculated that the probability of HIV transmission through oral sex during the early weeks of infection is considerably greater than at later stages in HIV infection. He based his calculations on the assumption of much higher viral load in semen during this period (see *The mechanisms of HIV transmission* for discussion of the evidence).

Koopman also argues that virtually all cases of HIV infection can be attributed to transmission during primary infection.

Koopman's statistical analysis does not allow for an increase in infectivity later in infection, and is also subject to potential bias because of the small size of the sample of seroconverters he used to calculate the probabilities of infection by different routes.

Nevertheless, the continuing low level of HIV infection through oral sex may be attributable entirely to infections acquired during primary infection or during symptomatic HIV disease. If this is the case, it raises a number of issues:

- HIV-positive people who have low CD4 counts and potentially high viral load should be aware that they can infect their partners if they ejaculate in their mouth during oral sex

- As greater numbers of people become symptomatic, the likelihood rises that infections will occur by this route

- The changing risk and reality needs to be acknowledged whilst still highlighting the relatively low risk attached to oral sex. Even if oral sex is risky during primary and symptomatic HIV disease, the remarkably low level of infections attributable to oral sex suggest that the risk remains small.

Lack of evidence of mouth to genitals transmission

Although it is well known that other sexually transmitted diseases, especially herpes, can be passed from the mouth to the penis, vagina or anus, no reliable report exists of a case where HIV was transmitted from the mouth to the genitals, except for a widely criticised French report describing two men who claimed to have no other risk factors for HIV infection apart from having been insertive in oral sex i.e. receiving a blow job (Rozenbaum).

There are a number of methodological problems with this report. First of all, the authors claim it to be part of a cohort study which was regularly monitored, yet data on this cohort has never subsequently been published in a peer-reviewed journal to allow independent validation of the methodology. The authors estimated that the chance of failure to recall or deception of the interviewers regarding sexual practices on the part of the five individuals reported to have been infected was minimal. The authors state:

We assessed the likelihood of these patients denying anal sex for psychological reasons, and concluded that it was unlikely: three patients had freely described participating in anal sex previously... .

There is, in other words, no evidence that the methodology was sufficiently adapted to account for lack of patient recall, or for a shame factor that could easily prevent someone confessing to unsafe sex. The fact that someone could happily admit to having unsafe sex before joining a safer sex study by no means precludes this kind of guilt at having unsafe sex after joining such a study.

One case of oral transmission has been reported in which a man who was impotent owing to diabetic illness claimed to have been infected after performing cunnilingus on a prostitute. It was subsequently established that the woman was HIV-negative, and that the man had in fact been infected through needle-sharing.

How oral transmission could happen

Although oral sex seems to be less risky than anal or vaginal intercourse, there are some factors which may increase the chance of HIV infection. These are:

- Taking semen into the mouth - all the credible reports of oral transmission (except for one) note that ejaculation did occur into the mouth of the individual reported to have been infected

- Bleeding gums, cuts or sores in the mouth

- Inflammation caused by common throat infections, allergies or sexually transmitted diseases such as gonorrhoea.

- The presence of genital piercings or lesions. A study in Sydney (Richters) judged that five gay male seroconverters out of 75 who were interviewed about their sexual behaviour had had oral sex as their only risk factor. Three of the men had had oral sex with men who had a genital piercing. The investigators commented that the possible transmission risk from genital piercings should be investigated.

Questions about oral transmission

Is oral sex safer than other forms of unprotected penetrative sex?

The evidence suggests that oral sex is less risky than unprotected anal intercourse. Oral sex is a common practice in both homosexual and heterosexual relationships. Although unprotected oral sex may be a less efficient means of transmitting HIV than unprotected anal or vaginal sex, the frequency of its occurrence may serve to increase its relative contribution to overall HIV transmission.

A case-control study nested within a large international cohort study of HIV-positive gay men has shown that having multiple partners for receptive oral sex increases the risk of seroconversion by one per cent (Page-Schafer).

Is HIV always present in semen?

Viral load testing suggests that traces of HIV can almost always be found in semen. Even if HIV is undetectable in blood it may still be present in high levels in semen. Viral load in blood may not be a good guide to the infectious potential of semen. See *Infectivity*, for further discussion of this issue. However, several studies have shown a trend towards higher levels of HIV in semen when plasma viral load is also high, and HIV can be isolated much more easily from the semen of individuals who have CD4 counts below 200.

Antiretroviral treatment has been shown to reduce HIV levels in semen in several small studies, but one study found detectable HIV in semen even after virus levels in blood became undetectable. This suggests that virus production in the genital tract may occur independently of virus production in the bloodstream and most other body tissues. This is because scientists describe the genital tract, and the testes, as an immunologically privileged site, where special immune processes take place.

Nevertheless, HIV levels are likely to be highest in the semen of individuals with CD4 counts below 200 not currently receiving antiretroviral therapy.

Is HIV always present in vaginal fluids?

Viral load testing suggests that HIV cannot be found in vaginal fluid with the same frequency as it has been detected in semen.

HIV levels tend to be highest around the time of menstruation, or if a genitourinary infection or candida are present.

HIV can be isolated more easily from the vaginal fluids of women with CD4 counts below 200.

Antiretroviral therapy has been shown to decrease levels of HIV in vaginal fluid 10-50 fold when two drugs are used in combination.

Is HIV absorbed through the undamaged tissue of the mouth? What about cuts, sores or damaged gums?

The mucous membrane of the mouth contains few cells which are vulnerable to HIV infection. In contrast, cells which are vulnerable to HIV infection (possessing receptors which enable HIV to bind onto them) are common in the walls of the vagina and the rectum (Lehner).

Furthermore, little is absorbed through the tissue of the mouth even if it is damaged. The mouth is an entry point into the digestive system where enzymes in saliva are secreted to begin the task of digesting food. It is very thick compared with the mucous membrane in the rectum, and fluids stay in contact with it for a very short time because swallowing clears the mouth regularly. Thus the likelihood of semen, blood or vaginal fluid coming into contact with cells such as dendritic or Langerhans cells (also identified as receptors for HIV) in damaged tissue is small. Nevertheless, two cases have been reported where bleeding gums or receding gums are speculated to have been the route of infection (Lifson).

Is HIV absorbed through the tissue of the throat?

The tissue of the throat (the oesophagus) is similar to that of the mouth - thick and fairly unabsorbent. As in the mouth, continuous swallowing or peristalsis ensures that anything ingested will be in contact with damaged tissue for only a short time. However, several cases have been reported where researchers speculate that HIV infection may have occurred as a result of inflammation of the throat, caused either by infections or allergies (Chen, Murray).

It is possible that HIV could come into contact with the immune system cells of the tonsils if semen or vaginal fluid come into contact with them, particularly if the tonsils are swollen or inflamed.

Even where there is an apparently normal mouth, it would be unwise to assume that HIV could not be transmitted through oral sex. Research has shown that the tonsils of rhesus monkeys act as an entry point for SIV (Stahl-Hennig). However infecting the monkeys via this route involved swabbing tranquillised monkeys' tonsils directly with monkey-adapted HIV after they had been given a mouth-drying agent. This is likely to have greatly increased the chances of infection compared with the normal oral environment.

Is HIV destroyed in the stomach?

There is no evidence to prove or disprove this. Researchers assume that as with other viral infections, HIV will be inactivated by the digestive enzymes and by changes in pH (acidity/alkalinity balance). It is not possible to say whether semen which enters the stomach may enter the bloodstream through stomach ulcers or other inflamed tissue, but it seems highly unlikely that HIV will have survived the process of neutralisation in saliva by the time it reaches the stomach.

Does saliva kill HIV?

There is strong evidence to suggest that an enzyme in saliva called secretory leukocyte protease inhibitor (SLPI) prevents HIV infection of lymphocytes, and therefore inhibits HIV infection in the mouth and throat. A 1989 study showed that even when greatly diluted, saliva was still capable of preventing HIV infection of white blood cells. It is still unclear how this happens and what agent inhibits infection (Fox).

The experiments showed that saliva taken from all 34 participants, nine of whom were seropositive, exhibited inhibitory effects (that is, it prevented infection); in 29 cases (85%) a complete inhibitory effect was observed. Inhibition is measured by incubating saliva with an equal quantity of HIV concentrate and then attempting to culture HIV over 18 days. If HIV cannot reproduce itself a 100% inhibitory effect can be reported. There was little correlation between health status, age or gender in the inhibitory effect of saliva (Fox). Previous experiments had shown that complete inhibition does not take place immediately, but this was more to do with the quantity of the virus than the infectivity of the saliva. Concentrations of HIV much higher than those occurring in blood were used.

Some researchers have also cited the presence of HIV antibodies in saliva as evidence of further protection, but since there is considerable ambiguity over the neutralising effect of HIV antibodies it is not possible to say that this is significant (Fultz).

Is HIV present in saliva?

One experiment took more than two months to culture HIV from the saliva of HIV-positive people, and in the four samples in which the virus was detected, the level was extremely low - one infectious particle per ml. This measure should be treated with caution but nevertheless suggests that saliva contains very low levels of infectious HIV (Piazza).

However, another study by the same research team found high levels of HIV in the saliva of several patients with AIDS when they used a more sensitive HIV PCR viral load test. Indeed, in several cases they found higher levels of HIV in saliva than in semen.

These findings should be treated with caution because the researchers tested only one sample from each patient, and the study was conducted in 1994, when PCR viral load testing was still at an experimental stage. The researchers reported that when they re-tested five patients two months later they found large differences in viral load from the previous study. This may be a consequence of changes in levels of virus production, or it may be due to variations which are a feature of the testing technology (Piazza 1995).

A more recent study found that infectious HIV can be detected at high levels in saliva during the early weeks of HIV infection (the 'window' period before antibodies appear), but levels fall rapidly after this point.

Free floating infectious viruses and virus-infected lymphocytes could be detected in saliva taken from individuals with primary HIV infection attending clinics in North Carolina. In 7 out of 8 cases, free floating infectious virus could be detected at an average level of 2,000 copies per ml, and in 5 out of 8 cases cell associated virus could be detected at an average level of 20,000 copies per ml.

The researchers said that virus levels in blood and semen were much higher, and it is not clear how much of a transmission risk the virus levels in saliva might pose, given that studies of transmission through vaginal intercourse have shown that transmission did not occur in serodiscordant couples when the infected partner had a viral load below 1500 copies . However, some individuals in this study had virus levels as high as 500,000 copies in saliva, suggesting that during the early weeks of infection some individuals may be 'super-excretors' of HIV, and may play a significant role in the ongoing amplification of the HIV epidemic (Pilcher).

Another point to bear in mind is that viral load of 500,000 copies is associated with a high risk of severe seroconversion illness. A person experiencing such a severe flu-like illness is unlikely to be interested in engaging in any form of sexual activity whilst so unwell.

What about blood in saliva?

An Italian study showed that while very small quantities of blood may be released into the saliva by kissing or eating, large quantities of blood can be released into saliva after brushing the teeth; at least ten times as much as after kissing or eating. Whether the HIV contained in blood would be diluted and inactivated by saliva is unclear (Piazza).

Is it safer to spit out or swallow semen or vaginal fluid?

It probably makes little difference, although it is often suggested that while swallowing semen or vaginal fluid keeps it away from any damaged tissue in the mouth, such as bleeding gums, swallowing also makes it possible for contact with any damaged or inflamed tissue in the throat to occur.

Is oral sex with a male partner safer if ejaculation does not occur in the mouth?

The evidence of all the case reports to date suggests that this is likely. Only two cases have been reported where ejaculation into the mouth did not occur.

What is the risk of infection from precum? Is there a lower concentration of HIV in this fluid?

Research suggests that high concentrations of HIV can sometimes be detected in pre-cum. Several studies show that HIV can be isolated from seminal fluid, and that in the event of male genital tract inflammation, much higher levels of the cells commonly infected with HIV (CD4 lymphocytes and macrophages) are likely to be present in semen (Borzy; Ilaria). The stage of disease does not seem to make a great difference to the level of HIV in pre-cum. Ilaria noted HIV in semen of some men with AIDS he studied, but not others, and found the same unpredictable distribution of HIV in pre-cum amongst asymptomatic men.

Despite this evidence, it is very difficult to judge whether pre-cum is likely to contain a sufficient quantity of HIV for infection to occur. Remember that contact with HIV alone is not sufficient to guarantee infection. The conditions for infection are discussed in *The mechanisms of HIV transmission*.

Is oral sex more risky with a partner who has AIDS?

Whatever risk is attached to oral sex is probably increased if the person who ejaculates into the mouth of his partner has a CD4 count below 100 and/or is symptomatic. The likelihood that someone with a low CD4 count has HIV in his semen increases as the CD4 count falls below 200; in one study 87% of those men with CD4 counts below 100 had HIV in their semen, compared with none who had CD4 counts above 500 (Vernazza).

What is the risk of infection from oralanal contact (rimming)?

It is possible that the presence of blood in the rectum (for instance as a result of fingering, fisting, having intercourse with or use of sex toys) may present a risk of infection for the person doing the rimming. Faeces may contain traces of blood containing HIV, and HIV infection of parasites found in faeces has been demonstrated in the laboratory. It is also possible that blood may be introduced into the rectum by the tongue, from bleeding gums. One case has been reported where a man rimming another man may have infected his partner by this route. The man who was infected was rimmed by an HIV - infected partner who is speculated to have had gum disease (Gill).

What are the risks of kissing?

There are no reported cases of HIV transmission through kissing, either social kissing or deep passionate kissing. Admittedly it might be difficult to separate out possible cases of transmission as a result of kissing, because it is rarely separate from other sexual activities. See *HIV in saliva* above for more detailed discussion of this issue, including reasons why transmission through kissing is unlikely.

How soon is it safe to have oral sex after brushing my teeth?

Brushing the teeth and gums often causes mild abrasions, and stimulates bleeding where gingivitis is present. Although a recent report by the Department of Health's Expert Advisory Group On AIDS suggested that such bleeding will probably stop within ten minutes, vigorous fellatio can easily stimulate bleeding in the unhealthy mouth. The best long-term precaution is to pay close attention to gum hygiene and change your toothbrush regularly. In the short term, if your gums normally bleed a lot when you brush your teeth, this means that you are at greater risk of infection if semen containing HIV gets into your mouth. If you are HIV-positive, it also means that you could pass on HIV to partners if you are sucking.

What risk is posed by mouth ulcers?

Mouth ulcers allow food particles and bacteria into the bloodstream, so they will let HIV in too. Mouth ulcers are most common in those under 30, and oral sex should be avoided if you have an ulcer or other cuts or lesions in your mouth.

Can HIV be passed from the mouth to the genitals?

There are no reliable reports in the scientific literature. An American report of a case in which a woman was alleged to have transmitted HIV through performing oral sex on a man with no other apparent risk factors was later shown to have been false. The man did have other risk factors which he didn't reveal to researchers in an initial interview. Similarly, doubts have been raised about the French report of two men infected through receiving oral sex (Rozenbaum).

Nevertheless, if a large amount of blood is present in saliva, there may be some risk.

Is HIV present in urine?

No. Although antibodies to HIV can be detected in urine, infectious HIV has never been isolated from urine (Skolnik). No cases of HIV transmission have ever been reported through taking urine into the mouth, or onto broken skin.

What role for the pharynx?

Whilst debate continues about exactly how risky oral sex really is, researchers from the University of Washington in Seattle and the Imapcta Salud y Educacion, Lima, Peru have successfully cultured infectious HIV from pharyngeal swabs from four men with high pharyngeal HIV RNA.

HIV-1 RNA can be detected in saliva, yet culture of HIV-1 from saliva is only successful in less than 1% of samples due to the inactivation of the virus by saliva. Tonsillar biopsy specimens have previously been shown to harbour both HIV-1 RNA and DNA. The researchers set about describing the predictors and variability of HIV-1 RNA in the pharynx and attempted to cultivate HIV-1 from oropharyngeal surfaces.

In total 64 HIV-positive men without bacterial STIs from Seattle, USA and Lima, Peru were evaluated prospectively at week 0, 2 and 4 to assess viral load in plasma and in swab specimens obtained from the pharynx. A subset of 17 men with high pharyngeal viral load were evaluated one year later for the recovery of infectious virus from blood, tonsil and buccal surfaces.

The median CD4 count of the 64 participants was 290 cells/ml and 45% were currently receiving antiretrovirals. The median baseline viral load was similar in plasma (4.24 log) and the pharynx (4.22 log). Each one log increase in plasma viral load was associated with a 0.323 log increase in pharyngeal viral load whilst both antiretroviral therapy and tonsillectomy were associated with reductions in pharyngeal viral load. There was a statistically significant study site effect between Seattle and Lima with respect to age, treatment, viral load and tonsillectomy; men were older in Seattle (median 39 vs 27 years), 24% in Seattle were using antiretroviral therapy compared with 5% in Lima, median viral in Seattle was 3.12 log compared to 4.75 log in Lima, and 42% of the men in Seattle had a tonsillectomy compared with 13% in Lima.

Infectious HIV was cultured from the pharynx of 4 of the subset of 17 men with high pharyngeal viral load but was not isolated from the buccal mucosa (the inside of the mouth) or the saliva of any of the men. The observation that the oropharynx appears to harbour higher levels of HIV than the buccal mucosa is likely due to the proximity of lymphoid tissue in the posterior oropharynx. Three of the four men were not using antiretroviral therapy and the other was taking dual nucleoside therapy which was not fully suppressive.

Median mucosal RNA was 5.85 log in the culture positive men versus 4.69 log in culture negative men.

Both tonsillectomy and use of antiretroviral therapy were associated with a reduction in pharyngeal viral load. Pharyngeal HIV shedding was higher among persons with tonsils and detectable viral load.

Whilst the detection of culturable HIV RNA in the posterior pharynx may indicate the potential for the oral transmission of HIV further behavioural data are needed if we are to understand the role sex acts such as "deep throating" may play in the oral transmission of HIV.

What role do the cells lining the mouth play?

When exposed to high levels of human immunodeficiency virus (HIV), the cells from the lining of the mouth can develop a low-level infection, according to research from Charles R. Drew University and the University of California, Los Angeles published in the March 2003 issue of the *Journal of Virology*.

In the study, the researchers tested the ability of HIV to infect oral mucosal cells known as normal human oral keratinocytes (NHOK) in the test tube. They found that when exposed to high concentrations of the virus, the cells established a low-level, productive infection that could subsequently transfer to activated lymphocytes.

"Human saliva contains several types of anti-HIV activity that may help protect an individual against a small virus inoculum. However, if individuals are exposed to inocula containing a heavy viral load, it is conceivable that the oral epithelium could be infected and thus serve as a beachhead for HIV-1 infection," say the researchers.

References

Borzy MS et al: Detection of human immunodeficiency virus in cell-free seminal fluid, JAIDS 1(5): 419-424, 1988.

Celum C et al. Recovery of infectious human immunodeficiency virus type-1 from the oropharynx: implications for oral transmission of HIV-1. Ninth Conference on Retroviruses, Seattle, abstract 379-M, 2002.

Castilla J. HIV transmission in a cohort of serodiscordant heterosexual couples. 14th International AIDS Conference, Barcelona, abstract no ThPeC7409, 2002.

Chen W. & Samarasinghe PL: Allergy, oral sex, and HIV (Letters), Lancet 339(8793): 627-628, 1992.

Del Romero, J et al. Evaluating the risk of HIV transmission through unprotected orogenital sex. AIDS 16(9): 1296-1297, 2002.

Department of Health. Review of the evidence on the risk of HIV transmission associated with oral sex, report of a working group of the UK chief medical officers' expert advisory group on AIDS, 12 June 2000.

Dillon B et al: Primary HIV Infections associated with oral transmission.   Seventh Conference on Retroviruses and Opportunistic Infections, San Francisco, abstract 473, 2000.

Fox PC et al: Saliva inhibits HIV infectivity, Journal of the American Dental Association 116: 635-637, 1988.

Fultz P N: Components of saliva inactivate human immunodeficiency virus, Lancet ii: 1215, 1986.

Gill SK et al: Transmission of HIV-1 infection by oroanal intercourse, Genitourinary Medicine 68: 254-257, 1992.

Grutzmeier S: HIV transmission in gay men in Stockholm, 1990-1992. IX International Conference on AIDS Po C02-2584.

HIV InSite. Risk of HIV Infection Through Receptive Oral Sex. Round table discussion, 14 March 2003. See http://hivinsite.ucsf.edu/InSite?page=pr-rr-05

Ilaria G et al: Detection of HIV-1 DNA sequences in pre-ejaculatory fluid, Lancet 340: 1469, 1992.

Koopman J et al: HIV transmission possibilities for oral and anal sex by stage of infection. Ninth International AIDS Conf, abstract PoC 4101, 1993.

Lehner T et al: Mucosal transmission of HIV, Nature 353: 709, 1991.

Lifson A et al: HIV seroconversion in two homosexual men after receptive oral intercourse with ejaculation: implication for counselling concerning safe sexual practices, AJPH 80(12): 1509 - 1511, 1990.

Liu X, et al. Human immunodefiency virus type 1 infection and replication in normal human oral keratinocytes. Journal of Virology, 77: 3470-3476, 2003.

Murray AB et al: Coincident acquisition of Neisseria gonorrhoeae and HIV from fellatio (Letters), Lancet 338: 830, 1991.

Page-Schafer K et al. Sexual risk and risk factors for HIV-1 seroconversion in homosexual men participating in the tricontinental seroconverter study 1982-1994, American Journal of Epidemiology 146: 531-542, 1997.

Page-Shafer K et al. Risk of HIV infection attributable to oral sex among men who have sex with men and in the population of men who have sex with men. AIDS 16(17): 2350-2352. 2002.

Piazza et al: Passionate kissing and microlesions of the oral mucosa: possible role in AIDS transmission JAMA: 244-245, 1989.

Piazza M et al: Quantitation of HIV-1 genome copy number in semen and saliva, AIDS 9(6): 651-653, 1995.

Pilcher C et al. In subjects with primary HV infection, high levels of HIV RNA are present in oral fluids, genital secretions, peripheral blood and CNS and are rapidly reduced with combination antiretroviral therapy. Seventh Conference on Retroviruses, San Francisco, abstract 556, 2000.

Pudney J et al: Pre-ejaculatory fluid as potential vector for sexual transmission of HIV-1, Lancet 340: 1470, 1991.

Richters J et al. HIV transmission among gay men through oral sex and other uncommon routes: case series of HIV seroconverters, Sydney. AIDS 17(15): 2269-2271, 2003.

Rozenbaum W, Gharakanian S, Cardon B et al: HIV transmission by oral sex, Lancet: 1395, 1988.

Skolnik P et al: Absence of infectious HIV-1 in the urine of seropositive individuals J Inf Dis 160(6): 1056-1060, 1989.

Stahl-Hennig C et al. The tonsil as a portal of entry for simian immunodeficiency virus (SIV). 15th Annual Symposium for non-human primate models for AIDS, Seattle, Washington, abstract 17, September 1997.

Circumcision

How does circumcision reduce the risk of HIV infection?

There is now a compelling body of epidemiological evidence, including results from three randomised controlled trials, which shows that male circumcision provides significant protection against HIV infection.

For more on this see **C is also for circumcision.** But briefly the 'per-protocol' reduction in the likelihood of HIV infection seen amongst circumcised as opposed to uncircumcised men in the three trials was as follows:

Orange Farm, South Africa (Auvert): 65%

Kisumu, Kenya: 53%

Rakai, Uganda (Gray, Wawer): 48%

The first ever randomised controlled trial (RCT) of male circumcision as an HIV prevention measure, presented at the 3rd IAS Conference in 2005, produced strong evidence of a protective effect (Auvert). There were only 35% as many infections in the circumcision arm as opposed to the control arm, implying that circumcision can prevent at least six out of ten female-to-male HIV transmissions, and possibly up to three-quarters of transmissions.

Previous cohort studies have shown that circumcised males are two to eight times less likely to become infected with HIV. Furthermore, circumcision also protects against other sexually transmitted infections, such as syphilis and gonorrhoea, and since people who have a sexually transmitted infection are two to five times more likely to become infected with HIV, circumcision may be even more protective.

It is worth remembering that the majority of men who are HIV-positive have been infected through the penis. Cells, called Langerhans cells, which line the inner surface of the foreskin. These cells have HIV receptors and are likely to be the primary point of viral entry into the penis of an uncircumcised man.

A 2002 report by the US Agency for International Development (USAID) was based on a systematic review of 28 scientific studies published by the London School of Hygiene and Tropical Medicine. *The Washington Times* reported that "a sub analysis of ten African studies found a 71% reduction among higher risk men". Edward G. Green, a senior researcher at Harvard University told the Washington Times that if all males in Africa were circumcised, the HIV/AIDS prevalence rate could be reduced from 20% in some regions to below 5%.

In one study of couples in Uganda where the woman was HIV-positive and her male partner was not, no new infections occurred among any of the 50 circumcised men over 30 months, whereas 40 of 137 uncircumcised men became infected during this time. Both groups had been given free access to HIV testing, intensive instruction about preventing infection, and free condoms (which were continuously available), but 89% of the men never used condoms, and condom use did not seem to influence the rate of transmission of HIV.

References

Auvert B et al. Impact of male circumcision on the female-to-male transmission of HIV. IAS Conference on HIV Pathogenesis and treatment, Rio de Janeiro, abstract TuOa0402, 2005

Gray R et al. Randomized trial of male circumcision for HIV prevention in Rakai, Uganda. Fourteenth Conference on Retroviruses and Opportunistic Infection, Los Angeles, abstract 155aLB, 2007. *Wawer M et al.* Effects of male circumcision on genital ulcer disease and urethral symptoms, and on HIV acquisition: an RCT in Rakai, Uganda. Fourteenth Conference on Retroviruses and Opportunistic Infections, Los Angeles, abstract 155bLB, 2007.

How sexually acquired HIV occurs

Most cases of primary HIV infection are thought to involve HIV binding initially to the CD4 and CCR5 receptors found on antigen presenting cells which include macrophages, Langerhans' cells, and dendritic cells in the genital and rectal mucosa.

The most widely accepted model for the sexual transmission of HIV is based on infection of the genital tract of rhesus macaques with simian immunodeficiency virus. After female macaques are inoculated intravaginally with simian immunodeficiency virus, the virus targets the Langerhans' cells located in the vaginal mucosa. Once infected, these cells fuse with adjacent CD4 lymphocytes and migrate to deeper tissues. Within two days of infection, the virus can be detected in the internal iliac lymph nodes and shortly thereafter in systemic lymph nodes. This ultimately leads to a fatal infection.

Infection in male macaques occurs when the penile urethra or foreskin is inoculated with simian immunodeficiency virus; the same sequence of cellular events involving the infection of Langerhans' cells is then likely to occur. Infected Langerhans' cells have also been detected in the penile mucosa of male rhesus macaques that have chronic simian immunodeficiency virus infection. In humans, histological studies have identified antigen-presenting cells in the mucosa of the inner foreskin and urethra. Therefore it seems likely that antigen-presenting cells at these mucosal sites are the primary target for HIV in men.

Test tube studies have shown that the CD4 receptor is generally necessary, although insufficient on its own, to permit HIV-1 to enter host cells. The entry of HIV-1 into cells requires an additional chemokine receptor, usually CCR5, although CXCR4 is used by cells that become infected during the later stages of the disease.

After primary infection occurs, the virus mutates, which allows it to utilise other chemokine receptors, such as CXCR4, and thus spread to a variety of cell types.

How does HIV enter the penis?

Through unprotected vaginal sex; a much smaller proportion have acquired HIV through unprotected anal sex. So it is fair to say that the majority of men globally who have acquired HIV have done so through the penis.

An uncircumcised penis consists of the penile shaft, glans, urethral meatus, inner and outer surface of the foreskin, and the fraenulum, the thin band connecting the inner foreskin to the ventral aspect of the glans. A keratinised, stratified squamous epithelium covers the penile shaft and outer surface of the foreskin. This provides a protective barrier against HIV infection. In contrast, the inner mucosal surface of the foreskin is not keratinised and is rich in Langerhans' cells, making it particularly susceptible to HIV.

There is debate over whether the epithelium of the glans in men who are not circumcised is keratinised; some authors claim that it is not, but examination of the glans of seven circumcised and six uncircumcised men, and found the epithelia to be equally keratinised. In circumcised males only the distal penile urethra is lined with a mucosal epithelium. However, this is unlikely to be a common site of infection because it contains comparatively few Langerhans' cells.

It is well documented that ulcerative or inflammatory lesions of the penile urethra, foreskin, fraenulum, or glans that are caused by other sexually transmitted infections may provide additional potential routes for HIV transmission.

What effect could circumcision have on the global HIV epidemic?

Essentially, condoms need to remain the first choice for HIV prevention, but acknowledging the many barriers to effective condom use; failure to use consistently or correctly, breaking during use as well as cultural or aesthetic objections to their use.

There are deeply held cultural and religious attitudes towards circumcision which cannot be ignored. However, in view of the growing body of evidence as to the protective effect of circumcision, circumcising men appears to be highly desirable, particularly in countries that have high background HIV prevalence rates.

A programme of neonatal circumcision would take 15-20 years to have any effect on HIV transmission rate - since it would, on average, take this length of time for those men to become sexually active. Circumcising pubescent boys and young adults would have a more immediate effect since it would be done before the young men become sexually active.

The WHO issued a strategy document on the rollout of circumcision programmes globally in response to the news from the African randomised controlled trials in March 2007. See **C is also for Circumcision** for details. The report may be downloaded from www.who.int/hiv/topics/malecircumcision/en/index.html

Women, gay men, circumcision and HIV transmission

The overwhelming majority of literature which suggests circumcision is protective against HIV infection has been carried out in heterosexual men, and predominantly in resource-limited settings. A cross-sectional study found that uncircumcised gay American men were more likely to have prevalent HIV infection, but it was not known whether they had been infected by insertive or receptive intercourse.

There is also at present conflicting evidence as to whether circumcising HIV-positive men has a protective effect on them passing on HIV to female partners and, by extension, receptive gay male partners.

A companion study of the Rakai circumcision trial continues at the time of writing. This randomised controlled trial will enrol approximately 800 HIV-positive men and will also study 1000 men from the original Rakai circumcision trial who declined to know their HIV test results when they were originally screened for this trial (and who were therefore ineligible for it). The hypotheses are that male circumcision will be acceptable to and safe in both groups and will reduce the rates of STI acquisition in both groups and of HIV acquisition in HIV-negative men. The study is also enrolling and following up to approximately 5,000 female partners of the men enrolled in this study

There is limited evidence that circumcision may have a role in protecting the female partner. A 2000 study from Rakai (Quinn) showed an overall protective effect of 26% to the female partner of HIV-positive circumcised, compared with uncircumcised, men. This was statistically significant (p=<0.05).

But this depended on the man's viral load. If men had viral loads of over 50,000 copies/ml, circumcision had no protective effect for women. But among men with viral loads under 50,000 copies/ml, there were zero transmissions from circumcised men, compared with 26 transmissions from uncircumcised men, and this was highly statistically significant. Circumcision also appeared to protect women from acquiring bacterial vaginosis and trichonomiasis, but not from other STIs.

One study has explored the relationship between circumcision and HIV transmission in gay men in Sydney, Australia. Between 1993 and 1999 a total of 74 gay men were interviewed soon after being diagnosed with recent infection. The men were asked to nominate a unprotected sexual encounter with a serodiscordant or HIV status unknown partner at which they believed they became infected with HIV. When there was more than one possible high-risk event, the researcher chose the most likely occasion. Participants were also asked to report all episodes of unprotected anal intercourse in the six months before their seroconversion.

The researchers hypothesised that if the presence of a foreskin was important in HIV transmission, those men who had been infected by insertive unprotected anal intercourse would be more likely to be uncircumcised than those infected by receptive unprotected anal intercourse.

Sixty-three of the men nominated an event as their highest possible risk activity. For 11 men this was insertive unprotected anal intercourse, for 52 it was unprotected receptive intercourse. All but one of the 11 men who reported unprotected receptive intercourse as the most likely source of HIV infection reported no receptive unprotected anal intercourse in the six months before seroconversion and one reported receptive unprotected anal intercourse with a regular partner who was definitely HIV-negative.

In total 20 of the men (27%) were circumcised. There was no association between circumcision and reporting insertive unprotected anal intercourse as the highest risk practice. Of the additional eleven men who denied unprotected anal intercourse as the event which they believed had led to their HIV infection, eight also denied having had unprotected anal intercourse in the previous six months. Of these eight, three were circumcised (38%).

The researchers found that 17% of gay men with newly acquired HIV infection reported insertive unprotected anal intercourse as their highest risk sexual activity. This suggest insertive unprotected anal intercourse is an important means of HIV transmission in this population.

The researchers found no association between circumcision status and infection by insertive unprotected anal intercourse. Additionally, men who had seroconverted despite no reported event of unprotected anal intercourse were also more likely to be uncircumcised. The researchers suggested that this would imply that the foreskin is not the main source of HIV infection in gay men who become infected by insertive UAI, and that other sites such as the distal urethra, must be important in HIV acquisition.

This study is limited by its small sample and it is possible that some men who reported receptive unprotected anal intercourse as their highest risk behaviour may have been infected by insertive unprotected anal intercourse. The researchers suggested that their data showing there is no difference in the circumcision status of men infected by receptive or insertive unprotected anal intercourse suggests that circumcision is not strongly protective against HIV infection in gay men. Further larger studies, preferably of prospective design are needed to confirm the absence of a relationship between circumcision and HIV infection risk in gay men.

Woman-to-woman transmission

Sexual identity and sexual practice

When considering the issue of woman-to-woman transmission it is important to draw a distinction between the risk of transmission by this route and diagnoses of HIV infection and AIDS in women who identify as lesbians. There have been only five reported cases of woman-to-woman transmission, and these reports need to be viewed with the same caution as any other above-mentioned reports of oral transmission.

The most thoroughly investigated report concerns a woman who had a monogamous sexual relationship lasting nearly two years with a woman who died of AIDS in 1989. Sexual activity consisted of mutual fingering and oral sex and use of a shared vibrator. Her partner had ceased menstruating and the woman could recall no instance when sexual activity resulted in a visible laceration or haemorrhage. In 1987 the patient developed vaginal herpes; her partner was not suffering from herpes. In April 1988 the woman developed what appears to have been a seroconversion illness. Upon the death of her partner in 1989 the woman tested HIV-positive. She had a relatively high CD4 count, suggesting that she had been infected recently. The woman denied any activity which could have put her at risk for HIV infection apart from sexual contact with her deceased partner (Rich).

It is sometimes argued that no large-scale epidemiological investigation of HIV prevalence amongst lesbians has taken place. However, three studies of the source of infection of all women with AIDS in the US have failed to identify any cases of woman-to-woman transmission (Chu; McCombs; Petersen). A 1992 follow-up of all 144 women identified as HIV-positive through the blood donation services in the US interviewed 106 women, and identified only three who had had sex with women. All of these women had other risk factors: either injecting drugs or intercourse with men. Of those who remained uninterviewed by the researchers, almost half had identified other risk factors in previous interviews following their diagnosis (Chu 1992).

These studies suggest that whilst lesbians may be infected with HIV through sexual intercourse with men or through shared injecting equipment, there is very little risk that they will transmit the virus to other women during sexual intercourse.

Petersen's study may have underestimated the number of lesbian or bisexual women who were infected with HIV because it was drawn from blood donors, who are asked not to donate blood if they are at risk for HIV infection.

An Italian study of 18 HIV-discordant lesbian couples who had been monogamous partners for at least three months prior to recruitment and who were followed for six months found no seroconversions occurred during this period. Three-quarters of the couples reported sharing sex toys and virtually all couples reported oral sex (Raiteri).

In January 2003 a case report of female-to-female sexual HIV transmission was reported in the journal *Clinical Infectious Diseases*. Doctors suggest the woman may have been infected through sharing sex toys after drug resistance tests found striking similarities between the genotypes of the woman and her female HIV-positive partner.

The case concerns a 20 year-old woman, from Philadelphia, who presented with HIV infection having had a negative HIV test result six months earlier. The woman had been in a monogamous lesbian relationship for the past two years, and denied having had any other sexual partners, male or female. She had never injected drugs or received blood products, and had no tattoos or body piercings.

The couple's sexual practices included the sharing of sex toys, and oral sex. These activities did not occur during menstruation, but sex toys had occasionally been used vigorously enough to draw blood.

A medical examination established that the woman was in good health with no evidence of injecting drug use, or nasal damage from cocaine snorting. The woman also had good oral health, which physicians took to mean that oral transmission could be ruled out.

Her bisexual partner was known to be HIV-positive, and is believed to be the source of infection because of similarities observed when the two women underwent genotypic drug resistance tests. The 20-year-old woman was infected with multi-drug resistant HIV, which carried the following mutations: T215Y (associated with resistance to AZT, d4T and abacavir), D30N (associated with resistance to nelfinavir), K103N (associated with resistance to NNRTIs), L63P (a polymorphism), V77I (also a polymorphism), and M41L (associated with resistance to AZT and d4T, and with resistance to other NRTIs in the presence of T215Y). Her partner's genotype carried mutations at each of these points, plus M184V (associated with resistance to 3TC).

The investigators note that this is the "first reported case of female-to-female sexual transmission of HIV supported by identification of similar HIV genotypes in the source patient and the recipient."

They conclude that whilst reports of woman-to-woman sexual transmission of HIV are scarce, lesbians in HIV-discordant relationships should be advised regarding safer sexual practices.

Risk factors which have been suggested in sex between women include:

- Oral sex (see above).

- Sharing of sex toys: although no cases have been reported, this cannot be ruled out.

- Fisting, particularly if blood is drawn (see next section).

References

Chu SY et al: Update: epidemiology of reported cases of AIDS in women who report sex only with other women, United States 1980-1991, AIDS 6: 516-519, 1992.

Chu SY et al: Epidemiology of reported cases of AIDS in lesbians, United States 1980-1989, AJPH 80: 1380-1381, 1990.

Kwakwa HA et al. Female-to-female transmission of human immunodeficiency virus. Clinical Infectious Diseases, 36, 1 February 2003.

Marmor M et al: Possible female to female transmission of HIV, AIM 105: 969, 1986.

McCombs SB et al: Epidemiology of HIV-1 Infection in Bisexual Women, AIDS 5: 850-852, 1992.

Monzon O and Capellan J B M: Female-to-female transmission of HIV, Lancet ii: 0-41, 1987.

Petersen L et al: No evidence for female-to-female HIV transmission among 960,000 female blood donors, JAIDS 5(9): 853-855, 1992.

Quinn T. Viral Load and Heterosexual Transmission of Human Immunodeficiency Virus Type 1. NEJM 342(13): 921-929 2000.

Raiteri R et al: No HIV-1 transmission through lesbian sex, Lancet 344: 270, 1994.

Rich JD et al: Transmission of human immunodeficiency virus infection presumed to have occurred via female homosexual contact, J Clin Inf Diseases 17: 1003-1005, 1993.

Ross MW et al: Sexually Transmissible Diseases, Injecting Drug Users, Genitourinary Medicine 67: 32-36, 1991.

Sabatini MT et al: Kaposi's sarcoma and T-cell lymphoma in an immunodeficient woman: a case report, AIDS Research 1(2): 135-157 (1983/84) The case of a 37 year-old lesbian who died of an AIDS related illness; both she and her female partner denied sexual contact with men or intravenous drug use; no explanation has been discovered for how either partner acquired HIV infection, but the means of transmission from one partner to another is assumed to have been orogenital contact.

Other sexual practices

Fisting

One case has been reported of infection as a consequence of fisting. A man who had not engaged in anal or oral intercourse for several years seroconverted eighteen months after beginning a sexual relationship with a man who was already symptomatic. Their sexual practice consisted only of dry kissing, mutual masturbation and fisting.

The subject of the report had frequent ulcers on his hand, and it was common for him to fist his partner without covering the cuts. He had a previous history of contracting syphilis by the same route.

Fisting received considerable attention as an 'AIDS risk' in the early years of the epidemic because many of those who practised anal intercourse were also likely to have been fisted. This case suggests that a small potential risk may be attached to fisting.

Being fisted and insertive fisting have both been identified as possible risk factors for hepatitis C acquisition among HIV-positive gay men, with this practice being one of the possible explanations for a recent increase in sexually-transmitted hepatitis C infections seen among gay men (especially Hiv-positive gay men) at clinic in London and other European cities.

For more on the possible link between fisting and hepatitis C, see the chapter on hepatitis.

References

Browne R et al. Increased numbers of acute hepatitis C infections in Hiv-positive homosexual men; is sexual transmission feeding the increase? Sex Transm Infect 80: 326-327. 2004.

Use of semen as a lubricant in mutual masturbation

One case has been reported. A South African man reported that his only possible route of exposure was by using the semen of his partners to lubricate his own penis whilst masturbating. It is possible that the man, who preferred not to have sex with fellow homosexuals and instead seduced 'heterosexual men' by getting drunk with them, and showing them erotic films, may have preferred to censor from his memory other sexual activities which put him at much greater risk of infection. See *Oral transmission*, earlier in this chapter, for further discussion of this phenomenon.

Common sense nevertheless suggests that a small risk might be attached to this activity.

Semen in the eye

One case has been reported where a man is believed to have been infected by getting his partner's semen into his eye. This case was reported by the same Swedish team which also reported six cases of oral transmission (Grutzmeier), see *Oral transmission* above. Two factors suggest that it is likely to be more reliable than some other case reports:

- The serostatus of the individual's sexual partners and confirmatory accounts of the sexual acts which took place has been obtained for each case through the Swedish compulsory partner notification scheme.

- The serostatus of the presenting patient was matched to his previous test result, obtained through clinics in Stockholm. Almost all cases had tested negative within the previous year; repeat testing by seronegative gay men is the norm in Sweden.

References

Donovan B et al: Brachioproctic eroticism and transmission of retrovirus, Genitourinary Medicine 62(6): 390-392, 1986.

Grutzmeier S: HIV transmission in gay men in Stockholm, 1990-1992 IX International Conference on AIDS Po C02-2584.

Sharing injecting equipment

Why infection occurs

Fewer than eight per cent of people with HIV in the UK acquired it through sharinginjection equipment and currently cases acquired via this route account for about two per cent of the annual total (up to four per cent in certain parts of the UK such as NW England). However it accounts for 24% of cases in the USA, more than half in Portugal and Spain, and 80% of cases in Russia.

It was one of the earliest routes of HIV transmission identified, because epidemiologists quickly noticed that HIV infection was following a pattern of prevalence in social groups similar to that of hepatitis B, another blood-borne infection also transmitted by shared needle use.

Transmission occurs through the injection into the body of blood from a previous user of a needle and/or syringe used to inject drugs - usually heroin, amphetamines or cocaine. This is an effective means of transmission because a large quantity of blood can be injected. But HIV infection will not automatically occur from a single incident of shared needle/syringe use. Two factors are likely to determine the chances of HIV infection from any single incident of shared needle/syringe use:

- The level of HIV present in the blood injected. Very low levels of circulating virus in the blood may make HIV infection less likely. But assuming fairly high viral load, it is thought that amounts of blood invisible to the naked eye may be sufficient to permit HIV infection.

- The quantity of blood injected. Evidence from the follow-up of needlestick injuries and other occupational injuries involving blood shows that the likelihood of HIV infection is dose-related - the more blood injected, the more likely it is that seroconversion will take place.

But HIV infection from blood can occur in other ways as a result of injecting drug use:

- Through the presence of blood on spoons used for heating up heroin.

- Through sharing water used to flush blood out of a needle and syringe.

- Through sharing syringes or 'works' which have been cleaned in a way that does not eliminate all the blood they contain.

- Through unsafe disposal of needles or syringes used for injecting drugs, leading to accidents in which blood gets into the body of another person.

For advice on how to take steps to prevent all these situations, see *Safer drug use*.

Remember that people who inject drugs - and their partners - are also vulnerable to HIV infection through sexual intercourse.

Medical and dental procedures and injuries

This section covers:

- Transmission through needlestick injuries: This information is likely to be particularly relevant to health care workers and those who work in needle exchanges where the risk of needlestick injuries is highest.

- Transmission during surgical and dental procedures, organ transplants, skin grafts, and accidents in clinical, healthcare and laboratory situations, including blood splashes and re-use of needles (for exposure by blood transfusion see *Blood transfusions and blood products* later in this chapter).

Needlestick injuries

The Health Protection Agency reports that to the end of 2004 there had been 106 needlestick injuries and other incidents in health care and laboratory settings around the world which had definitely resulted in HIV infection of health care workers.

While these figures probably do not provide an accurate picture of possible infections which have occurred in many countries in Africa, Asia and Latin America, they do reflect the rarity with which needlestick injuries result in HIV infection. It is noteworthy that only seven of these 109 infections have occurred since 2000.

A further 238 infections are presumed to have occurred through needlestick injuries. Although this route could not be proven definitively in these cases, no other risk factors could be identified.

In the UK five definite cases of HIV infection have occurred as a result of occupational needlestick injuries, and a further 14 cases are suspected to be the result of needlestick injuries (Evans). There had been no definite cases since 1993 until one case was reported in 1999, and none since then. Of the 'possible' cases, the five that have occurred since 2000 have all been among UK healthcare workers working in Africa and India.

Over the years from July 1996 to June 2004, a cumulative total of 2,140 initial reports of exposure to one or more blood-borne viruses have been reported to the HPA.

Of these, the majority of exposures were to a hepatitis C-positive positive source, accounting for 47% (997) of all initial reports, with HIV reports accounting for 26% (551 reports) and hepatitis B for 9% (181 reports).

Of the 551 workers exposed to HIV, 466 (84.5%) were put on post-exposure prophylaxis (PEP). Worldwide, there are 24 reports (form 1990 onwards) of PEP failing to prevent HIV infection via occupational exposure.

Percutaneous injury was the most frequently reported exposure route accounting for 75%.

Most exposures involved nursing professionals, accounting for 45% (962/2,140) of reports received, followed by medical professionals with 37% (793/2,140). The proportions of nursing and medical professionals reporting exposures have remained high compared to other occupational groups. Reports in professions allied to medicine and in ancillary staff are much lower and have not increased over time. However, the relative number of professionals in these groups should be taken into account. Importantly, it should be noted that 2% (39/2,140) of the exposures involved porters, security, and housekeeping staff, a group of staff who are not directly involved in patient care. The majority of exposures in ancillary staff involved injuries from needles in rubbish bins. Such injuries from inappropriately discarded sharps by other HCWs are a clear example of the consequences of non-compliance with universal precautions and safe disposal of clinical waste. In some cases however, ancillary staff are injured whilst directly helping in patient care, such as in restraining an agitated patient.

There were 1,597 (75%) six week follow-up reports returned out of the initial 2,140 reported incidents. Of these, only 1,066 [67% (1,066/1,597)] follow-up forms were received at six months follow-up. It is not known whether these health care workers may have been followed-up but the reporting centres did not return follow-up reports to the programme. Overall, six months follow-up reports were not received for 50% (1,074/2,140) of the initially reported incidents.

Percutaneous venepuncture remains the number one procedure reported, with suturing second.

Contributing factors were reported in 655 (32%) of reports. Non-compliance with universal precautions was the most frequent, followed by patients moving or being agitated.

Reported PEP regimes reflect those recommended by the HIV post exposure prophylaxis: guidance from the United Kingdom chief medical officers' expert advisory group on AIDS. Where PEP was discontinued and the source status was HIV-positive, side-effects was the most frequent reported reason. Overall the most frequently reported side-effect, regardless of source status, was gastro-intestinal disturbances. Where reported, PEP was commenced within an hour in 37% of HCWs prescribed PEP and 63% within two hours.

Follow-up is undertaken at six months for exposures to HIV and HCV. A total of 737 of these six month reports were received by HPA. Over the five-year period, seroconversions in four HCWs have been identified through the surveillance. One HCW seroconverted to HIV, despite triple PEP.

Surveillance on health care workers in England, Wales and Northern Ireland who have been exposed to blood born viruses has been carried out since 1984. By the end of June 2000 the PHLS Communicable Disease Surveillance Centre (CCSC) had received 827 initial reports of exposures to material from patients with antibody to HIV, or hepatitis C, or who were hepatitis B surface antigen positive. Two hundred and forty-two health care workers were exposed to HIV, (whilst 396 were exposed to patients with hepatitis C virus and 101 to hepatitis B virus). A further 83 healthcare workers were exposed to two viruses, whilst five were exposed to all three.

Nurses (337/827; 41%) and doctors (262/827; 32%) remain the two groups most frequently exposed.

The same surveillance programme also compiles data on the uptake and side-effects of post-exposure prophylaxis (PEP). Of 140 health care workers who were exposed to an HIV-positive source and given PEP, 100 were given AZT, 3TC and indinavir. Forty-four were known to complete the course. Fifty-seven discontinued PEP early, mostly due to side-effects.

As of March 2000 participants have been asked to report all incidents where PEP has been given, regardless of the HIV status of the source.

A six month follow-up report on infection status for all health care workers exposed to HIV or HCV was introduced in March 2000. Up until the end of June 2004 1066 follow-up reports (50% of all reports) related to exposure to HIV had been received, with one documented seroconversion, despite PEP.

A number of studies have calculated the risk of HIV infection from any single needlestick injury where HIV contaminated blood is involved is around 0.32% (Becker). Some studies have also calculated the risk of HIV infection on the basis of person-years, and show a similarly low chance of infection (Leentvar).

This is because the quantity of blood passed on from a needlestick injury is likely to be much smaller than that from an injection of blood when sharing injecting equipment. A 1991 study estimated that the volume of blood likely to be injected as a result of a needlestick injury was approximately one-seventh of the quantity passed on when sharing injecting equipment (Gaughwin). Although deep injection has been suggested as another factor which increases the likelihood of infection, reports of documented seroconversions fail to show a consistent pattern of type of needlestick injury which leads to HIV infection.

More on post-exposure prophylaxis (PEP)

For post-exposure prophylaxis after sexual exposure, see *Developing Prevention Technologies*.

New PEP resource from the Health Protection Agency

The UK's Health Protection Agency launched web pages offering guidance on occupational exposure to blood-borne viruses in healthcare workers in January 2003.

The web page address is www.hpa.org.uk/infections/topics_az/hiv_and_sti/hiv/occupational

The pages offer links to key guidance documents on occupational exposure issued by the UK Department of Health and other regulatory bodies.

Information on HIV, hepatitis B and hepatitis C is included in the web pages, and a poster *What to do if exposed* can be downloaded from the site. Data collected by the Communicable Diseases Surveillance Unit on occupational exposure to blood-borne viruses such as HIV are also available.

PEP for needlestick injuries

The risk of contracting HIV following occupational exposure to HIV is low. Epidemiological studies have indicated that the average risk of HIV transmission after percutaneous (passing through the skin) exposure to HIV infected blood in health care settings is about 3 per 1,000 injuries.

Following a mucocutaneous (via the mucous membrane) exposure the average risk is estimated to be less than 1 in 1,000.

Where intact skin is exposed to HIV infected blood, no risk of HIV transmission is considered.

A case control study amongst health care workers exposed to HIV has found that the administration of AZT for four weeks after exposure was associated with an 80% reduced risk of seroconversion.

AZT treatment at this stage is believed to block the infection of immune system cells by HIV, so prompt AZT treatment is likely to block the establishment of HIV infection in an individual who has been exposed to the virus.

It is assumed that a combination of two or three drugs may be even more effective than AZT at blocking HIV infection.

On the basis of these findings, US health authorities have recommended that healthcare workers who suffer certain types of injuries should be offered post-exposure prophylaxis with a combination of two or three drugs.

Those who received a deep injury from large diameter needle previously inserted in the veins of a patient with high viral load and/or advanced AIDS will be recommended to commence a combination of AZT, 3TC and indinavir or nelfinavir immediately. A three-drug combination is recommended in these circumstances because the risk of seroconversion is judged to be high.

Despite the benefits of PEP there is evidence that the standard regimen of AZT/3TC/indinavir is poorly tolerated. Nine of 18 healthcare workers at three London hospitals who commenced this regimen stopped or changed therapy due to side-effects within four weeks. Six of the 19 who started indinavir required more than two weeks off work; among the other 9 only one required more than 7 days' leave. There were no discontinuations among the five people who received saquinavir (Parkin).

Since the publication of the guidelines in 1998, according to the updated 2001 guidelines,

"Efavirenz, abacavir, and lopinavir/r (*Kaletra*) a PI, have been approved by FDA. Although side-effects might be common with the NNRTIs, Efavirenz might be considered for expanded PEP regimens, especially when resistance to PIs in the source person's virus is known or suspected. Abacavir has been associated with dangerous hypersensitivity reactions but, with careful monitoring, may be considered as a third drug for PEP. Kaletra, a combination of lopinavir and ritonavir, is a potent HIV inhibitor that, with expert consultation, may be considered in an expanded PEP regimen."

The 2001 guidelines were published before tenofovir became available. Protease inhibitors alone are not to be recommended as they only work after HIV has become integrated into the genome; they prevent viral proliferation but not necessarily infection.

Those who suffer blood splashes or other injuries may be offered a three-drug combination if the injury is extensive or the exposure prolonged. Otherwise, healthcare workers will usually be offered a combination of AZT and 3TC or tenofovir and 3TC/FTC.

It is recommended that post-exposure prophylaxis commence within 24 - 36 hours of injury, and preferably within a few hours of exposure.

UK guidelines issued by the Expert Advisory group on AIDS and the Department of Health recommend PEP be administered to health care workers if they have had a significant occupational exposure to blood or another high risk body fluid from a patient or other source either known to be HIV-positive, or considered to be at high risk of HIV infection, but where the result of an HIV test has not or cannot be obtained, for whatever reason.

Current UK practice

A telephone survey of 26 surgeons working in 13 hospitals in the South West of England found that only 8 out of 26 were aware of DoH guidance in September 1998, and only two out of 26 were aware of local recommendations, such as where to go for out-of-hours PEP (Duff). These findings suggest poor communication of policies on occupational PEP within NHS Trusts.

The July 2000 edition of the DoH guidance states that every NHS Trust or other health care setting should develop a post-exposure policy and protocol. In addition, it recommends that starter packs should be available on site for use following occupational exposure.

Data collection

Surveillance on health care workers in England, Wales and Northern Ireland who have been exposed to blood-borne viruses has been carried out since 1984.

Over the five years from July 1997 to June 2002, 1550 initial reports of occupational exposures to one or more blood borne virus were received by HPA. Of these 509 healthcare workers (HCWs), regardless of source status were prescribed post-exposure prophylaxis (PEP). Overall hepatitis C virus (HCV) represented 49% of all reports, HIV 30%, and hepatitis B 13%, and PEP with unknown source 8%. Percutaneous injury was the most frequently reported exposure route accounting for 72% (n=1125). Hollow bore needles accounted for 47% (n=734) of all reports. Occupationally, nursing related professions accounted for 42%, with doctors accounting for 35% of all reports.

For six-week follow-up HPA received 1064 reports. The most commonly reported location of exposures incident remains the ward. Exposure events occurring after the procedure or during or after disposal accounted for 36%.

Percutaneous venepuncture remains the number one procedure reported, with suturing second. Contributing factors were reported in 35% (n=369) of reports. Patients moving or being agitated was the most frequent, followed by non-compliance with universal precautions.

Reported PEP regimes reflect those recommended by the HIV post-exposure prophylaxis: guidance from the UK chief medical officers' expert advisory group on AIDS. Where PEP was discontinued and the source status was HIV-positive, side-effects were the most frequent reported reason to stop. Overall the most frequently reported side-effect, regardless of source status, was gastro-intestinal disturbances. Where reported, PEP was commenced within an hour in 37% of HCWs prescribed PEP and 63% within two hours.

Follow-up is undertaken at six months for exposures to HIV and HCV. A total of 737 of these six- month reports were received by HPA. Over the five-year period, seroconversions in four HCWs have been identified through the surveillance. One HCW seroconverted to HIV, despite triple PEP. Three HCWs seroconverted to HCV (one, which occurred in 1996 retrospectively reported).

The use of nevirapine

Nevirapine has been proposed as a suitable drug for PEP because it causes less nausea and is less disruptive to everyday life than indinavir, one of the protease inhibitors currently recommended in UK guidelines. There is a growing body of evidence from the use of two-dose nevirapine treatments in preventing mother-to-child transmission which suggests that nevirapine can be both safe and effective.

However, a recent study found that the use of nevirapine for post-exposure prophylaxis as a four-week course of treatment may carry an unacceptable risk of serious adverse effects.

Between 1997 and 1999 Camden and Islington Health Authority used d4T/3TC and nevirapine as its standard PEP regimen.

Researchers from the Royal Free and University College Medical School recently published an analysis of PEP including nevirapine prescribed to exposed healthcare workers and attendees at a central London GUM clinic. Data were collected from the case notes of 57 individuals (40 men and 17 women) who received PEP between January 1997 and November 1999 (Benn).

Of the 57 individuals, 33 reported that they had completed a full 4-week course of PEP. Five individuals had a major adverse event; two had a grade four rise in concentrations of liver aminotransferases and three had a grade three rise in liver aminotransferases. In all five of the patients nevirapine therapy was stopped.

A nevirapine-containing regimen was no better tolerated than an indinavir-containing regimen overall, although fewer minor adverse events were seen in the nevirapine group. The authors postulated that the study may have underestimated the occurrence of side-effects and overestimate tolerability due to the fact that only 41 of the 57 people who were prescribed PEP had any documented follow-up during the 4-week period on PEP.

The authors concluded that whilst there may be a biological argument for using a regimen that includes an NNRTI, the possible safety problems of such a regimen seen in their HIV-negative population might make alternative regimens preferable. One option might be to limit the nevirapine component to the first few days, but the impact of this on the incidence of side-effects is unknown.

US authorities recently reported 22 cases of severe or life-threatening side-effects such as rash and liver failure among people taking nevirapine as post-exposure prophylaxis. Some experts have suggested the risk of severe toxicity means that nevirapine should not be recommended for PEP in this context.

The problem of tolerability

Antiretroviral regimens prescribed for established HIV infection can be difficult to tolerate, those used immediately after exposure (PEP) are no exception.

Side-effects experienced during the course of PEP can have a critical influence on whether or not an individual is able to complete the course, which in turn has implications for the likely effectiveness of a combination.

The Italian Post-Exposure Prophylaxis Registry to the end of 1999 included data from 647 healthcare workers whose PEP consisted solely of AZT, and 341 who had taken a triple combination (191 of whom received indinavir).

Researchers found no significant differences in the proportion of health-care workers experiencing side-effects, though 10.5% of healthcare workers who had been prescribed a triple combination including indinavir did discontinue the indinavir and remain on double nucleoside analogue therapy after a median of seven days of treatment.(Puro)

Other reports have suggested that a regimen which includes a protease inhibitor may be particularly hard to tolerate.

Protocols for managing PEP requests

- Hospitals and other sites need to have protocols established in advance of any requests for post-exposure prophylaxis. Planners need to bear in mind:

- Confidentiality, both of the person who is exposed and of the patient or person who is the potential source of infection.

- Training on prevention of needle-stick injuries and post-exposure procedures, including AZT treatment.

- Speed of administration of PEP. It is assumed that PEP needs to be administered within 24 hours of exposure, and is most likely to be most efficacious if started within one hour of exposure.

- Counselling regarding the risks of seroconversion, the use of PEP, safer sex and other information on HIV transmission. Counselling should above all seek informed consent for the use of PEP and for post-exposure HIV testing. The worker should be informed of the diverse opinions amongst physicians regarding the post-exposure use of antiretrovirals. Further information on antiretrovirals is presented in the *HIV & AIDS Treatments Directory*, also published by NAM, and at aidsmap.com.

- Surveillance procedure, including recording of circumstances in which exposure occurred, dosage schedule, serological test results, reporting to relevant authorities.

PEP after sexual exposure

Further discussion of PEP after sexual exposure can be found in *Developing prevention technologies*. Several portions of this section appeared previously as a National HIV Prevention Information Service briefing on post-exposure prophylaxis.

References

Banatvala JE et al: HIV Infection: Hazards of Transmission to Patients and Health Care Workers during Invasive Procedures, Royal College of Pathologists Working Group.

Bell D et al: Zidovudine use after occupational HIV exposure: toxicity and failures reported to the CDC, Ninth International Conference on AIDS, abstract WS-C12-6, 1993.

Benn, P et al. Prophylaxis with a nevirapine-containing triple regimen after exposure to HIV-1. The Lancet, 357: 9257, 2001.

CDC: Public Health Service Statement on Management of Occupational Exposure to Human Immunodeficiency Virus, Including Considerations Regarding Zidovudine Postexposure Use, MMWR 39 Supp RR-1 Jan 26 1990.

CDC: Update: Provisional Public Health Service recommendations for chemoprophylaxis after occupational exposure to HIV MMWR 45: 468-472.

CDR Weekly Communicable Disease Report, Volume 10: 33, 2000.

Centers for Disease Control and Prevention. Public Health Service Guidelines for the Management of Health care worker exposure to HIV and recommendations for post-exposure prophylaxis. MMWR 47 1998.

Duff SE et al. Surgeons' and occupational health departments' awareness of guidelines on post-exposure prophylaxis for staff exposed to HIV: a telephone survey. British Medical Journal 319: 162, 1999.

Henderson DK. Post-exposure chemoprohylaxis for occupational exposure to the human immunodeficiency virus. Journal of the American Medical Association, 281: 931-936, 1999.

HIV Post-Exposure Prophylaxis: Guidance from the UK Chief Medical Officers' Expert Advisory Group on AIDS. Department of Health. July 2000.

Parkin J et al. Tolerability and side-effects of post-exposure prophylaxis for HIV infection. The Lancet 355: 9205, 2001.

Puro V. Post exposure prophylaxis for HIV infection. The Lancet, 355: 9214, 2000.

Transmission to healthcare workers through surgical and dental procedures

Apart from needlestick injuries, there have been a small number of other incidents which demonstrate the need for caution during medical procedures which might involve contact with blood. A handful of healthcare workers, almost all with previously damaged skin, have been infected through blood splashes. These have occurred when blood splashed into the eyes, onto damaged skin or into the mouth (CDC, Gionnini). Since it has been reported that the mucous membranes of the eye have been a route of infection in several cases, goggles should be worn in any situation where spattering of blood is likely.

Precautions

It is always in the nature of health care work to be at risk of infection. In the case of most other infections there are tried and trusted procedures to protect healthcare workers.

In the case of HIV it has been argued that the testing of patients is the best way of protecting health care workers. This would not be practical because it could never identify all HIV-infected patients. Instead, universal precautions need to be practised. These are discussed under *Infection control* later in this chapter. This section also summarises the danger-points - the medical procedures which have been identified as most likely to lead to injuries for healthcare workers.

Transmission from healthcare workers to patients

There have only ever been four documented cases of HIV transmission from healthcare workers to patients, though in all but one of these the exact route of transmission remains unclear. There has never been a case in the UK.

The most recent was reported in the 9 January 2006 issue of AIDS Journal (Mallolas). In this case a female patient was pretty certainly infected by a gay male obstetrician when he performed an emergency caesarean on her in 2004.

The woman came down with a feverish illness and showed signs of immune-system disturbance two weeks after her caesarean, and eight weeks later she tested positive for HIV. Neither her husband nor baby had HIV and she reported no other risk factors.

The surgeon, a gay man, did not know he had HIV and had never been tested. After it was realised he might have infected his patient, he said he recalled pricking his finger on a needle during the operation. He took an HIV test, which was positive, seven months after the caesarean.

Phylogenetic analysis of the HIV of both doctor and patient revealed that the viruses they had only differed by three per cent, whereas three unrelated samples taken for comparison were different by 23%. The three previous transmissions of HIV from a healthcare worker to a patient were:

- The 'Florida dentist', David Acer, who in 1990, somehow infected five of his patients

- A French surgeon who transmitted HIV to an elderly patient during a hip replacement operation in 1992.

- A French nurse who transmitted HIV to a patient during a hospital stay in May 1996, though it's not known exactly how.

The Spanish case is the first case where there appears to be relatively strong evidence for the exact route of transmission.

Almost all other follow-up studies of surgeons known to be HIV-positive have failed to find any cases of HIV infection from surgeons, despite fears that the surgeons might have cut themselves during operations and thus infected their patients (Grawshaw; Lowenfels; Porter). Up to several hundred patients have been followed up in some cases, both in the USA and in the UK. This provides us with a fairly good statistical sample, and should provide reassuring evidence.

However, in January 1997 French health authorities reported that an orthopaedic surgeon who had tested HIV-positive in 1994 had infected a patient during a lengthy hip-replacement and bone graft operation which took place in 1992 (Lot). The surgeon himself appeared to have been infected by a patient during an operation in 1983. Neither patient nor surgeon had any other known risk factors for HIV, and genetic sequences from the viruses of the surgeon and the patient were almost identical. The patient was the only positive diagnosis in 983 of the surgeon's former patients tested. Investigation of the surgeon's work practices revealed that he was in the habit of several practices that could have caused injuries such as palpating the needle tip when sewing up operation incisions and twisting sharp suture wires with his fingers.

In the third case (Goujon), a 61-year-old patient who had been admitted for surgery in May 1996 developed primary HIV infection the following month. No surgeons on the team were found to have HIV but two nurses who had cared for the patient were HIV-positive. One, a Zairean man, was ruled out on the basis of phylogenetic analysis. The source therefore appeared to be a 51-year-old female nurse, who was unaware of her HIV infection until, in June 1996, she was also hospitalised for hepatic insufficiency. A diagnosis of infection with both hepatitis C virus (HCV) and HIV-1 was established. HIV viral load was 1.8×10^5 copies per ml and her CD4+ cell count was 94.

Although the paper authors point out that "patient and nurse 2 might have independently acquired similar geographic local variants" of HIV, the nurse's low CD4 count implies longstanding HIV infection. However the nurse did not perform exposure-prone procedures such as venepunture on the patient and there is no indicaiton of how transmission might have happened in this case.

The only other case in which a healthcare worker is thought to have infected patients is that of a dentist. That case is discussed in detail in *Transmission from dentists and dental equipment*, below, because it is often used as a basis for warnings about the possible risks of HIV infection during surgical procedures. It is important to understand both the specific circumstances described in that report, and what lessons can be drawn from that report for minimising risk in all invasive surgical procedures. Other cases in which patients have been followed up are discussed immediately below.

Two studies provide evidence from extensive follow up programmes of the minimal risk associated with invasive procedures.

In June 1991 an orthopaedic surgeon who had been practising in the same community in New Hampshire, USA, for 16 years was found to be HIV-positive. He had probably been infected before 1979. As has been found for other orthopaedic surgeons, he had sustained quite frequent minor skin punctures, at least once a month. Following such injuries he used to remove and discard the instrument which had caused the injury immediately, to prevent it from subsequently coming into contact with the patient. He would also change his gloves. When injuries were caused by tiny fragments of bone, the patient's wound would immediately be washed with an antiseptic solution. The surgeon and theatre nurses were interviewed and none recalled any occasion when a patient was thought to have been exposed to the surgeon's blood.

Letters were sent to 2,317 former patients, who had undergone 2,652 invasive procedures between January 1978 and June 1991. 1,174 underwent HIV testing, all of whom were negative. None of the non-respondents or untested patients could be established to have AIDS through other medical records.

Despite practising for many years in a surgical speciality likely to have a higher than average risk of patient exposure, the surgeon was not found to have infected any patients (Von Reyn). This case suggests that when careful hygiene procedures are followed in situations where a risk exists, infection does not seem to occur.

A surgeon in Maryland, USA, died in November 1990, after which local newspapers demanded disclosure of the fact that he had died of AIDS. A trace-back exercise through his hospital followed, and 413 of the 1,012 patients known to have undergone invasive procedures were tested. One seropositive was subsequently identified. This person had previously received a blood transfusion from a donor who was traced and found to be HIV-positive, and who had probably already been infected at the time of the donation. The genetic sequences of viruses from the patient, the surgeon and the blood donor were compared. That from the patient was closely related to the blood donor's, but not to the surgeon's (Rogers). Researchers decided that the surgeon could not have been the source of infection.

Transmission through reuse of needles in clinics

A number of cases have been reported of multiple infections resulting from the re-use of needles in several hospitals. One focal infection may result in a large number of other infections. Cases have been reported in Russia and Romania, and such infections are believed to be commonplace in countries where the shortage of medical equipment makes the re-use of needles necessary. Unfortunately, little data on this subject have been gathered in recent years by researchers

The World Health Organization (WHO) estimates that worldwide, about five per cent of HIV infections come from the use of unsterilised needles.

In a series of papers published in 2002 and 2003, STI specialists David Gisselquist and John Potterat and psychologist Stuart Brody caused controversy by claiming that between 35% and 65% of HIV infections in Africa were caused by re-use of unsterilised needles rather than sex.

Gisselquist and colleagues based their theory on an analysis of early HIV infection reports received from countries in east and central Africa before 1990. They claimed to show that the number of medical injections reported by seroconverters were much better correlated with HIV infection than the number of sexual partners or STIs they had had.

Gisselquist also cited a South African study which found significant levels of HIV infection in children born to HIV-negative mothers, and evidence from Zimbabwe that falling STI rates were accompanied by rising HIV rates.

The work of Gisselquist and colleagues created enough controversy for the WHO to make an investigation of their theory. In an article published in the *Lancet* (Schmid) they reviewed Gisselquist and colleagues' arguments and refuted them:

- Transmission via unsterilised needles may possibly have contributed to the spread of HIV early on in the epidemic but Gisselquist had failed to review data since 1990 which showed an overwhelming *lack* of correlation between injections and HIV seropositivity (See, for instance, Lopman).

- Gisselquist was using 'reverse causality'; patients with HIV had had more injections because they had HIV-related illnesses, not HIV because they had injections.

- The South African study which found high rates of HIV infection in children of HIV-negative mothers was flawed, as the study authors admitted at the time; it had relied on oral HIV swabs self-administered by families and there was a lot of cross-contamination.

- More than twice as many injections with unsterilised needles are given in Asia (where the practice of getting vitamin shots from street-corner stalls is widespread) than in Africa. If HIV was largely spread by needles rather than sex, India would have the world's highest HIV prevalence.

- HIV has continued to increase in Zimbabwe and some other southern African countries as STIs have decreased because HIV prevalence is so high that most HIV infection is now occurring within marriage, where bacterial STIs are less likely to be commonly transmitted.

Transmission through reuse of medical instruments

A case has been reported in Australia of the sequential infection of four patients on the same day at an out-patient clinic where each received minor surgery. The first patient is believed to have been an HIV-positive man with a low CD4 count; four subsequent patients on that day were all discovered to be HIV-positive, although it still has not been established that they are all infected with the same strain of HIV. The cases are believed to have occurred as a consequence of a failure of infection control. The doctor re-used scalpel handles and disinfected rather than sterilised equipment (Chant).

Transmission through kidney dialysis equipment

A case has been reported from Colombia of the infection of at least nine patients who seroconverted within a four-month period during 1992 after kidney dialysis treatment at the same centre. The risk was eventually narrowed down to inadequate disinfection of dialysis equipment, including re-usable needles. It was noted by investigators that all those who had seroconverted had received treatment with needles soaked in the same disinfecting tray as the index case, in a solution of 0.16% benzalkonium chloride. The solution was changed only once a week, allowing considerable opportunities for cross-infection. Dialyser filters and bloodlines were sterilised between each patient with a solution of approximately 1.5% formaldehyde. What is surprising about this case is the viability of HIV in such a disinfectant solution and the relatively small quantities of blood likely to have been involved. The authors note that the anti-microbial activity of benzalkonium chloride is likely to decline over time, especially in the presence of organic matter from a large number of instruments.

Potential transmission through vaccination equipment

The US Centers for Disease Control and Prevention are currently investigating two cases in which doctors appear to have followed incorrect infection control procedures whilst conducting vaccination programmes. In one case a doctor was seen re-using needles; in the other case a doctor was seen puncturing vials of vaccine with needles already used to inoculate other patients. He did not re-use needles or syringes to vaccinate other patients (Levy). There is no evidence of HIV transmission in these cases.

Transmission through acupuncture needles

The case of a young man who had received acupuncture treatment and subsequently seroconverted has been reported (Vittecocq). He had no other identifiable risk factors. Although it was established that the acupuncturist had not sterilised needles between patients, the 1989 report could not provide information on whether other patients of the acupuncturist were indeed infected with HIV.

There was been a case of patients being infected with hepatitis B and C through unsterilised acupuncture needles by GP Dr

Madhusudan Shivadikar at his alternative therapy centre in Finchley in 1998. No HIV transmission occurred.

Transmission through organ transplants

HIV infection has occurred as a consequence of transplants of the liver, kidneys, pancreas, bone marrow and the heart, and also as a consequence of skin grafts. The most dramatic case occurred following the death of a donor who had tested HIV-negative at the time organ use was approved. Subsequently the donor seems to have seroconverted, because recipients of the heart, kidneys, liver and bone seroconverted after transplantation. Recipients of other processed bone and avascular soft tissue (tissue without blood supply), ligaments, corneas and the dura mater (the membrane which protects the brain and the spinal cord) did not become infected, indicating that it is vascular (blood bearing) organs which constitute the greatest risk (Simonds).

Grafted skin was also the source of HIV infection in an individual who had been treated for severe burns (Clark).

HIV has also been transmitted in semen donated for artificial insemination (Stewart).

Screening of donated organs and tissues

All donors of organs, tissues, eggs and semen are tested for HIV, but this does not completely rule out the possibility of infection, because of the 'window period' before antibodies form. However, people who donate organs are asked not to permit their organs to be donated if they believe themselves to have been at risk of HIV infection. Since this strategy has been fairly successful in screening out blood donations (which are far more commonly made), it is reasonable to assume that it will offer a very good degree of protection against the chances of HIV infection through receiving an organ transplant or skin graft. It is also possible that in some cases, hospitals will use PCR testing to check for HIV infection before antibodies appear. For an explanation of PCR testing see *HIV testing*.

Inactivation of HIV in donated organs and tissues

It is unclear whether any methods of HIV inactivation can be relied upon to make organs or tissues safe for use where doubts exist about the safety of transplanting the organs or tissues.

Transmission from dentists and dental equipment

Transmission reported in one dental practice: The Florida Dentist

One episode where transmission from a dentist to his patients is believed to have occurred has been reported. A dentist in the United States was identified as the source of infection for six of his patients. Infection was argued to have occurred during 1988-89 (Cieselski). This conclusion was reached after examining the DNA sequences of viral isolates from all patients found to be HIV-positive.

A very close correlation was found between the viral DNA of five patients and that of the dentist. In contrast, two other patients with other risk factors for HIV infection showed markedly different viral DNA patterns, as did 35 control samples taken at random from HIV-positive people in the same district.

Dentist doubted as source of infection

Subsequent analyses by another team have called into question a conclusive link between all five patients and the dentist (De Bry; Weiss). They argued that the similarity in viral isolates was not conclusive. In their own study De Bry and Weiss had recruited a control group of seropositive individuals who lived in the same area. Many of the control group recruited in the catchment area of the dental practice showed enough similarities in the genetic structure of their HIV isolates to cast doubt on the dentist as the irrefutable source. However, it should be borne in mind that HIV evolves rapidly, generating a mixed population of subtypes within each individual. The analysis of HIV genomes is still a new and experimental field, so scientific debate on the methodology for establishing sources of infection is likely to continue.

DeBry also argued that the exposure risk evidence of the five patients was open to question, since they were all aware of the dental transmission hypothesis (and by implication, could have falsified their accounts in order to make themselves eligible for compensation).

A subsequent investigation conducted on behalf of an insurance company has reported that all the patients may have had other risks for HIV infection which were not disclosed to the CDC investigators. Although this claim has been strongly refuted by the CDC, questions still hang over this unusual case.

For example, it is not clear from the insurance records of one of the infected patients whether she was ever treated by Dr Acer, and her insurance records do not tally with the information later provided to the CDC investigation. Indeed, her records suggest that she first visited the surgery nearly a year after the CDC investigators were told she first attended the practice.

A particularly unusual aspect of these cases is the very rapid development of symptoms following infection in some patients - in one case just 17 months after the assumed date of infection. This might have happened for several reasons. HIV infection through blood often leads to the development of AIDS more quickly. It may also be the case that patients were infected with an especially virulent strain of HIV, leading to faster disease progression. However, this question has not been addressed in any detail by the investigations which have taken place.

The case remains full of inconsistencies which are summarised and debated in two articles published by the *Annals of Internal Medicine* in 1996 (Barr; Brown).

How did transmission occur in this dental practice?

Cieselski reported that all five patients had invasive dental work after the dentist was diagnosed with AIDS and had evidence of severe immunosuppression. There were many opportunities for the dentist to have injured himself during invasive procedures such as tooth extractions (Lewis). Contrary to claims made in a BBC TV *Panorama* documentary, these injuries are common in dental practice.

All five patients received multiple injections of local anaesthetic, and sharps injury during anaesthetic administration could have resulted in contamination of the syringe apparatus with the dentist's blood, after which additional anaesthetic may have been injected into the same patient. A sharps injury could also result in direct contact of the dentist's blood with the patient's inflamed or damaged oral tissues during the invasive procedures. Although the dentist began to wear gloves routinely in 1987, gloves do not prevent most injuries caused by sharp instruments. Instruments were cleaned in accordance with guidelines intended to prevent HIV transmission after early 1987.

Instruments such as a high-speed dental handpiece, which might have facilitated cross-infection between patients (assuming, of course, that the dentist had first of all infected one of the

patients) do not appear to have been used on two HIV infected patients on the same day. Researchers reached this conclusion after examining the appointments book of the practice. If contaminated instruments or equipment are assumed to have been the route of transmission, one would expect to see a clustering of appointments of infected patients. However, it has been suggested that the dentist was treating HIV-positive patients who were his sexual partners (and therefore likely to be infected with the same strain of HIV) out of clinic hours. No official investigation has yet been able to substantiate this claim, or to correlate any alleged 'ghost' appointments with those of subsequently infected patients.

Another potential source of transmission remains uncertain, since it depends on anecdotal evidence. A practice nurse told investigators that the dentist was in the habit of cauterising his own mouth ulcers with dental instruments on an almost daily basis. CDC investigators remain uncertain as to whether these highly unhygienic episodes of self-treatment coincided with periods during which the HIV-infected patients were treated, and in their 1992 report suggested that sharps injuries were a more likely route of transmission.

Another school of thought, not addressed by the CDC investigation, takes the view that the infection of the six patients was deliberately planned and executed by the dentist, although there is no clear motive.

Lessons of this case concerning risks from invasive procedures

Whilst the CDC investigation points clearly to the potential risk attached to sharps injuries, there is considerable disagreement amongst dental experts over the risk posed by the inadequate sterilisation of dental equipment. A 1992 study showed that potentially infectious quantities of HIV may be present in water lines and other dental equipment not normally sterilised between each patient (Lewis).

Critics of Lewis's study point out that concentrations of HIV far in excess of those likely to be present in blood were used in combination with inadequate disinfectants, combining to give a misleading picture of the likelihood of infection because of inadequate cleaning of instruments. They also note that the failure to practise universal precautions, especially in regard to compliance with safety procedures for needle and glove use, continue to constitute a far greater area of risk than already adopted sterilisation procedures.

Whilst doubts about the dental transmission study persist amongst some experts, it is important to strike a balance between being overly cautious about the risks of HIV transmission through surgical accidents, and being less than cautious. The former is likely to result in panic; the latter in failures to observe sensible precautions.

Does this case show a potential risk of HIV infection through dental treatment?

The chief questions raised by this case are:

- Was the dentist the source of infection?

- Were dental handpieces the route of infection, and if so, how easily can they transmit HIV?

The answer to the first question is now widely agreed to be 'yes'. The second question remains debatable. It is by no means clear either that dental handpieces were the route of infection, or that they may harbour potentially infectious quantities of HIV despite autoclaving. Nevertheless, it seems clear that greater adherence to infection control guidelines is the only way to prevent a repetition of this incident and to allay fears of a repetition.

Transmission from healthcare workers - references

Arnold C et al: The case of the Florida dentist: an unusual mode of HIV transmission, PHLS Microbiology Digest 10:1, 1993.

Barr S: The 1990 Florida dental investigation: is the case really closed? AIM 124(2): 251-254, 1996.

Becker C et al: Occupational infection with HIV, AIM, 110(8): 653-656, 1989.

BrownD: The 1990 Florida dental investigation: theory and fact, AIM 124(2): 255-256, 1996.

Carson P, Goldsmith JC: Gay bashing as possible risk for HIV infection, Lancet 337 (8743): 731, 1991.

CDR Weekly Communicable Disease Report, Volume 10: 33, 2000.

Chant K et al: Patient-to-patient transmission of HIV, Lancet 342: 1548, 1993 & Lancet 343: 415-416, 1994.

Cieselski C et al: Transmission of human immunodeficiency virus in a dental practice, AIM 116:10: 798-805, 1992.

Clark JA: HIV transmission and skin grafts, Lancet i: 983, 1987.

De Bry RW et al: Letter to the Editor, Nature 361: 691, 1993.

Gaughwin MD et al Bloody needles: the volume of blood transferred in simulations of needlestick injuries AIDS 5(8): 1025-1027, 1991.

Giaonnini P et al: HIV infection acquired by a nurse, Eur J Epidemiology 4: 119-120, 1988.

Gisselquist D and Potterat J. Heterosexual transmission of HIV in Africa: an empiric estimate. International Journal of STD & AIDS 14: 162-173, 2003.

Goujon CP et al. Phylogenetic analyses indicate an atypical nurse-to-patient transmission of human immunodeficiency virus type 1. J Virol 74

Grawshaw SC: HIV Transmission during surgery (Letter), BMJ Sep 7 1991 303 (6082): 580, 1991. A follow-up of patients of an HIV infected gynaecologist did not reveal any cases of HIV infection.

Hill DW: HIV infection following motor vehicle trauma in central Africa, JAMA 261: 282-283, 1989.

Leentvaar AK et al: Needlestick injuries, surgeons and HIV risks, Lancet 335: 546-547, 1990. This study estimates that if a surgeon does 500 operations a year for 30 years, he will have 120 accidents during this period. If the transmission risk is 0.005 and seroprevalence is 0.002, the 30 year cumulative risk is 0.0012 - therefore routine HIV screening is not recommended.

Levy M et al: From the CDC: Improper infection control practices during employee vaccination programs-1993, JAMA 271(3): 182, 1994.

Lewis DL: Cross contamination potential with dental equipment, Lancet 340: 1252-1254, 1992.

Lopman BA et al. Individual Level Injection History: A Lack of Association with HIV Incidence in Rural Zimbabwe. PLoS Medicine 2(2): e37, 2005.

Lot F et al. Probable transmission of HIV from an orthopedic surgeon to a patient in France. Ann Int Med 130(1): 1-6. 1999.

Lowenfels AB et al: Risk of HIV transmission of HIV from surgeon to patient, NEJM 325(12): 888-889, 1991.

Mallolas J et al. Transmission of HIV-1 from an obstetrician to a patient during a caesarean section. AIDS 20(2): 285-299. 2006.

O' Farrell et al: Transmission of HIV-1 infection after a fight, Lancet 239 (Jan 25): 246, 1992.

Porter JD et al: Management of patients treated by a surgeon with HIV infection, Lancet 335, 113-114, 1990.

Rogers AS et al: Investigation of potential HIV transmission to the patients of an HIV infected surgeon, JAMA 269: 1795-1801, 1993.

Schmid GP et al. Transmission of HIV-1 infection in sub-Saharan Africa and effect of elimination of unsafe injections. Lancet. 363(9407): 482-488, 2004.

Simonds RJ et al: Transmission of human immunodeficiency virus type 1 from a seronegative organ and tissue donor, NEJM 326: 726-732, 1992.

Stewart GJ et al: Transmissions of human T-cell lymphotropic virus (HTLV-III) by donor, Lancet ii: 581-585, 1985.

Torre, D et al: Transmission of HIV-1 Infection via sports injury (Letter), Lancet 335 (8697) 1105, 1990.

Update: Transmission of HIV infection during an invasive dental procedure - Florida, MMWR 40(2), 1991.

Vittecoq D et al: Acute HIV infection after acupuncture treatments, NEJM 320 (4): 250-251, 1989.

Weiss SH et al: Analysis of reported HIV transmission in a dental practice, Ninth International Conference on AIDS, Berlin, abstract PO-A11-0186, 1993.

Blood transfusions and blood products

HIV transmission through blood transfusions

As of June 2005, 440 HIV infections had been identified in the UK as a consequence of blood/tissue transfer. Those infected through blood transfusions have been identified in the following ways:

- After a donor of blood was subsequently discovered to be HIV-positive and recipients of infected blood were traced

- After testing HIV-positive and where no other risk exists

- Upon the development of symptoms of HIV infection - either seroconversion illness or severe immunodeficiency.

Blood donations in the UK have been screened for HIV antibodies since October 1985 and people in high risk groups for AIDS have been requested to refrain from giving blood since 1983. Unlike Factor VIII, which is extracted from blood, whole blood for transfusion is not heat-treated.

Only two cases of HIV infection by blood transfusion were reported in the UK between 1985 and 1997, but two further cases were reported in 1997 by the Communicable Disease Surveillance Centre. They were traced to one donor who had given blood prior to seroconversion.

There have been 57 cases of patients testing positive whose risk factor was blood or tissue transfer between June 1999 and June 2005, but all of these patients acquired their HIV from blood transfusions abroad.

Rate of infection from HIV-infected transfusions

Not all recipients of HIV-infected blood seroconvert. A 1989 study of 220 recipients of blood from HIV-positive donors found that 85 were HIV-negative. Those who seroconverted were more likely to have received large quantities of blood and/or to have received blood from a donor who subsequently developed AIDS less than two and half years after giving blood.

Those who progressed to AIDS within seven years of the transfusion were more likely to have received large quantities of blood when transfused, and to have been more severely ill (measured by length of stay in hospital). After seven years 49% of the recipients of infected blood were estimated to have progressed to AIDS. Those who had received blood from donors who developed AIDS within two and half years of giving blood were more likely to have developed AIDS within four years than those who didn't (Ward).

Transfusing your own blood

In order to protect themselves against HIV infection, some people choose to have their own blood used in transfusions, a practice known as an autologous transfusion. This practice is becoming increasingly common in the United States and some European countries, and patients often say that it makes them worry less about the chance of HIV infection.

In fact, autologous transfusions are more important as a source of protection against other more common infections transmitted by transfusions which cause post-operative complications, such as CMV. Such transfusions also reduce the stress placed on the immune system by a transfusion of foreign proteins, so they may benefit people with HIV too. An infusion of foreign blood proteins can activate the immune system and boost HIV replication and infection of new cells. Unfortunately blood may not always be suitable for autologous transfusion; some people may be too weak or anaemic to benefit from autologous transfusions.

Blood transfusions abroad

In certain other countries infection through blood transfusion is a much higher risk.

The most up-to-date and reliable information about the risks of blood transfusion abroad is likely to be available from:

- MASTA at the London School of Hygiene and Tropical Medicine (0891-224100)

- The Foreign and Commonwealth Office Consular Department's Travel Office (020 7270 3000)

- If you are employed abroad, from your employer.

The UK NGO AIDS Consortium has published a manual for employment by voluntary organisations working abroad which includes material for employees.

References

Ward JW: The natural history of transfusion-associated infection with human immunodeficiency virus: factors influencing the rate of progression to disease, NEJM 321(14): 947-952, 1989.

Blood products

Awareness of people with clotting or bleeding conditions (i.e. Haemophilia) has existed for 2,000 years. It was not, however, until the early part of this century, that bleeding disorders were classified as haemophilia A or B (Christmas Disease) and Von Willibrand's disease (VW). VW can affect either men or women. Haemophilia A and B affect only men, although women carry the haemophilia gene, which will affect half their male offspring.

All three conditions are produced by an inability to produce a protein which causes blood to clot after an injury. The condition has varying degrees of severity. Some people with haemophilia only bleed after a severe injury, but some people will bleed very easily, even after a minor knock and many of these bleeds are internal. Bleeds in joints are particularly disabling as eventually the joints will seize up, causing severe arthritis. Many people with haemophilia have been disabled for some time and, even before the advent of HIV, 35% were receiving state benefits.

In the 1970s doctors started replacing the deficient protein (Factor VIII in haemophilia A and VW and Factor IX in haemophilia B) with blood products or factor concentrates. Such small quantities of protein are present in blood that donations from up to 30,000 people had to be pooled to produce one batch. The results of infusion with concentrates were excellent, and by the mid 1970s people with haemophilia were injecting themselves with Factor VIII at home with the onset of a bleed.

However these transfusions were often contaminated with the hepatitis B and hepatitis C viruses. By the late 1970s 100% of people with Haemophilia treated with pooled Factor VIII had come into contact with these viruses. The problem was blamed on imported Factor VIII and in 1977 the British government pledged to become independent in blood supplies.

The risk of HIV infection for haemophiliacs

Infections amongst haemophiliacs in the United States began as early as 1978, which explains why haemophiliac cases emerged so swiftly after the first cases in gay men. The first haemophiliacs were infected at the same time as the first wave of gay men in large cities like San Francisco. AIDS cases amongst haemophiliacs were never clustered in one area however, because Factor VIII concentrates were produced with blood from thousands of donors.

Studies have shown that those haemophiliacs who received the largest quantities of non heat-treated blood (invariably those suffering from more severe forms of haemophilia) were more likely to have been infected with HIV. Age was less significant than the quantity of clotting factor received (Gjerset). A small study amongst haemophiliacs in the UK has shown that immune suppression prior to being treated with a batch of HIV-infected Factor VIII increased the likelihood that an individual would be infected (Madhok). Subsequent studies have shown that a highly purified form of Factor VIII produced with the aid of monoclonal antibodies seems to reduce the level of immunological abnormalities (De Biasi).

Some commentators have interpreted these findings as proof that HIV does not cause AIDS in haemophiliacs, and that the syndrome is a consequence of the immunosuppressive effects of Factor VIII therapy. They argue that HIV antibodies correlate only with the highest level of exposure to Factor VIII.

This view is refuted by epidemiological study of HIV infection and AIDS amongst European haemophiliacs (Kroner). Clear differences can be observed in HIV prevalence and subsequent diagnoses of AIDS between haemophiliacs exposed to Factor VIII derived from United States donors and European donors. In Germany and Austria for instance, a large number of seroconversions are estimated to have occurred as a consequence of the continued use of US derived plasma throughout 1983. Furthermore, the introduction of heat treatment has eliminated the risk of HIV infection; there have been no recorded seroconversions in individuals seronegative up until the time that heat treatment was introduced, apart from the recipients of one batch of Factor VIII recalled by a manufacturer following the discovery that the clotting factor had been inadequately heat-treated.

Furthermore, a study of British haemophiliacs has shown that HIV-positive haemophiliacs followed between 1979 and 1992 had a tenfold greater chance of death than their HIV-negative counterparts, and the excess of deaths in the HIV-positive group was accounted for by AIDS-related illnesses and various forms of liver disease (Darby).

Claims that a large proportion of French haemophiliacs were infected whilst the French authorities used up stocks of non heat-treated Factor VIII are probably incorrect however; a 1994 study estimates that 93.2% of those French haemophiliacs who seroconverted had done so by the time this dispute began (Kroner).

The subsequent incidence of AIDS amongst HIV-positive haemophiliacs raises questions concerning the likelihood that AIDS will develop amongst this group. After having been infected for twelve years, haemophiliacs are less likely to have developed AIDS than those in other risk groups. There may be a number of explanations for this:

- it has been shown that treatment with very high purity Factor VIII slows or halts CD4 decline in several studies of HIV-positive haemophiliacs (de Biasi).

- age at seroconversion is a strongly associated with disease progression and survival: men with haemophilia in the UK under 15 at seroconversion are significantly more likely to be alive after twelve years than men with haemophilia aged 55 or over at seroconversion.

- It may also be the case that co-factors which affect other groups such as sexually transmitted infections or drug injecting are absent in this group.

The UK response to contamination of Factor VIII

In 1984 testing for HIV became available. By the end of June 2005, 1362 of the estimated 5,000 British people with haemophilia had been infected. This represents about one quarter of the entire haemophilia community. However, up to 60% of those with severe haemophilia had been infected.

At the end of 1984 all American Factor VIII had been heat treated to clear it of viruses. Britain followed suit in 1985, after which all people with haemophilia, regardless of HIV antibody status, should have been treated with heat treated product.

How safe is Factor VIII now?

Blood donations are routinely tested for HIV, and blood products are treated to destroy known viral contaminants.

Heat treatment has to be carried out carefully on account of the fragility of the Factor VIII molecule. Time has shown that heat treatment effectively eliminates HIV from blood products.

In 1984 an international committee stated there was a 'lack of uniformity and rational methodological approach of clinical evaluation' and since then, more useful studies have been conducted. British factor VIII is lyophilised (freeze dried - like coffee) and then heat-treated. A study of patients receiving this found none to be infected with hepatitis C - which was used as a marker for viral infection.

A more definitive test was done on German Factor VIII, which is pasteurised, and of 155 people with haemophilia given this, none were found to have become infected with HIV.

More modern technologies involving monoclonal antibodies or ion exchange chromatography have rendered blood products as safe as current scientific knowledge permits.

By 1989 the UK was largely self-sufficient in voluntarily donated heat treated product. Although 20% of product is still imported (by clinical choice) from international pharmaceutical companies, these concentrates are manufactured primarily from paid donors, but are tested and/or treated before use in the UK.

The risks of having been infected

The risk of having been infected with HIV for haemophiliacs is related to:

- Whether you received contaminated blood product concentrate; this is less likely after 1985 or before that date if you only received single donor agents like cryoprecipitate; your Haemophilia Centre should have a record of this.

- Whether you ever shared needles with someone who had HIV.

- Whether you have had unsafe sex with someone who has HIV.

References

De Biasi R et al: The impact of a very high purity factor VIII concentrate on the immune system of human immunodeficiency virus-infected haemophiliacs: a randomized, prospective, two-year comparison with an intermediate purity concentrate, Blood 78(8): 1919-1922, 1991.

Chelucci C et al: PCR analysis of HIV-1 sequences and differential immunological features in seronegative and seropositive haemophiliacs, Br J Haematology 81: 558-567, 1992.

Cuthbert RJ et al: Immunological studies in HIV seronegative haemophiliacs: relationships to blood product therapy, Br J Haematology 80: 364-369, 1992.

Gjerset GF et al: Treatment type and amount influenced human immunodeficiency virus seroprevalence of patients with congenital bleeding disorders, Blood 78(6): 1623-1627, 1991.

Kroner BL et al: HIV-1 infection among persons with haemophilia in the United States and Western Europe, 1978-1990, JAIDS 7: 279-286, 1994.

Ludlam CA et al: Human lymphotropic virus type III (HTLV-III) infection in seronegative haemophiliacs after transfusion of Factor VIII, Lancet 8449: 233-236, 1985.

Madhok R et al: Impaired cell mediated immunity in haemophilia in the absence of infection with human immunodeficiency virus, BMJ 293: 978-980, 1986.

Mother-to-baby transmission

Transmission routes

Transmission from mother to baby is known to occur in three ways:

- During pregnancy - the foetus is infected by HIV (in the mother's blood) crossing the placenta.

- During delivery - the infant is infected by HIV in the mother's cervical secretions or blood during childbirth.

- During breastfeeding - the infant is infected by HIV in the mother's breast milk or blood during breastfeeding.

The relative proportion of transmission occurring at these times is not yet clear, and may vary in different parts of the world.

How likely is mother-to-baby transmission?

The proportion of babies infected during pregnancy, delivery and breast feeding is not yet clear. Any congenital or infectious condition is not passed on at every occasion. In industrialised countries, overall estimates of the risks of HIV transmission from mother to child (in the absence of any preventative intervention) are about 15-20%: that is, roughly a one in seven to one in five chance.

Rates of up to 40% have been recorded from some studies in Africa, in other words double the European rates.

A 1995 review of 13 studies (Working Group on Mother-To-Child Transmission of HIV) found that the overall infection rate in Africa varied from 13% to 42%, and in the developed world from 14% to 25%.

A study of breastfeeding in Malawi (Miotti) found that the cumulative transmission rate due to breast feeding was 10.3% by 23 months of age, with a cumulative infection rate while breastfeeding, from month 1 to the end of months 5, 11, 17, and 23, of 3.5%, 7.0%, 8.9%, and 10.3%, respectively. This suggests that a quarter to a half of all mother-to-baby infections occur after birth.

It is important to bear in mind that these figures have been drawn from studies using differing methods. One explanation for the variation in rates between countries may be that different risk factors are found in different countries. For instance, women are more likely to breastfeed in Africa, (despite the transmission risk, because the alternative may prevent even greater health risks), than women in Europe or the USA. The lowest rates of transmission (14%) have been recorded amongst mothers in Europe (European Collaborative Study). In this study most of the women were asymptomatic and did not breastfeed, and as such were likely to record lower rates of HIV transmission. As is discussed later in this chapter, a range of medical interventions have been effective in reducing transmission rates dramatically, so that by 2000, policymakers in the developed world routinely talk about the 'elimination' of this form of HIV transmission.

What factors increase the chance of transmission from mother to baby?

Transmission of any infectious matter (including HIV) depends upon three factors:

- How infectious it is.

- How efficient the route of transmission is.

- How vulnerable the potential 'recipient' is.

Factors which increase the likelihood of transmission of HIV from mother to baby include:

- high viral load or low CD4 count.

- older age of mother.

- smoking during pregnancy.

- frequent unprotected sex or use of illicit drugs during pregnancy.

- no anti-HIV therapy during pregnancy or delivery.

- premature delivery.

- waters breaking more than four hours before delivery.

- prolonged or difficult labour, particularly in comparison to a planned caesarean section, which has been found to have a protective effect in women who receive no anti-HIV treatment, or who take AZT as a single treatment.

- cervical or vaginal infection (e.g. bacterial vaginosis).

- inflammation of the membranes which separate the foetus from the mother at the time of birth (chorioamniontitis).

- breastfeeding.

Pregnancy

HIV transmission during pregnancy is known to occur because:

- Terminated pre-term foetuses up to 14 weeks old have been found to be HIV-infected.

- PCR tests in the first days of life show that some infants have HIV, suggesting that they were infected in utero.

- Some infants develop HIV-related illness in the first months of life, suggesting that they were already infected in utero. However, this may have more to do with viral load and dose, rather than timing.

Can the risk be reduced?

The chance of HIV transmission increases if:

- the mother has more advanced HIV disease.

- mothers who have already experienced one AIDS-defining illness are more likely to transmit HIV to their babies.

- high viral load, especially during labour and delivery. A mother with high viral load is more likely to transmit HIV, and transmission is most likely to occur during labour and delivery. However, though transmission is rare in mothers with very low or undetectable viral load, which is one of the key reasons for using anti-HIV treatment during pregnancy, it does still occur.

- unprotected sexual intercourse during pregnancy. Women who had unprotected intercourse on at least eighty occasions (an average frequency of once every four days) had a four times greater chance of delivering an HIV-positive baby when all other risk factors (including an HIV-positive partner) were controlled for, according to a study which looked at children born in New York between 1986 and 1994.

- illicit drug use during pregnancy. The biological relationship between illicit drug use and mother- to-baby transmission is not understood, but a study of 525 women in the US showed that women who used heroin, methadone, crack or cocaine during pregnancy were almost twice as likely to transmit HIV to their babies when all other factors were controlled for (Landesman).

- low birth weight baby. Infants with a birth weight below 2.5 kg (five and half pounds) were almost twice as likely to be HIV-positive when all other factors were controlled for. This effect was seen in low birth weight babies born to mothers who did not use illicit drugs and who did not have AIDS. This association has also been seen in three other studies (Landesman).

It is difficult for studies to estimate the true likely risk of HIV infection from mother to baby if the mother is infected at the time of conception or during pregnancy, since it is difficult to locate and follow a group of just-infected pregnant women. It is possible that the higher rates of mother-to-baby transmission recorded in Africa are, in part, related to these factors.

HIV-positive women who wish to become pregnant, may be advised to choose to conceive at a time when viral load is likely to be low, or easily controlled by anti-HIV therapy. It should be stressed however, that all HIV-positive women retain the right to make their own choices about fertility and childbirth, regardless of their health, and can expect support from their doctors and health care workers in this regard.

Childbirth

HIV transmission during delivery is known to occur because:

- PCR tests on some infants have only become positive between one and three months after birth, suggesting that they were infected at delivery.

- Premature babies (earlier than 34 weeks gestation) have a significantly higher chance of being infected. As the baby's mucosa are very fine at this stage, it is suggested that they are highly susceptible to infection during delivery.

- Infants who are HIV-negative by PCR testing are frequently shown to have HIV DNA in their mouths and stomachs, indicating that they were probably exposed to the virus during delivery.

- A study of twins delivered to HIV-positive mothers has shown that the second twin to be delivered is less likely to be infected, especially where both were delivered vaginally. This could be related to the first twin having more prolonged contact with the mother's cervical secretions and blood.

- Prolonged rupture of membranes prior to delivery appears to be a risk factor. If the mother's waters break more than 24 hours before delivery the risk of HIV transmission is greatly increased. However, there does not appear to be a great difference in transmission risk between women whose membranes rupture less than 24 hours prior to delivery and those whose membranes rupture less than four hours prior to delivery (Landesman).

Can the risks be reduced?

The effects of antiretroviral therapy at the time of delivery are discussed in *Reducing the risk* below.

A review of 8,533 births in Europe and North America established that the risk of transmission was reduced from 7.3% to 2% by the use of a planned caesarean section before the rupture of membranes and onset of labour. The rate of transmission was reduced by 87% in women who received antiretroviral therapy plus elective caesarean delivery compared to women who delivered in other ways and had no therapy (International Perinatal Group). A Swiss population study also found caesarean sections reduced transmission (Kind).

In the French Perinatal Cohort, combined use of AZT and caesarean section before the onset of labour reduced the transmission rate to just 0.8% compared with 6.6% in women on AZT who had vaginal deliveries. However, this study reported that mode of delivery did not affect the rate of transmission among women not on anti-HIV therapy (Mandelbrot).

Preliminary data from a European randomised trial showed an 11% transmission rate for vaginal births, 3% for elective caesarean births and 4% for emergency caesarean births (Semprini 1998). The French study found a higher rate of transmission among the emergency caesarean group.

In 1999, results from the European Mode of Delivery Collaborative study reported reduced rates of transmission amongst women delivering by elective caesarean section than by vaginal delivery or emergency caesarean. In this study, the majority of women received antiretroviral treatment so it's not possible to say that the benefit conferred by this mode of delivery would necessarily be observed amongst untreated women. 436 pregnant HIV-positive women were randomised to deliver their infant by either elective caesarean section at 38 weeks of pregnancy or by vaginal delivery. Infection status was confirmed for 370 infants. 3 of 170 (1.8%) born to women assigned elective c-section, and 21 of 200 (10.5%) born to women assigned vaginal delivery were HIV-infected - a reduction in the rate of transmission of 80%.

Complications following delivery were uncommon, and there were no serious adverse events in either group. The women in the trial did not breastfeed. 69.7% of women allocated elective c-section took antiretroviral therapy during pregnancy (mostly AZT according to the 076 protocol), and 58.2% of women were allocated to vaginal delivery. One of 119 (0.8%) babies delivered by elective c-section to treated mothers was infected. Maternal CD4 count was evenly distributed between the two groups, and the lower rate of transmission associated with elective caesarean delivery was observed consistently across each CD4 count stratum (Parrazini).

Elective caesareans for all?

Though the strength of these data is unquestioned by many clinicians who work with mothers and children, there is some disagreement over whether they support the use of elective caesarean delivery for all pregnancies in HIV-positive women. A leading US commentator, Dr Lisa Frenkel, has proposed that c-sections may be unnecessary in women who have a good virological response to treatment.

In the ACTG 185 study which evaluated the use of AZT plus HIV hyperimmune globulin in pregnancy, there were no HIV transmissions amongst 48 women who had viral load below 500 copies (Lambert). In two other US studies, there were no transmissions observed in 89 and 73 women receiving HAART in pregnancy (Morris, Stek). However, it should be noted that these studies were not designed to investigate the role of elective caesareans in HIV mother-to-baby transmission.

An earlier meta-analysis of 1,115 mother-infant pairs found maternal viral load to be predictive of transmission, particularly so in untreated women. 696 of the women who participated were untreated, and 419 were treated. The rates of transmission for the untreated women whose viral load was below 1,000 copies was 5%; 15% for viral load between 1,000 and 9,999 copies; and 37% for viral load over 10,000 copies. Rates in treated women were 5%, 7% and 18% respectively (Contopoulos-Ioannidis).

Analysis of 373 mother-infant pairs enrolled in the European Collaborative Study similarly found that transmission rates rose with increasing maternal viral load levels, but that there was no threshold below which transmission did not occur. The majority of women in this study were untreated, though 21% received AZT. Delivery was by elective caesarean in 25%, by emergency caesarean in 8% and 62% gave birth by vaginal delivery. Overall, elective caesarean was associated with a 79% decrease in transmission, and delivery before 37 weeks doubled the risk compared with later delivery. In a subgroup analysis, women with higher viral load were less likely to transmit if they delivered by elective caesarean rather than other methods. In women with lower viral loads, the benefit did not reach significance however, perhaps because of the small sample size; only two of sixteen infected children in this group were delivered by elective caesarean section. Hence although this study confirms the relationship between maternal viral load and risk of transmission, it adds little to the continuing debate about mode of delivery in women whose viral load is maximally suppressed by combination therapy (European Collaborative Study).

It has been argued that across-the-board elective caesarean delivery may expose some women to an increased risk of postnatal complications. In an analysis of postnatal morbidity in 1,112 women in the US Women and Infants Transmission Study, researchers found an overall rate of 19% in women who had elective caesareans. Infectious morbidity rates (due to endometritis, urinary tract infections and wound infections) were 11% with elective caesareans, 21% in non-elective caesareans, 8% in women with vaginal forceps delivery, and 4% in vaginal delivery without use of instruments (Read 1999).

Similarly, in an analysis of 497 women from ACTG 185, infectious morbidity rates were 26% with elective caesarean; 40% in non-elective caesarean; 19% with assisted vaginal deliveries; and 13% with spontaneous vaginal delivery (Watts).

Following the publication of the findings of the European Mode of Delivery Collaboration in *the Lancet* in 1999, these issues were debated in correspondence published in the June 26, 1999 issue (Lancet 353(9171), 1999). Similar discussion also featured in correspondence to the July 15, 1999 issue of the *New England Journal of Medicine* (NEJM 341(3), 1999), and in an editorial in the May 26, 1999 issue of the *Journal of the American Medical Association* (JAMA 281:1946-1949, 1999).

For more on the rates of mother-to-baby transmission in the UK, see **Epidemiology**.

References

Contopoulos-Ioannidis DG et al. Maternal cell-free viremia in the natural history of perinatal HIV-1 transmission: a meta-analysis. Journal of Acquired Immune Deficiency Syndrome and Human Retrovirology 18(2): 126-135, 1998.

European Collaborative Study. Maternal viral load and vertical transmission of HIV-1: an important factor but not the only one. AIDS 13(11): 1377-1385, 1999.

The International Perinatal HIV Group. The mode of delivery and the risk of vertical transmission of human immunodeficiency virus type 1 - a meta-analysis of 15 prospective cohort studies. NEJM 340(13): 977-987, 1999.

Lambert J et al. Risk factors for perinatal HIV transmission in women/infants receiving standard zidovudine (ZDV) prophylaxis. Twelfth World AIDS Conference, Geneva, abstract 232265, 1998.

Mandelbrot L et al. Perinatal HIV-1 transmission, interaction between zidovudine prophylaxis and mode of delivery in the French perinatal cohort. JAMA 280: 55-60, 1998.

Mandelbrot L et al. Frequent detection of HIV-1 in the gastric aspirates of neonates born to HIV-infected mothers . AIDS 13(15): 2143-2149, 1999.

Miotti PG et al. HIV Transmission Through Breastfeeding: A Study in Malawi. JAMA 282, 744-749, 1999.

Morris A et al. A review of protease inhibitors (PI) use in 89 pregnancies. Sixth Conference on Retroviruses and Opportunistic Infections, Chicago, abstract 686, 1999.

Parrazini F for The European Mode of Delivery Collaboration. Elective caesarean-section versus vaginal delivery in prevention of vertical HIV-1 transmission: a randomised clinical trial. Lancet 353: 1035-1039, 1999.

Read J et al. Mode of delivery and postpartum morbidity among HIV-infected women: The women and infants transmission study (WITS). Sixth Conference on Retroviruses and Opportunistic Infections, Chicago, abstract 683, 1999.

Semprini AE et al. An international randomised trial of mode of delivery in HIV infected women. Twelfth World AIDS Conference, Geneva, abstract 23599, 1998.

Stek A et al. Maternal and infant outcomes with highly active antiretroviral therapy during pregnancy. Sixth Conference on Retroviruses and Opportunistic Infections, Chicago, abstract 687, 1999.

Watts H et al. Complications according to mode of delivery among HIV-positive women with CD4 counts <500. Sixth Conference on Retroviruses and Opportunistic Infections, Chicago, abstract 684, 1999.

Working Group on Mother-To-Child Transmission of HIV. Rates of mother-to-child transmission of HIV-1 in Africa, America, and Europe: results from 13 perinatal studies.J Acquir Immune Defic Syndr Hum Retrovirol. 15 (8): 506-510. 1995.

Breastfeeding

HIV transmission throughbreastfeeding is believed to occur because:

- HIV has been found in breast milk, and especially in colostrum.

- Transmission has been reported both in individual cases and in prospective studies.

- Infants' oral and gastro-intestinal mucosa are significantly more vulnerable than adults' and their immunity is less well developed.

- Blood, as well as breast milk may transmit the virus if the nipples are cracked or bleeding.

Researchers have suggested that there is a very high likelihood of transmission when the mother first becomes HIV-infected whilst breastfeeding (Van de Perre). In this situation, the risk of transmission from mother-to-child has been estimated to be about 30% (Dunn).

The breastfeeding and HIV International Transmission Study, which analysed data from over 5,000 children found that over a period of 6.8 months of breastfeeding, the best estimate is that a little over a third (36%) of infections were due to breas-feeding. As the overall infection rate was 25%, this suggests that 9%-10% of infants will be infected with HIV from seven months of breastfeeding.

Information from a number of studies (including the European Collaborative Study) has been used to estimate that the additional risk of transmission through breastfeeding for mothers who were already HIV-positive during pregnancy is an extra 14%.

Longer-term follow-up of mother-infant pairs involved in the African PETRA study has highlighted the potential for breastfeeding to undo the benefit which may be gained through the use of anti-HIV therapy. PETRA found that a short AZT/3TC regimen could reduce perinatal transmission, but within two years of birth, the risk of of HIV infection in infants exposed to treatment was no different than in untreated children - the treated children had effectively 'caught up' through the ongoing risk posed by exposure to breast milk (Gray).

Factors thought to increase the risk

A number of factors are thought likely to influence the chances of infection:

- Infection of the mother during the period of breastfeeding, resulting in temporarily higher levels of HIV in breast milk.

- The vulnerability of the child's oral and gastrointestinal mucosa and consequently their lesser immune function.

- Mixed-feeding practices where breast milk is supplemented by water, fluids, cereals, juices, etc.

Can the risks be reduced?

The risk of transmitting HIV through breastfeeding will be eliminated if the mother does not breastfeed. This includes not putting the baby to the breast immediately after delivery.

It must be remembered that in some countries where safe water is not available, the risk of other life-threatening conditions from formula feeding may be far higher and more immediate than the risk of HIV from breastfeeding. The high cost of formula may also be prohibitive, and in many societies, formula-feeding is stigmatised and may identify women as HIV-positive.

Whether or not to breastfeed

This decision should be made on the basis of local circumstances.

In the UK the Department of Health recommends that it is 'prudent' not to breastfeed, and has also issued instructions concerning the donation of breastmilk. Women who wish to donate breastmilk should follow the same self-exclusion criteria as for blood donors, and breastmilk banks are advised to pasteurise all donations by heating.

For women in countries where there is unsafe water and formula-feeding is therefore dangerous, the benefits of breastfeeding are, however, likely to outweigh the risks. Factors to consider include the following:

- Other forms of feeding can introduce other infections into the child's body.

- Breast milk contains immunoglobulin A, which hinders infection by viruses and micro-organisms through the walls of the gut.

- Maternal antibodies contained in breastmilk protect the child against many common infections.

- Breastfeeding may be psychologically satisfying to both child and mother, and a convenient and cheap source of nourishment.

However, these concerns must be balanced against the negative impact that breastfeeding may have on maternal health. A large Kenyan study found that breastfeeding women were three times more likely to die in the two years following delivery than women who formula fed their infant. Maternal mortality necessarily impacts on infant mortality - in this study, infants whose mother died during the period of follow-up were themselves eight times more likely to die consequently (Nduati).

A study involving women in Durban, South Africa, found an increased transmission risk associated with mixed-feeding - the use of supplementary liquids in addition to breast milk, compared to exclusive breastfeeding. It is suggested that mixed- feeding may have exposed babies to both allergens, causing inflammation and damage to gut mucosal barriers, and HIV, which in turn led to a higher infection rate (Coutsoudis 2000).

These data present health care workers with a significant challenge. Mixed-feeding is a very common practice in resource-poor nations. Only 26% of the women in the Durban study who chose to exclusively breastfeed their infants did so. A separate study involving women in rural Kwazulu Natal similarly found exclusive breastfeeding of very young infants to be uncommon. Of 124 infants followed for the first 16 weeks of life, 46% received supplementary fluid within the first 48 hours. 69% of mothers of these infants described a concern that their baby was unsatisfied as the reason for this. By 16 weeks, only 5% of babies were exclusively breastfed (Bland).

The 2005 Retrovirus Conference heard that the 'Mashi' trial, whose name means 'milk' in Tswana, included a phase which randomised babies to receive either formula feed, or breastfeeding plus AZT, up to seven months of age. All of the babies were given AZT until they were one month old.

There was little difference in the ultimate fate of the children in this trial. By the age of 18 months, 14% of formula-fed and 16% of breastfed babies were HIV-positive, including those who had HIV at birth.

However at seven months, when AZT was stopped, there was a larger difference, with 6% of formula-fed babies being positive, and 9% of those breastfed.

Set against this were higher mortality rates in the formula-fed babies. Nine per cent of formula-fed babies had died by eight months as opposed to 5% of breastfed babies. However by 18 months the 'mortality and morbidity' rates were similar: 14% in formula-fed and 16% in breastfed babies.

The original study design had also randomised mother / baby pairs to receive nevirapine or placebo at birth. The drug was given to the mothers during labour and to the infants no more than three days after birth.

This increased the difference between formula feeding and breastfeeding, with a 3% difference between breast and formula feeding in the placebo arm, but a 12% advantage to formula feeding by seven months in the nevirapine arm. Only 3% of babies given both formula feed and nevirapine were HIV-positive by seven months. This advantage disappeared during the second phase of the trial when all babies, but only half of the mothers received nevirapine. This seems to argue for continued measures to reduce the viral load in breast milk, especially in the immediate post-natal period.

One encouraging finding was that mothers were adherent to formula feeding. Only 9% of these mothers said they had sometimes breast-fed, despite 75% of trial participants having no mains electricity, 69% no fridge, and 45% no source of water on their premises. Formula-feeding mothers reported giving 95% of AZT doses to their babies, and breastfeeding mothers 86%. In contrast only 18% of women in the breastfeeding arm said they exclusively breast-fed up to 18 months and only 50% to seven months.

There was further bad news about breastfeeding at the 2007 Fourteenth Conference on Retroviruses and Opportunistic Infections in Los Angeles. The wisdom of advising mothers with HIV in resource-limited settings to avoid breastfeeding - or to abruptly wean their infants sooner than they normally would - in order to keep from transmitting HIV to their infants was called into question by several studies.

There was a report about last year's outbreak of diarrhoea among formula-fed infants in Botswana and more than one discussion of implications for infant feeding policy.

In addition, new reports from Malawi, Uganda and Kenya each documented that when HIV-exposed babies are weaned early and abruptly, they are at a very high risk of life-threatening diarrhoeal illnesses.

One prospective randomised study, the Zambian Exclusive Breastfeeding Study (ZEBS) reported a high rate of mortality after early weaning (at four months). The study concluded that

the strategy did not improve HIV-free survival at month 24. Weaning HIV-infected children early was especially harmful - with dramatically lower survival than the HIV-infected children who continued to be breastfed.

Dr Tracey Creek, of the US Centers for Disease Control, recounted a cautionary tale of a severe outbreak in diarrhoea and increase in infant mortality that followed within a month or two of flooding. Although Botswana's piped water is usually safe, the floods likely increased the risk of contamination of the water supply. In addition, latrines overflowed and standing pools of water nearby the homes served as possible sources of infection creating an environment that would be unsafe for any baby.

But the CDC analysis showed beyond any doubt that it was those infants who were not being breastfed, who were at greatest risk of being admitted into the emergency room with severe diarrhoea. Many infants were later readmitted with marasmus and kwashiorkor - severe malnutrition syndromes virtually unheard of in Botswana. And in the region of the outbreak, infant mortality for that period increased at least 25-fold over the previous year.

Other programmes in resource-limited settings have instead opted for encouraging women to exclusively breastfeed, but as per the previous WHO/UNICEF guidance to wean HIV-exposed infants as early as possible.

However, four new studies from Malawi, Kenya, Uganda and Zambia presented at the 14th CROI found that when you stop breastfeeding, you risk an acute episode of diarrhoea and gastroenteritis.

WHO held a technical consultation in October 2006 to consider this new evidence and came up with three recommendations to update and clarify the earlier guidance:

- The most appropriate infant feeding option for an HIV-infected mother continues to depend on her individual circumstances, including her health status and local situation but should take greater consideration of the health services available and the counselling and support she is likely to receive.

- Exclusive breastfeeding is now recommended for HIV-infected for the first six months of life, unless replacement feeding is AFASS before that, and

- When replacement feeding is acceptable, feasible, affordable, sustainable and safe, avoidance of all breastfeeding by HIV-infected women is recommended.

Further evidence to support a recommendation for exclusive breastfeeding by HIV-positive mothers in resource-limited settings was published on 30 March 2007 by South African researchers in *The* Lance (Coovadia)t. They said it was time to revise the UNICEF and World Health Organization (WHO) guidelines.

The new findings from the Africa Centre for Health and Population Studies define much more clearly the risk of mother to child transmission through breastfeeding during the first months of life, and also demonstrate the differences in transmission risk between women with advanced HIV disease and those with relatively intact immune systems. They also highlight the degree of risk attached to mixed feeding during the early months of life, especially the introduction of solid food alongside breastmilk.

The mucous membrane within the intestine is thought to act as an effective barrier to HIV infection. Breastmilk ordinarily strengthens and protects this lining. Exclusive breastfeeding is also associated with fewer breast health problems such as mastitis and breast abscesses, both of which can increase the amount of the HIV virus in the mother's breastmilk. It is unclear why adding solids may be particularly hazardous, though previous research has suggested that the larger, more complex proteins found in solid foods may lead to greater damage to the lining of the stomach, allowing the virus to pass through the gut wall.

The study recruited 1,372 HIV-positive pregnant women and 1345 HIV-negative pregnant women in KwaZulu-Natal, South Africa, and assessed feeding practices and the HIV status of their infants during six months follow-up after delivery.

Eighty-two per cent of HIV-positive mothers started exclusive breastfeeding, 7.9% replacement feeding and 2.5% started feeding with a mixture of breastfeeding and other fluids. All women were counselled on infant feeding in their homes three or four times during the first two weeks after delivery, and every two weeks subsequently until the infant was six months old. Mothers kept diaries on infant feeding and health. Complete feeding data for the first six months of life were available for 1,276 infants.

Exclusive breastfeeding was defined as breastfeeding only, but mothers were counted in this group if they had engaged in mixed feeding with liquids for a total of less than four separate or continuous days during the study. Giving porridge or any solid food on any occasion was counted as mixed feeding. Replacement feeding was defined as feeding that excluded breastmilk entirely, but could include mixed feeding, while mixed breastfeeding was defined as breastfeeding while giving other liquids or solid foods.

HIV testing using a viral load test was carried out on infants at four to eight weeks of age and again at 20-26 weeks of age. Fifteen per cent were infected at four to eight weeks (n=998) (presumably infected during pregnancy or delivery) and 21.6% at week 20-26 (n=962).

Among those infants exclusively breastfed who were HIV PCR-negative at week 6, the transmission rate through breastfeeding during the first six months of life was estimated at 4.04% (confidence interval 2.29 - 5.76%).

However when the transmission rate according to the mode of feeding was analysed, the risk of HIV transmission to infants who were initially breastfed but subsequently began to receive solids alongside breast milk (n=203) was nearly eleven times higher than among infants who were exclusively breastfed (hazard ratio 10.87, CI 1.51 - 78.0, p=0.018).

Infants who received both breast and formula milk at week 14 were twice as likely to become infected as infants given breast milk alone (HR 1.82, CI 1.07 - 3.06, p=0.057). In comparison infants who received only fluids in addition to breast milk were not at significantly greater risk of becoming infected with HIV by month 6 (HR 1.56, p=0.308).

Infants who were exclusively breastfed were significantly less likely to die by month 6 than those that received replacement feeding (6.1% vs 15.1%, HR 2.06, CI 1.00 - 4.27, p=0.051).

Multivariate analysis showed that the risk of transmission to exclusively breastfed infants was strongly influenced by the mother's immune status, likely representing a surrogate for virus levels in breast milk. Compared with infants born to mothers with a CD4 count above 500 cells/mm^3, infants born to mothers with a CD4 cell count between 200 and 500 were 2.2 times more likely to acquire HIV or die (CI 1.63-3.18, p<0.001), and infants born to mothers with CD4 cell counts below 200 were almost four times more likely to acquire HIV or die (CI 2.63 - 5.98, p<0.001).

Low birth weight (<2.5kg), prolonged labour (>12 hours duration after rupture of membranes) and caesarean section were also associated with decreased HIV-free survival.

The study shows, in contrast to large studies in South Africa and Zimbabwe, that with intensive community-based support it is possible for the vast majority of women to sustain exclusive breastfeeding for six months, even using a very stringent definition, say the authors.

The study also confirms that exclusive breastfeeding during the first six months of life carries much less risk of HIV transmission than mixed feeding.

Future guidelines on infant feeding will need to balance the well-established finding of an accumulating risk of HIV transmission with greater duration of breastfeeding against the mortality risk of weaning a child too early, a conflict which this study cannot shed light on.

"The key policy implication of the findings is that we provide definitive data showing that early introduction of solid foods and animal milks increases HIV transmission risks compared to exclusive breastfeeding," conclude the researchers,

"These data together with evidence of being able to successfully support exclusive breastfeeding in HIV-infected women warrant revision of the current UNICEF/WHO/UNAIDS infant feeding guidelines that were last revised in 2000. The need for this review is reinforced by the reported limitations of free formula milk and recent WHO recommendations for the provision of HAART to pregnant women with CD4 counts lower than 200 cells/mm^3."

References

Bland RM et al. Longitudinal infant feeding study: constraints to exclusive breast feeding. 13th International Conference on AIDS, Durban, abstract WeOrC497, 2000.

Bulterys M et al: Detection of HIV-1 in Breast Milk, Eighth International Conference on AIDS, Amsterdam, abstract ThC 1524, 1992.

Coovadia H et al. Mother-to-child transmission of HIV-1 infection during exclusive breastfeeding: the first six months of life. The Lancet, March 31 2007.

Coutsoudis A. Method of feeding and transmission of HIV-1 from mothers to children by 15 months of age: Prospective cohort study from Durban. 13th International Conference on AIDS, abstract LbOr6, Durban, 2000.

Creek T. A Large Outbreak of Diarrhea among Non-breastfed Children in Botswana, 2006--Implications for HIV Prevention Strategies and Child Health (http://www.retroconference.org/2007/Abstracts/30582.htm). 14th Conference on Retroviruses and Opportunistic Infections, Los Angeles, abstract 9, 2007.

Dunn et al: AIDS 7: 1064-1066, 1994.

Dunn DT et al: Risk of HIV-1 transmission through breast feeding, The Lancet 340: 585-588, 1992.

European Collaborative Study: Children born to women with HIV-1 infection: natural history and risk of transmission, Lancet 339: 1007-1212, 1992

Gray G et al. The PETRA study: early and late efficacy of three short ZDV/3TC combination regimens to prevent mother-to-child transmission of HIV-1. 13th International Conference on AIDS, Durban, abstract LbOr5, 2000.

Landesman S et al. Obstetrical factors and the transmission of HIV from mother to child, NEJM 334:25: 1617-1623, 1996.

Nduati R et al. Impact of breastfeeding on maternal mortality among HIV-1 infected women: results of a randomised clinical trial. 13th International Conference on AIDS, Durban, abstract WeOrC495, 2000.

Newell M et al: HIV-1 infection in mothers and babies. AIDS Care 2(3) 205-211.

Palmer G: Breast-feeding: the debate, WorldAIDS, Nov 1992.

Read JS et al. Breastfeeding and late postnatal transmission of HIV-1: an individual patient data met-analysis (Breastfeeding and HIV International Transmission Study). XIV International AIDS Conference, Barcelona, abstract TuOrB1177, 2002.

Sperling RS et al: Maternal viral load, zidovudine treatment and the risk of transmission of HIV type 1 from mother to infant, NEJM 335(22): 1621-1629, 1996.

Thior I et al. Breastfeeding with 6 months of infant zidovudine prophylaxis versus formula feeding for reducing postnatal HIV transmission and infant mortality: a randomized trial in Southern Africa. Twelfth Conference on Retroviruses and Opportunistic Infections, Boston, abstract 75LB, 2005.

Van De Perre P et al: Postnatal transmission of human immunodeficiency virus from mother to infant - a prospective cohort study in Kigali, Rwanda, NEJM 325 (9): 593-598, 1991.

Ziegler JB et al: Postnatal transmission of AIDS - associated retrovirus from mother to infant, Lancet i: 896-898, 1985.

Reducing viral load during pregnancy and delivery

How do antiretrovirals reduce transmission?

A woman with a high viral load appears more likely to transmit HIV to her baby, although a small proportion of women with very low or even undetectable viral load still transmit HIV to their infants. One way in which ARVs may work is by lowering maternal viral load.

ARVs may also reduce the risk of mother-to-baby transmission by reducing levels of virus in cervical and vaginal fluid.

It is estimated that up to 70% of mother-to-baby infections occur during the last weeks of pregnancy and during delivery.

However, there is also evidence that infection can occur as early as 8 weeks, and that up to a third of infections may occur during the second trimester (three to six months pregnancy). Current clinical practice is to avoid use of drugs during the first trimester unless the mother is already on treatment. In these circumstances it is feared that stopping and starting treatment, with its attendant risk of a rise in viral load, may actually increase the risk of transmission.

It is also likely that the treatment received by the new-born child during the first few weeks of life plays a substantial role. It could be acting like post exposure prophylaxis among healthcare workers who prick themselves on an HIV-exposed needle; the prompt use of ARVs after such accidents has been shown to reduce the risk of the worker becoming infected with HIV by 79%.

Real world impact since 1993

ARV use during pregnancy appears to have had a very significant impact on mother-to-baby transmission in countries where its use has been widely adopted. In France there has been a two-thirds reduction in mother-to-baby transmission since the adoption of a policy of offering maternal AZT treatment in 1994. In the US state of North Carolina researchers found that perinatal transmission declined from 21% of infants born to HIV-positive mothers in 1993 to 6.2% in the first half of 1996. During the same period the proportion of HIV-positive mothers who took AZT during pregnancy rose from 18% to 89%.

Three African studies bring transmission rate down to four per cent

Three trials of various regimens of nevirapine plus NRTIs to prevent mother-to-baby transmission of HIV presented at the 12th Retrovirus Conference in Boston in 2005 brought the infection rate among newborn babies in Africa down to below 5%.

The three presenters each finished their presentation with the declaration that "this is the lowest vertical transmission rate so far seen in Africa" - but the accolade actually went to the last presentation, the Mashi trial in Botswana, which achieved a transmission rate of 4%.

During questions after the presentations, Professor Charles Gilks of the World Health Organization said that in the light of the new data the WHO would convene a special meeting to discuss whether to modify guidelines for the prevention of mother-to-baby transmission of HIV. This was widely interpreted as a promise to reconsider its endorsement of nevirapine monotherapy.

The studies were as follows:

DREAM

A study in the Italy/Mozambique research collaboration DREAM (Palombi) provided the most comprehensive antiretroviral regime, giving mothers nevirapine plus either AZT/3TC or d4T/3TC from the 25th week of pregnancy or 60 days pre-delivery to six months post-delivery. Babies were not given ARVs. A total of 778 women were offered and completed taking the protocol. There was an overall rate of transmission at birth of 4.1% but a marked disparity between AZT and d4T regimens, which achieved transmission rates of 3.7% and 11.1% respectively. No explanation was offered for this discrepancy.

A total of 1.4% of babies were infected through breastfeeding in the first month and 0.6% after that leading to an overall transmission rate of 6.1%.

A total of 3% of women experienced grade four liver toxicity but there were no nevirapine-related deaths. Twenty women were selected for resistance testing and three (15%) turned out to have nevirapine resistance mutations.

DITRAME

The French DITRAME+ study (Chaix) in the Côte d'Ivoire gave 329 women AZT and 3TC from 32 weeks of pregnancy to three days after giving birth. During labour they were given a single dose of nevirapine and an extra dose of AZT/3TC. Babies received AZT for seven days after birth and a single dose of nevirapine two days after birth.

The transmission rate six weeks after birth was 4.7%. Viral load in the women who transmitted HIV was at that point 145,000 and their CD4 count 293; in the non-transmitting woman viral load was 28,000 and CD4 count 416.

This study made intensive investigations into drug resistance, genotyping the HIV of every transmitting woman and a third of the non-transmitters. One non-transmitting woman had nevirapine and 3TC resistance mutations and three transmitting women had the 3TC M184V mutation alone. One infected baby had nevirapine resistance and three had M184V even though babies were not given 3TC.

MASHI

The Botswana 'Mashi' study (Shapiro) was a complex randomised placebo controlled study giving AZT and nevirapine in various combinations to mothers and babies, combined with breastfeeding interventions, which are reported above (Thior).

Furthermore a third of the way through recruitment the protocol was changed. Originally the trial gave all mothers AZT from 34 weeks to delivery, and to the babies from birth to one month. It then randomised participants to single-dose nevirapine to the mother in labour and to the baby less than three days after birth, or a nevirapine placebo to both. The nevirapine placebo was judged unethical due to protocol revisions, and the revised protocol gave nevirapine to all babies as soon as possible (an average of 24 minutes) after birth, though half of the mothers still got nevirapine placebo.

During the first study period there were 485 births. The transmission rates at birth were 3.7% to babies given nevirapine and 4.5% to babies given placebo. A month after birth these rates had risen to 5.3 and 6.25% respectively.

During the second study period there were 694 births. The transmission rates at birth were 2.3% for mother/baby pairs who both received nevirapine and 3.8% where the mother received a placebo, rising to 3.7 and 4.3% respectively a month after birth.

During the second study period HAART became available and 71 of the 694 women involved took it. The overall transmission rate at birth over the entire study was 4%.

A resistance substudy found that 44% of women given nevirapine developed resistance mutations. This compares with 1.1% of women in the DITRAME+ study. Researchers were at a loss to explain how providing women with a 'tail' of three days' AZT/3TC after giving birth had cut the resistance rate forty-fold, knowing that nevirapine has a longer half-life than this in many women (Shapiro).

...but 50% of HIV-positive mothers giving birth in east London still have detectable viral loads

The real-world difficulties of achieving viral undetectability in mothers and therefore bringing intrapartum and peripartum HIV transmission down to no more than 2%, even in the UK, was underlined by a study presented at the Eighth Glasgow International Congress on Drug Therapy in HIV Infection in 2006 (Forbes).

The study revealed that during 2004-6 nearly half of HIV-positive pregnant women at one east London hospital give birth with a viral load over 50, and over one in seven with a viral load over 1000. The presenters, from the Greenway HIV Clinic at Newham University Hospital, commented that "the number of women delivering with a detectable viral load is a concern"

They attributed failure to achieve undetectable viral loads in the mother and minimise the HIV risk to the baby in part to late presentation and "the difficult socio-economic conditions many of these women experience."

There were 95 pregnancies in 84 women attending the Greenway Centre between March 2004 and March 2006, resulting in 88 live births, four miscarriages and three terminations. Of the women, 87% were from sub-Saharan Africa.

Fifty-six per cent of women knew they had HIV before they conceived, 41% did not and in 3% of cases it is not known if they knew. Of the women who knew they had HIV, half were already taking antiretroviral treatment.

Three-quarters of the women who were unaware of their HIV status were diagnosed in the second trimester (months three to six) of pregnancy and most of the rest in the third trimester but one was found to have HIV during labour, one did not volunteer her HIV status to the obstetrician despite being a Greenway patient, and in at least two other cases medical records are unclear about whether the women's status was known.

One-third of newly-diagnosed patients and nearly half of diagnosed patients took AZT monotherapy to prevent mother-to-child transmission, but this became a much less favoured treatment option over time. Of 59 women where the antiretroviral regimen was known, over half had AZT monotherapy in 2004 but only one (7.7%) had it in 2006. By 2006 the predominant ARV regime taken was protease-inhibitor-based HAART; this was given to a quarter of women in 2004 but two-thirds of women in 2006. Non-nucleoside-based regimens increased slightly from 20% to 30% of the total treatments.

Although the BHIVA pregnancy guidelines (published 2005) say that elective caesarean delivery is no longer necessary and vaginal delivery can be used with reasonable precautions, caesareans continued to be the primary mode of delivery. Elective and emergency caesareans declined from 91% of deliveries in 2004 to 75% of deliveries in 2006.

The maternal HIV viral load at delivery was available for 73 out of 88 live births. The mother's viral load was over 50 in 34 of these (47%) and over 1000 in 10 of these (14% or over one in seven).

Intravenous AZT was given to these women during delivery, although as the authors point out there is no data on the efficacy of this in reducing mother-to-child transmission.

Of the 34 mothers with viral loads over 50, five had vaginal delivery, eight emergency caesareans and 21 elective caesareans; 22 had intravenous AZT, two did not and no AZT information was available for the other eight.

Of the subset of 10 mothers with viral loads over 1000, all but one had caesareans (five emergency and four elective), six had intravenous AZT, one did not and no AZT information was available for the other three. One woman was diagnosed at the onset of labour and one presented in premature labour at 24 weeks and did not tell A&E staff she had HIV.

Why did so many women have detectable HIV at the time they gave birth? The authors suggest three reasons. Firstly, it takes longer to suppress HIV with protease-inhibitor-based regimens than with NNRTIs; secondly, with increased use of HAART there has also come an increased incidence of premature labour and hence of emergency caesareans and unplanned vaginal deliveries; and thirdly many women book into antenatal care very late and are therefore diagnosed very late, in part, the authors imply, due to fears about being entitled to care in the United Kingdom.

The use of anti-HIV treatment to prevent mother-to-baby transmission

AZT monotherapy

In the age of highly active antiretroviral therapy, some people have questioned whether AZT monotherapy is the best treatment option for mother and baby. Both UK and US guidelines recommend that a woman's health status should determine treatment. Only if a pregnant woman has a high CD4 count and low viral load, and does not require treatment for her own disease, should AZT monotherapy be considered.

One major concern about using AZT alone is that it is sub-optimal treatment for the mother herself, who may be at increased risk of developing resistance to the drug. In the ACTG 076 trial, however, few women developed resistance. Moreover, only one mother out of seven who transmitted HIV despite receiving AZT showed any signs of AZT-resistant HIV strains.

However, AZT-resistant HIV can be transmitted from mother-to-baby: a study in New York found that AZT-resistant virus was transmitted to two out of six infants born to mothers who themselves had AZT resistance. It is also possible for mothers to pass on drug-resistant variants of HIV to their children which are present only at a very low level in the virus population. In contrast, combinations of anti-HIV drugs reduce the chance of drug resistance developing, as well as having a more potent effect on viral load.

Using AZT alone may not be effective in reducing mother-to-baby transmission among women who have already taken AZT prior to conception. A review of all the women treated with AZT during pregnancy in France showed that 20% of the AZT-experienced mothers transmitted HIV to their children, compared with 5% of the AZT-naive mothers, even when all other factors (such as CD4 count and viral load) were taken into account.

Despite concerns about the effects of AZT monotherapy, fear of possible toxic effects of anti-HIV drugs means that some paediatricians remain unwilling to recommend multi-drug therapy to all HIV-positive pregnant women, whom are themselves often naturally concerned to strike a balance between risks and benefits when choosing treatment, and antenatal care options.

Ultra short course AZT

An ultra-short AZT regimen is just as effective as the longer AZT regimen used in resource-poor countries to prevent mother-to-child transmission, according to a Zimbabwean study presented at the Fourteenth World AIDS Conference in Barcelona in 2002.

By implication, the ultra-short course regimen may also be as effective as the single dose nevirapine regimen being implemented or advocated in many resource-poor countries, since the nevirapine regimen was originally tested against the same multiple dose AZT regimen used as the control arm in this study.

The investigators found that the AZT short-course regimen was just as effective as the AZT short course regimen previously validated by a placebo controlled study in Thailand. The Thai regimen used AZT twice daily from week 36 of pregnancy until birth, with AZT dosed three hourly during labour, and no AZT for the infant.

The ultra-short course regimen consisted of 300mg of zidovudine (AZT) every three hours during labour for the mother, while the infant received an AZT capsule dissolved in 30cc of water that had been boiled to sterilise it, divided into two hourly doses over the first three days of life.

The study randomised 222 women and infant pairs to receive either the Thai regimen or AZT during delivery, and both investigators and patients were blinded to which regimen they were receiving.

Data were available on the HIV status of 179 infants six weeks after birth The study found an 18.9% transmission rate in the Thai regimen arm versus a 15.7% transmission rate in the ultra short course AZT arm. Infant HIV status was established using viral load testing (Nuclisens, Organon Teknika) on dried blood spots.

At six weeks, 4.1% of infants were lost to follow-up, and at six months the lost to follow-up rate was 6.2%, a rate which compares favourably with other studies of interventions to prevent mother-to-child transmission carried out in Africa.

Michael Silverman of Health Canada, one of the study investigators, revealed that the study results suggested that it was possible to reduce the price of treatment to prevent mother-to-child transmission still further.

"This regimen costs $4 per mother paying full price for AZT, without any price reductions, compared to $6 for nevirapine."

However, resource-limited countries are currently offered nevirapine free by Boehringer-Ingelheim, so cost may not be the major attraction of this approach to preventing mother-to-child transmission if such programmes become more widespread. However, where nevirapine is not available free, AZT could be used in the way studied in Zimbabwe, and could be affordable for many families (especially if generic AZT is available).

The effect on the mother's future treatment options is also likely to make this approach attractive, at least in the short to medium term until triple therapy is available during pregnancy for mothers.

"The regimen reduces the risk of compromising the mother's future treatment options because the mother is exposed to AZT for such a short period, so there is less risk of resistance", said Michael Silverman.

In the Petra study, mothers who developed resistance did so after a week or more of AZT treatment, and in the 012 study women were effectively receiving a week of nevirapine monotherapy from one dose of the drug due to the long half-life of the drug.

The regimen is also easier to administer, said Michael Silverman, because it can be given when mothers attend the local hospital, does not require intravenous treatment of the child and does not require the use of a paediatric formulation that would be more expensive and require refrigeration. It is also more discreet when administered at home.

The study was conducted at the Salvation Army Howard Hospital in a rural area 80km north of Harare, the capital of Zimbabwe.

Nevirapine

Research in Uganda established that a single dose of nevirapine taken by the mother at the time of delivery and by the infant at delivery resulted in a lower transmission rate than a week of AZT, plus AZT for the infant (Owor). However, whilst this cheap and simple regimen may have a dramatic impact in the world's poorer nations, there is evidence that resistance can emerge even with such short exposure to the drug.

At the Fifteenth International AIDS Conference in Bangkok a Thai study showed that 41% of women exposed to nevirapine had evidence of resistance to the drug a median of 12 days after delivery, and multiple resistance mutations were associated with higher viral load (p<0.001). Subsequent studies have shown even higher resistance rates.

Given that drugs in the NNRTI class are a staple part of HAART therapy, women with access to anti-HIV therapy would not be advised to use nevirapine in this way, for fear of losing the chance to benefit from other similar drugs - resistance to nevirapine produces resistance to all other drugs in that class. A more detailed discussion of this study can be found in *Anti-HIV therapy: Options during pregnancy* at aidsmap.com.

Combination therapy & HAART during pregnancy

Observational cohort studies suggests that combination therapy does reduce mother-to-baby transmission of HIV, and that PI-containing HAART combinations are more effective than simpler regimens, although the extent of the reduction is yet to be fully determined (Blattner). Given that AZT monotherapy plus delivery by planned caesrean section has been shown to reduce transmission rates to as low as 2%, demonstrating a reduction from this level is challenging. Indeed, a US study found that the addition of nevirapine to a stable HAART regimen at the time of delivery had no clinical benefits and was likely to produce nevirapine resistance mutations (Cunningham). Detecting differences of say 1% would require very large numbers of women to take part in trials. Indeed, a large international study, ACTG 316, was abandoned in the summer of 2000 after an interim analysis found that given the very low transmission rate overall, any difference between protocol arms would likely be impossible to detect.

Combination therapy is now more widely used by pregnant women with HIV; however, AZT is the only drug formally cleared for use in pregnancy. Whether combinations of anti-HIV drugs are safe for use during pregnancy is not yet proven.

The choice of drugs for an HIV-positive woman who is pregnant will, in part, depend on the potential side-effects of the drugs for the woman. For example, one of the side-effects associated with indinavir is hyperbilirubinaemia, which is potentially more serious in pregnant women and may lead to complications. On the other hand, all of the protease inhibitors carry the risk of nausea during the first months of treatment, which may in any case be intense during the first 12 to 14 weeks of pregnancy.

Treatment in the early weeks of pregnancy

During the first 14 weeks of pregnancy, the foetus is most vulnerable to any toxic effects of drugs. Taking anti-HIV drugs during this time may increase the risk of birth abnormalities, although there is very little data on the effects of anti-retrovirals early in pregnancy. Some women on treatment at the time of conception choose to interrupt therapy for the first three months of pregnancy due to concerns about the possible toxic effects of drugs. However, recent American guidelines recommended that pregnant women should continue their treatment uninterrupted throughout their pregnancy.

Some experts have argued that the rebound in viral load which occurs when a person stops anti-HIV therapy, may in fact increase the risk of mother-to-baby transmission. It is worth noting that any of the toxicities associated with beginning a new treatment regimen may have to be endured all over again, because the body may no longer be adjusted to particular blood levels of the drugs.

Multivitamin supplementation during pregnancy

A study conducted in Tanzania has demonstrated that HIV-positive mothers who receive a multivitamin supplement have much less risk of bearing low birth weight babies, severely premature and/or small birth weight babies (Fawzi).

The study also found that women who received the multivitamin had substantial increases in CD4 and CD8 counts which were sustained for at least seven months after stopping multivitamin treatment. Although CD4 counts rose in all groups during pregnancy as expected, the multivitamin group had CD4 increases which remained more than 50 cells higher than the placebo group 7 months after ceasing treatment. Vitamin A alone was not associated with significant benefit.

The significance of these results is unclear for Europe and North America, because they may represent an improvement in nutrient status to the level normally seen in Europe and North America, so there may be no justification for supplementing at this level if dietary intake is adequate. Further supplementation may not result in a corresponding improvement in immune status.

The supplement used in the study contained 20mg of vitamin B1, 20mg of vitamin B2, 25mg of vitamin B6, 100mg of niacin, 50mg of B12, 500mg of vitamin C, 30mg of vitamin E and 0.8mg of folic acid, 30mg of beta carotene, 5,000 IU of vitamin A, 120mg of iron and 5mg of folate.

Safety issues

The frequency of adverse reactions to AZT in either mother or baby was very low during the ACTG 076 trial, and there is no current evidence that AZT leads to the development of birth defects in the doses used to prevent perinatal transmission. However, controversy persists about the possible long-term effects of anti-HIV drugs on children exposed in the womb, during birth or in the first weeks of life.

There has been surprisingly little research done on the teratogenicity of HIV drugs (their potential to cause birth defects). Efavirenz is not given to pregnant women, or certainly not in the first trimester, because in an animal study, of thirteen pregnant monkeys treated with efavirenz in doses comparable to those used in humans, three had progeny with serious birth defects, including a cleft palate and small eyes. One was born without a brain and missing one eye. However equivalent studies have not been done on some other drugs.

In a study presented to the 3rd IAS Conference in 2005 (Ekouevi), 24.7% of babies born to mothers receiving HAART throughout pregnancy had low birth weight compared with 1.5% of those whose mothers received a short-course AZT (or AZT/3TC) plus single-dose-nevirapine PMTCT regimen.

Research is conflicting regarding the use of combination therapy during pregnancy. There is some evidence that protease inhibitors increase the risk of premature delivery or of stillbirth. This was recently contradicted, however, by a US study involving over 2000 HIV-positive pregnant women found that there was no increased risk of premature delivery or stillbirth from using HAART combination containing a protease inhibitor. However the study did find that there was a risk associated with protease inhibitors of having a low birth weight baby (Tuomala).

Evidence has also emerged which suggests that irrespective of treatment, the infants of HIV-positive mothers may have an increased risk of heart irregularities. Investigators found that the babies of HIV-positive mothers had a faster heart beat and decreased left ventricle functioning, meaning that they were unable to efficiently pump oxygenated blood around their bodies. In HIV-positive babies such cardiac irregularities have been associated with an increased risk of heart failure and death. However, the heart irregularities in the HIV-negative babies of

HIV-positive mothers tended to be milder and improve over time (Lipshultz).

The long-term effects of antiretroviral drugs on children exposed during pregnancy, birth or the first weeks of life can only be assessed on a short-term basis. To date, however, children exposed to AZT during pregnancy show no evidence of an increased risk of cancers, development abnormalities or other problems.

Laboratory safety evidence

Experiments have shown no effects on the growth rates of rat foetuses exposed to AZT or to AZT/ddI combination therapy. However, rats exposed to AZT/ddC combination therapy did show evidence of retarded growth which was dose-related: the higher the dose and the longer it was taken for, the greater the growth retardation. It's important to note that this study did not simulate the effect of giving antiretroviral treatment only during the later stages of pregnancy. Birth defects related to drug treatment are most likely if the foetus is exposed to a mutagenic substance (one that induces birth defects) during the first 14 weeks of pregnancy.

Birth defects have not been observed in rats exposed to d4T, nor 3TC. Protease inhibitor studies are still not complete, but there is an indication that rats exposed to ritonavir during pregnancy gave birth to smaller litters with lower birth weights. Rats exposed to indinavir in the womb had a greater likelihood of being born with extra ribs.

Studies in monkeys have shown that foetal exposure to efavirenz can result in serious birth defects, and its manufacturers have already recommended that the drug should not be used during pregnancy.

References

Beckerman K et al. "Control of maternal HIV-1 disease during pregnancy". Twelfth World AIDS Conference, Geneva, abstract 12151, 1998.

Blattner W et al. Effectiveness of potent anti-retroviral therapies on reducing perinantal transmission of HIV-1. 13th International Conference on AIDS, abstract LbOr4, Durban, 9-14 July 2000.

Centers for Disease Control. "Administration of zidovudine during late pregnancy and delivery to prevent perinatal HIV transmission - Thailand, 1996-1998". Morbidity & Mortality Weekly Report 47: 151-154.

Chaix ML et al. Addition of 3 days of ZDV + 3TC postpartum to a short course of ZDV + 3TC and single-dose NVP provides low rates of NVP resistance mutations and high efficacy in preventing peripartum HIV-1 transmission: ANRS DITRAME Plus, Abidjan, Cote D'Ivoire. Twelfth Conference on Retroviruses and Opportunistic Infections, Boston, abstract 72LB, 2005.

Cunningham CK et al. Development of resistance mutations in women receiving standard antiretroviral therapy who received intrapartum nevirapine to prevent perinatal human immunodeficiency virus type 1 transmission: A substudy of pediatric AIDS clinical trials group protocol 316. Journal of Infectious Diseases, 186: 181-188, 2002

Ekouevi DK et al. Adverse pregnancy out-comes in HIV-infected women treated with HAART in Abidjan. Third IAS Conference, Rio de Janeiro, abstract TuFo0202, 2005.

Forbes KM et al. Use of antiretroviral therapy in pregnancy - how have BHIVA guidelines changed our practice? Eighth International Congress on Drug Therapy in HIV Infection, Glasgow. Abstract P382. 2006.

Le Coeur S et al. Perinatal HIV prevention trial (PHPT), Thailand: Simplified and shortened zidovudine prophylaxis regimen as efficacious as PACTG 076. 13th International Conference on AIDS, Durban, abstract LbOr3, 2000.

Lipshultz SE et al. Cardiovasular status of infants and children of women infected with HIV-1 (P2C2 HIV): a cohort study. Lancet, online edition, 18 June, 2002.

Owor M et al. The one year safety and efficacy data of the HIVNET 012 trial. 13th International Conference on AIDS, Durban, abstract LbOr1, 2000.

Palombi L et al. HAART in pregnancy: safety, effectiveness and protection from viral resistance: results from the DREAM cohort. Twelfth Conference on Retroviruses and Opportunistic Infections, Boston, abstract 67, 2005.

Shapiro R et al. Maternal single-dose nevirapine may not be needed to reduce mother to child transmission in the setting of maternal and infant zidovudine and infant single-dose nevirapine: results of a randomized clinical trial in Botswana. Twelfth Conference on Retroviruses and Opportunistic Infections, Boston, abstract 74LB, 2005.

Thistle P et al. Superiority of an ultra-short zidovudine regimen in the prevention of perinatal HIV transmission in rural Zimbabwe. Fourteenth International AIDS Conference, Barcelona, abstract MoD3680, 2002.

Tuamala RE et al Antiretroviral therapy during pregnancy and the risk of an adverse outcome. New England Journal of Medicine, 346, 24: 1863-1870, 2002.

Transmission from babies to their mothers

No convincing data exist on transmission from babies to their mothers. It was reported in 1990 that a number of women had been infected through breastfeeding babies, who themselves had been infected by the re-use of syringes to give injections in a Russian hospital.

It was suggested that the most likely route of transmission could have been through the babies' bleeding gums coming into contact with damaged tissue on the mothers' nipples. However, many researchers consider the data from this case to be unreliable.

Other risks to children

Several studies of close contact at school and between children and adults with HIV and their families and friends have established that casual transmission of HIV does not occur (Gershon, Berthier).

There is no evidence that children, no matter how roughly they play with other children, are likely to be at risk of HIV infection. One case of transmission between children has been suggested, but is inconclusive. Common sources of anxiety include:

- Biting. One case has been reported where no other route of transmission could be explained between two brothers. The authors of the report emphasise that the route of transmission is speculative, and it has since been suggested that both brothers were infected vertically. In this case the bite did not even break the child's skin, and other studies have shown no transmission where 39 bites from HIV-infected people have broken the skin (Gershon).

- Transmission through casual contact with HIV-positive adults. No known cases have been reported (see *The mechanisms of HIV transmission* earlier in this chapter).

- Exposure to large quantities of blood. One case has been reported where a child appears to have become infected after frequently sharing a bed with his HIV-positive brother, who was prone to severe nose bleeds.

- Blood-mixing or bonding. Although there are no known cases, this is a possible route of transmission best avoided by universal childhood education about the risks of a number of possible infections transmitted through shared blood.

- Scratching. There are no known cases.

- Sexual games with other children. There are no known cases, but this is a possible route of infection best avoided through sufficiently early and sufficiently frank safer sex education.

- Sexual activity. This is a likely route of infection for children and adolescents. There is no fixed age for the onset of sexual activity. As well as early consenting sexual activity, children may be vulnerable, they may be street children and/or involved in 'survival sex' for money. Again, this is a route of infection best avoided through sufficiently early and sufficiently frank safer sex education.

- Injecting equipment. There are no known cases, but this is a likely route of infection if children share equipment to inject drugs. There is a small risk of transmission through sharps injuries.

- Ear-piercing. There are no known cases, but infection could occur where the same ear-piercing equipment is used.

- Sports accidents. A potential very low risk exists in the light of a report of infection of an Italian footballer with no other known risk factors following a collision with another, HIV-positive, footballer.

Transmission of drug-resistant HIV

In the UK, the proportion of people becoming infected with HIV resistant to t least one drug increased from 8% in 1996-1997 to 16% in 2002 (previous reports that it was as high as 25% appeared to have been based on faulty methodology). However it appears since then to have gone into decline (see chart).

Resistance to nucleoside drugs increased between 1996 and 2002 from 7% to 11%, to protease inhibitors from 1% to 4%, and to non-nucleoside (NNRTI) drugs from 1% to 5%.

However in the two years following 2002, HIV drug resistance appeared to go into a decline, Overall, primary HIV drug resistance halved from

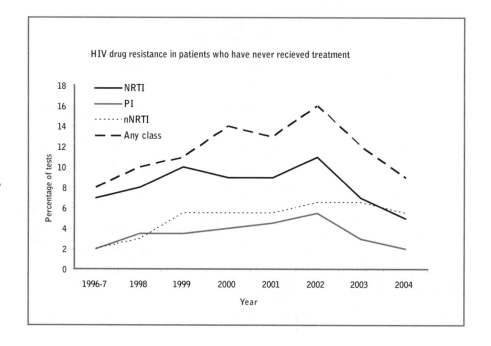

16% to 8&, NRTI resistance declined from 11% to 4%. And PI resistance from 4% to less than 2%. Only NNRTI drug resistance did not see a sharp decline, though there was a non-significant one.

This recent decline in transmitted HIV drug resistance may be a Europe-wide phenomenon.

Three studies from Europe presented to the Eighth Glasgow International Congress on Drug Therapy in HIV Infection in 2006 suggested that HIV drug resistance, especially to several drug classes, is in decline, largely due to improved treatment efficacy. However researchers and activists drew different conclusions about what this means for the future of drug development.

Jurgen Vercauteren of the Rega Institute at Leuven in Belgium analysed all 3093 HIV isolates from drug experienced patients that were included in the Portuguese Resistance Database between July 2001 and March 2006. These 3,093 samples of HIV came from 2,373 patients.

Vercauteren defined HIV with 'multi-drug resistance' (MDR) as virus whose genotype indicated susceptibility to no more than one HIV antiretroviral, with the exceptions of enfuvurtide (T-20), tipranavir and darunavir.

An approximately equal number of viral isolates was sent to the Database each year, but during the study period the proportion that were multi-drug-resistant declined from 5.7% in 2001-2 (33 out of 576 isolates) to 2.1% in 2005-6 (13 out of 490 isolates). The decline was steady, with an average 20% decrease per year, and highly statistically significant (p=0.003).

The two factors associated with having MDR virus were length of treatment (16% increase in likelihood per year on treatment) and having an uncertain date as to the start of therapy, which increased the chance of having MDR-virus nearly eightfold. This was taken as Vercauteren as being a 'surrogate marker' for having had early and suboptimal ARV treatment.

Vercauteren said that though his findings only showed that the incidence of MCR HIV had declined in one country - Portugal - he expected it to be replicated throughout Europe, telling conference delegates "it is up to you to show us that".

He said that his findings reflected the increasing efficacy of HAART and said that in the future new HIV drugs' ability to tackle MDR HIV might become less important compared with ease of use, tolerability and lack of toxicity.

Vercauteren's findings were questioned by some treatment activists. It is unlikely that in a country with the highest HIV prevalence in western Europe only 3,093 resistance tests have been performed since 2001 and the Database may not reflect reality. It is also important to note that the incidence of drug resistance is much easier to measure than its prevalence; resistance will remain archived in patients on successful HAART and may give trouble in the future, but will not show up as currently active resistance.

It is also the case that some of the drugs now increasingly used as first-line therapy, such as the boosted protease inhibitors, are chosen precisely because of a high resistance threshold and were initially designed as salvage therapies. This is still clearly a desirable attribute of any new therapy.

However Vercauteren's findings were backed up by two poster presentations on resistance, also from southern Europe.

A study from the HIV clinic at the Catholic University of Rome (Di Giambenedetto) looked at the incidence of resistance in patients tested for it between 1999 and 2005.

The number of patients treated at the clinic increased from 494 in 1999 to 1,429 in 2005, while the number with at least one viral load over 1,000 copies/ml declined during the same period from 59.5% to 9.4%.

Of these patients, the proportion genotyped for drug resistance increased from 35% in 1999 to 60% in 2005. However, because a decreasing proportion of patient had viral loads over 1,000 and could therefore be genotyped, this means that the actual number of genotypes performed declined from just over 100 in 1999 to 80 in 2005.

During this period the number of genotypes that showed any resistance mutation declined from 95% of samples to 55%, meaning that 45% of failed patients in 2005 did not fail because of drug resistance.

The percentage of treated patients regarded as having detectable viral loads due to drug resistance declined as follows:

- Any class, 57% in 1999 to 10% in 2005

- NRTI resistance, 53% in 1999 to 10% in 2005

- PI resistance, 39% in 1999 to 4% in 2005

- NNRTI resistance, 20% in 1999 to 1% in 2005.

Nearly all genotyped patients that had resistance had some nucleoside (NRTI) resistance, and this closely tracked total resistance, with 89% of genotypes showing NRTI resistance in 1999 and 50% in 2005.

The proportion of samples with resistance to non-nucleosides (NNRTIs) initially increased from 32% in 1999 to around 47% on the 2000-02 period. However it then declined to 32% in 2003-4 and 12% in 2005.

Protease inhibitor resistance showed a gentler decline from being present in 74% of samples in 2001 to 47% in 2003 and 27% in 2005.

Of note, both in terms of the total number of patients with resistance and the proportion of genotyped samples that showed evidence of resistance was the sudden and steep decline between 2004 and 2005. The proportion of genotyped samples with resistance declined from 82% in 2004 to 55% in 2005, with NRTI resistance from 81% to 50%, and NNRTI resistance from 32% to 12%.

Dr Di Giambennedeto ascribed this to changes in prescribing practice. The proportion of patients taking thymidine analogues (AZT or d4T) declined slowly from 90% in 1999 to 75% in 2005 and then suddenly to 41% in 2004.

Prescriptions for non-thymidine NRTIs (tenofovir, abacavir and ddI) increased from 22% to 49% in the same period. Non-boosted PIs were taken by 87% of patients in 1999 but declined to 16% in 2005. Concomitantly, boosted PI prescriptions increased from 1% to 71%.

Prescribing practice clearly favours boosted PIs over NNRTIs in Italy, because during the same period the proportion of patients on NNRTIs declined from 32% to 22%. This may be the reason for the generally dramatic decline in resistance, as studies from the UK, where NNRTIs are preferred for first-line therapy, indicate that although resistance in general may have undergone a modest decline, the proportion of resistance that is due to NNRTIs has increased.

A third study (Hernandez) did not look at resistance genotypes as such but did look at the 'proportion of patients with therapeutic failure susceptible to resistance testing', i.e. with viral loads over 1000. This proportion declined from 129 out of 1,201 patients in 2000 (10.7%) to 41 out of 1,204 patients in 2005 (3.4%). The proportion of failing patients who were new, i.e. experiencing first-line failure declined from around 60% of failures in 2000 to around 40% of failures in 2004-5.

Why is the transmission of drug-resistant HIV declining in Europe?

The last time this section was revised, data was only available till 2002. It therefore looked at this point as if drug-resistant HIV - as had been widely forecast - would inexorably increase as a proportion of HIV infections - a pattern seen in some parts of the world n other diseases such as TB.

There are several reasons why an increase in HIV drug resistance is not inevitable:

Firstly, studies that previously reported that up to 25% of HIV infections in the UK were drug-resistant may have been methodologically flawed. Studies of HIV drug resistance based on laboratory genotypes will always tend to overestimate resistance because resistance tests are more likely to be done on patients where resistance is already suspected - for instance, people whose source partner had drug-resistant HIV.

Secondly, HIV with drug-resistance mutations often has impaired replicative capacity compared to non-resistant 'wild type' virus and for this reason is less often transmitted, both because for this reason it tends to form a minority of differing viral strains within the source patient and because it finds it less easy to establish a new infection (is less virulent). When it is transmitted, however, the entire viral population in the recipient is drug-resistant, which means they are essentially resistant for life.

Thirdly and most importantly, however, drug resistance is not an inevitable evolutionary development in HIV: it is essentially a product of suboptimal therapy, The high levels of NRTI resistance, for instance, are partly legacies form the days of dual-NRTI therapy in the pre-HAART days. Similarly protease inhibitor resistance increased during the years when unboosted PIs were the predominant mode of therapy but are declining now most patients are taking boosted PIs, which are far less likely to produce resistance.

These improvements in treatment will also impact on the prevalence of resistance in patients who are already on HIV treatment. Firstly, as regimens improve in potency and tolerability the proportion of patients with detectable viral loads and who are infectious will go down. Secondly the proportion of patients who are failing on suboptimal therapies and therefore develop resistance will also go down. In fact resistance in patients on treatment peaked earlier, in 1999 when 80% of all drug resistance tests done on patients on treatment showed evidence of resistance. Since then resistance has gone into a less precipitous but still significant decline, to about 65%, meaning that a third of patients failing therapy due to suspected drug resistance are in fat doing so for other reasons such as poor adherence or malabsorption.

Reference

CDR weekly. HIV Drug Resistance in the United Kingdom: data to end of 2004. Vol 16 (4), 26 January 2006.

Di Giambenedetto S et al. Reduction in drug resistance prevalence in treatment-experienced patients; varied estimates according to employed methodologies in a clinical cohort study. Eighth International Congress on Drug Therapy in HIV Infection, Glasgow, abstract P212, 2006.

Hernandez B et al. Decline in the number of patients susceptible to resistance testing: 2000-2006. Eighth International Congress on Drug Therapy in HIV Infection, Glasgow, abstract P212, 2006.

Vercauteren J et al. Declining incidence of multidrug-resistant HIV-1 over time (2001-2006): which drugs do we really need? Eighth International Congress on Drug Therapy in HIV Infection, Glasgow. abstract PL5.5, 2006.

Transmission of drug-resistant HIV in resource-limited settings

Little surveillance evidence exists to date on the prevalence of drug-resistant HIV in resource-limited settings. However, the World Health Organization and the International AIDS Society have established a joint surveillance project to track prevalence of genotypic resistance in treatment-naïve people after the introduction of antiretroviral therapy in specific settings.

So far, the only such country in which resistance has been systematically studied in treatment-naive people is Brazil, where a national survey found that around 2% showed genotypic resistance to each of the three drug classes, and 8% showed resistance to at least one drug. A smaller pilot survey among 71 treatment-naive patients in Rio de Janeiro found only one case of drug resistance, associated with 3TC (Dias Tavares 2003).

Resistance in genital fluids

Resistance testing usually measures drug resistant HIV in the plasma. However, HIV also exists in lymph tissue, the genital tract and fluids, and the brain.

There is some evidence that resistance mutations in the blood plasma correlate with mutations in the lymph tissue. In contrast, there is strong evidence that resistance in the blood does not necessarily mean resistance in the genital tract. For example, a study of resistance mutations from blood and cervicovaginal lavage of two women found that response to therapy and resistance mutations differed in the two compartments (Eron 1998; Fang 1998). In addition, two men treated during primary infection had resistant virus in their blood, but undetectable virus in their semen (DePasquale 1999).

However, drug-resistant HIV has been detected in the genital tract (Hazelwood 1999). This case study confirmed that PI mutations not present in the blood may appear in the genital tract. Thus localised replication can lead to the development of resistance in the genital compartment. Whilst NRTIs such as AZT and 3TC may be present in much higher concentrations in semen than in blood (Periera 1999), PIs do not always appear to reach adequate concentrations in semen (Taylor 1999).

Transmission of drug-resistant HIV by different routes

A study of 21 recently infected injecting drug users and 56 individuals who contracted HIV through sexual activity found no difference in the rate of transmission, suggesting no difference in the transmissibility of drug-resistant viruses by blood or by sexual intercourse (Salomon 2000).

Resistance and reduced infectiousness

Although between 3 and 25% of seroconverters in countries with widespread access to antiretrovirals have contracted drug-resistant HIV, there is emerging evidence that resistant virus is less infectious. A study comparing the frequency of transmission of resistant virus with the prevalence of resistance among the HIV-positive community suggested that resistant virus has only a 25% capacity to infect others compared to wild-type virus (Leigh Brown 2003).

However, a study of eleven partner pairs carried out in San Francisco suggests that in each case where transmission of drug-resistant viruses took place, all the resistance mutations detected in the index case persisted in the infected patients (Hecht 2001).

Persistence of drug-resistant virus

A consensus appears to have emerged among HIV experts, based on a significant body of research, that resistance mutations present at the time of infection may remain present over many years in the absence of treatment. This is different to patients who develop drug resistance mutations during treatment. If these patients stop taking antiretroviral therapy, there is usually a reversion to the fittest strain of HIV in their body, the wild-type strain. However, in patients who were infected with a resistant strain, there is no wild-type strain archived in the body to become dominant, and random mutation of the virus to become wild-type is a very rare event.

Most recently, results of a large American study suggest resistance mutations persist over eight years of infection. The investigators from the Terry Beirn Community Programs for Clinical Research on AIDS (CPCRA) study team analysed the genetic make-up of HIV from 491 patients randomly selected from the Flexible Initial Retrovirus Suppressive Therapies

(FIRST) trial. None of the patients had taken any antiretroviral therapy. Their mean CD4 cell count was 269 cells/mm3 and 31% had a previous AIDS diagnosis, corresponding to an expected infection duration of seven to eight years.

Defining resistance according to the International AIDS Society 2003 guidelines, plus additional mutations at positions 215 and 69 of the reverse transcriptase enzyme, the researchers saw that 57 patients (12%) had at least one resistance mutation, and they estimated that 11% of the cohort had drug-resistant virus. The investigators estimated the prevalence of NRTI resistance mutations to be 8%. In contrast, it was 3% for NNRTIs and 1% for PIs, although only 'primary' protease mutations were included in the analysis (Novak 2005).

A British study of 14 people with primary HIV infection with a drug-resistant strain found that the vast majority of drug-resistant viruses persisted over two to 36 months follow-up (Pao 2005). Multidrug resistance in two of these cases was found to be stable for over 18 months. Key NRTI and PI mutations remained static but in two cases NNRTI mutations disappeared in the long term.

There is evidence that multidrug-resistant virus may be quite resilient when acquired through transmission. One study of six patients with multidrug resistant virus who were followed for a period of two to seven years from infection showed that the pattern of resistance mutations carried by their HIV scarcely changed. The only exception was that the M184V mutation reverted to wild type in two patients, and a viral load increase did occur associated with that reversion (Brenner 2000, 2002, 2004). Other studies have also confirmed the persistence of resistant virus, including multidrug-resistant virus, over time periods of up to seven years (Barbour 2004; Delaugerre 2003; Ravaux 2003).

Other cases of disappearance of the M184V mutation associated with 3TC resistance have been reported over six to twelve months after primary infection (Little 2004).

Despite the persistence of transmitted resistant HIV, use of genotypic testing can lead to choice of appropriate first-line treatment regimens, as recommended in current guidelines from the United Kingdom and the United States. An analysis of the international CASCADE collaboration showed that this selection of drugs results in similar outcomes in patients with and without primary resistance (Pillay 2004). However, it is possible that second- and third-line treatment options may be limited in these patients due to an exhaustion of effective drugs.

Implications for prognosis

At the Seventh International Congress on Drug Therapy in HIV Infection in 2004, Dr Mark Wainberg of McGill University AIDS Centre in Montreal, Canada, argued that the clinical consequences of infection with multidrug resistant virus were unpredictable, varying from repeated treatment failure to long-term non-progression. Low replicative capacity of multidrug resistant virus may correlate with low viral load and delayed progress, but this theory is yet to be proven.

Recent publicity given to the case of a man in New York who experienced rapid disease progression after infection with multidrug-resistant HIV. The man was diagnosed with HIV in December 2004, having previously received a negative test result in May 2003. However, he subsequently had unprotected anal sex with multiple male partners, often after taking the recreational drug methamphetamine. The man was infected with '3-DCR HIV', a strain of HIV resistant to three of the four classes of antiretroviral drugs.

However, experts discussing the case at the Twelfth Conference on Retroviruses and Opportunistic Infections in Boston in early 2005 said that this isolated case report does not indicate that the HIV strain found in this patient is aggressive, since disease progression is determined by the complex interaction between the virus and the host's genetic make-up (Markowitz 2005a,b). In addition, the probable source patient for this man's HIV strain who has recently been identified, did not experience rapid HIV

disease progression despite their viruses being over 99% identical (Blick 2005). This suggests that the host's immune response may be more important in determining the speed of progression than the virus's virulence.

The New York man had extensive genotypic resistance but phenotypic analysis of the virus revealed that it is fully susceptible to two antiretrovirals: efavirenz (*Sustiva*) and to the fusion inhibitor T-20 (enfuvirtide, *Fuzeon*), and he is currently on therapy.

In addition to the limited treatment options available to people infected with this strain of virus, two other factors suggest rapid disease progression is likely. First, despite the number of resistance mutations, this virus is able to replicate effectively, with a replication capacity by the PhenoSense assay 1.38 times greater than wild-type virus. Second, the virus is dual tropic (that is, it uses both co-receptors) and it produces 'clumping' of infected cells. This is associated with the CXCR4 co-receptor and advanced disease. Of note, the presumed source patient's virus was CCR5-tropic and less virulent, with a replicative capacity of less than half that of wild-type virus.

While coverage of high-profile case studies such as this might suggest that becoming infected with a multidrug-resistant virus spells doom, several studies suggest that infection with a resistant strain of HIV does not appear to influence the rate of disease progression nor does it mean an absence of treatment options.

Although people infected with drug-resistant virus may experience a slightly greater CD4 cell count decline in the first year after infection, a comparison with people infected with wild-type virus showed similar rates of CD4 T-cell loss thereafter in the absence of treatment (Bhaskaran 2004).

It is unclear whether unfit virus with little capacity to replicate will mean slower progression. A survey of 101 seroconverters found no evidence of a slower rate of disease progression, measured as time from estimated seroconversion date to a CD4 cell count of 350 cells/mm3 (Pillay 2002). Similar conclusions were reached in a three year follow-up of 46 Spanish seroconverters with available baseline genotypes (de Mendoza 2003). However, San Francisco researchers have produced contradictory findings to the UK Seroconverter Group. They identified 130 seroconverters diagnosed since 1996, and found that those with genotypic evidence of drug resistance or virus with reduced replication capacity had significantly higher CD4 cell counts after controlling for duration of infection (Grant 2002).

Of course, acquiring drug-resistant HIV is assumed to reduce treatment options but with resistance testing active regimens can be selected for many people in this situation. Furthermore, there is evidence that baseline resistance may also not affect the short-term efficacy of first-line antiretroviral therapy, according to data from the CASCADE study. However, experts suspect that second- and third-line therapy may be compromised by the acquisition of a drug-resistant form of HIV (Pillay 2004). Development of resistance to NRTIs and NNRTIs has been linked a greater risk of death in a large Canadian cohort followed between 1996 and 2003 (Hogg 2005).

References

Bhaskaran K et al. Do patients who are infected with drug-resistant HIV have a different CD4 cell decline after seroconversion? An exploratory analysis in the UK Register of HIV Seroconverters. AIDS 18: 1471-1473, 2004.

Blick G et al. "Patient zero": the Connecticut source of the multi-drug-resistant, dual-tropic, rapidly progressing HIV-1 strain found in NYC. Third International AIDS Society Conference on HIV Pathogenesis and Treatment, Rio de Janeiro, abstract MoOa0101, 2005.

Brenner B et al. Resistance to antiretroviral drugs in patients with primary HIV-1 infection. Investigators of the Quebec Primary Infection Study. Int J Antimicrobial Agents 16: 429-434, 2000.

Brenner BG et al. Persistence and fitness of multidrug resistant human immunodeficiency virus type 1 acquired in primary infection. J Virol 76: 1753-1761, 2002.

Delaugerre C et al. Persistence of HIV-1 multidrug resistance without any antiretroviral treatment 2 years after sexual transmission. Antivir Ther 8: S201, 2003.

DePasquale MP et al. Primary HIV infection: in vivo fitness of pre-therapy resistant mutants and potential for secondary spread of HIV from semen. Antivir Ther 4: S89, 1999.

Eron JJ et al. Resistance of HIV-1 to antiretroviral agents in blood and seminal plasma: implications for transmission. AIDS 12: F181-F189, 1998.

Fang G et al. Complete HIV pol sequence in plasma and genital tract of women: genital reservoir and differential drug resistance. 38th Interscience Conference on Antimicrobial Agents and Chemotherapy, San Diego, abstract I-122, 1998.

Hazelwood JD et al. Detection of RT and protease resistance in genital tract and plasma viruses from an HIV-infected woman receiving highly active antiretroviral triple therapy: a case report. Antivir Ther 4: S96, 1999.

Hecht FM et al. Transmission of specific antiviral resistance mutations within partner pairs. Eighth Annual Conference on Retroviruses and Opportunistic Infections, abstract 87, 2001.

Leigh Brown AJ et al. Transmission fitness of drug-resistant human immunodeficiency virus and the prevalence of resistance in the antiretroviral-treated population. J Infect Dis 187: 683-686, 2003.

Little S et al. Persistence of transmitted drug-resistant virus among subjects with primary HIV infection deferring antiretroviral therapy. Eleventh Conference on Retroviruses and Opportunistic Infections, San Francisco, abstract 36LB, 2004.

Markowitz M et al. A case of apparent recent infection with a multi-drug-resistant and dual-tropic HIV-1 in association with rapid progression to AIDS. Twelfth Conference on Retroviruses and Opportunistic Infections, Boston, abstract 973B, 2005a.

Markowitz M et al. Infection with multidrug resistant, dual-tropic HIV-1 and rapid progression to AIDS: a case report. Lancet 365: 1031-1038, 2005b.

Novak RM et al. Prevalence of antiretroviral drug resistance mutations in chronically HIV-infected, treatment-naive patients: implications for routine resistance screening before initiation of antiretroviral therapy. Clin Infect Dis 40: 468-474, 2005.

Pao D et al. Long-term persistence of primary genotypic resistance after HIV-1 seroconversion. J Acquir Immune Defic Syndr 37: 2004.

Periera A et al. Nucleoside analogues achieve high concentrations in seminal plasma: relationship between drug concentration and virus burden. J Infect Dis 180: 2039-2043, 1999.

Pillay D et al. The impact of transmitted resistance on time to CD4< 350 cells/ml. Antivir Ther 7: S147, 2002.

Pillay D et al. The effect of transmitted drug resistance on virological response to HAART regimens adjusted for genotypic resistance at baseline. Eleventh Conference on Retroviruses and Opportunistic Infections, San Francisco, abstract 685, 2004.

Ravaux I et al. Persistence in HIV-1 protease of resistance mutations in absence of drug selective pressure three years after sexual transmission of a multiclass drug resistant variant. Antivir Ther 8: S415, 2003.

Salomon H et al. Prevalence of HIV-1 resistant to antiretroviral drugs in 81 individuals newly infected by sexual contact or injecting drug use. Investigators of the Quebec Primary Infection Study. AIDS 14: F17-F23, 2000.

Taylor S et al. Poor penetration of the male genital tract by HIV-1 protease inhibitors. AIDS 13: 859-860, 1999.

Transmission: Low and 'theoretical' risks

Case reports of rare routes of transmission

There are a number of cases of transmission that have been reported which fit the known categories or modes of transmission but involve events that are extremely unusual.

Road accidents

Only one case has been reported where a blood spillage during a road accident was the source of infection (Hill). Fears about this eventuality need to be considered not only in the context of the likelihood of coming into contact with an HIV-positive person in this situation, but also the small risk of transmission from blood splashes, as established from the follow-up of health care workers exposed to blood. See *Transmission to health care workers* earlier in his chapter.

Traumatic accidents in sport

Only one case has been reported where a man was seemingly infected by another man as a result of bashing his head against another man's head during a football match (Torre). Blood was seemingly exchanged, but we cannot be certain that the man who believed he had been infected was uninfected beforehand, despite his failure to report any risk factors. Much greater risks in sport already exist, notably penetrative sex between men and the sharing of needles to inject steroids.

Contaminated blood transfusion getting through the screening system

Only two cases have been reported in the UK where HIV transmission has occurred after a blood transfusion, presumed to be negative, has been given to a patient. In both cases the blood came from the same source. This should be seen in the context of only 190 blood donations identified as HIV-positive out of 14.85 million donations during the period between the beginning of screening in 1985 and March 1991.

As long as the epidemic remains concentrated within certain core groups, it appears that the other safeguard in the blood screening system, asking people not to give blood if they perceive themselves to have been at risk, is working successfully despite early criticisms that it would not protect the blood supply.

A healthcare worker infecting patients through invasive surgical procedures

Various estimates have been produced of the risk of HIV transmission during an operation. They speculate on a wide range of levels of risk, leading to confusion.

The chances of a patient seroconverting after a one-hour operation performed by a known HIV-1 positive surgeon were estimated in 1991 to be between 1 in 28,000 and 1 in 500,000 (Lowenfels).

The US Centers for Disease Control (CDC) estimated in 1991 a risk of transmission during any invasive procedure by an HIV-positive surgeon of between 1 in 41,667 and 1 in 416,667. They also estimated that, assuming that a surgeon performs 500 procedures per year and that a surgeon's working lifetime after the acquisition of HIV infection was seven years, the risk of HIV transmission to a patient during this period ranged from 8.1% to 0.8%. They calculated that between 13 and 128 patients could have been infected during invasive procedures performed by HIV infected surgeons in the United States between 1981 and 1990 (CDC).

However, the only case yet identified is that of the Florida dentist, see above.

Biting

Several cases of HIV transmission have been attributed to biting. In one case a five year-old child infected with HIV by transfusion bit his eight year-old brother (Wahn). Infection was not detected until his death from AIDS three and a half years later. His brother was discovered to be HIV-positive. There appeared to be no other explanation for infection: the brother had not received blood and had not been sexually abused to the knowledge of his parents, but his mother had noticed a bite mark on his arm about six months before the younger child died.

In another case a man in the late stages of AIDS suffered a seizure and bit the finger of a neighbour who came to his aid. HIV antibody and antigen tests taken on the day of the incident were negative, but the man tested positive less than two months later. It is believed that the man with AIDS bit his tongue before biting his neighbour, and that blood was therefore present in his saliva (Widmar).

A third case is still under investigation. A man in Florida is believed to have been infected through multiple bites from a woman with bleeding gums. The US Centers for Disease Control have confirmed that they believe this case to be a case of blood to blood transmission, but no full report of their investigation has yet been published.

A fourth case is thought to be the first unequivocal case of HIV being spread by a human bite. The case involved a 31 year-old HIV-positive man who bit his 59 year-old mother on the hand during a seizure. The man, who had been previously unaware of his HIV status, was subsequently diagnosed with neurotoxoplamosis. Blood was present in the source patient's mouth since he had bitten his tongue and his mother's hand required stitching when she was taken to hospital.

Twenty-seven days following the incident the woman presented with fever and HIV antibody tests at that time were negative. Thirteen days later (40 days following the exposure incident) she was again tested for HIV infection by two ELISA (enzyme linked immunosorbent assay) tests, and a Western Blot test. The double ELISA testing strategy involved one sensitive and one less sensitive test and was deployed to detect recent HIV infection.

The less sensitive ELISA produced a negative result whilst the sensitive 'detuned' assay was found to be positive and this confirmed recent infection.

Researchers were also able to confirm epidemiological relatedness of the viruses infecting the individuals involved in the accident.

The authors commented "Although the possibility of transmission by human bite seems to be negligible because of the number of infecting particles and the inhibitors in saliva, cases with blood in the biter's mouth may deserve special attention".

In hospital environments, especially where healthcare workers are managing psychiatric, neurological, paediatric or combative patients this sort of exposure could be minimised by the use of gloves or arm protection.

A follow-up of thirty health care workers who cared for a patient with AIDS who bit them showed no cases of seroconversion (Tsoukas).

Fighting

Two cases of HIV transmission have been attributed to blood-to-blood contact as a result of fighting. Both these cases are open to question however.

The Queerbasher: A 49 year-old man tested HIV-positive after a 'routine' insurance screening. He was married but claimed to have been impotent for ten years and never to have had sex with another man. He admitted using intravenous drugs on one occasion but was adamant that he had used a clean needle. Following the suggestion of the doctor that he had indeed contracted HIV from needle use, the man enquired whether cuts on the hands might be a route for transmission. He said that at one time he had frequented gay cruising areas with work colleagues with the intention of beating up gay men. He had frequently sustained small lacerations on his hands, and got large amounts of his victim's blood on himself. Doctors noticed recently scabbed lacerations on his hands said to result from a recent fight (Carson).

It is not unusual for men who seek anonymous sex in cruising areas to be the same men who then beat up their sexual partners. Might the man have been lying about his sexual risk factors? We do not know because this line of questioning evidently was not pursued by the authors of this report.

The wedding brawl: A case was reported where a man was diagnosed HIV-positive following a blood donation. His only risk was identified as a fight with a man at a wedding party who was HIV-positive (O'Farrell). This case is an example of a combination approach to providing a case history, since the authors provided not only self-reported evidence, but also data from blood samples taken when the man was hospitalised for an unexplained viral syndrome approximately ten days after the fight. The blood samples taken during his hospital stay were subsequently tested for HIV, and seroconversion was shown to have occurred approximately two weeks after the onset of the illness.

However, these data do not prove that the wedding brawl was indeed the source of infection, although the timing is highly suggestive. It would be necessary to compare HIV sequences from the infected man and the intruder at the wedding.

Fighting between children

A case has been reported of a child contracting HIV from another child living in the same house and frequently sharing the same bed. The index case has a AZT-resistant strain of HIV which has subsequently been isolated in the infected child.

The children were both born to HIV-positive mothers. Child 1 was discovered to be HIV-positive and was diagnosed with AIDS at the age of eighteen months, but Child 2 was repeatedly found to be HIV-negative until acute lymphadenopathy was diagnosed. At this point sequences of HIV from Child 2 were compared with sequences from its mothers and from local HIV-positive control children. Sequences of HIV showed very strong similarities between Child 1 and Child 2, but much greater divergence when compared to the mother of Child 2 or other HIV-positive children, suggesting that Child 1 was the source of infection.

How is infection thought to have happened? Although no exposure of Child 2 to blood or body fluids of Child 1 was witnessed, there were numerous opportunities for exposure. Child 2 had an almost constant rash which was weeping or even bleeding as a result of scratching, whilst Child 1 had frequent nosebleeds and bleeding gums. Child 2 was bitten on more than one occasion by Child 1, as well as being hit so badly that he or she required stitches in the wound (Fitzgibbon). All these circumstances suggest that infection occurred as a consequence of Child 1's blood coming into contact with wounds or damaged skin on Child 2's body.

Child infected through household contact with mother

One case has been reported in which a child appears to have been infected through contact with his mother's ulcerated skin. The child had weeping skin rashes too, and it is speculated that the child may have contracted HIV as a result of close contact with his mother (MMWR Report).

Sharing razors, injecting equipment or unsafe sex

A final example should serve as a caution when examining unusual modes of transmission. A young man (Brother 1) who tested negative for HIV antibodies in 1989 and subsequently received only heat treated high purity Factor VIII had seroconverted by January 1992. His CD4 count had declined from 1,102 to 846/500 between 1985 and 1987, and had declined to 120-70 in 1992.

His brother (Brother 2) had tested positive for HIV antibodies in 1985, and had reported a possible seroconversion illness in 1983. His CD4 count ranged from 400 to 550 cells/mm3 between 1987 and 1991 to 110 cells/mm3 in 1992.

Nucleotide sequencing as used in the case of the two children discussed under *Fighting between children* above showed a strong similarity between viral isolates of Brother 1 and Brother 2. This finding suggests that the virus was transmitted from one to the other. If both brothers had been infected through Factor VIII infusions, researchers would expect to see significant differences in the virus strains carried by the two brothers. This evidence suggests that the brother who had seroconverted by 1992 had not been suffering from a long period of 'silent' infection.

Information on the route of transmission relies on self-report; the only means of transmission is said to be the sharing of a razor in 1988, over a year before the last negative test of Brother 2. Brother 2 was transfused with six units of red blood cells from seronegative donors during 1989 and 1990.

Discussion following the presentation of this report at the December 1993 First National Conference on Human Retroviruses and Related Infections centred on the possibility that the brothers had shared injecting equipment in order to self-administer Factor VIII.

The journal report evades the question of whether the virus might have been transmitted through sexual contact between the two brothers, but does note that the brothers routinely shared a bed during the period when seroconversion might have occurred (Brownstein). Transmission through the sharing of injecting equipment or sexual contact is more plausible than through the sharing of a razor.

See also *Medical and dental procedures and injuries* for discussion of further rare routes of HIV transmission.

'Theoretical' risks

Theoretical risks, such as the danger of people treading on syringes washed up on the beach, are distractions from the common routes of transmission and common dangers. In no other illness is there such constant displacement of attention from the real routes of transmission onto freak modes of transmission or minimal risks. The apparent abandonment of common sense in many people's assessment of the risks of HIV transmission suggests that fears of death, contamination and sexuality are being triggered. As if to confirm this, many people who understand the routes of HIV transmission very well nevertheless report irrational fears about HIV transmission, often in circumstances where they come into contact with people who have AIDS.

Many 'theoretical' risks emerge as sources of anxiety as a result of uncertainties about the length of time which HIV can survive outside the body. It is important to put these uncertainties in context.

Although HIV may be able to survive outside the body for several days, this has only been proved by collecting blood from needles and syringes, or else in laboratory conditions. Whilst small quantities of HIV may indeed be able to survive in syringes or needles for several days, if we correlate this finding with the evidence of the unlikelihood of transmission from needlestick injuries (in which large quantities of blood are often transferred without infection occurring), we can see why this evidence is not sufficient to justify fears about theoretical modes of transmission.

In fact, infection through blood has only occurred from needlestick injuries and blood spillages either where blood has splashed directly from the body of an infected person into open wounds or where blood stored for transfusion or laboratory research purposes has splashed into open wounds or mucous membranes such as the mouth or eyes.

Another reason why these theoretical routes are unlikely is that heat, light, cold, water and chemicals are all likely to damage the virus. Thus virus-laden syringes in the ocean or HIV in sewage are impossible routes of transmission on this score too.

Theoretical risks may also emerge as a source of anxiety because of doubts about the quantity of HIV needed to infect a person. Although virologists argue that it may only take one virus particle to infect a person, it is important to bear in mind that four factors have to be fulfilled if HIV transmission is to take place (see *The mechanisms of HIV transmission*). All 'theoretical' modes of transmission are very unlikely to fulfil these four factors.

Finally, theoretical routes of transmission may be given undue attention because of habitual public health concerns about the chances of the transmission of any infection by such a route. A good example of this is the repetition of fears about the transmission of HIV through food handling. This has been used to justify discrimination against people with HIV and gay men in catering on the 'theoretical' assumption that if someone cut his or her finger and bled into food while it is being prepared, and this food was then eaten by someone, it would constitute a risk.

References

Andreo S et al. HIV-1 transmission by human bite. Ninth Retroviruses Conference, Seattle, abstract 770-W, 2002.

Brownstein A et al: HIV transmission between two adolescent brothers with haemophilia, JAMA 271(4): 262-264, 1994.

Carson P: Gay bashing as possible risk for HIV infection, Lancet 337 (8743): 731, 1991.

CDC: Estimates of the risk of endemic transmission of Hepatitis B and HIV to patients by the percutaneous route during invasive surgical procedures, 1991.

Fitzgibbon JE: Transmission from one child to another of human immunodeficiency virus type 1 with a zidovudine-resistance mutation, NEJM 329(25): 1835-1841, 1993.

Hill DW: HIV infection following motor vehicle trauma in central Africa, JAMA 261: 282-283, 1989.

Keet IP et al: Short communication: Orogenital sex and the transmission of HIV among homosexual men, AIDS 6: 223-226, 1992.

Lowenfels AB et al: Risk of HIV transmission of HIV from surgeon to patient, NEJM 325(12): 888-889, 1992.

O' Farrell et al: Transmission of HIV-1 infection after a fight, Lancet 239: 246, 1992.

Piazza M et al: Passionate kissing and microlesions of the oral mucosa: possible role in AIDS transmission, JAMA 261(2), 1989.

Torre, D et al: Transmission of HIV-1 Infection via sports injury (Letter), Lancet 335 (8697): 1105, 1990.

Tsoukas C et al: Lack of transmission of HIV through human bites and scratches JAIDS: 1(5): 505 - 507, 1988.

Wahn V et al: Horizontal transmission of HIV between two siblings Lancet ii: 694, 1986.

Widmar L: Transmission of HIV by human bite, Lancet 347: 1762-1763, 1996.

Impossible routes of HIV transmission

The bottom line

The virus *cannot* be transmitted through

- Unbroken healthy skin, because cells vulnerable to HIV infection do not exist on the surface of the skin.

- Breathing in: (unlike the common cold, for instance, which can be spread through sneezing), because HIV cannot be airborne. It is not present in the tiny particles of moisture sneezed or coughed out of someone's mouth.

- A healthy, undamaged mouth, because cells vulnerable to HIV infection are not present in the mouth.

- Unbroken barriers, such as a latex condom or the female condom, because these barriers cannot be penetrated by HIV.

- Corneal transplants, because no blood vessels are present on the cornea.

- Mosquitoes, because although these insects suck blood, they do not regurgitate blood containing live HIV into the bodies of other victims.

- Sharing cutlery, plates or cups, because HIV cannot be transmitted in saliva.

- Over-broad and imprecise categories such as 'sex' or 'promiscuity' or 'drug abuse' are not in themselves a risk.

- Social contact with people with HIV, because HIV is not transmitted by touch or through the air

- Through animal bites, because animals do not carry HIV.

- By caring for people with HIV (but remember the guidelines on universal precautions, see *Infection control*, below).

- By association with blood (e.g. donating blood in the UK).

- By contact with small quantities of dried blood, because HIV will not be present in sufficient quantity (all infections through blood not injected or transfused have occurred where large quantities of blood splashed onto the broken skin of other people).

- Through swimming pools, showers, washing machines, because HIV will be killed by chemicals in disinfectant and detergent, or simply just washed away.

- By mouth-to-mouth resuscitation, because HIV is not present in saliva.

- By touching objects such as telephones, because HIV is not transmitted by touch.

- By using the same lavatory as people with HIV, because even if someone had bled into the lavatory, the water would immediately dilute the virus. Nor would HIV be picked up from blood on the lavatory seat.

Rarely, the virus may be transmitted through:

- The lining of the mouth if there are cuts, sores or ulcers or bleeding gums.

- The nipples, if bitten by a child with bleeding gums while breastfeeding.

- The mucous membranes in the eye, if splashed there in large quantities.

The vast majority of possible activities in life are not a risk. Sometimes people will be anxious about routes of transmission which do present a risk from other illnesses, but not HIV. So, apart from taking reassurance that these things are not a risk, it is also important to understand how transmission does occur, and why (see *The mechanisms of HIV transmission* earlier in this chapter).

Hype and misinformation

HIV/AIDS is not the only life-threatening disease; nor is it the only recently discovered infection; nor is it the only rapidly growing disease in the world; nor is it the only sexually transmitted disease. However, it has been subject to an unprecedented degree of fear, anxiety, prejudice and media hype in the modern world.

Yet, extraordinarily, although it is perfectly reasonable to be concerned about the modes of transmission of a life-threatening condition, the AIDS epidemic has been characterised by a special kind of topsy-turvyness. On the one hand, there continues to be widespread denial of its known, proven modes of transmission and, on the other hand, widespread perpetuation of theoretical, impossible, or highly unlikely modes of transmission. Why is this?

One explanation is that all this irrationalism is a consequence of pre-existing attitudes towards the particular groups of people first and most affected by HIV and AIDS: gay men, injecting drug users, and (to use an American term) 'people of color'. So by coincidence AIDS has encapsulated a number of key prejudices and fears of the modern world. This combination of a new and explosive epidemic together with homophobia, racism and other prejudices has tapped into the deepest symbolic terrors and uncertainties of our culture.

In other words, AIDS has been above all a political and cultural epidemic. A vicious circle has been created, where groundless fear has been piled upon groundless fear, and the impression has been forged that there must be grounds to all these fears because supposedly, there is 'no smoke without fire'.

Offering reassurance

It is essential for anyone seeking to provide reassurance for HIV/AIDS-related fears (no matter how groundless) to start from an understanding that facts alone (no matter how convincing) may not be enough to assuage such fears. Equally, it is important not to dismiss people with these anxieties as simply the 'worried well'. Such an approach is likely to   fail to reassure them.

What does usually work is to put those facts back into the context of the fears they came out of. A five-step guide to presenting the facts most persuasively is outlined below:

Anticipate hidden anxieties

For the cultural reasons mentioned above it is quite common to find that somebody's most important anxieties are not necessarily those they find most easy to articulate. The hidden ones (often to do with insecurities about their sexual identity) which may be at the root of their concerns may only emerge into the light of day if given sensitive encouragement by the counsellor.

Find out what they know or don't know about HIV transmission

There may be silent or implicit beliefs derived from old sources of information or from media misinformation which do not fit with and so prevent the assimilation of the new information that you are providing. Find out, then, what their sources of knowledge are, i.e. not only what they believe, but where they heard it from. This will help you pitch the tone and level of your advice and information.

Provide a basis for anticipating future anxieties

Simply giving someone the bare facts will only, at best, deal with past and existing fears. Given the number of future opportunities for coming across fresh misinformation it is much more effective in the long-term to furnish them with the tools to analyse those future situations for themselves. It doesn't do any harm at all to give examples of the kinds of misinformation or misplaced emphasis that we can predict will continue to arise in the mass media with wearying regularity.

Avoid being drawn into theoretical arguments

By definition, theoretical risks are possible in principle but highly unlikely in practice. It is better to address particular stated theoretical risks that are causing anxiety on a very practical level. For instance, if someone is concerned about the possibility of stepping on a used syringe on a beach, it may not be sufficiently reassuring to tell them that there is only a fraction of a fraction of a risk (not only is a needle-stick injury very unlikely to cause infection - a probability of less than 1% - but also any HIV there might have been will almost certainly have been diluted or degraded beyond likely infectiousness). It may be more effective to suggest practical precautions to set their mind at rest, such as wearing beach sandals. Better still, take it as an opportunity to help them re-focus upon safer sex and safer drug use since a denial of these often goes hand in hand with concern about theoretical risks.

Help put things into perspective

This can be done in two ways. One way is to encourage them to examine why they are worried about the kind of theoretical, extremely low-probability events that, in other areas of their lives don't concern them, such as the dangers of being killed by an airplane dropping on top of them out of the sky, etc. Another way is to look more closely at why AIDS means so much more to them than other much more likely threats, such as road traffic or heart disease. In other words it can be helpful to encourage them to compare their anxieties about AIDS with the general level of commitment they put into maximising their health.

Infection control

Universal precautions

The only infection control precautions which need to be taken against HIV in any job or any walk of life are the same as the usual proper standards of good infection control in that situation, known as 'universal precautions'.

HIV is known to have similar modes of transmission to hepatitis B but with one crucial difference - HIV is much less infectious than hepatitis B. Consequently, infection control procedures which protect against hepatitis B will also protect against HIV.

Universal precautions are the most effective way to ensure that the risk of HIV infection is minimised. The principle is the same as that of safer sex, where universal precautions such as condoms are far more effective at reducing risk than subjective methods such as 'choosing carefully'.

The dangers of relying upon screening

It is often suggested that the screening of patients in hospitals, the screening of health care workers, or the adoption of barrier precautions only against those identified either as HIV-positive or as identifiable members of risk groups, will prevent further cases of HIV infection. This is a fallacy for several reasons:

- It is impossible to identify everyone who is HIV-infected by HIV testing because of the 'window period' between infection and the appearance of antibodies

- It is impossible to identify everyone who is HIV infected on the basis either of questions about past behaviour or presumed membership of a 'risk group'

- It is impossible to judge the need for universal precautions on the basis of historical, retrospective knowledge about HIV prevalence in a particular area. For instance, many doctors and midwives were surprised to learn the extent of HIV prevalence amongst pregnant women in London as a result of anonymised seroprevalence studies. Although these data confirmed the extent of HIV infection amongst pregnant women, it could not have protected any health care workers at risk from blood during birth. On the other hand, universal precautions, if implemented at that time, would have protected midwives and doctors.

Universal precautions to protect patients

Even with very uneven adherence to universal precautions in the developed world, there have been only a handful of cases where a surgical procedure seems to have to led to infection (see *Transmission from dentists and dental equipment*, above). This suggests that universal precautions, coupled with the modification of working practices on the part of infected health care workers, are likely to be largely successful in protecting patients. Guidelines concerning the working practices of HIV-infected healthcare workers can be found in *Employment*.

Difficulties in adopting universal precautions

We continue to hear regular reports in the medical press of the un-systematic way in which precautions are adopted by health care workers, and the link between a failure to follow established infection control procedures and accidents which may result in occupational HIV infection. Accidents will always happen in health care settings, but the risk of accidents can be reduced by careful planning.

Universal precautions are least likely to be practised when:

- Patients are perceived to be 'low risk'.

- There is a lack of adequate time to complete procedures.

- Barrier precautions such as glove use interfere with manual dexterity.

A summary of infection control planning

Every event of occupational HIV transmission can be analysed for the purposes of prevention into five key components:

- A failure to assess risk accurately.

- A failure to identify protective procedures and supply what infection control resources (such as sharps containers and disposable equipment) are needed.

- A failure to implement effective procedures.

- A failure to evaluate working practices.

- A failure to develop procedures in the light of new information.

Consequently, avoiding infection involves preparing to avoid or minimise these risks in appropriate ways.

Accurate assessment of risks

This involves:

- Identifying real risks.

- Reassurance about groundless fears.

Identification of appropriate procedures

This involves:

- Identifying ineffective precautions such as testing.

- Identifying appropriate barriers such as gloves, goggles, etc.

- Identifying procedure specific risk reduction practices, such as goggle use in orthopaedic surgery.

- Establishment of reporting procedures for accidents in order to identify trouble spots.

- Identifying appropriate disinfection procedures. These will normally have three components: pre cleaning/decontamination so there is no visible contamination; safe disposal of sharps and other disposable materials; and chemical or heat sterilisation of re-usable instruments, materials and surfaces.

- Identifying precautions to prevent accidents, such as avoiding the practice of re-sheathing needles.

- Identifying care procedures following accidents.

A strategy for the implementation of procedures

This involves:

- A commitment to planning and implementing universal precautions by managers: this can easily be subverted through reasons of cost, difficulty of implementation and monitoring, or failure to accept the necessity of universal precautions.

- Identifying the implications for existing working practices.

- Addressing resource implications: whether or not precautions are universally observed, the introduction of equipment with the best possible safety features, such as automatic safety devices, should be part of such a programme. However it should not be seen as a substitute for procedures.

- Training for all: studies consistently show that the failure to practise universal precautions is often the result of a lack of training.

Monitoring and review

This is to ensure compulsory precautions for all situations. Even after training, there is often a failure to practise the precautions for the reasons noted above. Strict monitoring of precautions, and the support of senior staff is necessary to ensure their successful adoption.

Development

This will involve:

- Keeping up-to-date with the scientific literature.

- Regular 'refresher' courses and sessions for existing and new staff.

- Assessment and evaluation of the success of procedures.

- Infection control guidelines in developing countries.

Infection Control Guides

A short guide for employers and employees is probably the Health and Safety Executive's *Blood-borne viruses in the workplace: Guidance for employers and employees.* This can be downloaded from http://www.hse.gov.uk/pubns/indg342.pdf

A more comprehensive guide is *Protection against blood-borne infections in the workplace: HIV and hepatitis.* HMSO London: 1995. ISBN 0-11-321953-9. Price £12. This can be ordered from The Stationery Office, TSO Orders/Post Cash Dept, PO Box 29, Norwich NR3 1GN. Phone: **0870 600 5522**, email customer.services@tso.co.uk or order from the website: http://www.tsoshop.co.uk/

In the UK the most commonsense guide for health workers is the Royal College of Nursing's *Wipe it Out: Good Practice in Infection Prevention and Control.* This can be downloaded from http://www.rcn.org.uk/resources/mrsa/downloads/Wipe_it_out-Good_practice_in_infection_prevention_and_control.pdf

The British Dental Association has also issued its own infection control guide, *Infection Control in Dentistry.* This can be downloaded from http://www.udp.org.uk/resources/bda-cross-infection.pdf . Given reports that people with HIV find difficulty in obtaining treatment from dentists, it may be worthwhile quoting from this guide:

"Those with human immunodeficiency viruses (HIV), who are otherwise well, and carriers of the hepatitis viruses may be treated routinely in a primary care setting (general dental practice, community dental service, for example). The evidence indicates that, in the absence of an inoculation injury, the risk of infection to a dental health care worker during the dental treatment of HIV-infected individuals is negligible. HIV infected individuals need a high standard of dental care when they are asymptomatic to minimise dental problems. If they subsequently develop Acquired Immune Deficiency Syndrome (AIDS) it may be appropriate for them to be referred for specialist advice and care.

It is unethical to refuse dental care to those patients with a potentially infectious disease on the grounds that it could expose the dental clinician to personal risk. It is also illogical as many undiagnosed carriers of infectious diseases pass undetected through practices and clinics every day. If patients are refused treatment because they are known carriers of an infectious disease, they may not report their conditions honestly or abandon seeking treatment; both results are unacceptable. Those who reveal that they are infected are providing privileged information."

An excellent guide to infection control for workers in developing countries has been published by Healthlink Worldwide. Practical guidelines for preventing infections transmitted by blood or air in healthcare settings is available from Healthlink Worldwide, Cityside, 40 Adler Street, London, E1 1EE.

HIV survival outside the body

Questions regarding the survival of HIV are frequently raised by workers who may come into contact with spilled body fluids. Fears over the casual transmission of HIV have also led many people to be concerned over the risk of contact with spilled blood, dried blood or other body fluids, even in microscopic quantities.

It is important to bear in mind that whilst HIV may live for some time outside the body, HIV transmission has not been reported as a consequence of contact with spillages of blood, semen or other body fluids. Given the number of healthcare workers who come into contact with HIV-infected body fluids, it is reasonable to assume that infections by this route would have been detected by now if contact with small quantities of HIV in dried blood or other body fluids were possible.

Nevertheless it is important to be aware of the possible persistence of viable HIV in these fluids in order that proper infection control procedures are observed at all times.

Laboratory studies on the survival of HIV

Experiments which have looked at the survival of HIV have found that:

- HIV is sensitive to high temperatures but not to extreme cold. Experiments have shown that HIV is killed by heat, but temperatures over 60°C are needed to achieve reliable killing of HIV.

- Levels of virus remain relatively stable in blood at room temperature, and HIV may persist for at least a week in dried blood at 4°C. Blood containing HIV used for laboratory experiments is stored at -70°C without any loss of viral activity (Van Bueren; Tjotta).

- HIV may survive for up to four weeks in syringes after HIV-infected blood has been drawn up into the syringe and then flushed out (Abdala). A study of blood gathered from more than 800 syringes filled with small amounts of HIV-infected blood and stored for various periods found that HIV could be isolated from 10% of syringes after 11 days where the quantity of blood was less than 2μl, but 53% of syringes where the quantity of blood was 20μl. Longer survival of HIV was also associated with lower storage temperature (less than 4 degrees C); at higher temperatures (27-37 degrees C) survival was not detected beyond seven days.

- HIV is very sensitive to changes in alkalinity or acidity - pH level - and pH levels below 7 or above 8 are unsuitable for long-term survival of HIV. One reason why HIV transmission may be difficult in healthy women is due to the acidity of vaginal secretions (Tjotta; Voeller).

- HIV may survive in dried blood at room temperature for up to five or six days provided that the optimum pH level is maintained; drying of blood does not seem to affect the infectivity of HIV (Tjotta).

- Sewage is highly unlikely to pose a risk because infectious HIV has never been isolated from faeces or urine (ACDG). However, research by Thames Water has shown that HIV can survive for several days in sewage in the laboratory (Slade).

- HIV does not survive as long as other viruses in sea water (Slade)

- Infectious HIV has been recovered from human corpses between 11 and 16 days after death in bodies stored at the usual mortuary temperature of 2°C. It is unclear how long infectious HIV may persist in corpses left to decay at normal room temperature, but HIV has been cultured from organs stored at 20°C up to 14 days after death. HIV was not detected in significant quantities later than 16 days, implying that buried corpses or those preserved for long periods pose less of a risk to undertakers and pathologists (Anon; BMJ; Ball; Nyberg).

- No studies have investigated the survival of HIV in semen outside the body as such, but studies which have sought to culture HIV from semen in the laboratory have often found it difficult to do so, indicating the low quantities often present in semen.

These findings do not take into account factors such as the dose of virus necessary to establish infection (the tissue culture infectious dose or TCID) or the chance that the virus will reach target cells assuming that the skin is injured. Just because an individual comes into contact with tiny quantities of HIV in dried blood, it does not follow that infection will occur.

The effect of environmental conditions such as wind, rain etc. is not taken into account in these laboratory-based studies.

Concerns about contact with blood from corpses is more realistic given the quantities of blood present and the evidence for long-term survival of HIV after death. Guidelines have been produced by the Advisory Committee on Dangerous Pathogens (see *Infection Control*).

References

Abdala N et al. Survival of HIV-1 in syringes. Journal of Acquired Immune Deficiency Syndromes and Human Retrovirology 20: 73-80, 1999.

Advisory Committee on Dangerous Pathogens: HIV - the causative agent of AIDS and related conditions, Dept of Health, 1990.

Anon: BMJ report on Forensic Science International 60: 61-66 on post mortem, 1993.

Ball J et al: Long lasting viability of HIV after patient's death, Lancet 338: 63, 1991.

Nyberg M et al: Isolation of human immunodeficiency virus (HIV) at autopsy one to six days post-mortem, Am J Clin Pathol 94(4): 422-425, 1990.

Slade JS et al: The survival of human immunodeficiency virus in water, sewage and sea water, Water Science and Technology 21(3): 55-59, 1989.

Tjotta E: Survival of HIV-1 activity after disinfection, temperature and pH changes or drying, J Medical Virology 35(4): 223-227, 1991.

Van Bueren: Survival of HIV and inactivation by heat and chemical disinfectants, Eighth Int Conf AIDS, Amsterdam, abstract PoA 2401, 1992.

Voeller B: Heterosexual transmission of HIV, JAMA 267(14): 1917-1919, 1992.

First aid

There has been no known example of transmission as a result of giving or receiving first aid. The theoretical risk is very low in the context of ordinary good practice in delivering first aid.

Any theoretical risk from mouth to mouth resuscitation is extremely low indeed. But resuscitation using mouthpieces may be more effective if you are trained in their use and they are available.

The only risk would be from infected blood. But this would have to get inside your own bloodstream in order to infect you. The Red Cross has advised that 'safe handling of blood in first aid situations does not require 'space suits' or excessively high levels of protection.'

Existing standards of good practice are designed to protect both the giver and receiver of first aid from much more infectious germs than HIV.

These existing standards are also designed to protect you irrespective of who's involved. Remember, that for each person whom you know or think has HIV, there are going to be several others whom you don't know about. So relying on knowledge of peoples' antibody status is dangerously irrelevant. And it would be unethical to refuse first aid to anyone on those grounds.

Instead, the best precaution is making sure that:

- You're satisfied you've had adequate training.

- You understand the proper procedures.

- You're supplied with all the necessary infection control equipment such as disposable gloves and aprons, paper towels, bleach and other disinfectants, etc.

- You stick to the proper procedures.

- You report any incidents, problems or concerns to your supervisor or adviser.

Training in first aid is available from the British Red Cross or St John's Ambulance Brigade.

General healthcare workers' precautions

HIV is an infectious disease with a transmission pattern like that of hepatitis B.

However, it is much less infectious than hepatitis B. Consequently protection against HIV is automatically offered by 'universal precautions' against hepatitis B and other pathogens.

Most health care workers will already be familiar with these, so no extensive retraining is required.

Similar protocols are designed to protect against particular opportunistic infections, see below.

These existing protocols are designed to protect you irrespective of who is involved. Remember, that for each person whom you know or think has HIV, there are going to be several others whom you don't know about. So relying on knowledge of people's antibody status is dangerously irrelevant. And it would be unethical to refuse health care to anyone on those grounds.

Instead, the best precaution is making sure that:

- You're satisfied you've had adequate training.

- You have been immunised against hepatitis B.

- You understand the proper protocols.

- You're supplied with all the necessary infection control equipment.

- You stick to the proper protocols.

- You report any incidents, problems or concerns to your supervisor or manager.

- You take precautions against needle stick injuries and other accidents, see below.

Needlestick injuries and other accidents

The majority of needlestick injuries are reported by trainee doctors and nurses, so if you are just beginning work in the healthcare professions, make doubly sure that you receive proper training and that you understand the infection control procedures.

Why accidents happen

A US study of cases of occupational HIV infection amongst health care workers showed that the most common causes of events such as needlestick injuries and other sharps accidents were:

- Sudden or unexpected movement during a procedure.

- Improper disposal of needles or sharps.

- Recapping of needles.

Nearly half of the exposures in one study involved sharps penetrating rubber gloves (Cieselski 1993). But another survey found that the majority of needlestick injuries occurred when the needle and syringe were being prepared for disposal, often when an attempt is being made to re-cap or re-sheath the needle.

Needle type, size and depth of penetration are all determinants of the amount of blood injected; hollow bore needles tend to be the most likely to deliver large quantities of blood, and virtually all the needlestick accidents reported by Cieselski involved this type of needle. Obviously the medical procedure will determine the nature of the needle in use, but these findings may nevertheless serve as a useful rule of thumb to reassure anyone who has sustained a needlestick injury. These injuries are often described as percutaneous injuries.

Sharps injuries commonly occur during the stitching of wounds or whilst cutting tissue. They also occur frequently in situations where surgeons are operating without complete visibility - usually inside a patient (Gerberding).

It has been suggested that some basic changes in surgical practice and instrument design might significantly reduce the frequency of such injuries. These suggestions are discussed in detail in a supplement to the *Journal of Infection* published in 1991 (Raahave; Sim).

Sharps injuries appear to occur most frequently in gynaecological surgery and in heart surgery.

The frequency of such injuries in other less accident-prone forms of surgical practice is indicated by surveys of the frequency of needlestick and sharps injuries amongst orthopaedic surgeons, who have been identified as less prone than gynaecologists to such injuries. In the UK 49% of orthopaedic surgeons surveyed and in the USA 39% of orthopaedic surgeons had sustained such injuries in the previous month (Panlilio; Tokars).

Two US studies, of healthcare workers' occupational exposure to blood, showed that the majority of those exposed to blood were nurses - in one study only 19% were doctors and just 7% were laboratory personnel. This may well reflect under-reporting by doctors and medical students however. The rates of exposure amongst doctors and medical students are thought to be much higher.

Avoiding accidents

- Protect existing wounds: don't participate in invasive procedures if you have exposed lesions, cuts, chapped skin or weeping dermatitis.

- In other procedures: cover cuts and sores with waterproof plasters.

- Use disposable gloves and disposable aprons wherever appropriate.

- Wash hands to prevent the spread of infection.

- Take care in disinfection, mopping up blood and disposal of contaminated materials, see below.

- Prevent new wounds.

- Handle sharp instruments with care.

- Dispose of sharps with disposable tongs in puncture proof bins which can be clearly marked and then incinerated.

- Wear protective clothing or devices wherever recommended.

- Don't re-sheath or recap needles: about 40% of needle stick injuries occur as a result of this.

References

British Dental Association . Infection Control in Dentistry. Can be downloaded from http://www.udp.org.uk/resources/bda-cross-infection.pdf

British Medical Association: Bloodborne viruses and Infection Control: A guide for health care professionals. Harwood Academic Publishing, 1998. This is now an interactive CD-ROM costing £190.00, but is the most comprehensive guide around. ISBN 9057024047.

Cieselski C et al: Occupationally Acquired HIV Infection - United States, IX International Conference on AIDS, abstract Ws-C12-1, 1993.

Gerberding JL: AIDS and surgery: Reducing the risk, JAMA 265: 1572-1573, 1991.

Health and Safety Executive. Blood-borne viruses in the workplace: Guidance for employers and employees. Can be downloaded from http://www.hse.gov.uk/pubns/indg342.pdf

Jeffries DJ: Zidovudine after occupational exposure to HIV (editorial), BMJ 302: 1349-1350, 1991.

Panlilio AL et al: Blood contacts during surgical procedures, JAMA 265: 1788-1793, 1991.

Raahave D et al: New operative techniques to reduce surgeons' risk of HIV infection, Journal of Infection 18 Suppl A: 177-183, 1991.

Royal College of Nursing. Wipe it Out: Good Practice in Infection Prevention and Control. Can be downloaded from http://www.rcn.org.uk/resources/mrsa/downloads/Wipe_it_out-Good_practice_in_infection_prevention_and_control.pdf

Sim AJW: Towards safer surgery, Journal of Infection 18 Suppl A: 184-190, 1991.

The Stationery Office. Protection against blood-borne infections in the workplace: HIV and hepatitis.HMSO London: 1995. ISBN 0-11-321953-9. This can be ordered from The Stationery Office, TSO Orders/Post Cash Dept, PO Box 29, Norwich NR3 1GN. Phone: 0870 600 5522, email customer.services@tso.co.uk or order from the website http://www.tsoshop.co.uk/.

Tokars JI et al: Percutaneous injuries during surgical procedures, Seventh International Conference on AIDS, Florence, abstract TH D-108, 1991.

Morgan DR: Missing the point: preventing needlestick injury and exposure to HIV and other bloodborne viruses, Royal Society of Medicine AIDS Letter 42, 1994.

Guidelines for other accidents involving blood

First of all, physically wash away the contaminant:

- Blood in a cut or puncture: encourage the wound to bleed outwards by squeezing or pressing. Then wash it thoroughly with soap and water.

- Blood on the skin where there's no cut: wash with soap and water.

- Blood in the eyes: rinse while open with tap water and saline.

- Blood in the mouth: spit out, rinse with water and spit out again.

Then follow the Hepatitis B protocol, seek medical advice and report the accident.

Caring for people with specific opportunistic infections

There are rarely any extra precautions to be taken by carers and health care workers looking after people with HIV with specific opportunistic infections.

This is because, by the nature of the disease, the organisms that cause opportunistic infections such as candida, PCP, toxoplasmosis, MAI, CMV are prevalent everywhere and standard universal precautions are adequate to deal with them.

Some specific extra precautions for immunocompetent carers are probably only required in a few situations:

Herpes zoster (shingles)

If there's an attack, until the blisters or lesions settle down and dry out, people who have never had chicken pox (and especially pregnant women) should keep away. If contact has taken place protection is available in the form of immunoglobulin.

Herpes simplex

If there's an attack around the mouth kissing would be infectious at the time; if round the genitals touching could be infective, so wear gloves.

Cryptosporidiosis

The epidemiology isn't wholly understood: it could cause an acute diarrhoea-type illness in people with a normal immune system, or much more severe life-threatening illness in people with immune deficiency. The same precautions as for salmonella are advised.

'Active TB'

i.e. when coughing up TB organisms.

The chance of becoming infected with *Mycobacterium tuberculosis* if you have been in prolonged contact with someone who has active TB is approximately 50%. Prolonged contact means sharing a home, a ward or being in other close proximity for many hours. In other circumstances the chances of infection are very much lower - probably around 8-10% if you encounter TB organisms in the air. It is important to note that these risk estimates are derived from the USA, where the BCG vaccination is not given routinely at puberty, so the chances of infection in the UK are much lower for individuals who have received the BCG vaccination (it is believed to provide approximately 70% protection in immunocompetent people).   M.TB can linger on droplets in the air for several hours, so if you are caring for someone with TB and you haven't received the BCG vaccination, it is best to wear a mask.

Once treatment has begun, TB ceases to become infectious within a few weeks, and individuals can often be treated at home provided they can be relied upon to take the full course of medication. If the full course of medication is not taken the TB may relapse, with the additional danger that it will be multi-drug resistant: that is, insensitive to the commonly used cocktail of anti-TB drugs. If multi-drug resistant TB emerges it is frequently lethal, but it is not any more infectious than other strains of TB.

Unfortunately, active multi-drug resistant TB can persist for many months, and it is often difficult to determine if a patient has ceased to be infectious. For this reason people with MDR-TB are usually isolated in hospital until they are pronounced non-infectious, and the hospital will have infection control procedures to protect visitors.

Disinfection procedures

General principles

As in disinfection against any other germ, five basic steps need to be borne in mind in any HIV-related disinfection process:

- Wearing protective clothing and using protective devices.

- Physical cleaning: always make sure surfaces are clear of visible contamination. This needs to be effective because organic material provides a safe place for HIV. It blocks heat getting in and inactivates chemical disinfectants by reacting with them. So you have to be thorough to shift dried semen, blood, faeces, vaginal fluids etc.

- Heat or chemical treatment: follow recommended guidelines. Autoclaving is still the recommended means of sterilising most re-usable equipment. In some cases other specialised methods are necessary. For instance, ethylene oxide should be used to sterilise lensed instruments such as endoscopes or bronchoscopes.

- Careful disposal of contaminated materials and sharps.

- Reporting of any problems, concerns or incidents to your supervisor or adviser.

Domestic disinfection

- Clean up.

- Wear rubber gloves.

- Soak up any large spillages with absorbent paper or cloths which you then wrap up in plastic bags and throw away.

- Next give the spill a first going over with hot water and detergent.

Once you've cleared up all the visible blood or other organic material use a chemical disinfectant such as:

- Household bleach.

- Milton Fluid for cleaning babies' bottles (active ingredient 1.1% available chlorine)Boots' double strength Feeding Bottle Sterilising Fluid (active ingredient 2% available chlorine).

- Maws Simple Sterilising Tablets (active ingredient Sodium Dichloroisocyanurate) are very easy to use since you simply add a 500mg tablet to four pints of water (it is also available as granules which can be used to absorb any spillages of blood).

- Leave the disinfection fluid on the surface for as long as possible.

Dealing with sharps at home

If you need to use needles or Hickman lines (Hickman is a registered trademark of CR Bard Inc.) etc. at home, get hold of sharps boxes and yellow bags for safe collection and incineration.

Social workers or home care teams should be able to arrange this for you.

Laundry

A washing machine with a hot wash cycle at 70°C (ideally with a biological enzyme-containing detergent) will disinfect laundry.

Cleaning sex toys

- First check the toy for ageing: for instance, cracks or fissures in rubber are difficult to clean properly. If in doubt, get rid of it and buy a new one.

- Wear rubber gloves.

- Use a scrubbing brush and cold water first to remove any dried on bits (hot water would fix organic material to solid surfaces).

- Then wash it in washing up liquid and very hot water.

- Then soak it in one of the disinfectants mentioned above at room temperature for more than an hour, perhaps overnight. Air dry after soaking.

A toy which would get ruined by soaking can be disinfected in a different way:

- Pre-heat the oven to 140°C, 275°F, gas mark 1. Then put a small item in for at least 30 minutes. Larger toys may take longer to reach this required temperature.

- It may be worth checking your oven's thermostat with an oven thermometer, since not all oven thermostats are accurate!

Toys which cut or abrade the skin should ideally never be shared.

Further guidance on disinfection

Proper professional procedures in hospitals and laboratories automatically guard against HIV because they're designed with much more infectious agents in mind.

As always the challenge of HIV is that it acts as a spotlight showing up pre-existing problems.

Thus, if professional guidelines were always scrupulously followed, there would be minimal risk. The problem is that in some institutions these guidelines have not been properly implemented or clarified.

- The Department of Health issues guidelines through the Advisory Committee on Dangerous Pathogens and the Health and Safety Executive.

- The BMA publishes *A Code of Practice for Sterilisation and Control of Cross Infection*

- The BMA also publishes *Bloodborne viruses and Infection Control: A guide for health care professionals* - see above.

- For dentists the BDA publishes appropriate guidelines.

- COHSE publishes AIDS guidelines for health staff.

- Guidelines on disinfection in developing countries are regularly updated by the World Health Organisation and have been published in *AIDS Action* which is produced by Healthlink Worldwide.

HIV testing

The HIV antibody test

The HIV antibody test is the most common method of testing for HIV infection. It was devised in 1984, as soon as HIV was discovered, and has remained unchanged since then. The HIV antibody test detects the presence of antibodies to HIV in the blood or saliva, thus confirming the presence of HIV, and is widely used because it is easier and cheaper to detect HIV antibodies than it is to look for the virus itself.

Antibodies are one of the body's responses to infection. They are Y-shaped protein molecules that have the property of being immensely variable. The body can generate antibodies against a wide variety of foreign invaders: parasites, bacteria, viruses, poisons, allergens like pollen or nut protein, drugs, and even (when the response goes wrong) the body's own components. Antibodies do three jobs: they directly kill some pathogens; they render others harmless by neutralising them; or they 'tag' invaders for destruction by other components of the immune system.

Antibodies to HIV normally begin to appear in your blood 1-2 weeks after you become infected with HIV and will reach a plateau within 4-6 months of infection.

The HIV test is not a test for AIDS. If the test shows that you have HIV antibodies in your blood, you are said to be 'HIV-positive'. There is no way of knowing which, if any, HIV-related conditions you may develop, or when. Though HIV is the virus that can cause AIDS, not everyone who is infected with HIV has developed AIDS. In fact, about one in three people have no symptoms ten years after being infected.

However, without treatment, two-thirds of adults infected with HIV are likely to develop AIDS within ten years of being exposed to HIV. In countries where people are exposed to tuberculosis and parasitic diseases such as malaria, this period is likely to be shorter. It is also shorter for children born with the virus.

What a positive result means

A positive result means that your body has produced antibodies against HIV. Research shows that HIV can be found in almost everyone with HIV antibodies.

So it does mean you are infected with HIV, but because the course of HIV infection is so variable this doesn't tell you whether (without treatment) you will stay well, develop minor illnesses, or develop AIDS.

It almost certainly means you are infectious. This means that you should have safer sex with any sexual partners. If you use needles or syringes to inject drugs, you shouldn't share them. Taking these precautions will prevent anyone getting HIV infection from

you - and also safeguard your sexual health, as HIV is by no means the only serious and/or chronic STI you can get.

Further information about living with HIV infection can be found in the NAM booklet *Living with HIV*.

If you test positive for HIV antibodies, you will also undergo tests that can tell you and your doctor more about how much damage HIV has done to your immune system. Your doctor will almost certainly want to discuss with you the treatments currently available to fight HIV. These issues are discussed in more detail in *Treatment options and the newly diagnosed* later in this chapter.

What a negative result means

A negative test result means that antibodies against HIV have not been found in your blood. This probably means you don't have HIV infection.

However, it can take up to three months to produce antibodies after infection with HIV.

The window period

HIV antibodies don't appear the day after you become infected, so it is not possible to find out if you have been infected immediately after a possible risk. Antibodies usually take between two weeks to two months to appear in your blood. Ninety per cent of people have detectable antibodies within four weeks of infection and 99% of people by three months after infection (Lindback). The time between infection and the development of antibodies is called the window period.

During the window period, people infected with HIV may have no antibodies in their blood, but they are likely to have very high levels of HIV in their blood, sexual fluids or breastmilk. In fact, a person with HIV can be extremely infectious during this window period, before their immune system has tried to control the virus. So they could pass on HIV to another person, even though an antibody test would say they were HIV-negative.

Clinics generally recommend that you wait three months after a possible risk of exposure to HIV before being tested, to be sure that a negative result is truly negative. However, if you have been

at unusual risk or have good reason to believe you may have been exposed to HIV, you should not delay in seeking advice.

Note that if you are fairly sure you have been at high risk of acquiring HIV recently - but not recently enough to use post-exposure prophylaxis (see below) - other tests, such as Nucleic Acid Testing (NAT) or the p24 antigen test can find the infection as quickly as twelve days after exposure. Ask your clinic if they perform these tests on people with recent high-risk exposure. You will still need a confirmatory antibody test later, however.

A small number of people - probably one in a hundred of those who become infected - take more than two to three months to form antibodies, but it is highly unusual to take more than six months to form antibodies. A very tiny percentage of people with HIV infection - one in a hundred thousand - never seem to develop any antibodies at all.

Obviously a negative result offers you no guarantees for the future. So whatever the result of the test you need both to have safer sex (see *Safer sex*) and to avoid sharing needles and injecting equipment when injecting drugs (see *Drug use*).

References

Lindback S et al. *Diagnosis of primary HIV-1 infection and duration of follow-up after HIV exposure.* AIDS 14(15): 2333-2339. 2000.

Pros & cons of being tested

Medical reasons for having a test

The availability of HIV treatment has strongly shifted opinion in favour of identifying people who are HIV-positive before they start to develop HIV-related illnesses. Most doctors now think that starting antiretroviral treatment (combination therapy) while the immune system is relatively strong will improve the chance that treatments will be able to keep you healthy indefinitely. Indeed, at the moment (2007) the consensus seems to be moving in favour of starting treatment earlier, because studies have shown that HIV can adversely affect health even if people still retain a moderate degree of immune function, and because the treatments are getting easier to take, in terms of both convenience and of side-effects.

Antiretroviral therapies are used in conjunction with viral load tests, which monitor the amount of HIV in the blood. In HIV-infected people who are not on treatment, the level of HIV in the blood gradually increases, and, as it does, the health of the immune system gradually declines. As a result, the body becomes susceptible to a range of illnesses that it would usually be able to fight off - the so-called *opportunistic* infections.

The aim of antiretroviral treatments is to lower the level of HIV in the blood, and viral load tests can show very quickly whether or not an anti-HIV drug combination is working.

While you remain untested, you have no idea whether or not you are infected. If you are, in fact, infected with HIV, no one is monitoring you to see how HIV is affecting your health. You may not learn that you are infected until you become ill with some HIV-related illness, whereas if you had been tested earlier you might have benefited from treatments that could keep you healthy for a long time. Nowadays, the majority of people admitted to hospital with HIV-related illnesses are there because they had not previously known they were HIV-positive and had not been on treatments.

If you are actually ill, and a doctor who is experienced in dealing with HIV infection considers the test to be a useful part of the diagnosis, then the potential value of the result in terms of treatment almost always outweighs the drawbacks.

Give yourself time to consider all the issues

Give yourself a week or two to think about all these issues and decide if you really want to have a test or not. It's such an important decision that you must not rush into it.

You might find it useful to talk anonymously in confidence to a trained telephone advisor on one of the national helplines.

These are:

Terrence Higgins Trust Helpline

THT Direct: **0845 1221200**
Weekdays 10am - 10pm, Weekends Noon - 6pm

AIDS Treatment Helpline
0808 800 6013, Mon-Wed 12-4pm

National AIDS Helpline
0800 567123, Daily - 24-hour service

Some arguments against being tested

It is very difficult to construct a convincing argument against HIV testing - because of the availability of effective antiretroviral treatments, which can prevent disease progression and improve quality of life.

That said, it is still important for you to think about how you would cope with a positive result. The main reasons against being tested are not medical ones - they are social and psychological.

People may fear the stigma associated with HIV, or the obligation to tell a partner. In these circumstances, it is worth considering whether the anxiety of knowing you have HIV would be worse than the anxiety of suspecting you might have.

An HIV diagnosis is always a serious piece of news and some people may feel they are not ready to cope with it. It can cause a great deal of stress and, despite advances in treatments, people diagnosed with HIV infection may still experience psychological complications as a result of their diagnosis - or may have pre-existing problems that contributed to their becoming HIV-positive but are exacerbated by the result. A few people have become suicidal following a positive test result. Most clinics have access to psychological services for those who have received a positive diagnosis.

Some people are concerned about the effect of having an HIV test on future applications for life insurance or mortgages. Insurance companies now say that a negative test for HIV will not affect your chances of getting life insurance cover, but if you are considered to be at high risk of infection (for example, you are a gay man), you may be charged more for life insurance.

It is worth considering the possible adverse impact of a positive test result on your relationships, including those with family, partners and workmates. And there is the possibility of restrictions on those who are positive - for example, in international travel.

But the bottom line is that HIV-positive people who have been diagnosed and are receiving regular monitoring and decent treatment live longer, healthier and more fulfilling lives.

Testing after very recent exposure

In the last few years it has become evident that treatment with antiretroviral drugs during the early weeks of infection may have a significant effect on the course of HIV infection.

Exposure in the past 24-72 hours

In these circumstances you should consider **post-exposure prophylaxis (PEP)**, which is now generally available to people if they ask for it no more than one to three days after a possible exposure to HIV.

The sooner you take PEP after the exposure the more likely it is to be effective. A study of people exposed to HIV-infected blood through needlestick injuries showed that treatment with the drug AZT 24 hours after exposure reduced the risk of infection by 80%; animal studies suggest that it may be close to 100% effective if taken within 24 hours, but no more than 50% effective if taken more than 72 hours after an exposure to HIV and very much less effective if taken later than this.

PEP, if prescribed and taken properly, should be able to block HIV infection completely if treatment lasts one month, though there are cases of 'breakthrough' infections in which HIV became established despite PEP. Treatment does not need to continue for longer than one month, because the aim of treatment is to prevent HIV from entering cells in the body and establishing an infection.

Guidance from the Department of Health suggests PEP should be offered to healthcare workers exposed through needlestick injuries within one hour of exposure for maximum effectiveness.

In April 2006, the Chief Medical Officer for England, Sir Liam Donaldson, wrote to all NHS trusts emphasising that PEP was available and should be used according to the DoH guidelines in cases of non-occupational exposure too.

Clinics will not automatically offer this form of treatment to everyone who believes they have been at risk of HIV infection. They may use a number of questions to decide whether you have been at high risk of infection. These may include:

- Was your partner known to be HIV-positive?

- Was your partner in a high-risk group?

- What kind of sex did you have: anal, vaginal, or oral?

- Did ejaculation occur into your body, or were you the active partner?

- Did you inject blood into your veins if you were sharing needles?

- Was sexual intercourse violent, traumatic or due to sexual assault?

- Where did your partner come from - a metropolitan area with high HIV prevalence, or a small town with low prevalence?

- Are you able to adhere to a four-week course of treatment that might produce unpleasant side-effects?

See *HIV prevention: post-exposure prophylaxis* for more information on this subject. The use of post-exposure prophylaxis for sexual transmission is discussed in *Developing prevention technologies*.

Exposure more than 48 hours ago

Terminology varies, but the period of infection between exposure and seroconversion (the development of antibodies) is usually referred to as **Primary** or **Acute HIV Infection (PHI)**, while the period between seroconversion and about six months after infection, when antibodies have built up to their peak levels, is usually referred to as **Early HIV Infection.**

In people exposed to HIV more than 24-48 hours prior to seeking medical attention, and where signs of HIV infection have been detected, HIV p24 antigen testing can detect HIV infection within two to three weeks of infection. It is generally available as part of combination antibody/antigen tests; if one of these is positive but confirmatory antibody tests are negative, then either another p24 test or a viral load (RNA or NAT) test can be done.

Viral load or Nucleic Acid testing can detect the presence of HIV's genetic material even earlier, before antibodies have been developed. It can pick up HIV infection within a week to 10 days after exposure, which means that it can detect infection 10-14 days before an antibody test can.

The benefit of viral load or RNA testing during suspected acute (early) infection is largely a public health one: it maximises the number of HIV infections detected, particularly during a period when people have viral loads in the region of 100 times higher than they do during chronic infection (and so may be 100 times more infectious). By detecting primary infection it may be possible to inform partners and stop 'chains' or clusters of HIV infection happening. This is important because recent studies suggest that about 50% of all HIV infections are transmitted by people during primary infection.

Studies from North Carolina and Seattle in the USA have found that in high-incidence populations, viral load/RNA testing detects up to 10% more infections than are picked up by antibody testing. Viral load/RNA testing is considerably more expensive than HIV antibody testing, but by using a simplified version called Nucleic Acid testing (NAT) and by pooling 100 or so blood samples at a time and then re-testing individual samples only from those groups that test RNA positive, costs have been brought down to feasible levels.

There are other ways in which it may be possible to distinguish very recent infection with HIV from long-established infection: see the discussion of *Detuned tests* in *The scientific basis of HIV antibody testing*.

Other trials have been undertaken in which people are given antiretroviral drugs during primary HIV infection (PHI) in the hope, not that infection could be prevented but that by suppressing viral replication during the initial period when viral load is normally very high, further immune damage and disease progression could be delayed or even postponed indefinitely. However, these trials have shown disappointing and inconsistent results.

The current BHIVA guidelines say:

Longer-term follow-up of small numbers of patients treated during PHI with subsequent treatment interruption have not supported initial hopes that early treatment would alter the natural history of HIV infection. It is, therefore, the view of the panel that we should not change the recommendation that patients diagnosed during PHI should be offered recruitment into a clinical trial that will address the issue of whether treatment is beneficial in this setting.

In other words, treatment during primary HIV infection is not likely to be routinely offered at present, but this option is by no means a closed book and trials using new classes of drugs may produce better results in future. Some of the largest GUM clinics in London are running studies to follow people treated at this stage of infection. If you live outside London, call your local clinic and ask to speak to a consultant to find out whether they will consider embarking on an experimental course of treatment.

Some people may develop symptoms during this phase of infection before antibodies appear in the blood. Antibodies usually become detectable at the same time as these symptoms develop. This is known as seroconversion illness and symptoms may include:

- Prolonged fever (4 - 14 days) and aching limbs.

- Red blotchy rash over the trunk.

- Sore throat (pharyngitis).

- Ulceration in the mouth or genitals.

- Diarrhoea.

- Severe headaches.

- Aversion to light.

Other symptoms, such as paralysis, meningitis and opportunistic infections as a consequence of severe immune suppression are much less common. Symptoms of seroconversion may occur in up to 80% of people infected, but the severity of the symptoms varies. Some people report only a mild flu-like illness 30-60 days after a risk of HIV exposure, but others experience an illness severe enough to require hospitalisation. The longer the illness lasts, and the more severe it is, the more likely you are to develop AIDS within five years if you do not receive antiretroviral treatment at the appropriate time.

Remember that any symptoms you may have could be caused by other infections: flu, glandular fever, tonsillitis and a serious herpes attack have similar symptoms to those reported in seroconversion illness.

Testing after sexual assault

Many of the points made immediately above will also apply if you are concerned about HIV infection as a result of sexual assault.

If you are planning to take your attacker to court and it is possible that he has infected you with HIV, it may be wise to speak to a lawyer as soon as possible after the assault. The lawyer might advise you to have an HIV test straight away (including an RNA test), so that if a later test shows you have HIV you will have a better chance of proving that you did not have HIV at the time of the assault.

Testing and relationships

If you're in a stable relationship, knowing your antibody status may be important in deciding what kind of sex you can have with your regular partner. Many people would prefer not to use condoms with a regular partner, but the only way for both of you to be confident that this is a safe option is if you both have an HIV antibody test at the same time. Then you will have to make an agreement about what sort of sex either of you will have with other partners, in order to be confident that unprotected sex will continue to be safe. You also need to agree that if either of you uses needles to inject drugs, no sharing will take place with other people. This kind of arrangement has been termed 'negotiated safety'.

If you are thinking of having a test with a partner, you need to bear in mind that it is advisable to wait at least three months after the last occasion on which one of you had unprotected sex with anyone else. This is because it may take three months after

infection for antibodies to HIV to appear (although the majority of people produce antibodies within two months of infection).

This is an ideal scenario. A lot of people find that they start having unprotected sex with a regular partner without having gone through this process of testing together. An Australian study found that nearly 50% of gay men had been with their partners less than three months before they first had unprotected sex.

This may happen because you assumed that either you or your partner had not been at risk of HIV infection in the past. Or it may be that you stopped using condoms without thinking through all the implications, and now want to be reassured that this was the right decision. Or it may be that you stopped using condoms after a breakage or omitted to use them on some occasions. You may have assumed that if infection was going to occur, it would have happened immediately.

In all these situations, you will need to wait for at least three months after the last occasion on which you had unprotected sex, and resume using condoms, or else take a test immediately. Depending on the result of your test and your partner's test, you will then have the following options:

- If you have both tested negative, and neither of you have had unprotected sex with anyone else for at least three months prior to this test, you can carry on having unprotected sex confident that there is no risk of HIV transmission between you. You are both clear of HIV infection.

- If you have both tested negative, but at least one of you has had unprotected sex with someone else in the past three months, a risk of transmission still exists because the person who had unprotected sex less than three months ago may not have developed antibodies yet.

If this is the case, the person who has had unprotected sex with another person will need to be tested again three months after the occasion on which they had unprotected sex with another partner. If they are still negative, you can be confident at that point that you are both clear of HIV infection.

If the partner who has had unprotected sex with another person tests positive, you will need to wait at least three months after the last occasion on which you had unprotected sex together before taking another test yourself, and will need to use condoms. Remember, you may not have been infected with HIV at this point, so there is no sense in abandoning condom use.

Clearly this can be very complicated and stressful for both of you, and it is liable to arouse uncomfortable feelings in your relationship. It is at times like this that any negative feelings about sex outside your regular relationship are likely to be magnified, and resentments about previous incidents may be brought to the surface again. The support of a counsellor is likely to be especially important.

One study (Guzman) of negotiated safety amongst gay male couples in San Francisco underlined the difficulties of using negotiated safety as an HIV prevention measure.

The survey initially looked at 340 HIV-negative gay men in San Francisco. It found that 60% had no current steady relationship and that 10% had an HIV-positive partner. The other 30% had an HIV-negative boyfriend, of which 76 were "long-term" lovers, meaning for six months or more.

It found that 13 of these 76 men didn't have anal sex, and that 17 (only 22% of the entire group) practiced the supposed "gold standard" of safer sex, maintaining 100% condom use with their partner. Interestingly, six men had unprotected sex with casual partners but maintained 100% condom use with their boyfriend - behaviour that protected their partner, but not themselves.

Another eight of the men (11%) had unprotected anal sex within and outside the relationship and hadn't negotiated rules prohibiting it.

But the remaining 50% of the men had arrived at some form of negotiated safety agreement with their boyfriend. Nineteen of them, a quarter of the whole group, had negotiated total monogamy, i.e. no sex of any kind with men outside the relationship. Three disallowed anal sex of any kind but allowed other sex. And 16 allowed anal sex outside the relationship as long as it was with a condom.

Of the 38 men who had negotiated an agreement, 11 (29%) had broken their own rules in the previous three months: a quarter of the "monogamous" group and a third each of the "no anal sex" and "no unprotected sex" groups.

Three-quarters of the men who'd negotiated safety also had a rule that they must tell their partner if they'd broken their agreement. This rule did seem to help men comply - only 18% of those who had an "always tell" rule had broken their agreements, while 60% of those who had not made an "always tell" rule had broken their agreements.

Looking on the bright side, the study authors point out that there had been no campaign recommending "negotiated safety" in relationships - this was something HIV-negative men were working out between themselves. But two out of every five men who had such an agreement broke the rules they'd negotiated in as short a time as three months.

This study and others like it remind us that most of the advice about safer sex and HIV testing disseminated by health professionals ignores the emotional context in which decisions about unprotected sex and HIV testing take place.

Most relationships are plagued by some degree of mistrust and insecurity on the part of one or both partners. Most of us would like to believe that we are capable of putting these feelings to one side, but human behaviour repeatedly shows that this is very difficult for most of us to do. In relationships where a significant imbalance in power exists (for instance because of gender difference or age) it can be very easy for an individual to feel pressurised into unprotected sex and/or HIV testing against their better judgement. If you find yourself in this position, call on the counselling services available at GUM clinics and you will be helped to make the decision that is right for you. It may be particularly helpful for both of you to see a counsellor together if you are thinking of testing in order to give up condom use.

Testing in order to give up condom use requires an explicit agreement about whether or not it is permissible for either or both of you to have sex with other partners, and about what sort of sex you can have with other partners.

You both need to agree what you regard as *safer* sex with other partners, and you need to be confident that you can stick to these agreements.

If you're having the test together, how do you think this will affect your relationship? How would you feel if one of you tests positive and the other tests negative? Not only will one partner have to face up to living with HIV, but you will both have to cope with how this affects your relationship. Sometimes people cope well. They continue to practice safer sex and learn new ways to support each other.

At other times, the pressure is too much and the relationship breaks up. Another possibility is that you may both test positive. This could be very difficult to deal with, especially if you both fear that one partner infected the other.

References

Guzman R et al. *Negotiated safety relationships and sexual behavior among a diverse sample of HIV-negative men who have sex with men.* JAIDS 38(1): 82-86. 2005.

If you are thinking of having a baby

If you think you or your partner may have been at risk of HIV infection and you're intending to have a child, it makes sense to be tested. HIV can be passed from mother to baby in about 14-20% of pregnancies on average, and the transmission rate rises to around 30% if you breastfeed too. However, treatment during pregnancy with antiretroviral drugs cuts this risk very significantly. For more details see the section on *HIV testing, pregnancy and children* later in this chapter.

Travelling abroad

If you have to go and live in a country that enforces compulsory HIV testing for foreign residents (see **Travel** in the **Mental Health and Quality of Life**chapter), it may make sense to be tested in this country first if you think you have been at risk. But, if this is the case, you need to decide whether your trip is important enough to you for you to be, in effect, forced to be tested.

Similarly, if you need vaccination or immunisation with a live vaccine, it would be worth enquiring about the latest medical opinions about the risk to you if you were to be HIV-positive. See NAM's *HIV & AIDS Treatments Directory* for a full list of live vaccines.

Antenatal HIV testing

All pregnant women are now offered a test for HIV antibodies as a routine part of antenatal care. You will have a number of tests to make sure that you and your baby get the best possible care. An HIV test is one of these. The test is never done without asking you first, but if you do not want this test you must tell your doctor when asked, otherwise it will be carried out along with other routine checks on your health and your baby's health. You have the right to refuse this test, and you also have the right to be fully informed about the pros and cons of being tested so you can make up your mind about it.

Should I have an HIV test?

Unless you know that you have HIV, you cannot benefit from treatment that can prevent you from passing on HIV to your baby.

Around 0.45% (one in 230) pregnant women in London are HIV-positive, one in 900 in the rest of the UK, and one in 40 women from sub-Saharan Africa. Due to testing and the use of antiretrovirals to prevent mother-to-child transmission, the proportion of babies exposed to HIV from their mothers who are likely to have been infected has declined from 20% in 1997 to 3% in 2005. But because the number of HIV-positive women giving birth each year in the UK is increasing (it more than tripled between 1997 and 2004), there has not been a concomitant reduction in the number of infected infants born each year. Approximately 60 such babies were born in the UK in 1997 and reports so far for the last three years have been 25-30 a year.

However, unless you or partner have lived in sub-Saharan Africa, or you or your partner have injected drugs and shared needles in the past, your chances of having been infected with HIV are very low. Nevertheless, each year a small number of women - about one in 2500 - without any of these risk factors is diagnosed with HIV in the UK.

What happens if the test is positive?

If you are found to be HIV-positive, you could pass HIV on to your baby during pregnancy, during childbirth or by breastfeeding. Obviously an HIV-positive result affects your own health too.

However, very effective treatment now exists which can reduce the risk of passing on HIV to your baby. Without treatment, the chance of passing on HIV is around one in seven, but with the latest treatment, the risk falls to less than one in a hundred.

Babies are very vulnerable to HIV infection. About one quarter of children born with HIV will develop serious HIV-related illnesses or will die within the first year of life.

Tests to measure the amount of virus in your blood and the health of your immune system (your ability to fight off some serious infections) will be carried out.

Based on the results of these tests, you will be offered different treatment choices by your doctor:

- Immediate combination therapy with three drugs to protect your own health and your baby's health

OR

- Treatment with one drug (usually AZT because it is well-studied and does not cause birth defects) during pregnancy if your own health doesn't yet require you to take combination therapy, with treatment during childbirth and afterwards to protect your baby's health

AND

- Some doctors will suggest that you should have a caesarean section rather than a normal delivery, because there is some evidence that this further reduces the risk that your baby will be infected during delivery.

You will also be recommended not to breastfeed, because HIV can be transmitted through breastmilk. This is a highly contentious issue in the developing world, where the risks and benefits of bottle-feeding and breastfeeding by HIV-positivemothers are more complicated and it may sometimes be safest for mothers to breastfeed, but in the UK, where safe drinking water and adequate formula feed are universally available, choosing not to breastfeed is an effective way to keep your child HIV-negative and healthy.

If you don't start treatment right away, or you don't learn that you are HIV-positiveuntil late in your pregnancy, your baby can still benefit from treatment, because most cases of HIV infection are believed to occur during childbirth. This means you have time to make up your mind about what you want to do - you don't have to make the decision overnight.

After the birth

After your baby is born, the baby will have to receive a number of treatments and tests to make sure that HIV infection doesn't occur. This will mean quite a few extra hospital visits, and medication for your baby lasting six months. After six months it is usually possible to say for sure whether or not a child has been infected. Before this time, the child's blood may contain some antibodies to HIV that have come from its mother, but these disappear as the baby develops its own immune responses.

Telling people about a positive result during pregnancy

An HIV-positive result is likely to be a big shock for you. One implication of the result is that the father of your child may also be HIV-positive, and you will need to decide what to tell him and when. You may be angry because you fear that he has passed on HIV to you.

You may also be scared of what people will think if they find out that you are HIV-positive. It is important to discuss with the doctor, counsellor or midwife who gives you an HIV-positive result the question of who should be told. Your doctor and other people caring for you are not allowed to tell anyone without your permission, but the information will be written down in your medical record at the clinic where you are receiving your care.

What happens if the test is negative?

If you test negative for HIV, this means that no antibodies to HIV are present in your blood. In most cases this will mean that you and your baby are not at risk from HIV.

However, if you caught HIV less than three months ago, the antibodies may not have had time to develop. If you believe you were at risk of HIV infection recently you will need to discuss this with an HIV counsellor and decide when is the best time for you to be tested.

Further information

Further information is available in a booklet published by Terrence Higgins Trust called *Baby Matters*.

It is available from:

Terrence Higgins Trust
314-320 Gray's Inn Road
London, WC1X 8DP

Telephone: 020 7812 1600
Fax: 020 7812 1601
Email: info@tht.org.uk

There are two reports on pregnancy, childbirth and HIV issued by the Health Protection Agency.

Pregnant Women, available at
www.hpa.org.uk/publications/2006/hiv_sti_2006/pdf/Part%205/part5_pregnant_women.pdf

Reducing Mother to Child Transmission of HIV Infection in the United Kingdom, from www.fphm.org.uk/policy_communication/downloads/publications/reports/RCPCH_HIV_report.pdf

Practicalities of testing

Where to go for a test

Recommended

The best place to be tested for HIV is at a sexual health clinic (often called a genitourinary medicine, or GUM, clinic), because the result will be confidential and because trained and experienced counsellors will be available there to help you.

Not only that, but if you test positive, you will have the advantage of immediate monitoring, care and follow-up by doctors who are very experienced in treating people with HIV.

For details of your nearest clinic, use NAM's online search at aidsmap.com

GPs

The test is also available through your GP, and although many GPs will refer you to a GUM clinic rather than counsel or take blood themselves, some people prefer to be tested at their normal doctor's surgery than to attend a GUM clinic. Many GPs are unable to provide good quality pre- and post-test counselling, due to lack of time and training, but some have extra training in sexual health and are capable of providing as good an HIV service as a GUM clinic.

Remember, however, if you discuss or have an HIV test at your GP's surgery, it is likely to be noted on your medical record and this may have an impact later, for instance when you are seeking insurance, a mortgage, or employment.

Drugs agencies

Drug users may be able to have an HIV test through a local drugs agency. This may be a good idea, especially if the agency

has a regular clinical session for people with HIV - this means you will have access to doctors and nurses experienced in treating drug users with HIV. However, it's also important to know that not all drugs agencies provide the same standard of pre-and post-test counselling, particularly when it comes to safer sex.

Antenatal clinics

The test is routinely offered to all pregnant women through antenatal clinics see *HIV testing, Pregnancy and children.*

Non-residents or visitors to the UK

Even if you are not a British resident, you can still have an HIV test as long as you can provide an address in the UK. You will not be charged for it.

Choosing a clinic

You don't have to be referred to a sexual health clinic by your doctor, and you don't have to go to the one nearest your home. You can go wherever you want. If you have this choice - and it may be difficult for you to go anywhere other than your nearest hospital - there are several things you should look out for:

- Which clinic provides the quickest result?

- Does the clinic have its own health advisers or HIV counsellors?

- Does the clinic also have an HIV clinic, indicating that it has experience in treating people with HIV?

When you go to a sexual health clinic for an HIV test, you will usually be asked to register if you haven't already done so - the clinic will take your name and address. This information is confidential, but even so, you needn't give your real name and address. Just make sure you remember the false name you give, so that you answer when it is called.

The doctor will want to ask you questions about your sexual activities. This is also entirely confidential. The doctor should suggest that you have a check-up for other sexually transmitted infections - if you have had unprotected sex you may have picked up one of the very common sexually transmitted infections (STIs), and these are easily treatable in most cases.

There is a more detailed discussion of sexual health clinics in *Safer sex: sexually transmitted infections and sexual health.*

How the test is done

The test can be done in several ways. The most common method is to take a small sample of blood from a vein in your arm. The blood is sent away to a laboratory, where it is subjected to a procedure that quickly allows trained laboratory staff to recognise whether it contains antibodies. If the blood gives a negative reaction on the first test, it can be safely assumed that no HIV antibodies are present in the blood, and you are not infected. (Remember, however, that if you have been at risk within the previous three months, you will need to be tested again, three months after your last risk.)

If the blood appears to give a positive reaction to the testing procedure, however weak, a confirmatory test of a different sort is done to check the presence of HIV antibodies.

At most clinics you will need to make a second appointment to go back to the clinic to receive the result in person. HIV antibody test results should not be given out over the phone or sent through the post by sexual health clinics.

HIV antibody testing can also be done on a sample of saliva from the margin of the gums, but this method is only used for HIV testing with injecting drug users at present.

Waiting for a result: how long must I wait?

Test results may take up to two to three weeks in some cases, because sexual health clinics send their blood samples off to laboratories in batches. Some districts or regions are quicker than others, and some clinics may be able to supply test results more quickly if you are very distressed.

Same-day testing services now exist across the country on certain days of the week. These provide pre- and post-test counselling and some clinics may be able to offer a result within 15 minutes. Testing through these clinics can reduce the anxiety of waiting for a test result, but appointments may need to be booked several weeks in advance, so they may not provide instant answers. However THT now offers a walk-in testing service called FastTest on a first-come, first served basis at several locations in London and other large cities (see www.tht.org.uk for more details).

Does the test show when infection occurred?

Normal HIV antibody testing does not show when infection occurred, unless of course there are previous negative results. However, additional information - including the results of CD4 tests, clinical assessment, and other people's HIV status - may give clues.

Detuned antibody tests (discussed in *The scientific basis of HIV antibody testing*) may suggest recent infection, but these currently seem more appropriate for comparing populations, rather than for pinpointing exactly when individuals were infected.

See NAM's *The HIV & AIDS Treatments Directory* or **aidsmap.com** for further discussion of these issues.

Home testing

The sale of HIV testing kits is illegal in the UK, and there are no current plans to change this. However the sale of home *sampling* kits - where a blood sample is taken at home and then sent away for analysis - has never been illegal in the UK.

The UK attitude up until now has been that only qualified medical professionals should conduct HIV testing, and that testing should always be accompanied by counselling. However, HIV test kits are freely (if illegally) available on the internet, and in theory there is nothing to stop a UK resident or anyone else from buying a home-testing kit and getting themselves tested, though there is no guarantee that the test kit you are buying is reliable. If you were to home-test and get a positive result, it would be important to get a confirmatory test done at a sexual health clinic, as the result may have been a false positive.

In the USA, where there is more political backing for the extension of HIV testing to more settings, the Food and Drug Administration has been considering since 2005 whether to legalise home-testing kits. They have not made a decision yet.

For more information on this, see **The role of HIV testing in HIV prevention** in the **HIV prevention** chapter.

Rapid tests

Rapid HIV tests are widely used in resource-limited settings. The need for immediate HIV test results to make treatment decisions and to assist with prevention strategies portends their increased use in developed countries as well. Rapid HIV tests demonstrate sensitivities and specificities comparable to those of the enzyme-linked immunoassays (ELISAs) currently used for screening. Algorithms comprised of a combination of two or more rapid tests produce HIV test results with predictive values comparable to those of the ELISA-Western blot combination (see *The scientific basis for antibody testing* later in this chapter for more details). Rapid HIV tests offer the additional advantages of low cost and same-day results and are likely to gain increasing acceptance for HIV screening and diagnosis in both developed and developing countries.

The disadvantage of rapid testing is that a single rapid test may yield a false positive result, so positive results need a confirmatory test, preferably done by a different method. This problem was highlighted in December 2005, when the Los Angeles Gay and Lesbian Center announced that a higher-than-expected rate of positive results were being seen after the introduction of an oral rapid test.

The Los Angeles Gay Centre said it performed 600 oral HIV tests a month and normally found about 20 people who tested positive. False positives were rare till November 2005, when 13 people who had tested positive on the OraQuick test were later found to be negative on confirmatory testing.

A CDC survey of 17,000 results from the same oral test found a false-positive rate of only 0.2% compared with over 2% experienced by Los Angeles centre. No explanation was found for the unreliability of these results and no one ended up being falsely diagnosed HIV-positive, because confirmatory tests revealed people's true HIV status; but incidents like these are reminders of the importance of confirmatory testing.

Confidentiality

This is a brief guide: for more on confidentiality see **Confidentiality** in the **Law and HIV** chapter.

Confidentiality in the clinic

Sexual health clinics are the most reliably confidential parts of the Health Service. People attending sexual health clinics are legally protected under the VD Act (1974).

Informing your GP

Some clinics may wish to notify your GP if you turn out to be HIV-positive, even though you may have no symptoms of HIV infection. You may or may not want this to happen, depending on your relationship with your GP. Ask at the clinic whether they intend doing this.

If you are HIV-positive and have symptoms, then the clinic will want to tell your GP. This is medically advisable, to avoid any dangerous delay in diagnosis from now on. It is important to try to make sure that your GP is aware of the need for confidentiality and that your GP is sufficiently well informed to know that a positive test result does not mean that you have AIDS.

Informing other doctors in the hospital

If you are referred to any other departments within the hospital, the specialists there will probably be told that you are HIV-positive. This is then likely to go into your general hospital notes, which tend to be less confidential than those kept in the sexual health clinic. The result may then be available to any doctor, nurse, or anyone else who sees your case notes. Try to speak to a senior doctor to make sure how confidential your records will be in such situations.

Electronic Patient Records

The NHS is currently in the process of a huge programme of transferring patient records on to a dedicated NHS computer network so that patient records can be accessed by any suitably qualified healthcare professional with the right access permission, rather than being recorded in paper files. It is envisaged that Electronic Patient Records (EPRs) will exist in two forms: a **Summary Care Record** or **'National Spine'** which will be available to every qualified doctor in the UK, giving brief details of GP and hospital notes and treatments, and a more **Detailed Care Record** which will only be available to doctors involved in your care and members of the associated clinical network.

This represents a huge change to the way health records are stored. In some ways, EPRs will be more secure: only qualified professionals will be able to log in, and there will be a number of safeguards to ensure patient confidentiality and guard against unauthorised access. The problems this change should help avoid are those of loss of paper files and/or of files being read by unauthorised staff such as receptionists. Of course, the main benefit of EPRs is that care of patients, especially of those with complex conditions like HIV, will be better coordinated and rationalised.

However, EPRs inevitably imply that records that would previously remain in the files at your GP's surgery or your sexual health clinic will in future be available to a much wider range of healthcare professionals in a larger number of locations. Needless to say, HIV and sexual health records, along with similarly sensitive ones such as details of treatment for drug use or psychiatric health records, have proved to be the most problematic when it comes to deciding exactly which records should appear where.

In its 2007 *Standards for HIV Clinical Care*, the British HIV Association, the association of British HIV Doctors, proposed that the health records of patients with HIV should be treated the same as any others:

5.1.1. HIV care records

Information relating to HIV treatment and care should be recorded in ordinary NHS records alongside that relating to any other conditions and identified by the patient's name, NHS number and date of birth.

Information regarding a patient's sexual history (including circumstances of acquisition of HIV) and other STIs may be stored separately in genitourinary medicine records.

5.1.2. The electronic health record

Development of electronic health records (EHR) should proceed on the basis that HIV diagnosis and all current medication will ordinarily be included in the summary section of the EHR. The right of individual patients to opt out of record-sharing or to place this information in a sealed envelope should be respected, but clinicians should not encourage this practice.

Detailed HIV care records should be developed on the basis of the same access protocols as for other chronic diseases. Priority should be given to enabling network-wide access so that clinicians at HIV centres providing 24-hour advice can review the detailed records of individual patients attending any service within the HIV clinical network."

In other words, BHIVA is recommending that two pieces on information go into the Summary Care Record: your HIV diagnosis and your HIV treatment history. The mention of 'sealed envelopes' is a proposal that patients with particularly sensitive health conditions can ask that the information relating to these conditions is placed in a section of the Summary Care Record that requires explicit authorisation to access. However, the exact software specifications needed to make this arrangement work have not been finalised, exact consent protocols have not been established, and 'sealed envelopes' do not avoid the problem of 'deductive disclosure', namely that the presence of a sealed envelope in a patient's care record may itself be interpreted as evidence that they have HIV.

At the time of writing (April 2007) the first PCT (Bolton) is about to put all its patient records on to an electronic database, but many problems are yet to be sorted out - in particular, the issue of whether records from GUM clinics should be included remains completely unresolved. It has been established that, in the case of GPs at least, all patients will have to give explicit consent for their records to be transferred to the electronic database.

Using a false name

While there are indications that most patients will be relatively happy with the new file-sharing arrangements, some patients are particularly concerned about confidentiality and always have been. Examples include health workers who are HIV-positive and undocumented immigrants who are not entitled to free HIV care. Some people have an HIV test under a false name. It is not illegal to do this. But write it down so you don't forget it, and make sure the clinic can get in contact with you at whatever address you do give.

Who to tell

There is no obligation under the law to tell anyone you have HIV. The only exceptions are:

- You must tell your employer if you are a healthcare worker such as surgeon, anaesthetist, paramedic, dentist or midwife who may be involved in exposure-prone procedures.

- Most lawyers now think that case law has established that you are under a legal obligation to disclose to sexual partners before exposing them to the risk of HIV infection, which *probably* means before you have intercourse without a condom.

Disclosure has both benefits and risks. As an act, it doesn't only convey the information that you have HIV. Disclosure also carries with it two other pieces of information. Firstly, it implies that you trust the person you are telling not to abuse the information. Secondly, it can imply to the listener that you have processed the knowledge of your own HIV status sufficiently to be able to deal with their reaction. If you don't trust them or don't think you can cope with their reaction - think twice before telling.

Benefits

On balance, disclosure, in the absence of the risks outlined below, is probably a self-empowering and beneficial act when done to the right people, at the right time, and in the right way. Benefits include reduction in isolation, obtaining support, lessening of internal and, hopefully, external stigma, and reduction of the stress associated with concealment.

One recent paper suggested that disclosure - or the reduction in stress associated with it - may have positive health benefits too.

Researchers from Seattle in the USA found that in the research group studied, which was a group of 373 patients with HIV and psychiatric diagnoses, those who were totally open about either their HIV status or their sexuality experienced a 20% net increase in their CD4 count over a year, independent of any benefit from HIV treatment, their original CD4 count, or any other influence. Conversely, total concealment of either HIV status or sexual orientation led to a 10% fall in CD4 counts.

At the start of the study, patients had slightly poorer physical health than the average US citizen (a score of 44 against a national average of 50) and significantly poorer mental health (a score of 36). Being open was more common than being closeted, especially about being gay. Seventy per cent said they were open about their sexuality 'all or most of the time', and 48% said the same about their HIV status. However, about 14% said they concealed their sexual orientation all or most of the time, and a third concealed their HIV status to nearly everyone.

Over the study period there was, despite the majority being on HIV therapy, a net decline in CD4 counts amongst the patient group as a whole. Once all other considerations had been factored out, the only significant influences on final CD4 count were the patients' initial CD4 count, the length of time since the initial questionnaire, and, to a marginal extent, the initial severity of their mental health problems.

One these three factors were accounted for, there remained a 'disclosure effect'. This added, the researchers estimated, a bonus of about 45 CD4 cells to patients who were always or mostly open about their sexuality, and about 40 cells to those who were always or mostly open about their HIV status. On the other hand, being mostly closeted about either one's sexuality or one's HIV status led to a net deficit of about 10 CD4 cells over and above any other decline. These effects were the same regardless of whether or not people were on HIV therapy.

The researchers do not hypothesise about why disclosure should have positive health benefits, but they do note that a previous study (Cole) found that introverted individuals who were socially inhibited had considerably higher viral loads than did more extrovert individuals - and suggested that most of this difference was due to higher levels of stress hormones such as cortisol and norepinephrine. They suggest that comparing immune function in people with HIV who have attended workshops to help them disclose their status with people who have not may help test this idea further.

Risks

However, while disclosure may in general convey benefits, in individual cases certain risks may far outweigh these. This is particularly the case where people belong to small or tightly knit communities that might reject or ostracise them if it becomes known that they have HIV. Tragically, this is very much the situation in which many recent immigrants from sub-Saharan Africa find themselves, and studies have found that fear of being stigmatised within their community is one of the drivers behind the failure of African people with HIV to disclose their status or to access services. This is just one of many quotes from *Outsider Status* (Dodds), the Sigma Research project that investigated this phenomenon in the UK:

"There was a lady who lived with me in the hotel. She was from Zimbabwe. She was a great friend of mine. I asked her, 'Can't we go to [names African HIV support agency] or something together?' She said, 'Aye, I can't go there. I go there, and people know me, and maybe some people from home will see me, and they will know I am HIV-positive. I can't go.' She never came."

Disclosure of HIV status, once said, cannot be unsaid. People fear sexual and personal rejection, social ostracism and loss of jobs, housing or financial security. They fear they may become the target of gossip in the community and that people will make false assumptions about their sexual or drug-using behaviour. Another fear often expressed is that the person with HIV, seeking support, may end up having to support or educate friends about HIV.

While it is therefore very important to have someone to talk to, think carefully about which of your friends you can really trust. Try to decide before you get the result who you want to confide in. A positive result is always a shock and there is often a temptation to tell people, only to decide later that you'd rather they didn't know. But also consider the effect on your friendships if you decide to tell some people but not others.

There is no need for your employer or work colleagues to know that you are even having the test, let alone if the result is positive. Even knowing that you have been tested can make some people react badly because of ignorance or prejudice.

References

Strachan ED et al. *Disclosure of HIV status and sexual orientation independently predicts increased absolute CD4 cell counts over time for psychiatric patients.* Psychosomatic Medicine 69: 74-80, 2007.

Cole SW et al. *Psychological risk factors for HIV pathogenesis: Mediation by the autonomic nervous system.* Biological Psychiatry 54: 1444-1456. 2003.

Dodds C et al. *Outsider Status: Stigma and discrimination experienced by Gay men and African people with HIV.* Sigma Research, 2004. ISBN 1 872956 76 9.

Pre- and post-test counselling

Pre-test counselling

Recently, on both sides of the Atlantic, there has been a debate about the extent to which counselling is necessary for anyone contemplating being tested for HIV. This debate has been set within the wider debate about the 'normalisation' and universalising of HIV testing - see **The role of testing in HIV prevention** in the **Prevention** chapter.

In a way, it is presumptuous to assume that someone coming for an HIV test needs counselling (in the sense of needing to talk through with someone the situations that led to them wanting an HIV test or of wanting to make changes in their lives). A person may want to have an HIV test for reasons to do with managing their sexual health but do not need professional input; they may already have discussed it or thought about it deeply themselves before they came; and in some situations a professional sitting down with them and asking them, in effect, if they are quite sure they want to have an HIV test may act as a disincentive rather than a facilitator of testing.

The assumption that a person asking for an HIV test 'needs' counselling comes from the days when a positive result was a revelation of probably terminal illness, and even then the assumption that suicides or other dangerously maladaptive reactions to diagnosis would be common turned out to be largely unfounded. Repeated studies have also shown little relationship between whether a person has pre-test counselling and whether they subsequently go on to alter their risk behaviour.

Proponents for pre-test counselling, however, point out that there are few opportunities in life for someone to sit down with a trusted professional in a confidential situation and talk about their sex life and sexual health. In this view, the person seeking an HIV test will nearly always have issues, possibly long suppressed or difficult to articulate due to shame or embarrassment, and that counselling provides an opportunity to explore them.

However, this exploration need not happen prior to testing; even rapid testing involves a nearly 40-minute wait, which also provides an ideal opportunity for the patient to discuss issues and anxieties around the test.

A lot of pre-test 'counselling' is not in fact counselling, but assessment and education. Here the job of the Health Adviser or whoever is doing the test is essentially one of gathering and giving information. Assessment involves:

- Risk assessment. Has the individual actually been at risk? Is their understanding of the risks of HIV accurate or faulty?

- Have they been ill or had symptoms suggestive of HIV infection?

- Have they tested for HIV before, and if so when and how often?

- If the test involves a specific exposure to a known partner, have they told the partner? Is the partner HIV-positive?

While the educative part of testing may involve answering questions the client has about:

- The window period.

- The accuracy of HIV testing.

- Understanding of safer sex and safer drug use.

- The testing procedure, including how the test is done.

- The procedure for informing of the results

- Confidentiality: a discussion of the procedures to protect confidentiality.

- *IF WANTED:* Discussion of post-testing issues, including post-test counselling, how the individual might react to a positive result or a negative result, what clinical and social services are available, contact tracing.

In terms of any deeper therapeutic input, however, *pre*-test (as opposed to post-test) counselling is only likely to be required to help the client/patient think about their HIV risk and testing behaviour, in the case of two types of client not uncommonly encountered by HIV testing centres:

- The 'worried well'

- The 'repeat tester'

The worried well

This is a perhaps slightly pejorative term, or an inaccurate one (the 'worried well' person may be ill in other ways), so perhaps a better term might be the 'AIDS-anxious' person. The basic picture here is of a person who presents for testing, perhaps repeatedly, despite having been at extremely low or no risk of HIV. They may present with different anxieties:

- Anxiety about sexual contacts which posed very little or no risk, e.g. intercourse with a prostitute using a condom which remained intact. The individual then seeks a test 'just to be sure'.

- Anxiety about unlikely or impossible events which may have led to infection, e.g. being unaware of a supposed injection of HIV infected blood, for instance whilst asleep.

- Anxiety about the accuracy of test results, leading to repeated testing. This is usually connected with the anxieties already listed.

- A client who presents with one of the above scenarios because they are concealing a high-risk experience of which they are ashamed (e.g. a heterosexual man who has had a gay experience, a woman who has had anal intercourse, or someone who has been sexually assaulted).

In the first case, even though the person may be quite aware that the sexual contact they had carried little or no risk, they may present with intolerable anxiety about it which they insist can only be assuaged by a test. The anxiety the person feels is essentially a displaced anxiety; the thing they really fear is that they are a sinner, or have endangered their marriage, or may be gay, or are not in control of their behaviour. Alternatively, if the risk is minimal but not completely non-existent, the anxiety about HIV may be a more manageable way of feeling anxious about the extreme gravity of the loss the person feels they would suffer if they were to test positive - e.g. the break-up of their marriage.

If this is the first time the person has presented, then the simplest course of action may be to give them an HIV test and then 'chalk it up to experience'. As has been found with studies of post-exposure prophylaxis, going through the anxiety of having an HIV test may be a learning experience that helps the person avoid sexual encounters they feel bad about in the future.

But it is a questionable use of resources to test someone for HIV if they have essentially been at no risk, and the client may in fact be looking for something else - such as an opportunity to speak with someone of their feelings about sex. This is especially the case if the person repeatedly presents with a series of low-risk encounters.

If the person presents with the second kind of scenario or seeks repeat testing for a single incident of the first kind, then it's more likely their fear of HIV may have delusory or obsessional qualities and may be indicative of a mental health problem. Part of pre-test assessment is therefore trying to decide if the person may have unmet psychiatric needs. Therapeutic techniques for dealing with phobic states have been successfully employed to help people with obsessional fears about HIV infection. These fears cannot be successfully dealt with in the context of pre-test counselling or telephone advice, and referral to a clinical psychologist or counsellor who specialises in dealing with phobic states is the best policy. However, referral to a clinical psychologist is only likely to be of benefit if the psychologist is reasonably well informed about HIV infection. All too often people referred to psychologists for such help have found that the psychologist has given them contradictory information about HIV which has only made matters worse.

The fourth form of anxiety is often related to other issues. For instance, someone who feels guilty about having sex with another man, or having sex outside a relationship, may seek repeated tests to provide reassurance that what they did was not wrong and will not result in dire consequences.

It may, on the other hand, be related to a lack of confidence in the conflicting sources of information about HIV infection and testing. This may be very frustrating for advisers, since the repeated testing implicitly undermines the authority of advice. This is why it is important for advisers to be familiar with the latest information on transmission and testing, and to be able to explain clearly why we should have confidence in this information. See *The scientific basis of HIV antibody testing* later in this chapter.

All of these forms of anxiety can be accompanied by persistent and convincing symptoms, which tend to reinforce the anxiety of the client and encourage him or her to return repeatedly. The symptoms may well have a physical cause entirely unrelated to HIV infection, and suggesting to the client that such symptoms are psychosomatic may deny the genuine distress caused by the symptoms without offering any real form of relief.

The repeat tester

This is the opposite situation: the person comes in for HIV tests regularly and reveals a pattern of frequent high-risk behaviour in between tests.

This person is trying to manage the anxiety caused by their sexual risk-taking by having HIV tests as a form of reassurance - an irrational reassurance, because HIV tests are not a form of safer sex, and receiving a negative HIV result in no way reduces the degree of real risk they are running. At worst, the person may conclude that repeat negative tests are proof they are immune to HIV. They may also misunderstand the risks of HIV transmission or the meaning of the probabilities of transmission cited (for instance, a person who hears that the chances of HIV infection from a single act of anal intercourse is 'only one in 350' may misinterpret this to mean that their chances of infection are only one in 350 no matter how many times they have unprotected sex.

Repeat testers such as this should be encouraged to discuss their sexual risk management and whether they can adopt better strategies for safer sex than essentially subjecting themselves to a regular 'lottery' of HIV testing.

The accuracy of HIV testing

See also *The scientific basis of HIV antibody testing* later in this chapter.

A positive HIV test result in the UK will be accurate because the test has been done on two samples of your blood. In all, your blood will have been have tested by several testing kits (or assays) to show that it contains antibodies to HIV. The chances that this procedure could yield a false positive result are minute.

One paper (Chou) regarding the situation in the USA, where the same tests are used, put it this way:

"The use of repeatedly reactive enzyme immunoassay followed by confirmatory Western blot or immunofluorescent assay remains the standard method for diagnosing HIV-1 infection. A large study of HIV testing in 752 U.S. laboratories reported a sensitivity of 99.7% and specificity of 98.5% for enzyme immunoassay, and studies in U.S. blood donors reported specificities of 99.8% and greater than 99.99%. With confirmatory Western blot, the chance of a false-positive identification in a low-prevalence setting is about 1 in 250 000 (95% CI, 1 in 173 000 to 1 in 379 000)."

Other studies have shown the chance of a false positive on this method as being at most one chance in 143,000.

It is extremely important to emphasise that this degree of certainty is only achieved by confirmatory testing. A single HIV test done by the cheapest method, the ELISA assay (see below) may have a specificity of between 98.5% and 99.8%. This means that there is anything between one chance in 66 and one chance in 500 of it yielding a false-positive result when a sample is tested. Even with the Western Blot method, there is a chance of about one in 5000 of a single test yielding a false-positive result. This is why most clinics test all samples at least twice and why, if you do get a positive result, a confirmatory test is needed. This is one reason why there are reservations about licensing home testing. For more information, see *The scientific basis of HIV antibody testing* below.

Indeterminate results are also not uncommon. An indeterminate result is one which shows a weak positive reaction, because of some form of unknown antibody cross-reaction, or because of a technical error, or because only very low levels of HIV antibodies are present.

The latter is the most common scenario, and is usually because a weak positive result can occur if someone is tested soon after infection. This is due to the fact that a virus is composed of different proteins, and antibodies will form to each of those proteins. In the case of HIV, some proteins become detectable in the blood long before others. If antibodies to a single protein are detectable, rather than to a range of proteins, this is likely to trigger a weak positive result.

A negative result will be accurate if you have waited to test until at least three months after the last occasion on which you were at risk. This is because it takes most people weeks or occasionally even months for the body to form enough antibodies to give a positive test result. A test any earlier than this can produce a negative result, even though you are probably at your most infectious if you have just been infected.

A tiny number of people (estimates range from one in 35,000 to one in 100,000) never produce testable antibodies to HIV, but note that this means that there are no more than 30 people in the USA or two in the UK who would test false-negative because of this if HIV tests are done properly.

Reference

Chou R. *Screening for HIV: a review of the evidence for the U.S. Preventive Services Task Force.* Ann Intern Med. 2005; 143(1): 55-73. 2005.

Will I be tested for HIV2?

If you donate blood you will be tested for HIV-2 because all regional blood transfusion services now use a combined test for HIV-1 and HIV-2. Testing for HIV-2 began in June 1990.

This may not be the case at all GU clinics or other testing centres. The only way to establish this is to contact the clinic in question, since the form of test used by each district health authority is up to the virologist in charge.

The prevalence of HIV-2 in the UK is so low that a doctor may only consider it advisable for you to be tested for both viruses if you have had a sexual partner from West Africa or a blood transfusion in a West African country.

If you do test positive for HIV-2, this probably means that you are unlikely to develop any symptoms of immune system damage for up to fifteen years, if at all, since HIV-2 is thought to be considerably less virulent than HIV-1.

PCR testing/viral load testing/ nucleic acid testing

PCR stands for polymerase chain reaction testing, a form of test which looks for genetic material from HIV and then amplifies this material. PCR testing is able to detect the presence of the virus in the body even when it is not replicating. It is a highly sensitive test, which can cause problems in its use, since it is vulnerable to contamination.

Methods for PCR testing are developing, and false results are now less common. PCR is increasingly used to detect HIV infection in children before maternal antibodies clear (see *HIV testing, pregnancy and children*).

A simplified version of PCR testing, called Nucleic Acid Testing (NAT), is now increasingly being used in high-incidence populations in the USA in order to detect people in the 'window period'.

The testing procedure

A full description of the testing procedure is essential to obtaining fully informed consent. It should emphasise:

- That it isn't necessary to make a decision about testing on the spot.

- How long the client will have to wait for the results. The waiting period can be acutely stressful for clients, and the best way of alleviating this stress is by offering same-day testing or results within a few days. However, this shouldn't reduce the time available for counselling or consideration.

- How the results will be given. Results will usually be given face to face, but sometimes they can be given over the telephone or by post.

- Who will know the result - what records will be kept by the testing centre? Will the client's GP be informed?

Post-test counselling

A positive result

Whereas there is a debate about pre-test counselling, the extent to which it is really 'counselling' and whether it needs to be offered in all cases, there is agreement that anyone receiving a positive result is likely to need professional support, and should be offered that support by their clinic or by the other organisations that offer support.

However, some people may need time to get over the shock of diagnosis and may not be in the mood to talk immediately after receiving a positive result. Support should therefore be offered, but on the individual's own terms.

As with giving any other bad news, there is no easy way to do it. Any person receiving a positive HIV test result is likely to have some kind of emotional reaction to it and need a period of adjustment, but each individual will have different immediate and longer-term needs and will react to the news in different ways.

Characteristic reactions span a huge range of emotional responses:

- **Denial** or no apparent emotional reaction. This is probably indicative of shock and the need for a period of adjustment; the person may need to go away and think through their own reaction before discussing it with anyone. Lack of affect can also indicate depression.

- **Anxiety,** which may be more or less acute and managed in different ways ranging from coping behaviours (see below) to a need to acquire as much information as possible

- **Coping behaviours** such as drinking, taking drugs or - of concern - using sex as a 'fix'.

- **Anger** either at known or unknown persons who infected them or at themselves

- **Isolation,** indicative of depression or anxiety around stigma or, conversely, **needing reassurance.** In these circumstances people sometimes impulsively disclose their status to others and later regret it.

It can be tempting to reassure or overwhelm the client with information rather than giving them space to acknowledge feelings. Indeed, the person who requests large amounts of information may be trying to use this to quell feelings of acute anxiety that might be better expressed. Almost everyone who receives an HIV diagnosis will feel shock, which will make it difficult for them to deal immediately with complicated information on topics such as disease progression and safer sex.

It is important that you arrange to see the client again soon, as well as fixing other follow-up sessions. Does your client also need to arrange a clinical session? Make sure that you give your client helpline telephone numbers, and information about where they can contact you. It may be helpful to give the client some written material. It will be better not to give extensive details about the possible negative effects of HIV infection before the immediate information is understood.

Check that your client knows whom they can turn to immediately. If your client has brought a partner or friend with them, check if the client would like you to talk to them both.

- **For further information on issues for people who have been diagnosed HIV-positive, see *Living with HIV*.**

- **For treatment options for the newly diagnosed, see the *HIV/AIDS Treatments Directory*.**

A negative result

As with pre-test counselling, it should not be assumed that a person receiving a negative result 'needs' counselling. They may have had an accurate understanding of their degree of risk and may simply wish to walk away with a sigh of relief. A negative test result offers no guarantees for the future and does not mean someone will automatically adopt safer sex or safer drug use. Studies have not shown any link between offering pre- or post-test counselling to the HIV-negative and any subsequent behaviour change.

Even a negative result can be a shock, however, in certain circumstances. The person may have assumed they were positive and be at a loss to handle the unexpected discovery that they have 'escaped' HIV. They may even express disappointment or sadness about being negative. This is not necessarily pathological; someone who is themselves negative, if from a high-prevalence community such as gay men or sub-Saharan Africans, may know friends and family with HIV or AIDS, including people who have died, and may feel conflicting and painful emotions.

This is even more likely to apply if the person concerned is in a relationship with an HIV-positive partner, or is contemplating beginning such a relationship. Such emotions have been known to lead to risk-taking behaviour.

In this situation it is wise to be sensitive to whether or not the person wishes to discuss their negative result. For them, it may be that seeking an HIV test is an indication that they are poised to make changes to their behaviour, with encouragement.

Special issues for gay men

The experience of testing HIV-positive is now a common one among gay men in the UK, but it is important that counsellors do not make the assumption that all gay men are the same.

A positive result can reawaken feelings of self-hatred which many gay men thought they had dealt with, and for someone who still harbours such feelings, it can be especially devastating. Finding out how a client feels about being gay during pre-test counselling, if done sensitively, can often be helpful in preparing the counsellor for delivering a positive result. For example, some gay men may see a positive result as the inevitable consequence of their lifestyle or as a confirmation of the negative messages about gay men prevalent in our society.

For some gay men, a positive result may bring with it the fear of the loss of a particularly important part of their identity - their sexuality - or fear about the limiting of their potential for forming relationships.

Safer sex counselling with HIV-positive gay men must stress the need to protect against other sexually transmitted infections that could place a burden on the immune system. This may require the adoption of certain safer sex guidelines, which are discussed in *Safer sex: Safer sex for people for with HIV*.

Gay men who test positive may be in a relationship with a partner who is also HIV-positive, and may want to know whether unprotected anal intercourse is considered safe between men who are both infected. This question is discussed in *Safer sex for people with HIV*.

When discussing safer sex with men who identify as gay, it should never be assumed that their sexual partners are exclusively male. Although many gay men will not identify themselves as bisexual, they may have female partners too. The importance of safer sex with any female partners should be stressed.

People who are diagnosed with HIV and are also told that they have a low CD4 count may have an especially severe shock, since they will be faced with pressure to make immediate decisions about treatment. In these circumstances it may be better to

counsel caution rather than encourage an immediate rush to commence treatment. It is important that anyone who commences anti-viral treatment does so after a process of self-education, and not just because a doctor has recommended the treatment.

Some gay men may have reactions of guilt, shock or disbelief after a **negative** result. For many, this is the result of seeing many of their friends or peers affected by the disease. They may question why they are exceptional, and experience long-term feelings of guilt that they find difficult either to acknowledge or discuss with people close to them. This phenomenon has been labelled 'survivor guilt', and is a reaction that was also noted amongst those Jews who escaped the Holocaust, especially those who left Europe just before World War II. Sensitive acknowledgement of these feelings by a counsellor may be more helpful than an encouragement to go off and celebrate. Some gay men who test negative may be just as much in need of long-term counselling support as those who test positive.

However, these reactions are becoming less common as deaths due to AIDS are becoming less common, and younger gay men who are diagnosed HIV-positive may feel a sense of acute isolation from their peers because they know no one who is openly HIV-positive and have not discussed HIV with their friends. People like this may have an especially strong need to meet other HIV-positive people, especially younger ones or the newly diagnosed, to seek reassurance, gain information and tips on living with HIV, and find a non-stigmatising group of peers to relate to.

In this situation it is also possible that gay men will be unable to accept a negative test result, and will seek a repeat test. Others may seek repeat tests for reasons that cannot simply be labelled as 'worried well' behaviour. In a social group with such a high HIV prevalence, anxiety about coming into contact with HIV is likely to be heightened by anecdotal information - for instance about the safety of oral sex - and feelings of distress or horror at the effects HIV infection has had on friends.

Special issues for women

It is important to remember to give women information about sexual activity. Some women have found that in post-test counselling they are given advice about pregnancy (see *HIV testing, pregnancy and children* later in this chapter) but very little about their sex lives. Sex may be a more immediate concern. It is important to stress that an HIV-positive diagnosis does not mean an end to sex. In contrast to gay men, many women who are diagnosed HIV-positive will not be aware that many HIV-positive women continue to have sexual relationships.

If the woman is HIV-negative she may need support in adopting or maintaining safer sex. This could be particularly important, and difficult, if she cannot communicate easily with her partner(s), e.g. because of an abusive relationship or suspected infidelity.

If the woman is HIV-positive she will need information about how to protect herself from other STIs, and about sexual practices through which she could pass on the virus.

Not all women who have sex with other women will reveal this to their counsellor, but lesbian and bisexual women need information about any risks involved in sex with other women, see *HIV transmission: Woman-to-woman transmission*. Conversely, women who identify themselves as lesbians who inject drugs should be given information about the risks of sharing injecting equipment.

HIV-positive women will need special information about future clinical monitoring, such as the need for more frequent cervical smears.

Women with dependants, including children, may need encouragement and support to continue to address their health and need for support, as they may place the needs of their dependants before their own.

Special issues for drug users

It is important to use clear understandable language; it may be helpful for the client to have the result written down for them.

Is your client too stoned or drunk to be able to take in the information? Would it be better to reschedule the counselling to another day? Clients may use drugs or alcohol as 'Dutch courage' to find out their result, and it will be difficult to refuse to give them their result.

Remember to reinforce harm reduction techniques as a response to either a negative or a positive result (e.g. to remain negative or to protect one's health). Again, reinforce the client's own harm reduction strategies.

Be aware that drug users' primary concerns may not be around their health status and they may be initially resistant to the medical care you recommend to them.

The client will need to be reminded that a negative result does not mean they are immune to HIV infection.

For many people the information given to them during a counselling situation can be complicated and confusing, compounded by nervousness and drug- or alcohol-related factors. It is often helpful to reinforce verbal information by writing or drawing key points or through the use of a leaflet.

Many clients will use drugs as a result of either a negative or positive result. It can be valuable to discuss with them how to manage this celebration or commiseration 'hit'. There are reports of higher accidental death among people with HIV, which may be a result of people living more recklessly. The time immediately after a result is a particularly vulnerable time.

The result of an HIV test may motivate some drug users to reconsider their drug use. This may be to increase or reduce their use of drugs. For example, some drug users who test positive may see this as an opportunity to stop using, whereas others will see no point in going through the pain of stopping. It is unlikely that someone will embark on a definitive course of action immediately after receiving a test result.

Drug users who test negative may need advice about where they can access benefits and support outside of HIV services. Some drug users will have a number of friends who are HIV-positive, and may experience some of the same feelings of 'survivor guilt' as gay men can sometimes feel (see *Special issues for gay men,* above).

Special issues for people from ethnic minorities

It is not really possible to make a list of issues that are common to all people from ethnic minorities, since this term covers people who have had a very wide range of different cultural and personal experiences. However, there are a number of key issues that research has shown can particularly affect people from ethnic minorities.

One common finding is that people from ethnic minorities may be especially afraid of being stigmatised within their communities and may be much more reluctant, because of this, to seek support. This applies regardless of whether the community in question is one that has high or low HIV prevalence.

Language can be an especially important issue. People from ethnic minorities may need translation services, and without such a service, may have difficulty understanding what they are being told

about HIV testing and treatment. A further complication can be that some clients may be especially sensitive to the presence of a third party translator from their community, especially where that community is very small and they fear exposure.

Counselling in translation should not be conducted by someone who just happens to be able to speak the right language. It is important that it should be conducted by someone who understands HIV infection and the need for confidentiality.

Pre- and post-test counselling is likely to be especially important for people from cultures that value oral information-giving over written materials - for instance, people from Vietnamese backgrounds.

Men may have difficulty talking to women counsellors, as women may to men. This can be especially true for people from Muslim backgrounds.

Different cultures can have very different understandings of health and illness, and very different traditions around doctoring and medicine, and it is important to be aware of this.

It is also important to understand the differing experiences, fears and understandings of HIV/AIDS that clients from African countries may have.

In many African countries, an HIV diagnosis is likely to lead to stigmatisation, social rejection and ostracism, with the consequence that people with HIV can become depressed, isolated and fearful.

It is not uncommon for people from African countries who are diagnosed with HIV in the UK to assume that they are going to die very soon and simply retreat into their homes. It is especially important to make sure that your ethnic minority clients understand the difference between HIV and AIDS and, especially, that they know about any local support and information services they can turn to.

Having children is important in most cultures, but in some, it is regarded as being of the highest importance. Women and men from such cultures may seek a lot of information about HIV and conception, pregnancy and delivery.

Issues about planning for the future will need to be raised with mothers who are HIV-positive, in case they should die or become too ill to care for their children. Who will care for their children? If they are to be cared for within an extended family, what will the family be told about HIV infection, and how will this affect their treatment of the children?

Gay and bisexual men from ethnic minorities may have greater concerns about the consequences for their family relationships of an HIV-positive result, often due to the greater importance of family ties. It may also be difficult for men from ethnic minorities to acknowledge their bisexuality even to themselves, let alone to their female partners.

Many people from ethnic minorities seek HIV testing only after they have begun to develop symptoms. This is partly due to a lack of information about HIV infection and the available treatments, especially in refugee communities, and partly due to poor access to health care.

Refugees may also feel insecure about their status in the UK when presenting for testing, and uncertain of the consequences of a positive result for their residency in the UK. They will need special reassurance about the confidentiality of the HIV testing process and of follow-up procedures if they test positive.

They are more likely to return for follow-up care and counselling if such anxieties have been clearly addressed in pre-test counselling. This may involve asking blunt questions about the client's residency status, and giving reassurance that the information is absolutely confidential and will not be recorded anywhere.

The scientific basis of HIV antibody testing

Introduction to antibodies

The quickest and easiest way to find out if someone is HIV-positive is usually by testing for antibodies to the virus in blood or other body fluids. No single test is ideal for all uses. In practice, tests with different properties must be combined to get the information people need.

Beyond antibody tests, many other different tests are used in HIV medicine. Some of these are used to detect and measure HIV activity. CD4 counts and viral load tests are particularly important when taking decisions about antiretroviral treatment. These can incidentally provide a check on the accuracy of HIV antibody testing.

All antibody tests are based on the principle that antibodies are specific in what they will bind to. The 'antigen' to which an antibody binds is usually part of the surface of a protein made up of 'peptides' - particular sequences of amino-acids.

All HIV antibody tests must include HIV-related antigens. Many of them also include antibodies, which may or may not be HIV-related. The properties of each test depend on how the test antigens and any test antibodies are made and how they are used.

Some of the latest ('fourth generation') antibody tests include a test for an HIV protein called 'p24' and are therefore known as 'combined antibody/antigen tests'.

There is always a possibility of human error. Some of the tests described here are complex and depend on highly trained and competent operators. Beyond what happens in the laboratory, good systems for taking, handling and labelling samples are vital, with checks and safeguards built into the procedures.

How antibodies are made

Humans and other animals, such as mice, rats, goats or chickens, can make millions of different kinds of antibody protein or 'immunoglobulin'.

The cells that make these antibodies are white blood cells called B-cells, which originate in the bone marrow, from where they move to other sites, such as the lymph nodes. Their activation involves other parts of the immune system, including some of the CD4 cells that are directly affected by HIV.

Different kinds of antibody are created in B-cells by shuffling specialised DNA sequences, as they mature, to create B-cell-lines that each make just one kind of antibody. The shuffling is random, but the immune system selects and promotes the growth of cell-lines that happen to make antibodies, for example, against HIV in someone who is HIV-positive.

In a process called the maturation of antibody response, antibodies can be modified and improved over time. These modifications may include switching from producing antibodies of one class, such as IgM, to another such as IgG. ('Ig' is short for 'immunoglobulin'.) In all, there are five main classes of antibody, with different biological properties; others are IgA, IgD and IgE. (There are further sub-classes, especially within IgG.)

The same principles are now used in the laboratory to create cell-lines that make large quantities of useful antibodies at low cost.

Antibodies can be produced in the laboratory by injecting an animal with an antigen and then extracting antibodies from its blood. This method is used, for example, to create anti-venoms against snakebite.

A more reliable method is to find the cells that produce the antibodies and fuse them with tumour cells, to create long-lived cell-lines that make large quantities of antibodies.

Laboratory-produced antibodies based on a single cell line are called 'monoclonal antibodies,' in contrast to those extracted from blood - such as the human immunoglobulins used for the short-term prevention of viral hepatitis.

With genetic engineering, it is now possible to create libraries of artificial antibodies and to select those of interest, without having to use whole animals at all. It is even possible to put the DNA into plants and then grow antibodies that can be harvested for medical or scientific use.

Making antibodies visible

Early HIV antibody tests used antigens that bound to the non-variable parts of human antibodies. These antibodies were then linked to an enzyme - another protein - that drives an easily detected chemical reaction. The combined or 'conjugated' protein is then manufactured in large quantities.

An enzyme called horseradish peroxidase is commonly used because it is cheap and easy to link to other proteins. It drives a simple chemical reaction that is easy to see and to measure because it changes the colour of a test solution.

One alternative to enzyme-linkage is to label antibodies with a substance called fluorescein, which glows bright green under UV light. This is the basis for IFA tests (which are explained later in this section).

A limitation of the earliest HIV antibody tests was that they used antigens that only bound to IgG antibodies. Of the five classes, IgG is by far the most common in blood. However, the very first antibodies in the blood of someone who is HIV-positive are often of the IgM class.

The more modern tests, as we shall see, can recognise IgM as well as IgG, enabling detection of HIV antibodies approximately one week earlier in the course of HIV infection.

Mothers and babies

A mother's IgG antibodies cross the placenta during pregnancy into her baby, but not her IgA antibodies. Tests for IgA have therefore been used to identify HIV-positive babies. However, these tests don't work very well in the youngest babies. If viral load tests are available, as they are in the UK, they offer a better alternative (though it is best to make sure that the particular test works for the mother's strain of the virus, before relying on it to tell whether her baby is HIV-positive).

How antigens are made

To make an HIV antibody test, HIV-related antigens are always needed.

The simplest way to produce the antigens is from HIV virus particles grown in a cell culture. A centrifuge and detergent are used to extract around ten different HIV proteins, which can be used as the antigens in a test. (A centrifuge spins a sample at high speed to throw down any solids suspended in a liquid; the proteins will then be in the solution at the top of the sample container.)

One disadvantage of this is that HIV virus particles always include surface proteins from the cells in which the virus is grown. Any test based on them will therefore detect any antibodies that may be present against those human proteins. Such antibodies might arise from a blood transfusion, or from sexual exposure to a partner whose cells have those proteins on their surface.

Whole proteins or peptides?

Another way to create the antigens is to engineer them as proteins in bacteria. This makes the HIV proteins 'cleaner' and is safer and cheaper than growing the virus itself in a laboratory.

There is still a risk that the system may pick up some antibodies that are not specifically made in response to HIV, but 'cross-react' with some part of the virus.

So, finally, it is possible to choose parts of the virus to which antibodies commonly bind and to make them as peptides. Typically, parts of the envelope protein gp41 have been chosen by test-designers.

By including multiple peptides in the system, a range of antibodies against HIV can be identified.

However, someone might be infected with an unusual strain of HIV that doesn't have matching peptides anywhere on the surface of any of its proteins. So tests like this may not be appropriate for initial screening of blood samples.

Substrates

For use in a test, the antigens have to be fixed or 'bound' to a chemically inactive surface, called a substrate.

In an ELISA test (see below) this usually takes the form of polystyrene beads or could be the surface of a test plate with hollows to take test samples. In other tests, such as Western Blot, a flat nitrocellulose surface is used.

A basic ELISA test

ELISA stands for 'enzyme-linked immunosorbent assay'. Immunosorbent means it uses the principle of an antibody binding to an antigen. Enzyme-linked has been explained in *Making antibodies visible*.

When blood has been taken for an ELISA test, the next step is to separate the serum (a clear fluid present in blood, which will contain any antibodies present) from the red blood cells.

This serum is added to the substrate on which the antigen is fixed and incubated. If there are antibodies in the serum that recognise the antigen, they will bind to the antigen.

The substrate is then washed, to remove any antibodies that are NOT bound to the antigen.

The enzyme-linked antibody is then added and incubated, to bind to any antibodies that are still fixed to the antigen.

Once more, the substrate is washed to remove any enzyme-linked antibodies that are not bound to it.

Finally, a solution of the chemical on which the enzyme acts is added.

If the enzyme-linked antibody is present, a reaction occurs and a change of colour is seen. This is taken as a positive result.

If the enzyme-linked antibody has all been washed away, no reaction occurs. This is taken as a negative result.

Cross-reactions with malaria

In the very early years of HIV testing, the presence of antibodies to malaria was thought to lead to false positive results (Biggar). The tests had originally been designed without taking into account the prevalence of malarial antibodies in the populations of countries outside the United States, where the tests were first developed. By 1991, a study using newer antibody test kits failed to demonstrate any difference in the prevalence of malarial antibodies between seropositive and seronegative blood donors in an equatorial country, suggesting that people with malarial antibodies are now no more likely to test positive for HIV antibodies (Chattopadhya).

Competitive ELISA

In a competitive ELISA test the HIV antigen is exposed at the same time both to the test serum and to enzyme-linked antibodies chosen to bind to the HIV antigen.

What happens next depends on the outcome of a 'competition' between the antibodies, to see which binds more closely to the antigen. Weakly binding, 'cross-reactive' antibodies should not give a positive result, so this test should be more specific (see below) than basic ELISA tests. However, there is a risk that weakly binding genuine HIV antibodies might also be displaced, giving rise to false negatives and making the test less sensitive than basic ELISA tests.

This test should also detect antibodies, no matter what class of antibodies they are. Or, to put it the other way, it cannot distinguish between antibodies of different classes.

If the test serum has antibodies that bind to the antigen as well as or better than the test antibodies, these will prevent the enzyme-linked antibodies from binding. Otherwise the test antibodies, with their attached enzymes, will be bound.

The system is washed in the normal way for an ELISA test before the indicator chemical solution is added.

In this case, a colour change means a negative result and no change is a positive result.

The accuracy of this system does not depend on having highly purified antigen, because the only antigens that matter are the ones recognised by the enzyme-linked antibodies. The system has the further advantage that control tests are easy to run and will quickly show if the test system is working properly, as a check on operator error.

Sandwich tests

In practice, the ELISA tests previously described are being replaced by 'sandwich' tests, also known as 'third and fourth generation assays'.

These make use of the fact that antibodies each have more than one binding site. IgG antibodies have two binding sites and the IgM antibodies, which appear early in the course of infection, each have ten sites. This means that if one site binds to a fixed antigen, the other(s) can bind to a labelled antigen, holding them together in an 'immune complex'. This immune complex can be detected using the label on the antigen in the way previously described for detecting labelled enzymes. These tests are particularly good at detecting low levels of IgM antibodies, and can therefore detect antibodies earlier in the course of HIV infection than previous tests.

Another advantage of this system is that the sample can be added at the same time as the labelled antigen, reducing the number of washing steps involved. Technicians therefore have to spend less time on them and they are easier to automate, reducing costs.

Combined antibody and p24 antigen tests

Yet another advantage is that the same test system can include both an antibody test and a test for the HIV protein called 'p24' (Gag protein), which is the main component of the core of the virus. Testing for p24 detects some cases of HIV infection before antibodies are produced, further shortening the 'window period' in which people may test negative despite being able to transmit the virus. This is especially useful in blood transfusion services, although it adds costs if separate p24 or PCR (viral load) tests are done on samples which are positive in the initial screening test but antibody-negative in the Western Blot or IFA tests (described later), used to confirm positive results.

The p24 antigen test is a mirror image of the double antigen sandwich just described. Here, part of the test surface is coated with carefully selected monoclonal antibodies that recognise p24.

The sample is added to the test system together with a labelled antibody that recognises another part of the p24 molecule. If p24 is present in the sample, then a complex is formed which can be revealed in the same way as the label on the antigen in the antigen sandwich.

Using the same label on the antibodies and on the antigens in the combined system makes the test very simple to perform.

These combined antigen/antibody tests will NOT detect antibodies directed against p24. Fixed p24 antigens, needed to detect antibodies directed against p24, must be excluded, because they would also bind the labelled anti-p24 antibodies, making the test unusable.

One consequence is that if any vaccine were to be based on the p24 protein, then antibodies directed against that vaccine would not cause vaccine recipients to test positive in these tests.

Western Blot

The Western Blot test is a kind of ELISA test that distinguishes between antibodies that recognise different antigens in the test system.

So instead of serum being put (say) into a hollow well on a plate, it is spread over a nitrocellulose-coated plate to which the antigens have been bound in different places.

Because each plate is slightly different in the position of these bands of antigen, the test must use control sera and the results are read by looking at the depth of the colour change on each band.

The plates are expensive to make, and the test can give indeterminate results, when just one or two bands change colour or the colour change is not very marked. However, if the result shows that multiple HIV antigens are recognised by antibodies in the test sample, then the test is reasonably conclusive.

It is also possible to 'print' different antigens onto a strip in different places, to create a test that looks like a Western Blot and is used in the same way, but could distinguish between different antigens that wouldn't be separated on a real Western Blot - for example, because they were of the same molecular weight.

Limitations of Western Blot

Western Blot relies on a subjective judgement of the intensity of the bands of antibodies that form in response to particular antigens. It also relies upon well-trained technical staff, so false positive results are possible with this method just as with any other laboratory test. Early literature that describes Western Blot as a gold standard for antibody testing should be read with caution.

False positive results could arise as a result of similarities in the molecular weight of proteins derived from cellular material rather than from HIV.

Rare antibody cross-reactions have been documented in individuals with auto-immune illnesses such as lupus and multiple sclerosis, and in the case of people who have recently been vaccinated against hepatitis B, influenza and tetanus. Transient positive HIV antibody reactions after vaccination have been reported, but a positive antibody test for HIV has not been detected upon subsequent tests. Transient false positive results have also been seen in blood dialysis patients and recipients of blood transfusions. It should be emphasised that all these false positive results are isolated reports. In the case of multiple sclerosis, for instance, such reports are vastly outnumbered by studies which have failed to find HIV antibodies in large numbers of MS patients who lack known risks.

Particular antibodies considered to be specific for HIV sometimes appear in uninfected people as a consequence of other infections or auto-immune problems. For instance, 13% of people with warts were shown in one study to have antibodies to p24 but not to any other HIV antigens. In the same study 41% of a group of patients with multiple sclerosis were shown to have antibody to p24 but no other antibody (Ranki).

HIV may share similar genetic sequences to human retroviruses that have become encoded into human genes (endogenous retroviruses). These sequences are confined to the gag region alone, and do not include the env and pol regions (Haist). This may be another explanation for the greater frequency of false p24-positive reactions on the Western Blot test.

The p24 reaction may also be partly attributable to cross-reaction with cytomegalovirus (Landini). CMV does not generate cross-reactions to other HIV proteins.

Cross-reactions to other proteins such as gp41 have also been observed, but cross-reactions to all these proteins at once has never been reported.

Thus it is very important that HIV infection only be diagnosed upon the presence of a range of HIV antibodies: antibodies to p24 and p31 (HIV core proteins) are not sufficient without antibodies to either gp41, gp120 or gp160 (envelope proteins).

Western Blot should NOT be used as a stand-alone HIV antibody test, but only as part of a multi-test strategy.

IFA tests

IFA stands for 'indirect immunofluorescence assay'.

IFA tests are based on preparations of fixed HIV-infected and uninfected cells, supplied in wells on a microscope slide, to which test sera are added and incubated.

The idea is that anti-HIV antibodies will bind to HIV infected cells but not to uninfected ones. The test requires a skilled operator and an expensive piece of equipment, but gives faster results than Western Blot.

After incubation, the preparation is washed and fluorescein-labelled antibody against human immunoglobulins is added. This is again incubated and washed and then prepared for viewing.

When the slide is viewed under a fluorescent microscope, HIV antibodies are present if the infected cells in the test system glow green and the uninfected ones do not.

Rapid tests

All the tests described so far depend on having a laboratory with trained technicians to operate them. They often take more than an hour to carry out and some Western Blot tests have to be incubated overnight.

A number of companies have developed 'Rapid Tests' supplied as single-use kits that do not require laboratory facilities, although most of them do need to be kept in a refrigerator until they are used. Most of them use whole blood, not serum, which makes them much easier to use by health staff and, sometimes, untrained personnel.

These kits are a lot more expensive, per test, than ELISAs. They are therefore not suitable for use in mass screening, for example of blood donors. They have hardly been used in most Western countries. Only one has been licensed by the US Food and Drug Administration: the SUDS test made by Murex/Abbott [off the market at the time of writing, due to manufacturing problems].

However, evaluations by the World Health Organization and by the UK's Public Health Laboratory Service suggest that the best of these tests are comparable in performance to most ELISA tests. Individual tests give a comparatively high rate of false positives, but when used in combination these may still be a realistic alternative to ELISA and Western Blot tests.

The biggest advantage of Rapid Tests is, as their name implies, that they give results very fast - often in as little as 10 to 20 minutes. This means that people who may have travelled many miles to reach a test centre need not make another journey to get their results.

In the USA, it has been shown that a Rapid Test used as an initial screen can greatly increase the proportion of positive people who return for their test results. Unfortunately, when confirmation is delayed, many people are given an initial positive result that later turns out to be negative, causing avoidable distress.

How rapid tests work

One system uses antigen coated on the inside of a small tube through which the blood sample flows. If antibodies bind to the antigen, they block up the tube.

Another system uses a membrane on which the antigen is coated. If antibodies in a blood sample bind to this, they will hold a colloidal suspension of gold, which makes them visible as a dark spot on the membrane.

Risks and limitations

One disadvantage of Rapid Tests is their potential for misuse, if a single test is used without confirmation. The temptation to do this in a community where HIV prevalence is high, so that most positive results are genuinely positive, and where even $2 or $3 is a lot of money, must be considerable.

People working in the UK with migrant and refugee communities may come across individuals who have been tested in this way without proper confirmation of their test results. It is standard practice in the UK is to re-test any HIV-positive person who is seen for the first time by an HIV treatment service. If any test negative, they must obviously be treated with great sensitivity, as they will be at risk of losing confidence in treatment services which they or their family may still need at a later date.

Urine and saliva tests

Urine testing is more expensive and time-consuming than standard HIV testing, so it is used very infrequently. Saliva testing is used much more often, and involves chewing on cotton wool or using a small stick similar to a cotton bud to collect the fluid that lubricates the gums, in which HIV antibodies can be detected.

At first used largely for research and surveillance purposes, saliva tests are now becoming much more frequently used in rapid community testing situations, particularly in resource-poor settings. For more on this, see **How the test is done** above.

Detuned tests

For special purposes, it is possible to use tests in a different ways to get additional information on what is happening to the epidemic.

A good example of this is the development of 'detuned' ELISA tests to identify people who have only recently become infected with HIV.

This makes use of the observation that in the early stages of HIV infection relatively low levels of antibodies are present, which increase in quantity and quality (binding strength) over a period of months.

By taking a very sensitive test and making it less so, then using both tests on a part of each sample, it is possible to find some people who test positive on the sensitive test but negative on the less sensitive 'detuned' one. Complex maths then allows an estimate to be made of the proportion of people in a population who have seroconverted within the last year - the incidence of HIV.

This might help to identify populations where transmission is at its peak, to target HIV prevention efforts, such as help with partner notification, where they are most likely to be useful. However, at present detuned tests are largely used for research purposes rather than as a clinical tool, as there is no evidence that treatment in early (as opposed to acute) infection makes any difference to time to progression to AIDS. The most frequently used detuned assay is the STARHS (Serologic Testing Algorithm for Recent HIV Seroconversion) assay.

Test accuracy

The accuracy of any test is usually described using the ideas of 'sensitivity' and 'specificity'. However, the predictive value of the test - which is what most people would mean by its 'accuracy' - also depends on how common or rare HIV infection is in the population that is being tested.

Sensitivity

Sensitivity is the ability to detect all true positive results. A highly sensitive test should produce as few false-negative tests as possible. A test with a sensitivity of 99.9% will produce a false-negative result on one in 1000 blood samples tested. In other words, if you have 1000 blood samples from a high prevalence population, and 10% of them are from people who in fact have HIV (and are beyond the 'window period'), then there is a 10% chance that you may produce a single false-negative result and 99 positive results, and a 90% chance that you will produce all 100 positive results.

Sensitivity is most important for an initial screening test and it is where basic ELISA tests are strongest, in ruling out as HIV-negative all samples that are in fact so.

A basic ELISA test can be very sensitive, meaning that if antibodies are present, it will almost certainly detect them. It is also cheap to carry out on large numbers of samples, which makes it very suitable for initial screening. Commercial tests typically include a range of antigens to cover HIV-1 (group M) and HIV-2 and, increasingly, HIV-1 group O as well.

WHO currently recommends (in 2001) that ELISA kits should not be used unless they can detect 100% of known positive samples in a reference panel of 203 HIV-1 and/or 60 HIV-2 samples. For Rapid Tests, they require 99% sensitivity, reflecting the different use to which they tend to be put (telling individuals their status, rather than screening blood supplies).

The main limitation on the sensitivity of antibody tests is that it takes the body a while to mount an immune response to any infection. In the first few weeks, the antibodies may be at low levels in the blood and may not bind as well as antibodies produced later in the course of infection. These limitations have been partly overcome by improving the antigens used in HIV ELISA tests, but will always remain.

People who are infected with HIV will mostly test positive on modern antibody tests within six weeks of infection, and some in as little as one week, though the possibility of window periods of up to three months or, exceptionally, even longer, remains.

Specificity

Specificity is about the number of negative sera correctly identified as negative. WHO does not recommend the use of tests with a specificity of less than 95% when tested on a panel of African sera, but in practice most commercial tests are much better than this. One example is a test described as '99.8% specific'.

What this means is that 0.2% of samples - or one in 500 - will test positive when they are not.

Such a test must be used with another test, using different antigens, to confirm it. That second test need not be any more specific (though it helps if it is) to reduce the chances of a double-false-positive result to a very low level.

The tests most commonly used for this are a Western Blot test or an IFA test. Another way is to use other ELISA tests based on different antigens or to use a competitive ELISA test.

Predictive value

The specificity of a test varies in relevance inversely with the true HIV prevalence in the group studied. The lower the true HIV prevalence, the higher the chances that a positive result may, in fact, be a false positive result, to the extent that false positives may substantially outnumber true positives. Conversely, in a high-prevalence group, true positives will substantially outnumber false positives.

The specificity of a test relative to the prevalence within a particular group of samples is called its **predictive value**.

If the test mentioned in the previous example were used in a population such as UK blood donors - where the level of HIV infection has been around 1 in 100,000 donations - then, for every true positive result, there would be about 200 false positive results.

Consider, however, the opposite case, where the true level of HIV in a population is one in eight - which is the approximate prevalence amongst gay men in London. Here, there will be only one false positive result for approximately 63 true positive results.

It is important to confirm the test result in both cases, but if the people being tested are, for example, women about to give birth who have not received previous antenatal care, then in the second case one might not wait for confirmation before deciding to offer antiretroviral treatment to prevent HIV transmission to their babies. In the first case, all 200 donations would be kept out of the blood supply used in hospitals.

Sensitivity, in short, has a price - giving some false positive results. In the older kinds of test, as we have seen, these could occur because non-HIV proteins were included in the system. In the newer systems there is still a trade-off. Tests that are too precise can miss genuine HIV antibodies. This would, for example, be a disaster for a blood transfusion service. In practice, other tests are needed to confirm apparently positive results.

The window period

It is now clear that almost everybody forms antibodies to HIV within six months of infection, and that in the majority of cases, this happens within six weeks of infection.

Studies that have attempted to define the average length of time before seroconversion have taken two approaches.

One is to select a group of people likely to be at high risk of HIV infection, but who remain HIV antibody negative (for instance, gay men who have had unprotected anal sex with partners known to be HIV-positive), and to use polymerase chain reaction testing to detect proteins from HIV in the blood before the formation of antibodies. The other is to trace the recipients of HIV-infected blood donations, and to use a well-tried method of mathematical projection to estimate how long seroconversion took.

In 1988, Simmonds studied stored blood samples from 18 seropositive haemophiliacs; seroconversions were estimated to have taken place between 30 and 160 days from infection in this group.

In 1989, Horsburgh estimated that from a sample of 39 seropositive men for whom stored serum was available before and after seroconversion, the median time to seroconversion was 2.4 months; in other words, half the sample took longer than 2.4 months, with 95% of the total sample having seroconverted by 10.3 months. The researchers performed a similar analysis of data for other studies and concluded that the median time to seroconversion was 2.1 months, with 95% having seroconverted after 5.8 months.

This formed the basis of advice that anyone wishing to take an HIV antibody test should wait for between 3-6 months after the last occasion they might have been at risk of infection. However, past studies had a number of drawbacks. They used less sensitive antibody tests, and also employed PCR testing at a time when experience with the technology was still very limited. False results were much more common. Researchers also assumed that those exposed to the virus were likely to become infected after a small number of exposures. It's now known that some people may not become infected despite repeated exposures to HIV, and so what is assumed to be a lengthy delay between exposure and the formation of antibodies may be a combined result of erroneous PCR results and infection at a much later stage in the study than assumed.

A very small number of people may take longer than six months to form antibodies, as studies by Horsburgh, Wolinsky and Imagawa have noted. These studies all used polymerase chain reaction testing to detect genetic fragments of HIV, which appeared to be present despite no evidence of seroconversion.

However, in a follow-up to their original study, Imagawa and colleagues retested blood samples from gay men who had been seronegative despite evidence of infection by more advanced PCR methods, and discovered that only one of the sample still showed evidence of infection. They concluded that what they had previously observed were unsuccessful cases of infection, not latent infection. The phenomenon of unsuccessful infection is still poorly understood, but it is interesting to note that, in the period between the first and second test, all those who had shown earlier evidence of infection ceased having unprotected anal intercourse. This suggests that the earlier PCR result may well have been erroneous.

Ensuring uniform standards

It is important to know whether HIV testing is being conducted to the highest standards. The UK National External Quality Assessment Scheme for Medical Microbiology provides specimens of human serum, both positive and negative for antibodies to HIV, to participating clinical laboratories on a regular and frequent basis. The antibody content of the specimens is initially unknown to the participants, the purpose of the Scheme being to help laboratories to assess the accuracy of the results they obtain for patients' specimens.

The overall standard of performance in the Scheme obtained by UK clinical laboratories is very high. The Scheme has no sanctions on the very small number of laboratories who perform relatively poorly or do not respond, but help and advice is available from an Advisory panel of expert microbiologists. Participation in the Scheme is not mandatory, and the Public Health Laboratory Service's Quality Assessment Scheme for Medical Microbiology recommends that persons wishing to be tested for HIV antibodies should ascertain that the testing laboratory does take part in quality assessment exercises and has been granted provisional or full accreditation under the Scheme.

Since this is unrealistic for those seeking tests, it is clearly the responsibility of those providing and managing testing services within the NHS to check that the laboratories they use for HIV antibody testing are participating in the Scheme.

References

Biggar RJ et al: ELISA HTLV retrovirus antibody reactivity associated with malaria and immune complexes in healthy Africans, Lancet 8454 (II): 520-523, 1985.

Burke DS et al: Measurement of the false positive rate in a screening programme for human immunodeficiency virus infection, NEJM 319: 961-964, 1988.

Chattopadhya D et al: Antimalarial antibody in relation to seroreactivity for HIV infection in sera from blood donors, Journal of Communicable Diseases 23(3): 195-198, 1991.

Connell JA et al: Accurate assays for anti-HIV in urine, Lancet Jun 9 1990 335 (8702): 1366 -1369, 1980.

Gallo D et al: Comparison of detection of antibody to the acquired immune deficiency syndrome virus by enzyme immunoassay, immunofluorescence and Western Blot methods, Journal of Clinical Microbiology 23: 1049-1051, 1987.

Haist S et al: Reactivities of HIV-1 gag-derived peptides with antibodies of endogenous retroviral proteins AIDS Research and Human Retroviruses 8(11): 1909-1917, 1992.

Horsburgh CR et al: Duration of human immunodeficiency virus infection before detection of antibody, The Lancet 2 (8664): 637-640, 1989.

Imagawa D et al: Human immunodeficiency virus type 1 infection in homosexual men who remain seronegative for prolonged periods, NEJM 320: 1458-1462, 1989.

Imagawa D et al: HIV-1 in seronegative homosexual men, NEJM 325:17: 1250-1251, 1991.

Jackson JB et al: Human immunodeficiency virus type 1 detected in all seropositive symptomatic and asymptomatic individuals, J Clin Microb 28(1): 16-19, 1990.

Johnson AM et al: HIV surveillance by testing saliva, AIDS 2 (5): 369-371, 1988.

Landini MP et al: Non specific antibody reaction to HIV-p24 is partially due to antigenic cross reaction with the major structural antigen of human cytomegalovirus, Seventh International AIDS Conference, Florence, abstract No. WA 1321,1991.

Lee DA: HIV false positivity after hepatitis B vaccination, Lancet 339: 1060, 1992.

Lindback S et al. *Diagnosis of primary HIV-1 infection and duration of follow-up after HIV exposure.AIDS*, 2000; 14(15): 2333-2339.

Mackenzie WR et al: Multiple false-positive serologic tests for HIV, HTLV-1 and hepatitis C following influenza vaccination, 1991, JAMA 268 (8): 1015-1017, 1992.

Mortimer, PP and Parry, JV: Non-invasive virological diagnosis: are saliva and urine specimens adequate substitutes for blood? Reviews In Medical Virology 1, 73-78, 1987.

Ranki A et al: Interpretation of antibodies reacting solely with human retroviral core proteins, NEJM 318: 448-449, 1988.

Simmonds P et al: HIV antigen and antibody detection: variable responses to infection in the Edinburgh haemophiliac cohort, BMJ 296 (6622): 593-598, 1988.

Sloande E et al: HIV testing: state of the art, JAMA 266(20): 2861-2866, 1991.

Squire S et al: Early diagnosis of HIV infection, British Journal of Hospital Medicine, July 4 1990.

Wolinsky SM et al: Human immunodeficiency virus type 1 (HIV-1) infection for a median of eighteen months before a diagnostic western blot: evidence from a cohort study, AIM 111(12): 961-972, 1989.

HIV testing and consent

Testing in clinics

In principle, a clinic cannot test you without your consent. Any test or treatment done without your consent or knowledge is unethical and an assault upon you.

So, in the majority of cases, it doesn't happen. But if you do not want to be tested for HIV, it does no harm at all to be quite explicit and tell the doctor and clinic staff of your decision.

If you're worried because you had blood taken at a sexual health clinic, this is because they routinely do a blood test for syphilis, and not every doctor will explain this. So this is not in itself a sinister sign that you have been tested for HIV antibodies without your consent.

However, it would be very hard to check if a particular doctor had tested you without your consent. If you have good grounds to think this might have happened, make an appointment with the consultant and carefully explain your concern.

If this interview does not satisfy you, you should get help in making a complaint. Legal advice can be obtained from Terrence Higgins Trust.

HIV-negative certificates

For foreign travel

For the purposes of emigration to, or employment in, a foreign country, a statement from a GP or other qualified doctor will be satisfactory. It should be stamped with the official laboratory or practice stamp.

Most countries that require an HIV antibody test certificate will accept a statement from a GP or other qualified doctor. The GP or laboratory should prepare a statement saying when the test was carried out and indicating that the person tested was free from HIV antibodies at the time of the test. The statement should be drawn up on headed notepaper, signed and stamped with the official practice or laboratory stamp. The certificate should be dated as close as possible to the date of departure, or a second test might be required on arrival.

A few countries require a special certificate that may have to be obtained from either the Consular Department of the High Commission or Embassy of the country concerned, or the Consular department of the Foreign Office.

Most doctors will charge a fee for this service, as will all clinics, consultants and private clinics or laboratories, including NHS ones.

Our ethical objections to these practices

There are no justifiable reasons why anyone should be asked to certify their antibody status. Unfortunately, the attitudes of immigration authorities in many countries put many people in a very difficult position, whether or not they are aware of their HIV status.

You may well find that some doctors will provide HIV-negative certificates without performing a test to people who wish to work or travel abroad. Although this is fraudulent, the chances of being found out are minimal, and this is probably the easiest way of subverting these ludicrous regulations.

To show to partners

The opposite is the case here: if you are in fact HIV-positive but are looking for a certificate to 'show' you are HIV-negative to a prospective partner then most people would regard you as acting unethically. If you did get and show such a 'proof' to a sexual partner and then you subsequently transmitted HIV to them, you would be liable to prosecution and conviction in England and Wales, for reckless transmission of HIV. In other countries, you might be prosecuted just for exposing your partner to HIV, even if they did not become infected.

Blood Transfusion Service tests

The National Blood Transfusion Service tests all blood donations for HIV-1 and HIV-2, using a combined test for both. If a positive result is indicated by an ELISA test, a sample is sent away to the regional Public Health Laboratory for a confirmatory test. Those who have tested positive will be contacted by a letter sent to their home address. The letter will ask the donor to contact the regional blood transfusion centre because 'following your recent donation we have detected substances in your blood which may be important to your health.' This wording is also used for infectious diseases such as hepatitis and other abnormalities in the blood, indicating non-fatal conditions that may nevertheless require prompt treatment.

At the regional centre, the HIV-positive donor will be counselled by a trained consultant before referral to a local hospital.

This is a uniform policy throughout the country. There is also a uniform policy of asking some groups of people not to give blood.

Blood donors identified as HIV-positive

Between October 1985, when HIV testing of the blood supply began, and December 1999, 401 blood donors were identified as being HIV-1 antibody positive, out of 4,034,909 donations tested. During the same period, one donor was identified as being positive for HIV-2 antibodies. This shows that only a very small number of people infected with HIV donate blood having not been already excluded by the policy of asking people with identifiable risks to refrain from giving blood.

In 2002, a total of 33 HIV infected donors were identified in the UK out of a total of 2,844 465 donations tested - i.e. an approximate rate of 1.16 per 100 000.

Testing before surgery

Some surgeons are asking people whom they categorise as being in 'high risk' groups to be tested for HIV antibodies, on the grounds that the surgeons need to know for their own protection.

It is not true that they have a need to know. Standard good hygiene measures, if properly observed, will protect surgeons and their patients, even from diseases that are much more infectious than HIV. The problem should not be seen as your possible HIV status, but whether or not the recommended hygiene procedures are routinely carried out. After all, for every person whose antibody status is known, there will be many more whose status is unknown. As in any other workplace situation, the belief that HIV antibody testing can reveal everyone with HIV and thus minimise supposed risks, is dangerously misleading. In reality, just as with safer sex, everyone should proceed from the assumption that anyone, including him or herself, may be antibody positive. And in order to protect everyone, recommended standards of hygiene (universal precautions) should always be applied. Unfortunately, surgeons are not necessarily more rational about HIV than is any other section of the population.

In other words, you should refuse. This would be the worst possible way for you to be tested for HIV antibodies.

Remember, there's very little guarantee that your result would stay confidential in an ordinary surgical department. And you would receive little or no counselling and support.

Instead, you can insist that the surgeons take all appropriate precautions as if you were at risk of HIV infection. After all, if they don't take universal precautions, how are you being protected from infections like hepatitis B? There are clear professional guidelines on hygiene, sterilisation and disinfection for them to follow.

It would be unethical if they refused you treatment after this. But if you're being pressured, you need to get help in making a complaint.

The police

The police cannot make you have an HIV antibody test. Within the terms of the Police and Criminal Evidence Act, 1984, you are entirely within your rights to refuse any pressure from the police to have an HIV antibody test, at a police station or anywhere else.

However, there have been reports that pressure has been put on some individuals in some police stations to persuade them to be tested as a condition of earlier release.

As in any other workplace situation, there is no risk whatsoever of HIV transmission, except through unsafe sex or sharing needles. And any other anxieties individual police officers may have are evidence of their need for better HIV/AIDS education.

Insurance, employment and travel

Insurance

As soon as the insurance costs of HIV/AIDS became apparent, insurance companies moved to protect themselves against expensive claims. They argued that the 'general population' should be protected against the risk of an across-the-board increase in premiums, and that people in high-risk groups for HIV infection should be treated differently or surcharged, in the same way as smokers are subject to increased premiums, for instance. The way that insurers did this, however, was not merely to single out particular high-risk groups as an insurance risk (which has some epidemiological validity), but also to characterise the very process of HIV testing as a risk behaviour for insurance purposes. Thus, people who had been tested, even if the result was negative, were highly likely to undergo stringent questioning when applying for insurance and mortgages, on the basis that having an HIV test constitutes an admission of leading a high-risk lifestyle.

However, in 1994 insurers agreed to drop questions about negative HIV tests on insurance application forms, and in 2004 they agreed to drop questions regarded as intrusive or discriminatory about sexuality or sexual behaviour. The Association of British Insurers issued guidelines saying that in future, questions on life insurance or illness cover forms should no longer ask whether the applicant is gay or 'in a stable monogamous relationship', and that it would be regarded as 'bad practice' if they did. Insurers should instead ask a non-gay-specific question such as: "Within the last five years, have you been exposed to the risk of HIV infection?"

In some countries, every applicant for insurance over a certain amount is automatically required to have an HIV test. HIV-related discrimination by the insurance industry undoubtedly discourages some people from testing. While this has a questionable impact on HIV prevention, it undoubtedly affects the possibility of successful prevention of HIV-related illnesses among those already infected.

For further information on Insurance and mortgages, see *Insurance and HIV testing* later in this chapter.

Employment

Some employers also attempted to protect themselves, perhaps because of worries about insurance claims or misplaced fears about the way in which HIV infection would affect the ability of employees to perform their jobs. Outside medicine, the key example of this fear was in the airline industry. Following speculative and ill-founded reports that HIV-related dementia could be one of the earliest forms of HIV-related illness, several major airlines instituted testing of pilots and cabin crew. This was not primarily due to the large number of gay men working as cabin crew, but to fears that cognitive impairment related to HIV could affect passenger safety. This pointless panic was based on a speculation that turned out to be erroneous; HIV-related dementia and cognitive impairment are almost always late symptoms of HIV disease, and do not develop suddenly and without warning.

For further discussion of employment-related discrimination, see *Employment*.

Travel restrictions

International travel restrictions on people with HIV have been perhaps the most irrational application of testing as a prevention tool.

The countries of the European Union have taken the view that freedom of movement cannot be restricted on the grounds of HIV infection. This means that citizens of the Union are free to move from one country to another, but immigrants from outside the Union may be subject to testing if they seek residence in some EU countries. See *Mental Health and Quality of Life: Travel* for further details of restrictions country by country.

Mass anonymised screening

In 1989 the Department of Health announced plans for the introduction of a large-scale programme of anonymised HIV screening, in order to find out the prevalence (social distribution) and incidence (rate of new infection) of HIV in Britain.

The plans were drawn up for the DOH by the Medical Research Council, which is supervising the entire project. This is initially focused on a number of specific target groups, including pregnant women and people attending GUM clinics. The eventual aim is to extend the screening to include randomised samples from all general hospital admissions.

For example, women attending certain antenatal clinics will be informed that HIV antibody testing will be included amongst the other routine tests, unless an individual specifically objects.

The results of these tests will not be connected to the individuals by name, and are therefore anonymous. This also means that the results will not be available to the individuals concerned. Their sole use is meant to be statistical, in order to predict the likely future course of the epidemic.

Under these circumstances, there is no risk of a breach of confidentiality from the testing of the blood itself. However, some concern has been expressed that consent to this anonymised screening should not be sought from individuals in front of other people. Somebody who chooses to refuse, for whatever reasons, could be put in an awkward or embarrassing position.

Testing without consent

During 2003, two reports were published concerning people being tested for HIV without their knowledge or consent. The first concerned a private patient of the university clinic in Muenster, Germany who only discovered he had been tested for HIV when he received the bill for his care and saw that he had been charged 20 Euros for an HIV test. The man had signed a consent form to say he did not want the test. The local AIDS-Hilfe in North Rhine-Westphalia (NRW) said they were convinced this is not an isolated case.

Weeks after the man discovered that he had been tested for HIV, he was given a negative result.

The German doctors' magazine *Aerztezeitung* reported that the man is taking the clinic to court on the grounds of bodily harm and infringement of his personal rights.

The clinic spokesperson, Jutta Reising, said, "this should not have been allowed to happen." The clinic director has apologised to the patient and the clinic management drew the staff's attention to a 1988 clinical directive that stated that HIV tests couldn't be carried out without the consent of the patient.

AIDS-Hilfe NRW said they suspect that the university clinic often routinely tests patients' blood samples for HIV, irrespective of whether the patient is deemed to be from a high-risk group or indeed has requested the test. A spokesperson for the organisation said that they often receive reports of individuals who had been tested against their will, but this was the first incident in which the patient had made legal moves and was identifiable. Most patients, he said were unwilling to come forward and be identified. "Now, the case can be identified with an individual by name."

The March 7 2003 edition of the journal *AIDS* reported on non-consensual HIV testing by GPs in Belgium.

Data were recorded from 1993 to 2000 in the Belgian network of sentinel general practitioners (GPs). The network is representative of Belgian GPs, and has been a reliable surveillance system for more than 20 years. Since May 1988, every adult patient who has asked his GP for an HIV test has been recorded on a weekly registration form. Since 1993, questions about patient consent have been included.

In total, 292 GPs recorded 11,660 requests for an HIV test (52% by women). The mean age of the tested individuals was 33.2 years. Information about patient consent was available for 3628 tests. In total, 453 tests were performed without patient consent. This corresponds to 3.9% of all tests performed and 14% of the tests for which information is available about patient consent. The proportion of non-consented HIV tests decreased during the early 1990s from approximately 17% to less than 8%, and has increased since 1996 to approximately 12% in 2000. The proportion of non-consented HIV tests is 30% in the age group below 15 years, 40% in the age group above 64 years, and between 10 and 15% in the other age groups.

For 29% of the non-consented HIV tests, no risk behaviour was detected, and for 43% the existence of risk behaviour was unknown. In 28% of all non-consented HIV tests, the patient declared him or herself to be at risk of HIV. Eighteen per cent of the HIV tests among patients originating from an endemic region were non-consented HIV tests and 15% of the tests in gay men were non-consented HIV tests.

Twenty-three per cent of the non-consented HIV tests were performed on patients with suggestive symptoms. Non-consented

HIV testing was also popular as part of a check-up (21%) or during antenatal care (13%). Eleven per cent were carried out for an administrative reason, 8% in prospect of a new relationship and 8% among patients awaiting a surgical intervention.

Belgian law states that patients should be informed about the results of an HIV test. In this context, the proportion of non-consented HIV tests is astonishing. So is the proportion of physicians performing HIV tests without informed consent. In total, 36% of all GPs performed at least one non-consented HIV test. HIV tests returned positive for 1.5% (n = 7) of the non-consented HIV tests and for 0.5% (n = 23) of the consented tests.

Instead of performing HIV tests without consent, doctors should invest more time in pre-test councelling, especially in patients with a higher risk or with suggestive symptoms of HIV. In most of these cases, valuable opportunities to provide risk-reduction councelling were missed.

HIV testing, pregnancy and children

HIV testing in pregnancy - the background

In order to become pregnant, a woman may put herself at risk of HIV infection by having unprotected sex. If she is already HIV-positive, or becomes infected at the time of conception or later, there is a risk to her unborn child. This risk, in the UK, is currently a one in seven chance that the baby will be infected (assuming that no preventative measures were taken); that is, for every seven babies born to HIV-positive women, six will not be infected.

In the past there have been concerns about the value of testing for a disease that is highly stigmatised and for which there is no cure. However, interventions are now available which have proved highly effective at reducing the risk of transmission to the baby and which may be beneficial for the woman in her own right. These interventions are:

- Giving antiretroviral therapy to the mother during pregnancy and labour, and to the infant for one month after birth.

- Delivering the baby by Caesarean section rather than vaginal delivery. When Caesarean delivery was used alongside AZT, the risk of vertical transmission was further reduced by 50% compared with AZT treatment alone. When Caesarean delivery was used without antiretroviral therapy, it still resulted in a reduction in risk (10% transmission risk compared with 19% transmission risk amongst mothers who did not deliver by Caesarean and did not take AZT). However, some studies suggest that Caesarean section may be unnecessary if viral load is well controlled (below detection) during pregnancy.

- Advising against breastfeeding. Several studies have shown that women who breastfeed are more likely to transmit HIV to their babies than those who choose to bottle-feed.

However, while no one would dispute the desirability of preventing vertical transmission, some professionals believe that the rights of the pregnant woman could be compromised if HIV testing in the antenatal clinic is not introduced with care and sensitivity. The person being asked to consider having the test needs to have enough information to give informed consent. For a pregnant woman, the decision can be particularly complex. The

experience of being given an HIV-positive diagnosis is very painful at any time, even if it's been anticipated. During pregnancy, it is likely to be even more so.

Furthermore, such a diagnosis during pregnancy is likely to have a more profound effect on the family than it would at any other time. The father's HIV status will be in doubt, and the unborn child's status will be unknown. The HIV status of other children in the family might also be called into question. While there is still considerable stigma attached to HIV, many women are very fearful of the test, whatever the result might be. This fear can act as a disincentive to seeking or accepting antenatal care.

It is also the case that most babies born to HIV-positive women will be HIV-negative, even without any interventions. The interventions offered to reduce the risk of vertical (mother-to-baby) transmission are not without side-effects and do not offer 100% protection.

The long-term effects of anti-HIV drugs on an HIV-negative child are not known, although follow-up of mother-infant pairs treated with AZT has consistently shown no long-term effects. However, a review of 30 mother-infant pairs treated with dual or triple therapy demonstrated a higher than average rate of premature delivery, and nine cases of anaemia in infants exposed to AZT/3TC. Neither is Caesarean section risk-free for the mother. These risks must be balanced against the proven effectiveness of anti-HIV therapy in reducing transmission, and the well-established health consequences of being born HIV-positive.

See *The HIV & AIDS Treatments Directory*, or aidsmap.com, also published by NAM, for extensive discussion of research in this area.

The politics of antenatal testing

For a variety of reasons, HIV antenatal testing has been a political issue that has divided professionals. One reason that feelings have run high on this issue has been that for many people, the targeting of pregnant women has been seen as a tool to prevent babies becoming infected. There has been little attempt to prevent transmission of HIV to women. In addition, there have been few initiatives to target heterosexual men.

Research suggests that where women know their HIV status during pregnancy, counselling about the risks of vertical transmission results in a high uptake of antiretroviral therapy. In one study, in which 81% of the HIV-positive mothers were of African origin, 69% of mothers took the antiretroviral therapy offered. There was a transmission rate of 8% amongst this group, compared to a transmission rate of 22% amongst mothers who did not take antiretroviral drugs (Lyall).

Debate about how the test should be offered has been influenced by a randomised study in Edinburgh, where four different methods were compared. In this study, 3,024 pregnant women attending Edinburgh maternity clinics during 1996 were randomised either to:

- No pro-active offer of testing; the only information provided was a poster in clinic waiting areas.

- Provision of an HIV-specific leaflet describing the potential benefits of detection and treatment during pregnancy followed by an explicit offer of the test from a midwife.

- Provision of a blood tests leaflet that included a discussion of HIV testing followed by the explicit offer of a test from a midwife.

The two active intervention groups were further randomised to one of two forms of discussion:

- Detailed discussion with a midwife, who recapped the information in the HIV-specific leaflet.

- Minimal discussion to check that the leaflet had been understood.

There was a significant difference between the control group and the intervention groups in terms of uptake. However, other factors not directly connected with the study design were also significant. The uptake rates for testing varied between midwives irrespective of the intervention to which the patient had been assigned, suggesting that midwives' own attitudes towards offering the test affected the response of patients. It was also found that routine testing did not provoke any more anxiety amongst pregnant women than other routine blood tests offered during pregnancy. The authors of this study recommended that routine testing should be normalised (Simpson).

In 1998, the Department of Health endorsed an Intercollegiate Working Party Document that urged that pregnant women in areas of high HIV prevalence be offered and recommended to have an HIV test. This is part of an initiative to normalise the HIV test as one of many antenatal tests women are routinely offered. Although it will still be important for a woman to consent specifically to the test, it will be recommended in the same way as routine syphilis, rubella and hepatitis B tests.

This practice was extended to the whole of the UK by the Department of Health in August 1999.

It remains the case that some HIV infected pregnant women do not know, or do not disclose, their HIV status. One problem in offering this test is that many women feel HIV is not an issue for them. They may believe that HIV is a gay issue, despite the fact that the figures for infections in heterosexual women continue to rise, particularly in the sub-Saharan African population who are mainly living in London.

On the other hand, some women accept all antenatal tests believing they are of benefit to their baby and are totally unprepared for the impact of a positive result. It is vitally important that where HIV testing is routinely offered and recommended, midwives and other health care workers are prepared and adequately trained. Acceptance of the test depends on the manner in which it is offered. The follow-up care of women found to be HIV-positive, and their families, must also be adequately funded, both from treatment and psychosocial points of view.

Whilst HIV continues to incur stigma and discrimination, there will be a disincentive to HIV testing. Any attempts to normalise HIV antenatal testing must recognise this and strong measures to combat prejudice must accompany such efforts. Whilst testing is always a diagnostic tool, individual rights to treatment and risk-reduction strategies may be compromised if we do not constantly reassess the value of HIV testing.

References

D Gibb et al. Factors affecting uptake of antenatal HIV testing in London: results of a multicentre study. BMJ 316: 259-261, 1998.

EGH Lyall et al. Review of an uptake of interventions to reduce mother to child transmission of HIV by women aware of their HIV status. BMJ 316: 268-270, 1998.

W Simpson et al. Uptake and acceptability of antenatal HIV testing: randomised controlled trial of different methods of offering the test. BMJ 316: 262-267, 1998.

Pre-conception testing

Many women are advised to maximise their health before conceiving. They are often advised to increase their folic acid intake and try to make sure they are generally fit. For some couples, this might include having HIV tests. It should be stressed to both (would-be) parents that the HIV test will not show infection that might have taken place within the last three months. This might be important if the couple has only just begun having unprotected intercourse.

HIV testing in antenatal clinics

In August 1999 the government announced that HIV testing would be offered and recommended routinely to pregnant women in the UK. It was planned that all health authorities (as they were then called) should be offering the test on this basis by the end of 2000.

No woman who refuses HIV testing during pregnancy should receive different antenatal care from those who agree to be tested. Furthermore, the standard antenatal care of a pregnant HIV-positive woman should not be different from any other pregnant woman. The number of visits to see her midwife should not necessarily be different. She will probably see a specialist obstetrician more frequently, to discuss her mode of delivery - elective Caesarean or vaginal. In some hospitals a "minimal blood loss" Caesarean is offered. Her HIV care will normally be undertaken by specialist HIV physicians. Standard infection control and universal precautions are sufficient to protect health care providers from the risk of infection.

Reasons why midwives should be informed of HIV status

This is because appropriate care can be offered and certain procedures will be avoided.

A number of procedures may increase the risk of transmission, including:

- Amniocentesis.

- Use of foetal electrodes.

- Prolonged labour (4 hours +).

- Vaginal delivery.

- Breastfeeding.

A midwife will only be able to provide support for adherence to antiretroviral therapy during and after labour if she is aware of the mother's HIV status. Adherence can be particularly problematic at this time if other family members who are present at the birth are not aware of the mother's HIV status.

Adherence may also be complicated by extreme nausea experienced during labour. Once again, an informed midwife may be able to help.

Finally, mothers may need active assistance to bottle-feed after delivery, both in practical terms and in persuading other family members that this is good idea while preserving the mother's confidentiality.

HIV testing pregnant women in UK: still failing to meet targets

The latest figures from the Health Protection Agency show that during the first six months of 2002, clinics in the UK were still failing to reach government targets to diagnose 80% of HIV infections in pregnant women prior to delivery.

National Unlinked Anonymous (UA) monitoring of the prevalence of HIV infection in pregnant women, by testing for maternal antibody in infant dried blood spots, began in the UK in 1988. Since 1992, the survey has covered approximately 70% of UK births. The results of UA monitoring are aligned with reports of HIV-positive pregnant women made through the Royal College of Obstetricians and Gynaecologists (RCOG) to the National Study of HIV in Pregnancy and Childhood (NSHPC). This provides the best estimates of the proportions of HIV-positive pregnant women who have had their infection diagnosed prior to pregnancy or during current antenatal care.

In 1994 it became apparent that interventions implemented during pregnancy and in the perinatal period can reduce the risk of transmission of HIV from mother-to-child from one in seven to less than one in 50, and the uptake of such interventions by diagnosed HIV-positive pregnant women in the UK is high. There are also direct benefits to the woman's own health from having her HIV infection diagnosed earlier than might otherwise have happened.

Outside London, the prevalence of HIV infection among women giving birth has remained consistently low. Prevalence in the rest of England for the first half of 2002 is estimated to be 3.5/10,000, and in Scotland 4.8/10,000 women.

In 1999, national targets that offer and recommend HIV testing to all pregnant women throughout England were established by the Department of Health. It was intended that by increasing the uptake of antenatal HIV testing to 90%, and by increasing the proportion of HIV infections diagnosed prior to delivery to 80%, an 80% reduction in the proportion of children acquiring HIV infection from their mothers should be achieved by December 2002.

In London, up to the end of June 2002, 135 diagnosed maternal infections had been reported to the NSHPC by the end of the year, giving a minimum overall detection rate of 66% (135/205) and an antenatal detection rate of 53%. The data for the rest of England in the first half of 2002 show an overall detection rate of 81% (57/70), meeting the Department of Health target for the first time.

For Scotland, data show that at least 67% (8/12) of maternal HIV infections were diagnosed before delivery in the first half of 2002. The equivalent overall detection rates in the same period of 2001 for London, the rest of England, and Scotland were 73%, 33% and 75% respectively.

These interim half-year data are, however, subject to reporting delay and the estimated proportion of infections diagnosed is expected to rise further as late reports are received. In 2001, it can be estimated that there were about 560 births to HIV-positive women in the UK. Assuming a transmission rate of about 25% for undiagnosed women, and 2% for diagnosed women (allowing for late diagnoses and a small proportion of diagnosed

women declining interventions, about 50 infants would have acquired HIV infection from their mothers.

Continued improvements in detection rates before delivery have resulted in a decreasing proportion of HIV-positive women passing HIV infection on to their child and, despite an increase in the number of HIV-positive women giving birth, the number of maternally- acquired HIV infections was probably similar in 2001 to 2000.

Increase in prenatal testing rate in USA 1998-2001

The availability of increasingly effective antiretroviral drugs for prevention of transmission and maternal treatment has resulted in greater emphasis on prenatal HIV testing. In 2000, preliminary unpublished data from the Centers for Disease Control (CDC) in Atlanta indicated that 766 (93%) of 824 HIV-positive women in 25 states knew their status before delivery.

Each year an estimated 280-370 perinatal HIV transmissions occur in the USA.

In the USA and Canada three different prenatal HIV testing approaches have been implemented. The CDC reviewed prenatal HIV antibody testing rates to assess their effectiveness. Under the opt-in approach, women typically are provided pre-HIV test counselling and must consent specifically to an HIV test. Under the opt-out approach, women are notified that an HIV test will be included in a battery of prenatal tests and procedures and that they may refuse testing. Under mandatory newborn HIV testing, newborns are tested for HIV, with or without the mother's consent, if the mother's HIV status is unknown at delivery.

Medical record data suggest that the opt-in voluntary testing approach is associated with lower testing rates than either the opt-out or the mandatory newborn HIV testing approach.

Three different approaches were used to estimate prenatal testing rates among all women who delivered, regardless of whether they received prenatal care; firstly, eight US areas that participated during 1998-1999 in CDC's Active Bacterial Core Surveillance/Emerging Infections Program (ABC) Network assessed HIV testing during prenatal care. Secondly, public health investigators in each of the five Canadian provinces tallied the number of HIV tests among pregnant women that were submitted to provincial laboratories and divided the total by an estimate of all live and stillborn births in each province during the same year. Finally, CDC analysed weighted data collected in 1999 by interviewers in nine states for CDC's Pregnancy Risk Assessment Monitoring System (PRAMS) (an ongoing, population-based survey conducted in 32 states and New York City among women who had given birth in the preceding 2-6 months) who asked women if they had been tested for HIV during pregnancy.

HIV testing rates varied depending upon which approach was used. Rates for states using the opt-in approach to prenatal HIV testing included in the ABC Network ranged from 25% to 69%, testing rates in Canada ranged from 54% to 83%, and rates derived from the PRAMS data ranged from 61% to 81%.

Two US states, Arkansas and Tennessee, and two Canadian provinces (Alberta, and Newfoundland and Labrador) reported using an opt-out prenatal HIV testing policy. ABC Network data indicated that Tennessee had a testing rate of 85%. Canada's population-based data indicated a 98% testing rate in Alberta and a 94% testing rate in Newfoundland and Labrador. PRAMS interview data indicated a 71% testing rate in Arkansas, compared with a 57% testing rate in early 1997 before the law was implemented. Two states, New York and Connecticut, require HIV testing of newborns whose mothers were not tested during pregnancy.

Network review of medical records in the seven counties in the Rochester area of New York state indicated that the proportion of pregnant women who received a prenatal HIV test increased from 52% of 438 charts during January 1998-July 1999 to

83% of 112 charts during August-December 1999 after New York required that newborn HIV testing results be made available within 48 hours of specimen collection. PRAMS data for the state of New York in 1999 indicated that the proportion of women state-wide who reported having received an HIV test during pregnancy increased from 69% of 758 women during January-July to 93% of 502 during August-December.

Among the three prenatal HIV testing approaches assessed, opt-out voluntary testing and the mandatory testing of newborns appear to be associated with the highest testing rates. CDC is working with states with high HIV prevalence rates among women of childbearing age and high numbers of paediatric AIDS cases to ensure standardised monitoring of prenatal testing rates. The data suggest that jurisdictions that use an opt-in approach and that have low prenatal HIV testing rates should re-evaluate their approach.

References

HIV infection in women giving birth in the United Kingdom - trends in prevalence and proportions diagnosed to the end of June 2002. CDR Weekly, 17 March 2003.

Roome A et al. HIV testing among pregnant women-United States and Canada 1998-2001. Morbidity and Mortality Weekly Report 51: 1013-1016, 2002.

HIV testing during pregnancy - issues to consider

All HIV testing should be in the best interests of the person targeted for testing. In considering a test during pregnancy, the following guidelines might be useful:

- What prior knowledge of HIV does the woman have? Many people believe that all babies born to HIV-positive women will be HIV-positive too. This false assumption can be a disincentive to testing. It is important that women realise that testing, if they're found to HIV be positive, could be of benefit to them in terms of their own health, as well as that of their babies.

- Has the woman had a test previously?

- What are the risk factors involved - sexual partners, past or current IDU, blood transfusions?

- Does the woman/couple understand the significance of the window period?

- Does the woman/couple understand that discordant results between partners are common?

- What are the benefits of testing - reassurance if HIV-negative, preparation and intervention possibilities if HIV-positive, benefits for woman as person in her own right, as well as risk reduction for vertical transmission, health education opportunities?

- What are the disadvantages - impact on the woman, relationship, family, friends, work?

- Does the woman understand the potential problems with mortgages and life insurance if she is found to be HIV-positive? Does she realise that the insurance industry no longer penalises a woman who is tested as part of antenatal screening (as long as she is found to be HIV-negative)?

- Does the woman/couple know about safer sex/safer drug use during pregnancy?

It is also particularly important to recognise that the majority of women infected with HIV in this country are from sub-Saharan Africa. The pre-test discussion must be culturally appropriate. Antenatal screening is not common in parts of Africa, and, more importantly, the stigma of HIV is very great. For many African women, their immigration status, housing and social problems may seem more pressing than health concerns. The idea of HIV testing in pregnancy may be totally alien to them.

Issues for HIV-positive women deciding to have a child - see Women and HIV

Infection of the baby

The detection of HIV infection in children born to HIV-positive mothers is complex, and testing methods are changing rapidly. All babies born to HIV-positive women will have received HIV antibodies from their mother's blood, irrespective of whether they are HIV-infected themselves. These maternal antibodies persist for approximately ten months, and may last as long as eighteen months. HIV antibody tests on these young babies will only show if the mother is infected, and are not helpful in differentiating between infected and uninfected infants. Many parents want to have an early definitive diagnosis, as repeated observation and testing can be distressing and disruptive. Many doctors would like to be able to diagnose truly HIV-infected infants earlier in order to start treatment. There is an increasing availability of prophylaxes and therapies, and it is known that about 25% of babies who are HIV-infected develop clinical symptoms of AIDS or die within the first year of life.

When it is known that a child is at significant risk of HIV infection (e.g. when the mother is known to be HIV-positive), a number of measures should be employed to try to ascertain if the baby is HIV infected as quickly as possible, and before maternal antibodies clear. There are more sensitive tests, detailed below, which are carried out routinely at major centres experienced in dealing with children at risk of HIV infection. Most of these centres will be happy for less HIV-experienced centres to contact them for advice and assistance with care.

An accurate early diagnosis of HIV infection in infants depends on tests that establish the true presence of HIV virus, as opposed to HIV antibodies, in the baby. These tests are:

- p24 antigen or acid-dissociated p24 antigen tests.

- Virus culture.

- HIV DNA Polymerase Chain Reaction tests (PCR).

PCR and virus culture tests should be performed at repeated intervals: within 48 hours of birth (testing at this point identifies about 40% of infected children), at about 4-8 weeks, and at 3-6 months. US guidelines on testing state that if two or more IgG antibody tests (see below) are negative at least six months after birth, with a one month interval between the two tests, it is reasonable to assume that the child is not infected.

In addition, tests of the infant's immune system may help to make an early diagnosis. These tests are:

- High immunoglobulin levels (IgG, IgA, IgM).

- Inverted CD4:CD8 ratio.

- Persistent HIV antibody after 18 months.

Finally, many infants have some clinical manifestations of HIV infection by six months of age. In the USA, researchers suggest that the majority of children can be identified with currently available technology by 3-4 months old.

All infants born to HIV-infected mothers should ideally receive a six-week course of oral AZT, and should not be breastfed.

Healthcare workers should not treat a recently delivered mother who knows she is HIV-positive differently from any other mother. For some women (and families), this will be a time for planning for the future, despite the fact that the HIV status of the baby will not be known for some time. This will include decisions about any measures that might lower the chances of postnatal HIV transmission, such as not breastfeeding. It will also be important to consider how to cope with the uncertainty and monitoring of the baby in the first few months. This will also be a time to decide who needs to know about the baby's risk of HIV infection. Most women will find it helpful to inform their GP and Health Visitor, but only if these professionals are sympathetic to the woman's HIV status. Knowing that the baby might be HIV-infected can mean that appropriate care can more quickly be offered.

Although the majority of babies born to women with HIV are not infected, health care workers will understandably usually treat the baby as HIV-infected until their HIV status is clarified. The baby may be offered prophylaxis against Pneumocystis Carinii Pneumonia (PCP), an opportunistic infection commonly found in people who have comprised immune systems, while waiting for a definite diagnosis. The prophylaxis is known to be relatively safe in infants, and PCP is a significant risk to the baby in the first few months of life if she or he is HIV infected.

HIV disease in children is different from HIV disease in adults and different criteria are used to diagnose AIDS. About 25% of babies who are HIV-infected develop clinical symptoms of AIDS or die within the first year of life. Babies who survive the first year of life have a slow progression to AIDS comparable to adults. Out of all those children truly infected at birth, 70% are alive at six years and 50% at nine years old. There may be considerable psychosocial issues for children born HIV-infected when they reach their teens. These issues range from adolescent reactions to taking so many drug treatments to wanting to experiment sexually. Until recently, the life expectancy of children with HIV was not high. With combination therapy, life expectancy has been extended and these psychosocial issues are becoming more urgent.

See *Children, adolescents and families* for further discussion.

References

BMJ vol 316, 24 Jan 1998 Special issue devoted to HIV antenatal testing in the UK.

Intercollegiate Working Party for Enhancing Voluntary Confidential HIV testing in pregnancy, May 1998.

Kim L et al. Evaluation of sperm washing as a potential method of reducing HIV transmission in HIV-discordant couples wishing to have children. AIDS 13: 645-651, 1999.

Lorraine Sherr Of Mice and Women, http://iapac.org/clinmgt/women/mice.html.Summer 1997 DemiMondaine.

Semprini et al: Insemination of HIV-negative women with processed semen of HIV-positive partners, Lancet 340: 1317-1319, 1992.

The National HIV Prevention Information Service has published a Resource Guide on Antenatal HIV testing policy. This can be downloaded from www.hea.org/uk/nhpis

Insurance and HIV testing

Insurance and the law

An insurance company is not legally obliged to insure anyone, and an insurance company does not have to give reasons for refusing insurance.

Whenever you apply for any form of insurance (an application is called a 'proposal'), the insurance company will want you to answer some questions. If the insurance company then issues you with a policy, but later finds out that you have answered any question untruthfully, they can treat the policy as void, i.e. refuse to pay up for any claims, and can sometimes also keep any premiums you have paid.

As a general rule, you must also tell an insurance company - even if they do not ask specifically - about anything which might affect their decision whether or not to insure you, or on what terms. But what information you need to volunteer in any particular situation can be difficult to decide. It is best to seek professional advice if you are unsure about how to answer questions from an insurance company (see below).

Insurance, HIV and sexuality

Insurance company questions about HIV status and sexuality are usually asked when you apply for any form of life insurance or health insurance. These questions are asked primarily to identify gay men, who will often be refused insurance. Since other types of financial arrangement can also involve life or health insurance, you may come across these questions in other situations too, for example, when applying for:

- Mortgages

- Pension plans or company health and pension schemes

- 'Key man' policies

- Insurance against loss of income through ill health

- Credit card protection plans

HIV and AIDS issues also arise with other types of insurance. For example, travel insurance and motor insurance, see below.

When you apply for life or health insurance, the standard proposal form will always ask certain questions:

- Have you received medical attention recently?

- Has any proposal been refused or accepted on special terms (such as a higher premium)?

- You may also be asked at this stage whether you have ever had HIV or AIDS counselling, or an HIV antibody test (even if the result was negative). Following pressure on the insurance industry, life insurance companies should now be phasing this question out, replacing it with a question about positive tests for HIV and hepatitis and tests or treatment for other sexually transmitted infections. For other types of insurance, the old question will probably still be used.

In addition, you will be asked to consent to the insurance company approaching your doctor for a medical report (see below).

If you are a single man, you will probably also receive a separate, supplementary questionnaire. You may not get it if you are applying for a small amount of life insurance only. Sometimes others get this questionnaire too - for example, if you apply to be insured for a large sum of money.

HIV has made life and health insurance companies cautious about agreeing to insure various categories of people which insurance companies have classified as 'high-risk groups'. They wish to avoid insuring anybody who, in their view, may become infected with HIV. They have therefore developed a series of questions that they use to identify applicants they do not wish to insure, or who will have to pay higher premiums. These questions are not about your actual behaviour and whether or not it is risky.

Voluntary agencies and the Minister of Health have pointed out that the notion of high-risk groups is misleading when applied to individuals, since it is risk *behaviour*, not membership of a particular group, that is relevant. Attempts are being made by some voluntary groups to get insurance companies to change their practices. So far these attempts have not been successful, except for the change to questions about prior HIV tests and counselling.

The supplementary questionnaire, which contains these extra questions, will ask directly whether you are (or have been):

- A gay man

- A bisexual man

- A hæmophiliac

- An intravenous drug user

- A sexual partner of any of these

For insurance other than life insurance, this questionnaire may also ask (again) whether you have ever received HIV or AIDS counselling or had an HIV test, even if the result was negative.

Life insurance companies should be replacing this question with the new question that only asks about positive tests.

If you are HIV-positive

If you are HIV-positive, you will not get life insurance. If you get health insurance it will exclude any liability to pay for HIV-related illnesses.

Exceptions

This, at least, is the situation in the UK. In the USA, certain life insurance companies have been prepared to offer life insurance to people with HIV - though at such high premiums compared to the eventual payout that it was hardly worth taking out the insurance. One such company was the Guarantee Trust Life Insurance Company in Illinois, which has offered life insurance since 1997, though under strict conditions: applicants must be 21 to 49, be working, lead an "active life" and have a low viral load.

However in November 2004, African Life, a South Africa-based insurance company, announced that it was lifting HIV/AIDS exclusions on its life insurance policies, and in November 2005 the Netherlands became the first country to offer life insurance to people with HIV, at rates comparable to those offered to other members of the public. The six largest members of the Dutch Union of Insurers, who represent more than 80% of the Dutch market, decided to offer policies to some people with HIV. To qualify, people would have to be on stable anti-retroviral therapy, to have responded well to treatment, to not have any other medical complications, and never to have been intravenous drug

users. The decision was taken after the Dutch HIV Monitoring Foundation found that the risk of patients in this group dying had fallen to less than 0.5% a year. It was thought that about 25% of the 10,000 people living with HIV in the Netherlands will be eligible now and that this proportion will rise quickly.

So far, however, the Association of British Insurers has shown no inclination to respond with a similar initiative in the UK.

If you have tested HIV-negative

Insurance companies insist that they will not refuse you insurance just because you have already had a negative HIV test, and life insurance companies should not ask about prior negative HIV tests at all. They have also said that if you took the test as part of antenatal screening or for 'routine' purposes (e.g. at the request of another insurance company) this will be disregarded. But if you had a test on your own initiative they will use this as an indication of a risky lifestyle. It is likely nowadays that the company will take other things into account as well, but if they think you are at risk of HIV infection you will be refused insurance outright. If they do agree to insure you, it may well be at a higher premium.

If you are bisexual/gay

If you are gay, or the company thinks you might be, then you may possibly be refused insurance outright. Certainly if the company thinks you are 'promiscuous' this is what will happen. But such an outright refusal is less common than it used to be. If you are in a stable relationship, or if the company does not think you are particularly at risk for other reasons, it is likely that you will get insurance, provided that you take an HIV test first and it is negative. However you will probably have to pay a higher (sometimes much higher) premium. Different companies take different views about these matters. An independent financial adviser should be able to advise you on which companies to approach. See *Help and advice*, below.

Refusal of insurance

Life insurance companies always ask whether you have ever had a proposal turned down, or accepted on special terms (such as a higher premium). If you have, they will want to know why, or may turn you down on this ground alone.

For this reason it is best not to get in the position of being refused life insurance. If you think your proposal may be refused, it is better to withdraw it first, before they have the chance to refuse you. Do so in writing. You do not need to give a reason.

If you are refused life insurance or accepted on special terms for health reasons, you will be entered on a computerised list held by the British Association, called The Impaired Lives Registry.

If you later apply to any other company for life insurance, your name will show up. On occasions a person has found his or her name on this registry when it should not have been there - perhaps because of being identified as gay. Whenever this has been discovered, the company has said it was a mistake and the name has been removed.

Doctors and insurance

If your doctor's report says anything that is inconsistent with what you have told the insurance company they will be suspicious. They may wish to know more or they may turn down your application on this ground alone.

Your doctor may be asked questions about your lifestyle or sexuality. Many doctors refuse to answer this sort of question. If you are on good terms with your doctor you might like to consider discussing with him or her what sort of answers he or she would give. But if your doctor does not know about your lifestyle or sexuality, it might be better not to raise the matter at all.

You have the right to see a medical report on you written by your doctor before it is sent. You can ask for any mistakes to be corrected, and in the last resort you can refuse to allow it to be sent. There are rules about what you must do in order to exercise these rights (it doesn't happen automatically) and you should seek advice (see *Help and Advice* below).

If you do refuse to allow the report to be sent, withdraw your application at once, before it can be turned down.

Sometimes the insurance company will wish you to go to their doctor for a medical. You have no legal right to see a medical report on you prepared by a company's doctor.

Guidance to doctors on revealing HIV test and sexual history

The British Medical Association and the Association of British Insurers issued new guidance to doctors, patients and insurers on what information about HIV and sexual health can be supplied to insurers by GPs in December 2002.

In order to prevent people from being deterred from seeking advice and getting tested for HIV and other sexually transmitted infections (STIs), the guidelines state that doctors do not have to reveal all aspects of their patients' sexual health history.

The guidelines state that there is no reason to disclose single incidents of STIs, or even multiple episodes, provided there are no long-term health implications.

In addition, and in line with existing ABI guidance, insurance companies should not ask whether an applicant for insurance has taken an HIV or Hepatitis B or C test, had counselling in connection with such a test, or received a negative test result. Doctors should not reveal this information when writing reports, and insurance companies will not expect this information to be provided. Insurers may ask only whether someone has had a positive test result, is awaiting a test result, or is receiving treatment for HIV/AIDS or Hepatitis B or C.

In the event of applications for large amounts of life insurance cover (likely to be above £500,000, according to an ABI spokesman, although this figure may vary from one company to another), companies will reserve the right to ask for an HIV test and/or further medical information.

Mortgages and life insurance

There are several different types of mortgage. Some of them only work with life insurance. For others, life insurance is not necessary, but some lenders may insist on it (depending on how much you are borrowing and on the value of the property).

The most common mortgage for which life insurance is necessary is an endowment mortgage, which cannot work without it. Other types of mortgage for which life insurance cover is usually, if not always, required are pension-linked mortgages and foreign currency mortgages.

If you already have endowment life insurance, you can use it for a new endowment mortgage without any new questions being asked, provided you are not seeking to increase the sum covered in order to pay off your mortgage. For this reason, do not surrender a life insurance policy that you already have, unless you have no alternative.

Lenders often want you to take out a mortgage with life insurance because they are paid commission on the life insurance policy. But if they think you are likely to be refused life insurance, you should not apply for an endowment mortgage or any other mortgage that requires life insurance cover. This means you will need to apply for a different kind of mortgage, for example a repayment mortgage or an interest-only mortgage.

A straight repayment mortgage is available from many lenders (especially high-street building societies, or through a broker) without any life insurance cover. Sometimes, however, the lender wants you to have a mortgage protection policy as well, which pays off the mortgage if you die before all the borrowed money has been paid back.

A lender is more likely to insist on this if you are borrowing a large sum of money, or if the value of the property is nearly the same as the amount you are borrowing. But a mortgage protection policy is a form of life insurance and you should therefore not agree to apply for one if you are likely to be refused life insurance. Sometimes lenders also want you to pay for a mortgage guarantee policy, which the lender will claim on if they have to sell your property, and get less for it than they lent you: this is not life insurance and health questions will not be asked.

Apart from the question of whether you will get life insurance or not, the type of mortgage you decide to go for depends on your financial position and whether there is anyone you need to provide for if you die. You should seek advice from an independent financial adviser (see *Help and Advice* below).

Never exchange contracts on a property purchase until all the financial details have been worked out.

Travel insurance

See under Travel in Mental health and Quality of Life

Motor insurance

Some motor insurance companies ask questions about what medication you are taking and whether you have any illness or condition (whether it is relevant to your capacity to drive or not).

If you are asked a question which you do not want to answer, it would be best to try another motor insurance company that does not ask the same questions.

Help and advice

Financial advisers

An independent financial adviser, not attached to any particular insurance company, is the best place to go for financial advice. All insurance companies (other than Prudential) and all financial advisors should be members of the Personal Investment Authority (PIA). This information should be on their advertising material, business cards or letterheads.

Voluntary agencies

Voluntary agencies cannot give you financial advice, but will be able to give you advice about the law and problems in the area of insurance and mortgages generally. Advice is available from:

- Terrence Higgins Trust, 52-54 Grays Inn Road, London WC1X 8JU 020 7831 0330. Can help with legal questions concerning insurance and mortgages. The Advice Centre also publishes a leaflet on insurance.

- The Hæmophilia Society, Chesterfield House, 385 Euston Road, London NW1 3AU 020 7380 0600. Publishes leaflets that give advice on all aspects of insurance for people with hæmophilia.

Mortgage brokers

In general, mortgage brokers and independent financial advisers are ill-informed about the ways in which HIV-related insurance problems can be avoided. It will save a lot of time if you go to financial advisers who have developed expertise in dealing with such problems. You might get good advice from some of the brokers who regularly advertise in the gay press (*Pink Paper, Boyz, Gay Times*) or who are featured in directories of business services that target the gay community. London Lesbian and Gay Switchboard (020 7837 7324) may be able to provide details of brokers.

Complaints about insurance companies

If you have a complaint about the way an insurance company has treated you, the first thing to do is to complain to the company. If you get no satisfaction, the Insurance Ombudsman or the Personal Investment Authority Ombudsman may be able to help. The Ombudsmen cannot usually deal with complaints about the level of premium you are being charged, but they can deal with anything that shows bad or inefficient practice.

- Insurance Ombudsman Bureau, City Gate One, 135 Park Street, London SE1 9EA Tel: 020 7928 4488

- The Personal Investment Authority, Ombudsman Bureau, 6th floor, 1 London Wall, London EC2Y 5EA Tel: 020 7600 3838.

The Terrence Higgins Trust Insurance Working Party is also interested to hear about insurance company practices and your individual experience.

HIV prevention

The first thing that needs to be stated in any chapter on HIV prevention is that it works.

HIV has become a pandemic because it has a lethal combination of properties:

- transmission via that most taboo, intractable and instinctive of human activities, sex;

- and a long asymptomatic incubation period during which people are healthy, sexually active - and infectious.

Changing sexual behaviour involves revolutionising cultural attitudes, confronting taboos, reaching out to the most marginalised and despised populations and including them in dialogue, and helping people make rational decisions about their health at the very moments when they are least rational.

HIV prevention can include a myriad of activities, but falls into five broad classes:

- **Biomedical** approaches include HIV treatment, because antiretrovirals reduce people's infectiousness (a study in San Francisco (Porco) calculated that the average viral load, and therefore infectiousness, of gay men in the city had been cut by two-thirds since HAART). Post-exposure prophylaxis - taking HIV drugs immediately after a risky exposure to prevent HIV - is another intervention. Needle exchange is another, as is circumcision. Barrier methods like condoms are biomedical, though programmes to ensure their use are not,

and the same will apply to developing prevention technologies such as microbicides.

- **Individual** approaches include one-to-one counselling (including voluntary counselling and testing), cognitive behavioural therapy, face-to-face detached or outreach work, telephone helplines and certain internet interventions.

- **Group** approaches are those delivered to small groups of individuals, often from the same peer group, and are usually facilitated in some way. They include school sex education and small-group work that usually includes both information and risk reduction skills training.

- **Community** interventions are delivered to the whole population or (more frequently) a target audience; the difference from the previous interventions being that individuals do not need to seek out the programme. They include media stories and small-media resources (eg leaflets and posters), condom distribution schemes, the empowerment and development of communities (including communities of people with HIV), and some internet interventions like chat rooms.

- **Sociopolitical** interventions include legal change such as the decriminalisation of homosexuality or intravenous drug use; legal sanctions such as the criminalisation of transmission; and policy interventions which may permit other types of prevention work, such as allowing needle exchange.

It is tempting to conclude at times that only biomedical interventions such as treatment and vaccines can ever have an effect on HIV. But, to give just one example, a meta-reivew of prevention interventions for gay men in the USA (Johnson,2002) found that the overall effect of group- and community-level behavioural interventions targeted at gay men was a reduction in unprotected sex acts of 26%.

The largest meta-review of HIV interventions ever conducted (Albarracin, 2005) only measured condom use but found that 'active' interventions (getting people to practice skills) increased condom use by 38% relative to baseline and passive ones (where people just watched or listened to training) by 16%. Because baseline condom use was 32.3% this means that there was only an absolute increase in people who 'always' used condom by 7.8% and ones who started using them sometimes by 17%. (For other meta-analyses of the effectiveness of prevention programmes, see **HIV prevention - what methods work?**)

This may not sound like a great reduction. But no public health intervention is ever 100% successful. In addition public health measures may take decades to have an effect. For instance, in

the USA, the proportion of driving deaths caused by drunk drivers declined from 57% in 1982 to 45% in 1992. This 10% reduction was considered a major victory for public awareness campaigning and legal changes.

One paper (Stryker, 1995) put it this way: "Given experience in other health behaviour change endeavours, no interventions are likely to reduce the incidence of HIV infection to zero; indeed, insisting on too high a standard for HIV risk-reduction programs may actually undermine their effectiveness."

However small reductions in HIV incidence timed correctly may make a great deal of difference. To take an example: the first generation of topical microbicides are unlikely to prevent more than 50 to 60% of HIV infections when used. But, according to The Global Campaign for Microbicides, (2005) "Researchers have developed a mathematical model that shows that If even a small proportion of women in lower income countries used a 60% efficacious microbicide in half the sexual encounters where condoms were not used, 2.5 million HIV infections could be averted over 3 years."

Why prevention still matters

Prevention without treatment

A 2002 paper (Stover 2002) modeled mathematically what would happen to the global epidemic if a package of twelve prevention initiatives was adopted by each of 126 low- and middle-income countries. For the package and the assumptions built into it about effectiveness (which have been culled from different controlled trials of the interventions), see table 1 on the following page.

Stover and colleagues did a systematic review of published work on the prevention of HIV/AIDS and STDs in the developing

world, using a total of 86 studies to ascertain the effectiveness of interventions in reducing HIV transmission both through sex and needle-sharing. The effect for each activity was a pooled estimate of the results of these studies. They separately modelled the effect on 51 high-prevalence countries (comprising 92% of the HIV-positive population) and pooled the effect on the other 75 by grouping them into countries with common features to their epidemic, using 12 categories of likely response according to their current prevalence levels, whether HIV prevalence was increasing slowly or rapidly, and the predominant mode of transmission.

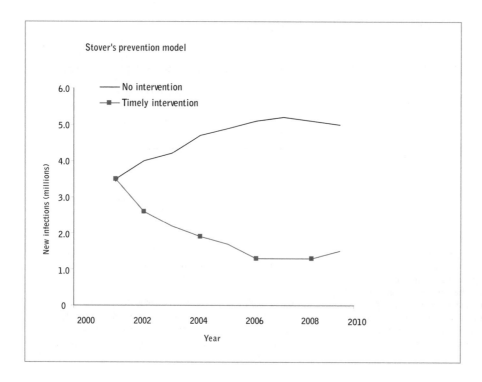

Stover calculated that the proportion of expected infections averted would range from a low of 40% in countries with stable or declining prevalence, such as Senegal and Thailand, to a high of 70% in countries with rapidly growing epidemics, such as Cameroon and China. This would cost an estimated $4.8 billion out of the $9.2 billion that UNAIDS calculated at the time would be needed to reduce HIV prevalence by 25% by the year 2005 (as pledged in the UNGASS Declaration of Commitment on HIV/AIDS in 2001), or about $1000 per infection averted. However it would cost $27 billion to sustain the programme to 2010 - prevention halted would result in a resurgent epidemic. Stover illustrated the results in a very simple graph (see chart on the left).

Success of interventions by method

Intervention	Condom Use (reduction in non-use)			Treatment for sexually transmitted disease (reduction in non-treatment)			Number of sexual partners (reduction in number of partners)			Age at first sexual intercourse (increase in age at first sexual intercourse)			Unsafe drug injections (increase in safe use of clean needles)		
	High Risk	Medium Risk	Low Risk	High Risk	Medium Risk	Low Risk	High Risk	Medium Risk	Low Risk	High Risk	Medium Risk	Low Risk	Low Risk	Medium Risk	Low Risk
Mass media campaigns		17%	17%												
Voluntary counselling and testing programmes for HIV/AIDS	50%	34%	16%												
Peer counselling - CSW	39%	42%					3%								
School-based programmes		34%						33%		0.30					
Programmes for out-of-school youths															
Workplace programmes	39%	34%	19%					23%							
Condom social marketing	21%	11%	5%							0.12					
Public sector condom distribution	57%	10%	5%	11%			35%								
Harm reduction programmes								33%					60%*		
Peer outreach to homosexual men	33%						-17%								
Treatment for sexually transmitted disease	54%	14%		47%		22%	50%								
PMTCT	50%	34%	16%												

* We assumed a 60% decrease in the average number of partners with whom needles are shared and a 60% increase in the fraction of shared needles that are cleaned.
CSW=commercial sex worker; PMTCT=prevention of mother-to-child transmission of HIV-1.

Prevention with treatment

Stover's paper was written just before the Barcelona World AIDS Conference and before treatment programmes started providing relatively widespread access to antiretrovirals in the developing world. It is an illustration of how prevention could affect incidence in a 'pure' epidemic where the infections that are *not* averted lead inevitably to AIDS.

As we have found in the developed world, the provision of treatment has had a paradoxical effect on HIV incidence - one explored three years later in a more sophisticated analysis.

In a paper in 2005 Joshua Salomon of the Harvard Center for Population and Development Studies demonstrated that effective HIV prevention programmes are essential for controlling the epidemic in the era of treatment. Using mathematical modelling, he found that, at least in situations of generalised epidemics as in Africa, relying on the scale-up of antiretroviral treatment alone would most likely not only result in increased HIV prevalence but in increased deaths due to AIDS, despite the effectiveness of antiretrovirals.

Salomon used an epidemiologic model of HIV and AIDS to investigate a range of possible positive and negative health outcomes under alternative scenarios

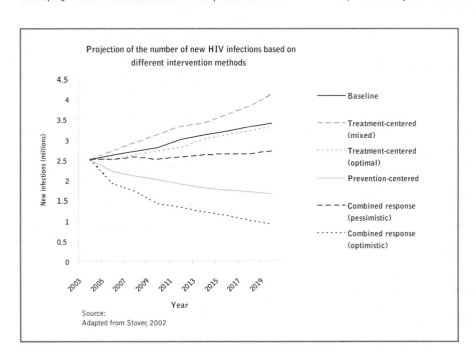

Projection of the number of new HIV infections based on different intervention methods

Baseline
Treatment-centered (mixed)
Treatment-centered (optimal)
Prevention-centered
Combined response (pessimistic)
Combined response (optimistic)

Source:
Adapted from Stover, 2002

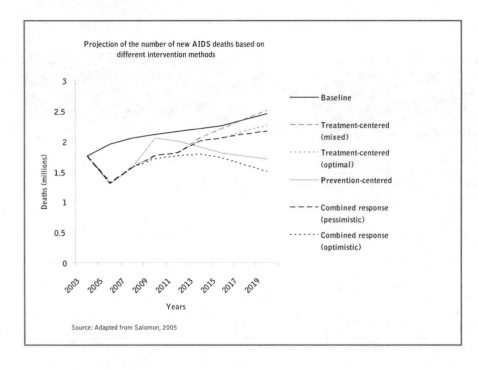

Projection of the number of new AIDS deaths based on
different intervention methods

— Baseline

– – – Treatment-centered
(mixed)

⋯⋯⋯ Treatment-centered
(optimal)

— Prevention-centered

– – – Combined response
(pessimistic)

⋯⋯⋯ Combined response
(optimistic)

Source: Adapted from Salomon, 2005

that reflected varying implementation of prevention and
treatment (see diagrams on this page).

The potential impacts of prevention efforts at a given coverage
level were based on Stover's comprehensive package of 12
interventions, although Stover and colleagues also included
interventions such as harm reduction for injecting drug users and
peer outreach for men who have sex with men, which Salomon
did not include in his model for Africa.

In the two scenarios representing treatment-centred strategies,
with different assumptions about the impact of treatment on
transmissibility and behaviour, the change in the total number the
number of new infections expected by the year 2020 ranged from
a 10% increase to a 6% reduction from the baseline level
expected at 2020.

But because the absolute number of new HIV infections in Africa
under a 'business as usual' scenario of no increased treatment
provision are expected to rise from 2.6 million in 2005 to 3.8
million by 2020, in both treatment-based scenarios there would
be a net increase in the number of people living with HIV. Indeed

annual incidence in Africa
would increase to 4.3 million
by 2020 if current rates of
treatment roll-out were
unaccompanied by effective
prevention strategies.

Similarly, the annual number
of AIDS deaths relative to the
expected 2020 baseline under
a treatment-only strategy
would decline by 9% to 13%
(meaning a net increase of
450,000 to 1.15 million AIDS
deaths) but would actually
increase if not-very-pessimistic
assumptions are made about
decreased condom use and the
increased longevity of people
with HIV resulting in
more transmissions.

In contrast, a prevention-only
strategy, based on Stover's
recommendations, with no
increased rollout of
antiretrovirals at all, provided
greater reductions in incidence
(36%) than using treatment.
It also provided and mortality
reductions similar to those of the treatment-centred scenarios by
2020, but more modest mortality benefits over the immediate
next five to ten years.

Salomon then looked at the potential synergy between treatment
and prevention. If they were to enhance each other in a combined
response, the expected benefits would be a 55% reduction in
annual incidence (a total of 29 million averted infections) and a
27% reduction in mortality (ten million lives saved) by 2020.

However, if treatment scale-up led to prevention efforts being
less effective (because of behaviour change or greater
infectivity), the benefits of a combined response would be
considerably smaller- a 17% reduction in incidence (nine million
averted infections) and a 16% reduction in AIDS deaths (six
million lives saved).

What assumptions did Salomon build into his model? The
number of people being treated in 2020 ranged from 9.2 million
in a treatment-only scenario, to 4.2 million in treatment and
prevention worked synergistically together to reduce new
infections.

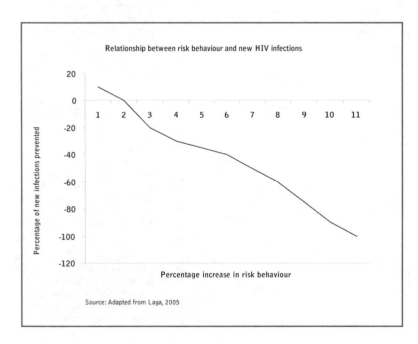

Relationship between risk behaviour and new HIV infections

Percentage increase in risk behaviour

Source: Adapted from Laga, 2005

It's worth noting that the 'pessimistic'
assumption for the effectiveness of
prevention campaigns assumed a 25%
effectiveness - pretty close to the figure
found in the Johnson study above. This
included assumptions such as the reduced
fear of death leading to a 10% reduction in
condom use - a pretty conservative estimate
given reductions seen among groups such as
gay men in the west.

Nonetheless, Salomon's model indicates
that, in a generalised epidemic at least, only
if prevention accompanies treatment can
there be control of HIV.

Why is this, given that some studies (Porco)
have found that, on a population level,
antiretroviral treatment, by reducing viral
loads, has reduced the average
infectiousness of the HIV-positive individual
by as much as two-thirds?

This is because it takes only a small
increase in sexual risk behaviour to
abrogate the effect of antiretrovirals. In a

paper presented at the 2005 IAS conference that quoted Salomon, Marie Laga of the Antwerp Institute for Tropical Diseases showed that anything more than a 5% increase in risk behaviour would cancel out the life-saving effects of antiretrovirals (see diagram).

This is because HIV transmission is not a simple, linear phenomenon. A disproportionate number (though exactly what proportion is disputed) of new infections occur due to transmission by people who are recently infected themselves and there for both have a high viral load and are ignorant of their infection.

There is also a non-linear relationship between the number of *concurrent* sex partners people have within a population and the frequency of HIV transmission. In a situation where people are serially monogamous - the predominant pattern among heterosexuals in the west - new HIV transmissions can only happen when one relationship stops and another starts. But in cultures where concurrent relationships are more common - as in some African and other non-western cultures, within the gay community, and among certain other groups such as sex workers and some young people - one person who is infected can quickly become the 'index case' for a cluster of infections.

Nicole Crepaz, in a 2004 meta-review of 21 studies, found that when individuals started taking antiretroviral therapy, there was no significant change in their sexual risk behaviour. However this does not include how the behaviour of people remaining off treatment in the same population may change when antiretroviral use becomes common in others, let alone how undiagnosed people may change their behaviour when AIDS is no longer seen as an inevitable death sentence.

In response to Salomon's paper, Stover wrote another (Stover 2006) in which he factored in an optimistic scenario of 80% global coverage of antiretroviral treatment by 2010.

His new estimate of the cost of his comprehensive prevention package was nearly five times greater than his previous one, reflecting new understandings about the complexities of sustaining prevention efforts. It would, he estimated, cost $122 billion to sustain comprehensive prevention from 2005 to 2010, or $3923 per infection averted.

However he estimated that the HIV treatment that would be necessary (as 80% coverage) for infections that would occur if the prevention package was *not* put in place averted would cost $4,707 per lifetime, leading to a net saving of $784 per infection averted or $24.38 billion in total.

The comprehensive prevention package could also prevent 30 million people becoming infected with HIV.

To summarise these modelling studies:

- We stand a chance of reversing the course of the HIV epidemic only if comprehensive prevention packages are combined with treatment access.

- Though costly, comprehensive worldwide prevention programmes could still be cost-effective.

Examples of success

The 26% reduction typical of prevention interventions found by Johnson is of course an average. Although it included many interventions that did *not* work, the history of the epidemic shows that specific interventions targeted accurately and at the right time can work much more dramatically.

To cite three of the two most widely-quoted examples:

- In **Uganda**, a countrywide programme of AIDS awareness-raising initiated by the Ugandan president in 1986 led to demonstrable reductions in risky behaviour and

at least contributed to a two- to four-fold reduction in HIV prevalence. Similar, more recent reductions have been seen in other African countries such as Kenya and Zimbabwe (see **The Epidemiology of HIV**)

- In **Thailand**, a single-minded campaign to institute 100% condom use in commercial sex establishments brought down the HIV incidence in young men from 2.5% in 1991 to 0.5% in 1993.

- The **UK** has its own major triumph. In 1986 HIV prevalence among injecting drug users in Edinburgh was approaching 50%. Reversing a police policy of confiscating needles and instituting needle exchange lowered annual HIV incidence among UK drug users to two per cent. Just seven per cent of Britons with HIV have caught it from needle-sharing, as opposed to 28% in the USA and 80% in Russia.

Why does prevention fail?

Given, then that (for instance) a combination of reduction programmes and HAART should have reduced HIV incidence in gay men in the developed world, why, in many cases, has it not - to the extent that many commentators talk of the 'failure' of HIV prevention?

Although it is important that a country's HIV prevention 'package' includes as wide a variety of interventions as possible (because what is appropriate to a heterosexual virgin teenager is not appropriate to a gay male sex worker), it's also important to be aware that HIV interventions are not necessarily synergistic (reinforce each other's effects). On the contrary, they may be antagonistic.

To take some examples:

- The advent of HAART has reduced fear of death among the community at large and gay men in particular, and has also increased the population of healthy, sexually active people with HIV. Between them, these contribute to cancelling out the net drop in infectiousness in the community, as show above.

- Opponents of condom distribution programmes say that providing condoms only encourages sexual activity.

- Doctors fear that providing post-exposure prophylaxis will lead to greater risks being taken.

- Some studies[4] of peer-led and facilitated group interventions have found that their effectiveness is compromised by the 'shame factor' - participants being reluctant to discuss times when they have deviated from the group norm of sexual behaviour.

In addition, the target audience dictates the message, and HIV prevention interventions devised for gay men in the pre-treatment era are no longer appropriate for a large proportion of the world's vulnerable population.

It is interesting to speculate how HIV prevention would have developed in the world's richer countries if the group most affected from the start had been young heterosexual women, as in Africa and other parts of the developing world, instead of gay men.

- Would an HIV prevention strategy based on an essentially male-controlled device - the condom - have been the primary focus of prevention?

- Would strategies encouraging sexual abstinence or monogamy have been more prominent?

- Would the invoking of criminal sanctions against infection have happened earlier?

- And would a general presumption of 'shared responsibility' in sexual relationships and negotiation have been tempered much earlier by questions of power and inequalities of gender, age and income?

These speculations were prompted by reading the previous version of this section of the AIDS Reference Manual, which was entitled 'Safer Sex' and concerned itself entirely with condom use and technique, the safety of specific sexual techniques, and sexually transmitted infections.

Because of the complex synergies and antagonisms possible between interventions, in the last decade HIV prevention, at least in the UK and the developed world, has been utterly transformed from what was essentially the social marketing of a simple message - 'Choose Safer Sex' - into a complex, contradictory and extremely politicised set of dialogues featuring heated debates between proponents of:

- abstinence versus comprehensive sex education

- the promotion of condoms versus the promotion of monogamy

- harm reduction versus risk elimination

- 'normalising' disclosure and HIV testing versus confidentiality and patient rights

- and whether HIV-negative or HIV-positive people are the best targets for - and the best originators of - prevention messages.

As well as becoming more complex, as an endeavour HIV prevention has also become by many to be seen as less effective.

HIV infection continues to climb in much of the developing world, and certain experts continue to forecast that countries like India and Russia are at the 'tipping point' for the development of generalised epidemics. Although prevalence has fallen in some African countries, there are fears that the cost of providing global access to antiretrovirals may impact adversely on community prevention initiatives - and there are equal fears that an American-led emphasis on abstinence as the mainstay of prevention rather than a balanced programme will lead to a resurgence of HIV. According to UNAIDS by July 2005 only one in five people needing HIV prevention had access to prevention programmes and only one in ten people had been tested for HIV.

These fears are best exemplified by the 2002 paper (Marseille, 2002) in *The Lancet* by Elliot Marseille and colleagues, who argued that HIV prevention is 28 times more cost-effective than providing treatment in the developing world, and that "funding HAART at the expense of prevention means greater loss of life."

Although Marseille's views were criticised as placing a false opposition between prevention and treatment, concerns continue to be expressed that over-emphasising treatment at the expense of prevention in not cost effective.

As recently as July 2005, in an opinion column in *Forbes Magazine*, economist Emily Oster said that the cost of global access to antiretroviral drugs in the developing world was $365 per life-year saved. In comparison, she said, a blanket programme of STI treatment would cost $3.65 per life-year saved and a national HIV education programme would cost $16.

There is also concern that treatment without proper education will lead to increased transmission of drug-resistant HIV in the developing world, with a resultant rapid loss of sustainability of cheap anti-retroviral regimens.

However these arguments ignore the fact that providing antiretroviral drugs provides hope, which is in turn a major generator of positive prevention behaviours such as increased testing, increased disclosure of HIV status, reduction of stigma, and an examination of community sexual norms. In one district in Uganda, for instance, the arrival of antiretrovirals in the area led to a 23-fold increase in the number of people coming forward for testing, and some studies (eg Holtgrave and Anderson) have

shown that, when diagnosed, people with HIV reduce the amount of unsafe sexual encounters they have by at least 50%.

In the developed world, HIV prevention work faces an uphill battle both against the loss of funding due to the cost of HAART and changes in behaviour leading to a greatly increased incidence of sexually transmitted diseases, especially among gay men, and, in some cases, HIV.

The USA has started to see an increasing degree of inequality when it comes to HIV vulnerability between ethnic minority and particularly African-American people and the white majority. A recent survey of gay men (Centers for Disease Control, 24 June 2005), for instance, found that HIV prevalence among Afro-American men who have sex with men it was more than twice what it was in whites; among Afro-Americans in general it is four times that of the general population: and four out of five women diagnosed with HIV (Centers for Disease Control, 16 June 2005) is black or Hispanic.

There has been a loss of certainty about how to do effective HIV prevention work with poor black women and also with men who, while having sex with men, may not identify as gay. With gay men in general there have been concerns that two decades of prevention success could be wiped away by recreational drug use.

Gay prevention campaigners are concerned that the global emphasis on HIV is obscuring the fact that men who have sex with men are still the most vulnerable population for infection in most developed countries. For instance, 80% of the people who acquired their HIV *in the UK* last year were gay men, and sexually active gay men, who form no more than one in 40 of the UK population, are at least 200 times more likely to catch HIV in the UK than heterosexuals (Health Protection Agency, 2005).

While European countries have not seen the same development of HIV health inequality as the USA, increasing HIV prevalence among immigrant populations who may have limited access to HIV treatment and to prevention messages has led to fears of a 'second generation' epidemic among minorities, though there are only very early signs so far that this is materialising.

This widely-held feeling that HIV prevention has lost its way and that we no longer live in a simple 'safer sex' world has led to an increased focus on the development and testing of new prevention technologies such as pre-exposure prophylaxis and microbicides.

The changes in HIV prevention work have been predicated upon two huge historical changes.

The 'feminisation' of AIDS. This has transformed HIV educators' views of the position of the HIV-negative partner in sex. Almost all countries have seen increased numbers of women diagnosed with HIV, to the extent of women now forming the majority of people affected in sub-Saharan Africa. The fact that for many of these women - a lot of whom are wives - it is quite simply culturally and personally impossible to negotiate condom use with male partners has led on the one hand to the drive to develop microbicides and other female-controlled technologies, and on the other for proponents of abstinence and monogamy to say that these are the only strategies that protect vulnerable women against male sexual dominance.

Post-HAART optimism. Although studies(Stolte, 2004; Huebner, 2004) have produced contradictory results as to whether 'treatment optimism' is responsible for the observed decreased condom use and increased levels of STIs, especially among gay men, it makes intuitive sense that when the extreme threat of a universally fatal disease that has killed lovers and friends is lifted, some people in vulnerable communities who might previously have maintained safer sex become prepared to take risks. The increased numbers and improved state of health of HIV-positive people has also meant that more continue to be sexually active, and for longer. This has led to a new and anxious concentration on people with HIV as sexual beings and vectors of disease.

In this chapter, we will therefore look at HIV prevention as a much broader set of techniques and messages than just 'choose safer sex'. To bring some order to a complex field we will use the template of the African 'A-B-C' prevention model, with a couple of additions, without implying that this is an endorsement of it as *the* HIV prevention approach.

A is for Abstinence will look at whether there is evidence that programmes which encourage sexual abstinence or delay sexual debut in young people help to reduce HIV infection.

B is for Being faithful and Behaviour change will look at the degree to which HIV prevention projects have changed sexual behaviour in general, especially in adults.

C is for Condoms and other barrier methods will look at the evidence for the effectiveness of male and female condoms in preventing HIV and other STIs and will review recent evidence on the effectiveness of programmes to encourage condom use.

D is for disclosure, negotiated safety and serosorting Will look at measures people with and without HIV take to reduce risk as an alternative to, or in addition to, using condoms

E is for Emergent technologies Will review available and potential new prevention technologies.

References

Albarracin D et al. A test of major assumptions about behaviour change: a comprehensive look at the effects of passive and active HIV-prevention interventions since the beginning of the epidemic. *Psychological Bulletin* 131(6), 856-897. 2005.

Centers for Disease Control. A Glance at the HIV/AIDS Epidemic. Centers for Disease Control. See http://www.cdc.gov/hiv/dhap.htm. 16 June 2005.

Centers for Disease Control. HIV Prevalence, Unrecognized Infection, and HIV Testing Among Men Who Have Sex with Men --- Five U.S. Cities, June 2004--April 2005. CDC Mortality and Morbidity Weekly Report. See http://www.cdc.gov/mmwr/preview/mmwrhtml/mm5424a2.htm.%2024%20June%202005.

Crepaz N et al. Highly Active Antiretroviral Therapy and Sexual Risk Behavior: A Meta-analytic Review. *JAMA* 292:224-236. 2004.

Elford, J et al. Peer education has no significant impact on HIV risk behaviours among gay men in London. *AIDS* 15(4) 535-538. 2001.

Global Campaign for Microbicides Factsheet: Frequently Asked Questions about Microbicides. See http://www.global-campaign.org/clientfiles/FS2-FAQs-May05.pdf. Revised May 2005.

Health Protection Agency Quarterly HIV/AIDS Surveillance tables. See http://www.hpa.org.uk/infections/topics_az/hiv_and_sti/hiv/epidemiology/files/quarterly.pdf.%20June%202005.

Holtgrave DR, Anderson T. Utilizing HIV transmission rates to assist in prioritizing HIV prevention services. *Int J STD AIDS* . 15(12):789-92. 2004.

Huebner D et al. A longitudinal study of the association between treatment optimism and sexual risk-behaviour in young adult men who have sex with men. 15th International AIDS Conference, Bangkok. Abstract D11585. 2004.

Johnson W et al. HIV prevention research for men who have sex with men: a systematic review and meta-analysis. *JAIDS* 30 (suppl. 1), S118-129. 2002.

Laga M. Synergy between prevention and care in Africa. Third IAS Conference on HIV Pathogenesis and Treatment, Rio de Janeiro. Abstract MoFo0104. 2005.

Marseille E, Hofmann PB, Kahn JG. HIV prevention before HAART in sub-Saharan Africa. *Lancet* 359:9320, 1851-1856. 2002.

Porco TC et al. Decline in HIV infectivity following the introduction of highly active antiretroviral therapy. *AIDS* 18(1):81-8. 2004.

Salomon JA et al. Integrating HIV Prevention and Treatment: From Slogans to Impact. *PLos Medicine*, 2(1), pp 50-56. 2005.

Stolte I et al. Homosexual men change to risky sex when perceiving less threat of HIV/AIDS since availability of highly active antiretroviral therapy: a longitudinal study. *AIDS* 18:303-309. 2004.

Stover J et al (2002). Can we reverse the HIV/AIDS pandemic with an expanded response? *Lancet* 360: 73-77. 2002.

Stover J et al (2006). The global impact of scaling up HIV/AIDS prevention programmes in low- and middle-income countries. *Science* 311 pp 1474-1476. 2006.

Stryker J et al. Prevention of HIV infection. Looking back, looking ahead. *JAMA* 273(14). 1995.

A is for abstinence

Delaying a young person's sexual debut, or at least the age at which they start having full intercourse, could be a very effective HIV prevention measure in certain populations.

In the developing world young women are much more vulnerable to HIV than young men. In southern Africa, for instance, HIV prevalence among young women ages 15-24 is three times higher than among young men, and among under-20s up to 10 times higher (UNAIDS, 2004.). This is attributed partly to culture - with a pattern of older men seeking out younger women for sex - but also partly to nature; the immature genital tract of young women is more susceptible to HIV and other STIs.

One population among whom delayed debut of intercourse would serve to reduce HIV infections is young gay men.

In the 2002 Gay Men's Sex Survey *Out and About* (Hickson, 2003), the authors comment on the finding that the median sexual debut age of young gay men is16 and the date of first anal intercourse is 17:

"The median age of first heterosexual sex among the male population in the UK is 14 years and median age of first vaginal intercourse is 18. This suggests that gay men have to wait longer before starting to experience sex with men than their heterosexual counterparts do with women, but proceed to intercourse quicker. This is congruent with gay men having been denied opportunities to 'date' or 'court' while a teenager and being left to enter the adult world of sexuality with little practice, support or guidance."

Unfortunately, lesbians and gay men are largely excluded from abstinence education programmes - explicitly so in the case of 'abstinence only till marriage'.

Abstinence in people with HIV

Another population that in some cases appears to be practising abstinence as an HIV prevention method is HIV-positive people. One US survey (Weinhardt, 2004), for instance, found that 18.5% of gay men and 26% of heterosexual men and women had not had sex in the three months prior to the survey. Although much of this lack of a sex life will be due to illness, stigma or fear of rejection, some individuals with HIV have taken a willed choice to remain sexually abstinent in order not to pass on their HIV. This appears to be particularly the case with women. The Padare Project (Chinouya, 2003), for instance, a survey of HIV-positive Africans living in London, found that while only 10% of men had not had sex in the pervious four weeks, among women the proportion rose to one-third.

Even some positive gay youth appear to be trying abstinence, in the absence of any encouragement to do so. A survey of HIV-positive gay men aged 15-24 in Los Angeles (Lightfoot, 2005) found that 12% of this group had had no sex with anyone in the three months preceding the study.

Another survey in 2006 looked at the sex lives of people with HIV from the US HIV Cost and Services Utilization Study (HCSUS).

Of the 1,339 HCUS respondents whose data were analysed, 415 participants reported being sexually inactive in the previous six months. Of those, 201 were deliberately abstinent. More women (18%) and heterosexual men (18%) were deliberately abstinent than gay/bisexual men (11 %).

The investigators found that the likelihood of deliberate abstinence was higher among women and heterosexual men, older participants, and those with a stronger sense of responsibility. It was lower among those with a primary relationship partner/spouse, those on antiretroviral therapy, subjects with CD4 counts of 50 or higher, and drinkers.

The researchers found that higher perceived responsibility for limiting disease transmission and non-drinking status were related to deliberate abstinence only among gay men. Worse health was associated with deliberate abstinence only among heterosexual men.

Does abstinence work to reduce HIV transmission?

Does encouraging abstinence work? And does it lead to lower HIV incidence? The data are contradictory, and clouded by differing interpretations of the data.

One study (Bessinger, 2003)found that the proportion of urban young women aged 15-19 in Uganda who said they had 'never had sex' increased from 44 to 60% between 1990 and 2000, with an even sharper increase in young men from 33 to 66%. The same study found similar declines in Zambia but not in Zimbabwe or among young women in Cameroon and Kenya.

However another study (Wawer, 2005). from the rural province of Rakai, Uganda found that abstinence rates in teenagers had *declined* from 60 to 50% in women and 32 to 28% in men between 1990 and 2002. The same study found that a decline in HIV prevalence from 17.6 to 11.4% during the same period was largely due to more people dying of AIDS than becoming infected with HIV. Rakai has a mature epidemic, being the first district of Uganda from which AIDS was reported, in 1982.

In the USA the Clinton administration was the first to set aside $50 a year specifically for abstinence education, though the Christian education centre had first mooted abstinence education as a way of reducing HIV and STIs in 1987 and programmes such as True Love Waits had been running since 1992.

By 2005 under George W Bush this money had risen to $167m, with an 18.5% increase promised for 2006 and $204 million for 2007, and with no comparative funding set aside directly for comprehensive, non abstinence-based sex education in schools.

Conservative think-tank the Heritage Foundation (Pardue, 2004) said this was still only one-twelfth the money spent on all condom provision and comprehensive sex education, and that a large proportion of the federal money was in fact being spent by 'abstinence plus' programmes which taught abstinence as the preferred option in a comprehensive sex education package.

In June 2006, however, more than 200 organisations, representing all 50 states and the District of Columbia, launched a nationwide *No More Money* campaign in an effort to stop federal funding for abstinence-only-until-marriage programs. The campaign was co-ordinated by the Sexuality Information and Education Council of the U.S. (SIECUS). Its vice-president, for public policy, William smith, said: "Now that it is clear that there is no sound research supporting these programs, no support in the public health community, and no support by the American people, we are asking Congress to stop funding these harmful programs." (see www.nomoremoney.org).

Whether abstinence programmes have made any difference is up for interpretation. One undisputed fact is that the teenage pregnancy rate - seen as an indicator of STI rates -declined in the USA during the 1990s from 117 per 1,000 in 1990 to 84 per 1,000 in 1999, and is now lower than the overall UK rate though it is still five times the rate in the Netherlands.

The national rate declined by 27% (Haddock, 2005) - but in California, which is the sole state to have refused federal funds for abstinence-only education, it fell by 40%, and the national rate has not declined further since 2000.

There is no definitive answer as to whether abstinence-only programmes will impact on HIV incidence in American youth.

Evidence against the effectiveness of abstinence programmes

The most rigorous published review to date(Kirby, 2001) of 28 sex education programs in the United States and Canada aimed at reducing teen pregnancy and STIs, including HIV, found that none of the three abstinence-only programs that met inclusion criteria for review demonstrated evidence of efficacy for delaying sexual debut. Furthermore, these three programs did not reduce the frequency of sex or the number of partners among those students who had ever had sex.

However, this same review found that nine abstinence-*plus* programmes (meaning abstinence education as part of comprehensive sex education) showed efficacy in delaying sexual debut, as well as reducing the frequency of intercourse and increasing condom use once sex began.

The largest study so far undertaken specifically of abstinence-only programmes (Bearman, 2005) also suggests that while they may significantly delay the age of sexual debut, the long-term effect on sexual health is neutral.

The study interviewed 20,000 teenagers aged 12-18 in 1995, and again in 1997 and 2002. At this point 11,550 of them also provided a urine sample so researchers could find any evidence of STI infections.

One in five teenagers said they had taken a virginity pledge. Despite this, 61% of 'consistent' pledgers had had sex before marriage or before the final 2002 interviews.

The study did find that youth who took abstinence pledges started having sexual intercourse on average 18 months to two years later than youth who did not - though without a proper longitudinal study with baseline attitudes measured, it's impossible to say whether they would have been the kind of young people who would have delayed sex anyway.

The study authors commented: "Pledgers have fewer partners than nonpledgers. Whereas the typical nonpledger male has had 2.4 partners, male pledgers have 1.5 partners on average ($p < .0009$). The same pattern holds for females as well, 2.7 for nonpledgers and 1.9 for pledgers ($p < .0009$).

"Nor are pledgers exposed to STI risk for as long as nonpledgers. The average number of years of sexual activity, or time of exposure, is shorter for pledgers than for others. Consistent pledgers were sexually active for an average of 4.2 years, compared with nonpledgers with 5.9 years ($p < .0009$). Thus, with respect to both the number of partners and cumulative exposure, pledgers are at lower risk to acquisition of an STI than nonpledgers."

However the same study found that 'pledgers' were one-third less likely to use contraception (barrier or otherwise) when they did have sex than 'non-pledgers'. It found that pledgers were slightly but significantly less likely to use a condom at first sex (55% versus 60% condom use, p= <.018). And teenagers' STI rates once they married were the same regardless of whether they had had premarital sex.

It also found that there was evidence that teenagers who took abstinence pledges were "technically" avoiding loss of virginity by having more oral and anal sex. Just two per cent of non-pledgers reported having no vaginal sex but having oral sex: in pledgers the proportion was 13%.

More worryingly, although the absolute figures were small, more pledgers had anal sex as an alternative to vaginal sex too: 1.2% of pledgers and 0.7% of non-pledgers.

Another survey, (Goodson, 2004) of five abstinence-only programmes from 59 schools in Texas, which interviewed 726 11-17 year olds, found that abstinence-only education apparently made no difference to the proportion of teenagers who were sexually active. It found that 23% of year 9 (14 year old) girls and boys were sexually active before attending an abstinence programme. Afterwards, 28% of girls were sexually active, and when boys were asked a year later at age 15, 39% were active. Other programmes have reported even more substantial increases in sexual activity after programmes, indicating that they have made little or even a negative difference to the natural tendency of more teenagers to start having sex as they get older.

Evidence for the effectiveness of abstinence programmes

The supporters of abstinence programmes, however, including the Heritage Foundation (Rector, 2002), pointed to studies which found that at least ten programmes had produced success, by some measures, though in some cases this was more to do with changing teenagers' attitudes towards abstinence than their actual behaviour. It did find, among other things, a steeper decrease in the teenage pregnancy rate in Monroe County, New York, where an abstinence-only programme called 'Not Me, Not Now' had been operating, compared with surrounding non-abstinence-only counties. It found that a programme in Little Rock, Arkansas "reduced the sexual activity rate of girls from 10.2 to 5.9% and from boys from 22.8 to 15.8%." And it found that 14 year-old boys who had not attended a programme in Georgia were three times as likely to have begun having sex by the end of eighth grade as boys who had attended it.

A study by Dr Robert Lerner published in *Adolescent and Family Health* evaluated the effectiveness of the Best Friends abstinence education programme. It found that students in it were significantly less likely than their peers to engage in high-risk behaviours.

The Best Friends program began in 1987 and currently operates in more than 100 schools across the United States. Its curriculum consists of a character-building program for girls in the fifth or sixth grade, including at least 110 hours of instruction, mentoring, and group activities throughout the year. Discussion topics include friendship, love and dating, self-respect, decision-making, alcohol abuse, drug abuse, physical fitness and nutrition, and AIDS/STDs. The predominant theme of the curriculum is encouragement to abstain from high-risk behavior, including sexual activities. A companion program for boys, Best Men, began in 2000.

Specifically, girls who participated the Best Friends program had:

- A 52% reduction in the likelihood that they would smoke;

- A 90% reduction in the likelihood that they would use drugs;

- A 60% reduction in the likelihood that they would drink alcohol;

- An 80% reduction in the likelihood that they would have sex.

The study compared several years of data on girls from Washington, D.C., who participated in the Best Friends program with data on Washington, D.C., girls of the same age from the Centers for Disease Control's (CDC) Youth Risk Behavior Survey (YRBS).

Using multiple logistic regressions, which controlled for grade, age, race, and survey year, the study found a significant decrease in the incidence of high-risk behaviours among Best Friends girls as compared to YRBS girls.

Abstinence supporters said that two other studies (Mohn, Santelli) supported the contention that abstinence was largely responsible for the decline in teenage pregnancy rates.

Mohn found that increased abstinence among 15- to 19 year-old teens accounted for at least two-thirds (67%) of the drop in teen pregnancy rates. Increased abstinence also accounted for more than half (51%) of the decline in teen birth rates.

Santelli found that 53% of the decline in teen pregnancy rates from 1991 to 2001 could be attributed to decreased sexual experience among teens aged 15-17 years old, while only 47% of the decline was attributed to increased use of contraception among teens.

Same data, differing interpretations

However Santelli also found that when teenagers had sex, condom use increased during this period from 40% to 51%, that teenagers who used no method of protection fell from 17% to 13% and that ones who tried to use withdrawal (without a condom) as their method declined from 20% to 13%. So these findings back the promotion of condom use as well as abstinence.

However although abstinence programmes may reduce rates of sexual activity, opponents of them say that many do so by spreading disempowering and negative messages about sex and condoms.

The Heritage Foundation document quoted above (Rector, 2002) documents significantly higher rates of depression and suicide in teenagers who have sex versus teenagers who don't, while failing to establish the direction of causation: does sex make teenagers depressed, or do depressed teenagers turn to sex for comfort or due to a history of sexual abuse?

And the fact that condoms prevent 85% of HIV infections if used consistently, and 30% of herpes infections (because herpes can be transmitted through touch) is used as evidence that condoms are not a 'safe' protection method against HIV and that they 'never or rarely' prevent herpes. This led to pressure on the US Centers for Disease Control and Prevention (the CDC) to take down temporarily from its website information on the effectiveness of condoms, and was the spur to various legislative changes, such as the State of Louisiana withdrawing all state-financed condom distribution in 2004.

Clearly, abstinence or at least delayed sexual debut could prevent a lot of HIV and STI infections in younger people if it was 'used properly' as a strategy, but equally clearly the evidence we have so far points to it being used more inconsistently than condoms.

Mindful of public controversy about the amount of money spent on abstinence-only programmes, the US government is currently conducting a large survey of their effectiveness.

Abstinence in Africa

Meanwhile in Africa, the lobbying group Human Rights Watch (Human Rights Watch, 2005) criticised an apparent policy shift towards abstinence-only programmes, saying that the Ugandan Government had removed critical HIV information from primary school curricula, including information about condoms, safer sex and the risks of HIV in marriage. Uganda's Minister of State for Primary Health Care was quoted as saying: "As a ministry, we have realised that abstinence and being faithful to one's partner are the only sure ways to curb AIDS. From next year, the ministry is going to be less involved in condom importation but more involved in awareness campaigns; abstinence and behaviour change."

Uganda's first lady, Janet Museveni, leads an abstinence programme called the National Youth Forum, describing her approach as "a blend of African and Christian values." However a spokesman for her husband, President Yoweri Museveni, said the government was merely being consistent in advocating for it's multi-pronged 'ABC' strategy against AIDS: "Those who are sexually active should be faithful to their partners, others who are single should abstain until marriage, and those who cannot abstain should use condoms."

There has certainly been an increase in the age of sexual debut in Uganda - see chart below - and this may have contributed to reports of declining HIV incidence (see 'Being faithful' below). But the sharpest decline happened in the mid-90s, long before abstinence-only as an approach had been adopted in this country, but around the time the HIV epidemic was maturing and large numbers of family members were dying. The fear of death may be a greater incentive to abstinence than exhortations to stay 'pure'.

(The Uganda charts in this section are all from "What Happened in Uganda? Declining HIV Prevalence, Behavior Change, and the National Response", Edited by Janice Hogle, USAID, 2002.)

HIV activist and prevention advocates in Uganda expressed concern that the new emphasis on abstinence-only programmes and restrictions in condom supply were reversing two decades of successful HIV prevention work, after a survey found that HIV prevalence was starting to increase again, according the The Lancet (Wakabi). The national serostatus survey for 2004/05 showed that average national prevalence was 6.4%, slightly up from 6.2% just over a year previously. Infection was shifting from the youth to adults aged between 30 and 40 years. Prevalence rates have traditionally been higher among younger people, so the new trend has baffled health workers. There are at least 1.4 million Ugandans living with HIV.

"Infection is high among adults now and we must ask ourselves why", said Vice President Gilbert Bukenya, a medical professor. He said the issue of condom use needs to be reviewed as the country seeks explanations for the rising prevalence rates. "The issue of condoms was politicised. Much as the religious sector is against it, I feel there are people who can't be left out. The issue must be re-addressed".

Two incidents had led to condoms being de-emphasised

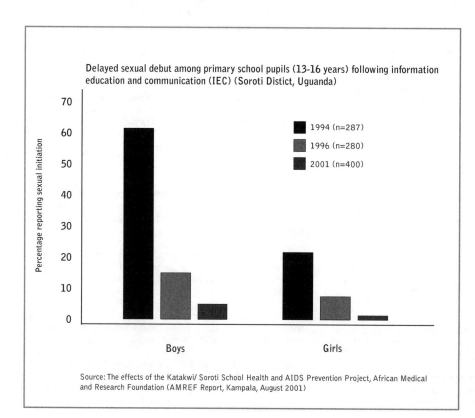

Delayed sexual debut among primary school pupils (13-16 years) following information education and communication (IEC) (Soroti Distict, Uguanda)

Percentage reporting sexual initiation

1994 (n=287)
1996 (n=280)
2001 (n=400)

Boys   Girls

Source: The effects of the Katakwi/ Soroti School Health and AIDS Prevention Project, African Medical and Research Foundation (AMREF Report, Kampala, August 2001)

as the main weapon in the fight against HIV/AIDS. The first was Janet Museveni's campaign.

Secondly, a recall of some brands of condoms in 2004/05 due to concerns about their quality led to a national shortage.

A 2005 study by researchers at the local Makerere University and the AIDS Information Centre showed that when condoms were used by most Ugandans aged 19-25, they were primarily considered contraceptive tools rather than protection against infections.

These findings have added weight to calls from local and international health groups for President Museveni and his government to commit to promoting the ABC strategy properly, rather than trying to downplay the utility of condoms in HIV prevention.

The U.S. Leadership against HIV/AIDS, Tuberculosis, and Malaria Act of 2003 which set up the President's Emergency Plan for AIDS Relief (PEPFAR) recommended that 20% of funds designated to fulfilling the law be designated to prevention. Of that 20%, the law mandated that 33% should be dedicated to abstinence-until-marriage programs.

In April 2006, the United States Government Accountability Office (GAO) released a report reviewing how the Office of the U.S. Global AIDS Coordinator (OGAC) administers funds for HIV prevention through PEPFAR. The GAO report found that 10 of the 15 PEPFAR focus countries had requested exemptions from fulfilling the abstinence 'earmark' between September 2005 and January 2006, citing the following challenges:

- reduced spending for Preventing Mother-to-Child Transmission (PMTCT):

- limited funding to deliver appropriate prevention messaging to high-risk groups:

- lack of responsiveness to cultural and social norms:

- cuts in medical and blood safety activities:

- and elimination of care programs.

The report found that OGAC was over-interpreting the abstinence-until-marriage earmark by applying it to all prevention funding although, by law, it only applies to funds appropriated to the Global HIV/AIDS Initiative account, which amounted to an additional $33 million in fiscal year 2006.

It found that the lack of clarity from OGAC on how to implement Abstinence, Be Faithful, Use Condoms (ABC) programs had caused major confusion and challenges for U.S. government staff and partners implementing programs in PEPFAR countries.

A lack of clarity about what is permitted in regard to "C" (condom activities) had created a culture of fear amongst PEPFAR implementing partners who are concerned about "crossing the line between providing information about condoms and promoting or marketing condoms." One PEPFAR partner NGO said that "although the organisation views condom demonstrations as appropriate in some settings it believes that condom demonstrations, even to adults, are prohibited under PEPFAR."

Seventeen of the 20 PEPFAR country teams interviewed reported that the earmark "presents challenges to their ability to respond to local epidemiology and cultural and social norms."

Despite the fact that OGAC's guidance on ABC programs requires the programs be integrated, "about half of the 15 focus country teams reported that meeting the abstinence-until-marriage earmark undermines their ability to

integrate ABC programs as required." Country teams went even further to say that segregating AB from other prevention funding compromises prevention programs for at-risk groups that need comprehensive messages.

In June 2006 the Protection Against Transmission of HIV for Women and Youth Act of 2006 (PATHWAY), a bill that would remove the abstinence-only-until-marriage funding earmark from PEPFAR, was sponsored by Republican and Democrat members of the House of Representatives. It required "the President and the Office of the Global AIDS Coordinator to establish a comprehensive and integrated HIV prevention strategy to address the vulnerabilities of women and girls in countries for which the United States provides assistance to combat HIV/AIDS, and for other purposes."

References

Bearman, P und Brückner, H. After the promise: the STD consequences of adolescent virginity pledges. Journal of Adolescent Health, 36.4:271-278. 2005.

Bessinger Ret al. Sexual Behavior, HIV, and Fertility Trends. A Comparative Analysis of Six Countries. Phase I of the ABC Study. Washington, DC: U.S. Agency for International Development, Measure Evaluation, 2003.

Bogart LM et al. Patterns and Correlates of Deliberate Abstinence Among Men and Women with HIV/AIDS. AM J Publ Health 96(6):1078-1984. 2006.

Chinouya, M. & Davidson, O. The Padare Project: Assessing health-related knowledge, attitudes and behaviours of HIV-positive Africans accessing services in north central London. African HIV Policy Network, February 2003.

Government Accountability Office. *Spending Requirement Presents Challenges for Allocating Prevention Funding Under the President's Emergency Plan for AIDS Relief. GAO report, April 2006. Can be downloaded from: http://democrats.reform.house.gov/Documents/20060404121414-18003.pdf*

Goodson P et al. Abstinence education evaluation phase 5: technical report. Department of health and kinesiology, Texas A&M University pp 170-172. College Station, Texas, 2004.

Haddock, Vicki. Key to Sex Education: discipline or knowledge - advocating abstinence and safe sex may both cut pregnancies. San Francisco Chronicle, May 22 2005.

Hickson F et al. Out and About: Findings from the United Kingdom Gay Men's Sex Survey 2002. Sigma Research, 2003.

Hogle J. What Happened in Uganda? Declining HIV Prevalence, Behavior Change, and the National Response, USAID, 2002.

Human Rights Watch. The Less They Know, the Better: Abstinence-Only HIV/AIDS Programs in Uganda. Human Rights Watch. See http://hrw.org/reports/2005/uganda0305/index.htm.%20March%202005.

Kirby D. Emerging Answers: Research Findings on Programs to Reduce Teen Pregnancy. Washington D.C.: The National Campaign to Prevent Teen Pregnancy, 2001.

Lerner P. Can Abstinence Work? An Analysis of the Best Friends Program. Adolescent and Family Health, 3(4):185-192. 2004.

Mohn J et al. An Analysis of the Causes of the Decline in Non-marital Birth and Pregnancy Rates for Teens from 1991 to 1995. Adolescent and Family Health, 3(1):39-47. 2003.

Pardue Melissa G. et al. Government Spends $12 on Safe Sex and Contraceptives for Every $1 Spent on Abstinence. Heritage Foundation backgrounder #718. See http://www.heritage.org/Research/Family/bg1718.cfm. 2004.

Rector Robert E. The effectiveness of abstinence education programs in reducing sexual activity among youth. Heritage Foundation backgrounder #1533. See http://www.heritage.org/Research/Family/BG1533.cfm.%202002.

Santelli JS et al. Can Changes in Sexual Behaviors Among High School Students Explain the Decline in Teen Pregnancy Rates in the 1990s? Journal of Adolescent Health, 35(2):80-90. 2004.

UNAIDS. AIDS Epidemic Update. See http://www.unaids.org/html/pub/gcwa/jc986-epiextract_en_pdf.pdf. , December 2004.

Wakabi W. Condoms still contentious in Uganda's struggle over AIDS. The Lancet 367 (9520): 1387-1388. 2006.

Wawer MJ et al. Declines in HIV Prevalence in Uganda: Not as Simple as ABC. 12th Conference on Retroviruses and Opportunistic Infections, Boston, 2005. Abstract LB27.

Weinhardt L et al. HIV Transmission Risk Behavior among Men and Women Living with HIV in 4 Cities in the United States. *JAIDS* 36(5), 1057-1066. 2004.

B is for being faithful and behaviour change

B, which stands in the original 'ABC' model for 'Be faithful', but also involves partner reduction as well as strict monogamy, has been called "The neglected middle child of 'ABC' (Shelton, 2004). It is difficult to gather evidence on whether HIV prevention programmes have influenced target populations in the direction of monogamy and reduction of the number of sexual partners, and there has been remarkably little research into, or co-ordinated campaigns promoting, partner reduction as an end in itself.

This is to be regretted, because the rate of spread of HIV in a population is more sensitively dependent on the rate of partner

monogamous. An example of the traps the faithful partner of an unfaithful one can fall into is illustrated by an April 2005 study (Thorburn, 2005) which found that among Afro-American heterosexual men and women, lower levels of condom use and contraception were found among people who agreed with the statement 'known partners are safe partners' than among ones who agreed that 'trusted partners are safe partners'.

In the developed world, far from the number of partners being reduced amongst the general population, the trend in the 1990s was the opposite way. For instance, in the UK, comparing the 1990 and 2000 National Surveys of Sexual Attitudes and

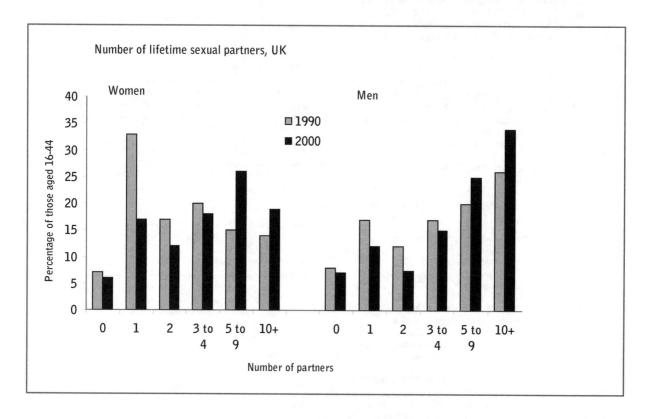

change, whether relationships are concurrent and consecutive, and whether partners are drawn from the local village or the global community, than on any other variable. The spread of HIV is crucially dependent on the establishment of sexual 'networks': remove a few links from those networks and the chain of infection can no longer be maintained. One paper (Garnett, 1998) put it this way:

"Heterogeneity in sexual behaviour is vital to generate a high sexual activity 'core group' within which HIV spreads rapidly. How far out of this core group the virus will spread depends on the patterns of mixing within populations."

Another important aspect of reducing the rate of partner change is that it reduces the number of times people are likely to come across partners in early HIV infection. One paper (Pilcher, 2004) calculated that, because people in acute HIV infection have much higher viral loads, up to a quarter of all HIV infections are spread by people within two months of themselves being infected, and the proportion could be even higher if concurrent STIs are taken into consideration.

One problem with research into monogamy and reduction in the number of sexual partners is that it takes two people to be

Lifestyles (NATSAL), the average number of lifetime sexual partners increased from 8.6 to 12.7 in men and from 3.7 to 6.5 in women, with a particularly sharp increase in the proportion of women reporting more than five lifetime partners, and an equally sharp decrease in the number reporting that they had only had one (see chart above).

In the developed world, several factors work against reductions in the number of partners and an increase in 'faithfulness'. An increasing sexualisation of 'pop culture' has gone hand in hand with increasing opportunities to access non-marital sex, via channels like the internet. Increasing numbers of people saying that they had had same-sex partnerships (both men and women) attest to this too.

The early 1990s may also have been an exceptional period with historically low points of sexual risk behaviour - as the data on sexually transmitted infections suggest - in that they coincided with the peak of public concerns about what was then an untreatable AIDS epidemic.

However it is probably true to say that monogamy or partner reduction, in itself (as opposed to abstinence till marriage and an assumption that marriage subsequently implies monogamy) has not been a target of HIV prevention campaigns in the developed world.

One of the few places where a reduction in the number of partners can be teased out as a contributor to lower HIV incidence and prevalence is, once again, in Uganda. That HIV prevalence has fallen no one disputes (except in the war-torn north of the country). But the evidence as to the contribution of partner reduction and increased monogamy to the decline in the figures is still indirect.

According to the USAID report cited above: "In the mid 1990s, two large randomised trials at Rakai and Masaka in Uganda attempted to look at the impact of STI treatment on reducing HIV prevalence. Although both interventions reduced the rates of some STIs, there was no significant reduction in HIV incidence."

"According to an expert panel at the 2002 World AIDS Conference in Barcelona, the main reason for the lack of effect on HIV from STI treatment was the large decrease in risky sex/multiple partner trends that had occurred in Uganda by the time the STI trials began. Most HIV transmission therefore now occurs within monogamous regular partnerships, where one partner has undiagnosed HIV, but where bacterial STIs tend to be rare."

Certainly a considerable reduction in the amount of 'casual sex' among the population had occurred by 1995, with 50-70% declines in the number of people reporting it (see top chart) and Uganda was the only country in the area to report such declines around that time (see chart below).

This decline appears to be evidence that it was not merely the ending of war and the restoring of civil order on Museveni's accession in 1986, which would involve men returning from the army and militias to their families, which created this change in behaviour patterns.

According to Stoneburner and colleagues (2000), "Ugandans are relatively more likely to receive AIDS information through friendship and other personal networks than through mass media or other sources, and are significantly more likely to know of a friend or relative with AIDS. Social communication elements, as suggested by these kinds of indicators, may be necessary to bridge the motivational gap between AIDS prevention activities and behavior change sufficient to affect HIV incidence."

In other words, Stoneburner is arguing that the social diffusion model (see *HIV Prevention: Which Methods Work?*) in which there is (a) a wide personal acquaintance

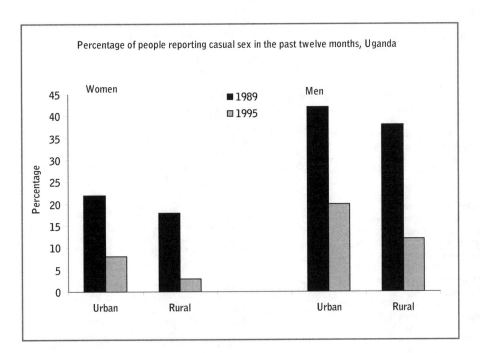

Percentage of people reporting casual sex in the past twelve months, Uganda

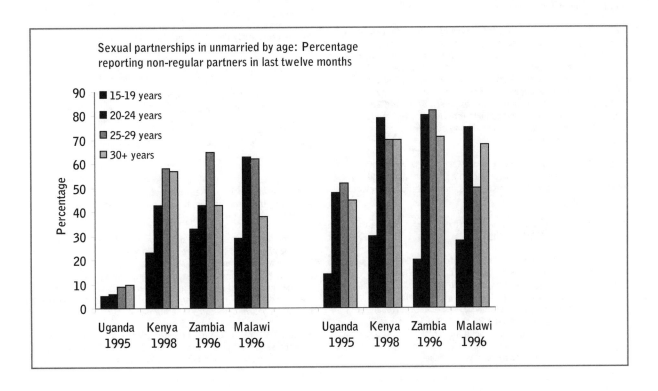

Sexual partnerships in unmarried by age: Percentage reporting non-regular partners in last twelve months

with HIV/AIDS in the population and (b) the encouragement and willingness to speak about it and pass knowledge on in informal social networks is the method that has worked to influence behaviour change, almost uniquely so far for an African country, in Uganda. The first is the inevitable consequence of a developing untreated epidemic: the second, however, can be influenced by political leadership and widespread awareness-raising work. Such work was, supporters say, initiated by Museveni when he started his AIDS awareness campaign in 1986, which included his famous 'Zero Grazing' policy, which urged monogamy on all Ugandans.

However there is recent evidence that this shift in behaviour in Uganda may have essentially happened in the decade from 1985 to 1995, but that in the last 10 years a more 'westernised' pattern of behaviour involving the resurgence of extra-marital sex, but an increased use of condoms, may be becoming more common.

In the Wawer study cited above (Wawer, 2005), which looked at behaviour change in the Rakai district from 1993 to 2004, the main driver of reduced HIV prevalence was found to be attrition of the HIV-positive population due to AIDS deaths, with a smaller contribution from increased condom use. During the study period, HIV prevalence had decreased from 17.5 to 11%, but the annual incidence of HIV had *not* declined, and may have even slightly increase, from 1.3 to 1.7% a year.

During the decade the age of sexual debut got younger again; 50% of 19 year old men had had sex in 2004 compared with 40% in 1994. The proportion of men reporting two or more sexual partners had gone up from 20 to 27%, and among who tested HIV-positive in the study from 40 to 68%. However condom used had doubled during the same time, from 19 to 38%, a high figure for Africa.

Is there evidence of partner reduction in other countries? In Zambia, there was a dramatic fall in HIV prevalence in young pregnant women (15-19) between 1993 and 1998, where the proportion living with the virus halved, from 28.4% to 14.8%. A study (Fylkesnes, 2001) found "a dominant declining trend in HIV prevalence that corresponds to declines in incidence since the early 1990s attributable to behavioural changes," which predominantly means a decline in casual sex.

More recently steep, and apparently real, declines in HIV prevalence have been observed in Zimbabwe - in contrast to neighbouring Botswana, where prevalence remains high.

The study (Gregson) that found the declines pointed to the multifactorial nature of the apparent reasons for the decline:

"We report a decline in HIV prevalence in eastern Zimbabwe between 1998 and 2003 associated with sexual behavior change in four distinct socioeconomic strata. HIV prevalence fell most steeply at young ages-by 23 and 49%, respectively, among men aged 17 to 29 years and women aged 15 to 24 years-and in more educated groups. Sexually experienced men and women reported reductions in casual sex of 49 and 22%, respectively, whereas recent cohorts reported delayed sexual debut. Selective AIDS-induced mortality contributed to the decline in HIV prevalence."

At the 2006 PEPFAR Implementers' Meeting in Durban, Dr Owen Murungifrom Zimbabwe's Ministry of Health and Child Welfare teased out some of the reasons for the decline (Gregson and Murungi).

The research is also available in a UNAIDS report published in November 2005 (UNAIDS 2005).

According to Dr Murungi, after the dramatic decline in HIV prevalence during 2004 was registered in Zimbabwe, nearly everyone was shocked. "The big question to all of us was, is this real? What's happened?" he said. A review was therefore conducted to determine whether other available data corroborated the finding, and whether the cause for the decline was due to high mortality rates or an actual decrease in incidence. Then, if there was a decline in incidence, could it be explained by natural dynamics of the epidemic or by behaviour changes.

The Ministry pulled together data from 30 different sources, all of which seemed to agree that the fall in HIV prevalence was real. According to antenatal clinic (ANC) data, in the year 2000, the HIV prevalence in Zimbabwe was 32.1% and in the following two years it hovered around 30%. No data were available for 2003 but in 2004 the HIV prevalence had fallen to 23.8% and the test for the trend was statistically significant (p<0.001). This trend was corroborated by data from the ZVITAMBO study, which included pregnant and post-natal women from Harare followed over several years. In this study population the HIV prevalence actually peaked around 1996 (at over 36%) and had been falling ever since (to somewhere around 21% in the middle of 2004).

A study from Manicaland in eastern Zimbabwe also looked at men between the ages of 17 and 44 years old, where there was also a decrease in prevalence, from 19.5% to 18.2% (p=0.01), with declines in all age groups except men over 35. Very few of the younger men were infected, but in the years 1998-2000 close to 50% of the men between the ages of 30-34 were HIV-infected, falling to around 40% in the next survey.

The data that Dr Murungi presented painted a complex picture for the decline in prevalence.

A very large part of the reduction in HIV prevalence was actually due to the very high mortality rate for people with HIV in the country. In Manicaland, the death rates in men peaked in the year 2000 at around 31-32 deaths per 1000 person years falling to around 26 deaths per 1000 person years in 2002/3. In women, rural death rates peaked in 2001, at just below 25 deaths per 1000 person years, falling to around 23 deaths per 1000 person years, although in both cases the confidence intervals overlap.

However, by itself, the mortality rate could not effect a reduction in prevalence unless there had also been a reduction in incidence of HIV infection. At some point in the last few years, people with HIV must have begun dying at a higher rate than new people were becoming infected.

Over the years, a number of studies have looked at HIV incidence in Zimbabwe. In the first one, Mbizvo et al., in 1993, the incidence was around 5% in antenatal women. Around the year 2000, the ZVITAMBO study observed an incidence that was around 3.6%. Among men, a survey in male factory workers, that the Zimbabwe AIDS prevention survey (ZAPS) conducted in 1994, found the incidence to be about 3.5%. Seven years later (2001), a similar survey in male factory workers reported an incidence of less than 2%.

So the cross-study data do suggest a falling incidence - at least between 1993/4 and 2001. If the current incidence is roughly around 2%, at the current mortality rate, the prevalence would decrease substantially each year.

Reductions in HIV incidence could be the result of natural dynamics of the HIV epidemic. Over time, any epidemic is somewhat self limiting. Mortality plays more than one part in this, because it doesn't only decrease prevalence directly, it can decrease incidence as well, by decreasing the pool of infectious individuals who can spread the infection.

But it can be due to behaviour change too. Dr Murungi said that colleagues at Imperial College in London had run simulations suggesting that other factors besides natural dynamics were needed to explain the changes in incidence observed in Zimbabwe.

Over the last few years, there does appear to have been a clear and substantial fall in the percentage of young men who reported having had sex during the last 12 months with non-regular partners. In the Manicaland study, statistically significant changes in reported sexual behaviour were observed for both males and females in 1) the age of sexual debut, 2) new partners in the last year/month and 3) the number of current partners.

The UNAIDS report did not find statistically significant evidence of increase in the age of sexual debut. But it found substantial evidence of partner reduction, especially in men under 30, where the proportion of men saying they had had 'non-regular' sexual partners in the previous 12 months declined from 58% in 1999 to 21% in 2003. Among women of the same age the trend was less significant but the proportion reporting non-regular partners declined from 17% to 8% in the same period. Since men are much more likely to have casual and commercial sex anyway, a decline in the number of partners men have is likely to have a larger effect on HIV incidence than a decline in the number women have, as we are usually starting from a much higher baseline.

However differences between the indicators of "faithfulness" used in the different surveys looked at meant that it was not possible to find a single indicator for which data were available over a wide range of time points. The charts below show the estimates that could be obtained for having one or more non-regular partners in the past 12 months. The data suggest a reduction in non-regular partnerships in the past 12 months occurred between 1999 and 2003, particularly amongst men. However, some caution is warranted since the indicator had to be calculated by combining responses to a number of different questions in 2003 whereas it was asked directly in 1999 and 2001.

Proportions of respondents aged 15-29 years at interview reporting a non-regular sexual partner in past twelve months:

	Men	Women
DHS data, 1999	≈ 58%	≈ 17%
PSI data, 2001	≈ 33%	≈ 18%
PSI data, 2003	≈ 21%	≈ 8%

Reported condom use with non-regular partners had also increased in the last five years. Dr Murungi noted that there has also been a steady increase in the number of condoms in circulation, particularly socially marketed condoms (rather than public sector condoms). A chart similar to the one above detailing increases in condom use in Zimbabwe is in **C is for condoms.**

What sort of prevention messages that were being spread in Zimbabwe in the late 90's and early 2000's - and who was doing it? It's interesting to compare and contrast what has happened in Zimbabwe with what is going on in Botswana, where despite massive efforts and funding spent on ABC-based prevention messages, the HIV prevalence in Botswana remains extremely high (38.5%).

Again the effects of such a high mortality rate in Zimbabwe need to be considered. History has shown that observing large numbers of people sick and dying of HIV can be a powerful motivator for changing behaviour. There could also be a host of other negative "enabling" factors that played a part in the reported behaviour change. Since the year 2000, Zimbabwe's economy has ground to a halt; the country suffered from floods, followed by severe drought and endemic food insecurity. As a result of Zimbabwe's economic contraction, many of the old hotspots for HIV transmission - near the factories and mines, at truck stops along the highway - could be dwindling or people no longer have a reason or the means to go there. Many of those with the means to get out and look for work have poured into neighbouring countries, including Botswana, and South Africa. Hundreds of thousands of adults in their prime working years (who may represent a substantial proportion of the sexually active and possibly HIV-infected population) have simply left the country. And yet, so far, no one has addressed what impact emigration might have had on Zimbabwe's HIV prevalence and incidence - and what might happen should they all return home for treatment (see below) which is increasingly available.

Dr Murungi stressed that Zimbabwe still has a long way to go "We acknowledge the fact that the prevalence rates are still very high in Zimbabwe. We still have a lot to do. 20% is still very, very high."

In Ethiopia (Mekonnen, 2003), a country with a more recent HIV crisis, the proportion of men who reported casual sex at two centres fell in just two years (1997 to 1999) from 17.5 to 3.5%, and the proportion reporting visiting sex workers from 11.2 to just 0.75%.

In Cambodia (UNAIDS, 2002), HIV prevalence halved between 1997 and 2002, as did the proportion of men who reported visiting a sex worker over the year, while condom use, already high, increased less dramatically (see chart below).

There is one paradox that one needs to be aware of in encouraging monogamous behaviour. In certain HIV prevalence situations it can make no difference to HIV incidence at all. For instance, in Zimbabwe and South Africa steep declines in the incidence of bacterial STIs like syphilis and gonorrhoea have not been accompanied by declines in HIV. This fact was noticed by an unorthodox researcher, David Gisselquist, who used it as evidence for his theory that the majority of HIV in Africa is being spread by unsterilised medical needles (Gisselquist, 2003).

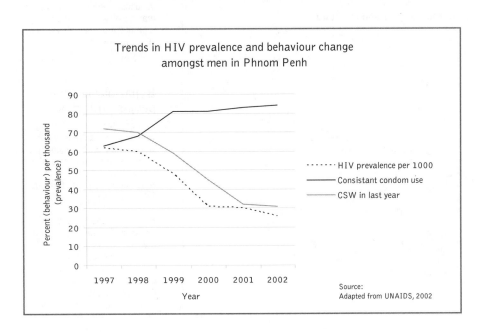

Trends in HIV prevalence and behaviour change amongst men in Phnom Penh

Percent (behaviour) per thousand (prevalence)

..... HIV prevalence per 1000
——— Consistant condom use
——— CSW in last year

Source:
Adapted from UNAIDS, 2002

But the real reason is probably to do with the fact that in these countries prevalence is so high that transmission within marriage or a monogamous relationship is now just as likely as it is during a casual encounter. A monogamous marriage only reduces HIV transmission risk if both partners going into it have the same HIV status, and in countries where HIV testing is the exception rather than the rule, encouraging monogamy may in certain circumstances have the effect of spreading HIV from a core group of sexually active men and their female partners into the female population at large.

What about vulnerable populations in the developed world? There is evidence from the early days of the epidemic(Low-Beer, 2003) that gay men rapidly adjusted their sexual behaviour as soon as the first reports of AIDS appeared. Rates of sexually transmitted diseases and HIV incidence started falling almost immediately, particularly among the more socially cohesive white gay community, though we do not know what proportion of these declines were due to condom adoption, having fewer partners, or abstinence from sex.

The comment of the authors of the paper from which the chart below comes comment that "These responses preceded and exceeded HIV prevention." However another way of looking at it, using a broader definition of prevention, is that they *were* the first examples of community-led HIV prevention. A chain of 'grapevine knowledge' spread by word of mouth through a closely-knit community is exactly the kind of response to AIDS President Museveni was trying to set up in Uganda.

In the post-HAART era, is a similar behaviour change in gay men possible? There is one intriguing piece of evidence that it might be. US researcher Thomas Dee (2005) used a mathematical model to relate changes in the rates of syphilis, gonorrhoea, TB and malaria in European countries to whether a country had legalised gay marriage or civil partnership.

Dee found a 24% reduction in syphilis incidence and a non-significant reduction in gonorrhoea compared with countries with no gay marriage legislation, and found that the reduction in syphilis started at the same time the marriage legislation was introduced. The rates of the non-sexually-transmitted diseases did not change at the same time: neither did HIV diagnoses, but being a non-acute condition, these are subject to a 'time lag'.

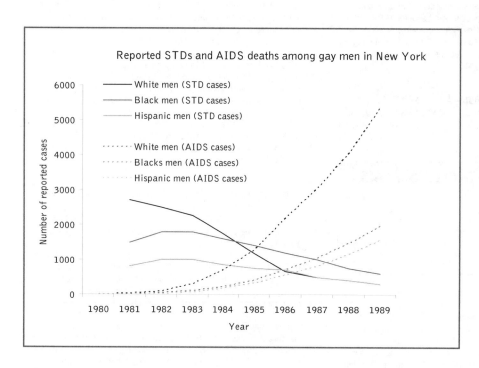

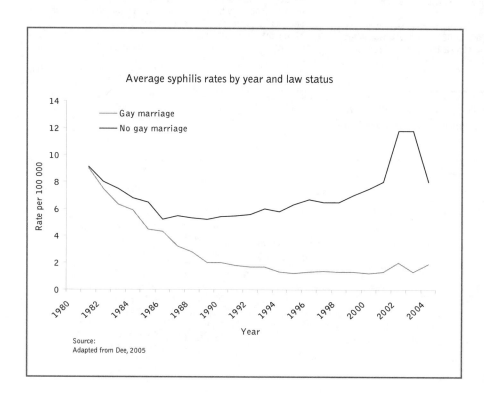

Source:
Adapted from Dee, 2005

This is obviously a highly indirect piece of evidence and cannot say directly whether gay marriage leads to fewer extra-marital partners. It also compares gay marriage with STI rates in the entire population, though in the case of syphilis, it was gay men during this era who were most affected. However Dee's analysis is conservative: he eliminated from his analysis every other possible variable such as improvements in other health and economic indicators which might also cause falls in STIs, and the difference in syphilis rates on the raw data alone is striking: the 'gay marriage' countries seem so far largely to have avoided the large increases in syphilis seen in countries like the UK.

If it really is true that, as Dee says "gay marriage will encourage [gay men] to form emotional and legal commitments.that will promote sexual fidelity and possibly reduce STI prevalence," then it again demonstrates that the activities which most successfully reduce HIV incidence and/or risk behaviour may be very far from ones that look like most people's idea of HIV prevention.

Behaviour change in people with HIV

In a country like Zimbabwe, where despite an increase in HIV testing, only a minority of people as yet know their HIV status, it is not possible to relate knowledge of status to behaviour change.

However in the developed world several surveys point to the fact that people with HIV, once diagnosed, substantially reduce their sexual risk behaviour. In the USA the CDC has estimated that people with HIV reduce the number of

HIV transmission risk incidents they take part in by 57% after diagnosis (Marks).

In Marks's 2006 study in *AIDS* (Marks) in was estimated that even if HIV-positive people did not reduce their average number of partners post-diagnosis, factors such as reduction in viral load due to HAART would reduce the proportion of HIV spread by people knowing their status such that only 46% of HIV transmissions would be spread by the 75% of people in the USA aware they had HIV, compared with 54% by the 25% of people unaware of their status. This means that a person with HIV who is unaware of their status would be over 3.5 times more likely to transmit HIV than a person aware of it.

However if HIV-positive people also reduced their number of partners generally, then this effect would be accentuated. For instance, if people with HIV reduced the number of HIV-negative partners they had unprotected sex with by 33% relative to the unaware group (or, to put it another way, if the unaware people had 50% more at-risk partners), then the 75% of people aware they had HIV would only be responsible for 37% of infections and the 25% unaware for 63% of them. This means that a person unaware of their status would be more than five times more likely to transmit HIV than a person aware of it.

A 33% reduction in partners was pretty much exactly what was observed in one study of how gay men's sexual behaviour changed after diagnosis (Gorbach).

Gorbach interviewed 113 HIV-positive gay men a month after diagnosis and then again three months afterwards. She found during that period that the average number of partners in the three months prior to interview had declined from 7.9 to 5.2 - a 34% decline. This was not generalised over the whole group, however. Nearly half (47%) of the men interviewed reported a decrease in the number of partners they had, a third reported an increase. However there was also a very significant shift among those who had unprotected sex to doing it with partners they knew had HIV - see **Disclosure, serosorting and negotiated safety** for details.

Refrences

Dee, Thomas. Forsaking All Others? The Effects of "Gay Marriage" on Risky Sex. National Bureau Of Economic Research working paper no. 11327. See http://www.nber.org/papers/w11327. 2005.

Fylkesnes K et al. Declining HIV prevalence and risk behaviours in Zambia: evidence from surveillance and population-based surveys. *AIDS* 15(7):907-16. 2001.

Garnett GP. The basic reproduction rate of infection and the course of HIV epidemics. *AIDS Patient Care STDs* 12: 435-49. 1998.

Gisselquist D et al. Let it be sexual: how health care transmission of AIDS in Africa was ignored. *Int J STD AIDS* 14(3):148-61. 2003.

Gorbach PM. Transmission behaviors of recently HIV-infected men who have sex with men. *JAIDS* 42(1):80-85. 2006.

Gregson S et al. HIV decline associated with behavior change in Eastern Zimbabwe. *Science.* 311(5761):664-6. 2006.

Gregson S and Murungi O. HIV decline accelerated by reductions in unprotected casual sex in Zimbabwe? Evidence from a comprehensive epidemiological review. The 2006 HIV/AIDS Implementers Meeting of the President's Emergency Plan for AIDS Relief, Durban, South Africa, Abstract 29.

House of Commons Select Committee on Health third report, 2002-3 session. See www.publications.parliament.uk/pa/cm200203/cmselect/cmhealth/69/6902.htm for details.

Low-Beer D, Stoneburner R. Behaviour and communication change in reducing HIV: is Uganda unique? *African Journal of AIDS Research* 2(1): 9-21. 2003.

Marks G et al. Estimating sexual transmission of HIV from persons aware and unaware that they are infected with the virus in the USA. *AIDS* 20(10):1447-1450. 2006.

Mekonnen Y et al. Evidence of changes in sexual behaviours among male factory workers in Ethiopia. *AIDS* 24;17(2):223-31. 2003.

Pilcher CD et al. Brief but efficient: acute HIV infection and the sexual transmission of HIV. J Infect Dis. 189(10):1785-92. 2004.

Shelton James D et al. Partner reduction is crucial for balanced "ABC" approach to HIV prevention. *British Medical Journal* 328:891-893. 2004.

Stoneburner R et al. "Enhancing HIV prevention in Africa: Investigating the role of social cohesion on knowledge diffusion and behavior change in Uganda." Paper presented at 13th International AIDS Conference, Durban, 2000. No abstract cited.

Thorburn S et al. HIV prevention heuristics and condom use among African-Americans at risk for HIV. AIDS Care 17(3):335-44. 2005.

UNAIDS 2002. Report on the global HIV/AIDS epidemic 2002. Geneva: WHO, 2002.

UNAIDS 2005. Evidence for HIV decline in Zimbabwe: a comprehensive review of the epidemiological data. ISBN 92 9 173461 6. Can be downloaded from http://data.unaids.org/publications/irc-pub06/zimbabwe_epi_report_nov05_en.pdf

Wawer MJ et al. Declines in HIV Prevalence in Uganda: not as simple as ABC. 12th Conference on Retroviruses and Opportunistic Infections, Abstract LB27. Boston, 2005.

C is for condoms

Efficacy and effectiveness

The crucial question to ask about condoms is not whether they work, but whether they get used.

This distinction is the difference between efficacy - whether an intervention works in ideal circumstances - and effectiveness - whether it reduces disease incidence.

Firstly, however, questions of efficacy have to be addressed, as in recent years condoms' ability to stop HIV has been brought into question by people opposed to their use on religious or moral grounds.

In one of the most highly-publicised statements (Bradshaw, 2003), in October 2003, the President of the Vatican's Pontifical Council for the Family, Cardinal Alfonso Lopez Trujillo, said: "The AIDS virus is roughly 450 times smaller than the spermatozoon. The spermatozoon can easily pass through the 'net' that is formed by the condom.

"These margins of uncertainty...should represent an obligation on the part of the health ministries and all these campaigns to act in the same way as they do with regard to cigarettes, which they state to be a danger."

These statements are quite simply untrue. When condoms are used consistently, their efficacy in preventing HIV and bacterial STIs is In the order of 85 to 90%.

The most rigorous review (Weller, 2002) of the evidence looked at 16 cross-sectional and 12 longitudinal studies and contrasted the HIV incidence rates between couples who said they 'always' used condoms and ones who said they 'never' did.

The more rigorous longitudinal studies followed condom user for an average of two years among serodiscordant couples and registered seroconversions among the negative partner. They were all among heterosexual couples (three of them people whose main HIV acquisition factor had been intravenous drug use).

The cross-sectional studies assessed HIV status among a high-risk group, and then asked them about their previous condom usage. Four of the cross-sectional studies were among heterosexuals, three of whom were also intravenous drug users. The other nine studies were of gay men. The cross-sectional studies will obviously tend to yield lower apparent efficacy rates, as HIV-positive people who report 'always' using condoms will tend to misreport or misremember their behaviour.

This yields the following efficacy rates for condoms, when the seroconversion rate among 'always used' is calculated as a proportion of the 'never used' rate:

- Gay men, retrospective: 63.6%

- Female to male, retrospective: 36%

- Female to male, longitudinal: 80.5%

- Male to female, longitudinal: 92.8%

- Hetero, direction not stated, longitudinal: 90.8%

This allowed the researchers to calculate a true **efficacy** rate from the longitudinal studies of **86.6%,** on the assumption that the 'always' users did use condoms consistently and correctly, and any seroconversions were due to the inevitable accidents such as slippage and splitting.

The **effectiveness** rate in gay men - that is, the degree to which condom use at the time of the surveys was reducing HIV incidence - can also be approximated. It can be seen that the seroconversion rate between 'sometimes' and 'never' users is very similar. If we assume that the 'always' condom users were gay men who *tried* always to use condoms, and the 'sometimes' gay men were so inconsistent as to make little difference to their HIV seroconversion risk, then this yields an **effectiveness** rate - among the gay community at the time of the surveys, namely from 1986 to 1992 - of around **60%.**

That is, at this early point in the history of the epidemic, condom use as a strategy might have been stopping a maximum of six out of 10 potential infections. This is a maximum, because some of those infections might have been stopped by men who use condoms also using other strategies like cutting down on the number of partners, having less anal sex, and so on.

Another study (Winer 2006) has found that condoms offer significant protection against a much more contagious virus than HIV, namely the genital wart- and cervical/anal cancer-causing human papilloma virus (HPV). This is a significant finding because it is a refutation of claims by anti-condom, pro-abstinence campaigners in the USA that condoms did not protect against this kind of infection, and previous studies had appeared to back this claim up (Winer 2003, Ho).

Winer and colleagues found that consistent use of male condoms effectively reduced the risk of male-to-female genital human papillomavirus (HPV) transmission. In contrast to the earlier studies, this was a longitudinal study designed specifically to look at the temporal relationship between condom use and HPV infection.

The authors followed a cohort of female undergraduates ranging in age from 18-22 years, who had either never had vaginal intercourse prior to enrolment or who had just started on their first (heterosexual) relationship.

A total of 126 incident HPV infections were identified in 40 of the 82 women eligible for analysis. The incidence of genital HPV when condoms were used 100% of the time was 37.8 per 100 patient-years, compared with 89.3 per 100 patient-years at risk when condoms were used less than 5% of the time.

Condom usage rates

The degree to which people have taken up the use of condoms during the HIV epidemic varies hugely according to a whole number of different factors. These include the following

- The degree to which people know that an activity carries an HIV transmission risk

- Whether they think their partner is likely to have HIV

- Whether they are having causal or commercial sex or are in a steady relationship

- Whether they are HIV-positive themselves

- Whether risky sex is linked to using alcohol or drugs, which impair people's ability to make healthy decisions

- Whether their behaviour is influenced by chronic mental health problems such as depression, low self-esteem or learned behaviour due to sexual abuse

- Whether they are in a position to insist on the use of condoms

The main factors that influence condom use (other than drugs and mental health) can be illustrated by taking, more or less at random, a selection of condom usage figures from different population groups and exploring the differences between them.

said they had anal sex, an even higher proportion did not use condoms - some 65%.

This prides an interesting insight into the under-researched world of heterosexual anal sex and condom use. Firstly, the figure for vaginal sex is quite close to the figures for UK gay men when it comes to consistent condom use for sexual intercourse. Secondly, it shows that a minority sexual behaviour which is in fact a higher HIV transmission risk can result in lower condom usage if HIV prevention messages do not acknowledge that risk. A similar survey from South Africa also found that among the minority of heterosexuals who had anal sex, condom use was lower (though of course, this may be because the kind of people who have anal sex may also be the kind of people who don't like condoms).

Thirdly, it also sheds light on how cautious one needs to be in interpreting condom usage results. The only other survey ever done among US adults in the general population (Erickson, 1995) found similar rates for anal intercourse but found that among those who has anal sex, only 40% did not use condoms.

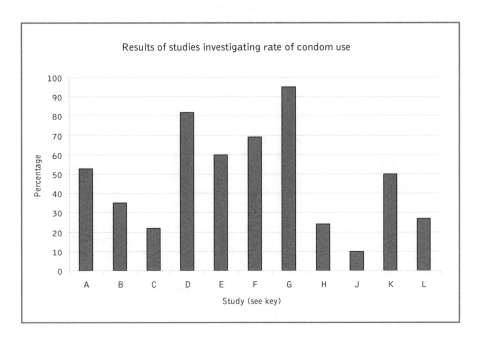

Results of studies investigating rate of condom use

KEY

A - US Heterosexuals under 35 - vaginal sex - 'always or often' (American Social Health Association, 2004)

B - US Heterosexuals under 35 - new partners - anal sex - 'always or often'(ibid)

C - San Francisco gay couples, seroconcordant (both HIV-negative) (Guzman, 2005)

D - US gay youth, serodiscordant (HIV+/HIV-)(Lightfoot, 2005)

E - UK gay men's sex survey 2003 - 'no unprotected anal sex' (Hickson, 2003)

F - UK gay mens's sex survey 2003 - 'probably not had serodiscordant unprotected anal sex'(ibid.)

G - Thai sex workers and clients (Mechai, 2004)

H - Thai teenage boys (Agence-France Presse, 2003)

J - Men, Rakai, Uganda - 1994 - wives and girlfriends (Najjumba, 2003)

K - Men, Rakai, Uganda - 2004 - wives and girlfriends (ibid)

L - Women, Uganda - 'ever used'(ibid)

Condom use is usually lower in long-term relationships

The next two columns (C and D) contrast condom use between two different populations of gay men. The first were HIV-negative men in long-term relationships living in San Francisco. Among them condom use was the exception not the rule, with only just over one in five couples always using them. Fifty per cent of couples 'allowed' sex outside the relationship, and the main purpose of the study was to see how couples negotiated rules around the safety 'extra-marital' sex and to what degree these rules were observed or broken.

In contrast, the second group of gay men - in column D - were gay youth (aged 15-25) living with HIV recruited in four US cities, who in the main did not have steady partners. The high condom use figure (82%) was in fact even higher when it came to sex that carried a risk of HIV transmission: with partners whose HIV status was negative or unknown, condom use was 93%.

Unprotected sex is not necessarily unsafe sex

The next two columns (E and F) come from the same data set, the UK Gay Men's Sex Survey of 2003. They represent (E) the proportion of gay and bisexual men who said they had not had unprotected anal intercourse with anyone over the last year (60.2%) and (F) the proportion who said they had 'probably or definitely' not had unprotected sex with someone of a different HIV status (69.3%).

A risk has to be seen as a risk

The first two columns (A and B) relate to a 2004 telephone survey of heterosexuals under 35 conducted by the US Association for Social Health. It found that 47% of respondents 'sometimes or never' used condoms for vaginal sex. It also found that of the approximately seven per cent of heterosexuals that

The nine per cent difference between these two figures represents people who were pretty sure they were having unprotected sex with people whose HIV status was the same as theirs, and were therefore not at risk of being infected or infecting someone with HIV (though they were at risk of other STIs). It might be asked how these men knew their partners' HIV status and whether many in that nine per cent were people making wrong assumptions about their partners' HIV status.

But this nine per cent also excludes the 24% or respondents who were less certain about whether they'd had unprotected sex with a person of differing HIV status. Only 10.3% of the men in the survey were fairly sure that had had serodiscordant unprotected sex, and thus represent the highest population at highest risk of HIV acquisition or transmission.

In recent years the emphasis on condom use has tended to change from a blanket insistence on 100 per cent condom use to a much more nuanced recognition that decisions as to whether or not to use condoms are often arrived at through a complex series of assumptions, calculations and conversations between people. This is discussed in the next section on disclosure, serosorting and negotiated safety.

However this is not an uncontroversial shift in emphasis. In the same way as opponents of condom distribution say that providing condoms only encourages more sex, some prevention experts worry that supporting harm-reduction strategies such as trying to only have sex with people of the same HIV status ('serosorting') spreads confusing messages and encourages people to rationalise about having unsafe sex. More on this below.

Risk populations change - prevention targets must, too

The next two columns (G and H) contrast condom use in Thai men visiting sex workers, which was as near to 100% as any use of condoms is likely to get, and the proportion of teenage boys in one province who used condoms during sex with girlfriends.

As cited already, the "100 per cent condom campaign" in 1990-92 in Thailand is often seen as one of the most successful HIV prevention programmes of all time. It slashed HIV incidence among young men from 2.5% a year to 0.5%, reduced prevalence among army recruits from 10% to 2.5%, and it is estimated that HIV prevalence in Thailand today is still - a decade after the campaign ended - 50% lower than it would have been if it had not happened.

Its success was partly due to good timing and an accurate perception that a widespread culture of commercial sex was responsible for the rapid growth of HIV at the time. It was also partly due to it being an easily enforceable target. The campaign put pressure on brothel owners to enforce 100% condom use in their establishments and ensured that ones not conforming to this rule were closed by the police.

Since then, however, the continued impact of tourism and the global media, and the growing affluence of Thailand, has led to a change in sexual behaviour. A pattern whereby men would marry young but also have extramarital commercial sex has given way to a more 'westernised' pattern of teenagers having pre-marital sexual relationships. The report that only 25% of Thai teenagers were using condoms led to a campaign to have condom machines placed in colleges and a counter-campaign resisting this - with both demands coming from students themselves. As sexual and drug-using cultures change, HIV prevention has to fight the same battle many times again on behalf of new populations.

Men can change...

That populations can adapt their safer-sex behaviour to continue to protect themselves when their habits change is evidenced by

the Wawer study quoted above (Wawer, 2005). In her study of adults in Rakai, Uganda Wawer found that although HIV prevalence had declined by 75% between 1993 and 2004, HIV incidence had not, and was running at a steady annual seroconversion rate of 1.5% or so. The decline in the number of people living with HIV in the area was almost entirely due to the thinning of the population by AIDS.

She found evidence that people were actually having more extramarital sex and having it younger in 2004 than in 1993, and that the behavioural changes of the early 1990s were being reversed. For instance, the proportion of 15- to 19-year-olds who were sexually active had gone up from 40 to 50%, and the number of adult men reporting two or more partners a year had increased from 20 to 27%.

What was keeping the incidence rate steady in the face of this 'liberalising' of sexual behaviour was an increased level of condom use. Condom use among men in general with casual partners had increased from 10% in 1993 to 50% in 2004 - a figure described by Wawer as 'incredibly high by African standards' (see columns J and K above).

This figure of 50% was skewed by a 95% rate of condom use in the few per cent of men who admitted having commercial sex. But even in male teenagers, who by and large did not use sex workers, it had gone up from 19 to 38%.

Other recent surveys have reported figures of about 50% of men in South Africa (Peltzer, 2000) and Uganda (Najjumba, 2003) saying they had 'ever' used condoms, with considerably higher usage in sex perceived to be risky.

Increased condom use is also apparently partly responsible for what appears to be a genuine, and marked, decrease in HIV prevalence in Zimbabwe in the last five years (UNAIDS 2005). A full investigation of the many possible factors behind the fall in Zimbabwean HIV prevalence is under **B is for Being Faithful.**

One of the factors, however, appeared to be increased condom use within casual sex. In 1999, men's condom use with non-regular partners was already high at about 75%, but by 2004 this had increased to 85%. Among women there was a much bigger rise: from around 50% in 1999 to at least 75% in 2004. Given that this is casual and non-regular relationships we are talking about, this may (hopefully) reflect and increasing ability of women to ask, or men to permit, the use of condoms within commercial and transactional sexual situations.

...but women can't always make them

The final column (K) represents the figure from the same Ugandan survey by Najjumba which reported 50% condom use among men. Surveys consistently show women reporting lower condom use than men. In this survey 51% of men and 36% of women who perceived themselves to be 'at high risk' or HIV said they had ever used a condom in sex. In those who saw themselves as low risk the figures were 36 and 11% respectively.

Are men lying about how often they use condoms? Or women forgetting about them? The answer is that men are using condoms in high-risk sexual situation such as in sex with sex workers and casual sex with men or women, but not using them with wives and regular partners. Since women in general have fewer partners and men, the average woman is less likely to encounter a man who wants to use a condom during sex.

Rates of condom use among married couples in Africa in fact vary from around 16% for regular or occasional use (in one study from KwaZulu Natal(Maharaj, 2005) to the Wawer study above, in which women reported using condoms 28% of the time with casual partners but only one per cent of the time with their husbands.

Similar results have been reported from other parts of the world. In a pioneering study of sexual risk among men who have sex with men in Andhra Pradesh, India, (Dandona, 2005) 42% of the MSM were married, half had had sex with a woman as well as a man in the last three months, but only 16% had used a condom in sex with a woman.

However even in India there is evidence that increased condom use in crucial populations may be having a positive impact on HIV transmission. A survey of four high-prevalence Indian states (Kumar) examined HIV prevalence among 294,000 women aged 15 to 34 attending antenatal clinics in four states in southern India and 14 states in the north, as well as prevalence among 59,000 men aged 15 to 34 attending clinics for sexually transmitted infections in the same regions.

The researchers found that among women ages 15 to 24 attending prenatal clinics in the southern states of Tamil Nadu, Andhra Pradesh, Maharashtra and Karanataka, HIV prevalence decreased from 1.7% in 2001 to 1.1% in 2004, a relative decline of 35%. Among men aged 20 to 29 attending STI clinics, the researchers recorded a 36% relative decline in HIV prevalence over the same time period.

The study found no significant decrease in HIV prevalence among women ages 25 to 34 or among men and women in the northern states, where the epidemic is driven by injection drug use. The researchers said the study's findings might signify a decrease in the number of new infections acquired through heterosexual contact in India, and they credited the decline among young people to an increase in condom use among commercial sex workers and their clients in the southern part of the country.

The researchers comment:

What could account for the reduction of HIV-1 prevalence in the South? Mathematical models of sex-work-based networks find that the prevalence is very sensitive to increases in abstinence from sex work or in condom use with sex work. Use of condoms between married couples is probably not relevant to the reductions seen in the south; it is well below 3% in the south and has changed little from 1992 to 1999. HIV-1 trends in young men attending STI clinics provide an imperfect snapshot of high-risk men, including those who have recently visited sex workers.

The fall in the south could be explained by increased condom use or increased abstinence, and is probably not due to STI antibiotic treatment, since reductions also occurred in men with ulcerative, and presumably viral, STIs.

In 2004, about 70-80% of female sex workers in Maharashtra and Tamil Nadu reported condom use with their last client, with lower percentages for all recent partners, and lower percentages still with regular non-paying partners. Data for male abstinence from sex workers are not well reported: indirect evidence from surveys of female sex workers in Tamil Nadu in 1996-2004 has shown increases in condom use, but no change in the number of clients per day (see AIDS Prevention and Control Project).

Why don't men use condoms, and why don't women make them?

Although this question is framed in a heterosexist way, the same question can just as well apply to gay men too, although there is more of a (possibly incorrect) assumption that in gay male relationships sexual roles are more fluid and the power to enforce condom use is more equally shared between the two partners.

However, we find that in gay men the same pattern applies as among heterosexuals: men in steady relationships, whether of the same HIV status or not, are far less likely to use condoms. This gives us a clue as to the primary psychological driver behind unsafe sex and the decision to use, or not to use, condoms.

Take two examples. A study from the Netherlands(Davidovich, 2000) found that 55% of gay men had unprotected sex with their regular partner but only 20% had it with casual partners.

A London study(Elford, 2001) a year later stratified the same results by HIV status of participants. It found that in HIV-negative men, 28.5% had unprotected sex within relationships but only five per cent with casual partners. HIV-positive men, by contrast, were just as likely to have unprotected sex with regular and casual partners (22.2 vs. 20.6%). The researchers argued that HIV-negative men cannot be sure of the HIV status of partners without mutual testing HIV-positive men, on the other hand, can find out their partners' HIV status by the simple act of mutual disclosure. However it was not ascertained whether disclosure was what was driving up higher rates of casual unprotected sex in positive men.

We will look at evidence like this in the next section to understand how gay men are using disclosure to minimise HIV transmission risk. For the time being we are looking at the psychology of what condoms symbolise and why they tend not to get used in primary relationships.

An interesting insight into this was provided by a study from New York (Simoni, 2000) which examined whether HIV-positive women had safer sex and if so, whether they did so more often in primary relationships. The authors hypothesised that women would be more likely to maintain condom use in steady relationships in order to protect partners.

They found the opposite to be the case. Forty-six per cent of women maintained condom use in all sex (in this study oral sex without a condom was counted as 'unprotected'). But of the remainder, 61% had had at least one episode of unprotected sex in the past 90 days with a steady partner compared with 16% who had done it with a casual partner. Women in steady relationships were three times more likely to have unprotected sex with a steady than with a casual partner.

Was this because steady partners were more likely to be known to be HIV-positive themselves? No, because unprotected sex was just as common with HIV-negative male partners as HIV-positive ones.

On further investigation, condom use had a bipolar distribution. Condom use was significantly higher in women who had casual partners - but also within the *most* committed relationships, when these were defined by length (over one year), by being within a legalised marriage, or by partners living together. Condom use was a lot lower with primary partners who were new or who did not live with the women.

The researchers theorised: "Women in our study who were married and in the longest, most supportive relationships may have possessed the power to broach or insist upon consistent condom use."

Conversely, they add: "Perhaps in [more recently established] steady partnerships, condom use implies, not primarily protection, but mistrust, suspicion, lack of emotional and physical intimacy, or denial of potential motherhood."

Ugandan President Yoweri Museveni used almost the same words when he address the Bangkok World AIDS Conference in 2004: "The best way to fight AIDS is with relationships based on love and trust, instead of institutionalised mistrust, which is what the condom is all about."

Museveni's words were attacked at the time by activists such as fellow-speaker Mabel van Oranje of the Open Society Foundation, who commented that his opinion "seems slightly drawn by ideology rather than an assessment of needs on the ground."

But he may have been saying something more perceptive about human psychology as the reason why condoms can only ever form part, rather than the whole, of HIV prevention.

A more recent study among gay men in the UK provides similar insights. The INSIGHT study (Elam) is the name of the study conducted by the UK's Health Protection Agency (HPA), which aims to tease out differences in the behaviour and motivations of gay men who catch HIV and ones who stay negative.

The HPA's Dr Gillian Elam took a group of 75 gay men who had tested positive within two years of a previous negative test and compared them with 159 men whose most recent test was negative, again within two years of their previous negative one.

Unsurprisingly, she found that the HIV-positive ones had taken more sexual risks.

Eight out of ten of the positive men had had unprotected sex as the passive partner since their last test, and seven out of ten as the active partner: just under half of the HIV-negative men had done the same.

But it was the interviews Elam did with a subset of men about their reasons for having unsafe sex that were really revealing. They showed that gay men have a multiplicity of reasons for taking sexual risks, so that no one prevention strategy will fit all.

Elam divided gay men into various groups:

Men who had caught HIV within a steady partnership, of whom:

- Some caught HIV through being mistaken about their partner's or each other's serostatus

- Some caught HIV through being in a serodiscordant relationship and taking a positive decision to risk unsafe sex

- Some caught HIV when one partner seroconverted during the relationship and the couple was faced with the decision of whether to start using condoms

Men who had caught HIV in casual sexual situation, of whom:

- Some took a positive decision to have and even seek out unprotected sex

- Some ended up having unprotected sex even tough they had tried not to and it was contrary to their health beliefs

First there were men who'd caught HIV while in a steady relationship. A common theme was that condoms were seen as a barrier to intimacy, love and trust. Men made comments such as: "We've got this thing in the way", "It makes it feel like a process", "it takes away a lot of the emotion".

There were steady partners who thought each other was negative. Here the risk was where men thought their partner was monogamous and he wasn't, or where they decided to drop condoms too soon in a relationship to really establish trust. A common theme was that people didn't think they or their partner was the 'type' to get HIV. One said: "It shouldn't have really been me...my friends have lots of sexual partners and take drugs . I'm the most reserved out of the people I know."

There were couples where one knew he was positive from the start, and the negative partner decided to risk unsafe sex. Here having unprotected sex was a conscious trade-off between the risk of HIV and the need for intimacy. People also rationalised that repeated negative test results meant they were 'immune'.

Then there were couples where one partner seroconverted during the relationship. One common finding here was that the other partner suddenly felt 'distant' from them. One said: "There was no 'fuck me without a condom, I want to be positive sort of thing'. It is the intimacy . We had that intimacy and then it was just suddenly taken away."

Then there were people who caught HIV through casual sex. Elam divided these into men who had intentionally not used condoms and ones where they felt they should have done, but had allowed unprotected sex to happen without one in the heat of the moment.

Intentional non-users were seeking positive things through not using condoms: they saw it as a signal of love and trust, at least potentially. Elam commented that the need for 'love and trust' and for 'submission, sleaze and adventures' often went together. One said: "There's sort of hope for something," meaning that having 'bareback' sex was a sort of signal that he was emotionally available. Men rationalised their way into unsafe sex. Younger men told themselves that if a partner was well-groomed and 'fit', he would not have HIV. Older men told themselves that HIV would not have such a negative impact because HIV would have no worse an impact than other facets of ageing.

Then there were the 'accidental' non-condom-users. There were men who normally tried to use condoms but who had accidents, not in the sense of condoms splitting, but in giving up their normal safer-sex behaviour in the heat of the moment. Some talked about wanting to please a particularly attractive or confident partner. This was the group who were most likely to talk about depression, drink and drugs as being factors in HIV infection. One said: "Depression really influenced my sexual behaviour. You go out, you want to be abused, almost. you might as well let anybody do what they want to do to you."

Elam said there were themes common to all. Many men talked of condoms reducing intimacy, about not being the 'sort' who caught HIV, and about negative test results giving a sense of false security. Many 'tops' thought they were at no risk, not lower risk. Above all was the sense that giving people more information about HIV risk was not the answer: Elam's interviewees had high levels of knowledge about HIV transmission.

If there was a common theme, it was that catching HIV often involves a conscious decision to trade safety for the possibility of love, approval and fun.

Has condom use declined in the developed world?

The decade during which HIV/AIDS was both widespread and untreatable in the developed world - roughly 1985 to 1995 - marked a historic low point in diagnoses of sexually transmitted diseases in countries like the USA and UK. See below, for instance, for gonorrhoea diagnoses, which peaked briefly after world war two and then for a prolonged period from 1970-85. (see chart next page)

HIV incidence has also increased among risk groups. For instance, according to UNAIDS (UNAIDS, 2001), HIV incidence (new diagnoses) in gay men increased from 0.6% a year in the late 1990s in Vancouver to 3.7% a year in 2000; from 1.16% in 1996 in Madrid to 2.16% in 2000; and from 1.1% in 1997 in San Francisco to 1.7% in 2000. Increases were also reported in London

But was this due to decreased condom use? Among the UK population in general, the 1990 and 2000 National Surveys of Sexual Attitudes and Lifestyles (NATSAL)(Johnson, 2001) found that consistent condom use among the sexually active population as whole increased from 17 to 24% during the 1990s, even as the rate of STIs also increased.

NATSAL found that the effect of increased condom use had been more than cancelled out by other demographic changes - to which the increased condom use was probably consequent.

- The mean number of lifetime partners had increased from 8.6 to 12.7% in men and from 3.7 to 6.5% in women

- Concurrent relationships - which are an extremely important factor in the spread of STIs, and which are cited as an important contributing factor to the HIV rate in Africa - increased from 12% to 14% in men and from 5% to 8% in women

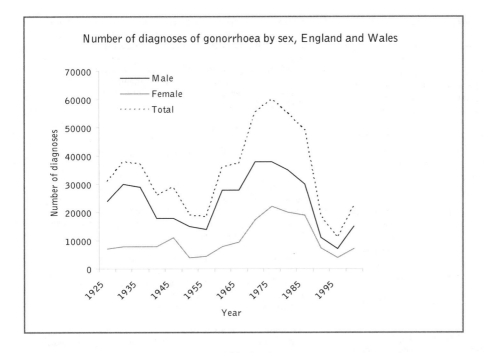

Number of diagnoses of gonorrhoea by sex, England and Wales

1990s, this increased from 1997 onwards and reached a peak of 45% in 2000.

Since then, however, there is some evidence that the amount of unprotected sex among gay men has reached a plateau, at least in the relatively unmarginalised gay populations of US urban centres. A more recent survey from San Francisco (Prabhu, 2004) found some evidence of a levelling-off of unprotected sex after 2001. More importantly, the amount of unprotected sex which was or could potentially be between partners of different HIV status (serodiscordant) showed a more distinct decline since that date.

An annual survey of gay men using London gyms (Elford, 2005a) found that the percentage of gay men reporting 'high risk behaviour' with a *casual* partner increased from 6.7 to 15.2%

- Age at first sex declined from 21% in women and 17% in men in the 1990 survey to 16% for both sexes fir teenagers included in the 2000 survey.

- The proportion of British men who had a male partner increased from 3.6% to 5.4%.

between 1998 and 2001 but remained stable after that, with the figure for 2004 being 14.7%.

This is a reminder that many other risk factors, some of them modifiable and others hardly so, or which it would be difficult to change, produce changes in the rates of STIs.

But condom use in gay men certainly declined during the late 1990s, with the rates of unprotected sex increasing almost as soon at combination therapy became available in 1996 (in the USA) and in 1997 (in Britain). A survey in San Francisco (Centers for Disease Control, 1999), for instance, found that the proportion of gay men who sometimes did without condoms when having anal sex increased from 30.4% in 1994 to 39.2%in 1997.

These figures were almost exactly mirrored, with a year's time lag, by the figures in the annual UK Gay Men's Sex Surveys(Gay Men's Sex Surveys, 1999-2003) and their predecessors. From about 33% of gay men who had anal sex doing it unprotected in the early

The evidence from the large annual UK Gay Men's Sex Survey is harder to interpret as questions are not always asked in standardised ways. But this appears to indicate a continued increase in unprotected sex between gay men in general, rather than a levelling off, from 33% in 1993 to 54.4% in 2003. UAI in itself does not imply HIV transmission, but there is also incomplete evidence that rates of potentially and definitely serodiscordant sex are increasing.

However an unpublished study by Jonathan Elford (Elford, 2005b) suggests that rates of serodiscordant sex between gay men in London are levelling off, and may be falling in HIV-positive men - see the next section for details.

One consistent finding from all these surveys has been that HIV-positive men have a great deal more unprotected sex than HIV-negative men. Data from the 2004 San Francisco Department of Public Health HIV Epidemiology Annual Report(2004) show that the increase in unprotected anal intercourse among gay men since 1998 is entirely among HIV-positive men.

We will revisit the subject of exactly why HIV-positive gay men have more unprotected sex, who they are having it with, and what the implications are for HIV, in the next section.

Condom controversies

Condoms as a method both of contraception and of reducing the transmission of HIV have always been controversial. Opponents of condoms, when not simply against their use for religious reasons, consistently suggest (either explicitly or implicitly) that the free or subsidised provision of condoms will simply encourage people, particularly young people, to have sex and take sexual risks they might not otherwise have done.

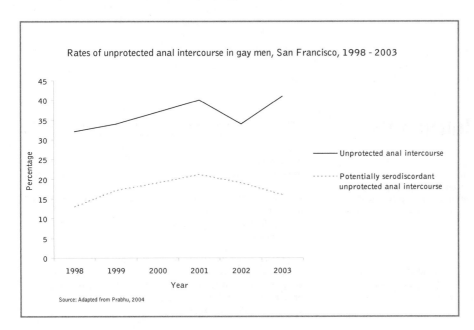

Rates of unprotected anal intercourse in gay men, San Francisco, 1998 - 2003

Unprotected anal intercourse

Potentially serodiscordant unprotected anal intercourse

Source: Adapted from Prabhu, 2004

As we see above under **A is for abstinence**, the opponents and proponents of comprehensive sex education and condom promotion often use the same data to reach different conclusions about the relative contribution of their favoured prevention method on HIV and STD incidence. In fact, all types of behaviour change are more likely to work together to reduce HIV incidence and should ideally be promoted together in a comprehensive package, rather than narrowly focusing on one. See, in particular, Santelli 2004, where the contribution of sexual abstinence to lower teenage pregnancy rates in the USA was calculated to be slightly higher than increased condom use (a finding seized on by pro-abstinence campaigners), but where increased condom use among teenagers who *did* have sex was also a significant factor.

We will not spend a great deal of time on the arguments for and against condoms here, many of which are conducted from positions informed by ideology rather than evidence. What opponents of condom use have lacked, however, is a 'smoking gun' study that shows that in some circumstances condom provision can increase rather than decrease HIV risk.

Such a study may have been provided by a team from Makerere University in Uganda (see Kajubi).

It found that providing young men with condoms and lessons on how to use them certainly increased condom use, when compared with a control group of men who just had a general talk on HIV and AIDS. However, it also found that the young men had a greater number of sexual partners and more unprotected sex than the control group.

The researchers took 378 young men aged 18-30 from two urban communities near Kampala and split them randomly into two groups. One group attended a three-hour workshop teaching them about how condoms stopped HIV and STDs, how to put on a condom, strategies for negotiating condom use with partners and talking about barriers to having safer sex. They were then given vouchers to redeem for free condoms provided by young people in their local community

The control group was just given a general lecture on the HIV situation in Uganda and given the free vouchers but no condom tuition.

The men taught how to use condoms certainly used more - 110 per man in the 6-month period after the study compared with 13 per man in the control group.

However the public health benefit of this was potentially offset by the fact that they had an increased number of partners, whereas the control group reduced their partners.

Men taught condom use increased their average number of partners from 2.13 to 2.44 in the six months whereas the control group decreased their number of partners from 2.20 to 2.03. This was highly statistically significant.

The control group ended up having fewer regular and casual partners; the condom group reduced their number of casual partners slightly but had considerably more regular partners.

This would not matter if condom use was consistent; but while the amount of unprotected sex the control group had was reduced with both regular and casual partners, the condom group only reduced unprotected sex with all partners slightly and actually slightly increased the amount of unprotected sex they had with casual partners.

After adjusting for the fact that men in the condom group were on the whole somewhat older and more likely to be married, the researchers calculated that providing the men with condom lessons actually led to them having 48% more unprotected sex relative to the ones without lessons.

The study had many limitations. It was small and the two groups compared were not identical. And of course it does not show that providing condoms makes you have unsafe sex. But it may demonstrate that condom provision in the absence of other measures encouraging behaviour change is an incomplete answer are an incomplete answer to HIV transmission, at least in the African situation.

The researchers commented: "Prevention interventions in generalised HIV epidemics need to promote all aspects of sexual risk reduction to slow HIV transmission."

Meanwhile, however, despite all the above reservations and complexities of behaviour, it is important to remember that **condoms remain the most effective and most widely used HIV prevention method by sexually active people,** and that in high-risk populations where condoms are widely available, half of all acts of sexual intercourse take place with a condom.

It's also important to know, as we said above, that properly implemented **HIV prevention programmes** have been shown to consistently increase condom use. For more on this see **HIV prevention: which methods work?**

This leads us to the best way to use them.

Safer sex

Condoms and lubricants

Using condoms

There are many other kinds of sexual activities which you can enjoy other than penetration, but if like many people you want to keep on having penetrative sex, either anally or vaginally, then learning to use condoms properly, and using them consistently, is the major step in adopting safer sex.

Reliability of condoms

Condoms do not make sex totally safe. Remember that, according to the statistics quoted above, they stop 85 to 90% of STIs (with the exception of contagious viruses like herpes and HPV, which can be spread via the fingers). Experience with birth control shows that over a period of a year, about six per cent of women who use condoms as their sole form of contraception will get pregnant. Although this is not all down to condom failure (a proportion of those pregnancies are no doubt due to failure to use condoms every time) it is still quite a high failure rate.

However, the main reason that condoms fail is because they are used incorrectly - they may be torn during opening, oil-based lubricants may be used, or they may be put on incorrectly, for example.

In general, condoms provide an effective barrier against HIV and other STIs, and, given that so many people practice penetrative sex as part of their sex lives, it is important that they are used properly. They are still the most effective barrier to HIV transmission during sexual intercourse.

In this section, we outline how to use condoms and lubricants most effectively, which cuts down on the already small risk of something going wrong.

Condom reluctance

Condoms can be uncomfortable, they can reduce the sensation during sex, and can often interrupt your fun when you have to find a condom, open the packet, find the lubricant and put it on. Nobody is saying that condoms are perfect, or that sex will be just as good if you use them. But, frankly, they are the best thing we have now to cut down on HIV transmission during sex.

A lot of blame has been placed on men's reluctance to use condoms. This ignores the fact that many women also prefer condomless sex, and, as indicated by the Simoni study above (Simoni, 2000), there may be deep psychological reasons to do with the demonstration of trust and closeness why both sexes may find them difficult to use consistently.

It also does not explain the deeper reasons for specifically male reluctance. One clue was given by a recent study of 78 HIV-positive gay men (Cove, 2004) in London. It found that while 38% of the men reported some degree of erectile dysfunction. But this went up to 51% in the context of trying to use condoms - in other worlds, more than half of the men experienced difficulty in getting or sustaining an erection when trying to put a condom on. Furthermore 90% of the 37 men whose erectile dysfunction was associated with condom use reported inconsistent condom use during insertive sex, compared with 28% of those who did not report condom-related erectile dysfunction.

If other groups of men have anything in common with gay men, we may be underestimating performance anxiety and the terror of impotence (often disguised with bravado) as a driver of men's reluctance to use condoms.

Strategies for women whose partners will not use condoms

Women cannot control condom use. Women who perceive themselves at special risk of acquiring HIV should consider the following strategies:

- Ask their partner to wear a condom and use water-based lubricant which does not contain nonoxynol-9

- Use a female condom (vaginal pouch) and lubricant. Although women may insert the female condom, this is not like a female-controlled prevention technology (such as the diaphragm). It is not discreet - your partner will always know you are using it - and it's possible to insert the penis between the wall of the vagina and the female condom, in which case it will offer no protection

- The effectiveness of the female condom with regard to preventing HIV infection has not been established

- Withdrawal: the European Study Group on Heterosexual Transmission of HIV(De Vincenzi, 1994) reported in 1994 that HIV-positive men who always withdrew before ejaculating had not infected their partners, even after 18 months. This suggests that if loss of sensation is the problem, intercourse without condoms may not present a significant risk unless ejaculation takes place, and may in some cases be an agreeable solution for both partners. However, Australian AIDS organisations have mounted specific campaigns to warn gay men against this strategy, after research suggested that a significant proportion of (an admittedly small number) of new infections were occurring among men who were using this technique instead of condoms.

Using condoms properly

Although everyone is happy to talk about condoms, very few people can tell you how to use them properly. The best demonstration of condom use that most people get is seeing a rubber placed hurriedly onto a banana. That kind of prudishness is no help to anyone, and can lead to people taking needless risks when they use condoms.

Using a condom properly is easy, once you have learnt how. And one of the best ways you can improve your safer sex life is to spend a little time getting it right. Although condoms will not let HIV pass through them under laboratory conditions, they can break, leak, or (and this is the most common reason for failure) *slip off* during sex, and if they do, they offer much less, or no, protection.

Golden rules of condom use

Later in this section we give a full explanation of how to get used to, and use, condoms, as well as explaining why they can break, what brands to choose and what lubricants to buy. But if you want a quick, easy shorthand to condom use, try to remember the Golden Rules we've listed below. Remember, condoms are not difficult to use, but do take a bit of practice to learn.

- Practise and be prepared

- Choose a condom which carries the British Kitemark

- Use the right kind of lubricant (water-based) and not the wrong kind of lubricant (oil-based)

- Always expel any air by holding the teat between thumb and forefinger

- Apply lubricant over the outside of the whole condom, re-apply if necessary

- Look after the condom - do not leave unused condoms in direct sunlight, be careful of tearing, using old condoms, leaving space or air in the condom, or not using enough lubrication

- Unroll the condom all the way to the base of the penis after it is hard and before starting sex

- When pulling out, hold the condom tight to the base of the penis, to prevent leakage

- Never re-use a condom. Once it is used, throw it away and put on a new one if you start again.

Step-by-step guide to using a condom

Open the packet carefully to avoid damaging the condom (jewellery, long fingernails or careless teeth could tear it). The condom comes out rolled up forming a ring which will fit over the penis

- Put the condom on after the penis is hard and before any kind of penetration begins

- Check the condom is the right way up; you can test with a finger that it rolls out and down

- Keep the penis completely free of grease and lubricant for best 'holding power'

- Squeeze the closed end between the thumb and forefinger to expel the air. Air bubbles can make condoms break

- Hold the condom over the tip of the penis and with the other hand carefully unroll it down to the base. It may help to stretch the condom width-ways in order to ease it down the penis and to ensure that it remains in place once sexual intercourse begins. But be careful not to pierce the condom with your fingernails when doing this

- If you have a foreskin, pull it back before covering the head of the penis with the condom. Don't try to cover the testicles with a condom

- Smooth the condom to eliminate any air bubbles

- Some men withdraw to check the condom, occasionally. If you need more lubrication (and you should use plenty), use more water-based lubricant

- **Never use two condoms at once.** This more is likely to lead to breakage because of rubber rubbing against rubber

- If you lose your erection the condom may slip. ***This is the biggest single cause of condom failure.*** Fingers held round the base of the condom will help it stay put

- If the condom does break or slip off withdraw as soon as you find out! Obviously you will need to use a new one if this happens

- A condom is more likely to break if sex lasts a long time, (longer than 45 minutes). Consider changing the condom during a long sex session

- After coming (ejaculation) withdraw the penis before it becomes soft (otherwise semen could leak out of the condom). To prevent the condom slipping off your penis at this stage, hold it firmly round the base as you withdraw

- Throw used condoms away. Dispose of them thoughtfully, e.g. wrapped up in tissue paper and then thrown in the rubbish. They shouldn't be flushed down the loo, since this may cause blockages in sewage disposal, according to water companies

- Never use a condom more than once

- Never use the same condom on two people in succession.

Practise and be prepared

Practise putting a condom on when you are masturbating on your own. Making it part of masturbation will help you to get used to the feel and look of a condom, and can be a turn-on in itself. You can take your time, following instructions step-by-step, so that you know exactly what you are doing. That way, when it comes to using condoms during sex, you will know what to do.

You can also practise putting a condom on your partner, on a banana or on a dildo. Some people like to put condoms onto their partner's penis during sex, and this is a way of getting used to it. But never use a condom that you have practised with by inflating or stretching. Use a new one instead.

You never know when you will strike lucky. Carry some around with you all the time. Remember that this is not 'loose' but responsible behaviour. And leave condoms around your flat - in the bedroom, the bathroom, in fact wherever you have sex at home. They will also advertise the fact that you expect to use condoms when you have sex.

Types of condoms

Which condom is safest?

Unfortunately we cannot give an easy answer to this question. There is no national watchdog agency overseeing the safety of all condoms sold in the UK. There is no independent comparative sampling and testing of condoms as actually sold in packets. And it is not illegal to market condoms which don't measure up to the British Standard BS EN600, which lays down requirements for good quality condoms.

Which condom should I choose?

The best advice is to choose a condom which carries the Kitemark. The Kitemark indicates that the condom brand is recognised under the British Standards Institution's (BSI) scheme. The BSI is responsible for drawing up the British Standard (known as BS4074:2002) and its testing division polices the scheme. A manufacturer who wants their brand to carry the Kitemark has to agree that BSI inspectors may regularly test samples of the brand and ensure that those samples will pass the tests laid down in the British Standard.

It's not compulsory for condoms to comply with the British Standard. What's more, any condom manufacturer can claim that his product conforms to the British Standard, but not sign up to the Kitemark scheme to have the claim checked by the BSI. Even if this claim appears to be backed up by a set of laboratory test results, the testing may not have been independent and may reflect only a one-off testing of a sample of condoms from one given batch at one given moment, rather than regular checking of multiple batches over time. So consumers can only be confident that a brand does meet the British Standard on an ongoing basis if it does carry the Kitemark.

During the 1990s, standards organisations throughout Europe have been working together to agree a pan-European condom standard. This was finally approved in early 1996, and European Union member states are obliged to replace their existing national standards with the new European one (known as EN600:1996).

HIV/AIDS organisations usually recommend consumers to stick to Kitemarked brands, but this can cause confusion when they also endorse certain brands such as HT Special that don't have a Kitemark. That's because Kitemarking is a British scheme, and condoms that are not formally marketed by their manufacturer in the UK are unlikely to be submitted for Kitemarking regardless of their quality.

Standard thickness condoms

The only difference between condoms listed in this section and the thicker condoms listed below is the thickness of the rubber. On average the condoms listed below are 30% thinner than the thickest brands such as HT Special and Durex Ultra Strong, and around 25% thinner than the other brands listed above.

Durex
- Gossamer

Hypoallergenic, non-spermicidal, regular-sized condom

- Close fit

Narrower condoms designed for a closer fit for those who have problems with regular-sized condoms. Non-spermicidal.

- Comfort Fit

Extra-long and wide, non-spermicidal

Condomi
- Nature

Lubricated with silicon-based lube, regular-sized

- Ultra THIN

Ultra thin, non-spermicidal, regular-sized condom

- XXL

Longer and wider than the average condom, lubricated with a silicone-based lubricant.

Confident
- Classic

Non-spermicidal, slightly longer condom

- Feelings

Non-spermicidal, slightly longer, ribbed and textured.

Mates
- Crystal

Dermatologically tested, thinner, with a straight profile, and non-spermicidal lube. Mates Crystal condoms have undergone a unique treatment to reduce the risk of an allergic latex reaction and are thinner.

- Conform

Non-spermicidal, one of the narrowest brands on the market.

- Large

Flared shape at the closed end of the condom, to provide comfort for those who find condoms too tight. Non-spermicidal lube

- Pleasure

An oversize tip on a uniquely shaped condom. Non-spermicidal lube

Boots
- Ultra safe

Non-spermicidal lube, slightly thicker for extra reassurance.

- Multi-ribbed

Textured to enhance stimulation for ultimate intensity, non-spermicidal lube with reservoir.

RFSU
- Okeido

Longer, wider and slightly fuller than our other condoms. Non-spermicidal

- Profile

Non-spermicidal, regular-sized

Trojan
- Ultra Pleasure

Extra thin, non-spermicidal, wider than average from top to bottom

EX S
- Natural

Non-spermicidal, regular-sized

SAFEX
- Natural

Non-spermicidal, regular-sized (non-spermicidal)

- Sensitive

Fine sheath for increased sensitivity, non-spermicidal

Not recommended (lubricated with nonoxynol-9)
- Condomi Supersafe
- Trojan Supra
- Safex Natural Spermicidal
- Mates Ultra Safe
- Mates Ribbed

The thickest condoms
Since the introduction of the harmonised European standard, condoms that claim to be extra strong have had to pass more a more stringent tensile breaking force test than those that do not make such a claim. There is no difference between the air-burst test requirements for standard versus strong condoms.

In early 1996 Rubberstuffers commissioned the British Standards Institution's laboratories to test condoms that claimed to be extra strong to the new standard. Over 200 condoms from each brand were subjected to tests for holes by filling with water, stretched until broken and inflated until they burst. In late 1996 the Consumers Association published in *Health Which?* the results of tests on a range of condom brands including some (but not all) of the brands tested by Rubberstuffers. Both sets of tests reached the same conclusions. There was little difference in strength between any of the following brands:

Extra strong condoms
Condomi
Strong

- Non-spermicidal lube, recommended for gay men

Durex
- Ultra strong

For maximum security. Lubricated with non-spermicidal lubricant. Made from natural rubber latex.

- Avanti

Non-allergenic, non-spermicidal polyurethane condom, which is much thinner than the latex condom

EX S
- Boys Own

Independently tested and approved for gay men's use. Silicone lubricated and manufactured to EN 600 and certified to the ec directive mark, non-spermicidal

- Ultra Strong

non-spermicidal

Another brand marketed to gay men in the UK is SAFEGUARD FORTE. In both sets of tests, these condoms just failed to meet the tensile breaking force requirements for condoms that claim to be extra strong, as defined in the British Standard. Safex Supplies claim that they have since improved their manufacturing processes, but there have not yet been any independent tests to verify this claim.

Notwithstanding their name, the Dutch GAY SAFE condoms performed poorly in both Rubberstuffers' and the Consumers Association's tests, and cannot be considered an extra-strong brand.

Both these brands were also thinner than the others, reinforcing the impression that the thicker condoms are generally the stronger.

Which strength condoms for anal sex?

It is one of the scandals of this epidemic that only in recent years have any of the condoms available in the UK been marketed for anything other than vaginal use. For example, only Boys Own and Safeguard Forte condoms are currently promoted by their manufacturers towards the gay community.

Naturally, they are regularly used in very large numbers for anal sex as well as for vaginal sex. But because there are no standards for anal sex condoms, nor any guidelines on how to use them for this purpose, those using 'vaginal' condoms for anal sex may not be using the best brands, or using them in the safest way.

It may be that in the same way the female condom will also serve as an anal condom, though the same issues that apply to women using female condom also apply to gay men being penetrated with one. See the section on female condomsfor further detail.

At the 13th International AIDS Conference in Durban, a team of researchers from London's City University (Golombok 2001, Harding, 2000) presented data from a study of 283 gay male couples who had been randomised to use either standard or thicker condoms for anal sex and additional water based lubricant. Each couple were provided with nine condoms and completed a questionnaire after each sexual act.

The researchers found that condoms broke for the same reasons as previously identified in studies among heterosexual couples; unrolling the condom before fitting it to the penis, longer duration of intercourse (longer than 45 minutes), and absence of additional lubricant. Use of additional inappropriate, (oil-based lubricant or saliva) was also associated with condom breakage. Penis length was also associated with condom breakage, yet girth was not.

The study found **no significant differences** between the two types of condoms with respect to breakage or slippage. Condoms were more likely to slip if lubricant was placed on the penis under the condom. A low incidence of clinical breakage was reported for both condom types during appropriate use.

In order to use standard condoms most effectively, the researchers recommended that gay men be reminded of the following:

- unroll the condom *after* fitting it to the penis

- use additional lubricant

- apply the lubricant to the *outside* of the condom only

- apply the lubricant in and around the anus.

The findings of this study call into question the long-standing UK recommendation that gay men should use extra-strong or thicker condoms wherever possible. The researchers have proposed that gay men should be advised to use Kitemarked condoms, and note that inexperience in the use of condoms and use of inappropriate lubricants were far more important factors in explaining condom failure.

In North America and Australia (yet not in Europe) HIV prevention messages have always offered the alternative of standard condoms for anal sex. This trial has seemingly offered the first piece of evidence to confirm this approach to HIV health promotion.

The authors concluded that the data concerning the predictors of failure should be used in health promotion "to reduce the incidence of condom failure among gay men".

For the past 15 years one of the cornerstones of gay men's HIV prevention in the UK has been the recommendation to use extra-strong condoms for anal sex.

However, this view is not universally shared. Around the world, the UK is almost unique in recommending extra-strong condoms to gay men, with HIV prevention agencies in both the USA and Australia happy to say that it's okay for gay men to use standard strength condoms for anal sex. Only Germany and the Netherlands share the UK's insistence on extra-strong condoms.

Based on this research GMFA designed and launched a mass media campaign which says that standard strength condoms are just as reliable for anal sex as extra-strength ones.

Not everybody involved in UK HIV prevention agreed, most notably and vocally, the then Team Leader of Camden and Islington's HIV and Sexual Health Promotion Service, who now run Freedoms. This meant that gay men in the UK were being offered conflicting advice on condoms by two equally well respected HIV prevention agencies. A debate organised in 2002 between the two sides failed to reach a resolution.

The advice now (2005) offered by Camden and Islington and Freedoms is still that they recommend extra-strong condoms for anal sex, and extra-strong condoms are described as 'gay condoms' on their shop site. But David Smith the current team leader says: "We're cautious about changing that advice. Nut the important thing is to have people using condoms correctly, not failing to use them because they can't find an extra strong one or don't like them."

Warning: Spermicides

A spermicide is a chemical substance which is designed as a form of birth control by inactivating sperm to prevent conception. Some are also effective against HIV in some circumstances (see *Uncertainty about spermicidal lubricants* below). Spermicides may be introduced in lubricant on condoms, lubricating gels, pessaries etc.

The most frequently used spermicide is nonoxynol-9. CONDOMS THAT CONTAIN NONOXYNOL-9 ARE NO LONGER RECOMMENDED FOR ANAL SEX OR FOR WOMEN THAT HAVE A LOT OF VAGINAL SEX, LIKE SEX WORKERS.

Several scientific trials have now shown that that nonoxynol-9 may actually facilitate HIV transmission rather than provide added protection. The clinching trial was the COL-1492 trial nonoxynol-9 as a candidate microbicide in West Africa in 2002. This showed that using N-9, which kills HIV in the test tube, in fact doubled the rate of HIV transmission in frequent users because it damaged the mucous membrane lining the vagina (and has an even worse effect on anal and rectal membranes).

There is now a consensus among organisations concerned with sexual and reproductive health that nonoxynol-9 has no role in preventing HIV and other sexually transmitted infections, and its use should be discouraged by anyone perceived to be at risk. At the same time, there continues to be a role for spermicides containing N-9, as readily-available but moderately effective non-hormonal contraceptives, for women and couples who are at very low risk of HIV or other STIs.

It is particularly important that products containing N-9 should not be used for anal sex.

There has been resistance from condom manufacturers to calls to remove 'spermicidal lubrication' with N-9 from their products, as they perceive that it 'meets a demand' for 'extra safety' from some users. Expert opinion is that the low dose of N-9 in that lubricant does not add to their contraceptive value and might even distract women from the need for emergency back-up contraception if condoms fail. Durex have now removed sprmicidal lubrication from all their condoms, but some Mates brands still contain it - see list above.

The dose of N-9 in spermicidally lubricated condoms might still cause problems if such condoms are used for anal sex. Since many heterosexual couples practise anal sex on occasion, it seems unreasonable to expect them to decide in advance, when buying condoms, on what sort of sex they are going to have.

There is an even greater risk for gay men, since in many settings they are more likely to be exposed to HIV, yet there is evidence that gay men continue to use N-9 products despite publicity that these are dangerous.

A survey of gay men in San Francisco was carried out in 2001, a year after the publication of data showing that nonoxynol-9 increased the risk of HIV transmission. This found 349 men out of 573 had heard of nonoxynol-9. Among these, 55% had used products containing it in the previous year, for anal sex. In fact, it had been used in a median of 50% of acts of anal sex in the past twelve months. 23% had used it without a condom in the belief that it reduced their risk of HIV infection. On being informed that N-9 exposure caused disruption of the rectal mucosa, the great majority said they would be less likely to use it.

Brands to use if you are allergic to rubber

The vast majority of condoms are made of latex. If you are allergic to latex:

- Try Durex Allergy: it contains less of what makes you allergic to rubber condoms

- Try Femidoms which are made of plastic rather than latex

- Try polyurethane condoms if they are available.

There is no evidence that lambskin condoms prevent the transmission of HIV.

Teatless condoms

Some condoms are manufactured without a teat at the end. In the past the teat has always been considered necessary to contain semen and prevent the condom from bursting under the force of ejaculation. However, there is no conclusive evidence that teatless condoms are more prone to bursting, and research in Holland during the development of a stronger condom suitable for anal sex showed that a teatless condom was more acceptable to gay men (it looked less artificial) and performed just as well in strength trials.

Larger and snugger fitting condoms

Men who have experienced difficulty in using condoms quite often complain that condoms split because they are not large enough, or that they slip off because they do not fit snugly enough. There are quite considerable variations in penis size amongst men in the UK which are related to some extent to ethnicity. It was recently estimated that a third of penises in the UK exceed the size designated as 'average' in the UK condom standard. A London GUM clinic recently investigated this variation and found that black men experienced the problem of condoms splitting more frequently, whilst Asian men were more likely to report problems with condoms slipping off.

This list above notes differences between the length and width of the standard strength condoms tested by the Consumers Association.

If you cannot afford condoms

- Free supplies are often available from:

- NHS Family Planning Clinics

- Brook Advisory Centres

- Needle exchanges and drugs agencies

- Some GUM clinics

- Some local HIV/AIDS services and self help groups

- And increasingly from some GPs

- Gay pubs and clubs in London participating in the health-authority funded free condom scheme Freedoms.

All these sources should also be able to supply you with free water-based lubricant.

Lubricants

Why use plenty of water-based lubricant?

Condoms are vital to safer sex. They act as a barrier to body fluids, and help to protect us from HIV. But often people use condoms 'dry', that is without any lubricant on them, and this can create problems. The condom is more likely to slip, or tear, because of increased friction.

Anal sex without lubricant can not only be hugely painful, it also greatly increases the risk of tears and cuts to the lining of the rectum as well as the risk of breakage of the condom.

During vaginal intercourse, a woman produces natural lubricating fluids, but these may not be enough for safer condom use. The amount of fluid a woman produces changes throughout the menstrual cycle, and is influenced by several factors. It is quite natural for women to need additional lubrication for comfort as well as for safer sex.

The most important thing to remember is: - don't use oil-based lubricants with condoms: they weaken condoms drastically and dangerously within minutes! Often an oil-covered condom will split whilst you are having sex, so that you never realise it is burst or torn until after the event. If you are desperate to have sex, and only have oil-based lubricant to hand, then still don't use it. Spit is preferable.

On the other hand it is important to ensure that you are not having 'dry sex'. The increased friction from this puts extra strain on the condom. Adequate lubrication can sometimes be ensured in vaginal intercourse by means of plenty of 'foreplay' but this is not always effective. Spit or water are not very good lubricants.

The wrong lubricants: oil-based

Anything made of rubber, from tyres to condoms, begins to rot and split when it comes into contact with anything oil-based. For many years, people have used oil-based 'lubricants' that are found in any home as an aid to sexual intercourse.

But if you want to practice safer sex, or help to avoid pregnancy, by using condoms, then you should switch to using water-based lubricants. Examples of the wrong lubricants are:

- Oil

- Baby oil

- Corn oil

- Butter

- Margarine

- Crisco and other 'vegetable fats'

- Vaseline

- Petroleum jelly

- Hand cream and body lotion.

It is important not to rely upon whether the lubricant will wash off your hands or not. There are certain lubricants that are oil-based which will wash off, giving the false impression that they are water-based.

Many ointments, creams, gels, vaginal pessaries or suppositories come in an oil-based medium as well. Your doctor will be able to tell you which prescribed treatments are oil-based. A leaflet detailing which ones are oil-based is also produced by Durex.

If you want to keep having sex, but have to use oil-based products, then you may want to consider using a Femidom instead of condoms (see *female condoms and spermicides* below).

The right lubricants: water-based

Liquid Silk

Doesn't contain glycerine, available in sachets/pump

Eros

Silicone-based, oil-free formulation - safe for use with all condoms

ID

Millennium
Silicone-based

Pleasure
Silicone-based, contains amino acid Arginine

Glide
Water-based

Wet Stuff

Water-based lubricant, available in bottle/tube/pump/sachets

Oncore

Homeopathic, water-based gel, available in tube/pump

Boots Lubricating Jelly

Water-based

K-Y Jelly

Water-based

K-Y Liquid

Water-based, ideal for use with condoms

You can buy water-based lubricants, such as KY, Wet Stuff, Comfort, Probe, Astroglide or 121 at many chemists.

The new **silicone-based** lubricants such as Millennium ID and Eros are more expensive than water-based ones. But they are also condom-friendly, do not feel sticky or dry out so fast, and are economical (a little goes a long way).

There are also lubricants, such as Boots's own brand which explain that they are water-based on the packaging. Some people like different lubes because they stay wet for longer, and you might want to experiment.

Replens

A recently-launched product on the market, Replens is a 'super lubricant', designed to help post-menopausal women who find that their vaginal juices are too limited to help with the intercourse, or who are generally dry and need lubrication. Replens lasts for a long time, and although based on palm oil, it does not affect rubber. Tests by Durex on Replens with condoms registered no damage.

Don't use nonoxynol-9 coated condoms

In September 2002 the Global Campaign for Microbicides launched a public 'Call to discontinue nonoxynol-9 for rectal use'. This is based on concerns, set out by the US Centers for Disease Control and Prevention and the World Health Organisation, that this widely-used spermicide causes damage to the lining of the rectum when used for anal sex, significantly increasing the risk of HIV and other STI transmission.

The call has been backed by leading scientists in the field and by many HIV, AIDS, gay and women's organisations including all of the main microbicide advocacy groups, the American Foundation for AIDS Research (amFAR), the Family Planning Association (UK), International HIV/AIDS Alliance, International AIDS Vaccine Initiative, National AIDS Trust, Terrence Higgins Trust, and the US Gay and Lesbian Medical Association.

The call demands that manufacturers discontinue the sale of condoms and sexual lubricants containing nonoxynol-9, while continuing to supply over-the-counter spermicides containing nonoxynol-9 in forms designed for vaginal use. The argument is that a public education campaign, to persuade individual consumers to check the labels and avoid products containing nonoxynol-9, would not be as effective in bringing about change as a simple change to the products.

While gay men may generally be at the highest risk of HIV transmission through anal sex, there are many heterosexual couples who sometimes have anal sex and therefore many women who are also potentially at risk.

Female condoms

The most effective method to prevent HIV acquisition and transmission, the condom, is worn by men. Many women do not have relationships of equality with the men they have sex with, and they can experience difficulties 'persuading' men to use condoms. This can be particularly difficult in situations where HIV is not the priority concern (for example, when the woman experiences violence). However, it is also problematic for women in more equal relationships, since many men find condoms unpleasant, and as women are more vulnerable to HIV than men from vaginal intercourse, they may not afford the same priority to condom use.

The female condom is the first product which has been developed to offer women more control over HIV prevention methods. However, it is not a method entirely within women's control. Although, in general, the woman inserts the device, it requires compliance and consent from the man for it to be used. It is extremely visible - many would say unattractive - as it extends beyond the labia. It is possible for the man to avoid it and penetrate between the female condom and the vaginal wall, and it is unlikely that the woman would be aware if he was doing this.

Since there are no methods entirely within women's control, and as the vulnerability to HIV from vaginal sex increases for women, the need for new prevention methods is urgent. Microbicides (previously known as virucides) have been spoken about for several years, and are now receiving a fair degree of attention from some policy makers (such as WHO) and sectors of the research community. Currently no proven safe and effective microbicides are available, but research is underway. Microbicides are also beneficial because they offer the potential to protect against sexually transmitted infections, which are a significant contributor to death, illness and infertility around the world.

For more information on the development of microbicides see *Microbicides* in *Emergent prevention technologies*.

Advantages

Since it does not fit the penis snugly like a male condom, several men report that it is more pleasurable because it is not constricting. The female condom can be inserted before sexual activity begins and so it may be less of an interference than the male condom. Because it is made of polyurethane, the female condom can be used with oil-based or water-based lubricants.

It has been suggested that some women (for example, sex workers) would find the female condoms an easier way of practising safer sex, by keeping it in for a period of time. However, women who have tried this report that it can be uncomfortable, and it is also important to check the female condom at regular intervals for tears in the plastic. Using a female condom on a number of occasions may present few problems with a single sexual partner, but it is clearly different if used for multiple partners (e.g. for a sex worker). There would be risks to multiple partners who came into contact with infected semen in the female condom deposited by previous men.

The manufacturers also warn against taking out the female condom, washing it and then re-inserting it, since this doesn't guarantee hygiene, and the product would need re-lubricating. They advise using a new female condom on each occasion. There are plans to develop the product so that it can be used on several occasions, like the diaphragm.

The female condom is expensive, although it is increasingly available for free from outlets, such as health clinics, which also provide free male condoms. You may need to ask for the female condom if you don't see it on disply at some clinics, since they may prefer to give out male condoms, which are cheaper.

There are some reported problems with using the female condom. Some women report losing the inner ring inside their vagina whilst others fear that, because the female condom is seamed, it may be more liable to tearing. Some cases of tearing have been noted.

Trials not sponsored by the company have tended to show a lower rate of acceptability. The female condom is very visible, and many women find it unattractive (and comic) because the appliance hangs down beyond the labia. Some women experience irritation to the vulval area because of the outer ring, which fits over the labia to hold the device in place.

The sound of trapped air in the female condom has irritated some users. Other activities, in particular oral sex, are not feasible with it in place. Some men have found the inner ring uncomfortable as they thrust into it - this problem can be solved by either removing the inner ring, or inserting the female condom on the penis (rather than the woman inserting it like a diaphragm).

Use of the female condom in the developing world

Studies conducted in Africa, Asia, Latin America, Europe and North America have found good initial acceptability of the device. A recent review by the World Health Organization of 41 acceptability studies indicated that the degree of acceptance varies widely, from 41% to 95% of study participants. Research indicates that counselling helps overcome women's initial difficulties in using the device, that directing promotion campaigns to men and providing women with negotiation skills are important to overcome men's resistance to use, and that over time, use tends to become concentrated among a subset of women or couples with high motivation to use it.

Among the many acceptability studies, recent UNAIDS-supported research in Costa Rica, Indonesia, Mexico and Senegal found that women who introduced the female condom into a relationship reported it allowed them to communicate more successfully about safer sex. In a study involving 377 women in the Dominican Republic, Mexico and United States, about four of every five women liked the device and said they would recommend it to others.

In Zambia and Zimbabwe, mass marketing campaigns and some educational support have made the female condom available in urban areas. A year after the Zimbabwe campaign began, a survey of more than 1,600 people at retail outlets concluded that single women and men with partners outside of marriage seemed to benefit most from the female condom introduction. After six months in the Zambia campaign, a random sample of 1,570 persons at 52 retail outlets found that those who had already discussed the female condom with a partner were more likely to use it in the future.

Nine hundred women were provided with both male and female condoms at STI clinics in the U.S. After six months, eight percent had used only the female condom. Another 73% had used both the male and female condom. About a third of those used 10 or more female condoms. The researchers concluded that women at risk of STIs find the female condom acceptable, with many using either the male or female condom consistently over time.

Two studies among women at high risk of HIV infection indicated successful sustained use. A study in Zambia found that the devices were used in one quarter of coital acts at three, six and 12 months. In a study among sex workers in Thailand, some 250 women offered both male and female condoms used female condoms in 12% of all sexual acts, a level that continued for the entire six-month study period.

Instructions for use

1 Find a comfortable position, for example, lying down, sitting with your knees apart, or standing with one foot up on a chair

2 Open the female condom packet by tearing down from the notch, and remove the product. You will see that the female condom is pre-lubricated. Make sure that the flexible inner ring is at the closed end of the female condom

3 Squeeze the lower half of the inner ring between your thumb, index and middle fingers. This should give you a confident grip and narrows the inner ring to ease insertion

4 With the other hand, spread the labia (folds of skin around your vaginal opening). Insert the squeezed ring of the female condom into the vagina, and push inside as far as you can

5 Then put your finger inside the female condom until you can feel the bottom of the inner ring. Push the ring up into the vagina

6 You can tell if it is in place when the inner ring is up past the pubic bone. You can feel your pubic bone by curving your finger (towards the front) when it is a couple of inches inside your vagina

7 The outer ring and a small part of the female condom will stay outside your vagina. This is quite normal so don't worry

8 Another method is to use the female condom as a penile (male) condom. It may be best to leave the inner ring at the far end of the Female condom, as this will hold it around the cervix. Since the ring helps to guide the device when it is inserted first into the vagina, and it can cause discomfort, another option is to remove the inner ring. This method could also be used for anal sex

9 Add extra lubricant during sex if one of you needs it. If the outer ring is being drawn into the vagina, or if the penis starts to enter between the vagina and the female condom, then stop. The man should withdraw and add extra lube to the inside of the female condom

10 Removing the female condom: because the female condom lines the inside of the vagina the man doesn't have to withdraw immediately after coming. You can remove the sheath when it suits you, making sure that no semen is spilt. Twist the outer ring to keep the semen inside, then pull gently. Throw away the used female condom. Do not throw it down the toilet as it may cause a blockage.

It is also possible to use the female condom like a baggy penile condom (see below). Although it would make sense for this method to be as safe as the one described, trials have not been conducted to assess the efficacy of using it in this way.

Female condoms for anal sex

Like condoms, it appears that, although not designed for the purpose, female condoms do work as an effective barrier during anal sex. A study in the United States of 14 male couples using the equivalent of the female condoms found that, although no leaks or tears were found in any of the sheaths used, all of the men found design and usage difficulties, 'which were primarily due to lack of experience and knowledge' of the product.

Provisional guidelines for anal sex with female condoms

1 The easiest way to use the female condom for anal sex is to wear it like a 'male' (penile) condom. Put lubricant in the female condom and then place it over the penis (or a dildo). Use plenty of lubricant on the outside of the female condom or around your partner's rectum before sex.

2 Alternatively, you could try to insert the female condom in the rectum first, as for vaginal intercourse. Use plenty of lubricant around the anus, and loosen it with a finger in readiness for the female condom. Make sure your fingernails are cut short.

3 After removing the female condom from its wrapper, hold the inner ring between your thumb, index and forefinger, and squeeze it so that it forms an oval. Don't remove the inner ring, as this will lead the female condom to become tangled, and could lead to breakage.

4 Push the female condom up into your rectum as far as you can, using the inner ring as a guide, whilst spreading your anus with your other hand. You may find this easier if you raise one leg onto the side of the bath, or a stool.

5 Then put your index finger inside the female condom, until you feel the bottom of the inner ring. Push up as far as you can, but do not insert the outer ring.

6 You will find that the outer ring, and perhaps a small part of the female condom, are on the outside of your rectum. That's meant to happen, and should stop the female condom from slipping inside.

7 Use more lubricant inside the female condom, to keep it moist, and add it whenever you need it during sex.

8 Check every now and again during sex that the outer ring of the female condom hasn't slipped inside your anus, or that his penis hasn't slipped between the female condom and your anus. If it has, stop, remove the female condom, and use a new one before starting again.

9 Don't re-use the female condom. Some gay men are reported to have used a female condom as a semi-permanent barrier to HIV, being penetrated by multiple partners. The female condom is designed for vaginal sex and for single use. If you use it more than once for anal sex, we don't know the strains that it could put on the sides of the sheath, which might easily tear. And if you get a lot of semen in the female condom, we don't know how effective it is in holding it in, or whether any seepage into your rectum could take place. It is likely that penetration in somebody else's cum would also be dangerous for your partners

10 Removing the female condom. Because the female condom lines the inside of the rectum, your partner doesn't have to withdraw immediately after coming. You can remove the sheath when it suits you, making sure that no semen is spilt. Twist the outer ring to keep the semen inside, then pull gently. Throw away the used female condom.

Gay men's use of female condoms

Female condoms were the first product developed to offer women more control over HIV prevention methods. The *Reality* condom was approved in the USA in 1992 for vaginal contraceptive use. Latex male condoms have been associated with usage problems including, breakage, slippage, latex allergies and lack of control by receptive partners. Although female condoms are essentially not designed for the purpose, some gay men have used them and it seems they do provide an effective barrier during anal sex.

A 1999 study (Renzi, 2001) among gay men in San Francisco gave *Reality* condoms to 100 men attending an STI clinic. Eighty-six men said they would use the *Reality* condom again and 54 said they preferred it to penile condoms. Acceptability was greatest among HIV-positive men and men in serodiscordant relationships or non-monogamous ones. Problems cited included difficulty inserting (33%), irritation (17%), bunching up (12%), unpleasant texture (10%), and noise (9%). Breakage was reported three times in 334 episodes of use.

Research published in the March 2003 edition of the journal *AIDS* has assessed the safety and acceptability of a brand of female condom called *Reality* for anal sex among gay men. The study enrolled 56 monogamous seroconcordant gay male couples who had not used condoms in the past three months were randomised to use latex male condoms or the *Reality* female condom for anal sex. On study entry the men were given 10 *Reality* or lubricated male condoms to use with lubricant during the following six weeks. In the second six weeks the couples crossed over and began using the other condom type.

The *Reality* condom has two polyurethane rings and a thin, loose-fitting polyurethane sheath which in laboratory studies has been shown to be impermeable to viruses and less likely to rupture than latex condoms. Since it is made of polyurethane it can be used with both water-based and other kinds of lubricant. In this study couples were advised to remove the inner ring to reduce potential rectal trauma and bleeding.

Receptive partners were more likely to report pain or discomfort with the *Reality* rather than the male condom. Both partners were significantly more likely to report *Reality* condom slippage during use or withdrawal. Rates of condom breakage were similar for Reality and male condoms.

After using both sets of condoms , both active and passive partners were significantly less likely to be willing to use *Reality* condoms in the future with partners of unknown HIV than they were to be willing to use male latex condoms; (21% of receptive and 26% of insertive partners would be willing to use *Reality* condoms, compared to 61% of both receptive and insertive partners who were willing to use latex condoms. The main reason reported by those who would be willing to use the *Reality* condom with future partners of unknown HIV status were that the *Reality* condom was more comfortable, easier to use, and perceived to be stronger and safer.

The researchers suggested that gay men who are considering using the *Reality* condom might require training relating to slippage and methods for avoiding semen spillage that might expose the anal mucosa. They added "further work is warranted on design modifications, safety and acceptability of the *Reality* condom in HIV-negative gay men".

References

Agence-France Presse. THAI TEENAGERS SHUNNING CONDOMS, HEALTH MINISTRY WARNS. 16 November 2003.

AIDS Prevention and Control Project. Voluntary health services: executive summary of BSS report wave IX report. Tamil Nadu. India, 2005.

American Social Health Association Press Release: SURVEY SUGGESTS LACK OF AWARENESS HEIGHTENS RISK FOR SEXUALLY TRANSMITTED DISEASES. See http://www.planetout.com/health/hiv/?sernum=2778. 6 April 2004.

Bradshaw S. Vatican: condoms don't stop Aids, *The Guardian, 9 October 2003*. See http://www.guardian.co.uk/aids/story/0,7369,1059068,00.html

Centers for Disease Control and Prevention, Communicable Disease Weekly, January 29, 1999. 148(03):45-48.

Cove J, Petrak J. Factors associated with sexual problems in HIV-positive gay men. *Int J STD AIDS*. 15(11):732-6. 2004.

Dandona L. Sex behaviour of men who have sex with men and risk of HIV in Andhra Pradesh, India. AIDS. 19(6):611-9. 2005.

Davidovich U et al. Assessing sexual risk behaviour of young gay men in primary relationships: the incorporation of negotiated safety and negotiated safety compliance. *AIDS* 14(6) 701-706. 2000.

De Vincenzi I. A Longitudinal Study of Human Immunodeficiency virus Transmission by Heterosexual Partners. *NEJM* 331(6), 341-346. 1994.

Elam G et al. Intentional and unintentional UAI among gay men who HIV test in the UK: qualitative results from an investigation into risk factors for seroconversion among gay men who HIV test (INSIGHT). *HIV Med* 7 (supplement 1), abstract 027, 2006.

Elford J et al. HIV-positive and negative homosexual men have adopted different strategies for reducing the risk of HIV transmission. *Sexually Transmitted Infections* 77:224-225. 2001.

Elford J. High Risk Sexual Behaviour among London gay men: no longer increasing? 11th Annual BHIVA Conference, Dublin. Abstract O14. 2005a.

Elford J et al. High-risk sexual behaviour among London gay men: no longer increasing. *AIDS*, 2005 (in press). 2005b.

Erickson P. Prevalence of anal sex among heterosexuals in California and its relationship to other AIDS risk behaviours. *AIDS Education & Prevention* 7(6):477-93, 1995

Gay Men's Sex Surveys 1999-2003: See www.sigmaresearch.org

Golombok S et al. An evaluation of a thicker versus a standard condom with gay men. AIDS 2001, 15:245-250.

Guzman, R et al. Negotiated safety relationships and sexual behaviour among a diverse sample of HIV-negative men who have sex with men. *JAIDS* 38(1), 82-86. 2005.

Harding, R et al. A clinical trial of a thicker versus a standard condom for gay men. Thirteenth International AIDS Conference, abstract WePpC1395, Durban, 9-14 July 2000.

Hickson F et al. Out and About: Findings form the UK Gay Men's Sex Survey 2002. Sigma Research, 2003.

Ho GY et al. Natural history of cervicovaginal papillomavirus infection in young women. *N Engl J Med* 338(7):423-428. 1998.

Johnson AM et al. Sexual behaviour in Britain: partnerships, practices, and HIV risk behaviours. *Lancet* 358(9296):1835-42. 2001.

Kajubi P et al.Increasing Condom Use without Reducing HIV Risk: Results of a Controlled Community Trial in Uganda. *JAIDS* 40(1):77-82.2005. 2005.

Kumar R, et al, for the International Studies of HIV/AIDS (ISHA) Investigators. Trends in HIV-1 in young adults in south India from 2000 to 2004: a prevalence study. *Lancet* 367: 1164-72. 2006.

Lightfoot M et al. The Influence of partner type and risk status on the sexual behaviour of young men who have sex with me living with HIV/AIDS. *JAIDS* 38(1), 61-68. 2005.

Maharaj P and Cleland J. Risk Perception and Condom Use Among Married Or Cohabiting Couples in KwaZulu-Natal, South Africa. *International Family Planning Perspectives* 31 (1), 2005

Najjumba M. Risk Perception and Condom Use in Uganda. African Population Studies 18(1). 2003.

Peltzer K. Factors affecting condom use among senior secondary school pupils in South Africa. *Cent Afr J Med. 46(11):302-8. 2000.*

Mechai Viravaidya. Personal communication with author, 2004.

Prabhu R. et al. The bisexual bridge revisited: sexual risk behavior among men who have sex with men and women, San Francisco, 1998-2003. *AIDS* 18(11), 1604-1606. 2004.

Renzi, C. et al. Safety and acceptability of the Reality™ condom for anal sex among men who have sex with men. *AIDS* 17(5) 28: 727-731. 2003.

San Francisco Department of Public Health - HIV Epidemiology Annual Report 2004 - see http://www.dph.sf.ca.us/Reports/HlthAssess.htm.%202004.

Santelli JS et al. Can Changes in Sexual Behaviors Among High School Students Explain the Decline in Teen Pregnancy Rates in the 1990s? Journal of Adolescent Health, 35(2):80-90. 2004.

Simoni J M et al..Safer sex among HIV+ women: The role of relationships. *Sex Roles*, 42, 691-708. 2000.

Weller S, Davis K. Condom Effectiveness in Reducing Heterosexual Transmission. *The Cohrane Database of Systematic Reviews*, issue 1, 2002.

UNAIDS: AIDS Epidemic Update, December 2001.

UNAIDS 2005. Evidence for HIV decline in Zimbabwe: a comprehensive review of the epidemiological data. ISBN 92 9 173461 6. Can be downloaded from http://data.unaids.org/publications/irc-pub06/zimbabwe_epi_report_nov05_en.pdf

Winer RL et al. Genital human papillomavirus infection: incidence and risk factors in a cohort of female university students. *Am J Epidemiol* 157(3):218-226. 2003.

Winer RL et al. Condom use and the risk of genital human papillomavirus infection in young women. *N Engl J Med* 354(25):2645-2654. 2006.

C is also for Circumcision

There is strong biological and epidemiological evidence that circumcised men are less vulnerable than uncircumcised men to HIV infection via heterosexual intercourse. Circumcision is believed to reduce the risk of male infection because it removes the vulnerable tissue inside the foreskin, which contains Langerhans cells (a type of cell particularly vulnerable to HIV infection). The mucosa that covers the inside of the foreskin contains more Langerhans cells than almost any other part of the body except the gut. These are a type of dendritic cell whose job is to ferry foreign particles to the lymph nodes for recognition by the immune system, and which HIV hijacks as part of its infection strategy. In ex-vivo explant models, foreskin mucosa was found to be nine times more vulnerable than cervical tissue to HIV infection.

The area under the foreskin is also vulnerable to trauma, and is more likely to become abraded if vaginal lubrication is not present. Also, uncircumcised men may be more vulnerable to sexually transmitted infections, because the area under the foreskin can retain bacteria acquired during sex, thus increasing the chance that an infection will become established

Epidemiological studies

In Africa, the countries in which less than 20% of the male population are circumcised form a broad swathe that extends from the Central African Republic and southern Sudan in the north, through the former British colonies of east Africa, and down to Botswana, Zimbabwe, and Swaziland (Halperin). The only country that has high (>10%) levels of HIV prevalence alongside rates of male circumcision greater than 20% is South Africa, whose very mixed cultural, sexual and racial background may make it a special case.

Kenya is a special and more studied case. The general HIV prevalence in 1999 was estimated at 11%. But among circumcised men prevalence was about 3%. In a study of Nyanza province on the shores of Lake Victoria, prevalence in circumcised men was 2% and in uncircumcised men 21%.

Most ethnic groups in Kenya practice circumcision. The main tribe that does not is the Luo people, who live in the east of the country and are concentrated in Nyanza. In a paper for the World Bank, Beegle and Özler found that HIV prevalence in Luo men aged 15-49 in Nyanza was 20.4% and amongst non-Luo men it was 0.8%. In women aged 15-49 it was 25.6% and 7.0% amongst Luo and non-Luo women respectively.

In countries where less than 20% of the male population is circumcised, HIV prevalence ranges from 25% in Zimbabwe to around 12% in Rwanda (these are figures from Halperin's 1999 paper and in some cases have been revised downwards now). In countries where levels of male circumcision are greater than 20%, HIV prevalence ranges from 7.6% in Congo (Brazzaville) to 2% in west African countries such as Guinea and Benin. Circumcision is probably not the whole explanation for these differences, and Halperin argues that countries that have low circumcision rates also tend to have cultures in which people commonly have non-commercial concurrent sexual partnerships. These two factors taken together, he says, are in themselves sufficient to explain differences in HIV prevalence.

Conversely, in many countries that have higher circumcision rates, such as Guinea and Ghana, though non-primary-partner sex tends to happen with sex workers, among whom HIV prevalence is very high, there has been little spread into the general population, possibly because the circumcised clients are at low risk of infection and so do not carry HIV home to their wives (as has been observed in countries where circumcision is less common, such as India).

The same patterns regarding HIV prevalence and circumcision are observed in Asia, though with HIV prevalence figures an order of magnitude lower. Countries where less than 20% of the male population are circumcised range from Cambodia (HIV prevalence 2.4%) to China (0.1%). In countries where more than 20% of men are circumcised, HIV prevalence figures range from the Philippines (0.1%) down to Bangladesh (0.03%) and what HIV these countries do have tends to be concentrated among sex workers and injecting drug users. In Muslim countries, there is a near-100% circumcision rate - which is at least part of the explanation for the continuing low HIV prevalence figures in middle-eastern countries.

Critics of the circumcision theory have suggested that Islam's prohibition of concurrent sexual partnerships may be the explanation, with circumcision a passive marker for being Muslim. As Halperin suggests, the two factors may work synergistically together but this does not explain the relatively low prevalence rates in largely Christian countries such as Ghana.

Non-randomised trials had already found that circumcision has a significant protective effect. In the one with the most dramatic findings, Thomas Quinn, who reported on circumcision at the 13th Retrovirus Conference in 2006, found that 40 of 137 uncircumcised male partners of HIV-positive women became infected. In contrast, there were no infections among the 50 circumcised men with HIV-positive partners.

Not all studies have shown such a dramatic protective effect, but there are virtually none that have shown no effect. A meta-analysis of 16 different circumcision studies by the UK's Medical Research Council demonstrated a protective effect identical to that seen in the Orange Farm study below - just over 70% (Weiss 2000). Individual study effects ranged from over 95% in the Quinn study (which was a comparatively small one) to around 30%. Only one study had findings that were not statistically significant.

The randomised controlled trials

The above is all that was known, in terms of epidemiological and non-randomised studies, until mid-2005. However, HIV prevention researchers had been sufficiently interested in the possibility of using circumcision as an HIV prevention tool that three randomised controlled trials of circumcision in (largely young) HIV-negative adult males were initiated in three different countries in Africa: one in the peri-urban township of Orange Farm in South Africa, one in the urban setting of the largely Luo city of Kisumu in Kenya, and the other in the rural setting of Rakai Province in Uganda on the opposite shore of Lake Victoria.

In each case, the trial was stopped early because the results were so conclusive (demonstrating that circumcision has anything between a 50% and a 75% protective effect against HIV infection in men) that it was considered unethical not to offer circumcision to the control group in advance of the trial's planned end date.

The South African trial

The first to report was the South African trial (Auvert), whose preliminary findings were announced at the Third International AIDS Society Conference on HIV Pathogenesis and Treatment in Rio de Janeiro in July 2005. This trial, conducted by the French research organisation INSERM, randomised 3,273 men aged 16 to 24 to be circumcised at the start of the trial or to be offered circumcision at the end of it, 21 months later.

At the point the trial was stopped, it had become apparent that there were only 35% as many infections in the circumcision arm as in the control arm, implying that circumcision can prevent at least six out of ten female-to-male HIV transmissions.

However, when the results were analysed according to true circumcision status rather than by intervention group, the protective effect went up to 75%. This is because there were 'crossovers' between the intervention and control arms in that some men randomised to be circumcised were not, and some in the control arm were.

Circumcisions in the intervention arm were carried out by a surgeon under local anaesthesia, and post-operative pain relief was also given. There had been no deaths or permanent adverse effects in any participant. Thirty-one per cent complained of pain and 15% initially had problems with the changed appearance of their penis.

HIV incidence was measured at three and twelve months into the trial and, finally, at 21 months (though the average follow-up period was in fact 20 months, due to the premature termination of the trial). Although all participants received intensive safer sex counselling and condoms, there were 51 HIV seroconversions in the control arm versus 18 in the circumcision arm. This translates as HIV incidences of 2.2% and 0.77% per year respectively. In the control arm there were nine, 15 and 27 new infections at three, 12 and 21 months and in the circumcision arm two, seven and nine.

"This is the first RCT demonstrating a strong protective effect of safe male circumcision," said Auvert. He added that, as a short-term study, it could not predict the long-term effect of circumcision, but that its compelling results demanded discussions on the use of circumcision as a public health measure.

Two more trials stopped early

The other two trials, involving 2784 men in Kisumu and 4996 men in Rakai, had not expected to finish data collection till February 2007 and December 2007 respectively.

However, the US National Institute of Allergy and Infectious Diseases (NIAID), part of the National Institutes of Health (NIH), halted both trials on 12 December 2006 because an interim review of trial data revealed similarly convincing results, though not quite such a strong protective effect as found in the INSERM trial. In the Kisumu trial the per-protocol protective effect was 53%, while in Rakai it was 51%.

An analysis using data from UNAIDS and the South African study published earlier in 2006 had estimated that if the full effect seen in the South African study were to be replicated when circumcision was taken up widely, three million HIV infections could be averted in Africa by 2026.

The World Health Organization and UNAIDS announced on 13 December that they would rapidly convene a consultation to examine the results of these trials to date and their implications for countries, particularly those in sub-Saharan Africa and elsewhere, that have high HIV prevalence and low male circumcision levels.

The Kisumu trial

Results from the Kisumu trial were published in TheLancet on 23 February 2007 (Bailey). By the time the trial was stopped, with an average follow-up time of 24 months after circumcision, 22 men out of 1391 in the intervention group and 47 out of

1393 in the control group had tested positive for HIV. The two-year HIV incidence was 2·1% in the circumcision group and 4·2 in the control group (p=0·0065); the relative risk of HIV infection in circumcised men was 0·47, which corresponds to a reduction in the risk of acquiring an HIV infection of 53% (95% confidence interval, 22%-72%).

Adjusting for non-adherence to treatment and excluding four men found to be HIV-positive at enrolment, the protective effect of circumcision was 60% - the same as that seen in the Rakai trial (see below). Adverse events related to the intervention (21 events in 1·5% of those circumcised) resolved quickly.

A study of the way infections accumulated after follow-up seemed to show that the beneficial effect of circumcision was only seen after 12 months - before this time infection rates in the intervention and control arms were identical, but then started to diverge. This supports other data cited below that people may be at elevated risk of HIV acquisition or transmission in the period immediately after circumcision.

There were some signs of behavioural disinhibition in circumcised men. One was the number of partners reported in the previous six months. There was a linear decrease across visits in the proportion of men in the control group reporting two or more partners in the previous 6 months, whereas the proportion reporting this same behaviour in the circumcision group fell from month 0 to month 6, but did not fall thereafter. This was statistically significant (p=~0.03).

Differences between the study groups were also found for unprotected sexual intercourse (p=0·0349) and consistent condom use (p=0·0326), with individuals in the control group practising the safer sexual behaviours. The researchers say that 'notably greater' numbers of circumcised men reported other risky behaviours, but that the differences were not significant.

Details of the Rakai trial

Ronald Gray, lead investigator of the Rakai trial, gave more details of this trial to the Fourteenth Conference on Retroviruses and Opportunistic Infections in Los Angeles in February 2007 (Gray and Wawer 2007). He said that the benefit of circumcision was probably greater than the preliminary efficacy of 51% would indicate. This is because the benefit, for reasons as yet unclear, appears to grow over time and because the highest-risk men, namely those who have multiple partners and/or genital ulcer disease, appeared to particularly benefit.

In the Rakai study the 4996 men randomised were aged 15-49, a wider age range than in the other two trials, which only randomised men aged 25 and under. They were randomised either to immediate circumcision or to be offered circumcision at the end of the two-year study. Fifty per cent of the men reported extramarital partners and 40% reported (inconsistent) condom use. Men who turned out to be HIV-positive on screening were referred to a parallel and ongoing study, looking at the effect of circumcision on HIV transmission by positive men.

The study was stopped early when interim analysis showed that in an 'intent-to-treat' analysis, the incidence of HIV infection in the circumcision group was reduced by 51%. It was 0.66 per 100 person years in the circumcised men and 1.33 per 100 person years among uncircumcised men. This difference was statistically significant (p = 0.007).

Gray told the conference that the protective effect of circumcision appeared to increase over time. HIV incidence for circumcised men was 1.19% a year from 0-6 months after circumcision, 0.42% from 6-12 months and 0.40% from 12-24 months. This reduction over time was statistically significant too (p=0.0014). The corresponding incidence rates in uncircumcised men for the same time periods were 1.58%, 1.19% and 1.19%.

Gray said he "had no idea" why the protective effect of circumcision appeared to increase over time, but speculated that it was due to increased keratinisation of the glans of the penis.

However, he added that, because of the premature stoppage of the trial, 73% of person-time had accrued, but only 44% of the men were in the second year of follow-up. If the study had continued as planned, the protective effect of circumcision over time might have been found to be stronger still.

There were also 'crossovers' between the intervention and control arms of the trial. There were 146 crossovers in the intervention arm, i.e. men who were randomised for circumcision but then did not go ahead with it, and 33 in the control arm, i.e. men who decided not to wait and got circumcised elsewhere. This means the 'as treated' efficacy of circumcision was greater that the 'intent to treat' efficacy.

Taking both these factors together and taking the 'as-treated' figures as if all men had stayed in the trial for 24 months, Gray calculated that the true efficacy of circumcision was 60% rather than 51%.

Gray added that circumcision appeared to offer greater benefit to higher-risk men.

The efficacy was 45% in men with one partner but 70% in men with two or more; it was 36% in men whose only sex was with their wives but 66% in men who had extramarital partners.

"It may be more efficacious in higher-risk people," he said. "This is possibly due to induced mucosal immune response in regular partners." In other words, because men acquire a degree of immunity to the HIV of regular partners, as other studies have demonstrated.

Effects on other STIs

Gray said that circumcision appeared to protect against some, but not all, other sexually transmitted infections.

Three per cent of circumcised men experienced genital ulcers, compared to 6% of uncircumcised men, a 47% difference which was statistically significant (p < 0.0001). However, rates of urethral discharge were identical between the two arms of the study, at 2%, as were rates of urethral pain at 3%. Gray commented that circumcision appeared to be protective against cutaneous skin lesions but not against internal STIs that attacked the urethral mucosa.

Genital ulcers were associated with a considerably increased risk of HIV acquisition. In men without genital ulcers, HIV incidence was 0.63 a year in circumcised men and 1.1% a year in uncircumcised men - an efficacy for circumcision of 34%. But HIV incidence in men with genital ulcers was 1.8% a year in circumcised men and 6.3% a year in uncircumcised men - a circumcision efficacy of 71%. Men with genital ulcers were 2.89 times more likely to get HIV if circumcised but 5.89 times more likely to get HIV if they were not circumcised - which again shows that circumcision offers more protection to men at higher risk of HIV.

Safety and side-effects

The circumcision operation takes 20-25 minutes. Moderate or severe side-effects following circumcision were reported by 4% of the men who remained HIV-negative and 3% of the men who became infected with HIV.

Gray said that adverse events reported in the Gates-funded trial of HIV-positive men were similar.

Eighty-one per cent of men reported that the operation wound was completely healed within 30 days, and 89% of men did not resume sex until the wound was certified healed.

After the trial closure, no less than 80% of the men in the control arm elected to be circumcised.

Just five (0.2%) of the men developed 'severe' side-effects, meaning they had to be recalled to hospital.

'Behavioural disinhibition' not so far seen in Rakai - seen in Kisumu

One great concern of the effect of circumcision - or indeed of any novel HIV prevention method - is that it might simply cause people (in this case men) to abandon previous risk-management behaviour such as partner reduction or condom use.

One study discussed at the 2006 CROI Conference (Quinn) found that if circumcision led to a perception in men that they were protected from HIV and could go back to having multiple partners, all the benefits of the measure would be lost. Using the same projections, if the average number of partners men had increased by 50% post-circumcision, HIV prevalence would increase by 40%, and if the average number of partners doubled, prevalence would more than double and would be higher than it was pre-circumcision.

Circumcision did not appear to affect sexual activity - there were no consistent or substantial differences in reported sexual risk behaviour between the two arms. In fact, condom use, though inconsistent, was slightly higher in circumcised men and alcohol use was slightly higher in uncircumcised men. This suggested that circumcision was not "disinhibiting" men, though Gray stressed that the men received much more intensive monitoring and support than they would if circumcision were to be rolled out as a national programme.

The Kisumu trial, however, did report some evidence of behavioural disinhibition. This may be related to the younger age of the men in the Kisumu trial, and may point to the need for additional post-operative safer-sex counselling for younger men.

The investigators believe that one strength of their study was the setting in which it was conducted - a public health facility where circumcision is provided, as opposed to the "highly controlled research settings where circumcision studies have been conducted."

The study was conducted between 2002 and 2004 among men attending the Siaya and Bondo district hospitals in Kenya. It involved 324 men undergoing elective circumcision and an equal number of demographically matched men remaining uncircumcised. Men joining the study provided sexual histories at enrolment to the study and returned for follow-up visits at which they provided details of their sexual activity throughout the first year following circumcision. The investigators defined "risky sex" as sexual intercourse with an individual other than the patient's wife or regular partner, and "unprotected risky sex" was sex without a condom with an individual other than a wife or regular partner. Data were also gathered on the frequency of sex acts.

The investigators found that men who chose to be circumcised were significantly more likely than men who chose to remain uncircumcised to have had risky sex in the three months *before* entry to the study (p = 0.025) and to have had unprotected risky sex during this period (p = 0.03).

In the month following circumcision, men undergoing the procedure were 60% less likely to report risky sex than men remaining uncircumcised, and 87% less likely than uncircumcised men to report unprotected risky sex. This is hardly surprising, and is probably due to healing of the penis following the circumcision operation and to the counselling about safer sex that the men received.

However, in the year following circumcision, there ceased to be any differences in the amount of risky or unprotected risky sex reported by circumcised and uncircumcised men. The investigators stress that: "at no point during this year was there any appreciable reported excess of risky sex or unprotected risky sex among circumcised men."

The most common reason cited for circumcision was protection from HIV/sexually transmitted infections (47%). Yet the investigators found that men who reported this motivation for circumcision were no more likely than those citing hygiene (24%), the avoidance of injuries during sex (14%), or the influence of friends (10%) to have risky or unprotected risky sex in the year after the operation.

Increased risk possible immediately post-operation

In March 2007, there was an interim analysis from the Data and Safety Monitoring Board of the complementary trial taking place in Rakai, which has been circumcising HIV-positive men and looking for possible effects on HIV incidence in their female partners.

It found that there *was* an increased risk to female partners of HIV-positive men if they were *not* sexually inhibited post-operation and had sex before the operation wound was certified as healed. There was even tentative evidence that this risk might extend beyond the time the wound was certified as healed.

These findings could not demonstrate if the opposite might also apply - if HIV-negative men would be at increased risk of infection if they had sex with an HIV-positive woman immediately post-circumcision - but it seems at least possible.

This trial involves 997 couples from the Rakai district of southern Uganda and the interim analysis looked at 124 discordant couples in which the man was HIV-positive. The risks, benefits, and safety of circumcision regarding the male partner were looked at, as was circumcision's impact on HIV transmission to the female partner.

In 25% of the couples that engaged in sexual activity before a physician had "certified" the man as being healed, HIV transmission took place (3/12 women). In those couples that abstained from sexual activity until wound healing was complete, transmission took place in 11% (6/55 women). In those couples where the man was not randomised to undergo circumcision, ~9% of the women became HIV-infected in this six-month study period (4/46 women).

Dr Maria Wawer, the study's principal investigator, said that because the total number of men who resumed sex before certified wound healing was so small, the finding of increased transmission after surgery may have occurred by chance alone.

"However, we need to err on the side of caution to protect women in the context of any future male circumcision programme," she added. "Women make up a majority of people living with HIV in Africa, and these results demonstrate that women need to be educated about the risks and benefits of male circumcision."

Many studies undertaken in Africa have shown that the risk of acquiring HIV, or any other sexually transmitted infection, is lessened for men who have undergone circumcision. These preliminary results caution that circumcision may not be effective in preventing male-to-female transmission and may even result in an increased risk of transmission, particularly in the first months after surgery.

"While male circumcision has extraordinary potential to prevent HIV infection, these new findings remind us that we must proceed with thought and care in developing strategies to expand male circumcision in Africa," said Dr Kevin De Cock, the head of the WHO's HIV/AIDS department. "Circumcision of adult males is a surgical intervention that needs to be performed by trained medical personnel, and issues such as wound healing, condom use, other prevention approaches, and HIV testing must be considered very carefully. Even under the best of conditions, male circumcision must be implemented as part of a comprehensive programme for HIV/AIDS prevention, treatment and care."

Might circumcision benefit women in the long term?

The question of whether circumcision might have an indirect protective benefit for women in the long term (more than six-12 months after surgery) remains to be answered.

There was tentative evidence from the Rakai trial that it might have some protective effect. In a study presented to CROI in 2006, Ronald Gray said that there was indirect evidence that circumcision might reduce female sexual partners by approximately one-third.

In an observational study involving individuals from the Rakai cohort in Uganda, the incidence of HIV infection was measured in 44 women with circumcised HIV-positive partners and 299 women with uncircumcised HIV-positive partners. Data were also collected on the incidence of syphilis, herpes simplex virus-2, gonorrhoea/chlamydia, human papilloma virus, bacterial vaginosis and trichomonas.

The incidence of HIV infection was just under seven infections per 100 person years for women with circumcised male partners compared to ten infections per 100 person years for women with uncircumcised partners.

However the difference was not statistically significant (p = 0.22).

The female partners of circumcised and uncircumcised men were equally likely to be infected with syphilis, gonorrhoea and chlamydia. However, the investigators noted that the partners of circumcised men had a lower risk of human papilloma virus, herpes simplex virus-2, trichomonas and bacterial vaginosis.

Circumcision may reduce the risk of HIV transmission because removal of the foreskin mucosa reduces the exposure of sexual partners to HIV, the investigators speculate. Another explanation could be that circumcision reduces the risk of genital ulcerative diseases such as herpes, a known risk factor for HIV infection. Conversely, it does not seem to reduce the transmission of diseases where urethral inflammation is a major symptom.

An earlier study from Rakai (Quinn 2000) had found statistically significant evidence that circumcision might have a role in protecting the female partner - but also that the effect of viral load may be crucial too. This suggests that the effects of circumcision and antiretroviral therapy might be synergistic in reducing HIV transmission.

This study showed an overall protective effect to the female partner of HIV-positive circumcised, compared with uncircumcised, men of 26%. This was statistically significant (p=<0.05).

But this depended on the man's viral load. If men had viral loads of over 50,000 copies/ml, circumcision had no protective effect for women. But among men with viral loads under 50,000 copies/ml, there were zero transmissions from circumcised men, compared with 26 transmissions from uncircumcised men, and this was highly statistically significant. Circumcision also appeared to protect women from acquiring bacterial vaginosis and trichomoniasis, but not other STIs.

Might circumcision benefit gay men?

There is not much literature on whether circumcision might reduce the risk of acquiring HIV in gay men. The HIV Network for Prevention Trials Vaccine Preparedness Study (Buchbinder) enrolled 3257 gay men in six US cities from 1995 to 1997. This was a longitudinal study, and HIV incidence was 1.55 per 100 person-years over 18 months of follow-up. Interestingly, the biggest difference in HIV seroconversion risk was between men who had had receptive *oral* sex to ejaculation with an

HIV-positive partner and men who had not. This difference was greater than the difference between men who'd had receptive anal sex and men who hadn't, though oral sex was responsible for a smaller number of infections (adjusted odds ratios 3.88 and 3.4).

Other significant risks were unprotected receptive anal sex with an HIV unknown serostatus partner (AOR 2.7), *protected* receptive anal sex with an HIV-positive partner (AOR 2.2), nitrite/poppers use (AOR 2.2), and not being circumcised (AOR 2.0). However, the biggest risk of all was having lots of partners - there was a 14% increase in the risk of HIV seroconversion with each additional partner.

The 'population attributable risk' or proportion of HIV infections that might be ascribed to a particular factor were 28% each to having multiple partners and using poppers, 25% for having receptive anal sex with a positive or a status-unknown partner, 10% to being uncircumcised and 7% for receptive oral sex because, although having receptive oral sex was considerably more risky than not having it, it was still not in itself associated with a lot of seroconversions.

The big surprises in this study were the findings on oral sex and on how significant poppers use was, but it's the first big study to show a doubling of HIV risk amongst uncircumcised gay men. However, this is not a randomised controlled trial and although the results are suggestive, they don't rule out differences in behaviour between circumcised and uncircumcised men as the cause.

One study (Grulich) has explored the relationship between circumcision and HIV transmission in gay men in Sydney, Australia. Between 1993 and 1999, a total of 74 gay men were interviewed soon after being diagnosed with recent HIV infection. The men were asked to nominate an unprotected sexual encounter with a serodiscordant or HIV status unknown partner during which they believed they became infected with HIV. When there was more than one possible high-risk event, the researcher chose the most likely occasion. Participants were also asked to report all episodes of unprotected anal intercourse in the six months before their seroconversion.

The researchers hypothesised that if the presence of a foreskin was important in HIV transmission, those men who had been infected by insertive unprotected anal intercourse would be more likely to be uncircumcised than those infected by receptive unprotected anal intercourse.

Sixty-three of the men nominated an event as their highest possible risk activity. For eleven men this was unprotected insertive anal intercourse, for 52 it was unprotected receptive anal intercourse. Ten of the eleven men who reported unprotected insertive intercourse as the most likely source of HIV infection reported no receptive unprotected anal intercourse in the six months before seroconversion and one reported receptive unprotected anal intercourse with a regular partner who was definitely HIV-negative.

In total, 20 of the men (27%) were circumcised. There was no association between circumcision and reporting insertive unprotected anal intercourse as the highest risk practice. Of the additional eleven men who denied unprotected anal intercourse as the event which they believed had led to their HIV infection, eight also denied having had unprotected anal intercourse in the previous six months. Of these eight, three were circumcised (38%).

The researchers found that 17% of gay men with newly acquired HIV infection reported insertive unprotected anal intercourse as their highest risk sexual activity. This suggests that insertive unprotected anal intercourse is an important means of HIV transmission in this population.

The researchers found no association between circumcision status and infection by insertive unprotected anal intercourse. Additionally, men who had seroconverted despite no reported event of unprotected anal intercourse were also more likely to be uncircumcised. The researchers suggested that this would imply that the foreskin is not the main source of HIV infection in gay men who become infected by insertive UAI, and that other sites, such as the distal urethra, must be important in HIV acquisition.

This study is limited by its small sample and it is possible that some men who reported receptive unprotected anal intercourse as their highest risk behaviour may have been infected by insertive unprotected anal intercourse. The researchers suggested that their data showing there is no difference in the circumcision status of men infected by receptive or insertive unprotected anal intercourse suggests that circumcision is not strongly protective against HIV infection in gay men. Further larger studies, preferably of prospective design, are needed to confirm the absence of a relationship between circumcision and HIV infection risk in gay men.

The WHO/UNAIDS recommendations

Whatever the effect on women and gay men, The World Health Organization (WHO) and UNAIDS recommended on 28 March 2007 that circumcision programmes should become part of HIV prevention programmes in countries seriously affected by HIV, following an expert consultation earlier that month.

Experts warned, however, that circumcision must not be relied upon as the sole means of protection against HIV. Dr Kevin De Cock of the World Health Organization's HIV department said that it will take "a number of years" before money spent on circumcision programmes will translate into any slowing of the epidemic.

Circumcision provides "important but incomplete protection" against HIV, said Dr De Cock, and is an "important but additional strategy" for HIV prevention programmes.

Dr Catherine Hankins of UNAIDS said: "It is partial protection for men and it's not to be scoffed at. We haven't had news like this in a long time. But it does not replace the need for promotion of safer sexual practices."

"High HIV prevalence, low circumcision prevalence countries with high rates of heterosexual transmission should consider adopting circumcision as a priority," said Dr De Cock. "We are primarily talking about the countries of southern and eastern Africa."

"The first consideration should be to scale up circumcision for adolescents and young sexually active men. Although circumcision in babies and young children is an important consideration, it will take 15 to 20 years to see the benefits."

"Scale up will take a long time and for this to have a population-level effect, coverage will have to be very high - we're talking about [rolling this out over] the next ten to twenty years," Dr De Cock went on.

Asked whether circumcision should be recommended for all HIV-negative men, not just men in countries with high HIV prevalence, Catherine Hankins said: "For individual men there can be a real benefit immediately."

Widespread changes in cultural attitudes would be needed, said Kim Dickson of WHO. However, it was important that any changes did not affect the human rights of males.

"It's very important that we don't create a new stigma around circumcision status," said Catherine Hankins. "In the case of adolescents, it's important that parents and health care providers recognise their evolving capacity to assent or withhold consent for the procedure."

Spokespersons for WHO and UNAIDS stressed that it would be up to individual countries to decide how to implement circumcision programmes. Once national assessments have been conducted, said Catherine Hankins, "PEPFAR, the Global Fund and the World Bank have all indicated they would be willing to fund."

WHO and UNAIDS are recommending that circumcision should be provided at no cost or at the lowest possible cost, and that it should be performed by medically trained personnel in order to reduce the risk of complications.

The possible public health benefits

A 2006 scientific modelling study (Williams) suggested that the widespread adoption of male circumcision throughout Africa could avert up to 5.7 million HIV infections by 2026.

If male circumcision reduced the risk of male acquisition of HIV by 60%, and did not encourage men to believe that they can have multiple sexual partners without taking precautions, African countries could begin to see marked reductions in HIV incidence within a few years of promoting adult male circumcision for all, the study suggested.

Male circumcision could avert two million new infections and 0.3 million deaths over the next ten years. It could avert a further 3.7 million infections and 2.7 million deaths by 2026.

One quarter of all infections and deaths averted would be in South Africa, the country with one of the lowest circumcision rates in Africa among the black African population.

Because circumcision reduces male vulnerability to HIV infection, the proportion of HIV-positive people who are women in sub-Saharan Africa would continue to grow, reaching 58% by 2026.

Among circumcised men in South Africa, HIV prevalence would be one-fifth lower than in uncircumcised men.

The study used data from UNAIDS on country HIV prevalence and from a 2004 survey of male circumcision in Africa, and made the following assumptions based on evidence from African research:

- Each case of HIV infection would generate approximately six further cases, assuming an average age of 27 at infection and a life expectancy of approximately ten years.

- 52% of those infected would be women

- Men were twice as likely to pass on HIV to women as women were to men

The authors of the study, who included epidemiologists from the World Health Organization, UNAIDS, the University of California, South Africa and France, warned that better data would be needed before these figures could be used to make public health policy decisions. In particular, better information was needed on HIV prevalence: UNAIDS prevalence estimates have a margin of error of up to 30%. Information on the prevalence of circumcision, the age at circumcision and the safety of current circumcision practices would also be needed.

However, the study was published before the announcement of the results from Rakai and Kisumu. The Rakai investigators used the findings from their trial to make further predictions as to the efficacy of circumcision in April 2007 (Gray 2007).

Gray worked out that as long as circumcised men don't start having more sexual partners because they feel safer, only half of the men targeted in mass circumcision programmes would have to undergo the operation if it was 60% effective, and only three-quarters if it was 50% effective, in order for a magic number called R_0 to become less than one. R_0 is important because it is the so-called Reproductive Number of an epidemic. It means the average number of people someone infects with a disease before they die of it.

In explosive epidemics such as flu, the R_0 is huge: in slow ones like AIDS it is smaller, but still has to be above one in order for the epidemic to grow. Below one, and the number of people with HIV will start to decline and the HIV epidemic will gradually wither away.

Gray found that the R_0 in areas of Africa likely to benefit from circumcision was currently 1.44. But it would go below one even if circumcision was only 40% effective, if more than three-quarters of uncircumcised men got circumcised.

In terms of cost, Gray calculated that a single circumcision operation would cost $US69.00. The number of surgeries per infection averted over 10 years would be 19-58, and the costs per infection averted would be $1269-3911, depending on the efficacy of circumcision for either or both sexes, assuming 75% service coverage.

"However," warned Gray, "behavioural disinhibition could offset any benefits of circumcision."

This may not necessarily be the case, according to two studies presented at the World AIDS Conference in Toronto in 2006. According to mathematical modelling done by Kyeen Mesesan of the Yale University Department of Public Health, if more than 63% of potential HIV infections are stopped by the widespread adoption of male circumcision - a rate consistent with that seen in the INSERM study - then there would be a net positive effect on HIV incidence in the population even if a 50% rate of consistent condom use went down to zero. This, at least, would be the situation in Soweto, South Africa.

Mesesan said that if the protective effect of circumcision were ignored, there would be 318,000 new HIV infections among the 823,000 sexually active adults in Soweto over the next 20 years. The overall HIV prevalence would increase from 16 to 23%.

If, however, a 35% rate of circumcision amongst the male population is assumed - that seen at baseline at Orange Farm - then 20-year prevalence would go down to 17% - a 1% increase - and the number of new infections over that period would decrease by 23%, to 244,000. If an additional 20% of men were circumcised in a mass prevention programme, then an additional 53,000 infections would be prevented - a further 22% decrease - and the 20-year prevalence rate would be 14%, or 2% lower than it is today.

If overall condom use (currently about 50% in South Africa, according to other surveys) decreased to 35%, then such a mass programme would only prevent 18,000 new infections. However the protective effect of circumcision is such that if the protective effect seen in the intent-to-treat analysis of the Orange Farm was the true effect, then condom use could fall to 3% before the benefit of such a 20% circumcision programme was completely lost. If the protective effect was 63%, all men could stop using condoms and there would still be a neutral effect on new HIV infections.

Jim Kahn of the University of California, San Francisco said that assuming a cost per circumcision of $55.75, the cost of a mass male circumcision programme where HIV prevalence was 8.4% - regardless of the programme's actual coverage - would be $550 per HIV infection averted, but that when antiretroviral and other treatment costs were taken into account, there would be a net saving of $753 per circumcision. He said that circumcision would be a cost-saving measure at any efficacy above 21%.

However, these mathematical models are dependent on there being a high baseline incidence in the population and they might not work in lower-incidence areas.

Reactions in Africa

The news from the trial caused huge debate in Africa, with widely different reactions from country to country.

In Swaziland, where a third of the entire population has HIV, there has been soaring demand for the operation, even in advance of the news from the randomised controlled trials.

The Swazi health ministry is keen to roll out a mass circumcision programme, and is waiting for advice from the World Health Organisation on how best to do it. The problem is not publicising circumcision. The news is already out, and desperate Swazi men are besieging the clinics, which are already offering mass 'circumcision days'. However clinics have to turn away more than half the men who present for circumcision, due to lack of trained personnel, according to newspaper reports.

But in Uganda, where near-Swazi levels of HIV prevalence in the late 1980s have declined to around 6.5%, the country's president said in February 2006 that he had fears that circumcision would give people licence to "behave recklessly".

President Yoweri Museveni told the PLUSNEWS Agency that he was worried that the news about circumcision would dilute the message that the only way to protect yourself from HIV was to "avoid all risky sexual behaviour".

Referring to reports that HIV prevalence in Uganda has started to creep up again and that the annual new infection rate has doubled since 1993, President Museveni said: "I am worried that HIV infections have started to rise, and people think HIV is no longer there. So abstain till you get a regular partner."

He added: "These days there are many confusing messages: one of them is that if you are circumcised, you are less likely to catch AIDS even if you behave recklessly - now what sort of message is that?"

Would circumcision be accepted in African countries? Studies done between 2002 and 2005 in six African countries found that between 40% (Zimbabwe) and 65% (south Africa, Botswana, Kenya) of men said they would be willing to be circumcised if it protected them from HIV. In South Africa, Botswana and Kenya, parents were asked about their sons. South African fathers weren't sure: 50% said they would have their sons circumcised. But 70-75% of fathers in Botswana and Kenya said they'd be willing to have their sons circumcised, as did 75-85% of mothers.

Circumcision in the developed world

There has been relatively little consideration so far of whether circumcision has a part to play in the more focal epidemics in the developed world. Gay men are likely to wait to see if randomised controlled studies show circumcision has any protective effect for the receptive partner in anal sex - if such studies ever get done.

The only country where there has been a level of public debate is the USA - ironically, as about 70% of men in the USA are already circumcised. However, only 42% of non-US born men living in the USA are circumcised and, perhaps significantly, fewer African-American (65%) and Hispanic (58%) men.

In Europe, circumcision rates are less than half of those in the US, and are only about 20% in the UK, with only 12.5% of boys circumcised as infants and the others getting circumcised when older, usually for medical reasons.

On 5 April 2007, however, the *New York Times* reported (McNeil) that the city's Department of Health and Mental Hygiene was planning a campaign to encourage men at high HIV risk to get circumcised - though this was denied in a letter a week later.

In the USA there is also a vocal anti-circumcision lobby. These self-dubbed 'intactivists' regard circumcision as 'male genital mutilation' and regard the risks of circumcision as outweighing the benefits - a debatable position in countries where circumcisions are performed safely.

They also say that being circumcised reduces sexual pleasure, and here they have some evidence to back them up. Some studies in both developed countries and Africa show a higher rate of sexual dysfunction in older circumcised men compared with uncircumcised men.

One recent study (Sorrells) subjected men to a "Semmes-Weinstein monofilament touch-test." In other words, they stimulated circumcised and uncircumcised men's penises with a fine probe and mapped the relative sensitivity of different areas "to map the fine-touch pressure thresholds of the penis", in the words of the researchers. They found that uncircumcised men had significantly lower pressure thresholds, i.e. were sensitive to a much lighter touch.

Sorrells found, furthermore, that "The transitional region from the external to the internal prepuce is the most sensitive region of the uncircumcised penis and is more sensitive than the most sensitive region of the circumcised penis." In other words, they found that parts of the foreskin are more sensitive than the glans and that circumcision "ablates the most sensitive parts of the penis".

Whether circumcised men compensate for this by trying other sexual techniques - as some other studies suggest they do - was not within the remit of the study. But it does add fuel to the considerable controversy about circumcision that is building up in the USA.

References

Auvert B et al. *Impact of male circumcision on the female-to-male transmission of HIV.* IAS Conference on HIV Pathogenesis and treatment, Rio de Janeiro, abstract Tu0a0402, 2005.

Bailey RC et al. *Male circumcision for HIV prevention in young men in Kisumu, Kenya: a randomisedcontrolled trial.* Lancet 369: 643-56. 2007.

Beegle K, Özler B. *Young Women, Rich(er) Men, and the spread of HIV.* Development Research Group, The World Bank, Unpublished paper.

Buchbinder SP et al. *Sexual risk, nitrite inhalant use, and lack of circumcision associated with HIV seroconversion in men who have sex with men in the United States.* JAIDS 39(1):82-9. 2005.

Gray R et al. *The impact of male circumcision on HIV incidence and cost per infection prevented: a stochastic simulation model from Rakai, Uganda.*AIDS 21(7):845-850.2007.

Gray R, Wawer M et al. *Randomized trial of male circumcision for HIV prevention in Rakai, Uganda* and *Effects of male circumcision on genital ulcer disease and urethral symptoms, and on HIV acquisition: an RCT in Rakai, Uganda.* Fourteenth Conference on Retroviruses and Opportunistic Infection, Los Angeles, abstract nos. 155aLB and 155bLB, 2007.

Grulich AE et al. *Circumcision and male-to-male sexual transmission of HIV.* AIDS 15: 1188-89. 2001.

Halperin D, Bailey R. *Male circumcision and HIV infection: 10 years and counting.* Lancet 354:1813-15. 1999.

Kahn JG. *Cost-effectiveness of male circumcision in sub-Saharan Africa.* Sixteenth International AIDS Conference, Toronto. Abstract TUAC0204. 2006.

Kawango EA et al. *Male circumcision in Siaya and Bondo districts, Kenya: prospective cohort study to assess behavioural disinhibition following circumcision.* J Acquir Immune Defic Syndr 44: 66 - 70, 2007.

Laumann EO et al. *Circumcision in the United States: Prevalence, Prophylactic Effects, and Sexual Practice.* JAMA 277(13): 1052-1057.

McNeil DG. *New York CityPlans to Promote Circumcision to Reduce Spread of AIDS.* NewYork Times, 5 April 2007.

Mesesan K et al. *The potential benefits of expanded male circumcision programs in Africa: predicting the population-level impact on heterosexual HIV transmission in Soweto.* Sixteenth International AIDS Conference, Toronto, abstract TUAC0203, 2006.

Quinn T. *Viral Load and Heterosexual Transmission of Human Immunodeficiency Virus Type 1.* NEJM 342(13): 921-929 2000.

Quinn T. *Circumcision and HIV transmission: the cutting edge.* Plenary presentation. Thirteenth Conference on Retroviruses and Opportunistic Infections, Denver, abstract 120, 2006.

Timberg C. *In Swaziland, science revives an old rite: circumcision makes a comeback to fight AIDS in virus-ravaged African nation.* Washington Post, 26 December 2005.

Sorrells ML et al. *Fine-touch pressure thresholds in the adult penis.* British Journal of Urology, 9 9, 8 6 4 - 8 6 9. 2007.

Weiss H et al. Male circumcision and risk of HIV infection in sub-Saharan Africa: a systematic review and meta-analysis. AIDS14(15):2361-70, 2000.

Williams BG et al. *The potential impact of male circumcision on HIV in sub-Saharan Africa.* PloS Medicine 3 (7): e262, 2006.

D is for disclosure, serosorting and negotiated safety

Compare the two charts below from the San Francisco Department of Public health's 2004 HIV Epidemiology Report (2004):

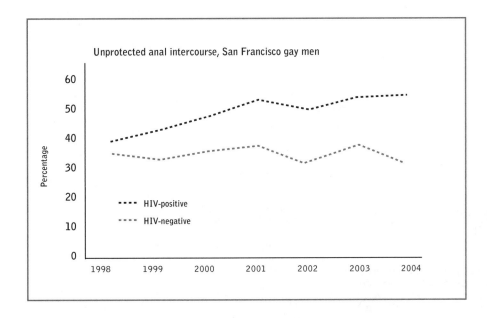

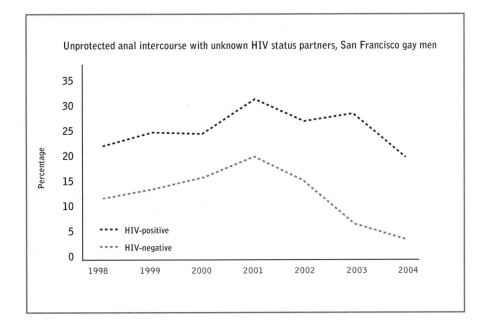

among a community - has declined from a peak in 2001 among both positive and negative men.

Similarly, in the UK, a decline in serodiscordant unprotected sex may be starting to happen too, and amongst gay men. and among positive men the decline appears to be more dramatic. The annual survey of gay men using London gyms (Elford 2005b) between January and March each year, in which so far more than 5,000 gay men have participated, found last year that the amount of serodiscordant unprotected sex increased between 1998 and 2002, but has remained stable since then or slightly declined among HIV-negative men, and has declined significantly (p=<0.05) in HIV-positive men, from a peak of 41% in 2002 to 20% in 2005 (see chart next page).

How can gay men be having *more* unprotected sex while at the same time having *less* sex of the kind that could spread HIV?

Clearly, by increasing the proportion of unprotected sex they have with men with the same HIV status.

The phenomenon by which HIV comes to be brought under better control by people seeking out sex partners with their own HIV status has become called **Serosorting,** and is usually applied specifically to situations where unprotected sex is being sought.

Serosorting may be one reason why an increase in STIs in gay men, especially syphilis, has not led to a concomitant increase in HIV infections. This has shaken an assumption previously used by many HIV epidemiologists - that increases in STI rates can be used as surrogate markers or predictors of increases in HIV.

The first shows that unprotected anal sex (any episode over the previous six months) was practised by about a third of HIV-negative men consistently from 1998 to 2004, with very little change. In contrast the proportion of HIV-positive men having unprotected sex went up during the same period from 38% to 52%.

The second chart, however, shows that these high and (in positive men) increasing levels of unprotected sex did not translate into increasing levels of unsafe sex. The amount of *potentially serodiscordant* sex - the true measure of the degree of HIV risk

This has found not to be the case. In the US huge increases in syphilis in gay men have not coincided with equally big increases in HIV. (Conversely, in certain African countries like Zimbabwe, STI rates have gone down while HIV incidence has not, because more HIV infections are now occurring within marriages and fewer within casual encounters (Gisselquist, 2003).

This was first noticed in 2003 when two US cities, Seattle and San Francisco, noticed that HIV incidence among gay men attending for HIV tests was starting to decline even though syphilis rates had increased 25-fold (Buchacz, 2004). At the time this was partly put down to a lot of syphilis being spread via oral

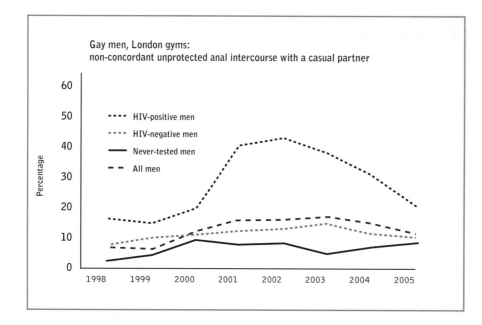

Gay men, London gyms:
non-concordant unprotected anal intercourse with a casual partner

- - - - HIV-positive men
- - - - HIV-negative men
——— Never-tested men
- - - All men

In a backroom or anonymous sex situation, people's HIV status is deduced by their status. The lack of insistence on a condom is assumed by a positive man to be a sign that the other is positive ("He must be positive or he wouldn't let me do that"). A negative man makes the opposite assumption ("If he was positive he would protect me and use a condom").

The 2002 UK Gay Men's Sex Survey *Out and About* makes the false assumptions gay men make about other's status very clear - and underlines the disincentive many HIV-positive men have to disclose.

A summary of the survey's findings on **aidsmap** says:

sex, and particularly among gay men, as they were unaware of this transmission route. However only 25% of syphilis, it was thought, was being spread orally. Syphilis is also more contagious than HIV so can spread more rapidly through a connected network of sexual partners.

But Dr Jeffrey Klausner, San Francisco Health Department's Director of STI Prevention, commented at the 11th Retrovirus Conference where these findings were presented that there was a lot of evidence that much of the lack of a rise in HIV was due to serosorting.

This phenomenon - of concentrating the unprotected sex you have with people of the same HIV status - was previously thought to be rare.

Serosorting is one example of 'negotiated safety'. In the previous edition of the AIDS Reference Manual it was thought, as an HIV prevention strategy, to be quite uncommon, particularly in the UK. It quoted findings from Edinburgh and Glasgow that negotiated safety in the light of full knowledge about HIV status was still rare. Research conducted in 1996 showed that only 16% of men questioned were having unprotected anal sex in a relationship were doing so in the light of knowledge about both partner's HIV status, compared with 60% of men in Australia.

However serosorting may be an important way by which HIV-positive men attempt to reduce the risk of their passing on HIV to others. In one US study (Lightfoot, 2005) of young US gay men (most of them black or Latino) aged 15-24, about 34% of youth with multiple partners and 28% with one primary partner had unprotected anal intercourse.

However they were overwhelmingly more likely to have unprotected sex with other partners *perceived* to be HIV-positive than with partners whose HIV status was negative or unknown.

In some cases the perception was probably accurate. The estimated number of instances of unprotected sex was 32 times greater among youth in a committed relationship if their regular partner was thought to be positive than if he was thought to be negative but at high risk of having other STIs (eg in an open relationship), and 18 times more if he was thought unlikely to have STIs (eg if thought monogamous). In at least some of these cases, the HIV status of the partners must have been known, rather than just a perception.

However, it is the word 'perceived' that has made HIV prevention workers very wary of encouraging serosorting as an HIV prevention technique. Attempting to guess a partner's HIV status, many studies have shown, is doomed to failure, especially as many so-called 'negotiations' do not take place with words.

"Of the participants whose most recent HIV test was negative, two-thirds (65.3%) said they would expect an HIV-positive man to disclose his status before having sex. Even more men who had never tested for HIV had the same expectation (77%). In contrast only just over a third of HIV-positive men expected that a partner would disclose their HIV status.

44% of HIV-negative or untested men said they would not want to have sex with the man who'd just disclosed his HIV status to them - and this rose to 56% of men who had never had an HIV test.

Report authors Sigma Research comment: "Expectations that men with HIV will tell a prospective sexual partner their HIV status are still widespread. Over a third of men not tested [HIV] positive both expected a positive partner to disclose their status prior to sex and would not want to have sex with them if they did.

"In this climate, it is difficult to see what incentive men with HIV have for disclosing their status."

In addition, significant numbers of gay men do not know their HIV status. In the year 2000 Gay Men's Sex Survey (*Time for More*), 44% of respondents had never tested for HIV, but of those only 1.3% thought they were 'probably or definitely positive'.

Even if a lot of the others are correct that they are negative, this is still only an eighth of the 10.9% prevalence reported from another survey of gay men in UK cities (Dodds, 2004). Of the HIV-positive men in this survey, who were tested anonymously with an oral saliva test, a third (32.5%) were unaware of their infection and over one in five (21.2%) said their last HIV test was negative.

In these circumstances, how can making safer-sex decisions on the basis of a partner's HIV status possibly be a way of not being infected or infecting someone? The idea that serosorting or making other safer-sex decisions on the basis of a partner's HIV status can possibly contribute to HIV prevention is a challenge to orthodox HIV prevention approaches, and makes many people deeply uneasy:

- As above, people may be making decisions on the basis of assumptions or inaccurate information

- It relies on disclosure - something still practices by a minority of gay men with HIV. In one unpublished survey by Gay Men Fighting AIDS, only 20% of respondents said they always disclosed their HIV status (positive or negative) to partners, forty per cent said they sometimes did, and forty per cent said they never did.

- It is seen as diluting the 'use a condom' message and providing ways for men to rationalise unsafe behaviour

- 'Serosorting' men can do things that at first look like ways of wilfully increasing their HIV risk rather than reducing it. For instance, gay men who advertise for 'bareback' sex may seem to be nothing other than irresponsible. If however 'bareback' is a code for 'HIV-positive', or if bareback discussions lead to disclosure of HIV status, the net result may be a paradoxical isolation of HIV within a specific group.

- Even if this is the case, HIV-positive men having unprotected sex together are still vulnerable to other STIs and possibly (especially during the first three years of infection) to infection with a second strain of HIV ('superinfection').

- All 'negotiated safety' unprotected sex strategies between men of differing HIV status are likely to involve a considerably greater risk or HIV infection than protected sex does.

However there is indirect evidence that a lot of HIV-positive men, in particular *are* at least attempting to restrict their unprotected sex to other HIV-positive men. The debate around this kind of 'negotiated safety' centres on this dilemma:

- Should prevention messages concentrate on the fact that these practices still involve considerable HIV risk, and should therefore be discouraged?

- Or, since the gay men (and heterosexuals, though negotiated safety among heterosexuals is less well studied) who use these strategies to minimise HIV risk are unlikely to be persuaded back to consistent condom use, should prevention messages encourage behaviours that enable them to happen, such as disclosure of HIV status?

In one analysis of the ongoing survey of gay men attending London gyms (Elford, 2001), the authors detected two very different strategies being adopted by HIV-positive and negative gay men to avoid infection.

In HIV-negative men what the authors call "concordant UAI" and we call serosorting was mainly restricted to main partners. Over one in four (28.6%) practised it with their primary partner and only five per cent with casual partners.

In HIV-positive men concordant UAI was equally practised with main partners (22.2%) and with casual partners (20.6%).

These unprotected sexual encounters were those restricted to ones where men were fairly sure their partner was of the same HIV status. If all men had an equal tendency to be uncertain or to be making decisions on the basis of assumption, the authors argue, one would expect the lower proportion of unprotected encounters with *casual* partners to apply to both HIV-negative and positive men. The significantly greater difference can only be explained, at least in part, by the fact that it is possible for HIV-positive men to disclose their status with certainty:

"Seroconcordance among negative men can only be established with confidence if both men test for HIV together. For this reason it is difficult for HIV-negative men to establish concordance with a casual partner.

"On the other hand, HIV-positive men can establish concordance, be it with a casual or regular partner, simply by mutual disclosure. This requires no confirmatory test."

They add a caution: "Although seroconcordant UAI among positive men carries no risk of HIV transmission to an uninfected person, it raises the possibility of reinfection and drug resistance for the men themselves."

But is this disclosure actually taking place?

The internet as disclosure venue

Concern has been expressed in recent years that the huge increase in sexual encounters being arranged on the internet may be facilitating an upsurge in unprotected sex. This concern has been fuelled by the rise in the number of explicit 'barebacking' sites.

In a more recent study by the same group of researchers (Bolding, 2005), four groups of gay men (internet chatroom users, London gym users, HIV-positive men attending clinics, and HIV-negative men attending for an HIV test) were asked about their patterns of unprotected sex and internet use.

HIV-positive men in the clinic and gym samples who used the internet to look for sex were significantly more likely to report unprotected anal sex with men of the same HIV status than were other men (p < 0.05).

The investigators also established that in both the clinic and gym samples, HIV-positive and HIV-negative men who used the internet to find sex were more likely to report non-concordant unprotected anal sex with a casual partner than other men (p < 0.05).

So far, this looks as if the internet is facilitating increased levels of unsafe sex.

But the investigators found that internet users were also more likely to have *concordant* unprotected sex, i.e. to 'serosort'.

In all samples, HIV-positive men who looked for sex through the internet were significantly more (p <0 .05) likely to report concordant unprotected anal sex with a partner they met online rather than off-line. For example, 10% of the clinic sample reported concordant unprotected unprotected anal sex with a man they met on-line, and only four per cent said they had had concordant unprotected sex with a man met off-line.

What's more, the investigators found that amongst the HIV-positive clinic sample, men said that they were more likely to disclose their HIV status to men met online (24%) than men met off-line (14%, p < 0.001).

They also found that the apparent causal link between internet use and *serodiscordant* unprotected sex was an artefact. When asked directly about *how they met* partners they subsequently had unprotected sex with, there was no evidence that gay men, whether HIV-positive, negative or untested, were more likely to meet partners for discordant unprotected anal sex online rather than off-line.

For example, among HIV-negative men in the internet sample, 10% reported non-concordant unprotected anal sex with men met online only, 11% with men met off-line only, and six per cent with men met on- and off-line. "In fact," note the investigators, "for HIV-negative men in the clinic and gym samples, the reverse pattern was seen; they were more likely to report non-concordant unprotected anal sex with a casual partner met off-line."

In other words internet meets were more likely to result in unprotected sex which was concordant: serodiscordant unprotected sex was at least as likely to occur during casual encounters.

"What is new about this study is that we can establish whether the excess risk of HIV and sexually transmitted infections seen among gay men who looked for sex through the internet actually occurred with the men they met online", write the investigators.

"In our study, HIV-positive men who looked for sex through the internet were more likely to meet other HIV-positive men with whom they had (concordant) unprotected anal intercourse online rather than off-line ", note the investigators. They add "Men who looked for sex through the internet were no more likely to meet their non-concordant unprotected anal intercourse partners online than off-line. This was seen for HIV-positive, HIV-negative and never-tested men alike."

The investigators suggest that the internet may provide a safe space for HIV-positive men to disclose their health status, 'thus facilitating "filtering" or "serosorting' of sexual partners'.

This is not the only study that suggests the internet is being used by HIV-positive men as a safe place in which to disclose and negotiate the level of sexual safety they want.

A study presented at the 2005 Retrovirus Conference (Chiasson, 2005) of users of 14 US-based gay websites found that 28.5% of men had unprotected sex during their last encounter.

However twice as many instances of unprotected sex happened after casual offline encounters that after internet meets.

And online meets, however, were more likely to involve discussion of HIV status. More than half of the men who had met online had discussed their HIV status before sex as opposed to a third of partners who met offline.

The authors comment: "The large number of men on-line and the diversity of their risk and ways of meeting partners show that the Internet provides a unique opportunity for far-reaching behavioural interventions."

Does serosorting work?

No rigorous longitudinal study has yet been done to find out if HIV-positive serosorters transmit HIV less often, and given that research on serosorting has mainly been carried out on gay men who may have multiple casual partners, this may be difficult to establish. However there is epidemiological evidence that serosorting has *some* impact on HIV incidence - or, at least, has done so in San Francisco (Russell).

This impact, however, is relatively slight and may be cancelled out by other demographic or behavioural changes.

In March 2006, San Francisco Department of Public Health epidemiologist Dr Willi McFarland concluded that estimates of ongoing HIV incidence among gay men in the city should be reduced by a 'disappointing' 10% per year.

This was disappointing because 2005 results from HIV clinics (see Centers for Disease control) had suggested that HIV incidence in among gay men in the city had declined from 2.2% a year - an estimate unchanged since 2000 - to 1.2% in 2004, a difference attributed to the increased practice of serosorting.

"It hasn't changed that much," McFarland told the *San Francisco Chronicle*, "but the fact is, we've reversed a trend. There is some evidence that our efforts at prevention are working."

In fact, the new estimates did conclude that the actual infection rate among gay men in San Francisco had declined substantially, by about 20% since 2001. However it also found that this decrease has been offset by a 25% increase in the city's gay male population during those five years.

Hopes were raised in June 2005 that the city's rate of new infections might be lowered as much as 40% after the Centers for Disease Control study came out. However, after months of analysing fresh data from a dozen programs that track the epidemic in the city, McFarland opted for a more conservative revision.

Since 2001, the city's official estimate has been that each year 1,084 residents become infected with HIV, the virus that causes AIDS. The new estimate is 976 - 87% of them gay men.

McFarland stressed that the science of making these estimates is far less precise than the un-rounded numbers might suggest. Into the mix of data used to make these estimates are new HIV cases reported from public clinics, scattered reports from private doctors and centres that provide anonymous tests, and findings that track trends in sexual behaviour that may affect future infection rates.

McFarland said the most surprising finding in his analysis was the increase in the population of gay men in San Francisco. Because there are no census data based on sexual orientation, it has always been difficult to come up with a number. Based on nine surveys, the health department estimates that the number of gay men living in San Francisco is 58,000, a 25% increase from 47,000 in 2001.

It is easier to make an estimate of the degree to which 'serosorting' - most of which might more properly be called negotiated safety - works in HIV-negative people, as one can ask HIV seroconverters about whether they had attempted to restrict their sexual risk behaviour to other HIV-negative people.

At a study presented at CROI, Matthew Golden of the University of Washington, Seattle Center for AIDS and Sexually transmitted Diseases came up with a figure: he estimated that serosorting among HIVV negative gay men was reducing the number of infections that might otherwise have occurred by about 40%.

Golden looked at what he called "The practice of preferentially choosing sex partners, or deciding not to use condoms with selected partners, based on their disclosed, concordant HIV status."

Data from Golden's clinic found that HIV-positive patients were particularly likely to serosort. Forty and 49% of his HIV-positive patients, respectively, had unprotected receptive and insertive sex with HIV-positive partners but only 3% and 6%, respectively, with HIV-negative partners.

In his HIV-negative patients 31% and 37%, respectively, had unprotected receptive and insertive sex with HIV-negative partners, and 19% and 15% respectively had unprotected receptive and insertive sex with HIV-positive partners - less, though still a surprisingly high figure.

"Where the whole system breaks down," however, Golden commented, "is where the other partner is of unknown status." Here partners were almost equally likely to have unprotected insertive sex regardless if their own status or if the partner's was unknown. In the case of receptive sex, there was some evidence that positive gay men were attempting to adopt 'strategic positioning'. HIV-positive men were somewhat more likely (31% vs 24%) to have unprotected receptive rather than insertive sex with partners of unknown status; conversely HIV-negative men were somewhat less likely (16% vs 22%. Golden did not say whether any of these differences reached statistical significance.

Golden then investigated whether serosorting was actually reducing the number of serodiscordant partners that gay men had, regardless of condom use. The answer was yes. In a population like Seattle where 15% of gay men have HIV (not dissimilar to London), if gay men chose partners completely at random, and if they all had the mean number of partners rather than a few having many and many having a few, you would expect 54% of gay men to have at least one serodiscordant relationship per year (with the figure obviously lower for people with few partners and higher for those with many).

In fact about 35% of gay men had had at least one serodiscordant partner, so serosorting appeared to be reducing the number of serodiscordant relationships by about 40%, though Golden also suggested some of this was due to the fact that gay men tend to have sex with men fairly near their own age, and that because young men are less likely to have HIV than older men, some of this concordance was purely due to age similarity. Golden also found that 13-18% of gay men were 'exclusive serosorters', i.e. only had unprotected sex with seroconcordant partners.

Is serosorting actually protective? When it comes to HIV-negative men, Golden found that the rate of new HIV diagnosis among patients who had unprotected sex but tried only to do it with same-status partners (2.6%) was intermediate between men who had unprotected sex regardless (4.1%) and men who attempted always to use condoms (1.5%).

Adjusting for the number of partners, whereas condom use was 76% effective in preventing new HIV infections, serosorting was about 40% effective.

As a 'control', Golden also looked at the rate of STIs and in this case, as you would expect, there was no difference in the STI rates between serosorters and non-serosorters.

Viral load and negotiated safety

HIV status is not the only thing that can be disclosed by men attempting to minimise their HIV risk. Several recent studies have found that gay men are questioning each other about their HIV viral load in order to try and establish if they are infectious. "Are you undetectable?" is becoming as common a chatroom question as "are you poz?"

In a study from San Francisco (Goldhammer, 2005) 78% of 507 gay men questioned were familiar with the term 'viral load' and one third (111 of the total sample) had discussed viral load with a partner of a different HIV status during the previous year in order to make decisions about which sexual practices to engage in.

Of those who had discussed viral load, more than half estimated that they used viral load disclosure to guide sexual decision-making in at least 70% of their sexual encounters. In another study from Sydney (Van de Ven, 2005) researchers asked 119 men who were in an HIV-serodiscordant regular relationship about whether they used viral load as a basis for their decisions on condom use. Twice as many (39.4%) reported unprotected anal intercourse when the partner's HIV last viral load test was undetectable as when it was detectable (20.8%).

HIV-negative couples and negotiated safety

Another major way in which HIV testing is already affecting sexual behaviour has been described as 'negotiated safety' by Australian researchers. (This has also been called 'serosorting' or 'HIV-negative serosorting').

'Negotiated safety' refers to an agreement between partners about sexual practices which takes into account the HIV antibody status of both partners. Australian and British researchers observed that gay men who had taken the HIV test were having unprotected sex, and doing so with other men who also knew their antibody status. These men had worked out agreements about sexual activity outside the relationship that were designed to minimise the risk of infection within the relationship if it was not sexually exclusive.

These strategies were a consequence of the availability of HIV antibody testing from 1985 onward, but they were not promoted by HIV prevention campaigns. Indeed, most HIV prevention campaigns around the world have consistently promoted the message "Positive or negative, it's all the same" as a means of encouraging solidarity between infected and uninfected men.

Nevertheless, despite such messages, a significant minority of gay men adopted 'negotiated safety strategies' because they were preferable to the continued use of condoms.

Since such strategies were first identified many people have argued that it is unreasonable to assume that long-term condom use is sustainable for the majority of gay men (Odets; King). A proportion of gay men will still continue to have unprotected sex, and the job of HIV prevention ought to be to facilitate the safe practice of unprotected sex, they argue.

This has been a difficult notion to accept in some quarters, for it appears to undermine the continued promotion of condom use. Yet research suggests that in practice gay men in particular are already using information about their HIV status to guide sexual practice, and that many gay men are much more careful about condom use with casual partners than they are with primary partners (Coxon). In his review of the SIGMA cohort data, Tony Coxon identified a number of worrying trends that are particularly important to consider in relation to debates about 'negotiated safety':

- Those who engage most frequently in unprotected sex generally restrict their unprotected sexual activity to one partner who has the same HIV status

- But, nearly 50% of all men interviewed invert any notion of 'negotiated safety' by having unprotected sex with casual partners and regular partners, or else using condoms with their regular partner whilst having unprotected sex with one-off casual partners

- Those not tested tend to have the highest-risk sex, primarily with those known to be negative.

However, Coxon also observes:

- The non-use of condoms is often as much a matter of waiting for the partner to object as it is a pre-negotiated condition (i.e. it happens by default)

- "paradoxically the group which overwhelmingly exhibits close conformity to the ideal of choice, responsibility and negotiation...are those already diagnosed HIV- positive."

These findings present a number of significant problems. They suggest that much unprotected sex is unnegotiated (verbally, at least), and whilst it may not lead to HIV infection with any greater frequency than unprotected sex with regular partners, it will present significant problems to anyone trying to develop 'negotiated safety' approaches to HIV prevention.

For example, negotiated approaches rely on trust. One of the major criticisms of this approach is the degree to which it relies upon the honesty and trust of both partners. Given the degree to which personal relationships are bedeviled by problems of honesty and trust, it is a little difficult to imagine such agreements working well for some people.

Many partnerships have agreements about no sex outside the relationship, but these agreements are broken frequently. Sometimes the other partner will find out, but often they will not, because the partner who has been 'playing away' is scared of the consequences for the relationship. If any agreement about unprotected sex outside the relationship is tied up with an agreement about no other sexual activity outside the relationship, this may reduce the incentive for honesty if a lapse in the agreement does occur.

When does negotiated safety work?

Australian researchers recently looked at whether making explicit agreements about unprotected sex had any effect on the likelihood that men would have unprotected sex outside their primary relationship. They looked at 165 men in seroconcordant HIV-negative relationships. 61% had engaged in unprotected anal intercourse at some point. The researchers found that amongst this group the following factors were associated with a lower likelihood of having unprotected sex with casual partners and with a primary partner (Kippax).

- Having an agreement about unprotected sex outside the relationship

- Agreement included no anal sex with casual partners.

Men who found condom use unacceptable were more likely to have unprotected anal sex with their casual partners. No other demographic or behavioural factors were found to be significant.

HIV-negative serosorting?

There is also some evidence from Australia that HIV-negative men may be beginning to find it possible to engage in what one might call 'true serosorting' rather than negotiated safety. That is, increasingly disclosing and attempting to establish their partner's status in casual as opposed to committed unprotected sex situations.

Limin Mao and colleagues from Sydney looked at the serosorting behaviour of gay men known to be HIV-negative between 2002 and 2005. Although these men were not explicitly asked if they had "serosorted," this behaviour was inferred from information they provided about unprotected sex with casual partners.

The 302 men enrolled in the study were asked to provide details of the total number of casual partners they had unprotected anal sex with in the previous six months, and to provide information on their partner's HIV infection status.

Although there was an overall decrease in the amount of unprotected anal sex with casual partners in the six months before the study interview, the investigators noted that when they looked at the results according to the HIV status of casual partners, the mean number of HIV-negative casual partners who individuals had sex with actually increased (p < 0.001). The proportion of casual unprotected anal sex partners reported to be HIV-negative increased from 6% in 2002 to 25% in 2005.

The proportion of casual unprotected sex partners whose status was unknown also reduced, from 85% to 60%: butthe investigators emphasised that this still meant that the majority of casual unprotected sex among HIV-negative men was occurring with partners of unknown status.

"Serosorting.especially is used as a deliberate strategy to replace consistent condom use with casual partners, is highly problematic", write the investigators. They note that even if both partners are indeed HIV-negative there is still the risk of other sexually transmitted infections.

Talk, Test, Test, Trust

Australian approaches to negotiated safety have used the slogan 'Talk, Test, Test, Trust' to highlight the issues involved in making such a commitment. This approach is useful because it highlights the issue of trust, and makes it a talking point amongst the target audience. It implies that an agreement about unprotected sex is a serious matter.

The Australian approach has also used advertising about the testing procedure to follow if you want to come to an agreement about unprotected sex. This advertising emphasises that negotiated safety is a complex process, and shouldn't depend on assumptions about HIV status or short-cuts to abandoning condom use.

Several other factors are likely to distort the strategy of negotiated safety:

- Ability to negotiate and assert: some individuals may find it less easy to assert their doubts about the chosen strategy

- Pressures on the gay scene to have sex outside the primary relationship, increasing the potential for slip-ups

- Unwillingness to wait long enough to go through a demanding testing procedure: unprotected sex may become the norm very quickly in a relationship as a signal that the relationship is intensifying

- Lapses in condom use before the HIV test window period is over.

Negotiation when testing uptake is low

A significant difference between the UK and Australia is the level of HIV testing within the gay population. In Australia nearly 90% of gay men are thought to have been tested at least once, but in the UK the proportion is closer to 50%. SIGMA Research has found that the proportion of gay men under 30 who have taken an HIV test is greater than the proportion of those over 35, and hence it may be reasonable to assume that this group may already be practising strategies of negotiated safety more frequently than their older counterparts (Weatherburn).

Yet it has also been reported that gay men over 35 are more likely to report unprotected sex with both regular partners and with casual partners (Coxon).

A consequence of the lower rates of HIV testing in the UK, in the view of some researchers, is the tendency of gay men to make assumptions about their own and their partner's HIV status. It should be noted that this 'optimistic bias' is also likely to be a function of low HIV prevalence in comparison with the US and Australia. In such circumstances 'negotiated safety' strategies need to be approached carefully in order that they do not promote more 'guessing' about HIV status (based on the assumption that HIV testing is a community norm). This could occur if campaigns appear to communicate a primary message that unprotected sex within relationships is preferable to condom use, rather than focusing on the issue of how to make unprotected sex within a relationship as safe as possible.

Recent research in Edinburgh and Glasgow suggests that 'negotiated safety' in the light of full knowledge about HIV status is still very rare. Research conducted in 1996 shows that only 16% of men questioned were having unprotected anal sex in a relationship were doing so in the light of knowledge about both partner's HIV status (Hart). This compares with around 60% in the Australian study discussed above.

Approaches to 'negotiated safety' also need to take into account widespread psychological resistance to the suggestion that it is permissable for some gay men to stop condom use. The use of condoms has become inextricably linked with the idea of sexual interocurse for many gay men, and it can seem threatening to suggest that 100% condom use is no longer necessary when some people have worked so hard to achieve it. For many, 100% condom use may be part of what constitutes being a good, responsible gay man.

Negotiated safety agreements are also used by HIV-negative couples to attempt to reduce the chance of HIV entering the relationship. In one study(Guzman, 2005) of 76 HIV-negative gay men with HIV-negative steady partners, 17% of the men did not practice anal sex and 22% maintained 100 % condom use in all anal sex, inside or outside the relationship.

Another 11% had unprotected sex within and outside the relationship and had not negotiated any rules prohibiting it.

But 39 of the men (51%) had some sort of negotiated safety agreement in place in their relationship. Nineteen (25%) had unprotected sex with each other but had negotiated total monogamy. Three (four per cent) disallowed anal sex with partners outside the relationship but allowed other sex. And 16 (21%) allowed anal sex outside the relationship as long as it was always protected.

This left six (eight per cent) who had protected sex *within* the relationship but allowed unprotected sex outside it - a stance protecting their partner but not themselves.

However these negotiated safety agreements were often broken. Eleven (14% of the whole group, 29% of those who had an agreement) had broken it in the previous three months. However they were less likely to break it if there was a requirement that they 'must always tell' if it had been broken; only 18% of those who had an agreement had broken it if the rule was always to say if they had.

Disclosure: an HIV-positive-controlled safer sex strategy?

There are two necessary conditions for any of these attempts to reduce HIV risk. Men have to know their HIV status. And disclosure (of HIV status, or in the case of the HIV-negative couples, HIV risk behaviour) has to happen.

The recent upsurge in studies of negotiated-safety behaviour has led to the asking of a question. In most of these situations the partner (or partners) with HIV is the one in possession of the knowledge that makes a difference to behaviour.

Drives to get more high-risk people to test for HIV have been based on the assumption that, once they test positive, people will moderate their behaviour. In fact, as we have seen, HIV-positive people end up having *more* unprotected sex rather than less. This has led to anguished questioning among HIV prevention experts and a lot of hostile media and intensified stigma against the perceived irresponsible behaviour of people with the virus.

If, however HIV-positive people are at least attempting to inform and protect their sexual partners, should more HIV prevention money be directed towards enabling them to do so? After all, HIV-positive people form 50% of any risky sexual encounter and 100% of those with the knowledge to reduce its risk.

An illustration of the paradoxes around disclosure and serosorting comes from the publicity surrounding a study of 'Poz parties' in New York (Clatts).

Researchers interviewed 115 men attending an HIV-positive-only sex party in New York. The primary reasons cited by the men for attending were "Not having to worry about disclosing my HIV status (35% citing this as their primary reason) and "I like having uninhibited or unrestricted sex' (also 35%), with 14% citing 'Not having to worry about infecting others'.

The majority of men indulged in unprotected anal sex: 59% receptive and 72% insertive. 47% and 50% respectively had receptive and insertive anal sex to ejaculation.

The men were on average relatively old (median 42) and relatively long-term diagnosed (nearly ten years), though the youngest attendee was 20 and the most recently infected had been so for two months. A third of men said they had had an STI other than HIV diagnosed in the past year.

In contrast to concerns that the use of recreational drugs was fuelling unprotected sex among gay men, only a small number (nine out of 86) used 'hard' drugs such as ecstasy, methamphetamine or ketamine, or sexual enhancers like *Viagra* or poppers.

Although the researchers acknowledged that the serosorting involved might be a public health benefit, they added that attendees had also had sex with status-unknown partners on other occasions.

They also cited the dangers of HIV superinfection, but as yet there is conflicting evidence as to exactly how often this happens or - more to the point - whether it often causes adverse clinical consequences.

Superinfection may turn out to be quite a frequent occurrence (see Smith 2004), but at present the cases that come to the attention of researchers do so *because* of adverse consequences, such as a person with wild type virus contracting resistant virus (see, for instance, Smith 2005). If superinfection is in fact common, one would also expect more evidence that it was damaging, though this evidence might be disguised as treatment failure attributed to other reasons.

However the choice of entitling the paper "An emerging HIV risk environment" may have been unfortunate in that it is easier to argue that on balance 'poz parties' are a risk environment for every STI *except* HIV. Media outlets, however, mainly picked up on the 'HIV risk' angle, with headlines such as "POZ parties may spread HIV superstrain" (Mitchell).

A similar controversy, though restricted to the HIV sector, arose in the UK around a London public-sex venue for gay men called Pigpitmen. This fortnightly sex club started off as an underground sex club in members' homes, but soon moved to an established gay venue.

Members are required to state (though not to prove) that they are HIV-positive to join. There was considerable debate in the HIV-positive press and websites as to whether the involvement of HIV prevention programmes in this club (some nights they set up stalls) was condoning behaviour destructive to the health of the participants or whether, being a space where HIV-positive men had their status 'predisclosed' for them, it was an HIV containment measure.

Such debates will continue to happen until it can be shown that disclosure and negotiated safety actually are helping to contain the spread of HIV among high-risk populations.

References

Bolding G et al. Gay men who look for sex on the internet: is there more HIV/STI risk with online partners? *AIDS* 19: 961-968, 2005.

Buchacz K et al. Trends in Primary and Secondary Syphilis and HIV Seroincidence among Men Who Have Sex with Men in San Francisco, 1998-2002. 11th Conference on Retroviruses and Opportunistic Infections, San Francisco, 2004. Abstract 88.

Centers for Disease Control and Prevention HIV Prevalence, Unrecognized Infection, and HIV Testing Among Men Who Have Sex with Men - Five U.S. Cities, June 2004-April 2005. *MMRW Weekly* 54(24): 597-601, 2005.

Chiasson M A et al. A Comparison of On-line and Off-line Risk among Men Who Have Sex with Men. 12th Retrovirus Conference, Boston, 2005. Abstract 168.

Chinouya, M. & Davidson, O. The Padare Project: Assessing health-related knowledge, attitudes and behaviours of HIV-positive Africans accessing services in north central London. African HIV Policy Network, February 2003.

Clatts MC et al. An emerging HIV risk environment: a preliminary epidemiological profile of an MSM POZ party in New York City. *Sex Transm Infect* 81:373-376. 2005.

Dodds JP et al. Increasing risk behaviour and high levels of undiagnosed HIV infection in a community sample of homosexual men. *Sex Transm Infect* 80:236-240. 2004.

Elford J et al. High-risk sexual behaviour among London gay men: no longer increasing?. Eleventh Annual Conference of the British HIV Association, Dublin, oral presentation abstract O14, April 20 - 23, 2005.

Gisselquist D et al. Let it be sexual: how health care transmission of AIDS in Africa was ignored. *Int J STD AIDS* 14(3):148-61. 2003.

Golden M. HIV serosorting among men who have sex with men: implications for prevention. Thirteenth Conference on Retroviruses and Opportunistic Infections, Denver, abstract 163, 2006.

Goldhammer H et al. Beliefs about viral load, sexual positioning and transmission risk among HIV+ men who have sex with men (MSM): Shaping a secondary prevention intervention. 2005 National HIV Prevention Conference, Atlanta, USA, presentation W0-D1201.

Guzman R et al. Negotiated safety relationships and sexual behaviour among a diverse sample of HIV-negative men who have sex with men. *JAIDS* 38(1) 82-86. 2005.

Lightfoot M et al. The Influence of partner type and risk status on the sexual behaviour of young men who have sex with me living with HIV/AIDS. *JAIDS* 38(1), 61-68. 2005.

Mao L et al. "Serosorting" in casual anal sex of HIV-negative gay men is noteworthy and is increasing in Sydney, Australia. *AIDS* 20: 1204-1206, 2006.

Mitchell S. POZ parties may spread HIV superstrain. UPI release, 28 September 2005. **See** http://www.aidsmap.com/en/news/930CCABC-A29F-4CCC-B7A9-52D93402E765.asp

Russell S. Decrease in new HIV infections smaller than expected. *San Francisco Chronicle,* 31 March 2006.

Smith D et al. Incidence of HIV Superinfection Following Primary Infection. 11th CROI, San Francisco, abstract 21, 2004

Smith DM et al. HIV drug resistance acquired through superinfection. *AIDS* 19: 1251 - 1256, 2005

Van de Ven P et al. Undetectable viral load is associated with sexual risk taking in HIV serodiscordant gay couples in Sydney. *AIDS* 19(2): 179-184. 2005.

Weinhardt L et al. HIV Transmission Risk Behavior among Men and Women Living with HIV in 4 Cities in the United States. *JAIDS* 36(5), 1057-1066. 2004.

E is for emergent prevention technologies

Common themes

Two illustrations

1.A vaccine against cervical cancer

On the 8th June 2006, the US Food and Drug Administration announced that it had given approval to *Gardasil*, a vaccine that had demonstrated 100% protection against four of the most common subtypes of the human papilloma virus (HPV), including the two most common types that cause cervical (and anal) cancer. Another cervical cancer vaccine, *Cervarix*, is expected to be licensed soon.

HPV is the most common sexually-transmitted infection in the United States. The Centers for Disease Control and Prevention (CDC) estimates that about 6.2 million Americans become infected with genital HPV each year and that over half of all sexually active men and women become infected at some time in their lives. On average, there are 9,710 new cases of cervical cancer and 3,700 deaths attributed to it in the United States each year. Worldwide, cervical cancer is the second most common cancer in women; and is estimated to cause over 470,000 new cases and 233,000 deaths each year.Anal cancer, though rare, is 35 times more common in gay men and at least 70 times more common in people with HIV.

Shortly before licensing Alan Kaye, chairman of the National Cervical Cancer Coalition, had told the *NewRepublic* (Groopman): "I don't think anyone wants to stop a cancer vaccine."

However the vaccine caused unease among conservative groups. *The Chicago Tribune* reported that "conservative groups promoting abstinence say they will fight recommendations that children get shots," while the *Los Angeles Times* warned of a "clash between health advocates ... and social conservatives."

The HPV vaccines are not the first ever to be developed against a sexually transmitted disease: the first was the hepatitis B vaccine. But whereas sexually-transmitted hepatitis B mainly affects the same high-risk groups as HIV, HPV infection is so common that 60% of American women and gay men will have at least one strain after just five sexual encounters, and 80% of Americans eventually get infected (Jansen).

The vaccine would therefore have to be given to adolescents or, to be on the safe side, children (in whom it produced similar immune responses) before they start having sex.

It was this that worried the conservative groups. They were concerned that giving the vaccine would endorse promiscuity rather than their favoured method of STI prevention, abstinence till marriage. "We feel people should have the choice of abstinence as a means to avoid HPV," a spokeswoman for Christian Medical & Dental Associations told me. "Our concern is this vaccine will be marketed to a segment of the population that should be getting a message about abstinence," says the Family Research Council.

After meetings between the vaccine manufacturers and groups such as the Family Research Council, conservatives softened their outright opposition. However they still opposed the vaccine becoming mandatory. "Because parents have an inherent right to be the primary educator and decision-maker regarding their children's health, we would oppose any measures to legally require the vaccination or to coerce parents into authorizing it," said the Family Research Council.

However for any vaccine against a common infection to be effective, it has to be as close to mandatory as it can be. The upsurge in measles cases in the UK when scare stories about the MMR vaccine caused a temporary drop in uptake is a case in point. In the USA this usually means adding the vaccine to the vaccinations that states require before students can enrol in school - a list that in the USA includes the hepatitis B vaccine.

HPV is transmissible through touch, so can be caught through sexual activities other than intercourse. Even those who remain fully abstinent until marriage could contract it from their spouses. In short, HPV is a significant public health threat and there should be the strongest possible steps to inoculate the entire population.

The Centers for Disease Control issues recommendations in the USA as to which vaccines should be distributed universally and added to regular immunization schedules, and doctors follow guidelines closely. Even if conservative groups back such a recommendation, state governments would face a decision about whether to require that students be vaccinated - which public health advocates fear that Christian conservatives will oppose vigorously. At the time of writing, the widespread provision of the new vaccines remains in the balance.

2. Circumcision to prevent HIV infection

At the 2005 International AIDS Society Conference in Rio, the results of the first-ever randomised controlled trial (RCT) of the circumcision of adult men as a method of reducing the risk of HIV infection were announced (Auvert). They were conclusive. Circumcision reduced the risk to men of contracting HIV through heterosexual intercourse by at least two-thirds and possibly by as much as three-quarters. Even in advance of two other RCTs whose results are expected in 2006/7, men in high-prevalence countries like Swaziland heard the news and were reported to be besieging clinics asking for the operation.

At the Retrovirus Conference in Denver six months later, evidence was presented (Quinn) that circumcising men offered a smaller, but real, protective effect against HIV infection to the female partners of HIV-positive men too, reducing their risk of infection by about 30%.

In a best-case scenario, if 100% of men in a country were circumcised and circumcision prevented 70% of male infections, HIV incidence in the whole population would be reduced by one-third even if it had no protective effect on women. However if the protective effect on women was included, HIV incidence would fall by two-thirds if all men were circumcised and by 40% if half of them were.

However the presenter had a warning up his sleeve. If circumcision produced a perception in men that they were protected from HIV and could go back to having multiple partners, all benefits of the measure would be lost. Using the same projections, if the average number of partners circumcised men had increased by 50%, HIV prevalence would increase by 40%; if the average number of partners doubled, prevalence would more than double and would be higher than it is today.

International bodies like the World Health Organization are waiting for the results of the two other RCTs before they make a decision on whether to recommend circumcision as a widespread HIV prevention measure. But confounders such as behaviour change may render predictions literally incalculable.

The need for better protection

While HIV treatment has been revolutionised, we still have essentially the same prevention tools that we had at the very start of the epidemic. Using condoms for sex and sterile needles for injecting; sexual abstinence or delay of sexual debut; reducing the number of sexual partners; and measures enabled by disclosure, such as serosorting.

Behind these are strategies to ensure and support their wider use such as education for knowledge and skills; challenging or reinforcing traditional patterns of behaviour; and safer-sex promotion activities.

All of these measures have two features in common. Firstly, if they're to be effective they require the continued maintenance of the behaviour - for life, in most cases - and a conscious effort of will. They are more like avoiding alcohol when driving than having an airbag in your car.

Secondly, they're options which, for reasons to do with personal and social inequality, simply aren't available to a large proportion of the people most vulnerable to HIV in the world. This especially applies to women, and in particular married women. A married woman isn't expected to have sex using condoms and can't enforce their use; abstinence is an irrelevant concept for her; and, while she may be monogamous, she can't ensure that her partner or husband is.

These are the negative reasons why HIV prevention often doesn't work and why we need new answers. But there are positive ones too. Many people, and especially people in long term relationships, don't want to spend their entire sex lives using barrier methods; condoms symbolise lack of closeness and trust; women (and men) want to have children. Current prevention methods all work by somehow blunting or modifying the experience of sex. The emergent prevention technologies hold out a promise of being either completely invisible and out-of-mind during the actual process of sex or, in the case of microbicides, even enhancing it. An HIV prevention intervention that actually made sex more fun and less anxiety-provoking might be extremely effective.

The unavailability, unenforceability and irrelevance of the traditional HIV prevention methods have led to increased calls for development of what are usually called New Prevention Technologies. Some of these, if developed, will be truly new, such as an effective microbicide or vaccine. But some are ways of pressing older interventions into the service of HIV prevention. Circumcision is as old as history; antibody testing and the option of disclosure has existed since 1985; the possibility of post-exposure prophylaxis since the development of AZT soon afterwards.

For this reason, we prefer to call them Emergent Prevention Technologies, partly for alphabetical neatness, but also to make the point that many of these possible solutions to the continued spread of HIV were already out there.

The Emergent technologies are a mixed bag of techniques and approaches that aim to answer one or both of the current deficits of prevention. Some, like circumcision and (hopefully) a vaccine, are or would be one-off medical interventions that would involve no further effort of will on the part of the person concerned - they would decrease the person's vulnerability to HIV infection or its consequences to a specific degree and that would be that.

Others, like microbicides and pre-exposure prophylaxis (PREP), will require at least as much attention to 'adherence' as condoms do. But PREP can be taken hours in advance of sex and in secret; microbicides, while they may be much more difficult to use without a partner's knowledge, are being touted as a prevention method that puts women firmly back in control of keeping themselves safe during sex. Even campaigners for post-exposure prophylaxis have stressed that making this 'backstop' option available will decrease anxiety of sex between sero-different people.

No magic bullet

However, as the above illustrations show, the development of new prevention technologies and the exploitation of existing ones are not unproblematic areas. There is no single intervention among them which in itself is likely to be able to turn round the course of the HIV epidemic. This is for a number of reasons:

1. Efficacy

None of the new prevention technologies outlined below is likely to match the 85-95% efficacy of properly - and consistently - used condoms in preventing HIV infection if used as the sole method of protection.

Universal HIV testing is contingent upon effective prevention support for people with HIV for its success. Circumcision, as outlined above, will still fail to stop one in four infections in men and will only have a small protective effect on women. Post-exposure prophylaxis will only ever be an emergency 'backstop' measure. For pre-exposure prophylaxis the scientific evidence for efficacy is highly contradictory, and we have no idea how to best use it. Even the most enthusiastic advocates of antiviral treatment to prevent sexual transmission would see it as a back-up to other methods for use in extreme circumstances, such as when condoms fail, or to protect victims of sexual assault, or to cover limited periods in a person's life when they are at greatest risk of HIV infection.

Even optimistic microbicide researchers do not expect the first generation of products to have more than 65% efficacy and 'adherence' will be a crucial issue. The first generation of vaccines may not even prevent HIV infection but may work by slowing or preventing the development of AIDS in infected people; if they do prevent infection they may also only have partial efficacy.

This means that the evaluation of these technologies must always be undertaken alongside and in combination with existing approaches.

2. The safety problem

Any prevention intervention that involves administering a substance to people for internal or topical use must be rigorously tested for safety, and the safety barrier such a product must 'jump' in order to be approved needs to be higher than it is for treatments.

In a trial of a drug or other intervention for a disease, the risk/benefit calculation being made is whether the treatment will do more or less harm to the individual than the untreated disease. In a trial of a prophylaxis method, the risk/benefit calculation being made is whether using the intervention will do more or less harm than doing nothing. In the one case you are trying to fight an active process that is harming the individual and the more harmful the disease the more toxicity may be allowed in the treatments for it. In the second case you are trying to build in an additional layer of safety against a disease that might well have been avoided anyway. In the worst-case scenario you may even make people more vulnerable to infection with your prevention intervention. On an obvious level this happened in the COL-1492 trial of nonoxynol-9 as a candidate microbicide, where twice as many regular users of the intervention caught HIV as users of the placebo. On a more subtle level, your prevention intervention may do more net damage in the long run if its effect on behaviour change is not taken into account.

3. Behaviour change

Because none of these interventions are 100% effective, the risk behaviour of people who use them will be crucial for them to make a difference. If they create a false sense of security or cause people who would otherwise have refrained from sex or used condoms to have unprotected sex, their effect could be negative rather than positive. 'Condom migration', meaning the abandonment of condom use by people using alternative methods, is a continued concern of researchers into the new methods.

The effect of behaviour change depends sensitively on both the efficacy of the new intervention and the degree of use of old ones that might be abandoned. One of a number of mathematical models (Foss) developed to predict the effect of microbicides found that in situations where previous condom use was less than 50%, where condom efficacy when used was 95%, and where the microbicide was 50% effective then "any amount of migration can be tolerated if microbicides are used whenever condoms are not." The crucial part of that sentence is obviously the second half; for microbicides to succeed they will have to be both more available and more appealing than condoms.

Conversely, however, if condom use is already high then switching to a less effective microbicide would increase HIV incidence. This concern has been particularly expressed with regard to sex workers, who may have commercial incentives to find alternatives to condoms, but by doing so may put themselves in more danger. The same concerns have been expressed around PREP.

4. The statistics problem

Methods of preventing disease are inherently more difficult to research than methods of treating it. In a trial of a drug for an illness, the illness (whether fatal or not) will occur if you don't provide a treatment, or at least surrogate parkers like immune dysfunction that predict that disease is going to occur will deteriorate. You are stopping something happening.

In a trial of a prevention method, there is no telling what would have happened on an individual level if you hadn't provided the intervention. Even in extremely high-risk populations, HIV incidence is in the order of 5 - 10% a year. Two per cent a year is the approximate HIV incidence in western urban gay men, and this is seen as high. You are trying to prevent something happening that, on the balance of probabilities, wouldn't have happened anyway to the majority of trial participants. HIV seroconversion will only happen to a minority of individuals with or without your intervention, so what you are hoping to find is usually the difference between a small percentage of individuals who become infected and an even smaller one that doesn't. For your findings to reach statistical significance, you need a large study group.

Then there is the ethical question of what you do for your control group. It is unethical to withhold existing prevention methods from them when available, and in a blinded RCT it is equally unethical to give the impression to the intervention group that your method *will* work. Existing methods of HIV prevention such as free condoms and safer-sex advice should therefore be given to all trial participants, and this may in fact be a better 'standard of care' than is normally available - for instance, you may have to offer free condoms in countries where people normally buy them. This may further confound trial findings. The most extreme development of this problem was when community activists in Thailand objected to a trial of PREP among injecting drug users on the grounds that researchers should be offering all participants the best proven prevention, namely needle exchange, and that it was unethical to offer the choice between an unproven intervention or nothing when a proven one existed.

The problem was that needle exchange is illegal in Thailand, so participants would have been getting something denied to other drug users. Researchers countered that this would not only confound findings, it would be a possibly unethical incentive for people to join the trial.

Phase III trials of prevention methods therefore need to be much bigger - ten to 50 times bigger - than treatment trials. A lot of the argument (see below) about the trials of pre-exposure prophylaxis was to do with the choice of trial population. Researchers insisted they could only do trials in populations where HIV incidence was sufficiently high for a feasibly-sized trial to produce a meaningful result. Community campaigners insisted that such groups did exist in the developed world.

Trials need to be bigger still if results are confounded by participants already using other prevention methods. For instance, in some microbicide trials, it already looks as if a meaningful result will be difficult to extract as the most

consistent microbicide users are also the most consistent condom users. Then there is the question of what happens if a first-generation microbicide is partially but suboptimally effective. It will be unethical then to use an inert placebo in a trial of a hopefully more effective second-generation product; the partially effective microbicide should be used instead. But if this offers, say, 33% protective power then you are going to have to use a concomitantly larger number of trial subjects to detect any superiority in your new product.

The same effect applies between trials of different technologies, and concerns have been expressed that the introduction of new prevention methods (and of HIV treatment) may make it increasingly difficult to recruit 'pure' populations for vaccine trials.

5. The medicalisation of prevention

Prevention has always been talked about in the same breath as words like 'choice' and 'empowerment'. No one (except AIDS denialists of the garlic-will-cure-you variety) sees the treatment of HIV disease as the sole responsibility of the person with it; it is understood even at best as a collaboration between patients and medical professionals who have the drugs and the knowledge to relieve their condition, and at worst as the administration of medicine to an essentially passive sufferer.

Prevention has always operated from the opposite paradigm. Increased use of condoms, better choice of partner, decision-making ability about whether to have unprotected sex and with whom, will, it is assumed, only result from situations in which people have greater power and control over all areas of their lives. Because of this, along with preventing HIV and AIDS, much HIV prevention work has other goals. These may include changing gender relations, to increase boys' respect for girls and women and the confidence of girls and women in their ability to achieve their ambitions. Campaigners seek to increase the self-respect and social standing of people who have been marginalised in many societies, such as men who have sex with men and injecting drug users.

Some, though not all, of the emerging prevention technologies, however, are much more like treatments in that decisions as to availability may well be made by professionals in collaboration with, or instead of, members of affected communities. This is seen most starkly in the area of antiretroviral prophylaxis where the perception (whether real or not) that the medical profession is unwilling to provide PEP after sexual exposure has led to campaigns and legal action. The same will be doubly true in the case of PREP, which will not and should not be available 'over the counter'. Doctors or other health workers will be making decisions about who should and should not get it, and there are fears that these decisions may be clouded by prejudice, discrimination or ignorance. We have, after all, already seen this happen on a national scale in countries that refuse to provide needle exchange or substitution therapy for drug users.

The same may apply in the initial stages to microbicides, though it has always been the intention that formulations should in the end be commercially available or, in resource-poor settings, free, though then we run into the same problems and arguments about access as we do with HIV treatment. And the whole argument about the introduction of universal HIV testing in the USA has been about replacing a community-education and empowerment model of HIV prevention with a 'medicalised' one.

Proponents of emergent prevention technologies, however, would counter this by saying that in situations where people do *not* have power, whether because of cultural or institutional inequality or personal incapacity such as mental illness, then the only humane and compassionate thing to do is to medicalise HIV prevention and provide people with 'mechanical' methods of HIV prevention that will work regardless of whether they have personal choice or not. Individuals change their behaviour slowly and cultures change more slowly still; HIV infection can happen fast and we need interventions that will stop it no matter what the circumstances of vulnerable individuals.

6. Personal belief systems

In addition to, or masquerading as, the above rational concerns about the new prevention technologies, lie political, moral and religious belief systems that may cause people to prefer one prevention method over another. This is already so familiar in the case of the debate around abstinence programmes versus comprehensive strategies including condom distribution that there is no point in repeating it here, but these debates are bound to arise every time a new prevention method is suggested or becomes available, as in the case of the HPV vaccine above.

7. The importance of community consultation

The idea that new prevention technologies may negatively affect use of the strategies we already have may also occur to the communities among whom trials are done, and they may react negatively to what they see as a medicalised method that takes away their control over infection. We already have an example above with the PREP trial in Thailand.

The controversy that blew up so unexpectedly around trials of PREP in Cambodia, Cameroon and Thailand in 2004-5 was a salutary lesson to researchers that genuine consultation with trial subjects, members of their community, activists and advocates and other stakeholders such as political leaders was vital if laege prevention trials were not to cause controversy.

There is a detailed list of the issues that arose in the section on PREP, but in brief what activists objected to were what they saw as undue pressure from researchers on candidate participants to join the trial and the lack of provision for compensation and/or treatment in the case of trial failures (seroconversions) and side-effects.

Organising prevention research as a clinical trial opens the way to formal review by ethical committees, providing important safeguards to trial participants, and increasingly, those organising prevention trials have seen the need for and value of a Community Advisory Board. Most of the work that has been done on Community Advisory Boards has been in the context of preventive vaccine trials, and this is reflected in the UNAIDS ethical guidelines. Here, the main point to make is that the same considerations apply to all of the prevention research discussed here. Most of the ethical guidance set out by UNAIDS for vaccine trials is equally applicable to microbicide trials or trials of antiretrovirals used to prevent HIV infection.

One of the critical roles of the Community Advisory Board should be, to decide on the nature of the HIV prevention efforts that should be directed at all trial participants, aside from the use of the product that is being evaluated. It is also vital that the standard of care to be provided to any trial participant who becomes HIV-positive should be discussed and agreed in advance of the trial.

However one lesson of the PREP trials is that the Community Advisory Board model is insufficient for truly comprehensive consultation as it begs the question: 'who is the community?' If a CAB consists of a group of self-appointed activists, or even more so in countries without a strong civil society tradition if it consists of paid NGO members, then there is no guarantee that the concerns expressed by the CAB are in any way representative of the concerns of all stakeholders or are uninfluenced by other considerations, or that the consultations with the CAB will be fed back accurately to the people they represent.

The PREP trials have therefore provided a sharp learning curve both in what truly comprehensive community consultation needs to look like and in the development of truly 'informed' consent in what may be highly marginalised and even illiterate people. An object lesson in how to do this is provided by the Peruvian PREP trial among gay men - see below.

Many questions may need to be asked. How do people understand the role of this new technology? How can they integrate it into their other strategies? Does it open up new strategies to them? Does it change the way they perceive the epidemic and their own and other people's relationship to it?

To answer such questions requires the active involvement of social researchers in evaluating new biomedical technologies. When it comes to HIV prevention, medicine is far too important to be left only to medical scientists.

Conclusion

So, all in all, there is no 'magic bullet' in prevention interventions which is likely to make as dramatic a difference to HIV infection as antiretrovirals have made to HIV disease.

However, this is not in any way an argument that trials of new prevention methods should not be attempted. We already have a result in the shape of the circumcision trial, and demographic evidence from countries with high and low circumcision rates - which tend to match neatly up with whether they have high or low HIV rates - suggest it could possibly be a turning point in the worldwide prevention of HIV, even with all the above considerations taken into account. In practice, as more experience is gained with *Phase III trials* of vaccines, PREP and microbicides, some concerns may disappear.

Even when a trial has a 'negative' result it should not be seen as an unqualified failure. The COL-1492 microbicide trial, discussed later on, was an impressive demonstration that it is possible to show the superiority of one product over another (even if it was the placebo that came out ahead), despite a successful campaign to promote increased condom use among trial participants.

Similarly, the VaxGen trials showed that it was possible to recruit, motivate and retain a large group of volunteers at continuing high risk of HIV without adding to their risk-taking. (Reported risk-taking behaviour declined during the course of the trial and HIV infection rates were stable.)

This highlights the importance of feasibility studies, to identify populations in which there is continuing HIV risk despite the wholehearted promotion of the best available means of HIV prevention.

It may also point to the need for multi-agency as well as multi-disciplinary projects, in which some or all of the prevention education can be provided independently of the researchers.

References

Auvert B et al. Impact of male circumcision on the female-to-male transmission of HIV. IAS Conference on HIV Pathogenesis and treatment, Rio de Janeiro, abstract TuOa0402, 2005.

Foss AM et al. Will shifts from condom to microbicide use increase HIV risk? Model projections. International AIDS Conference, Barcelona: abstract WeOrD1319, 2002.

Groopman S. Conservative Christians and HPV: Blind Faith. *New Republic*, 10 March 2006.

Jansen K. Vaccine Protection against Human Papillomaviruses (http://www.retroconference.org/2005/cd/Sessions/032.htm). Twelfth Conference on Retroviruses and Opportunistic Infections, Boston. Abstract 126. 2005.

Quinn T. Circumcision and HIV transmission: the cutting edge. Plenary presentation, 13th Conference on Retroviruses and Opportunistic Infections, Denver, abstract #120, 2006.

The role of HIV testing in HIV prevention

It might seem strange to start with a section of HIV testing as a prevention method. After all, the role of HIV testing is to find out whether prevention has failed, isn't it?

This, however, is to ignore the contribution people with HIV can make to HIV prevention.

While there is very little evidence that HIV testing in itself leads to behaviour change in people who remain negative, there is abundant evidence that, once diagnosed, people with HIV reduce their risk behaviour. Maximising the uptake of HIV testing and detecting early infections should therefore, in theory, lead to a significant decline in HIV infections.

It has been known since the early 1990s that people diagnosed with HIV modify their risk behaviour. In previous years this fact tended to be obscured by researchers citing it as evidence that some people with HIV *continued* high-risk behaviour in studies whose primary aim was to quantify that figure so that prevention programmes could be directed at these people.

But it was eventually realised that the majority of people with HIV tended to reduce their risk behaviour and that, because of this, ensuring that as many people knew their status as possible could be an effective prevention method.

To take a recent example: a study of recently-diagnosed gay men in the USA (Gorbach) interviewed 153 men an average of 4-6 weeks after diagnosis and then again three months later. It found that between the first and second interviews nearly a half (47%) of the 91% of men who remained sexually active men reported that they had reduced the number of sexual partners they had had in the previous three months, a third reported no change and a fifth reported that they had increased their number of partners. The average number of partners within three months went down from 7.9 to 5.2, a 34% decrease.

Nonetheless, 54% of the newly-diagnosed HIV-positive men had unprotected anal intercourse (UAI) during the three months before the second interview. In the past this might have been regarded as a failure of prevention methods. However, the researchers found that, of the men who did have UAI, the majority switched to HIV-positive partners if they had unprotected sex. In other words, there was considerable evidence of serosorting.

At the baseline interview the men reported that nearly half (48%) of their UAI partners had been HIV-negative, a third of unknown status and less than a fifth (18%) HIV-positive.

Three months later the proportion of UAI partners who were negative had declined to 30% of the total (a 37% decline). The proportion who were positive had nearly tripled to 52% of the total (a 188% increase). And the proportion of unknown status had halved, to 18%. This is strong evidence both for disclosure (since fewer partners were of unknown status) and for serosorting.

These figures may underestimate the behaviour shift, since the first interview took place 4-6 weeks after diagnosis, and therefore during a third to a half of the preceding three months the men would already know they had HIV and might have already started to change their behaviour.

This evidence of behaviour change is nothing new. In a 1994 survey (Wenger) half of a group of HIV-positive men had UAI with HIV-positive partners but only a sixth with HIV-negative ones - exactly the same proportions as in the 2006 survey. The difference was that in this survey 41% had UAI with partners of unknown status, but that by 2006 this proportion had more than halved. Although obviously we are talking about two different groups of gay men who cannot be compared directly, this seems to provide some evidence of both increased knowledge of status and increased willingness to talk and ask about it.

The Centers for Disease Control in the USA (see CDC) has calculated that on average people with HIV once diagnosed reduce their risk behaviours (i.e. potentially serodiscordant unprotected sex and needle-sharing) by 70% by a year after diagnosis.

The difference HIV diagnosis may make could be even larger than this. The CDC used this figure and what it knew or suspected about the relative infectiousness of people with HIV and different disease stages to calculate that as many as a two-thirds of HIV infections could be transmitted by people unaware of their HIV status. This takes into account not only the behaviour change in people with HIV but the fact that because a proportion will be on treatment, their average infectiousness will decrease.

In 2004 Holtgrave and Anderson used these figures to claim that more than one in nine of people in the USA who don't know their HIV status pass on their virus in a year compared with only one in 58 of people who do know their status - over six times as many.

This may exaggerate the difference. A presentation at the 2006 13th CROI Conference suggested that although people in acute HIV infection were on average 28 times more infectious than people in chronic infection, because the period of chronic infection was so much longer, transmission during acute infection only accounted for one in eight infections. However, the fact remains that diagnosis allows people in both acute and chronic infection to reduce their risk behaviour, to seek treatment so they become less infectious, and to considerably reduce their chances of passing on their HIV infection.

Making HIV testing routine

Emboldened by this, the CDC in April 2003 announced its Advancing HIV Prevention Initiative (see MMWR). This was a strategic remodelling of prevention in which much more emphasis was to be laid on increasing HIV test uptake and diagnosing as many people as possible, and working with those who were diagnosed to reinforce safer sex messages. What was also implicit, though not declared, in the new policy was that federal funding for old-style community-based HIV awareness-raising and prevention initiatives was to be downgraded.

Advancing HIV Prevention had four strategic aims:

1. Make HIV testing a routine part of medical care

The CDC said that screening all persons in high-prevalence medical settings, regardless of what if any HIV risks are reported, made sense because testing based on reported or perceived risk alone was failing to identify many people with HIV. Acceptance of HIV testing, as demonstrated among pregnant women, was greater when it was offered routinely than when it was based on risk assessments. Furthermore, routine HIV screening met the three generally accepted principles that apply to screening efforts:

- HIV infection is a serious disease that can be detected before symptoms occur using a reliable and inexpensive test.

- Treatment given before symptoms develop is more effective than waiting until after symptoms develop.

- The cost of screening is reasonable compared with the anticipated benefits.

2. Use new models for diagnosing HIV infection outside of traditional medical settings

The CDC said that HIV testing programs outside of traditional medical settings were more likely to reach racial/ethnic minorities and 'people who report increased risk for HIV but do not have access to medical care', such as people without insurance and undocumented immigrants. It also said that evidence had shown that testing programmes conducted in some non-traditional settings produced higher rates of seropositivity. For instance, it was estimated that nearly a quarter of the HIV-positive people in the USA at some point passed through the prison system, but fewer than half of prisons routinely tested inmates on entry.

Recently approved rapid HIV tests could be done outside a traditional laboratory setting and could reduce the time it took to process tests from two weeks to 20 minutes. The availability of these tests meant that testing could be implemented in diverse settings and essential health information can be provided quickly in settings where people may be unlikely to return to receive test results.

3. Prevent new infections by working with people diagnosed with HIV and their partners

The CDC said that each person living with HIV who adopted safer behavior could prevent many potential transmissions of HIV infection. It cited the figure already quoted above, that people with HIV once diagnosed reduced their sexual risk behaviour by as much as 70%.

The CDC said: "Studies suggest that working with HIV-infected persons will result in greater reductions in risk behaviors and HIV transmission than working with HIV-negative persons."

It explicitly portrayed the specialised counselling of people who sought tests and turned out to be HIV-negative, however high risk their behaviour, as a waste of resources. It said that among persons testing negative for HIV, those receiving enhanced risk reduction counseling had only 18% fewer sexually transmitted infections at one year after testing compared with persons receiving standard counseling.

The CDC also said that it would "increase the emphasis on assisting HIV-infected persons in notifying partners of their recent exposure and ensure voluntary testing of partners," pointing out that when partners were referred, from 8% to 40% turned out to have previously undiagnosed HIV infection.

What help with preventing onward transmission would the newly diagnosed people get? The CDC said that prevention interventions included

- ongoing case management

- focused risk-reduction counselling

- medical interventions (leaving these undefined)

- support for other psychosocial stressors (leaving these also undefined, though in another paper they specify as examples of stressors homelessness, and drink and drug problems).

4. Continue to decrease perinatal HIV transmission.

This speaks for itself; the CDC said it would continue to recommend that all pregnant women be screened for HIV in order to take advantage of medical interventions to reduce the risk of mother-to-baby transmission. It strongly supported an "opt-out" testing strategy for prenatal HIV screening, doing HIV tests as routinely as, and with the same consent forms, as other medical tests.

This policy was received with suspicion by existing HIV prevention workers and advocates for people with HIV. Opinions were voiced that the main driver behind the new policy was the distaste that the George W Bush government had for traditional community HIV prevention programmes, with their often bold and 'sex positive' campaigns and their explicit work with marginalised communities such as gay men of colour (or indeed any gay men) and sex workers.

Exactly a year after the CDC's policy was adopted Terje Anderson, Director of the National Association of People with AIDS (NAPWA), criticised its approach (Anderson). He said the narrow emphasis on testing and individualised counselling was inherently stigmatising:

The lack of any mention of anything that isn't an individual level intervention delivered behind closed doors in a doctor's or social worker's office - the lack of any mention of anything that happens in the community - lays individual responsibility for transmission on each person with HIV, lays no responsibility on their negative partners, makes possible no conversation about the social context that puts people at risk, and treats people with HIV as vectors of infection and not as full people.

In fact, the Expanding HIV Prevention initiative made surprisingly little difference to diagnosis rates in the USA. By 2002, an estimated 38-44% of people in the USA had been tested at least once for HIV; but despite this, the proportion of people with HIV who were unaware of their status stayed stubbornly at 25% of the total.

With the exception of routine testing for pregnant women, and despite repeated recommendations in support of routine risk-based testing in health care settings, the number of people at risk for HIV infection screened in acute-care settings remained low. In a survey (Fincher-Mergi) of 154 healthcare providers in ten hospital emergency departments, providers reported caring for an average of 13 patients per week with suspected STDs, but only 10% encouraged these patients to be tested for HIV infection in the emergency department. Although 35% referred patients to confidential HIV testing sites in the community, such referrals had proved ineffective because patients did not turn up.

Reasons cited for not offering HIV testing in the emergency department included lack of established mechanisms to assure follow-up (51%), lack of the certification perceived as necessary to provide counselling (45%), and belief that the testing process was too-time consuming (19%).

With routine HIV screening in some hospitals and emergency departments, the percentage of patients with positive tests (2% to 7%) often exceeded that observed nationally in publicly-funded HIV counselling and testing sites (1.5%) and STD clinics (2.0%) serving 'high-risk' people.

Should we test everyone for HIV?

In February 2005 the New England Journal of Medicine published two cost-effectiveness estimates (Paltiel, Sanders) of what would happen if there was universal screening for HIV - that is, at least one test performed on the entirety of selected populations ranging from high-risk people to the entire US population.

David Paltiel of Yale University divided the US population into a 'high risk' group (meaning an *undiagnosed* HIV prevalence of 3%, similar to gay men in London) and an annual incidence on 1.2%; a 'CDC threshold' group meaning populations the CDC had recommended for routine testing in its Advancing HIV Prevention strategy (undiagnosed prevalence of 1%, annual incidence of 0.12%); and the general US population (undiagnosed prevalence 0.1%, annual incidence 0.01%).

If everyone in 'high risk' populations (though how you discovered who was 'high risk' was a question left unaddressed) was given a routine one-off HIV test in addition to whatever voluntary HIV tests some of them may have, the average CD4 count at diagnosis would increase from 154 to 210, though there would be very little additional benefit in survival time.

Testing all these people at least once routinely would cost $36,000 per quality-adjusted life-year (QALY) gained, testing them everyfive years would cost $50,000 per QALY gained, and testing every three years would cost $63,000. One-off testing of the CDC Threshold group would cost not much more - about $38,000 per QALY gained. But if you tested the entire adult US population at least once, it would cost $113,000 per QALY gained.

Paltiel said his modelling showed that "In all but the lowest-risk populations, routine, voluntary screening for HIV once every three to five years isjustified on both clinical and cost-effectiveness grounds." The threshold for what is regarded as a 'cost-effective' treatment is set at about £30,000 by the National Institute for Health and Clinical Excellence (NICE) in the UK, which translates to about $60,000 given the generally higher costs of health in the USA.

Gillian Sanders of Duke University found somewhat lower costs with her model than Paltiel. She found that one-off screening of the CDC threshold population would cost $15,078 per quality-adjusted life-year gained and that screening in any population with a prevalence of over 0.05% (a quarter of UK prevalence and one-twelfth of US prevalence) would cost less than $50,000 per quality-adjusted life-year. Screening the entire adult population every five years would cost $57,140 per QALY gained, "but was more attractivein settings with a high incidence of infection."

Sanders said her results were 'sensitive to the efficacy of behaviour modification', meaning that if the resultant newly-diagnosed people significantly reduced their risk behaviour, universal screening might be more cost-effective.

She concluded that "The cost-effectiveness of routine HIV screening in healthcare settings, even in relatively low-prevalence populations,is similar to that of commonly accepted interventions, and suchprograms should be expanded."

Encouraged by this, the CDC announced a much bolder move - they would push for a policy of universal screening. All adults in the USA should take at least one HIV test.

In a talk at the 13th Retrovirus conference in early 2006, Timothy Mastro of the CDC quoted the startlingly high prevalence and incidence figures among gay men and particularly black gay men in cities other than San Francisco. In a large sample of gay men in five US cities 25% of gay men had had HIV and 48% were unaware of their infection; 46% of black gay men were positive and 67% did not know it. Late testing was also common: 45% of AIDS diagnoses were among people who had been diagnosed less than 12 months previously.

He said that HIV testing in the USA had not been increasing in recent years despite the launch of the Advancing HIV Prevention strategy in 2003.

He said that only about one in 500 visits to hospital emergency departments involved an HIV test despite the fact that, when tested, rates of previously undiagnosed HIV among A&E patients varied from 1.3% to 3.2%.

In Texas, which adopted opt-out testing in its STD clinics back in 1997, the proportion of STD patients tested for HIV increased by over 50% (from 78% to 97%) in one year and the number of positive tests had gone up 60% from 168 to 268. He showed a notice from a Dallas STD clinic which said that "All patients seen in this clinic will be tested for gonorrhoea, syphilis, Chlamydia and HIV."

He said that before opt-out testing had been adopted in pregnant women in the UK only 35% had tested because they feared it indicated high-risk behaviour whereas 88% accepted opt-out testing.

"We think the need for extensive pre-test counselling is less because it's 2006 and people now have a high level of knowledge about HIV," he said.

The CDC had therefore decided to revise its HIV screening guidelines and from June 2006 would be recommending routine, voluntary screening for all persons aged 13-64 in healthcare settings, *not* based on risk, and annual HIV testing for people with risk behaviour. Pre-test counselling would not be required.

'Healthcare settings' includes all hospital in-patient and out-patient departments and community clinics as well as STD clinics. An exception would be made of prisons, where it was recognised that receiving an HIV diagnosis created profound difficulties both for inmate and institution.

This is a radical proposal which would require revising a myriad of local regulations, including ones mandating pre-test counselling and written consent.

Mastro was faced with a battery of questions after his presentation by questioners with numerous concerns. Among them were:

- How would the CDC move from recommendation to implementation? It had recommended names-based reporting years ago but it had taken the threat of the removal of federal funds for states to move towards this.

- If the information given in pre-test counselling and discussion around informed consent is removed, where are patients going to get any option to talk about HIV and harm reduction?

- How real is the 'voluntary' nature of the testing when the photo he showed said 'You *will* be tested for HIV?'

- How is the opting-out process to work and how will it be recorded? Without adequate recording, patients could say they were tested without consent.

In an article on the universal test recommendation (Young), the *Atlanta Jounal-Constitution*, home-town newspaper of the CDC, pointed out that the CDC's ambitious plan was not backed by the force of law, and said that whether it would become reality remained a question.

It also pointed out that the guidelines conflicted with an influential federal task force's conclusion the previous year that widespread voluntary testing has no direct evidence of benefits. In July 2005, the US Preventive Services Task Force, the nation's leading independent panel of private-sector experts on prevention and primary care, issued its own findings on HIV testing. That group found there was not enough evidence to recommend for or against routine HIV screening.

Dr Bruce Calonge, task force chairman, said his group looked at the state of the scientific evidence to decide whether actions had documented benefits. They could not find documented benefits for universal screening.

The difference between the two recommendations, Calonge said, may point to the different missions of the task force and the CDC. The task force looks at benefits to the patient sitting in front of a clinician; the CDC is focused on public health and improving the overall health of a population.

The task force's recommendations are what the nation's health insurers generally look to when deciding coverage issues, and they are also influential with family physicians. The conflicting recommendations raise questions about whether universal testing will be adopted by family doctors and whether private and government health programs will pay for the tests. In general, Medicare will not pay for routine screening tests unless specifically authorised by Congress.

Private insurers are studying the proposal, said Susan Pisano, spokeswoman for America's Health Insurance Plans, which represents them. "Generally speaking our member companies follow recommendations of the U.S. Preventive Services Task Force," she said.

Dr Carlos del Rio, chief of medicine at Grady Memorial Hospital in Atlanta, said he was concerned the new recommendations would go the way of the CDC's 1993 call for universal HIV screening of people going to hospitals in areas with high rates of HIV. He said that he and others had called it "the most ignored recommendation ever made by CDC."

Jeff Graham, senior director of advocacy and communications for the Atlanta-based AIDS Survival Project, said more testing is important. "However, the devil is in the details." He said his greatest concern was the plan to do away with pre-test counseling because it was one of the few opportunities for medical professionals to educate people on preventing HIV.

He said: "Our greater concern is not legal issues, but the personal sense of stigma."

At CROI, a presentation by Tom Coates of the University of California, San Francisco, had looked at drives to normalise HIV testing in Africa (where opt-out testing has been a policy in Bostwana since 2004 and where, in 2005, Lesotho announced a plan to HIV-test its entire population). His findings underscored these concerns. Africans were in general in agreement with normalising HIV testing (82% of Batswana, for instance, think that the routine testing introduced by their President Festus Mogae is 2004 was a good thing). However this contrasted with their individual distress at contemplating a positive result and the stigma and societal rejection it might bring.

In one qualitative survey, one said: "I have a dream of having children; if I test positive my dream will be shattered." Another said: "My father will chase me away from the house and call me Satan."

Despite these concerns, AIDS activists in the USA, who had previously been suspicious of recommendations for universal testing, broadly welcomed them. *Aidsmeds.com* founder Peter Staley, writing in the *New York Times*, said:

"AIDS groups should be screaming for expanded testing, and many of them are. But some are fighting any change, as though the epidemic hasn't evolved since the 1980's. In those days, there were important reasons to protect people getting tested for AIDS. There were no drugs to treat the disease. A positive test meant that you were just waiting to die.

"That's why AIDS groups argued that H.I.V. infection was very different from, for instance, diabetes, and that we needed to treat it differently. New York, along with other states, adopted policies that came to be known as 'H.I.V. exceptionalism.' The state passed laws to protect patients from unwanted testing.

"But today, treating H.I.V. can delay, sometimes indefinitely, the onset of AIDS. That has made H.I.V. testing - the first step toward dealing effectively with the disease - a lot more important. Testing itself has become less stressful as well. While older tests required patients to wait two weeks for results, new technology gives them an answer in 20 minutes.

The rigorous demands of H.I.V. exceptionalism are limiting the widespread availability of the H.I.V. test. And oddly enough, treating H.I.V. infection as a secret that must be kept at all costs makes it seem more shameful than other diseases. Right now, state legislation is "protecting" people so much that one in four H.I.V.-positive New Yorkers have to get sick to find out that they are ill. We can do better than that, and we should."

Staley quoted Dennis deLeon, president of the Latino Commission on AIDS, on his own change in attitude about testing. DeLeon said he had spoken with a pregnant woman who had no idea she was at risk for HIV - she had been married and monogamous, and had never used drugs. When her test came back positive, she was shocked.

"I had strongly opposed this testing program, but when I encountered this woman, I realised that I had been wrong," he

said. "My activism may have served to deprive other women of knowing their status during pregnancy. That troubles me a lot."

An illustration of the difficulties the CDC policy may encounter came from San Francisco where Jeffrey Klausner, head of the San Francisco Public Health Department's HIV programme, introduced a policy saying that doctors no longer had to obtain written consent from patients taking an HIV test.

Klausner came under criticism for his efforts to make "a simple administrative change bringing some city [testing] facilities in line with what was already standard practice at most hospitals."

As a result of Klausner's actions on HIV testing reform, the San Francisco Board of Supervisors considered an emergency ordinance specifically mandating informed written consent as well as pre-test counselling at city-funded HIV testing sites. However, as the 'Bay Area Reporter' also pointed out, "...terms like 'informed consent' and 'counseling' rarely have a uniform statewide legal definition."

Michael Weinstein, President of AIDS Healthcare Foundation said that "Dr Klausner's remarks on HIV testing in San Francisco led to widespread confusion as to what he actually intended to accomplish. Unfortunately, the confusion around his remarks led many in the Bay Area to weigh in, not surprisingly, on the side of perceived potential civil rights infringements versus prudent public health policy.

The position in the UK

Surveys in the UK have found that a large proportion of gay men and Africans who turn up at GUM clinics for sexual health checkups and even with acute sexually transmitted infections were going away without being offered an HIV test.

For instance, the 2004 HIV Prevalence and Sexual Behaviour Survey among gay men in London, Brighton and Manchester (Dodds) found that, of the gay men who turned out to have HIV when tested anonymously, 44% in London, 33% in Brighton and 37% in Manchester had told the questionnaire they were HIV-negative or untested. The survey divided the men up into those who had had an STI checkup in the last year and those who had not. In London, one in five GUM clinic attendees had HIV, but 30% of those were unaware of it, implying that opportunities to test them had not been taken.

In contrast, only seven per cent of London men who had *not* had an STI checkup turned out to have HIV. But one in five of these (42 men) were positive, despite the majority presumably thinking they had been at low risk.

In terms of Africans, during 2003, according to data from GUM clinics participating in the unlinked anonymous survey, the prevalence of previously undiagnosed HIV infection among heterosexuals born in sub-Saharan Africa was high, with 3.6% (137/3787) of those in London and 8% elsewhere in England, Wales and Northern Ireland, infected and unaware of their infection. This regional disparity probably reflects the recent dispersal of migrant populations to areas outside London, and highlights the increasing burden being placed on GUM clinics outside of London.

Current UK policy is to encourage clinics to make 'opt-out' HIV testing a routine part of care for anyone visiting a GUM clinic with an acute sexually transmitted infection.

The Sexual Health and HIV Strategy for Scotland says that "Lead Clinicians must develop a framework to ensure that HIV testing is offered to all GUM clinic attendees not known to be HIV-infected who present with a new STI.

"This offer should be made in the context of the HIV test being presented as a routine recommended test. Reasons for non-uptake should be recorded."

Although the Sexual Health and HIV Strategy for England and Wales was written before the greatly expanded use of HIV testing was being recommended as a strategy, the most recent guidance issued by the Department of Health says that "All GUM clinic attendees should be offered an HIV test on their first screening for sexually transmitted infections (and subsequently according to risk).

It adds: "Attenders at genitourinary medicine clinics are considered to be at increased risk of HIV infection because of their behaviour. Most clinics routinely offer an HIV test only to those in recognised high-risk groups, namely homosexual men, current/former injection drug users and people from or with close links to high prevalence countries (currently those in sub-Saharan Africa). We know from unlinked anonymous surveys of HIV infection carried out in a network of GUM clinics across the country that this selective strategy has not reached all those who have been at risk. A high proportion is still unaware that they have HIV infection after their visit."

Studies have shown that where opt-out testing is offered, the number of HIV tests taken immediately increases. One English clinic to do this early was the GUM clinic at the North Cumbria Hospital in Carlisle. In a paper in the *BMJ* in 2001 (Stanley), the clinic performed 154 syphilis tests in August 2001 and 70 'opt-in' HIV tests (i.e., patients had to specifically ask for an HIV test).

The clinic changed to 'opt-out' consent in September 2001. That month 148 syphilis tests were performed and 130 HIV tests - an 85% increase.

There were similar experiences in Scotland. At Glasgow's Sandyford Clinic opt-out testing was introduced at the start of 2004. Every person coming for an STI screen, whether symptomatic or not, would be offered an HIV test and consent would be taken verbally. Objections to the test would be recorded and patients would be told they had the option to return if they changed their minds.

In May to August 2003, from 400 to 470 HIV tests were performed a month at the clinic. During the same time period in 2004, 710-880 tests were performed a month, with an upward trend (the highest figure was the last recorded for the paper presented, in August 2004). This represents a 78-87% increase in HIV tests being performed from one year to the next.

Current UK policy on HIV testing has been established as a result of a number of factors:

- Desire to avoid compulsory testing

- Desire to avoid discrimination and stigmatisation

- Qualified medical support for widespread testing

- Lack of support from the voluntary sector for widespread testing.

Debates about HIV testing have tended to focus on the complex decision-making process which faces individuals who are considering whether or not to test. Many doctors and voluntary organisations continue to argue that HIV testing is an individual decision. The outcome of such a consensus is that the wider social consequences of not promoting HIV testing are never discussed because this would be seen to undermine individual choice.

However, it is important to discuss the negative consequences of not promoting HIV testing more aggressively. These include:

- Avoidable morbidity and mortality

- Avoidable mother-to-baby transmission

- Frequent incorrect assumptions about HIV status in sexual relationships

- Underestimates of the size of the infected population and of the costs of the HIV/AIDS epidemic.

Home testing

Home testing kits

Home testing for HIV antibodies became available in the United States in 1996. Two different testing kits - more accurately, home sampling kits, which enable people to send blood away for testing - have been approved for sale by pharmacists. There are no indications that such kits will become available in the UK in the near future, and strict regulations exist regarding who can perform HIV tests. Major AIDS organisations in the UK have consistently opposed the idea of any form of home testing, arguing that HIV testing should always be conducted with full pre- and post-test counselling.

However, US authorities decided that the potential benefits of home testing services outweighed the disadvantages, and that the systems proposed by the makers contained enough safeguards of confidentiality and the client's emotional reactions to the test result.

The home tests available in the USA

Neither of the testing kits available now in the US are true 'home tests' in the way that pregnancy testing kits are understood to be. Both require individuals to send off a sample of blood to a laboratory and phone in for a result. Their chief advantages are anonymity and accessibility rather than speed.

The Confide testing kit

Confide is manufactured by Direct Access Diagnostics, a subsidiary of Johnson and Johnson. The testing kit is an over the counter product which consists of a blood specimen collection kit, pre-test counselling booklet and a personal ID number. The test kit can also be ordered by credit card phone line. They cost between $35 and $50 depending on point of sale.

The purchaser uses a retractable lancet to prick a fingertip and place few drops of blood on a paper test card. The card is then sent to the laboratory in a pre-paid envelope.

At the laboratory the sample is tested using a standard ELISA antibody test, with a confirmatory test using another form of test kit if the result is positive. False positives have not been reported in trials of this methodology, and the false negative rate is comparable with standard ELISA testing (5 in 1000). Results are available in seven days by telephone. The caller gives their ID number to obtain the result. If the result is negative the caller has the option of speaking to a counsellor or recorded information. If the caller is positive or the result is indeterminate, he or she will be referred to a counsellor. Counsellors can refer to treatment centres and callers may use the telephone counselling service for up to two years after diagnosis. There is no way that the testing service can follow up callers if they opt out of the counselling process at any point.

The Home Access test

The Home Access kit is also available from pharmacies or by mail order, price ranging from $40 to $60. The test kit consists of a lancet and a filter paper circle which must be completely filled with blood. The sample is then sent to the laboratory, where it is tested by several ELISA kits. If a sample is positive by two ELISA tests, another test method will be used to confirm the result.

A trial has shown that the test method resulted in no false positive or false negative results when 756 individuals at high risk of HIV infection were tested. However, almost 7% of test kit users had problems providing the blood sample in such a way that it could be tested.

Results are available within three to seven days. Some people with negative results will be referred automatically to a counsellor. Others will be given the option. All callers with positive results are referred directly to a counsellor, who will give them referrals and post-test counselling. As with the Confide test, callers can opt out of the counselling process at any time.

Advantages and disadvantages

These testing kits offer a number of advantages over current methods of testing.

- Anonymity: many people may be put off attending HIV testing sites by embarrassment or the wish to remain anonymous

- Accessibility: testing sites may be inaccessible to some people either because they are too far away or because they are not open at convenient times.

However, there are several disadvantages:

- Lack of face-to-face counselling

- No guarantee that those who test positive will remain engaged with the counselling process once they have received a positive result

- Cost: those with very low incomes may be unable to afford the testing kits, and may continue to be underserved by free, anonymous testing sites.

However, it is generally agreed that the availability of such testing kits is likely to increase the level of HIV testing. It will be important to see the results of post-marketing studies into questions such as:

- Do a higher proportion of self-test kit users return for their results? In the US it has been reported that up to 50% of those tested do not return for their results at some conventional testing sites

- Does the system of referring people to physicians and treatment centres work?

- Is the quality of the advice people are getting about treatment options, safer sex and referrals up to scratch?

- What are the psychosocial consequences of receiving results in this way compared with conventional testing?

- What is the false positive and false negative rate in much larger sample group?

In the longer term home testing may be an important element in encouraging the early diagnosis of HIV infection. However, the introduction of such a system raises specific issues for the UK. For example, the UK has a very good system of GUM clinics which also function as HIV treatment centres and sexual health clinics. Home testing might damage the useful relationship between these services, which does not exist to the same extent in other countries.

Home testing also calls into question the right of British residents to free treatment and diagnosis under the NHS. It would be part of the creeping 'privatisation' of NHS services, and ought to be considered as part of the debate about how health services should be funded. Would it be a good thing if many people at lower risk of HIV infection ceased to use GUM services and took up home testing instead? Should people not at high-risk be charged for HIV testing anyway, as is the case in the Australian state of Victoria?

HIV testing has not been as widespread amongst gay men in the UK as it has in the United States. Would companies manufacturing the kits be permitted to market them in the same way as they do in the US, over the counter and backed up by advertising campaigns? Would this advertising be targeted at high risk groups or the general population? How would this affect health promotion activities targeted at gay men, who have much lower testing rates than injecting drug users (approx 50% of gay men vs 85% of IVDUs in contact with drugs services)?

Rapid self-testing

A further generation of home tests is likely to be offered in the next few years. These tests will use rapid, on the spot diagnostic techniques already developed for use in medical settings, testing saliva, urine or blood. These tests could be true *home tests*.

Such tests raise more difficult ethical issues. For example, how would people react to discovering a positive result without even having telephone support to talk about their diagnosis? Is there any guarantee that they would read or understand any counselling material supplied with the test kit?

There may also be a particular danger of false positive results with the technologies which could be employed for self-testing at home. This is especially problematic, since test kit users may not fully understand the need for confirmatory testing.

Home testing may also be used in confused or even abusive ways. For instance, it may be used to test new sexual partners without a clear understanding of the potential window period. Partners or adolescent children may be forced to test, and it might be possible to test people surreptitiously with such test kits, particularly if they are based on a saliva or urine assay. This raises particular issues in the workplace, where compulsory drug testing is becoming increasingly frequent. If home testing became sufficiently routine, companies might be able to argue that the testing of employees did not constitute a discriminatory practice.

However, some doctors and policy makers in the US argue that self-testing would be good thing if it encouraged more people to come forward for HIV treatment earlier. They say that whilst it was appropriate for testing to be carried out on a restricted basis when treatment options were less promising, and the implications of a positive result very serious, it is now imperative that people are encouraged to test. However, this view pre-supposes that the resources will remain available to treat all the newly diagnosed people. At present this appears unlikely, especially if home testing achieved what some of its proponents hope: a large increase in people from minority communities coming forward for treatment. It is this group of the US population which already has the poorest access to state of the art treatment, due to cuts in AIDS Drug Assistance Programmes, lack of health insurance, or restrictive health insurance.

A possible setback to extending HIV testing, especially home testing, happened in late 2005.

In November 2005 the FDA had met to give consideration to approving the oral *OraQuick* HIV test for over-the-counter sale in pharmacies. Currently the OraQuick test is only sold officially to doctors and nurses, although it has been unofficially available from Internet suppliers for some time.

Freya Spielberg, a researcher at the Centre for AIDS Research at the University of Washington, said the availability of a rapid, at-home HIV test "is the most powerful strategy we have to bring down HIV infections". She pointed out that about 8,000 people who test positive for HIV annually at health clinics in the USA never return to pick up their results.

The FDA was thought partly to be guided by the change of heart among HIV treatment activists. Two years ago Gay Men's Health Crisis (GMHC) in New York, the country's oldest HIV organisation, opposed home testing. But in November 2005 it said it supported it - with reservations.

"For people who don't have access to a clinic or make a decision not to go to a clinic, this is better than nothing," said GMHC's Gregg Gonsalves. "But it's not a magic bullet."

So-called 'home testing' kits have in fact been legal in the USA since 1996, but the two tests available till now, Confide® and the Home Access Test® have in fact been blood sampling kits where you take a fingertip blood sample with a lancet and send it off on a card for laboratory testing. However the OraQuick test has been unofficially available on the internet for some time.

However plans to make the test available over the counter were thrown into reverse after certain community centres using the OraQuick 20-minute HIV test reported ten times the expected number of false-positive test results.

A provision to direct the US Department of Health to purchase one million of the tests for distribution to pharmacies was unexpectedly stripped from a Senate Bill on 14 December 2005.

The problem first came to public attention when the Los Angeles Gay and Lesbian Center announced on the 8th of December that there had been a large number of false positive tests among people using OraQuick.

The centre said it performed 600 oral HIV tests a month and normally found about 20 people who tested positive. False positives were rare till November, when 13 people who had tested positive on the OraQuick test were later found to be negative on confirmatory testing.

Barbara Adler, the project's testing programme manager, said "It was excruciating for our clients and our staff to be getting these results, not knowing whether they were accurate." She said the project has gone back to using the pin-prick blood test it was previously using. Clinics in New York had also noticed an increase in false positives from 10 in October to 30 in November - about a quarter of all positive test results.

Dr Bernard Branson of the Division of HIV Prevention at the US Centers for Disease Control said he could offer no explanation for the rise in false positives in recent months. A CDC survey of 17,000 results found a false-positive rate of only 0.2% compared with over 2% experienced by the Los Angeles Gay Center.

In the UK selling HIV tests to anyone but medical professionals is illegal and likely to remain so for some time, even though a lower proportion of gay men test in the UK than in the US. In the last UK Gay Men's Sex Survey 56% of gay men had ever taken an HIV test.

UK activists have traditionally been more concerned by the ethical implications of the availability of home tests, not just in terms of whether people could face the shock of an unexpected positive result, but by whether repeat home testing could be used as a substitute for safer sex and even whether someone could surreptitiously test another family member for HIV without their knowledge.

References

CDC. Advancing HIV Prevention: New Strategies for a Changing Epidemic --- United States, 2003. *Mortality and Morbidity Weekly Report* (MMWR) 52(15);329-332. April 2003.

CDC. Advancing HIV prevention: the science behind the new initiative. See http://www.cdc.gov/hiv/topics/prev_prog/AHP/resources/qa/AdvancingFS.pdf%20.%20 September%202003.

Dodds JP (http://www.ncbi.nlm.nih.gov/entrez/query.fcgi?db=pubmed&cmd=Search&itool=pubme d_Abstract&term=%22Dodds+JP%22%5BAuthor%5D) et al. Increasing risk behaviour and high levels of undiagnosed HIV infection in a community sample of homosexual men. *Sex Transm Infect.* (javascript:AL_get(this,%20'jour',%20'Sex%20Transm%20Infect.');) 2004 Jun;80(3):236-40.

Fincher-Mergi M, Cartone KJ, Mischler J, et al. Assessment of emergency department professionals' behaviors regarding HIV testing and referral for patients with STDs. AIDS Patient Care STDs 2002;16:549-53.

Gorbach PM. Transmission behaviors of recently HIV-infected men who have sex with men. *JAIDS* 42(1): 80-85. 2006.

Holtgrave DR and Anderson T. Utilising HIV transmission rates to assist in prioritising HIV prevention services. *International Journal of STD & AIDS* 15: 789-792. 2004.

Paltiel AD et al. Expanded Screening for HIV in the United States - An Analysis of Cost-Effectiveness. *NEJM* 352(6): 586-595. 2005.

Sanders GD et al. Cost-Effectiveness of Screening for HIV in the Era of Highly Active Antiretroviral Therapy. *NEJM* 352(6): 570-585. 2005.

Staley P. Why It's Right to Test. *New York Times,* 02 June 2006.

Stanley R. Uptake of HIV screening in genitourinary medicine after change to 'opt-out' consent. *BMJ* 326:1174. 2003.

Wenger NS et al. Sexual behavior of individuals infected with the human immunodeficiency virus. The need for intervention. *Arch Intern Med.* 154(16):1849-54. 1994.

Using antiretrovirals for HIV prevention

How can ARVs prevent HIV transmission?

Antiretrovirals (ARVs) can theoretically be used to prevent HIV transmission in two ways:

Firstly, when taken by people with HIV, they might suppress the virus in the person's body in a way that makes it harder to transmit to others.

Secondly, when taken by people who do not have HIV, they might prevent the virus from establishing itself in the body.

The first effect certainly exists. In one San Francisco study (Porco) it was estimated that, averaged over population of people with HIV, people on HAART were one-third as infectious as people not on treatment.

In one study of 415 members of the Rakai cohort in Uganda (Quinn), which is one of the most reliable guides we have to exactly how and how often transmission occurs(at least within heterosexual sex), no person transmitted HIV out of the 51 whose viral load was under 1500.

However it is usually thought unwise to rely on viral load as a means of HIV prevention. Why not?

For one thing, viral load tests do not measure virus that is present inside cells. These can be transmitted through blood transfusions or through needle-sharing, and may be transmissible sexually, so an 'undetectable' viral load is not going to prevent transmission in this way.

Also, viral load in blood may not match that in semen or vaginal fluids, especially when a sexually transmitted infection or other reproductive tract infection is present. See **HIV transmission** for more on this. Some ARVs are more effective in suppressing viral load in seminal fluids than others. While some ARVs are concentrated in semen, others appear unable to enter it.

Even if viral load in the blood were an accurate guide, it would only be as good as the last viral load test. Any virus that is transmitted in the context of a rising viral load due to treatment failure be drug-resistant.

There has already been a report of HIV transmission occurring to a steady sexual partner during a treatment interruption. Paradoxically, this does suggest that the treatment was previously a factor preventing HIV transmission (Tubiana).

One context in which further research on this effect is planned is in the provision of ARVs to women who are breastfeeding. WHO has developed a protocol for international clinical trials that will seek to find out whether, and to what extent, ARV treatment for mothers can prevent breast milk transmission to their children. This could have major advantages in settings where formula feed is unsafe and unaffordable: in fact, the cost of ARVs for the mother is equivalent to the cost of formula feed for the baby and - it may be argued - could be a better use of limited resources.

The uncertainties about using viral load as a guide to whether a person is infectious or not has not stopped this being used 'informally' as a way for partners, predominantly gay men, to decide whether to risk unprotected sex or not.

Several recent studies have found that gay men are questioning each other about their HIV viral load in order to try and establish if they are infectious. "Are you undetectable?" is becoming as common a chatroom question as "are you poz?"

In a study from San Francisco (Goldhammer, 2005) 78% of 507 gay men questioned were familiar with the term 'viral load' and one third (111 of the total sample) had discussed viral load with a partner of a different HIV status during the previous year in order to make decisions about which sexual practices to engage in.

Of those who had discussed viral load, more than half estimated that they used viral load disclosure to guide sexual decision-making in at least 70% of their sexual encounters.

In another study from Sydney (Van de Ven, 2005) researchers asked 119 men who were in an HIV-serodiscordant regular relationship about whether they used viral load as a basis for their decisions on condom use. Twice as many (39.4%) reported unprotected anal intercourse when the partner's HIV last viral load test was undetectable as when it was detectable (20.8%).

So it is possible to regard the provision of treatment to people with HIV as a preventative measure, and this is often factored into mathematical models of the likely future development of the epidemic.

However this is not what is generally thought of when we mention antiretrovirals in this context. In the vast majority of cases we are talking about:

- HIV drugs being given to HIV-negative people as emergency protection after a possible exposure event has already occurred (**post-exposure prophylaxis** or **PEP), or**

- HIV drugs being given to HIV-negative people as a general prophylactic regimen before any exposure occurs (**pre-exposure prophylaxis** or **PREP**).

The value of prophlyaxis being given to HIV-negative people to prevent HIV being established, is best illustrated in the case of two-dose nevirapine prophylaxis, used to prevent transmission from mothers to babies.

Here, the dose taken by the woman at the onset of labour does nothing to suppress her virus. The only way in which it can act is by reaching the baby across the placenta, from where it has been shown to reach levels sufficient to prevent HIV infection (a 'PREP' dose). A second dose of nevirapine, given to the baby 72 hours after birth, extends this protection long enough to ensure that any virus to which the baby was exposed during birth is unable to establish itself (a 'PEP' dose). This is discussed further in the context of preventing mother-to-child transmission.

Post-exposure prophylaxis

The case for providing antiviral treatment as 'post-exposure prophylaxis' after sexual exposure is an extension of the case for providing it in occupational settings. Much of the section on needlestick injuries in *HIV transmission* is relevant here.

PEP using AZT was in use by as early as 1988 in health-care settings (Henderson and Gerberding).

The argument is based on a comparison of per-exposure risks. Estimates of these rates based on studies show that unprotected receptive anal sex with an HIV-positive partner is probably at least twice as risky in terms of the likelihood of infection from a single exposure as a needlestick injury, and may be 10 times more risky if the partner has a high viral load. And although a single needlestick injury is probably three to four times riskier than a single act of receptive vaginal sex (unless the partner has a high viral load), factors such as trauma during rape may make this as risky too (Vittinghof - and see the table of per-exposure risks in **HIV transmission**).

It is obviously far more difficult to give prompt access to medical treatment when exposure occurs in the community, than it is when accidents occur in a hospital. The usual occupational exposure target, of starting treatment within four hours of an exposure incident, is unlikely to be achieved.

A recent UK survey by the Health Protection Agency (Delpech) of PEP provision at ten London HIV clinics found that for people seeking post-exposure prophylaxis after non-occupational exposure, the average time elapsed between exposure and taking PEP was 23 hours, whereas for occupational exposure it was two hours.

It has not been possible, and may never be, to organise a randomised controlled trial of antiretroviral treatment to assess its effectiveness. The HPA survey above was originally designed as a case-control study but the control arm had to be abandoned because people who turn up for PEP are very unlikely to decline it. It is clearly unethical, when someone has just experienced what may have been a traumatic and worrying event, to allocate them to a control or placebo instead of giving them PEP.

Another reason is the comparative rarity of events that require PEP, so it is hard to predict in advance who will need it. One precondition for offering PEP is the widespread availability of HIV antibody testing, so that people at risk are aware of their own HIV-negative status. This would be especially important if the treatment option provided were inappropriate for treating HIV-positive people, for example, single dose nevirapine and/or short course combivir (AZT and 3TC).

Finally, a large trial would be needed. Delpech estimated that 2.6 transmission events would occur in 300 people in the population studied in the HPA trial if PEP was not used. The study audited 1500 cases in which PEP was given but was only able to find full details on 333 and had a 42% lost-to-follow-up rate, meaning that only 170 people could be traced later to see if there had been any seroconversions. A zero rate of seroconversions in a group this size would therefore have no statistical significance. In fact, there were two seroconversions among the 170 people who'd taken PEP. But both people had gone on to risk further exposures to HIV subsequent to taking PEP.

This underlines another of the big problems with assessing the effectiveness and desirability of PEP. No less than 27% of the whole group, and 34% of the gay men, had, after taking PEP, then gone on to risk further exposure within three months of taking it!

People are not necessarily rational about assessing the degree of risk they have been exposed to and may form very different estimates of the 'riskiness' of an incident even where the external circumstances are the same. The desire to seek PEP may also wax and wane according to several factors:

- whether the source partner is known to be positive;

- whether the source partner is judged to be a 'high risk' person if their serostatus is unknown;

- whether the source partner recommended PEP;

- whether the exposure was consensual or non-consensual or involved trauma;

- whether it occurred while the person was under the influence or drink or drugs;

- whether it occurred within a casual encounter or within a primary relationship;

- and psychological factors such as depression or fatalism among the person at risk.

All of these factors may influence the decision whether or not to seek PEP (or not decide to seek it until too late).

There is another unresolved question, whether treatments which are clearly inadequate for treating HIV may be perfectly adequate for preventing infection. Animal studies which used a form of tenofovir, and the mother-to-child prevention with two doses of nevirapine mentioned above, strongly suggest that this is the case. There are precedents from other diseases, such as tuberculosis and malaria, where single agents in relatively low doses are successfully used for prophylaxis whereas treatment requires much higher doses and/or combinations of effective drugs.

It is also argued that when antiviral drugs are given to people who are HIV-negative, the level of toxicity that can be tolerated is far lower than when drugs are used to treat a life-threatening illness.

The UK guidelines recommend 28 days of two nucleosides plus either nelfinavir or a boosted protease inhibitor. Didanosine (ddI) is excluded from the nucleosides for possible liver or pancreatic toxicity; abacavir and the NNRTI nevirapine are excluded because of the well-known risk of acute hypersensitivity reactions to these drugs; and efavirenz is excluded because it also causes rash and because it "causes short-term psychostimulation, which is possibly less well tolerated in anxious patients receiving PEP than in patients with established HIV infection." This leaves Either *Combivir* (AZT/3TC), *Truvada* (tenofovir/FTC), or d4t/3TC as the nucleosides plus either a protease inhibitor in the shape of nelfinavir, or a boosted PI such as *Kaletra* (liponavir/r) or saquinavir/r.

The UK is one of the few countries in fact to recommend a three-drug regime. Many others continue to recommend two nucleosides except in very high-risk exposures or there is evidence that the transmitted virus could be drug-resistant.

A poster at the 13th CROI Conference in 2006 (Rabaud) discussed the tolerability of PEP regimens given at nine hospitals in France. The regimens compared were AZT/3TC (*Combivir*) plus nelfinavir (*Viracept*); *Combivir* plus lopinavir/ritonavir (*Kaletra*); *Combivir* plus tenofovir (*Viread*); and tenofovir/3TC plus atazanavir/ritonavir.

The regimen containing nelfinavir was significantly less well tolerated, with 34.5% of patients discontinuing a 28-day course of PEP due to adverse events, compared with an average of 20% with the other regimens.

Commentators at the poster session said that they had found AZT-free regimens were better tolerated; questioned the usefulness of Kaletra due to its poor genital penetration; and aired the ever-controversial topic (in PEP terms) of whether to provide two or three drugs. A survey of occupational antiretroviral post-exposure prophylaxis among health workers in Canada uncovered a major hidden cost. Time off work due to side- effects of the drugs cost the health service as much as providing the drugs for the treatment. This time off work appears to have doubled, from an average of 7.0 days to 15.8 days in the year 2000, when the protease inhibitor nelfinavir was added to the regimen, previously d4T plus 3TC (McLeod).

Experience to date with PEP

Large-scale prospective, placebo-controlled trials have not been carried out for PEP, and so a definitive answer regarding its effectiveness cannot be given at this time.

A much-cited 1997 case control study (Cardo) of health care workers from France, Italy, the UK, and the US came to the conclusion that PEP (in this case AZT monotherapy) reduced the risk of becoming infected with HIV by 81% (with a confidence interval of 48-94%.) This was equivalent to reducing the risk of infection from 1 in 200 to 1 in 10,000 risk However, there is much less solid data on PEP's effectiveness after sexual exposure.

The San Francisco study

A 2005 study in San Francisco (Roland 2005) evaluated 702 subjects who took PEP twelve weeks after their exposure. Seven subjects became HIV-positive despite PEP but in four of these there were either additional exposures to HIV after PEP had been initiated or HIV was found in blood specimens given at the start of PEP, meaning they either sought it too late or were already infected with HIV and did not know it. Three seroconverters reported having no exposures after PEP initiation and probably represented evidence of PEP failure.

Of course, given that the chance of getting HIV from a single occasion of receptive anal intercourse is in the region of one chance in 30 to one in 250, many of the men taking PEP would not have been infected with HIV anyway. Because of this, among 702 men, one would only expect about six infections if they only had one risky encounter each. But because only three got infected who had definitely only had one encounter, the study implies that PEP prevents at least one in two infections.

The average time delay between the sexual exposure and taking PEP was 32.5 hours, but among men who became HIV-positive it was 45.5 hours - nearly two days - indicating that initiating PEP within a day of exposure is probably necessary to ensure it has the best chance of working.

Researcher Michelle Roland from the University of California, San Francisco, said that the example of the four men who went on to have unsafe sex soon after taking PEP was a reminder that it could not be a stand-alone prevention method.

"It provides an important HIV prevention opportunity when exposed individuals may be especially receptive to assistance with reducing their HIV risk...but is only one part of that prevention activity," she said.

"Sexual exposures are usually not isolated, and helping people stay HIV-negative requires response to both the presenting exposure and attempts to reduce subsequent exposures."

The Brazil study

One of the more convincing studies was conducted in Brazil and reported two years ago at the 9th Retroviruses Conference in Seattle (Schechter). Here, 202 HIV-negative gay men were enrolled and followed for an average of two years. At the time of enrolment, 57% of the group reported "high-risk behaviour". PEP, consisting of four weeks of AZT/3TC, was used 100 times by 73 (36%) of the participants, 91% of whom completed the course. Most men took it just once or twice during the two years of the trial, but one man took it nine times.

There were 11 seroconversions among the group; however, only one occurred in someone who had taken PEP. Analysis of the strain of HIV that infected him despite using PEP showed that it harboured the *M184V* mutation which is likely to lead to high-level resistance to 3TC.

The researchers calculated that PEP reduced the seroconversion rate by 83%, from 4.1 cases per 100 patients a year to 0.7 cases.

However the study also found that although quite a high proportion of the study population took PEP, they were bad at evaluating risk and did not take PEP nearly often enough, or did not take it at the times it was really needed. As a result, there was almost no difference in the infection rate observed in the study population as a whole and what would have been expected if PEP had not been available.

During the trial eleven men (5.5%) became HIV-positive, representing 2.9 infections per 100 men a year. While the researchers were able to conclude that PEP, if used properly, could prevent at least 70% of sexual infections, the predicted rate of HIV infection among this group if they had not had PEP available was 3.1 infections per 100 men a year - meaning PEP had actually made almost no difference to the average HIV infection rate.

The reasons PEP was not taken were either that gay men mistakenly assumed their partner was faithful and HIV-negative, or that they caught HIV through routes they considered low risk, such as oral sex. This seems to bear out findings from the UK about gay men's estimation of risk.

The 2005 Gay Men's Sex Survey, *Risk and Reflexion*, found that gay men tend to see sexual risk in terms of risky actions rather than risky partners.

Sigma Research comment: "Overall, 89% of descriptions of risky sex given to the survey by respondents featured information about sexual acts or condoms, whereas only 15% mentioned the status of the partner or alluded to their potential sero-discordancy. The things that constitute risky sex give an insight into where men go wrong when they have sex they consider secure but which results in HIV transmission. The problems seem to be more with misreading the presence of HIV infection (exposure) than underestimating the potential for transmission when it is present."

When the reasons for not taking PEP were looked at in the ten Brazilian men who seroconverted, three thought they were at no risk from their partners. Two mistakenly assumed their boyfriend had been faithful, while another's partner had lied about his HIV status. One didn't want to be seen to be taking HIV drugs, and the reasons were unknown for one man.

This left five who considered their exposure low risk. This worryingly included three - nearly a third of the HIV infections - who said they had only had oral sex.

This study highlighted one of the central dilemmas of PEP. Unlike the other interventions considered in this section, its availability may be crucial to individuals who need it but, as an emergency measure only used by a minority of gay men, it is unlikely to make much difference to HIV incidence on a population level. This has led to controversy about exactly how much it should be promoted as a prevention method - see more below.

However because persons seeking PEP are highly motivated to avoid infection, they may be in a window period in which education and counselling will have significant influence.

Several other interesting findings came from this study. One was that "high-risk" behaviour declined during the study from 56% to 40%. Although it has been suggested from other studies that people reporting declines in risky behaviour may sometimes not be reporting the whole story due, possibly, to guilt at being a 'study failure', this finding may help allay fears that the widespread availability of PEP for sexual exposure will cause an increase in condomless intercourse.

Furthermore, 92% of the time, PEP was taken appropriately, i.e. after an exposure that researchers considered "high risk". This seems to offer a degree of assurance that PEP will not be abused by the 'worried well' concerned by very low-risk incidents.

Finally, the study issued people with 'starter packs' - ready-wrapped doses of AZT/3TC with instructions that participants should take them immediately following exposure. Other PEP schemes have relied on people reporting to A&E departments after weekend incidents. Since one of the key components to successful PEP is prompt treatment - ideally within 24 hours - this may explain some of the difference between the reported effectiveness rate of 83% in the Brazil study and the 53% rate in the cost-effectiveness study detailed below (Pinkerton).

An earlier study in San Francisco has investigated the safety and acceptability of PEP after possible sexual or IDU exposure to HIV. Individuals who have experienced this type of exposure within the previous 72 hours are offered one month's treatment with AZT and 3TC in the form of one tablet twice a day (also known by the trade name Combivir). Other drugs (ddI and d4T) are being offered in cases where it is believed that a risk may exist of exposure to AZT and/or 3TC-resistant virus (Kahn).

The study collected data on the number of cases, the types of risk exposure, the uptake of PEP, side-effects, adherence, the development of drug-resistant HIV strains, and subsequent risk behaviour. The study is not large enough to provide statistically significant evidence of PEP's effectiveness, although it is collecting data on the number of seroconversions.

In total 401 requests for PEP were received between December 1997 and March 1999. 91% of participants were men and the median age was 32 years.

375 of the 401 participants sought PEP because of sexual exposure and only 2% reported sharing of IDU equipment. Receptive anal intercourse was reported in 40% of the exposures.

PEP was supplied within 72 hours of exposure.

Certainty of source partner's HIV-positive status was expressed by 174 (43%) of participants. For the majority of participants exposed during sexual activity, the sexual exposure that prompted enrolment represented a lapse in safe sex practices rather than habitual high-risk behaviour.

In total 309 (48%) of participants completed 4 weeks of treatment. Complete adherence to medication in the four days before the clinic visit was reported by 84% to 78% of participants, despite high levels of self-reported side-effects, including; nausea (52%), fatigue (44%), headache (24%) and diarrhoea (15%).

This study is one of the first to provide data on the actual practice of providing PEP after sexual and IDU exposure. It demonstrated that people with sexual exposures will seek PEP. For the majority of individuals, the episode represented a lapse in safer sexual practices. The study demonstrated the feasibility of identifying persons with a sexual exposure to HIV as well as that exposed persons can be reliably and safely treated with a four-week course.

Completion rates were high at 78%. This was most likely due to several factors including, the provision of one-to-one medication adherence counselling, dispensing only a limited supply of medications at each visit which required individuals to make regular contact with staff and finally, the majority of participant took a dual nucleoside analogue regimen which was dose twice daily. Such a regimen is associated with fewer side-effects and greater ease of use than triple combinations including a protease inhibitor.

The study was not designed to evaluate efficacy, though no individuals were observed to develop antibodies to HIV at six months after exposure.

In New York, seven patients were enrolled via a 24-hour telephone helpline to receive an individualised antiretroviral regimen. An NNRTI was given alongside AZT and 3TC, and those patients presenting between 48 and 72 hours after exposure were given nelfinavir. One patient discontinued nelfinavir due to elevated lipid levels, otherwise side-effects were limited to GI disturbances and did not require treatment modification or discontinuation. The researchers found that with adequate counselling and support, participants were able to demonstrate excellent adherence (Torres). This was the first nonoccupational post-exposure prophylaxis (PEP) pilot program in New York City and aimed to enroll 120 participants over the first twelve months.

Several other preliminary studies have reported poor rates of adherence and follow-up; for example, only three out of eight sexually exposed patients completed a PEP course at the

Chelsea and Westminster Hospital in London (Easterbrook), and only one out of eight returned for all follow-up visits. At St Vincent's Hospital in New York, none of the six individuals who received PEP after sexual assault returned for HIV testing when the course was completed (Opio). It is worth remembering that numbers in these studies are low.

The cost-effectiveness of PEP

A major concern about PEP is cost. It could be argued that offering everybody anti-HIV drugs as a preventative measure is a lot more expensive than offering condoms. However, it could also be argued that PEP is HIV treatment rather than HIV prevention, and should therefore be paid for out of treatment budgets. A universal policy of prescribing PEP for people who have experienced any significant HIV risk exposure could never be cost-effective, even though at around £750 the cost of a month's triple combination therapy PEP for a single individual seems to compares extremely favourably with the likely life-time costs of treating the same individual should he or she become infected with HIV. The cost-effectiveness of an intervention such as PEP can only be meaningfully calculated in terms of the amount of money that would need to be spent to prevent a single infection. On average, no more than about one out of every three hundred people who have a single episode of unprotected receptive anal sex with an HIV-positive person becomes infected as a result (Katz). So if all 300 came forward for PEP after their risk exposure, 299 would be treated 'unnecessarily', because they would not have become infected regardless of whether or not they received PEP. If doctors have to treat 300 people in order to prevent the one single infection, the cost of preventing that infection would be three hundred times £750, which makes £225,000. In blunt financial terms, this no longer compares so favourably with the life-time costs of medical care.

The cost-effectiveness of PEP could be improved by using fewer or cheaper drugs; for example, if only two nucleoside analogue drugs were used (or if an additional protease inhibitor was reserved only for specific cases of the greatest risk) the cost per course of PEP would be approximately halved. Moreover, PEP would also be more cost-effective if it were delivered only to people whose circumstances meant that they were most at risk of becoming infected (effectively reducing the proportion of recipients who are being treated 'unnecessarily').

Possible criteria for prioritisation might include limiting PEP to cases in which people had a risk encounter with someone who was known for sure to be HIV-positive - even though the US guidelines for occupational use do not carry such a restriction. PEP would also become more cost-effective if offered only to people whose risk had been substantial, such as unprotected receptive anal or vaginal sex or shared drug injecting equipment.

A study published in January 2004 (Pinkerton) attempted to calculate the cost-effectiveness of PEP. Here, Pinkerton and colleagues looked at 401 people who had sought PEP in San Francisco.

The group included men and women who sought PEP for incidents of unprotected anal and/or vaginal intercourse and needle-sharing. The researchers concluded that PEP reduced expected HIV infections by 53% by calculating that, according to types of risk reported by the study participants, an average of 2.36 HIV infections would have been expected: PEP reduced this to 1.1 infections.

This 53% reduction saved 11.74 quality adjusted life years (QALYs). This measurement, frequently used in cost-benefit calculations, means that, for those that used it successfully, PEP should lead to an extra 11.74 years of reasonable health. This in turn, it was calculated, would save a total of US$281,323 in future HIV-related medical costs. When all factors were taken into account, the cost of PEP per QALY saved was US$14,449 - approximately £9,500 at the time of the study or £7,950 now.

This may sound a lot, but in the US programmes costing $40,000 - $60,000 per QALY are seen as cost-effective. By comparison, similar cost-effectiveness studies (Freedberg) showed that HIV combination therapy resulted in a cost of US$23,000 per QALY saved. There is no official figure for the UK, but it is thought that the National Institute of Clinical Excellence (NICE), which guides Primary Care Trust spending, considers anything below £30,000 per QALY saved to be cost-effective.

By including a varied population with different risks, this study found that PEP, given to the general at-risk population, did work out to be much less cost-effective than other HIV prevention methods. One risk-reduction programme for at-risk women (Holtgrave 1996) attending an urban primary health care clinic was successful at increasing condom use and cost about US$260 per client or about US$2,000 per QALY. A similar programme for gay men, (Holtgrave 1997), although costing US$470 per client, was not only cost-effective but actually cost-saving: the cost of likely future treatment and care of those infected without the programme outweighed the cost of delivering the programme to the whole group. This compares with an average cost of US$8,607 per QALY saved for PEP for gay men as a whole as reported by Pinkerton.

However, when it came to gay men who had been on the receiving end of unprotected anal sex (i.e. 'bottoms'), the Pinkerton study found that PEP was not merely cost-effective, but actually cost-saving. The cost per infection averted for this group was US$177,293 - which is less than the likely cost of their lifetime HIV treatment if they had not received successful PEP. On the other hand, PEP for gay men on the insertive end of unprotected anal sex (i.e. 'tops') was not considered cost-effective.

The variation seen in cost-effectiveness between subgroups of different populations is not surprising, given that you need to provide PEP to the people most at-risk for it to be cost-effective. The Health Protection Agency (HPA) estimates that gay men who are the passive partner in unprotected anal intercourse have a 1-in-33 risk of being infected with HIV if they are certain their partner is HIV-positive, but a 1-in-222 risk if they do not know the HIV status of their partner. They estimate that gay men who are the active partner in unprotected anal intercourse have a 1-in-555 risk of being infected with HIV if they are certain their partner is HIV-positive, but a 1-in-11,111 risk if they do not know the HIV status of their partner. However, other factors such as geographical location, STIs, viral load and bleeding may affect the risk estimate, so there is likely to be a range of risk of transmission rather than an exact value.

In short, if PEP in the UK is offered to gay men who have been the passive partner in unprotected anal intercourse and/or who have known HIV-positive partners, PEP could potentially save as much money as providing condoms and safer-sex education, as long as PEP is not routinely relied upon as a substitute for these other safer-sex practices.

Putting PEP into practice

The Australian policy on PEP for sexual exposure - the first of its kind - was first written in 1998, though a decision to actively promote PEP as a prevention tool was not taken until June 2000. The high-risk groups targeted initially were gay men and people in serodiscordant relationships; subsequently, IDUs and sex workers were also targeted.

A phoneline with the number 1-800-PEP-NOW was publicised, posters were placed in community press and information was issued in leaflets and on the web. There were 493 calls for the January-November 2001 duration of the helpline, of which 88% were direct requests for PEP. Sixty-one percent met guidelines for PEP prescription; 28% did not because they were considered low risk, and 11% fell outside the 72-hour time limit.

Interestingly, and contrary to some other surveys, only 7.2% of callers were seeking PEP for exposure with regular partners.

In terms of community awareness of PEP, 64% of those polled in the target groups had not heard of PEP in February 2001. Six months later, 58.5% *had* heard of PEP. Triple combination therapy was prescribed at the start of the programme, but cost pressure meant that HAART was reduced to the dual nucleoside therapy, AZT/3TC.

Following on from the Australian experience, the Terrence Higgins Trust (THT) in the UK mounted an awareness raising campaign about PEP directed at gay men in 2004.

In the 2005 Gay Men's Sex survey (data collected 2004), when gay men were asked about what they considered 'risky' sex, no respondent mentioned anti-HIV treatments, viral load or post-exposure prophylaxis (PEP) as moderators of risk, suggesting these do not feature in men's perceptions of sexual risk and safety.

However, following the campaign, according to data released early from the 2006 National Gay Men's Sex Survey, gay men in the UK in 2005 were twice as likely to be aware of PEP than they were in 2003 - an increase from 22% to 39%. Awareness of PEP significantly increased in every demographic subgroup and in every area of the country, although the rise was greatest in London and Brighton, the cities most targeted by the THT's campaign.

The campaign also had a significant impact on the numbers of gay men seeking PEP, and the numbers of men being prescribed the drugs. In the UK, the proportion of gay men who had ever sought PEP increased significantly from 1.0% in 2003 to 1.4% in 2005, and the proportion who had ever actually taken PEP rose from 0.6% in 2003 to 1.2% in 2005.

Seeking PEP and taking PEP rose in all demographic groups and in all areas and remained highest in London and Brighton, among men with higher numbers of sexual partners and those with higher incomes.

Ford Hickson of Sigma Research, who conducted the research, said: "The proportion of those men who sought the treatment who went on to take it also rose significantly from 59% in 2003 to 74% in 2005, suggesting an on-going improvement in access to this service which is clearly necessary."

However, taking PEP is still very rare even among the group most at risk from HIV in the UK. Although 7.5% of men not tested HIV-positive said they thought they had been involved in sexual HIV exposure in the last year, only 1.2% of men, or 16% of those who thought they had definitely been at risk, had ever taken PEP.

Ethical and practical issues

Providing PEP after sexual or IDU exposures, then, presents different challenges than for occupational or perinatal exposures. Persons exposed to HIV from sexual or IDU activities often do not accurately assess their risk for infection and may delay seeking treatment.

Identifying a person's source partner and determining his or her HIV status after sexual exposure may be problematic.

Concerns have been raised that if PEP were provided for sexual or IDU exposure, individuals would experience unacceptable side-effects or would inadequately adhere to the treatment regimen or refuse to return for follow-up HIV testing.

Additionally, there is the concern that PEP would fail to fully suppress the virus and rapidly induce resistance to the drugs

used. This risk is greatest, if people take it in the belief that they are HIV-negative when in fact they are already HIV-positive.

The point has been raised that the availability of PEP for sexual and IDU exposures might paradoxically increase risk behaviour. For this reason the San Francisco study described above included a number of sessions of risk reduction counselling.

In the study, only 10% of people seeking PEP reported an increase in risk behaviour following a PEP consultation. This compares with 74% reporting a decrease in risk behaviour and 16% no change. Health-related interventions such as PEP may therefore help capitalise on 'close calls' to motivate and sustain risk reduction.

A US survey of gay men in 1998 (Kalichman) attending a large Pride festival in Atlanta found that 3% of those surveyed had used PEP, 26% planned to use it, and 74% doubted if they would need to use PEP.

However, those planning to use PEP were more likely to have had unprotected receptive anal sex. They were also younger, less educated, more likely to have used recreational drugs and have a history of IDU.

This user profile could be seen either as a problem or as an opportunity. Does the availability of PEP mean that young, drug-using gay men have an 'excuse' not to try to maintain safer sex habits? Or, conversely, are they taking a realistic look at their behaviour and its likely risks and seizing upon a technology that may protect them?

There are also concerns about the potential cost (as opposed to cost-effectiveness) of PEP if taken up as a mass prevention measure. One of the implications of the San Francisco study is that if the entire annual US HIV prevention budget was used for PEP, it would fund 550,000 treatments and prevent a mere 880 new infections, or 2.2% of the estimated US annual incidence.

It will be difficult to define the boundary between cases of sexual risk which are high enough to justify offering PEP, and those in which the risk of infection is sufficiently low that the financial cost of PEP and the risk of drug side-effects is felt to be unjustifiable. For instance, the CDC guidelines indicate that combination therapy may be reasonable for health-care workers who experience mucosal exposure to semen even where there are only grounds for suspicion, rather than certainty, that the source patient is HIV-positive. How does this differ from the situation of any gay man who is penetrated without a condom in a large city in the UK?

A 1998 review of ethical and clinical implications of PEP for non-occupational exposure concluded that it would be prudent to consider local HIV prevalence rather than relying on per-exposure risks calculated for very high prevalence cities when considering the likely need for PEP (Lurie).

How soon should PEP be used?

When used, PEP should be initiated promptly. Animal research suggests that PEP may be ineffective if started later than 24 to 36 hours after exposure. The animal study upon which these estimates is based comes from macaque monkeys given tenofovir as the sole PEP drug (Tsai 1998).

In this study, 24 macaque monkeys were divided into six groups of four. They were all given a dose of SIV (monkey HIV) 10 times larger than the dose which would be expected to infect 50% of monkeys - a dose that should have infected all of them. They were then treated with tenofovir starting various times after infection and continued for various time periods. The results were as follows:

A: Control group (treated only with saline, not tenofovir: 100% infected: all seroconverted by week four).

B: Tenofovir started 24 hours after exposure and continued for 28 days: probably none infected (one monkey eventually showed antibodies to SIV after 32 weeks but free or cell-associated virus was not detected in any monkey).

C: Tenofovir started 48 hours after exposure, continued for 28 days: all seroconverted to SIV by week 16, though virus was only detectable in 50% of monkeys.

D: Tenofovir started 72 hours after exposure, continued for 28 days: all seroconverted by eight weeks, though virus only detectable in 50%.

E: Tenofovir started 24 hours after exposure, continued for ten days: 50% eventually seroconverted, though virus only detectable in one (25%).

F: Tenofovir started 24 hours after exposure, continued for three days: all seroconverted by eight weeks, virus detectable in 50%.

It is this study that is the basis for the recommendation that PEP should be started within 24 hours of exposure, though it may be 50% effective up to 72 hours after exposure.

A recent discussion of PEP for non-occupational risks recommends against initiating treatment more than 72 hours after the exposure (Katz), although the CDC guidelines argue that starting even one to two weeks post-exposure may be justified in cases of the highest risk. The protocol used at San Francisco General Hospital notes that "after an exposure, most health-care workers are upset and find that decisions about treatment are very hard to make. We recommend that the exposed person start therapy. Therapy can be stopped later, after the exposed person has had a chance to talk with their clinician and loved ones. Once the immediate crisis has passed, it is usually easier to make the best decision." (San Francisco General Hospital Epi-Center). If PEP is ever to become a practical option for non-occupational exposure, a new system of 'rapid response' clinic services may be required to provide prompt access to treatment - as has indeed happened in San Francisco, where all patients seeking PEP are referred to one central clinic.

UK guidelines - the draft

In December 2004, HIV prevention experts and community activists met in London to discuss a draft of the BASHH guidelines at a round table session organised by Terrence Higgins Trust (THT). The first guest speaker was Dr Martin Fisher of Brighton and Sussex University Hospitals, who is lead author of the guidelines writing group.

There was a wide variation in the availability of PEP at STD clinics, he told the meeting. For example, one HIV-negative partner of a serodiscordant couple who sought (and received) PEP at Brighton had been refused by three other clinics.

The guidelines would cover, among other things:

- The scientific basis for recommending PEP

- A guide to calculating the risk of a given exposure

- The pros and cons of PEP as a prevention measure

- Recommended protocols

- Pathways for access

- An emphasis that PEP is only one strand in HIV prevention

The draft recommendations were as follows:

	Partner status HIV-positive	Partner status unknown
Receptive anal intercourse	Recommended	Recommended if partner high risk
Insertive anal intercourse	Recommended	Consider if partner high risk
Receptive vaginal intercourse	Recommended	Not recommended
Insertive vaginal intercourse	Recommended	Not recommended

Other factors to consider include whether either partner has a concurrent STI, the viral load in the HIV-positive partner, and whether there was sexual assault/trauma.

Draft recommendations for PEP regimens are:

	plus *either*	or
Combivir (zidovudine, AZT + lamivudine, 3TC)	*Viracept* (nelfinavir)	*Kaletra* (lopinavir/ritonavir)
or		
Zerit (stavudine, D4T) + *Epivir* (lamivudine, 3TC)		
or		
Truvada (tenofovir, TDF + emtricitabine, FTC)	*Note: Viracept temporarily withdrawn from market in Europe, June 2007*	

Although *Combivir* was suggested as one of the nucleoside components, this may be ruled out due to high rates of pre-existing HIV strains resistant to both drugs that are currently circulating within the UK. NNRTIs are not recommended because of the likelihood of short-term side-effects: central nervous system problems such as sleep disturbance and depression with efavirenz and liver toxicity with nevirapine.

Other draft recommendations included:

- 24-hour access and expertise via A&E

- Baseline HIV test mandatory

- Rapid GUM/HIV clinic referral

- Weekly follow-up during PEP period

- Three- and six-month HIV antibody test

- No limit on repeat requests, but an appointment with a psychologist or health advisor should be mandatory after several repeats.

This last recommendation contrasted with Australia's 'three strikes and you're out' policy. France and Spain allow a maximum of four and five repeats respectively.

Campaigns and controversy

The increased awareness of PEP did not go down well with some clinicians. An editorial in the journal *Sexually Transmitted Infections* in June 2005 by London HIV doctor John Richens opposed the idea of publicising PEP among gay men, saying it would increase sexual risk-taking. In the article, Dr Richens, from the London-based Centre for Sexual Health and HIV Research, said that promoting PEP could have the unintended consequence of encouraging gay men to take greater risks.

He told Reuters Health: "Promoting PEP may bring unintended and undesirable consequences that have not been sufficiently considered by those who have worked on PEP guidelines."

In the journal article, Dr Richens says: "There is a distinct danger that the promotion of PEP after sexual exposure could reinforce rising trends in risky sexual behaviour and might add to, rather than lessen, HIV transmission.

"My ideas create discomfort and may be interpreted as anti-gay," he continues. "But I have no hostility to gay men and enjoy looking after a large cohort of gay men in my HIV clinic."

Richens also cites the cost of PEP as a reason to be concerned about its promotion.

Prescriptions of PEP after sexual exposure grew from 48 in 2003 to 119 in 2004 at one London clinic, the Mortimer Market Centre. Richens says that the projected drug cost to the clinic for PEP will be £180,000 at a time when sexual health clinics are already financially stretched. Dr Richens' views have been dismissed by another prominent HIV doctor, and lead author of the BASHH PEP guidelines (see below). Dr Martin Fisher of Brighton's HIV clinic said: "All available data suggests that the opposite behaviour occurs - high-risk sexual acts actually declined over time in the two studies that have examined behaviour after PEP."

He continued: "Clearly more work needs to be done on the possible effects on risk behaviour, though what work has been done to date suggests that there is not a deleterious effect."

However, Richens' views were soon to be contradicted from another quarter. In December 2005 it was announced that a groundbreaking legal action was to be launched that accused the government of denying people who have been sexually exposed to HIV one month's anti-HIV treatment which can prevent HIV infection.

A gay man, known by the pseudonym of Robert Jenkins, who firstly caught HIV from one partner and then inadvertently passed it on to another, was granted legal aid on public interest grounds to seek a Judicial Review try to force the Department of Health to implement a national policy for PEP and get the guidelines being written by BASHH to say that PEP should be available 24 hours a day at casualty departments and should be provided for all who have been at significant risk.

Jenkins said that widespread public ignorance of PEP for sexual exposure to HIV is leading to unknown numbers to be unnecessarily infected with HIV. Jenkins passed on the virus to his partner after a condom split. Both were unaware of PEP and say that had they been, at least one and possibly both of them would not have been infected.

His solicitor, Frances Swaine of Leigh, Day & Co, said: "We are asking for guidelines for all members of the population, for publicity along the lines of the old Aids campaigns, and training for all general practitioners and accident and emergency departments. Obviously we can't ask for everybody to be given the drugs, but we are asking for guidelines so anyone who wants to can make a request."

She argued that the £1,000 cost of PEP needed to be set against the £1m it may cost to provide lifetime care for someone infected with HIV.

Jenkins said: "The only reason my partner has HIV is because they didn't tell me when I was diagnosed that PEP existed. That's how it's spreading."

PEP-related counselling

Kindrick's paper was just one of five discussed in the poster forum. Michelle Roland's own paper (Roland 2006) discussed not PEP itself but the sexual risk reduction counselling that

accompanied it. Her paper studied outcomes, in terms of reduction in unprotected sex acts twelve months after counselling compared with baseline, in 457 people given PEP in 2001-2002. Previous practice had been to offer five risk reduction counselling sessions during which clients were asked to discuss circumstances around the exposure, contrast it with times they had felt in control of their sexual safety, and determine what level of risk they were happy with.

Her study found that two sessions of counselling achieved a statistically significant reduction in risk exposures among 'lower risk' patients (defined as having had risky sex no more than four times before the request for PEP), but that it took five sessions to achieve a reduction in risk among patients who had had more exposures. Roland commented that despite very active outreach during the study period to high-risk environments such as sex parties and a documented increase in risky behaviour during that time, there was no increase in requests for or provision of PEP.

She said "I am very supportive of PEP as an emergency provision patients deserve, but I actually think it is of interest to only a few."

The BASHH Guidelines

In February 2006 the guidelines were eventually issued. They recommended that should be provided on a 24-hour basis at casualty departments.

Any gay man presenting who was the passive partner in anal sex without a condom should be provided with PEP, they recommend, regardless of whether the partner is known to have HIV. The same would apply to heterosexuals having vaginal or anal sex who are from groups that have a high risk of having HIV, particularly people from sub-Saharan Africa.

Where the partner is known to have HIV, PEP should be provided for any sexual intercourse without condoms or where there has been a condom accident, whether the sex was anal or vaginal, active or passive, and PEP should also be 'considered' for oral sex where ejaculation into the mouth has occurred, again regardless of the partner's HIV status.

It is not recommended for oral sex without ejaculation, cunnilingus or any sex other than being the passive partner in anal sex where the partner's status is unknown and they come from a group with low HIV prevalence, such as white UK heterosexuals.

Here is a summary of the full recommendations as they eventually appeared:

Source individual is known to be HIV-positive	
Receptive anal sex	Recommended
Insertive anal sex	Recommended
Receptive vaginal sex	Recommended
Insertive vaginal sex	Recommended
Fellatio with ejaculation	Considered
Splash of semen into eye	Considered
Fellation without ejaculation	Not recommended
Cunnilingus	Not recommended

Source individual is of unknown status and from a group or area of high HIV prevalence (>10%) *Attempt should be made, where possible, to establish the HIV status of the source individual (according to appropriate guidance on HIV testing and cosent) as early as possible.	
Receptive anal sex	Recommended
Insertive anal sex	Recommended
Receptive vaginal sex	Recommended
Insertive vaginal sex	Recommended
Fellatio with ejaculation	Considered

Source individual is not from the group of area of high HIV prevalence	
Receptive anal sex	Considered
Insertive anal sex	Not recommended
Receptive vaginal sex	Not recommended
Insertive vaginal sex	Not recommended
Fellatio with ejaculation	Not recommended

The drug regimens recommended were the same as in the draft guidelines, with the exception that boosted fosamprenavir (*Telzir*) or boosted saquinavir (*Invirase*) are added to the boosted-PI column alongside *Kaletra*.

PEP "is only recommended where the individual presents within 72 hours of exposure," the guidelines say, though they add that PEP "may be considered after this time if the exposure is 'high risk'". Whether PEP prevents HIV infection taking place after risky exposure tails off the longer starting treatment is delayed. Sooner is much better than later and hours matter.

The importance of 24-hour access is underlined by the fact that the average time to giving PEP after an occupational exposure such as a needle-stick accident to a medical worker in the UK is only two hours, whereas in cases of sexual exposure it is 23 hours.

Studies in animals have shown that PEP can be up to 100% effective if it is given within 24 hours and a course of tablets is taken for four weeks. It failed half the time if it was taken three days after exposure or where the course was only for 10 days. HIV is found in the lymph nodes 2-3 days after transmission and after five days in the blood, which is generally seen as evidence of established infection.

People who visit casualty should be given 'starter packs' consisting of *Combivir* (AZT/3TC) and nelfinavir or *Truvada* (tenofovir/FTC) to tide them over the first few days till a proper assessment can be made of their degree of risk, the guidelines say. All people coming forward for PEP must be tested for HIV in case of previous infection (and because giving PEP could cause drug resistance), and "strong efforts" should be made to establish the HIV status of the source partner if this is not known for certain.

The guidelines say that people who present repeatedly for PEP should not be penalised but should be "considered for repeat courses.according to the risk of HIV acquisition at the time of presentation," particularly if their life situation means they are exposed to a degree of regular risk (such as the negative partner of a positive person, a sex worker, or someone unable to get their

partner to use condoms). However all repeat presenters should be encouraged to see a health advisor or psychologist, and people who present more than once a year "who do not otherwise have prevailing circumstances for doing so" should be told that PEP is conditional "on their attendance for discussions around future safer sex strategies"

The guidelines end by setting targets for PEP: at least 90% of prescriptions should be filled within 72 hours and should fall within the 'recommended' criteria; at least 75% of individuals should complete their four-week course; and at least 60% should get HIV tests done three and six months after presenting themselves.

PEP will never replace other HIV prevention strategies, the authors emphasise. They say: "It is crucial to consider PEP.as only one strategy in preventing HIV infection and, as such, it should be considered as a last measure where conventional, and proven, methods of HIV prevention have failed."

The 2006 UK Guidelines for PEP after sexual exposure can be read at http://www.bashh.org/guidelines/2006/pepse_0206.pdf

It is a good idea for people seeking PEP to print them out and take them with them if they need to ask for PEP at a hospital A&E department, and they may help at some GUM Departments. When the GUM clinic is open, patients should tell reception they need to be seen immediately as an emergency appointment for PEP because of exposure to HIV. If the GUM clinic is not open, patients should go as soon as possible to the hospital's A&E department with the guidelines or take a piece of paper with the web address of the guidance.

THT Direct can advise patients who have problems getting PEP while they are still at the A&E or GUM. They can also ask the hospital worker to speak to THT Direct if this would help you - 0845 12 21 200 [open Monday to Friday 10.00am - 10pm, Saturday and Sunday 12.00 noon to 6.00pm]

The campaign continues

In February 2006, Jenkins gave an interview to the BBC. He said that he was motivated by wanting to spare others the 'hell' he went through when he was diagnosed. Robert said that there was very little knowledge of a treatment that could stop HIV infection and that the government had failed in its duty to inform the public of its availability. He said that after he was diagnosed he went through 'hell'.

"I had a massive breakdown, lost friends, and could not speak to my family. I distanced myself from them for three years."

Adding to his distress was the knowledge that he accidentally infected a partner. He says he only found out about PEP by reading about it on the internet last year.

"To be turned into a nervous wreck and then find out there was a treatment I didn't know about.now people maybe can understand how angry I feel."

He added: "The Terrence Higgins Trust told me that it was down to the department of health and certain senior clinicians saying, 'We're not going to prescribe PEP to gay men for sexual exposure'. "It shouldn't be a moral question. It should be about saving people's lives."

Robert's barrister, David Wolfe, said that he was helping him to pursue a Judicial Review to force the government to publicise and provide PEP on the basis of Article two of the European convention of Human Rights - the right to life.

He said: "My client accepts that the DoH funded the THT to run a limited campaign to run in focused communities - ads in the gents' toilets of some clubs, and so on. But this hasn't caught the generality of the community at risk."

He said that people contacting NHS Direct or GUM clinics worried they had risked HIV were still not being told about PEP, but to wait three months before they could take an HIV test.

"My client will argue the same publicity should be given to PEP as to condoms in the late 1980s. I do not expect the judges to say there should be five minute ads on TV - but I do expect them to say the government has not done enough."

One gay man, 'Tom', told the BBC he was so convinced he would not get PEP after having had unsafe sex that he pricked himself with a needle and pretended he had injured himself on a hypodermic in a dustbin.

There are certainly doctors opposed to PEP. Dr Trevor Stammers of the Christian Medical Fellowship said that publicising PEP could "open the floodgates" and work against the encouragement to have safe sex.

HIV consultant Dr David Hawkins said that he had not come across many people who needed PEP and hadn't got it, "but that clearly some people feel this is the case."

He said that people should go to the nearest GUM clinic and ask for it.

Admitting that GUM clinics are not open 24 hours, he said that "if people have had the very riskiest sex - say receptive anal sex with a positive partner - then they should go to a casualty department."

The new DoH guidelines should help to ensure better availability, he added. However he said he was concerned that publicising PEP did not raise anxiety too far.

"Even if you've had sex with someone known to be HIV-positive it's important to remember that the chances of infection through a single exposure are in the order of one to two per cent."

However Jenkins's most controversial campaigning aim - one he said was supported by the BASHH guidelines - was that people seeking PEP should be entitled to receive it as even if they approached clinics as long as one or two weeks after exposure. He used the prefatory remark in the guidelines that PEP "may be considered after [72 hours] if the exposure is 'high risk'" as evidence for this claim.

As we said above, it is not really known what the cut-off point for the use of PEP is in humans. However the evidence from the Tsai monkey studies, coupled with the indirect evidence from the Roland study in San Francisco, suggests that PEP should be taken within 24 hours of exposure if it is to have a high chance of success, that it is likely to have a less than even chance of success if taken more than three (or possibly two) days after exposure, and that it is unlikely ever to work more than four to five days after exposure.

Government backing

It was perceived as an acknowledgment of the effectiveness of Jenkins's campaigning when in April 2006 all primary care and hospital trusts in the UK were sent a letter by the Chief Medical Officer, Sir Liam Donaldson, asking them to make sure that PEP against HIV infection through sexual exposure was routinely available to those that needed it.

As the government's top doctor, Donaldson is in a powerful position to influence health policy. Lisa Power, THT's Head of Policy, said: "Terrence Higgins Trust is extremely pleased that the Chief Medical Officer agrees with our campaign to ensure that PEP is available to all those in genuine need within a reasonable time limit."

In his letter, Donaldson says: "I would ask you to ensure that PEP is part of the spectrum of sexual health services for your local populations.

"Provision of PEP for non-occupational exposure is not a replacement for evidence-based HIV health promotion, but it can have a contribution to make in preventing transmission of HIV.

"I would be grateful if you could bring this advice to the attention of your clinical and public health teams to that they can

take any necessary action to safeguard the health of you local population."

However Donaldson reiterated the 72-hour limit for PEP, saying that "after 72 hours it is unlikely to be effective," which most health authorities will take as a limit to prescription.

Access is still difficult

However Jenkins's other contentions were supported by research from Sigma Research presented at the 2006 9th CHAPS gay men's HIV prevention conference in Leeds in England.

About one in six gay men who seek PEP after an HIV risk may still be getting turned away 'inappropriately', according to Sigma Research (see Delpech for reference).

Sigma's Cathy Dodds told the conference that five out of 30 PEP seekers Sigma interviewed about their experiences was turned away. Four of the five were denied it by A&E staff but a fifth was told flatly by a GUM clinic health advisor that 'There was no such thing as PEP'. Most interviewees had sought PEP in the six months previous to Dodds' presentation, so this was not an old phenomenon.

Altogether eight out of the 30 people Sigma interviewed in detail were turned away for PEP. In three cases, Dodds commented, the refusals were probably appropriate as the men had not understood that were at low risk, and there were still cases of people getting PEP inappropriately too (for instance following oral sex without getting semen in the mouth).

However most gay men who sought PEP did so for good reasons. Four of the five who were turned away had had unsafe anal sex as the passive partner - in one case with someone known to be HIV-positive. In the fifth case, the seeker was the active partner with a known positive person.

Even when given PEP, some men found the experience humiliating: "The GUM doctor said 'You know it costs a lot of money; if we give it to you this time, we won't give it to you again,'" said one person.

Three others had phoned the NHS Direct helpline to clarify their risk and were met with advisors who had never heard of PEP.

Kay Orton, head of HIV and Health Promotion Services at the Department of Health, was in the audience and said the training deficit at NHS Direct had already been addressed and that she hoped the publication of the BASHH guidelines would lead to better decision-making by casualty staff.

In general, however, both gay men's awareness of PEP and their success in getting it has improved.

Another survey suggested doctors in the USA were also prescribing PEP inappropriately or misunderstood their own guidelines. The 13th CROI Conference was told that the majority of calls to a helpline set up to advise doctors about non-occupational post-exposure prophylaxis (PEP) against HIV were made too late to offer much or any benefit to the person exposed

Amy Kindrick of the National HIV/AIDS Clinicians' Consultation Centre reviewed all calls regarding sexual exposures made to the National Clinicians' PEP Hotline between January 2004 and September 2005. She said that 55% of calls were made more than 24 hours after the patient's exposure to HIV and that 28% of them were made more than 72 hours after exposure. Only 32% were definitely made within 24 hours of the exposure.

Altogether 918 calls concerning specific sexual exposures, excluding follow-up calls, were made to the helpline during the study period. Although the majority (58%) were made by doctors, these physicians were in the main not experienced in giving PEP: only 12% had ever managed more than ten cases. Nearly a third of calls were made from A&E departments.

Clinicians did appear to assess exposure risk reasonably accurately. 54.6% of calls were made about exposures deemed by the investigators to be 'high risk' and only 4.8% were low risk. In 30.4% of cases the source partner was known to have HIV. The main types of sexual risk were receptive vaginal intercourse (38.7%) and receptive anal intercourse by a man (21.3%). However calls concerning oral sex (9.6%) were more common than ones concerning insertive anal intercourse (5.1%) even though this is probably more risky, and nearly as common as all calls concerning insertive sex (9.8%).

However it was the fact that only a third of calls were made within time to start PEP optimally that mainly concerned the investigators.

In a poster discussion on several studies concerning PEP and exposure counselling, chair Michelle Roland, author of the San Francisco study cited above, commented: "People still get the wrong message, which is: 'You have 72 hours to start PEP'. The message should be: 'You should start PEP as soon as possible'. You can always stop taking PEP if the risk is re-assessed; you can't 'have started' it." She commented that in San Francisco the experience that requests for PEP so often resulted in 'panic' by inexperienced physicians meant that all referrals were now made to a single emergency clinic

International guidelines

This topic also came up in a review (Vitoria) of guidelines for the use of both occupational and non-occupational PEP from 41 countries, conducted by the World Health Organization.

All but one country had developed PEP guidelines, though 28% had only done so for occupational exposure. Forty-three countries had a national register of PEP use.

Sixty per cent of countries recommended dual or triple regimens with only 40% recommending only triple ones.

Fifteen per cent did not specify a four-week course as optimal and 10% did not specify a 'window' after exposure in which to prescribe PEP.

Vitoria commented that "We did not ask if countries were actually implementing PEP," and asked if there were audience members from developing countries who had done so. A physician from a clinic in Cameroon he described as 'remote and rural' said that although they were fully aware of PEP and the country had guidelines, in many cases access to antiretrovirals had not been possible within 72 hours in cases of occupational exposure.

European guidelines

Guidelines for post-exposure prophylaxis (PEP) following non-occupational exposure were published by the European Project on Non-Occupational Post-exposure Prophylaxis in June 2004 (Almeda).

The guidelines recommend PEP following unprotected receptive anal sex and needle or syringe exchange when the source person is known to be HIV-positive or from a group with high HIV prevalence. They state that it should be considered after vaginal sex or insertive anal sex with someone known to be HIV-positive, as well as following receptive oral sex with ejaculation or a splash of semen into the eye from an HIV-positive source. However, following rape or other high-risk factors, such as bleeding, ulcers around the genitals or in the mouth or sexually transmitted infections, PEP should be used more readily.

Unlike British guidelines, the European guidelines state that any combination of drugs licensed for HIV-infected patients can be used, with the simplest and least toxic combinations being preferred. Triple-drug combinations are preferred, two drugs may

be an option. They also recommend efavirenz (*Sustiva*) for people who are not pregnant, despite the drug's possible side-effects. However, if the source is known to be HIV-positive and treatment history can be obtained or a resistance test carried out, the results may be used to determine the best choice of drugs for PEP.

PEP should be started within 72 hours of exposure, starting as early as possible and lasting four weeks, with recipients receiving medical attention and counselling for at least six months.

United States guidelines

The United States government announced new public health guidelines for the use of non-occupational post-exposure prophylaxis (PEP) in January 2005 (Smith). The guidelines recommend treatment for people who seek treatment no more than 72 hours after a high-risk exposure to an HIV-positive person, such as through unprotected sex or sharing injecting equipment.

Unlike the United Kingdom guidelines, the guidelines from the United States state that any triple-drug antiretroviral regimen approved by the Department of Health and Human Services may be used. They also suggest that a dual nucleoside reverse transcriptase inhibitor (NRTI) regimen may be sufficient, as there is no evidence for the increased effectiveness of an extra drug, particularly in the face of increased risk of side-effects.

Preferred regimens include efavirenz (*Sustiva*) with 3TC (lamivudine, *Epivir*) or FTC (emtricitabine, *Emtriva*) and AZT (zidovudine, *Retrovir*) or tenofovir (*Viread*), and ritonavir-boosted lopinavir (*Kaletra*) with AZT and either 3TC or FTC. This may be modified if details of the source patient's treatment history or resistance profile are available. The United States guidelines recommend the avoidance of nevirapine and efavirenz in women of childbearing age.

As in other guidelines, the United States recommendations include care for patients for up to six months following exposure, to determine whether HIV infection has occurred, as well as tests for hepatitis B and C co-infection, sexually transmitted infections and pregnancy.

While European and United States guidelines agree that treatment should be given for 28 days and when the source is known to be HIV-positive, they differ when the source's HIV status is unknown. European guidelines recommend treatment following unprotected receptive anal sex or following unprotected anal, vaginal or oral sex with ejaculation with a person from a group or an area of high HIV prevalence (more than 15%). If the source is not from a group or an area with a high HIV prevalence, PEP is only recommended following unprotected receptive anal sex (Blackham). In contrast, the United States recommendations suggest deciding whether to administer PEP on a case-by-case basis.

The US non-occupational PEP registry

Following the US Centers for Disease Control (CDC) issuing specific recommendations concerning occupational PEP. The suggestion was made that PEP should also be offered to people with unanticipated sexual or drug-related exposures.

A recent CDC statement on the management of non-occupational exposures to HIV concluded that since no data exist regarding the efficacy of PEP for non-occupational exposure, recommendations for or against its use cannot yet be made.

In order to collect needed information, the US National non-occupational HIV post-exposure Prophylaxis Registry was created back in 1999. Data presented at XIV International AIDS Conference in Barcelona in July 2002 showed 219 cases in the registry up to March 2001.

US clinicians are invited to provide information on potential HIV exposure within 60 days of the event occurring, so long as the exposure was sexual, or involved drug use or some other known HIV transmission pathway- for example needlestick injury, so long as it did not occur in the occupational setting. The objectives of the registry are to;

- determine the characteristics of the exposures for which PEP is prescribed

- assess the completion rate of prescribed PEP regimens, and to assess the impact of side-effects and adverse events on early discontinuations

- identify differences in PEP practice in different clinical settings (i.e., emergency rooms, private practice)

- evaluate and compare HIV infection rates between those who sustain exposures and are treated with PEP and those who are exposed but untreated

- monitor the occurrence of acute retroviral syndrome

- monitor repeat use of PEP by those receiving an initial course reported to the registry.

The initial report will ascertain patient and provider demographic characteristics; the nature, extent, and timing of the reported exposure; HIV status and risk behaviors of the reported source (if known); whether antiretroviral treatment was offered and accepted; and what treatment (if any) was given.

Follow-up reporting will provide additional information;

- at 4-6 weeks

At 4-6 weeks following the initial visit, data will be collected to document the HIV status of the patient at the time of exposure, whether treatment (if given) was completed, altered, or discontinued before 28 days, and the HIV status of the patient 4-6 weeks after potential exposure. Information on side-effects and adverse effects of therapy, and any symptoms of acute retroviral syndrome will also be collected.

- at 6 and 12 months

Information collected at the 6-month and 12-month follow-up will include information about HIV test results and HIV exposures reported since the 4-6 week follow-up visit, and whether or not an additional course of PEP was given.

References

The 2006 UK Guidelines for PEP after sexual exposure can be read at http://www.bashh.org/guidelines/2006/pepse_0206.pdf

Ackers ML et al. Post-exposure prophylaxis among HIV-uninfected participants in a phase III HIV vaccine efficacy trial. XIV International AIDS Conference, Barcelona, abstract WePpD2105, 2002.

Almeda J et al. Proposed recommendations for the management of HIV post-exposure prophylaxis after sexual, injecting drug or other expsoures in Europe, Euro Surveillance 9: 35-40, 2004.

Blackham J et al. Differences between new United States recommendations and existing European guidelines on the use of postexposure prophylaxis (PEP) following non-occupational exposure, Eurosurveillance Weekly 10: 3, 2005

Cardo DM et al A case-control study of HIV seroconversion in health care workers after precutaneous exposure to HIV-infected blood: clinical and public health implications, N Engl J Med 337: 1485-1490, 1997

Delpech V. PEP: the bigger picture. Presentation at 9th CHAPS Conference, Leeds, UK. March 2006.

Dodds C et al. PEPSeekers: Men's experiences of accessing PEP following sexual exposure. CHAPS 9, Leeds, March 2006.

Easterbrook P et al. Post-exposure prophylaxis for occupational and sexual exposures to HIV: experience in a London hospital. Twelfth World AIDS Conference, Geneva, abstract 33176, 1998.

Freedberg KA et al. The cost effectiveness of combination antiretroviral therapy for HIV disease. N Engl J Med 344:824-831. 2001.

Henderson DK and Gerberding JL. Prophylactic zidovudine after occupational exposure to the human immunodeficiency virus: an interim analysis. J Infect Dis. 160(2):321-7. 1989.

HIV Post Exposure Prophylaxis: Guidance from the UK Chief Medical Officers' Expert Advisory Group on AIDS. Department of Health. July 2000.

Holtgrave DR, Kelly JA. Preventing HIV/AIDS among high-risk urban women: the cost-effectiveness of a behavioral group intervention. Am J Public Health 86: 1442 -1445. 1996.

Holtgrave DR, Kelly JA. The cost-effectiveness of an HIV prevention intervention for gay men. AIDS Behav 1: 173 -180. 1997.

Jackson JB et al. Nevirapine prophylaxis for prevention of sexual/blood HIV transmission in HIV uninfected subjects. XIV International AIDS Conference, Barcelona, abstract MoOrD1105, 2002.

Kalichman SC. Post-exposure prophylaxis for HIV infection in gay and bisexual men: implications for the future of HIV prevention. Am J Prev Med. 15(2): 120-7. August 1998.

Kahn J et al. Feasibility of post-exposure prophylaxis (PEP) against human immunodeficiency virus infection after sexual or injection drug use exposure: The San Francisco PEP study. Journal of Infectious Diseases 183; 707-714, 2001.

Katz M et al. Postexposure treatment of people exposed to the human immunodeficiency virus through sexual contact or injection-drug use. New England Journal of Medicine 336: 1097-1100, 1997.

Kindrick A et al. HIV post-exposure prophylaxis following sexual exposure is started too late for optimal benefit. Thirteenth Conference on Retroviruses and Opportunistic Infections, Denver, 2006. Abstract #906.

Lurie P et al. Postexposure prophylaxis after nonoccupational HIV exposure: clinical, ethical and policy considerations. Journal of the American Medical Association 280: 1769-1773, 1998.

Mauss S et al. Rapid development of central adiposity after postexposure prophylaxis with antiretroviral drugs: a proof of principle? AIDS 17: 944 - 955, 2003.

McLeod A et al. Absenteeism adds significant cost to HIV needlestick prophylaxis. XIV International AIDS Conference, Barcelona, abstract TuPeE5167, 2002.

Opio G et al. Post-sexual exposure prophylaxis with HAART after sexual assault. Twelfth World AIDS Conference, Geneva, abstract 33174, 1998.

Pinkerton SD et al. Cost-effectiveness of Postexposure Prophylaxis after Sexual or Injection-Drug Exposure to Human Immunodeficiency Virus. Arch Intern Med 164:46-54, 2004.

Rabaud C et al. Post-exposure prophylaxis of HIV infection: comparison of tolerability of 4 PEP regimens. Thirteenth Conference on Retroviruses and Opportunistic Infections, Denver, 2006. Abstract #905.

Roland ME at al. Seroconversion following nonoccupational postexposure prophylaxis against HIV. Clin Infect Dis. 15;41(10):1507-13. 2005.

Roland ME et al. A randomized trial of standard versus enhanced risk reduction counseling for individuals receiving post-exposure prophylaxis following sexual exposure to HIV. Thirteenth Conference on Retroviruses and Opportunistic Infections, Denver, 2006. Abstract #902.

Sigma Research. Risk and reflexion: findings from the United Kingdom Gay Men's Sex Survey 2004.Sigma Research, 2005 (ISBN 1 872956 81 5).

Smith DK et al. Antiretroviral postexposure prophylaxis after sexual, injection-drug use, or other nonoccupational exposure to HIV in the United States. MMWR Recomm Rep 54: 1-20, 2005

Stephenson J. PEP talk: treating nonoccupational HIV exposure JAMA 289: 287-288, 2003.

Tsai, CC et al. Prevention of SIV infection in macaques by (R)-9-(2-phosphonylmethoxypropyl)adenine. Science 270:1197-1199. 1995.

Tsai CC et al. Effectiveness of postinoculation (R)-9-(2-phosphonylmethoxypropyl)adenine treatment for prevention of persistent simian immunodeficiency virus SIVmne infection depends critically on timing of initiation and duration of treatment. J Virol 72: 4265-4273. 1998.

Torres R et al. Preliminary report on nonoccupational post-exposure prophylaxis utilizing an NNRTI/NRTI regimen. Thirteenth International AIDS Conference, Durban, abstract TuPeB3204, 2000.

Vitoria M et al. Guidelines for post-exposure prophylaxis for HIV in developing countries. Thirteenth Conference on Retroviruses and Opportunistic Infections, Denver, 2006. Abstract #904.

Vittinghoff E et al. Per-contact risk of human immunodeficiency virus transmission between male sexual partners. American J of Epidemiology 150: 306-311, 1999.

Pre-exposure prophylaxis: the challenge

The most challenging option that is emerging is to use ARVs to prevent sexual transmission, by giving them for extended periods to HIV-negative people at high risk.

In some populations, the risk of HIV infection may be so high that even with some of the current ARV drugs, people may choose to take the drug if it can prevent HIV transmission. PREP is envisaged to be used solely by people who may be at frequent risk for HIV. This includes high-risk behaviour groups such as commercial sex workers, injecting drug users and people who have unsafe sex with a multiple partners.

As their names suggest, with post- and pre-exposure prophylaxis we are doing something very similar in both cases; using chemoprophylaxis to prevent an HIV infection establishing itself.

When Che-Chung Tsai did his original experiments using tenofovir to block HIV infections in monkeys, he gave his monkeys the drug at four different times relative to injecting them with SIV. He gave 10 of them PEP five or 24 hours after infection. But he also gave 15 of them PREP, 24 or 48 hours before infection.

Within these boundaries, the timing didn't greatly matter. In Tsai's initial experiments, all the macaques were protected.

And yet 'before' is a lot more controversial than 'after'. When we move from PEP to PREP we are crossing a huge gulf in terms of how much we already know about whether the concept can work and about its eventual implications.

As we have seen, PEP itself is not an area lacking controversy. But it is an established, short-term emergency use of antiretrovirals by the already exposed that will probably make never make more than a minor contribution to HIV prevention on a population scale. Also, as an emergency measure, PEP escapes some of the moral complexity that attends some other prevention methods; everyone can understand why someone might seek help to avoid the consequences of accidental exposure.

But to take expensive antiretrovirals *in anticipation* that you will indulge in risky behaviour? As Bill Gates said at the Seattle CROI Conference when first introduced to the concept in 2002, "Wouldn't it just be simpler if they used condoms?"

PREP, which has never been properly tried except in an 'underground' way (see below), is an idea that even its advocates acknowledge is radical and fraught with potential difficulties. It would mean giving HIV-negative people potentially toxic antiretroviral drugs, not in order to prevent an infection they have been exposed to, but in order to prevent an infection they might *never* be exposed to - or which they could avoid by other means.

With vaccines we are talking about a one-off medical intervention (or, at worst, a series of shots that might need boosting now and then) which then requires no further 'adherence' by the subject in order to be effective.

With microbicides we are talking about something that will require adherence but which, it is intended, will be a benign substance that can be bought over the counter or given out. Even microbicides that contain antiretrovirals will be rigorously tested to make quite sure that they do not create any topical or systemic toxicity and that they do not penetrate enough to create the possibility of resistance, should a person who is already HIV-positive use them.

But with PREP we are talking about a highly medicalised intervention, dispensed by a healthcare worker, that has the potential both to create systemic toxicity and HIV drug resistance and will therefore never (or should never) be sold over the counter.

It's also an obviously expensive prevention option (or it is if you take it all the time).

This begs huge questions:

- Who would get it?

- Why not help them use other interventions instead, like condoms?

- Who would decide who gets it?

- How would it be distributed?

- What would be the consequences of a proportion (probably the most high-risk proportion) of the HIV-negative population being on antiretrovirals?

- Which drugs should we use?

- Do we have *any* antiretrovirals currently whose safety we are sufficiently comfortable with to allow them to be given to HIV-negative people as a preventative measure?

- What is the potential for drug resistance, given that it will be almost impossible to ensure that people who are seroconverting never take it?

- What are the cost implications, not just of the drugs but of things like viral load test, which are implied in order to make sure we give PREP to as few seroconverters as possible?

- As we have already explored, the usefulness of a New Prevention Technology will vanish if people abandon other proven, and possibly safer, measures such as condoms in favour of the new idea. If PREP is not 100% effective, how do we explain to vulnerable populations?

- How do we do ethical trials of the concept?

The need for PREP

And yet PREP is also an obvious idea. What could be simpler - if it works - than popping a pill which could proof you against HIV? *If* such a measure was highly effective, *if* it was economically feasible, *if* it was safe and *if* the right people took it at the right time.we might have something as effective as a vaccine, but here and now, in the shape of a pill you can hold in your hand.

There are historical precedents for the idea of PREP. The classic one is the use of quinine against malaria.

Henry Hobhouse's book *The Seeds of Change* describes how six crucial plant products have shaped the history of colonialism. He gives pride of place to quinine, the anti-malaria drug which, as an ingredient of the 'tonic water' sipped by colonial Colonels, enabled the white man to conquer parts of the world where previously his life had made impossible by malaria.

There would be a sense of historical justice if we could find a drug that could protect the developing world's native people from a deadly disease that retards economic development as effectively as quinine protected its colonisers.

There are good reasons why testing PREP as a concept should be an urgent priority.

The main reasons are those that also apply to microbicides. Condoms are frequently not used even by high-risk populations; women are unable to enforce condom use by men or may be unaware they are at risk. The most frequent number of sex partners young women under 20 in South Africa with HIV have had is just one. A recent survey from Andhra Pradesh in India showed that half of men who have sex with men there had unprotected anal sex both with other men and with their wives.

PREP has additional advantages. It involves using a pill that exists right now rather than developing new compounds and methods of application. It would be more discreet and user-controlled than either a condom or a microbicide. It could be taken well in advance of any sex or even afterwards.

In addition, the efficacy of the first generation of microbicides is forecast even by the most optimistic researchers to be no more than 60%.

There is a crucial kind of sex those candidate microbicides are not designed for - anal sex. Microbicides for rectal use pose considerably greater design, toxicity and testing challenges than vaginal ones. They are also an even less popular target for research funding. So far only a few small animal trials have tested the concept, and one acceptability trial, using a neutral gel, has taken place in gay men in Boston.

In addition, PREP could maybe prevent transmission through needle sharing, which a microbicide could not.

There are, in short, populations who, like the intended users of microbicides, cannot or will not use condoms for social, economic or psychological reasons, but who are also unlikely to benefit from at least the first generation of microbicides, One argument for testing PREP is that to do otherwise would be to disrespect the human rights of sexual and drug-injecting minorities who would get left behind if vaginal microbicide use becomes widespread.

'Doing a T' - underground PREP

Some of the urgency around getting the concept of PrEP tested is fuelled by evidence that members of high-risk communities are already trying the concept out.

A study presented at the IAS Conference in Rio, 2005 of gay men attending minority-ethnic gay pride events in four US cities (Kellerman) found surprisingly high numbers of HIV-negative gay men who had taken antiretrovirals in order to try and avoid HIV.

The researchers asked 1,046 people attending gay pride events in San Francisco, Oakland, Baltimore and Detroit: "Have you ever used AIDS medicines before engaging in risky behaviour because you thought it would reduce your chances of getting HIV?"

Researchers also asked if they had heard of the PREP concept at all.

The group questioned was quite mixed, with 7% being women, 18% saying they were heterosexual and 17% bisexual. Over 40% were black, reflecting the events where the research was done, with other ethnic groups represented evenly.

A quarter of those questioned had heard of PREP and seven per cent had actually taken it (presumably 'borrowing' HIV-positive friends' pills).

The figures were higher in San Francisco and Baltimore, where nine per cent had taken PREP, and only three per cent had taken it in Oakland.

There was evidence that PREP was an 'underground' phenomenon used by people who didn't believe everything they heard about HIV. People who'd taken it were more likely to believe that they had been tested for HIV without being told, or that HV is a man-made virus. They were also less trusting of HIV information from official prevention agencies.

The researchers comment that the percentage of gay pride attendees who had taken PREP was "surprising".

They add that further surveys should be done to find out "what medications are being taken, on what schedule they are being taken, from where they are obtained, and whether their use is associated with higher-risk sexual behaviours."

The Centers for Disease Control in the USA explicitly cited safety concerns around this practice as one of the reasons to mount the study of tenofovir PREP in 400 gay men it is currently conducting in San Francisco and Atlanta (see below).

A piece in the Los Angeles Times in December 2005 (Costello) said that tenofovir was being sold in packets along with Viagra and Ecstasy in gay dance clubs.

Costello interviewed one physician who already prescribed tenofovir to very high-risk patients. Marc Conant, an HIV doctor in San Francisco, said he recently began prescribing tenofovir to two uninfected men after they told him they were very sexually active and would not use condoms. Though troubled by the fact that the drug had not been proven effective for such a use and that his patients might be increasing their risky behavior while using it, he told the LA Times that using the drug was better than taking no precaution at all.

"What choice do I have? Forty-thousand people are still getting infected every year," he said. "Everyone knows condoms work, but they're not using them. All I am trying to do is reduce the risk that people harm themselves."

Part of the problem with this kind of use is that even if tenofovir is more effective than some animal studies might suggest, no trial so far has tested the efficacy of occasional use - so-called 'disco dosing' or 'taking a T'. While this might be advantageous in terms of reducing toxicity and the possibility of resistance, it is also as dependent as condom or microbicide use is on patients' estimates of the risk they are running or likely to run - one of the factors continuous PREP use was supposed to avoid.

The evidence so far

However, while it is crucial to start preparing answers for these questions now if we are to turn PrEP into a reality, we have to answer another question first. Does it work?

The answer is that we simply don't know. The few trials of the idea mounted so far have given contradictory results.

Back in 1994, the 15 (out of 35) macaques that were given tenofovir pre-exposure prophylaxis by Tsai were completely protected. This created strong initial hopes that it might be a very effective prevention measure indeed

Ten years later, at a study presented to the 12th Retrovirus Conference (Subbarao), these hopes appeared to be dashed.

The US Centers for Disease Control gave 12 rhesus macaques either placebo, a daily dose of tenofovir, or a weekly dose.

They also mimicked human anal sex more accurately than Tsai had done. He injected his macaques with a single massive dose of SIV. Subbarao introduced SIV repeatedly - as a weekly 'rectal inoculation'.

In this study, tenofovir delayed but did not stop infection in any monkey. Half the non-treated monkeys were infected after the first inoculation of SIV, whereas it took seven inoculations to infect half the treated monkeys. However, all the monkeys were infected after 15 inoculations, and all but one after 12.

The researchers put an optimistic spin on the results by saying that the study 'delayed infection by 85%'. But another way of saying it would be that it stopped zero per cent of infections.

Which study is more likely to reflect the effectiveness of PrEP in the real world? We don't know. There were about 400,000 SIV viral particles in each millilitre of the rectal inoculation. This is a 'viral load' three to five times higher than the maximum normally recorded in people who have acute HIV infection, when they are at their most infections, and 26-60 times higher than the usual viral load in chronic infection. We also don't know if the results would be the same for a vaginal sex model.

The following year at the 13th Retrovirus Conference, the pendulum swung back again. As with HIV treatment, there is a scientific rationale that using more than one drug may confer a higher level of protection than single-drug pre-exposure prophylaxis (PrEP). The benefits of this approach, often called 'combo-PrEP' have yet to be proven in humans.

A study (Garcia-Lerma) by the United States National Institutes of Health (NIH) tested daily intramuscular injections of high-doses of tenofovir (*Viread*) combined with the nucleoside reverse transcriptase inhibitor (NRTI) FTC (emtricitabine, *Emtriva*). All six macaques given tenofovir and FTC were protected following four rectal challenges with simian / human immunodeficiency virus (SHIV). Even after ten further exposures, all of the treated monkeys remained uninfected. In contrast, five of the six control monkeys, which received no treatment, seroconverted. This supported the effectiveness of the combo-PrEP used in this study.

Interestingly, when the experiment was repeated with FTC alone, two of the six monkeys became infected, demonstrating a weaker protective effect with FTC as monotherapy. It is important to remember that these animals were injected with treatment at higher doses than the normal oral therapeutic dose and so is not directly analogous to the response that may be expected in humans. However, it is an important first study of the effectiveness of a combination of tenofovir and FTC in this monkey model. Trials in humans will be essential to validate these initial findings.

PrEP has, of course, been tried successfully on that most vulnerable of populations, new-born babies. As we point out above, in any single-dose nevirapine strategy, the drug is working not by suppressing HIV in the mother but by crossing the placental barrier and acting as prophylaxis in the foetus.

However among a large number of mother-to-child-transmission prevention studies have been some that included giving antiretrovirals to the baby after birth but not the mother. This effectively represents PrEP for infants against HIV transmission through breast milk.

The SIMBA trial in Southern Africa, for instance, gave AZT+ddI to the mothers from 36 weeks of pregnancy to one week after giving birth.

It then gave nevirapine or 3TC to the babies from birth till four weeks after weaning, with the mothers committing to breastfeed for only six months.

The 'late transmission rate' in babies (meaning infection from four weeks to six months after birth) was only one per cent, compared with a usual rate of around nine per cent, thus reflecting a PrEP efficacy in this case of around 80%.

Efficacy trials

So, thus far, the evidence for PREP has been very conflicting. As a result several US-based institutes - Family Health International, the Centers for Disease Control, and the National Institutes of Health -started trials of tenofovir as HIV prophylaxis in nine different countries - the USA and Peru (in gay men), Malawi (in 'high risk' men), Thailand (in injecting drug users), Botswana (young adults) and Cameroon, Nigeria, Ghana and Cambodia ('high risk' women including sex workers).

These nine trials between them would have involved 9,000 volunteers. This may sound a lot, but they are distributed among several risk group (female sex workers, injecting drug users, and gay men) and none are as big as any of the phase III microbicide trials currently recruiting or about to start.

In fact some of these trials were halted prematurely, for reasons we explore below. What we have left at present are three studies of tenofovir as PREP:

- A study of high-risk women in Ghana, sponsored by Family Health International and funded by the Bill & Melinda Gates Foundation (800 volunteers, expected to report 2007)

- A study of injection drug users in Thailand, sponsored by the United States Centers for Disease Control and Prevention (CDC) (1,600 volunteers, expected late 2007).

- A study of gay men in the United States, also sponsored by the CDC. This with 400 volunteers, is too small to produce a meaningful result as an efficacy study and is purely intended as a safety study.

Following recent promising data in monkeys, two other studies are being considered to test the combination of tenofovir and FTC (emtricitabine, *Emtriva*) to prevent HIV transmission. These include a CDC-funded study in Botswana focused particularly on sexual transmission in young adults, and a trial in Peru involving 1,400 gay men. These could be the first trials to test combination PREP in humans.

It is hoped that these trials will help determine whether tenofovir, with or without FTC, is safe to use in uninfected individuals and whether it helps to prevent HIV. However, there is a risk that they may be too small to provide definitive answers, particularly

since ethical considerations dictate that trial participants be counselled on how to reduce their risk of contracting HIV.

Trial problems

So we need more trials. But in fact, two trials have now been stopped permanently, two others are currently not recruiting more volunteers (though it is following up those already recruited), and another has gone ahead in the teeth of bitter activist opposition.

Trials of tenofovir PREP were prematurely halted at two sites, Cambodia and Cameroon, because activists were concerned that trial participants may not be offered antiretroviral therapy should they become infected during the study. Concerns were also raised about the provision of independent counselling on safer sex and injection practices and the availability of condoms and sterile needles.

Tenofovir trials at two further sites were stopped on different grounds. In Nigeria, the sites were not able to comply with the appropriate laboratory and clinical conditions needed for the safe conduct of the trial, while in Malawi, there were broader concerns regarding the ability of the government to implement PREP if it were proven effective.

The first time the wider world became aware of trouble was when Womyn's Agenda for Change, an advocacy group for Cambodian sex workers, supported by the French activist group ACT-UP, demonstrated against the Cambodian trial at the Bangkok World AIDS Conference in 2004.

On 12 August 2004, after an intervention from the Cambodian Prime Minister, the trial was stopped.

On 31 January, a community meeting between Thai drug users and the researchers broke up after protests that people were being coerced to participate and that tenofovir was being offered as a second-best to needle exchange.

On 3 February 2005, after a French TV documentary questioning the ethics of the trial in Cameroon and demonstrations by ACT-UP Paris outside the Cameroon embassy, this trial was suspended, with the country's health minister saying he was going to investigate the trial. On 22 February participant follow-up resumed, but no further recruitment.

On 16 March Family Health International itself cancelled the Nigeria trial (leaving only the Malawi and Ghana arms of the trial intact) saying that local researchers had failed to meet "necessary scientific standards."

On March 30, the Centers for Disease Control announced that the Botswana and Bangkok trial was 'to start soon'.

In April, the trial among drug users in Bangkok began recruiting. The small US trial in gay men (only 200 volunteers apiece in Atlanta and San Francisco) has been recruiting for some time. The Peru trial is yet to start.

The Malawi trial, among high-risk men, was due to start in September 2005 but was halted by the government very soon after recruitment started due to concerns that it would foster HIV resistance to tenofovir, which they are now using in treatment.

Lessons learned

What happened here? Among accusations and counter-accusations, a number of issues stand out.

In some cases the scientific reservations that cause trials to be cancelled are valid. Tenofovir resistance, for instance, is a real concern.

Many studies have shown that tenofovir resistance is not easily transmitted and may decrease the capacity of the virus to replicate efficiently. More recent studies, however, have not been so positive. A study presented in 2006 found that four out of eleven monkeys dosed with high levels of tenofovir rapidly developed the K65R mutation within just one week. Another seven animals in the study developed resistance but over a longer period of six to nine weeks (Johnson).

Whether these results are significant for humans remains unclear: many of these studies involve infecting monkeys with extremely high levels of virus which are administered through more efficient routes than might be expected in the normal course of sexual interaction in humans.

Although trial recruiters made great efforts to consult with 'the community', there is a difference between consulting with well-informed activists in NGOs and ensuring ethical treatment of actual trial participants. Nigerian activist Rolake Nwagwu said: "In Nigeria, sex work is illegal. These women have no human rights and are not organised, so I don't see how sex workers will be involved in any meaningful way."

In Cambodia, there was a political dimension. US government policies had resulted in the withdrawal of USAID funding from local sex worker support groups in 2003. They were, unsurprisingly, disinclined to co-operate when asked to help by the same people in 2004.

Stories were widespread about local recruiters misinforming participants in order to get them on the trials. A Cameroon participant and several Cambodian participants were quoted as saying they thought that tenofovir was a 'vaccine' which would mean they 'no longer had to use condoms'. Karyn Kaplan of the Thai drug Users' Network said: "The trial looked beautiful on paper, but there has been a lot of coercion by local staff who implemented it."

Whether these accounts are true or not they represent a failure to communicate the potential benefits and risks of the trials in a clear way. Recruiters have failed to correct an impression that PREP is all about forcing a biomedical prevention tool on HIV-negative people in order to make profits for drug companies.

One complexity of a prevention trial is that in order to demonstrate the effectiveness of a new intervention (such as PREP) older interventions (such as condoms) have to 'fail', and yet ethically researchers have to offer safer-sex advice and condoms. This can been seen as a conflict of interest on the part of researchers, who need to make it clear that they do not *want* participants to take risks, they just have evidence that risks get taken (in fact risk behaviour tends to fall during prevention studies).

It can also be seen as a distraction from campaigning for prevention measures that communities *do* want. In the case of the Bangkok trial, drug user activists saw tenofovir as a politically acceptable alternative to their own preferred prevention intervention, needle exchange. The ethical question then becomes: will more lives be saved by holding out for an intervention we know works, or will more be saved by accepting a trial of one of unknown effectiveness?

Activists in the four countries where trials have been suspended expressed frank disbelief that tenofovir would ever be made available to the local population. In Cambodia, Womyn's Agenda for Change said: "Obviously, there is a benefit to anyone whom tenofovir prevents from HIV infection, if it proves able to do that. But it is not likely that many Cambodians would be able to use it.it seems clear that tenofovir is being tested mainly in poor countries because that is cheaper than doing it in rich countries."

HIV prevention trials in general have focused attention on the issue of researchers' responsibility to care for people who are infected with HIV or suffer drug side-effects during the trial. There is a complex ethical debate around whether the standard of care offered for people infected with HIV should be the best possible, the same as that on offer in the host country, or something in between. There is also the issue of whether

researchers have the ability or power to offer anti-retroviral treatment that might not be needed until ten years after the trial ends.

It is in the nature of trials that more people can be harmed than helped. The classic example of this in a prevention trial was the COL-1492 trial of the spermicide nonoxynol-9 in West Africa. This showed that using N-9, which killed HIV in the test tube, in fact doubled the rate of HIV transmission in frequent users because it disrupted the vaginal epithelium. While this trial proved that you could put on a large, double-blinded placebo-controlled trials for a microbicide, it ended up causing more women to become HIV-positive than would have otherwise.

Given some of the above points, it is legitimate to ask why so far PREP research in the developed world has been restricted to a small US trial in gay men. Talks are underway about a possible trial among gay men in Europe and Australia, but these are at a very early stage.

The Seattle Consultation

A meeting between stakeholders involved in every current trial took place on 19-20 May 2005 in Seattle, convened by the International AIDS Society.

Participants included the Bill and Melinda Gates Foundation, which has sponsored the trials, the CDC, the NIH, and over 50 stakeholders representing participants in Botswana, Cameroon, Ghana, Malawi and Thailand.

The meeting's recommendations took note of a lot of the above points. Many country-specific recommendations were made, but broad ones that applied to all the trials included:

- In immediate review to ensure that the level of counselling participants receive is significantly improved;

- Ensure access to male and female condoms;

- Ensure that there are proper support mechanisms for individuals screened for enrolment in the trials who are found to be HIV-positive;

- Establish national guidelines to inform and improve civil society engagement - efforts so far were acknowledged to have been "at times ill-informed and inconsistent";

- Clear mechanisms for feedback and conflict resolution at trial sites.

This has now become part of an ongoing dialogue to ensure that future studies are properly planned and proceed with the support of the local and international communities. Since existing international ethical frameworks do not provide detailed guidance on the criteria for prevention research, this should empower and protect vulnerable populations, as well as ensure rigorous standards for the ethical design and conduct of future research.

Who is 'The Community'?

At the 2005 IAS Conference in Rio, Renée Ridzon of the Bill and Melinda Gates Foundation expressed frustration at the opposition to the trials mounted by some activists.

She said: "The trials will not be all-answering. But PREP can only be tested in humans, and the derailment of prevention trials and the loss of focus on the urgent need for prevention interventions show that 'the good can be the enemy of the perfect'. The definition of 'community' can be elusive, and we have heard many voices from the community on this issue, rather than one."

In an attempt to avoid the controversies excited by other trials, the researchers behind the trial of PREP for gay men in Peru conducted a comprehensive community consultation process in 2004/5, the results of which were presented at the 13th Retrovirus Conference in February 2006 (Goicochea).

The researchers conducted an informed consent review process with a community advisory board and an institutional advisory board. They conducted a series of open forums on the trial with HIV and non-HIV civil society activists and with academics. And they conducted 20 focus groups in the two cities that were trial sites with activists and with possible trial participants or people who would be interested. This included participants in existing HIV prevention trials, and three classes of men who have sex with men: 'buses', who are men who may or may not self-identify as gay but are mainly MSM who maintain a "straight" demeanour; 'deschavados', who are generally effeminate MSM who self-identify as gay; transvestites; male sex workers; and 'mostaceros', who are men who have sex with transvestites or deschavados but do not identify as gay.

They asked each group their opinion on five topics:

- How to obtain truly informed consent in vulnerable populations

- Adverse events and whether participants should be compensated for them

- Whether there should be financial compensation for trial participation and whether this would act as coercion to join the trial

- Whether the trial would lead to 'condom migration' or sexual disinhibition in participants

- Their general opinions on HIV prevention research and whether they might participate.

A wide range of opinion was expressed by the different stakeholders. For instance, while opinion leaders, academics and 'buses' expressed reservations about there being any financial compensation to participate and thought it would be coercive, activists wanted the allowance doubled, and sex workers wanted to be compensated for lost work time and opportunities. Academics and 'buses' were concerned that PREP might lead to sexual disinhibition, while 'deschavados' recognised that high-risk behaviour already existed. Potential participants expressed a variety of unexpected concerns about the health implications of the trial. Would tenofovir interfere with female hormones taken by trangendered participants? Would the monthly blood sampling have a weakening effect? One opinion leader asked if compensation would extend as far as paying for dialysis of someone got renal toxicity from tenofovir.

The stakeholders' different comments were then used to write the final trial protocol. This exhaustive exercise delayed the t=start of the trial for nearly two years, but is probably an example of the kind of good practice in community consultation that prevention trials need to adopt in the future.

Designing second-generation trials

After the results presented in the 'combo-PREP' trial, the trials in Botswana and Peru have now switched from using tenofovir to using *Truvada* (tenofovir/FTC).

Plans for second-generation trials into pre-exposure prophylaxis are already underway. A number of approaches are being considered including the use of other antiretroviral agents including protease inhibitors and entry inhibitors, which stop viral entry into cells. Since some of these drugs remain effective for a long time achieving high plasma or cellular concentrations, it may be possible to dose people at risk of infection less frequently. However, this remains hypothetical and no current studies are underway to evaluate less frequent dosing.

A further strategy may be to combine different types of drugs to prevent infection such as the use of topical microbicides together with oral drug treatment to prevent infection.

Access

Even if PREP proves safe and effective in human trials, distributing it in the community will face an enormous economic barrier. The US price of *Truvada* is about $10,000 per year, and of tenofovir $7,000. Both are made by Gilead Sciences, which supplies the drugs free of charge for the PREP trials but does not otherwise participate.

Gilead also has a "Global Access Program" that theoretically applies to 95 resource-poor countries, which offers to sell Truvada and tenofovir in these countries for $360 and $300 yearly, but which has been severely criticised by groups such as Médecins sans Frontières for slow progress, especially in tackling the licensing bureaucracy of some developing countries. In any case, if PREP were to be adopted widely as a prevention strategy, $300-$400 a year would probably still be too high a price.

The answer lies probably in generic provision with a licensing fee paid to Gilead. But it throws up a second problem. PREP should never be sold over the counter: the potential for misuse (for treatment as well as prevention) and resultant widespread HIV resistance is just too great.

But in that case, what would be the procedures for access and dispensing? We have seen in the example of PEP that some people seeking it have come across discriminatory attitudes from healthcare staff. Would the stigmatisation of marginalised, high-risk communities lead to PREP being denied to the very people who need it most? These power inequalities and a comprehensive training programme for probable providers would have to be addressed in advance of any move to make PREP widely available, regardless of other considerations.

Conclusion

As with many of the biomedical approaches being studied at this time, including vaccines and microbicides, we may have to anticipate that PrEP might not provide complete protection against HIV. PrEP may supplement condoms rather than supplanting them.

Generally, the PrEP trials have happened historically at a time when a stronger activist movement is starting to develop in the host countries that is wary of further trials that provide no benefit to local people.

One example given was the AIDSVAX gp120 HIV vaccine trial in Thailand, which was widely criticised as pointless at the time by researchers as the vaccine had already proven effective. The Thai Drug Users' Network's comment was "At the time we weren't organised enough to resist the AIDSVAX trial. Now we are."

Researchers involved in all trials of new prevention technologies should take account of the above concerns and establish maximum clarity of communication with trial participants and their communities, without overstating the benefits or fluffing the risks of a trial.

If they do not, they could make prevention technology trials far more difficult to put on and delay or even prevent implementation of vitally needed new weapons against HIV.

- An excellent summary of the issues involved in the PrEP trials was published by the AIDS Vaccine Advocacy Coalition (AVAC) in March 2005. It can be found at http://avac.org/pdf/tenofovir.pdf

- The Community HIV and AIDS Mobilization Project (CHAMP) published a useful update on both PrEP and microbicides in May 2006. It can be found at http://www.champnetwork.org/media/HHSWatch0506.doc

References

Garcia-Lerma J et al. Prevention of rectal SHIV transmission in macaques by tenofovir/FTC combination.13th Conference on Retroviruses and Opportunistic Infections, Denver, abstract 609, 2006

Goicochea P et al. Finding the Community in "Community Consultation" to Prepare for Biomedical HIV Prevention Trials. 13th Conference on Retroviruses and Opportunistic Infections, Denver. Abstract 898. 2006.

Johnson J et al.Rapid emergence of drug-resistant SIV in tenofovir-treated macaques: implications for tenofovir chemoprophylaxis against HIV.13th Conference on Retroviruses and Opportunistic Infections, Denver, abstract 609, 2006

Kellerman S. Knowledge and use of pre-exposure prophylaxis asmong attendees of minority gay pride events, 2004. Thrid IAS Conference on HIV Pathogenesis and Treatment, Rio de Janeiro, 2005. Abstract WePe10.3P03.

Subbaro S et al. Tenofovir delays but does not prevent infection in rhesus macaques given repeated rectal challenges of SHIV. Twelfth Conference on Retroviruses and Opportunistic Infections, San Francisco, abstract 41, 2003

Tsai CC et al. Prevention of SIV infection in macaques by (R)-9-(2-phosphonylmethoxypropyl) adenine,Science 270: 1197-1199, 1995

Microbicides

An introduction to microbicides

What is a microbicide?

Microbicides are any substances which protect people against infection by microbes, such as viruses or bacteria, on contact with those microbes. They might do this by directly killing microbes or physically preventing them from entering the body. The term 'microbicides' has replaced 'virucides' to embrace products that could be active against a wide range of infections, not just viruses.

Microbicides are still at a developmental stage, and no proven safe and effective products are currently available. However, the prospects are good for products with at least some efficacy and there is a growing body of opinion supporting their development. The main focus is on microbicides for vaginal use, which is seen as technically simpler than providing protection during anal sex. Ideally, microbicides are needed for anal sex to protect heterosexuals as well as gay men. However acceptability studies of rectal microbicides in humans and animal studies have taken place.

Microbicide research began by analogy with spermicides (contraceptives which kill sperm). Some microbicides may also be spermicidal. The big difference is that while spermicides only act to 'protect' women against sperm, a microbicide may be able to act in both directions. It could be used by HIV-positive women to protect uninfected men, as well as by HIV-negative women to protect themselves. Microbicide development advocates have called for sub-studies of microbicide effectiveness to prevent transmission as well as infection in the development of all candidate products.

Microbicides could take the form of a cream, pessary, film, sponge, foam or jelly. The first products to be tested are gels which closely resemble the lubricants used with condoms.

In reality, some products would have much broader activity than others, raising issues in public education. There is already a great deal of confusion around the meaning of 'safe' or 'safer' sex: safe from what? Pregnancy, HIV, other infections? Such questions must be answered as microbicides are evaluated and, it is hoped, made widely available.

A study commissioned by the Rockefeller Foundation has projected the impact of microbicides in four subpopulations in 73 lower income countries. In particular: sex workers and their clients; sexually active youth; injecting drug users and their sexual partners; women in regular partnerships. Numbers were estimated for those in each of these groups in contact with services that could distribute microbicides.

Using conservative estimates of product efficacy (40-60% vs. HIV, 0-40% vs. STIs), coverage (10% of populations) and usage (50% of sexual acts), it was possible to show that over three years several million HIV infections could be averted (Watts).

Who supports microbicide development?

- The first advocacy group specifically for microbicides was formed at an eight-day consultation in 1993 when the International Women's Health Coalition, the Population Council and individual held an 8-day consultation on microbicides in New York for women's health advocates; Group decided to form the Women's Health Advocates on Microbicide (WHAM). This body organised a panel on microbicides at the 9th International Conference on HIV/AIDS in Berlin that year.

- An **International Working Group on Microbicides (IWGM)** was set up in 1994, which has sought to stimulate research and build consensus on future directions. IWGM is an inter-agency coordinating body which works to facilitate the development and approval of safe, effective, affordable and acceptable microbicides to prevent the sexual transmission of HIV and other STIs.

- The US **National Institutes of Health** have been major sponsors of microbicides research. The NIH issued its first grants in 1995, and at the Vancouver AIDS Conference that year, US health and Human Services Secretary Donna Shalala announced a $100 million initiative to support microbicide research.

- WHAM disbanded in 1997, to make way for two organisations, both founded in 1998, that have since driven the advocacy and research agenda:

- The **Alliancefor Microbicide Development (AMD -www.microbicide.org)** is a global, non-profit organisation whose sole mission is to speed the development of safe, effective, and affordable microbicides to prevent sexually transmitted infections, especially HIV. It maintains a database of current research and candidate products; monitors the progress of microbicide projects that are being pursued by research groups and biotech companies; and produces regular surveys of the state of the field. It also brings together those companies that are involved with interested scientists and activists, conducts conferences and meetings; builds alliances between developers; and advocates for funding.

- Advocacy has been pursued by the **Global Campaign for Microbicides (GCM - www.global-campaign.org).** The Global Campaign for Microbicides is a broad-based, international effort to build support among policymakers, opinion leaders, and the general public for increased investment into microbicides and other user-controlled prevention methods. It raises awareness and mobilises political support for microbicide development, creates a supportive policy environment for the development, introduction and use of new prevention technologies, and ensures that as science proceeds, the rights and interests of trial participants, users, and communities are fully represented and respected.

- In 2000, CONRAD (Contraceptive Research and development established the Global Microbicides Project (www.gmp.org) to help develop new microbicidal agents that specifically address the needs and perspectives of women. The main objective of this project is to develop vaginal methods that would protect women against sexually transmitted infections, including HIV/AIDS.

- Between the two of them, the AMD and the GCM helped to create a cohesive approach to the development of microbicides that avoided some of the fragmentation of the vaccines development field and some (though not all) of the controversies about trial ethics that have dogged the development of both PrEP and vaccines. However there was still frustration that microbicide development was underfunded in comparison with vaccines and that a truly coherent programme to research and deliver an effective microbicide was needed.

- So in 2002 **the International Partnership for Microbicides(IPM - www.ipm-microbicides.org)** was established. Initial funding was provided by the Rockefeller Foundation which was also an early supporter of the International AIDS Vaccine Initiative. IPM, headed by Dr Zeda Rosenberg and based in the USA, is setting out to create public-private partnerships to expand the pipeline of products in development, ultimately licensing them to industry in return for guarantees of access for users in developing countries. Similar in mission to IAVI, its goal is to deliver a safe and effective microbicide for women in developing countries as soon as possible. IPM both conducts its own research and works in partnership with other researchers. It identifies the most promising technologies and invests its resources to help develop them into usable products. Through its partnerships, IPM aims to accelerate and increase the efficiency of product development at every stage, including formulation and drug delivery research, clinical trials and manufacturing.

The need for a microbicide received powerful endorsement in the 2001 declaration issued by the UN General Assembly Special Session on AIDS.

There are many barriers to the development of a successful microbicide. To maximise access, a product would need to be sold cheaply or distributed widely without medical supervision. This militates against the involvement of major research-based pharmaceutical companies that are geared to developing prescription medicines. There has been even less private investment in microbicides than in vaccines.

Microbicide research has mainly been pursued by academic and charitable organisations, and a few small companies. The main funders have been the US National Institutes of Health (Reichelderfer) and private philanthropists, although increasing interest is being shown by other governments and the European Commission. The UK's Department for International Development and the Swedish International Development Agency have both funded work. Private funding has come from the Gates Foundation, the American Foundation for AIDS Research and the Rockefeller Foundation among others.

The microbicide development process

The earliest stages of microbicide development can be carried out in cell cultures and small animals. Increasingly elaborate models of the tissues that are exposed to HIV containing a mixture of different cell types, some vulnerable to HIV, are being constructed.

The Global Microbicides Project has collaborated on a screening system with investigators at the Pennsylvania State College of Medicine. This uses cell-cultures to test the ability of microbicides to interfere with binding by two distinct strains of HIV-1, one binding to CXCR4 and one to CCR5 receptors. It tests cell-free virus inhibition and cell-to-cell transfer of HIV. It also tests mammalian cell toxicity. Compounds that pass all of these tests are then assessed for their ability to protect human peripheral blood monocytes from clinical strains of HIV. It is then possible to use a wider range of tests to measure possible protection against other (non-HIV) pathogens, before taking products forwards into clinical trials (Claypool).

Mice are susceptible to herpes (HSV-2) and this can be used for studies of broad-spectrum microbicide candidates. Another mouse model has been developed, using immunodeficient animals implanted with human vaginal tissues and allowed to heal (Kish). Some studies have been carried out in female monkeys, using HIV-related virus strains developed for vaccine research.

The two basic questions throughout the process of development:

- is it safe or does it damage healthy tissue?

- can it prevent HIV or other microbes from entering the body?

Phase I and Phase II trials of microbicides address the first of these questions. Initially, a small number of low-risk women, abstaining from sex, are asked to volunteer to expose themselves to the substance and report any reactions they suspect may be related to it. Increasingly detailed protocols have been developed for vaginal and cervical examinations, including standardised systems for reporting injuries and inflammation.

Studies of the safety of microbicides for anal use may be justified at an early stage although for protection, it may be necessary to have entirely different formulations as the area of mucosal tissue at risk in the rectum is much larger and is open-ended rather than a closed space as in the vagina.

Can early clinical evaluation be accelerated? A three-day dosing schedule and a seven-day dosing schedule have been compared for C31G, a candidate microbicide that was compared to N-9 and found to be **more** irritating. Unfortunately, N-9 itself is now considered unacceptable, so any test which makes it look good is of limited value (Bax).

In the later stages of these trials, women who are sexually active with regular partners may be enrolled, along with their partners.

Discussion of efficacy trials for microbicides has emphasised their potential value in protecting HIV-negative women from infection by men, but the fact that they would be used by HIV-positive women must be considered in designing clinical trials. Involvement of HIV-positive people in these early tests of the safety of the product is therefore important.

While the COL-1492 study of nonoxynol-9 (see below) was greeted with dismay because it showed that nonoxynol-9, far from working, actually facilitated HIV transmission if used regularly, it did show admirably that these challenges can be met and paved the way for the current phase III trials.

There is a full review of the issues raised by such trials in Elias (see references).

For more on this issue, see **challenges to microbicide development** below.

References

Bax R et al. Use of a rapid screening study to predict long term tolerance. 14th International AIDS Conference, Barcelona, abstract TuPeF5305, 2002.

Claypool LE et al. Evaluating the in vitro anti-HIV-1 activity and cytotoxicity of compounds for potential use in topical microbicides: the CONRAD/GMP algorithm. XIV International AIDS Conference, Barcelona, abstract MoPeD3649, 2002.

Elias L et al. Challenges for the development of female-controlled vaginal microbicides. AIDS 8: 1-9, 1994.

Forbes AS. Microbicide advocacy and mobilization: three models from the global north. XIV International AIDS Conference, Barcelona, abstract MoPeG4270, 2002.

Reichelderfer PS et al. National Institutes of Health microbicide development. XIV International AIDS Conference, Barcelona, abstract TuPeF5304, 2002.

Watts C et al. The public health and economic benefits of microbicide introduction: model projections. XIV International AIDS Conference, Barcelona, abstract TuPeF5307, 2002.

Do we already have a microbicide?

Natural defences against HIV infection

While breastfed infants can clearly be infected with HIV by mouth, the mucosal surfaces in the mouth do not seem to allow adult human infection so readily. It has been argued that the rarity of transmission of HIV through oral sex may be due in part to substances in saliva, which inhibit the growth of HIV (Baron).

Another key observation is that the per-exposure risk of HIV infection through vaginal sexual contact is generally low. Important exceptions apply where STIs are present and possibly where girls are young and physically immature.

Natural human defences against HIV and other microbes, especially at mucosal surfaces, may therefore be important in preventing even more rapid HIV transmission. There is some evidence that these include local HIV-specific immune responses. In all microbicide research, it is necessary to be on guard against the possibility that a product will undermine natural protection - or the protection gained from future vaccines - and so make the situation worse, not better. This is an area where microbicide and vaccine researchers can work together and are increasingly likely to need to exchange ideas and experimental results (Kaul).

Sexual lubricants as microbicides

Researchers at the University of Texas set out to assess all vaginal lubricants sold commercially in the USA for their ability to inhibit the growth of HIV in cell cultures, in the presence of seminal fluid. They also looked at the ability of these mixtures to protect against cell-free HIV. After excluding products containing nonoxynol-9 (N-9), and others thought most likely to cause irritation, they reached the conclusion that three of the 22 commercial products they examined could, indeed, greatly inhibit HIV. Specifically, AstroGlide (made by Biofilm of Vista, California), Vagisil (Combe, White Plains, New York), and ViAmor (WomenFirst Healthcare Inc). They have not, however, shown activity against other viruses or sexually transmitted infections (Baron).

Unfortunately, this does not automatically mean that these products can or should be promoted for HIV prevention. Experience with N-9 has shown that laboratory studies can be misleading.

The Global Campaign for Microbicides has observed that these products have not been evaluated for their effect on vaginal or rectal mucosa, especially when used regularly in the quantities that might be needed for microbicidal use. Their US licensing is only as cosmetics, not as medicines, which requires a lower level of safety testing.

The only way to assess the value of these or other products would be through conducting clinical trials specifically designed to assess their safety and efficacy. If their manufacturers are able to sponsor such trials, this may yet happen. Otherwise, the current consensus is that there are more scientifically interesting and promising candidates which should be evaluated first.

Some have asked if the 'placebos' used in microbicide trials are themselves protective (for example, in the COL-1492 trial discussed below, Replens was more effective than the N-9 formulation). Did that mean Replens had a neutral effect and N-9 a harmful one, or that Replens actually had an actively microbicidal effect? Others argue that such products are clearly of only marginal value for HIV prevention and it is reasonable to demand that any microbicide shows a substantial improvement over them (Stein).

Two tales of possible microbicide candidates that turned out no be either useless or actively harmful serve as lessons that what may appear on the surface to be a promising microbicide may be nothing of the sort, and underline the crucial role of safety trials in these products: the use of lemon or lime juice as a 'natural' microbicide, and the tale of the spermicide nonoxynol-9.

Lesson one: Lemon juice as a microbicide

A Melbourne-based researcher, Professor Roger Short, has called for consideration of lemon juice as a possible anti-HIV microbicide. The basic principle, that acids - such as lemon juice - can inactivate both sperm and HIV, has been known for some years.

Current microbicide research does include products - BufferGel and Acidform -based on the principle of keeping the pH of the vagina low during sex, though the goal has been described as 'acidifying the semen, not acidifying the vagina'. BufferGel is set for full-scale international clinical trials sponsored by the US National Institutes of Health through its HIV Prevention Trials Network. However, a study which combined Acidform and N-9 found that the acid increased the damage done by N-9 to an unacceptable level.

In an in vitro study by Roger Short of the University of Melbourne presented at a poster at the Fifteenth International AIDS Conference in Bangkok, a solution containing 20% lemon or lime juice was found to inactivate 90% of HIV reverse transcriptase activity within two minutes. A phase I safety study of using citrus juices as topical microbicides is now planned.

Obviously, finding that something as cheap and universally available as lemon juice could be an HIV preventative is an exciting idea, and Short mooted the idea of using it as a microbicide

At the Bangkok Conference he explained to **aidsmap.com** that the idea had come to him during a conversation with Senator Mechai Viravaidya, Community Co-Chair of the Bangkok Conference and architect of Thailand's '100% Condom' campaign.

"I had been aware that women had used it as a folk contraceptive for centuries. And since then I have learned that sex workers in Nigeria and possibly other high-prevalence countries are using lemon and lime douches regularly as a post-coital contraceptive and anti-infective precaution. This means that we can design an ethical placebo-controlled study, whereas previously the possibility that the approach could cause damage would have made this very difficult."

Prevention researchers had urged considerable caution about Short's ideas, given the previous experience when the spermicide nonoxynol-9, which inactivates HIV in vitro, was found to actually facilitate HIV transmission in vivo because it damages the epithelial cells lining the vagina (and rectum).

However nonoxynol-9 is a surfactant, not an acid. Short said that the environment of the vagina is normally acid and that citric acid is a major component of semen. "The vagina is no stranger to an acidic environment," he said. One of the candidates in the efficacy studies of microbicides due to start in the second half of this year, BufferGel, uses the same principle.

Short's poster says that daily intravaginal administration of neat lime juice to macaque monkeys for one month caused no discernible epithelial damage.

Short then investigated the degree to which different dilutions of lime and lemon juice inactivated HIV replication and the viability of HIV-infected cells in a test-tube cell culture.

Short says he was optimistic "because if you can get the pH in ejaculate down to 4" (the lower the pH of a fluid, the higher its acidity) you can efficiently immobilise 100% of sperm cells within 30 seconds." The pH of neat lemon or lime juice is about 2.4.

Short exposed peripheral blood mononuclear cells (PBMCs) to different dilutions of lemon or lime juice. He them cultured HIV within the cells for two weeks and measured HIV replication by measuring reverse transcriptase activity.

A 5% lemon juice solution in culture halved HIV replication within an hour, while a 10% solution cut it by two thirds. Both of these were non-toxic to the PBMCs in culture. A 20% solution, while it reduced HIV replication by 90% within two minutes, also killed off 25% of the PBMCs, indicating possible toxicity limits to the approach.

However several studies presented in 2006 put paid to the hopes that lemon juice could be a good microbicide.

In one, conducted by Dr Anke Hemmerling, of the University of California, Berkeley, concluded that the practice was relatively safe - at lower concentrations.

In her trial, twenty-five women were randomly assigned to apply a tampon soaked either without juice or with a 10% or 20% concentration of lime juice for 14 consecutive days. Tests for genital infections, measurement for signs of inflammation and a colposcopy were performed before and after treatment.

None of the participants showed signs of severe vaginal irritation, although more than 70% of women in all groups reported minor and temporary side-effects such as dryness. No other significant problems were observed. However, in light of the preclinical activity studies, these concentrations would be unlikely to affect HIV transmission.

Dr Christine Mauckof CONRAD did a study enrolling 48 sexually abstinent women volunteers. She divided the women into four groups: those using 100% lime juice ("neat" juice with no water), 50% (half water, half juice), 25% (one part water, three parts juice) and one group using plain water.

Each group inserted their assigned test fluid twice daily for six consecutive days during two menstrual cycles. In one cycle, it was inserted via a douche and, in the other, via a modified tampon soaked in lime juice.

The result showed that some women got small but serious abrasions in the walls of their vaginas after using 50% and 100% lime juice. The women who used 25% juice or plain water didn't get these abrasions. So the juice had a dose-dependent effect, and the likelihood of damage increased as the concentration of juice increases. Among the women using 100% lime juice with no water, more than 65% experienced genital irritation, 50% experienced deep epithelial abrasions and more than 70% reported experiencing pain.

Carol Lackman-Smithof the Southern Research Institute did a laboratory study comparing the cytotoxicity (cell-damaging effect) and anti-HIV activity of lemon and lime juice to that of the spermicide nonoxynol-9 (N-9).

She tested these three substances on cervical explant tissue (human cells obtained from routine hysterectomies and kept alive in lab cultures) to find out what impact they might have on the same kinds of cells in the human body. She found the amount of

cell damage caused by lemon and lime juice was similar to the damage caused by N-9.

Lackman-Smith also looked at how much lemon or lime juice was needed to stop HIV and found that it was the same concentration (50% or greater) that also caused cell damage. She concluded that, when the juice is diluted to a point where no cell damage occurred, it also had little or no effect on HIV.

This research suggests that, in real life use (in the vagina along with semen), a 50% concentration of lime juice is needed to stop HIV, but that this concentration is also likely to cause damage to the vagina - and possibly the penis. This damage could make it easier for HIV infection to occur.

As the Economist magazine wrote on 29 April, 2006, "as a microbicide, lime juice is safe when it is ineffective and effective when it is unsafe."

References

Baron S et al. Practical prevention of vaginal and rectal transmission of HIV by adapting the oral defence: use of commercial lubricants. AIDS Research and Human Retroviruses 17: 997-1002, 2001.

Economist, the: Bitter Fruit: Another Idea for Stopping AIDS Falls Flat. Print edition, 27th April 2006.

Hemmerling A et al. The safety of lime juice used vaginally. Microbicides 2006 Conference, Cape Town, abstract PB28, 2006.

Kaul R. Mucosal immunity and HIV-1 transmission. Microbicides 2002, Antwerp (http://www.itg.be/micro2002/downloads/presentations/3Tuesday_May_14_2002/Plenary_session/Rupert_Kaul.pdf), 2002.

Lackman-Smith C et al. Preclinical evaluations of lemon and lime juice as microbicide candidates. Microbicides 2006 Conference, Cape Town, abstract PA93, 2006.

Mauck C. 6-Day safety trial of intravaginal lime juice (in three concentrations) Vs. water, applied twice daily. Microbicides 2006 Conference, Cape Town, abstract OB3, 2006.

Short RV et al. Lemon and lime juice as potent natural microbicides. 15th International AIDS Conference, Bangkok. Abstract TuPeB4668. 2004.

Stein Z et al. Appropriate controls in microbicide efficacy trials: the continuing search. XIV International AIDS Conference, Barcelona, abstract TuPeC4834, 2002.

Lesson two: nonoxynol-9

The most thoroughly studied candidate microbicides have been based on the spermicide nonoxynol-9, also known as N-9. This is a detergent which was chosen for research on the basis of laboratory findings that it disrupted HIV and other STIs, even at very low doses, and because it was already in widespread use, including in lubricants for condoms. Animal studies confirmed that N-9 protects female monkeys against challenge with HIV-related viruses (Miller, Weber). Unfortunately, N-9 causes damage to human tissue, leading to inflammation and ulceration, which is dose related (Niruthisard).

Research into N-9 as a rectal microbicide has been minimal and where it has occurred, has produced even more worrying results than in trials as a vaginal microbicide: the use of nonoxynol-9 caused the rectal lining to slough off in both mice and humans, prompting a warning about the popular use of N9-containing lubricants during anal sex. Far from protecting against HIV and other viral infections, N-9 leaves the rectum more susceptible to it (Phillips).

It was nonetheless hoped that low-dose N-9 products, used vaginally, might be able to protect against HIV without causing excess inflammation.

However, the results of the most extensive clinical trials carried out on any microbicide are clear-cut: N-9 increases HIV transmission to women who are at high risk of HIV when they use the product frequently, and appears to have no protective effect either against HIV or other STIs when used less frequently. There are better candidates available for evaluation, and the consensus is that future research should focus on those.

The most important evidence that nonoxynol-9 is ineffective - or has a negative value - as a microbicide came from a randomised, placebo-controlled trial of a low-dose nonoxynol-9 vaginal gel, COL-1492 (Van Damme).

This study enrolled 892 female sex workers in four countries: Benin, Cote d'Ivoire, South Africa and Thailand, all of whom were supplied with condoms and encouraged to use them, as well as having enhanced access to diagnosis and treatment of sexually transmitted infections. 765 women were included in the analysis of the results, of whom 376 were on N-9 and 389 on placebo. Among these women, a further distinction was made between frequent users and less frequent users, with a threshold mean value of 3.5 uses per day.

The N-9 product was made by Columbia Laboratories as *Advantage S* and the placebo, which was provided in identical packaging, was a vaginal lubricant called *Replens*. The women were asked to keep a diary of their activities (although this was replaced by interviews after some women were seen to complete their diaries in the clinic). All women were provided with condoms (free of N-9), which they were advised to urge their partners to use.

The findings were that among less frequent users, HIV rates were not significantly different between N-9 and placebo groups. However, among more frequent users, HIV rates among N-9 users were twice the rate among placebo users. There was no effect of N-9 on rates of gonorrhoea or chlamydia infection.

The Phase III study was double blinded, so neither the researchers nor the participants knew whether they were receiving Advantage S or placebo.

The researchers had anticipated that those receiving the placebo would have higher rates of infection than those who received Advantage S. Several safety studies carried out using this formulation before the start of the phase III trial failed to show any side-effects usually associated with N-9 such as genital sores and irritation.

The use of placebos as an alternative to active treatment (rather than to disguise which of two active treatments is being given) has become increasingly controversial in HIV clinical trials and is inappropriate as soon as a standard of treatment is established. Some commentators have extended this concern to argue that placebos should not be used in prevention trials either. However, until we have a microbicide of proven effectiveness, placebos must continue to be used. The COL-1492 researchers have drawn attention, however, to the challenge this represents in explaining to trial volunteers precisely what placebo use means. (Ramjee).

Similarly, concerns that the promotion of condoms might prevent a valid finding of difference have not been borne out by these results. While condom use varied between the trial sites, it was clearly higher in the trial. This may help explain the finding that HIV infection rates among women receiving N9 were lower than in women who did not take part in the trial. But surely, this is what we should all want to see in every trial?

The most reasonable conclusion would seem to be, that N9 will not be the answer to the need for a microbicide but the trials show that other more promising candidates can and should be evaluated with the utmost urgency. There are many unanswered questions and the experience with N-9 has made microbicide researchers wary of premature adoption of untested products.

References

Miller C et al. The effect of contraceptives containing nonoxynol-9 on the genital transmission of simian immunodeficiency virus in rhesus macaques. Fertility and Sterility 57: 1126-1128, 1992.

Niruthisard S et al. The effects of frequent nonoxynol-9 use on the vaginal and cervical mucosa. Sexually Transmitted Diseases 18: 176-179, 1991.

Ramjee G et al. Challenges in the conduct of vaginal microbicide effectiveness trials in the developing world. AIDS 14: 2553-2557, 2000.

Van Damme L et al. Effectiveness of COL-1492, a nonoxynol-9 vaginal gel, on HIV-1 transmission in female sex workers: a randomised controlled trial. Lancet 360:971-977, 2002.

Weber J et al. 'Chemical condoms' for the prevention of HIV infection: evaluation of novel agents against SHIV 89.6 PD in vitro and in vivo. AIDS 15: 1563-1568, 2001.

Current microbicide efficacy trials

Three principles, multiple products

The candidate microbicides which are now closest to publicly funded full-scale clinical trials are based on three principles, two of which at least may end up being combined in a single product.

BufferGel (produced by Reprotect LLC) is based on the observation that vaginal fluids are naturally acid, whereas seminal fluids are alkaline. HIV and other sexually transmitted infections (and also human sperm) are inhibited by the natural acidity of the vagina, so the idea of *BufferGel* is to maintain this (below pH 5) even in the presence of seminal fluid.

Following successful US phase I trials (Mayer) the US National Institutes of Health has sponsored preliminary international clinical trials of this product (and also PRO 2000, see below) through its HIV Prevention Trials Network. These have shown that it is at least as well tolerated as dextrin 2 sulphate and other credible candidate microbicides.

PRO 2000 (originally made by Procept but sold to Interneuron), cellulose sulphate, and carrageenan (*CarraGuard* or PC515, backed by the New-York based Population Council) are three of the leading products in development, based on very large, stable polymers. Carrageenan is a natural product derived from seaweed; the others are also inherently easy and cheap to make.

These coat cell surfaces, preventing the binding of viruses or the entry of microbes into tissue. In addition, dextrin sulphate and PRO 2000 are sulphonated polymers, whose sulphur-containing components have a great affinity for the receptor molecules on the surface of the cells HIV infects within the genital tract such as dendritic cells and preferentially latch on to them.

This activity has been confirmed in a range of laboratory studies using cell-cultures and there is evidence that PRO 2000 and dextrin 2 sulphate can protect female monkeys from vaginal infection with large quantities of HIV-related viruses (Lewis, Weber).

None of these products has the inflammatory problems that go with N9; Phase I and II clinical trials have shown that these products are all very well tolerated.

Their molecular size makes them unlikely to be absorbed into the bloodstream, which increases confidence in their safety.

A third class of microbicides still being tried are the surfactants like nonoxynol-9, which disrupt cell and viral membranes. The only one still persisting into efficacy trials is C31G (*Savvy*), a compound found to be more cytotoxic than N-9 is previous trials. Two trials are continuing in Nigeria though one has been discontinued in Ghana, though not for reasons of toxicity - see below.

By the time of the 2006 Microbicides conference in Cape Town, eight large clinical efficacy studies of microbicides had begun. Although one was discontinued, mounting so many trials in such a brief period is a logistical triumph and testimony to the dedication of the researchers involved. The trials include:

- The *Carraguard* study is one of the furthest along in implementation. *Carraguard* contains a seaweed extract that acts as an HIV fusion or entry inhibitor. Formulated as a gel, the microbicide is being compared to placebo in a randomised controlled trial by the Population Council at three sites in South Africa (Cape Town, Durban and Limpopo). The study will be unblinded for final efficacy analysis in the second quarter of 2007.

- Cellulose Sulphate (CS) is another entry inhibitor formulated as a gel that is being compared to HEC gel (a non-active gel placebo) in two randomised controlled trials. Trial #1 is in Uganda, South Africa, India, Benin and Burkina Faso. The last follow-up in this study is expected be in July 2008, data analysis should occur in December 2008, with results in March 2009. Trial # 2 is in Lagos, and Port Harcourt, Nigeria. The last follow-up in this study is expected to be in January 2008, with results due sometime later that year.

- HIV Prevention Trials Network (HPTN) study 035 is comparison of 0.5% *PRO 2000* and *BufferGel* versus two controls -- a placebo gel and open label no gel arm. The trial is looking at safety and efficacy against HIV and also bacterial vaginosis, a number of sexually transmitted infections (STIs) and pregnancy at six sites in Malawi, South Africa, Zimbabwe, Zambia, and one site in the United States. The trial is currently in still in a safety analysis phase, but will roll over uninterrupted into the efficacy phase in October this year, with primary effectiveness results expected by early 2009.

- Microbicides Development Programme (MDP) 301, is a study funded by United Kingdom's medical research council and DFID looking at two strengths of *PRO 2000* (0.5%, and 2.0%) versus placebo at six sites in South Africa, Uganda and Tanzania. The trial is expected to continue until March 2009 with results due later than year.

- Methods for Reproductive Health in Africa (MIRA) is conducting a study of the Ortho All-Flex diaphragm containing *Replens* gel (an acidifying buffer) in Harare, Zimbabwe, and in Soweto and Durban, South Africa. The study is fully enrolled, and final results are projected for the fall of 2007.

- Two trials of *Savvy*, a surface active agent formulated as a gel that provides a protective coating within the vagina, have begun: *Savvy* Nigeria, conducted in Lagos and Ibadan, Nigeria, began in October 2004 and is expected to continue until May 2007.

Savvy Ghana was discontinued when it was discovered that the HIV incidence among trial participants (in both placebo and microbicide arm) would be too low to reach any clear conclusion about the effectiveness (or lack of effect) of *Savvy*.

As the latter example attests, the fact that so many studies have begun is no guarantee that they will conclude successfully. Researchers at the meeting discussed various challenges with conducting these trials, some anticipated and some not, including:

- Problems of study design and size - especially in light of lower than expected incidence rates.

- Recruitment of high risk women.

- How to provide a high standard of HIV care to women who test HIV-positive at screening or during these clinical trials?

- What to do when women in microbicide trials become pregnant?

- The benefits and challenges involved in measuring a microbicide's effect on other sexually transmitted infections.

- Poor adherence to the studies' experimental arms.

- Finally, if a somewhat effective microbicide is identified, approved and makes it to the market, how will this affect other ongoing or planned clinical trials?

References

Johansson E. *Population Council phase III study of the efficacy and safety of the microbicide Carraguard in preventing HIV seroconversion in women.* Microbicides 2006 Conference, Cape Town, panel discussion talk, 2006.

Karim SA. *HPTN 035 phase II/IIb safety and effectiveness study of the vaginal microbicides BufferGel and 0.5% Pro 2000/5 Gel for the prevention of HIV infection among women.* Microbicides 2006 Conference, Cape Town, panel discussion talk, 2006.

Van Damme L. *CONRAD Randomised controlled trial of 6% Cellulose Sulphate Gel and the effect on vaginal HIV transmission.* Microbicides 2006 Conference, Cape Town, panel discussion talk, 2006.

McCormack S. *MDP International multi-centre, randomised, double-blind, placebo controlled trial to evaluate the efficacy and safety of 0.5% and 2% Pro 2000/5 Gels*

for the prevention of vaginally acquired HIV infection. Microbicides 2006 Conference, Cape Town, panel discussion talk, 2006.

Halpern V. *FHI Phase II/III study of cellulose sulfate in 2 Nigerian cities.* Microbicides 2006 Conference, Cape Town, panel discussion talk, 2006.

Padian N. *MIRA Latex diaphragm to prevent HIV acquisition among women: a female controlled, physical barrier of the cervix.* Microbicides 2006 Conference, Cape Town, panel discussion talk, 2006.

Feldblum P and Peterson L. *FHI Phase II/III study of C31G in 2 Nigerian cities and in Ghana.* Microbicides 2006 Conference, Cape Town, panel discussion talk, 2006.

Microbicides in development

At the microbicides 2006 conference in Cape town, professor Ian McGowan provided a summary of current human microbicide trials thus, showing that there were only five candidate substances in current efficacy trials, with a few more (some already discredited, and some where the exact formulation and mechanism of action is either unknown or a closely commercially-guarded secret) in smaller safety and dose-ranging studies (see table on next page).

However he also provided another slide giving a much larger list of candidate compounds (see table on next page).

So although scientists have identified a great number of ways to disrupt HIV transmission, the near term pipeline of microbicides ready to enter early clinical studies is fairly modest and needs to be expanded rapidly. The handful of microbicides that have advanced into large scale human trials have relatively low potency against HIV compared to antiretroviral drugs - and there is no guarantee that they will actually work in practice.

Fortunately, many ways to prevent HIV and other sexually transmitted diseases (STIs) in the vagina or rectum have been identified - each with its own set of strengths and challenges for development.

Surface active agents

Surface active agents (or membrane disruptive agents) could prevent HIV and STI transmission and pregnancy by forming a protective barrier in the vagina or rectum. Surface active agents are also cheap to make.

Nonoxynol-9 (N-9) was an early surface active microbicide that has been abandoned because it was abrasive to mucosal tissue and actually increasing transmission risks. Newer surface active products have been shown to have very low toxicity. However, such compounds are not specific for HIV and their effectiveness will depend on how thoroughly they coat the vagina or rectum, as well as how consistently they are used.

Furthermore, these products need to be applied shortly before coitus (and may not be on hand when intercourse has not been planned). If too closely linked to sex, products could be stigmatised in some cultures in the same way that condoms have been - although a study of 200 people in Nigeria presented at the conference suggested that this may not be a problem for the leading product, *Savvy*, and that acceptance of this microbicide was very high (90%). Even so, there were complaints about excessive wetness, and in other cultures where dry sex is the norm (such as parts of Southern Africa), men may insist that women not use such products.

USAID-sponsored efficacy trials of *Savvy* are ongoing - however, a major *Savvy* study in Ghana had to be discontinued when observed rates of HIV transmission were determined to be too low in both the *Savvy* and placebo-controlled arm for the study to reach a statistically significant conclusion. A related study in Nigeria is still continuing, however, while a study comparing *Savvy* and tenofovir (*Viread*) gel vs. placebo is being planned.

Two other new surface active agents in development include cellulose acetate 1,2-benzenedicarboxylate (CAP), a polymer

Microbicides in development

Phase	Membrane Disruption	Defence Enhancers	Entry Fusion Inhibitors	Replication Inhibitors
1		*Acidform* Lime Juice Lactobacillus	*VivaGel* Cellulose acetate	PC-815 UC-781 TMC-120
1/2	*Invisible Condom*			
2	(Praneem)			Tenofovir
2/2b	C31G	*BufferGel*	PRO-2000 (0.5% & 2%)	
3			*Carraguard* Cellulose Sulfate	

Preclinical microbicide candidates

Uncertain	Defence Enhancers	Entry/ Fusion Inhibitors	
Ciclopiroxolamine Praneem polyherbal	MucoCept HIV Lime Juice Acidform gel	Cellulose sulfate Cellulose acetate Carraguard VivaGel Dextrin-2 sulfate Cyanovirin-N C85FL K5-N, OS(H) SAMMA Invisible Condom Novaflux Porphyrins PSC Rantes BMS-806 BMS-378806 CMP D167	C52L Tobacco-derived antibodies/ fusion proteins Anti-ICAM-1 Ab mAb B12, 2G 12 mAb 2F5, 4E10 CD4 IgG2 T20 T-1249 SCH-C, D UK-427, 857 TAK779 AMD3100 SFD-1 Bicyclams Aptamers
Membrane Disruption	**Replication Inhibitors**		
Alkul sulfates Savvy (C31G) Beta cyclodextrin	Tenofovir TMC-120 UC-781 MIV-150 MC1220 C-731, 988		

mixture, with a long history of safe use in humans as enteric coating for capsules and tablets, and octylglycerol (a naturally occurring antimicrobial lipid found in human breast milk). Preclinical studies in tissue models and macaques presented at the conference demonstrated that these products should be safe in the rectum (for octylglycerol) and vagina (for both products).

Acid/buffering agents

The environment of the vagina is on the acidic side, but semen contains strong alkalinising properties to protect sperm from the vagina's natural defences. Unfortunately, increasing the pH in the vagina also protects microbes such as HIV and increases the likelihood of their transmission. Acid or buffering agents, such as leading products, *BufferGel* (which has a pH of 3.9), and *Acidform* are sometimes called vaginal defence enhancers because they restore the vagina to its naturally acidic state. Buffering agents may also protect against both pregnancy and sexually transmitted infections by killing sperm and by inactivating acid-sensitive pathogens.

Many women try to restore their pH by using acidic washes (such as vinegar or juice), but as we have seen, are too toxic to use in effective concentrations. But the buffering agents in commercial development have low local toxicity and no systemic activity. They are active, in vitro, against bacterial vaginosis (BV) and several sexually transmitted infections. However, their potency is rather low, although it could be improved by combining them with other products such as cervical barrier delivery devices.

A clinical study comparing *BufferGel* to *PRO 2000* and placebo is underway in Zimbabwe, Zambia, Malawi and South Africa.

Fusion/entry inhibitors

Most of the products in advanced clinical trials are simple entry or fusion inhibitors such as cellulose sulfate, *PRO 2000* and *Carraguard*. In test tube studies, the negatively charged active molecules in these gels have been shown to interfere with the binding of HIV, HSV-2 and other enveloped viruses to CD4 and other receptors on macrophages and dendritic cells.

Though these compounds are more directly microbicidal than surface active agents, they are fairly non-specific for HIV and may have a relatively low potency in the presence of seminal fluid and vaginal flora. While they may persist in the vagina longer than surface active agents, they are still generally formulated in gels which have to be applied (with plastic a prior to sex.

But thus far they appear to be quite safe and have moved into large clinical efficacy studies. Researchers believe(Hillier) that if any of these products are shown to work in clinical trials, they are likely to only be "mildly" effective (reducing transmission by 30-40%). and may wind up being considered as secondary actives for combination products.

Antiretrovirals

One solution to the low potency potential of the previous microbicides would be to use antiretrovirals (ARVs), which already have proven efficacy as therapeutics. As we have seen, drugs such as oral tenofovir are being tested in advanced studies worldwide as pre-exposure prophylaxis (PrEP) to prevent HIV transmission, but tenofovir and many other ARVs can also be formulated as topical microbicides. Tenofovir gel is already moving forward into expanded phase 2 testing (HPTN 059).

One drawback of formulating ARVs into microbicides is that they only work against HIV (and, in the case of tenofovir, probably hepatitis B) - with no activity against other STIs or other benefits for vaginal health or contraception. Another potential weakness for ARV microbicides, at least for those containing only a single ARV compound, is drug resistance. For example, if a woman's partner has HIV which is resistant to the ARV in her microbicide, she may not be as protected as she thinks.

In the case of PrEP, if a woman who is unaware that she is HIV-infected takes a single drug like tenofovir, she could develop resistance to the drug and possibly limit her future treatment options. It is unclear, however, whether that would happen with a microbicide containing a single ARV that is not systemically absorbed. Drug levels would probably be too low to select for drug resistant virus - research is ongoing into this question.

Another issue is that the barrier to ARV resistance development may be lower for some subtypes of HIV. For example, in a presentation later during in the conference, Professor Mark Wainberg, of Toronto, Canada, noted that the K65R mutation that confers resistance to tenofovir may be more common in people with HIV clade C. Prof. Wainberg conducted a laboratory study with HIV-1C isolates showing that resistance developed after only twelve weeks exposure to the drug (compared to more than a year for HIV-1B). If tenofovir becomes commonly used for treatment in southern Africa (and at present it is too expensive), its potential for microbicide use could be limited here.

One possible solution to the resistance problem would be to use combination ARVs in the microbicide.

Fortunately, there is a host of ARV compounds to choose from, including many whose clinical development as oral drugs was halted when they were found to have poor systemic absorption. Many of these ARVs have been licensed to the International Partnership for Microbicides (IPM). IPM identifies the most promising ARV candidates for microbicidal development, licenses them from the big pharmaceutical companies and handles their clinical development. If the microbicides are shown to be effective, IPM has the right to distribute the microbicides at affordable prices in the developing world while the originator pharmaceutical company retains the right to market the products in the western industrialised countries.

The first one, TMC120 (dapivirine), a non-nucleoside reverse transcriptase inhibitor (NNRTI), was   licensed through an agreement with IPM and Tibotec's owners Johnson and Johnson (who also make sexual lubricants such as KY jelly) in 2004. Now a gel formulation of the is slated to enter a very large (10,000+ participants) efficacy study in 2007. IPM is also studying a sustained release formulation of drug (see below). A benefit of such delivery forms is that ARV-containing microbicides can be effective even when applied or delivered long before (or even shortly) coitus.

CCR5 antagonists

CCR5 antagonists, including PSC-RANTES, aplaviroc, maraviroc and Merck-167, are a new class of highly potent ARVs that could be effective even when applied as a topical microbicides days before coitus. CCR5 antagonists bind to CCR5 receptors and specifically block HIV fusion to cells for up to five days - and the virus finds it difficult to develop resistance to them.

Some CCR5 antagonists have had toxicity problems when used as therapeutic agents, but at the Microbicides 2006 conference Prof Hillier said the thought that that, since there are a number of these compounds to choose from, with careful preclinical selection, there is a good chance that a safe and effective product can be identified for further development as a topical microbicide.

None of these compounds are in human trials as topical microbicides yet. However, PSC-RANTES has been shown to protect against transmission in the macaque model and is being developed specifically for vaginal application. However, the formulation challenges are considerable because it is a rather large molecule and could be expensive to manufacture. Meanwhile, Merck 167 and two related molecules have recently been licensed for development by IPM.

gp120 binders

Although some microbicides in clinical development may block fusion by binding to gp120, a number of more sophisticated and potent HIV fusion inhibitors have been identified including Cyanovirin-N, SPL, *VivaGel*, and a couple of BMS compounds that have now been licensed to IPM. Most are members of the molecular class called dendrimers - large, many-branched almost globular molecules that trap HIV and other viruses within their branches.

Cyanovirin, which is derived from blue-green algae may be difficult and expensive to formulate. However, it can be expressed in a number of different genetically altered organisms such as tobacco and potentially even in intestinal and vaginal flora (see below). The dendrimers SPL and *VivaGel*, which have also shown activity against herpes virus 2, are in phase 1 clinical trials and beginning studies for STI prevention.

Microbicide-expressing bacteria

The most radical idea in microbicide formulation is to genetically engineer naturally-occurring gut bacteria so that they manufacture microbicidal substances themselves.

Several researchers have investigated this possibility. Dean Hamer of the US National Institutes for Health described one approach at the third IAS Conference in 2005. He had devised a way of getting 'friendly' bacteria to colonise the gut and to produce bits of HIV proteins - which, in the test tube at least, have provoked enough of an immune response in gut-surface cells to stop HIV infecting them.

Hamer took a harmless but vigorous strain of the E. coli bacterium called Nissle 1917. This particular microbe has been used as a 'probiotic' in digestive supplements for over 50 years, so is known to be safe.

He spliced into it HIV genes that caused the bacterium to make HIV antigens - protein fragments of HIV that gut-surface 'recognise' and mount an immune reaction to that would repel a complete virus.

So far, in experiments in mice, the bacteria have colonised the gut and have out-competed other friendly bacteria without disturbing the digestive system. And in test-tube experiments the HIV fragments produced by the bacteria effectively stopped cells from being infected with HIV.

Once the E.coli bacterium was dosed, it colonised the mice's guts for weeks to months. So, in theory, a probiotic drink - or at least an enema - given every few weeks might provide enough protection against HIV.

At the 2006 Microbicides Conference Hamer gave a presentation on a strain of *E. coli* genetically engineered to secrete gp41 (which stably binds gp120) in the gut. Studies have demonstrated that it can colonise the rectum in mice following ampicillin treatment, and Dr Hamer presented new data showing that it effectively colonised the intestinal tract of rhesus macaques, protecting about half of them from rectal challenge with SIV.

Several other teams have shown that organisms that make up part of the normal vaginal or intestinal flora, such as *Lactobacillus* and *Escherichia coli*, can be genetically modified to continuously produce and release molecules with anti-HIV activity, such as soluble CD4, cyanovirin or gp41. A number of products have already been formulated including *MucoCept HIV*, a vaginal *Lactobacillus* which can secrete cyanovirin that is now being studied in pig-tailed macaques.

However it is a long way before we can find out if test-tube effects are reproduced in real live humans, and some researchers are sceptical that the bacteria will express enough viral protein to produce an immune response. Such vectors could also be delivered long before sexual activity, but it would be nearly impossible to ensure delivery of an effective dose. For one thing, the genetically modified organisms may not be as adaptable as the native flora, and it would be difficult to know whether successful and sustained colonisation had indeed occurred within an individual. Finally, the immune system may react against the organism or the protein which it is secreting.

The next step will be a trial in Rhesus monkeys and pig-tailed macaques to find out if this 'natural microbicide' can offer protection.

Combination and multi-purpose products

Combinations have a lower risk of breakthrough infections and have a proven therapeutic approach in a number of diseases. There are some challenges though because the complexity of formulating such products can be great. Furthermore, the regulatory approval process of combination products can be tedious. For example, in the United States, the current Food and Drug Administration (FDA) regulatory pathway requires that combination products be evaluated in clinical trials with as many arms as there are individual drugs and combinations, plus placebo, creating daunting recruitment requirements. So a study of two new agents would have to be studies in an 'A versus B versus A+B versus placebo' design, unless one of the compounds was already shown to have limited efficacy as a microbicide, in which case it would be the standard of comparison. Clinical trials that are trying to measure small improvements (20 to 30%) in an infrequent clinical marker (HIV seroconversion) can wind up being enormous and exorbitantly expensive - see **challenges to microbicide development** below. Licensing issues can also be complex - the great hope here, though is IPM, which controls the rights to combine the products that they have licensed any way they like.

Despite these difficulties, many researchers believe that combinations are the long term future. In the nearer term future, if proven efficacious, combinations of cervical barriers and non-specific microbicides will be the first available. Combinations based on acid buffer gels plus a high potency active ingredient may be developed because they have lower regulatory barriers.

Given the difficulty in moving combination products through clinical trials and towards regulatory approval, it becomes all the more important to give early consideration of formulation and pharmacology challenges.

How will microbicides be delivered?

Most of the leading microbicides have been formulated as gels. To make certain that enough microbicide is delivered, plastic applicators have been developed prefilled with a set volume of gel that a woman must insert into her vagina. A number of studies at the Microbicides 2006 conference addressed the acceptance of these devices and the uptake of this process.

Cups or diaphragms that are used in contraception protect the cervix and could be adapted for use with different microbicides, concentrating the formulation on target cells in the cervix. A few of these are in development. Use of such cervical barriers is more common in industrialised nations and there is some question as to how well they will be as accepted in other cultures. According to one study from Brazil, diaphragms were the least popular of three delivery devices (comparing to plastic applicators and intravaginal rings). Some women complained of difficulty inserting them and of local or mechanical irritation. At US $0.25 per unit, they are also more expensive than standard plastic applicators.

Intravaginal rings are another commonly used device for contraception in industrialised countries that are relatively unknown in resource-limited settings. However, rings are a sustained release mechanism that could potentially deliver a variety of microbicides (with contraceptive, antibiotic, anti-STI or anti-HIV activity) over a long period of time. Rings increase compliance and acceptability because they can be inserted weeks before sex - and are usually undetectable to the male partner. The downside to this is that the woman is exposed to more drug so there is a greater potential for side-effects. Also, if a woman should seroconvert while using rings containing ARVs, this would be the optimal method for inducing ARV resistance. IPM has conducted phase I trials with rings containing TMC120 that have demonstrated good safety and tissue levels of drug. IPM is also looking at a variety of other new ring technologies which can deliver multiple drugs.

Perhaps the most innovative microbicide delivery research is being conducted by Dr. Patrick Kiser and colleagues in Utah (of all places), who are looking at a number of technologies to optimise microbicide delivery in the vagina in the presence of semen. Polymers containing ARVs could be delivered in a long lasting gel that stays inert in the normal pH of the vagina. However, with exposure to semen, the gel turns into a liquid. Semen contains high levels of natural proteases that then free the ARVs (bound to a molecule which looks like the proteases' natural substrate or target). The ARVs are then immediately available to combat HIV present within the semen. This gets the drug exactly where it needs to go, when it is needed, and protects the woman from systemic effects of the drug when not having sex. Somewhat different gels could also be formulated for rectal deployment.

References

Primary reference

Hillier SL. *Microbicides: State of the Art and Its Evolution*. Microbicides 2006 Conference, Cape Town, Monday oral plenary, 2006.

Other references

Ballagh SA. *BufferGel® Duet: Safety and Acceptability Study of a Novel Product Combining a Mechanical and Chemical Barrier in the Vagina*. Microbicides 2006 Conference, Cape Town, abstract OB23, 2006.

Barnhart K T. *BufferGel® with diaphragm found to be an effective contraceptive in two Phase II/III trials*. Microbicides 2006 Conference, Cape Town, abstract OB22, 2006.

Cosgrove-Sweeney Y, Patton D. *Cellulose Acetate Phthalate (CAP): Vaginal Safety Evaluation in the Macaque Model*. Microbicides 2006 Conference, Cape Town, abstract PA57, 2006.

Hamer D. *Using live microbes as anti-HIV microbicides*. Third IAS Conference on HIV Pathogenesis and Treatment, Rio de Janeiro. Abstract MoPp0101. 2005.

Hamer D, Henry K. *Live Microbial Microbicides for HIV*. Microbicides 2006 Conference, Cape Town, abstract OA30, 2006.

Hardy E. *Devices for the administration of a vaginal microbicide: use difficulties, adherence to use and preferred device*. Microbicides 2006 Conference, Cape Town, abstract PC23, 2006.

Kilbourne-Brook M. *SILCS Diaphragm: acceptability of a single-size, reusable cervical barrier by couples in three countries*. Microbicides 2006 Conference, Cape Town, abstract PC33, 2006.

Kiser P. *Novel Delivery Systems for Microbicides: Semen Triggered Release and In Situ Gelling Polymer Carrier*. Microbicides 2006 Conference, Cape Town, abstract OA32, 2006.

Lagenaur L. *Vaginal lactobacilli for mucosal delivery of the anti-HIV microbicide, cyanovirin-N*. Microbicides 2006 Conference, Cape Town, abstract OA33, 2006.

Mosier D. *Lack of resistance to a candidate topical microbicide targeting CCR5*. Microbicides 2006 Conference, Cape Town, abstract OA8, 2006.

Oladele D et al. *Acceptability of savvy (C31G) gel in phase III randomised clinical trial in Lagos, Nigeria*. Microbicides 2006 Conference, Cape Town, abstract PC57, 2006.

Patton D, Cosgrove-Sweeney Y, Rohan L. *0.5% Octylglycerol Gel: Vaginal Safety Evaluation in the Macaque Model*. Microbicides 2006 Conference, Cape Town, abstract PA54, 2006.

Trifonova R, Pasicznyk J-M, Fichorova R. *Biocompatibility of solid dosage anti-HIV-1 microbicides and vaginal products with the mucosal cytokine network*. Microbicides 2006 Conference, Cape Town, abstract OA35, 2006.

Wallace G. *HIV-1 nucleocapsid zinc finger inhibitors (zfi's) impede HIV-1 trans infection in cellular and explant models*. Microbicides 2006 Conference, Cape Town, abstract OA25, 2006.

Rectal microbicides

Rectal microbicides, it is realised by many researchers working in the field, are also an urgent priority for research and development, but for many reasons have lagged behind the development of vaginal microbicides.

HIV is transmitted about ten times as easily rectally as vaginally, with a frequency (from partners with chronic HIV infection) of about 0.8% per act of intercourse compared with 0.08% (Vittinghoff, Wawer). Obviously in many countries where the epidemic is concentrated among men who have sex with men it is the major route of transmission but both homosexual and heterosexual anal sex may also contribute disproportionately to infections in countries where heterosexual vaginal sex is presumed to be the main transmission route. The taboo nature of both homosexuality and anal sex makes if difficult to establish its exact contribution here.

HIV incidence among gay men is, at the very least, not decreasing in many countries and may be increasing.

One major concern of researchers and microbicide advocates is that once a vaginal microbicide is available it may well be used for anal sex too. Because the rectal mucosa is more delicate than the vaginal mucosa and cervix, this has alarming safety implications. A microbicide that is safe for vaginal but not rectal use could even hasten transmission.

It is also extremely important to realise that anal sex is not restricted to sex between men. In one study of women 'at high risk of HIV infection' (Gross), a third of the women had had anal sex. In another (Erickson) researchers conducted telephone interviews with sample of 3,545 California adults (undersampling those age 44 and older). Seven per cent of the sexually active respondents, 8% of males, and 6% of females, reported having anal sex at least once a month during the year prior to the survey. Of these, most engaged in anal sex from one to five times per month, and about 60% reported never using condoms.

Because sexually active gay men probably form at most 3% of the population, this implies that anything from two to six times as many heterosexuals may have anal sex as gay men do - though of course they may not do so often, or with am many partners.

Rectal microbicides - the design challenge

Rectal microbicides need to pass more stringent safety tests than vaginal microbicides because of the fragility of the rectal mucosa. The vaginal mucosa is made up of a so-called 'stratified epithelium" of cells arranged in layers some 10-12 cells deep. Infection through vaginal tissue is thought to take place only when dendritic cells patrolling the mucosal surface actively transport HIV into the body, or through tears and abrasions in the vaginal wall (the reason for nonoxynol-9's toxicity). The only area with a thinner mucosa than this is the cervix.

In contrast the rectal mucosa is made from a 'columnar epithelium' of just one layer of cuboidal cells. Infection is facilitated by several processes. As well as though tears and abrasions and transport by dendritic cells, HIV may travel passively through the cell in vacuoles (so-called transcytosis) or may actively infect cells which then discharge viral particles into the bloodstream. For all these reasons HIV finds it easier to get through - and microbicides may cause more damage. In addition, though this has yet to be proved, there may be more potential for antiretrovirals in a microbicide to get into the body systemically, with implications for resistance described above.

The other big challenge for rectal microbicides is that a much larger surface area has to be covered. Whereas the vagina is a closed pouch, the rectum is the bottom of an open-ended tube. Craig Hendrix of Johns Hopkins University has done some fascinating experiments subjecting volunteers to simulated sex (both vaginal and anal) within MRI scanning machines. In the case of rectal sex he found that four hours after simulated intercourse and ejaculation, the semen surrogate had travelled up the rectum and colon as far as the splenic flexure - where the colon takes a right-angled turn under the diaphragm to become transverse instead of descending, a distance of about half a metre.

This implies a rectal microbicide might need to have a very different formulation to a vaginal one - possibly in the form of an enema or douche - or at least might need greater volume

Exactly how much gay men were prepared to tolerate was measured by US researcher Alex Carballo-Diéguez in a study reported to the third IAS Conference in Rio in 2005.

He got 18 gay men to insert measured amounts of a neutral gel rectally and then to say how much felt comfortable. He used a women's vaginal gel called Femglide similar to the placebo gels used in vaginal studies. The discomfort index was measured by how highly the men scored the gel on scales called 'leakage', 'bloating' and 'soiling'.

The upshot was that 20 millilitres (four teaspoons) was acceptable to all 18 men and one of 35ml to all but three. He then got 14 of the men to use the gel while having anal sex. This reduced the satisfaction scores so that only nine of the 14 found 35ml acceptable, though there was still a 100% acceptability rating for 20ml.

The question is, would this be enough gel to carry a microbicide and to get it everywhere it is needed? The answer is possibly not, given that it would have to get halfway up the colon. Microbicide-expressing but bacteria may be a long-term solution, but this may never prove to be feasible.

Carballo-Diéguez is planning a second-line trial in 100 men to establish the acceptability of a thicker gel versus a suppository.

Commenting on his studies, Carballo-Diéguez said that part of the challenge of introducing gay men (or anyone) to a microbicide was that it introduced a new behaviour during sex - very much like persuading people to use condoms who hadn't done so before.

"You can't just put on a microbicide like a dab of lube," he said. "You have to put it right up the rectum with an applicator or it doesn't get to where it's needed."

He said the answer might be to put HIV-blocking substances into enemas devised for douching.

Before we can start testing microbicide candidates rectally, even for safety, we need to know about the safety of sexual lubricant gels when used rectally. Although gay men and others have been using these for decades, we know virtually nothing about their potential for cytotoxicity or irritation.

David Phillips of the Population Research Council assessed the safety of 17 different commercial 'lubes' in two studies he presented at Microbicides 2006. In the first study he compared five commercial lubricants (Vagisil, Viamor, Astroglide, Delube, and KY-plus) for cytotoxicity with a candidate microbicide, Carraguard and with the neutral gel methylcellulose both on rectal explants (cultivated pieces of rectal tissue) and by looking at the infectivity of herpes viruses delivered rectally to mice in the presence of the gels (human herpesvirus infection is lethal in mice).

He found that two of the lubes (Delube and KY-plus) were very cytotoxic and all the others mildly so except for Viamor. In the case of KY-plus this is not surprising as it includes nonoxynol-9.

He extended his work for the Microbicides 2006 conference. Products assayed were Forplay Gel-PLUS, Liquid Silk, Maximus, Wet Classic, Wet Platinum, Elbow Grease Light Gel, Eros Bodyglide, Probe Thick Rich, Slippery Stuff, Toys in Babeland, KY Jelly, O'My Natural.

Methylcellulose and saline were used as the control.

None of the products tested proved to be safer or more protective than the controls. Overall the safest lubricants were found to be Toys in Babeland, Elbow Grease, Slippery Stuff and O'my. The least safe were Probe, Anal Lube and Forplay Gel Plus. Results for Maximus showed that although it did not cause significant sloughing of rectal epithelial cells, it did enhance rectal infection by HSV-2 more than any of the other products.

Although Phillips' work may seem only tangentially connected with microbicides, it is essential to get an understanding of what introducing *any* gel or lubricant up the rectum in order to have baseline criteria for the measurement of the performance of microbicides.

Animal studies

Nonetheless, rectal microbicides have shown evidence of efficacy in animal studies. The proof-of-concept study took place in 2003 when Che-Chung Tsai (who also did the pioneering animal studies in PEP and PrEP) used the dendrimer protein cyanovirin-N to inhibit HIV infection in male rhesus macaques challenged rectally with a 100% infectious dose of a virulent human/monkey chimeric virus, SHIV89.6P.

Four out of four untreated macaques and three out of three treated with a placebo gel were infected and experienced CD4+T cell depletion. In contrast, none of the ten macaques that received either 1% or 2% cyanovirin-N gel showed evidence of SHIV89.6P infection. The researchers reported that neither CV-N nor placebo gels produced any adverse effects in any macaque following the rectal application.

It the microbicides 2006 Conference in Cape Town, a gel formulation of 1% tenofovir demonstrated protection in four out of six monkeys who were challenged with SIV rectally.

Rhesus macaques received 3ml of 1% tenofovir gel rectally and then 15 minutes or two hours later an infectious dose of SIV. Infection in CD4 and CD8 cells in the blood was monitored for 20 weeks.

In four out of four untreated macaques and three out of four macaques given a placebo gel SIV virus was recovered every time point tested from a week after infection.

In contrast, in only one out of six animals receiving Tenofovir gel 15 minutes prior to virus challenge was virus recovered persistently and in this animal virus was not recovered until two weeks after challenge. In one other monkey, SIV was recovered only at weeks 2 and 6 and the other four animals appeared to be completely protected from overt infection.

Two out of three animals receiving the tenofovir two hours prior to virus challenge showed no evidence of circulating virus and in the third animal virus isolation was delayed until week 12.

Preparing for human studies

Although teams elsewhere, including the UK, are studying rectal microbicides, the strongest development pipeline for a rectal microbicide comes from the team led by Ian McGowan at the University of California, Los Angeles. The US National Institute of Health granted $16.5 million towards this research and other rectal microbicide research. McGowan's trials will work gradually towards the development of a microbicide whose active ingredient is the NNRTI antiretroviral drug UC-781 (thiocarboxanilide), a drug whose extreme non-bioavailability orally led to it being dropped as an anti-HIV treatment but which makes it ideal for a microbicide.

The first experiments, which are already underway, will compare the performance of gels containing UC-781, tenofovir and TMC120 on cell cultures, cell explants and in monkey challenge studies similar to the tenofovir one above. The second set of trials will research anal sex behaviour in women and men and do more acceptability studies.

Only if results from these are acceptable will McGowan move to a phase I safety study in human volunteers of the actual microbicide. If all goes to plan, this is due to start in HIV-negative subjects in mid-2007 and in HIV-positive subjects in mid-2008.

If safety proves to be acceptable, rectal microbicides could enter a phase II or even phase II/III study in 2010 - around the time the first generation of vaginal microbicides is expected to hit the market, if they prove efficacious.

Political unpopularity

The $16.5m granted for rectal microbicides is only 6% of the $280 million (£156.3m) spent on vaginal microbicides and only 1% on what has been spent on the search for an HIV vaccine.

Part of the problem is the stigma against anal sex and its extreme political unpopularity as a subject for research.

Dr Alex Carballo-Diéguez told a meeting of the US Rectal Microbicides campaign that he had had to call his study 'topical microbicide acceptability in high risk men'.

"We have to play this infantile game," he commented, "Avoiding all mention of works like 'gay', 'MSM' and 'rectal'. It gets past people who are hostile to gay men's work, but it means well-intentioned people trying to find out about rectal microbicide research can't find the paper."

Carballo-Diéguez criticised European funders for putting no money into microbicides for anal sex at all

A report issued at the 2006 microbicides conference in Cape Town (Feuer) urged more investment into research for microbicides for use in anal sex.

It is estimated that to bring a vaginal microbicide to market, funders need to double the $140 million a year currently being invested in research.

But the report issued by the International Rectal Microbicides Working Group (IRMWG), the first one ever issued on this area of research, finds that this amount dwarfed what has been spent so far on research into rectal microbicides

Although some vaginal microbicide research will further the search for a rectal one, the report could only find $34 million that had ever been spent on rectal microbicide research, and that annual funding, after a promising start, was going down, not up.

In 2006 $7.1 million was granted for research, mainly by US public health bodies, but the US National institutes of Health, which fund the bulk of the research, estimated that only $5.5 million would be granted in 2007.

The IRMWG could find no European funding specifically directed at rectal microbicide research at all, though some is being done with general microbicide funding.

The group estimates that to develop even one rectal microbicide candidate over the next 10-15 years would cost $70 million and that to develop enough to find a really good one $350 million - meaning that 2006 funding would have to be multiplied fivefold.

Researchers are convinced that the underfunding of the area is due to political prejudices against gay men and the taboo area of anal sex.

Anna Forbes, of the Global Campaign for microbicides, said: "A receptive sex partner is a receptive sex partner. We need rectal microbicides, just as we need vaginal microbicides, to help receptive sex partners save their own lives."

References

Carballo-Diéguez A. *Rectal microbicide acceptability: results of a volume escalation trial.* Third IAS Conference on HIV Pathogenesis and Treatment, Rio de Janeiro. Abstract MoPp0206. 2005.

Hendrix C et al. *Imaging the distribution of a rectal microbicide gel and semen surrogate in the lower GI tract.* Microbicides 2004 Conference, London, Abstract 02685.

Erickson PI et al. *Prevalence of anal sex among heterosexuals in California and its relationship to other AIDS risk behaviors.* AIDS Educ Prev. 7(6):477-93. 1995.

Feuer C. Rectal Microbicides: Investments and Advocacy. International Rectal Microbicides Working Group. 2006. Available from http://www.aidschicago.org/prevention/lifelube.php

Gross, M. et al. *Anal sex among HIV-seronegative women at high risk of HIV exposure.* JAIDS 24:393-398. 2000.

Patton D, Cosgrove-Sweeney Y, Hillier S. *Rectal Safety Studies Conducted in the Pigtailed Macaque.* Microbicides 2006 Conference, Cape Town, abstract PA59, 2006.

Shattock M. *Protection of macaques against rectal SIV challenge by mucosally-applied PMPA.* Microbicides 2006 Conference, Cape Town, abstract OA15, 2006.

Vittinghoff E. Per-contact risk of human immunodeficiency virus transmission between male sexual partners. *American Journal of Epidemiology* 150(3), 306-311. 1999.

Wawer M J et al. HIV-1 Transmission per Coital Act, by Stage of HIV Infection in the HIV+ Index Partner, in Discordant Couples, Rakai, Uganda. Tenth Conference on Retroviruses and Opportunistic Infections, Boston, abstract 40, 2003.

Challenges to microbicide development

Where microbicide trials differ from vaccine trials and even drug efficacy trials is that there is no obvious 'surrogate marker' for efficacy, in line with immune responses that can be measured for a vaccine or blood levels of a drug that can be compared with those that block the virus in cell cultures. While these may not translate into clinical benefit, candidate vaccines that do not produce such immune responses can be eliminated. With microbicides, there is no measure of success so far other than the incidence of HIV in the study population.

For this reason, microbicides need to progress relatively early to full-scale ('Phase III') trials of their effectiveness.

Phase III trials of microbicides (to test efficacy) are complex and expensive, and raise many of the same ethical issues as preventive vaccine trials. Microbicides must be provided alongside and in combination with other means of protection, including counselling, condom provision and medical treatment of infections.

For these reasons, studies have to be very large. Andrew Nunn of the Medical Research Council told the 2004 Microbicides Conference that a 12-month randomised study recruiting 2,000 women in a country with 5% annual HIV incidence (possibly high, even for Africa) would have a one in three chance of failing to detect a halving of the incidence.

This is because the actual difference in numbers between 50 and 25 women infected hovers very near the boundary of statistical significance. If the microbicide was 40% effective and the incidence 4%, no meaningful data could be generated, Nunn said.

The Carraguard study, for example, has enrolled 5,620 women so far, but there are plans to accrue 6,639 women to measure a 33% reduction in HIV incidence.

There are numerous behavioural problems that could confound the data. One of the most significant is adherence. Norman Hearst of UCSF pointed out that a theoretical efficacy of 98-99% for condoms had never translated into a 'real world' actual effectiveness of more than 85-90%, due to the difficulty of maintaining 100% use. Given that an optimistic prediction for the efficacy of the first generation of microbicides is 60%, the actual proportion of infections prevented could be small enough to be undetectable except in the most high-powered studies.

Because adherence tends to weaken over time, opinion is turning away from huge trials lasting two to three years. If the aim of the first phase III trials is to demonstrate the efficacy of the compound under ideal conditions, more meaningful data would be generated by a group of very high-risk women receiving intensive monitoring for a shorter period. For this reason, a couple of the phase III trials changed their follow-up period from two years to one year or, in the case of the South African MDP

trial of PRO-2000 and dextran sulphate, nine months (this is also the biggest trial, with a planned recruitment of 12,600 women in six countries).

Microbicide trials are also a thorny ethical area. There is the problem of providing enough monitoring and support to participants to ensure adherence while not providing so much that condom use increases enough to make results meaningless.

Conversely, over-confidence by participants because they are using the microbicide could lead to 'condom migration'; and this could result in the trial producing more, rather than fewer, cases of HIV.

There is also the problem of placebo control. We may only have one 'go' at placebo-controlled microbicide trials, because if a compound produces marginally significant results it would not then be ethical to re-test it in a second placebo trial. It would have to be tested against another active compound and this would require an even larger trial.

Another area regarding the design of phase III trials that has caused great controversy, and not been properly resolved, is whether to include a no-treatment or 'condom-only' arm in trials. The US Food and Drug Agency has insisted on a three-arm design: a) microbicide plus condom b) placebo plus condom c) condom only.

A 'condom-only' arm is desirable, firstly because some placebo gels might have slight anti-HIV properties themselves and this can be measured against a condom-only arm; and secondly because it would then be possible to measure whether the microbicide/placebo becomes a disincentive to condom use.

But it is essentially adding an unblinded arm to a blinded trial. There is no guarantee that trials would not be biased by the fact that one group is receiving no compound changing their sexual behaviour. People in the microbicide and placebo arms could give trial compound to the no-treatment people (this has confounded results in trials of breast-milk substitutes before). And, of course, another arm either adds to the size of the trial by 50% or reduces its power by 33%.

It is thought that the HIV Prevention Treatment Network 035 trial of *Buffergel* and *PRO-2000*, which is regulated by the FDA, was delayed and had to be scaled down into a less powerful phase II/III trial (where safety is pre-assessed in a small preliminary study) because the FDA insist on a condom-only arm as a condition of any product receiving a licence.

Microbicide trials involve screening people for HIV, and in high-prevalence countries this results in a lot of women finding out they have HIV. Some presenters commented that this was leading to counsellor burnout and stretched support resources, particularly in rural areas with poor infrastructure.

Anal sex (a subject just beginning to be researched in Africa) could confound results, as could IV drug use and other high-risk activities. However, the exclusion of people who report these activities could simply lead to people concealing them in the 'coital diaries' that are a feature of many of the trials.

Finally there is the question of 'standard of care', which was the subject of a whole plenary. What are researchers' obligations to trial participants who become HIV-positive or suffer adverse events? Are researchers were obliged to offer the best possible care, the standard of care in the host country, or something in between?

A consensus arrived at the 2004 conference was that developed-world care standards were not realistic and that the best that could be hoped for was that the process of doing a trial would 'ratchet up' local skills and infrastructure enough to benefit the whole population as well as trial failures. however the increasing but patchy provision of antiretrovirals in trial countries means that these care standards have to be constantly recalculated rather than set in stone at the start of a trial that may last several years.

Estimates for the cost of bringing a successful microbicide or choice of microbicides to market from the current pipeline range from $750m to $1bn; and that is without accounting for unforeseen events like trial failures or new classes of compound.

At the 2006 Microbicides Conference in Cape Town, some of these concerns came into sharper focus.

Poor adherence to condoms means poor adherence to microbicides

Women randomised to microbicides in the phase III studies reported that they did not always use the products as consistently as they should, and in one study, adherence to the microbicides was lower without condoms than when condoms are being used.

Self-reported behaviour, particularly around microbicide and condom use (and sexual behaviour in general), is not always reliable but if these trends continue, it could make it more difficult for those studies to provide clear answers as to whether the products work or not. Numerous presentations at the Microbicides 2006 Conference focused on ways to improve acceptance, encourage longer-term adherence - and to verify whether the products are being used or not in the ongoing trials.

The investigators in the clinical efficacy trials of microbicides are in the awkward position of needing to encourage participants in their studies to use both the product to which they've been randomised (microbicide or placebo) *and* practice safer sex and use condoms - but the trials would have a better chance of reaching a clear conclusion about the effectiveness of the microbicide if people did not actually use the condoms.

According to Dr Elof Johansson of the Population Council, which is conducting the phase III trial of the microbicide, Carraguard, consistent condom use probably works better than the microbicide:

"For ethical reasons we have to promote condom use within the trial. In my 35 years of experience working with clinical trials, I've never been in such a difficult situation were you have to promote another treatment that will work **as good, and probably better,** than the product you are testing. So we have to rely on non-compliance on the condom side and compliance on the gel."

Yet just the reverse - better adherence to condoms than the microbicide - is being reported in some studies.

For example, in the Cellulose Sulfate trial in Nigeria, participants reported using a condom for 90% of sexual acts in the past week, but women reported using the microbicide less frequently for 83% of the sex acts in the past week. Reports from the *Savvy Nigeria* study are similar (88% using condoms, 78% using gel for sexual acts in the past week). Such high condom use rates, if true and sustained, would mean that very few women in the study may become infected - and that the trials may be too small to reach a clear conclusion.

And muddying the picture even further, women in HPTN 035, which compares *Pro 2000* and *BufferGel* to a gel placebo or no gel, are reporting that they use the microbicide less frequently when they don't use the condoms, which could confound the study's ability to measure the effect of the microbicide.

According to the study's protocol chair, Dr Salim Karim: "In many ways, we spend so much time within our trial promoting a highly efficacious prevention method in the form of condoms, and we have depended to some extent upon the fact that a condom will simply not be used on every occasion; and in those particular instances where condoms are not used, that we would have a high proportion of those women adhering to the gel. So in a way we are looking for two conflicting things, non-adherence to the condom and adherence to the gel and you can see the hazards and problems that that particularly poses." See table.

Among participants assigned to gel, number of last vaginal sex acts reported by 422 participants

	With gel	Without gel	Total
With condom	82%	18%	70%
Without condom	57%	43%	30%
Total	74%	26%	100%

"In the last sex acts of 422 participants, we only have 30% of sexual acts where there is no condom being used. If you look at adherence to gel, you'll see that 74% of the sexual acts included gel. But one of the issues however, is that if we look at how well adherence to gel tracts with adherence to a condom. In women who used condoms, adherence to gel is very good (82%); however, of the women who did not use condoms, only 57% used the gel. So what we have is a situation in which even when the condom is not be used, we still have a problem with at adherence to gel," he said.

What if HIV incidence is too low?

Savvy is a surface active microbicide which entered into a phase III efficacy study in March 2004 at two sites in Ghana (Ampofo). The researchers estimated that there would be at least five infections per 100 person years in the placebo group, and that they would observe at least 66 incident infections.

However, halfway through the study, an interim analysis found that only 17 total seroconversions had occurred: nine on placebo and eight on *Savvy*.

This HIV incidence was dramatically lower than anyone anticipated, and the trial was closed on the recommendation of the Data Safety and Monitoring Board because HIV incidence in the study population was too low to demonstrate whether or not the microbicide had an effect.

"We cannot make any conclusion about product effectiveness using this protocol in the Ghana cohort," said Dr Leigh Peterson of FHI, who presented these results.

So what happened? No one is exactly sure but there are a number of theories.

- One is that the HIV epidemic in Ghana, or at least these parts of Ghana, has matured and that the incidence in the area is simply on the decline.

- Another is that the high rate of pregnancy - about four times as common as HIV seroconversion in this study - decreased the likelihood of the study to reach a result, because the women who were most likely to become infected simply became pregnant first, and then either dropped out of the study or changed their sexual risk taking behaviour for the sake of the pregnancy.

- A final possibility (that might be even more problematic for the conduct of these studies) is that simply participating in an ethical patient-centred prevention trial reduces the risk of HIV acquisition dramatically. It's important to remember that these women get the best available safer sex counselling and support, which is reinforced with every clinic visit. The stress of being repeatedly tested for HIV may be a fairly effective motivator to reduce one's risk taking behaviour.

In fact, self-reported condom use has increased significantly in several of the microbicide studies. For example, in *Savvy* Nigeria, participants reported that condoms were used for 66% of their last sex acts. After follow-up, however, participants reported that they now used condoms for 88% of their sex acts within the last seven days (gel use, however, was not as high). In the CS #2 study, self-reported condom use during the last week went up from 58% at screening, to 90% at follow-up.

There is also another answer, for "when a placebo is not a placebo?" When you receive free medical treatment to which you previously didn't have access, including treatment of sexually transmitted infections (STIs). Treatment of STIs directly impacts the likelihood of HIV acquisition.

If simply conducting a good HIV prevention study dramatically lowers HIV incidence, it would be a happy outcome for the trial participants, but many of these studies could find that they are underpowered.

Mess and awkwardness

The adherence issues in the MIRA study diaphragm study are even more complicated because the experimental arm has two components: the All-Flex diaphragm with *Replens* gel (a vaginal moisturiser). Overall, adherence in the study overall is lower than expected but if that weren't trouble enough, women often don't use the gel provided with the diaphragm. Participants in the trial reported using condoms at last sexual contact about 70% of the time (in both arms), while in the diaphragm and gel arm, only slightly more (76%) of the sex was covered by diaphragm, but the gel was only used in 50% of the last sex acts. Such low adherence could indicate that there is a problem with product acceptability in this setting, for both the diaphragm and for the gel.

More women in the study wanted to remove the diaphragm immediately after sex - but to be effective, diaphragms need to remain within the vagina for 6-24 hours after sex, depending upon the model.

Acceptability studies are usually conducted in the early stages of product development and clinical testing, in order to understand

Messiness or excessive wetness has frequently been cited as another drawback of some of the gels, and could be part of the problem with poor adherence in a number of the studies.

"Not surprisingly, gels increase lubrication" said the key note speaker on acceptability studies, Professor Joanne Mantell, a public health and social scientist from Columbia University, "but preferences regarding lubrication vary. Some studies show that women do not like a product that is too messy or drippy, although it is difficult to know what the underlying meaning is of excessive vaginal fluids."

In a Brazilian safety study (Hardy), participants said that would like to use a smaller amount each time, and that this gel should be less fluid to prevent excessive lubrication or messiness.

It should be pointed out that most of the various microbicides in advanced studies have specifically been designed to be less messy. Even so, the lubrication does not go unnoticed - including, often, by the male partner.

While lubrication may be desirable for sex in Western society, in some African cultures, men prefer dry sex. Male partners may interpret too much lubrication, especially before sexual intercourse, as meaning that the woman is unfaithful, has a sexually transmitted infection or has poor vaginal hygiene. Several studies noted that regular male partners are occasionally problematic for adherence in some studies - particularly if they were not informed of the woman's participation or involved in the study from early on. (LINK)

But the acceptability or adherence problems in these studies could also simply be due to logistics, e.g., having access to and being able to insert the gel before sex occurs could be the issue. Several studies noted that storage and disposal of gel applicators and privacy needed to assemble the applicator and apply the gel in advance of sexual activity can be problematic in resource-limited settings.

Product adherence in clinical trials is generally higher than when products are on the market, so getting to the bottom of these problems is crucial in order to anticipate problems in up-take and adherence that could occur and actually be worse once an effective product goes to market.

Counselling messages

One of the reasons why there is usually higher product use is because of high levels of staff support and the desire to please staff. But another possibility is that the staff counselling participants in the studies could be communicating the mixed messages about using the microbicides.

Although there's only been a limited number of studies looking at the role of providers (from doctors to counsellors who are providing safe sex counselling), they have found that "providers say that they are reluctant to counsel people to use a 'half-safe method' especially when condoms offer a higher level of protection. The concept of harm reduction has not been incorporated into sexual risk reduction counselling in most settings, especially among family planning providers, who typically aim to promote the most effective contraceptive methods," Prof Mantell said.

Preliminary indications are that this could at least be part of the problem. According to Dr. Karem, in HPTN 035, "the team's initial exploration suggests that there may have been some misunderstanding of counselling messages among study staff and participants. So we're looking at how to address this challenge and refine the kinds of messages that might be used to improve adherence to gel. Over the weekend before the conference, the protocol team got together to develop enhanced adherence counselling messages and scripts for immediate use at all the sites."

Likewise, in the MIRA diaphragm study, they are focusing on the study staff, conducting in-person meetings trying to reinforce the importance of using the gel. They discuss how staff should respond to a patient who reports that either she or her partner does not want to use some/all products, stressing the importance of use for study results with role-playing and so on.

Such adaptability over the course of the study may overcome the adherence challenges faced in these studies - but in case it doesn't always work, performing on treatment or on-adherence analyses could salvage the ability of these studies to determine whether the microbicides are effective in the subset of women who actually use the products.

But since self-reports are not always reliable, some of the studies are looking for more concrete evidence that the products have been used. In the MDP301 study they are looking at gel returns after a pilot study found that, if asked, women will return virtually all their used and unused applicators. This practice also allows the pharmacy staff to flag the participants whose gel use is low, who then receive intensive counselling to achieve overall higher gel adherence.

Who will control microbicides?

The recurring motif of the Microbicides 2006 conference, represented everywhere on conference bags, programmes, and banners, was an illustration of a beautiful African woman in traditional dress, with hands outstretched as if receiving a gift - presumably, given the conference theme - of a way that she controls to protect herself from exposure to HIV. This is in contrast to condoms, which, although highly effective if used properly and consistently, require negotiation with her male partner - a negotiation that the woman is likely to lose in many situations in the developing world.

Microbicides have been billed as a female-controlled HIV prevention method; but even though most women like the idea that they could use such a product without informing their partners, most would nevertheless prefer to tell their regular partners if they are using a microbicide, according to studies presented at the Microbicide 2006 conference. Some want to disclose the use of microbicides to enhance intimacy while others believe that gel-based lubricants would be detectable to their partners - and fear negative consequences.

Such consequences have already been observed in some of the clinical efficacy studies as researchers reported that failure to involve men in the clinical trials of microbicides has sometimes contributed to poorer adherence to microbicide use and has even led to some women dropping out of the studies. As a result, researchers are increasingly looking at ways of involving regular male partners in the trials from early on.

"Microbicides are branded to be female-controlled or aimed at empowering women in sexual encounters which threatens the traditional gender roles and societal norms", Zoë Bakoko Bakoru, the Ugandan Minister for Gender, Labour and Social Development, told the conference.

"But the development of microbicides could be seen as a venture leading to taking power away from the men. And within your societies, you know who is in charge of sex and how it is played, and who enjoys it most and who doesn't." Minister Bakoru mentioned dry sex, a practice which increases women's vulnerability - and which could conflict with gel-based microbicides that increase lubrication. "Dry sex is not a pleasure for the women but for the man."

Even when the context of partnership and sex appears to be loving and trusting, women are at risk

"Ironically, trust and affection within marriage and other long-term relationships are sometimes part of the problem," said Minister Bakoru. "We have been preaching a lot about the use of condoms, but the use of condoms is also decided by the man. And research has also shown that when people have used condoms three or four times, then the question comes 'don't you trust me?' and the condom is thrown to the side." A number of studies suggest that the desire for love and trust within a relationship will lead to microbicide use being negotiated in much the same way as is condom use.

"The majority of studies show that women want to tell their partners about using a microbicide," said Professor Joanne Mantell, a public health and social scientist from Columbia University. "There are a number of reasons why. Communications may enhance intimacy, and women want to share the responsibility for protection with their partners."

Even when women know better than to trust their regular partners, studies suggest it may not be easy to use a gel-based microbicide without him knowing.

"Covert use or the ability to use a prevention method without the explicit knowledge of male partners is one of the main reasons for developing microbicides," said Dr Hoffman. However, many participants in HPTN 050 (a US trial) felt that it would be difficult to keep using gel-based microbicides a secret. In the study, 86% of the women reported increased vaginal lubrication with the gel and some women were pretty sure that their regular partners would know. Other studies with gels also report increased vaginal lubrication. In one African study, even though HIV-positive men were supportive of their partner's microbicide use, the majority (51%) of the men reported that the women could not hide its use as they were able to feel the gel's wetness during sex.

Thus, since the use of a gel microbicide may be impossible to keep as a secret from their regular partners, studies show that some woman will disclose use to avert potential negative repercussions, such as preventing accusations of infidelity and avoiding the possibility of being abandoned by partners.

Future studies within the community at large will be essential to get the exact picture of how male involvement could affect microbicide use - and what sort of community-based marketing might be necessary to change attitudes. In the meantime, the job might be made easier if the microbicidal products that eventually go to the market have broader applications than simply being anti-HIV or anti-STI (sexually transmitted infections). Combination products that are seen being for female hygiene or contraception might raise fewer eyebrows and allow women more freedom to use a product without raising suspicion. Also, slow-release technologies such as intravaginal rings or even oral PrEP may better deliver on the promise of women-controlled devices.

Finally, Lori Heise of the GCM thinks that the development of microbicides present an opportunity to "begin the discussion about sex and power. But it can't end there. Successful microbicide introduction also requires working on the underlying gender power imbalances that condition women's risk.

"I think we need to embed our work on microbicides into women's protection strategies [which] also include the need for social power and economic opportunities, and if we don't [address these other factors], it's not going to matter if we have a safe and effective microbicide."

References

Ampofo W et al. *Randomized controlled trial of SAVVY and HIV in Ghana: operational challenges of the Accra site.* Microbicides 2006 Conference, Cape Town, abstract AB4, 2006.

Bakoru ZB. *Vaginas and applicators: expanding the national discourse on microbicides, sex and sexuality.* Microbicides 2006 Conference, Cape Town, Plenary talk, 2006.

Hardy E, Hebling EM, De Sousa MH. *Devices for the administration of a vaginal microbicide: use difficulties, adherence to use and preferred device.* Microbicides 2006 Conference, Cape Town, PC23, 2006.

Hebling EM, Hardy E, De Sousa MH. *Devices for the administration of a vaginal microbicide: suggestions on how to make three devices more attractive.* Microbicides 2006 Conference, Cape Town, OC6, 2006.

Heise L et al. *The WHO multi-country study on women's health and domestic violence: implications for microbicide development.* Microbicides 2006 Conference, Cape Town, OC12, 2006.

Kilbourne-Brook M et al. *SILCS Diaphragm: acceptability of a single-size, reusable cervical barrier by couples in three countries.* Microbicides 2006 Conference, Cape Town, PC33, 2006.

Manickum S et al. *Challenges in introducing vaginal diaphragm among women in a phase III HIV prevention clinical trial.* Microbicides 2006 Conference, Cape Town, PB44, 2006.

Mantell J. *Acceptability research: Outcomes & future direction.* Microbicides 2006 Conference, Cape Town, key note address #1, 2006.

Nunn A. *Criteria for advancing into phase III.* Microbicides 2004 Conference, London. Speaker presentation CT-03.

The search for an HIV vaccine

The day the discovery of the Human Immunodeficiency Virus was announced in 1984, the then US Health Secretary Margaret Heckler forecast that a vaccine against the newly-discovered virus should not be too difficult to develop. She said: "We hope to have such a vaccine ready for testing in approximately two years.*yet another terrible disease is about to yield to patience, persistence and outright genius"*.

We know an HIV vaccine must be possible. For example, on average ten years elapse from the time one is infected with HIV to when the virus has done enough damage to warrant AIDS diagnosis. This means that the immune system has some ability to control HIV, albeit temporarily. The role of a vaccine could be to boost these defences to where they can contain an HIV infection permanently.

Additionally, there are individuals who exhibit an exceptional ability to shrug off HIV infection, and analysing what is different about their immune systems yields ideas for vaccines. For example, some female sex workers and partners of gay men have remained HIV uninfected, or infected but able to control infection so it is harmless, for many years, despite repeated sex without condoms. Researchers are building and testing vaccines designed to stimulate the immune cells that are believed to be responsible for these people's apparent acquired immunity to the virus.

Already experimental vaccines against SIV, a close cousin of HIV that infects monkeys, have been shown to prevent AIDS (Shiver). What works in animals does not always translate into humans; still this is an exciting proof of concept, and the results from these experiments have led to the development of only the second large human trial of a candidate vaccine, the STEP trial of the Merck trivalent adenovirus-5 vaccine, which started in May 2006.

When Heckler made her original announcement, the experts listening already knew better than to expect a vaccine in a couple of years. Several scientists seated in the packed auditorium "blanchedvisibly" at Heckler's declaration, according to Randy Shilts' history of the early epidemic, *And the Band Played On.*

They were right to be cautious. After all, it had taken 105 years after the discovery of the typhoid bacterium to develop a vaccine for typhoid. For whooping cough (pertussis) it had taken 89 years;for polio and measles 47 and 42 years.

But the time lag was getting shorter. It had only taken 16 years from the discovery of the hepatitis B virus to the development of a vaccine against that disease. Margaret Heckler may have been naively optimistic, but surely HIV, probably the most intensively-researched pathogen of all time, would yield to an effective vaccine within a decade or two?

Far from it. Twenty-two years after the discovery of HIV, we appear nowhere near the development of a truly preventative HIV vaccine. About the furthest we have got are experiments in which some monkeys given a vaccine and then challenged with SIV, though still infected, showed signs of not progressing to AIDS: they maintained their CD4 counts and had lower-than-average viral loads

Even researchers previously optimistic about a vaccine have tempered their optimism in the last few years.

At the Barcelona World AIDS Conference in 2002, for instance, Jose Esparza, then of the WHO Vaccine Initiative, advised caution about the then much-publicised first-ever large efficacy trial of an HIV vaccine, the AIDSVAX trial. (he was right to be: six months later it was found to be ineffective). Nonetheless, he predicted that at least one phase III trial of a workable vaccine would be underway within the next three years - and that there should be at least one effective HIV vaccine available by 2009.

Two years later at the Bangkok World AIDS Conference, Esparza, by this time seconded to the Bill and Melinda Gates Foundation, was much less optimistic.

He said: "When HIV was discovered.we all expected that an HIV vaccine would be very quickly developed. And we were wrong because this virus proved to be much more complex than we had thought at that time." Developing an HIV vaccine, he added, was "one of the most difficult scientific challenges that biomedical science is confronting."

Esparza pointed out that the search for a **first generation** of HIV vaccines - ones that elicit antibodies to neutralise HIV (see below) - was started soon after HIV was discovered in 1984. It appeared to have finally run into the ground 20 years later in February 2003 when the first-ever (and still effectively the only) large phase III efficacy trial of an HIV vaccine ended with failure with the demonstrating that the AIDSVAX gp120 vaccine was ineffective.

He said that the search for the **second generation** - vaccines that elicit a cellular immune response and stimulate anti-HIV CD8 cells - started about 1990. The first study that stands a chance of showing whether a CD8 vaccine offers significant protection to humans, the STEP study of the Merck adenovirus-5 trivalent vaccine, started in 2006 and may produce results by 2011/12. It may therefore take at least two decades to find out if this approach yields an effective vaccine.

There are many reasons to suspect it won't, or that it will only produce a vaccine that moderates the course of infection rather than prevents it.

Esparza therefore advocated for the development of a **third generation** of HIV vaccines, ones that include both a CD8-stimulating component but which also stimulate elusive 'broadly neutralising' antibodies that will act against fleetingly-exposed 'conserved' parts of HIV that cannot evade immune control.

The first serious experiments describing these broadly neutralising antibodies took place in 2000/1 (see Stiegler).

Given the time taken to show proof-of-concept (or lack of it) for the previous two generations of vaccine candidates, therefore, Esparza forecast that an effective HIV vaccine might now not be available till 2017-2021.

Why had Esparza's estimate of the time for the arrival of a vaccine jumped 10 years forward in the space of two years? To answer that question we will have to look at what an HIV vaccine would have to do in order to work.

What an HIV vaccine would have to do

A vaccine is essentially a 'fake infection'. It is a way of priming the body by getting it to mount an immune response to essentially harmless microbes - or to parts of microbes called antigens - so that these immune responses also work against a similar but disease-causing microbe later on. The principle is essentially unchanged since Robert Jenner observed that dairymaids exposed to the relatively harmless cowpox virus (though he didn't know it was a virus then) were later immune to the ravages of the smallpox virus.

Vaccines set in motion an immune response the body would mount against the dangerous pathogen (disease-causing organism) anyway.

The reason most diseases kill is not that the body mounts no fight against them but because there is always a timelag between an invasion by a previously-unknown infection and the immune system learning how to fight it.

In a few cases the invader will win and kill or cripple - either by directly causing damage before the immune system can stop it, or by generating an immune response so extreme that it starts to damage the body's own cells (this is what is thought to happen in illnesses like SARS and bird flu, and it is also the cause of the liver damage in chronic hepatitis B infection).

In most cases the immune system will eventually win and the invader will be driven out. What a vaccine to most diseases does is to prime the immune system to an invader so that when it eventually arrives, it is already 'known' to the immune system and there is a much shorter timelag between infection and the generation of an effective immune response.

Vaccines do this in the same way that infections do. Once an antigen of any sort - a bacterium, a virus, a parasite, a vaccine, even chemical, drugs and dust - enters the body for the first time, the immune system sets about devising an immune response that will, in future, defeat this invader. It does this in several ways - with **innate** immunity (a set of chemicals that non-specifically attack invaders) - with **humoral** immunity (a set of free-floating proteins called antibodies that either chemically neutralise invaders or tag them for destruction) or with **cellular** immunity (a set of roving cells that destroy infected cells).

In the latter two cases, the initial attack leaves behind a few **memory** cells. These are cells that have 'learned' the signature of the invader to that when the same one (or apparently the same one) turns up again, the immune system can spring into action far faster and contain an infection before it has any time to do damage.

It is this memory effect that vaccines exploit, and the goal of an HIV vaccine would be to produce enough broadly-effective memory B-cells (which make antibodies) and T-cells (which direct and operate the cell-killing mechanism) to recognise any strain of HIV when it arrives and quickly neutralise it.

Vaccination happens all the time naturally, in the spirit of Nietzsche's saying "That which does not kill us, makes us stronger."

Malaria, for instance, is a particularly tricky infection because, like HIV, it constantly changes its shape in order to fool the immune system. However children in Africa who do not die of repeated malaria infections within their first three years will eventually develop a broad-enough immune response to malaria to either repel further infections or develop only mild symptoms.

One theory as to why allergies like asthma are so much more common in the modern world is the so-called 'hygiene hypothesis'. This states that children these days are not exposed to *enough* allergens and germs when they are young. As a result, their immune system does not 'learn' to respond appropriately to certain foreign substances and mounts a disproportionate response when it finally encounters them.

This provides the clue as to why it has proven so difficult to develop a vaccine against HIV. The body *does* mount an immune response to HIV - indeed, without one, the virus would destroy the average person's immune system within weeks rather than years.

However in the case of HIV infection the immune response is sufficient neither to prevent infection in the first place nor to prevent the virus circumventing the body's immune defences in the long run.

An HIV vaccine, therefore, would have to do 'better than nature' - and that is why is has proven so difficult to develop.

An HIV vaccine would have to do one of three things.

Humoral immunity

It could prevent infection in the first place by generating so-called **'sterilising immunity'**.

Sterilising immunity, broadly speaking, happens when the body mounts an antibody or humoral response to the infection. Antibodies are extremely variable Y-shaped protein molecules that are produced in huge quantities by the B-cells of the immune system. They either destroy invading microbes themselves or tag them for destruction by other components of the immune system. If the invader is one the body already recognises, an antibody response can be generated so fast that an infection never becomes established. If it is not recognised, it may take some time for enough antibodies that 'fit' the invader to be generated.

Some vaccinations, so-called **passive** ones, actually consist of antibodies rather than of antigens that generate an antibody response. Passive inoculation with anti-hepatitis B antibodies, for instance, is used to strengthen the immune response and augment the regular vaccine, especially in cases where exposure may have already happened as in a needlestick injury. However passive inoculation is similar to using a drug - the antibodies quickly disappear from the body and no permanent immunity is generated.

Antibodies generally only recognise the surface molecules of bacteria, viruses, parasites etc. The first generation of candidate HIV vaccines, therefore, used this principle. They consisted of parts of HIV's envelope - the outer viral covering. In particular, they used the gp120 protein that forms the 'knobs' on the surface of HIV that are the virus's mechanism for entering cells.

Hope that an envelope vaccine might work died when the AIDVAX vaccine trial (see below) proved ineffective in February 2003 (rgp120 HIV Vaccine Study Group), and were finally buried when the second AIDVAX trial in Thailand (Pitisutithum) proved equally ineffective two years later.

Why did they not work? The answer lies in the hyper-variability of the HIV envelope.

The gp120 protein, and in particular the part of the molecule called the V3 loop that actually makes contact with cellular receptors, is the most variable part of the HIV virus. Not only is the antibody sequence that makes up the core chain of the protein more variable than any other part of HIV, but it is also heavily 'glycosylated'. This means that HIV, as it evolves, coats its envelope protein with an immensely variable 'fuzz' of sugar molecules that frustrate the attempts of antibodies to latch on to it.

What this means, essentially, is that an HIV envelope vaccine would produce an antibody response - but only one that worked against the *exact* strain of virus that the vaccine was developed from, or imitated. The first generation of vaccines did not work because they were uselessly specific.

Cellular immunity

The other thing a vaccine could do is to delay or halt the damage that an established infection can do.

It would do this by stimulating the other branch of the immune system - the **cellular** immunity.

The prime movers in the cellular immune system are the cytotoxic T-lymphocytes, otherwise known as the CD8 cells. This branch of the immune system developed to deal with the problem that once a virus is inside a cell, it essentially becomes invisible to the humoral immune system.

However cells have a mechanism whereby the 'advertise' their contents by displaying tiny fragments of their internal constituents, called epitopes, on their surface. This is the way the body distinguishes between self and not-self - and between healthy cells and ones subverted into virus-making factories.

Cells infected by viruses and other pathogens display tiny pieces of the viral proteins on their surface. When the immune system senses the presence of foreign epitopes, a cascade of immune activation is generated which ends with the CD8 cells destroying the infected cell.

The advantage of this kind of immunity is that the cell displays protein fragments from all parts of the invading virus and not just its envelope. In the case of HIV, this means that an immune response can be generated against deeper, more 'conserved' parts of HIV that cannot afford to vary so much genetically if the virus is to work.

The disadvantage of the cellular immune response is that it does not prevent an infection, but acts against already-infected cells.

In most illnesses, this does not matter; the cellular immune response wipes the body clean of sick cells and the disease is gone. Serious damage only occurs if so many cells are infected that the immune response itself becomes harmful.

However in the case of retroviruses like HIV and the HTLV viruses, the virus becomes incorporated into the cell's genetic code itself - as proviral DNA.

By the time this has happened, the virus has essentially lost its identity as an independent entity and become so much part of the cell that it is not recognised as foreign. It is only when the cell is activated and starts producing new viruses that the immune system can recognise it as infected.

For this reason, a vaccine that generated cellular immunity could have immensely variable effects depending on whether it acts in time to prevent the incorporation of HIV's genes into the human cells' DNA.

At best, it might be able to turn people into 'exposed seronegatives'. The majority of exposed seronegatives remain little-studied and we don't know how many there are and why they did not develop HIV infections. They are people who remain HIV antibody-negative but where extremely sensitive tests detect signs of a historical infection by HIV - one that remains so well-contained that not enough virus is ever present to trip the humoral immune response and induce antibodies to HIV.

Even though exposed seronegatives do not have antibodies to HIV, immune experiments showed that their T cells 'recognise' HIV in the test tube - so they must have seen it before (see Shearer). The types of cellular responses detected included both CD4 and CD8 cell responses to HIV and the production of immune-activating cytokines in response to HIV. These CD4 and CD8 responses have been reported in sexual partners of HIV-infected individuals, as well as in seronegative health care workers who were accidentally exposed to HIV-infected blood via a needle stick.

At the time of the above study, no HIV was detectable within these people by PCR viral load testing. Subsequent extremely sensitive PCR testing, however, has found that many exposed seronegatives may have extremely small viral loads - in the order of 0.05 copies This means that they do have some cells that have been infected by HIV and contain proviral DNA.

What appears to be the case with most of them, however, is that by good luck, good genes or good timing, their immune system developed a CD8 response against actively-infected cells so efficient that it nips any productive viral infection in the bud.

One fascinating example of this phenomenon was a study by Tuofu Zhu presented at the Bangkok International AIDS Conference. Zhu was studying long-term exposed seronegative partners of HIV-positive gay men. The group consisted of the HIV-negative partners of HIV-positive men who had been diagnosed between 1994 and 1998.

Out of 94 HIV-negative regular partners of positive men, he found 14 who had in fact become HIV-positive - a rate of only 15%, despite regular unprotected sex with their partners over a period of years.

Two of the partners appeared to have caught HIV from their partners early on in their relationship, but to have mounted a successful immune response to it. They had no antibodies to HIV and therefore did not test HIV-positive. The fact that they had HIV at all could only be detected by hypersensitive viral-load testing, which picked up HIV in their blood at a count of 0.05 copies - one thousandth of the amount usually called "undetectable" by standard "ultrasensitive" tests.

The ultimate goal of a CD8 vaccine, therefore, would be to turn people into 'fake' exposed seronegatives.

However no CD8 vaccine has come anywhere producing this effective an immune response, and the exposed seronegatives - or at least the ones that have been studied, who are mainly multiply-exposed people that somehow do not become HIV-positive - remain with their immunity secrets tantalisingly elusive (it appears now that they may also generate broadly neutralising antibodies - see below).

What CD8 vaccines have done up till now, at least in animal studies, is to blunt HIV infection. Though the vaccine-generated immune response may not be able to stop people becoming HIV-positive, it may be enough to slow down viral production by interfering with the chain-reaction of viral infection and reproduction. A vaccine of this kind might not be able to prevent people becoming HIV-positive (and in many cases would actually generate a 'false positive' result itself). But it might be able to contain HIV reproduction and enable people to develop a much lower viral load; so low, possibly, that progression to AIDS might never happen.

This kind of vaccine essentially blurs the distinction between a **preventative** vaccine and a **therapeutic** one. The latter are not the subject of this chapter as they are a treatment. But the object of scientists who are trying to develop therapeutic vaccines is essentially identical: by manipulating parts of the immune system of people with HIV in such a way that their anti-HIV CD8 responses are amplified, they are aiming to contain HIV infection to the point where it becomes non-pathogenic.

The other very important thing therapeutic or cellular vaccines could do would be to do what HIV treatment can also do - they would act to prevent onward HIV infection by lowering the average viral load in the infected population.

Mucosal immunity

There is a third kind of immunity a vaccine might be able to generate, but it's not one that previous vaccines have attempted to stimulate. This refers to humoral or cellular immune responses that are concentrated at the mucosal surfaces where most HIV transmission takes place, such as the vagina and rectum. Vaccines may be able to induce immune responses acting only at these surfaces, to prevent HIV transmission through sex or breast milk. They would not work against infection by injection, but since the majority of HIV in the world is spread through sex or from mother to baby, they would potentially contain the epidemic.

What would a mucosal vaccine look like? It might look a lot more like a microbicide than a vaccine, though it would be one that generated an immune response. It does not take a big leap of science to move from the idea of a microbicide that would work by getting genetically-altered versions of natural gut and genital bacteria to develop microbicidal substances like cyanovirin-N to getting genetically-altered bacteria to develop bits of HIV proteins that would then generate an immune response.

Such an approach has indeed been developed by Dean Hamer of the US National Institutes of Health. Because its method of delivery is more like a microbicide than a vaccine, it is described under **microbicide-expressing bacteria** in the **Microbicides** section.

In December 2005 one of the leading exponents of both microbicide and vaccine technology, Dr Robin Shattock of St George's Hospital, London, told a vaccines meeting organised by the National AIDS Trust that the first effective HIV 'vaccine' to be developed might indeed look more like a microbicide or a long-acting contraceptive device than a standard injection. He said that the first vaccines might also only work for months at a time, and his talk was a useful summary of the challenges HIV throws at vaccine developers and why this might be so.

"With an HIV vaccine we are trying to do something science has never done before," he said. "Most vaccines mimic the successful immunity the body mounts against an actual infection. With HIV this response does not work, so we have to do better than nature."

"And most vaccines work for years against a virus that changes very little over time. But HIV changes rapidly. In an untreated person a billion subtly different copies of HIV are produced every day.

"There is more genetic diversity in the HIV in a single patient than there is for influenza over the entire world."

Shattock added that most diseases for which a successful vaccine had been developed got into the body via the lungs or the digestive system. Apart from hepatitis B we had little experience of a vaccine against something that usually gets in through the genital tract. He said that the direction his own research was taking might not be a truly preventive vaccine, but one that blunts the huge surge in viral load people get when they are first infected with HIV (within the first six weeks). It is estimated that because people are so much more infectious at this time, anything from 30-60% of all HIV is transmitted by people who have just got it themselves.

He said: "If we could do this it might give infected individuals a better prognosis - and it would have a major impact on transmission within the community."

However he warned that it might require "regular and repeated vaginal [or rectal] exposure" to have an effect.

So he was looking at technologies like intravaginal rings and caps that could deliver a sustained-release dose of a substance that would stimulate HIV-specific immunity. Such devises might reinforce or potentiate the effect of a more conventional injected vaccine.

Shattock said he was not pessimistic about the eventual discovery of a vaccine against HIV. "We have found out that conventional approaches don't work against HIV, but we only know that because of 20 years of intensive research," he said.

Broadly neutralising antibodies

As we said above, exposed seronegative people have also been found that have antibodies that are broadly effective against a wide range of different strains of HIV infection rather than just very specific ones.

Researchers such has Robert Gallo (see below) have argued that CD8 vaccines will not prove to be enough to prevent HIV and that a completely new 'third generation' approach to an HIV vaccine should be developed using a combination of CD8 stimulation and broadly neutralising antibodies.

Broadly neutralising antibodies extremely rare and so far only a few have been isolated from the blood of exposed seronegative individuals. A study in 2004 (Binley) found that just one antibody, 4E10, neutralised every one of a panel of 90 HIV viruses with moderate potency. One called 2F5 neutralised 67% of isolates, but none from clade C of HIV, the most common type in Africa. An antibody called b12 neutralised 50% of viruses, including some from almost every clade, while one called 2G12 neutralised 41% of the viruses, but none from clades C or E.

Experiments with these antibodies have so far mainly involved using then as passive inoculations and studying how they are eliminated in the body. Here they act more like potential long-lasting anti-HIV drugs, as they are eliminated from the body over a timescale of one to three weeks. Some artificially-created antibodies such as the experimental drug TNX-355 use the same principle.

Developing a vaccine which induces the body to generate them will be much more difficult. The reason these antibodies work against so many types of HIV appears to be because they act against highly 'conserved' parts of HIV that have to retain the same configuration in order to infect cells. In the main these are parts of the viral infection mechanism that are only exposed for a fraction of a second during the intricate unfolding and insertion process that happens during the infection of a cell. It is therefore challenging to establish what the epitopes that elicit the antibodies are.

Vaccines against viral proteins

Vaccines can be made against toxins that bacteria and viruses produce as well as against parts of the mature virus. An example is the tetanus toxoid vaccine. It is an inactivated version of the bacterial toxin the tetanus bacterium produces, and it induces antibodies against the toxin itself.

HIV produces several harmful proteins that could be vaccine targets. The most promising so far is the tat protein, which is produced early on in the viral lifecycle and stimulates the host cell's genes to become active.

The tat protein is so important to HIV that it is highly conserved. A small trial involving 47 volunteers in Italy ending in 2006 produced a strong immune response in 80% of subjects given it. The Italian team studying it is trying to get funding for a large African trial scheduled to end in 2011.

The hurdles to climb

In a paper in the Lancet in November 2005, Robert Gallo summarised the barriers to developing a vaccine and made recommendations as to future directions for research.

He said HIV vaccine development was difficult because of the following factors:

- **An HIV vaccine cannot consist of attenuated, actively replicating (live) HIV** (as the measles vaccine does). See below for more on live attenuated vaccines: although the best vaccines for other viral diseases have usually used live viruses, there is an inherent danger that attenuated HIV could cause AIDS.

- **Killed whole virus** (like the polio vaccine) might also be dangerous because one could not be sure one has killed all viral particles and it had worked poorly in animal tests.

- **HIV vaccines therefore had to use subunits** of HIV. There are successful vaccines that use subunits of viruses such as individual proteins: an example is the hepatitis B vaccine. However medical science was less experienced with them.

- There is **no truly useful small animal model for studying HIV infection.** Vaccines have to be developed using SIV or the artificial monkey/human virus SHIV in monkeys. SIV infection tends to follow a different path in monkeys and they are, says Gallo, "both expensive and available to very few investigators."

- **We do not know with certainty which immune response will provide protection.** This is a major problem. Pre-efficacy studies of vaccines in monkeys and humans use correlates of immunogenicity such as CD8 cell response, and in particular use the production of cytokines. The most rigorously evaluated approach is the ELISpot assay, which counts the number of T cells making the cytokine interferon-gamma. However at the 2004 AIDS Vaccine Conference in Lausanne, Switzerland, studies found that immune-stimulated cells might respond by producing other cytokines such as interleukin-2: and whatever they produce, we do not know enough about whether this immune response will translate into a protective one.

- **HIV is extremely variable** and as we have already seen with the broadly neutralising antibodies, a vaccine may not work for all subtypes of HIV. Because of this, bodies such as IAVI are supporting the development of vaccines against different subtypes.

- **HIV is a retrovirus** and we have never before attempted to develop a vaccine against a retroviral infection. This, Gallo believes, is the most important obstacle of all. As detailed above, it means that a vaccine has a small 'window' of opportunity in which to prevent infection and will have to be extremely effective if it is to prevent viral DNA from being integrated into the host genome and establishing a permanent infection.

- **HIV produces viral proteins** such as tat that actively interfere with the immune response of both infected and uninfected cells They may do with   a cellular vaccine response too. For this reason, Gallo believes that an effective vaccine would have to include an anti-tat component.

- **CD8 cellular vaccines** do not block infection because they act at too late a stage. They are therefore acting against a continued infection rather than stopping one happening. Because of this, in some monkey studies, the virus mutated and acquired immunity to the CD8 cellular response. In other words, HIV may become 'vaccine-resistant' in the same way it becomes drug-resistant. CD8 vaccines, if they work, largely do so by reducing the viral load in chronic infection, but would not necessarily do much to reduce the peak level of viremia in the early burst of viral reproduction that occurs in acute infection, so they might not do much to control infections transmitted by people in acute infection.

Gallo concludes by saying that "Instead of focusing on finding the elusive correlate [of effective immunity], obtaining or approaching sterilising immunity should be the goal; both conceptually and experimentally we know of only one practical way to accomplish this, namely - by eliciting neutralising antibodies that are broadly reactive against various HIV strains and that are expressed for long periods."

He therefore makes a plea that much more research should be aimed at developing vaccines that stimulate broadly neutralising antibodies, and that include an anti-tat component.

Gallo has been a notable sceptic about more conventional approaches to HIV vaccines, but has proven right in his predictions that the first generation of antibody-eliciting vaccines would be ineffective. Despite his scepticism, however, research into the second generation of cellular-immunity vaccines continues apace, with some indications that they may be more effective than the previous generation. What methods are being used?

Types of HIV vaccines

To date, over 40 different HIV vaccines have been tested in several thousand volunteers. Most of this research has consisted of early safety and efficacy studies of recombinant proteins, produced in a variety of different systems. Despite some encouraging evidence of immune responses in people, it is unclear whether many of these would prevent HIV infection.

Typically, vaccines are administered to large numbers of people at high risk of infection. After a certain time, the vaccinated participants' experiences are compared to those of people who received a placebo. This may involve assessing the antibodies present in their blood, or the response of their CD8 T-cells to HIV in the test tube, or looking for HIV seroconversions in the trial participants.

Researchers have explored a number of strategies that they hope will produce protective immune responses. These include:

- Live attenuated vaccines.

- Inactivated vaccines.

- Recombinant vectored vaccines.

- Recombinant sub-unit vaccines.

- DNA vaccines and replicons.

Several studies have examined the use of combination or 'prime and boost' vaccines, in which two or more different vaccines to broaden or intensify immune responses. Examples include a vector virus to prime a T-cell response with a subunit booster to produce antibodies, or two different vector viruses expressing the same gene sequence.

Live attenuated vaccines

One of the most powerful ways to create vaccines is by weakening or 'attenuating' the pathogen. These defective viruses are harmless to people, but stimulate the body to produce an immune response. Creating live attenuated vaccines normally involves deleting genes that protect the virus against the immune system, but which are not essential for its reproduction. The measles vaccine is an example.

Live attenuated HIV vaccines are considered unsafe, after research in monkeys indicated that can a live attenuated vaccine, made by deleting the nef gene, protected monkeys against SIV, but caused AIDS, albeit more slowly than the normal virus (Baba, Daniel)

Inactivated vaccines

Creating vaccines based on inactivated or 'killed' viruses is another classic technique, which was used in creating the world's first successful polio vaccine. However, the technique is considered risky, as vaccine recipients could easily be infected with HIV if the inactivation process should fail. There have been no claims of a significant level of success with these types of vaccine for HIV, although some, such as Remune, an HIV preparation with envelope protein gp120 removed, are being pursued as therapeutic vaccines for people already infected with HIV.

Recombinant vectored vaccines

Recombinant vectored vaccines are made by incorporating fragments of HIV into established vaccines made from harmless viruses, such as the canarypox viruses or adenovirus. These vaccines aim to stimulate the immune system to recognise the fragments of HIV, protecting the vaccinated host from future infection. Vector vaccines have been shown to produce HIV-specific cytotoxic T-cell responses in animals and humans. Adenovirus vectors appear to be among the best of those tested so far, but the first and most widely used strain, Ad5, has problems because of widespread natural immunity to the virus.

Pox virus vaccines

The most advanced vectors used for HIV vaccines are pox viruses, using relatives of the smallpox virus. One attraction of these is that they induce strong cytotoxic T-lymphocyte (CTL) immune responses. Researchers are working on the bird viruses fowlpox and canarypox, and bird-adapted strains of vaccinia, such as NYVAC and modified vaccinia Ankara (MVA).

Canarypox

Canarypox is known to be safe since it is already the basis of a commercial rabies vaccine. Aventis Pasteur has developed a range of canarypox vaccines in their ALVAC range. The first ALVAC product, vCP125, consisted of gp160 inserted in the vector, while a second product, vCP205, which also contains env, gag and protease appear to generate greater cell-mediated immune responses.

The most extensively tested candidate is vCP1452, which incorporates sequences from the *env*, *gag*, *nef* and *pol* genes. Unfortunately, however, since the cellular immune responses seen with canarypox constructs appear to be weak, transient and only seen in a minority of trial volunteers, little research is currently being carried out into their use alone.

However, they are being tested in prime-boost strategies with subunit vaccines. The controversial RV144 phase III trial, which at the time of writing is still ongoing in Thailand and which is due to finish in 2008 (see below), uses the ALVAX vCP1521 vaccine as the prime and the AIDSVAX gp120 envelope subunit vaccine as the boost.

Modified vaccinia Ankara

MVA was given safely to tens of thousands of people in the 1970s [55]. MVA has long been studied in animals, but its first clinical use as the basis for an HIV vaccine is as a booster in a 'prime-boost' strategy. Other MVA-based vaccines are being developed and tested in further trials.

Adenovirus vaccines

Adenovirus is a relatively harmless and common human virus associated with cold-like illnesses. Despite two large companies developing HIV vaccines based on adenovirus, a problem is that adenovirus 5 (Ad5) is widely distributed across the world and a substantial proportion of the population are naturally exposed to it, leading to high levels of natural immunity. This renders Ad5-based vaccine useless, as all they can do is re-awaken natural immunity to Ad5 (Isaacs).

However, recent research results have indicated that Ad5-based vaccines may in fact generate immune responses even in people with pre-existing immunity to the virus. Merck & Co. is currently running a large phase II trial, the STEP trial (see above), of an Ad5-based vaccine that contains the HIV genes gag, pol and nef.

Other vectors

Other viral vectors currently being studied with HIV or simian immunodeficiency virus (SIV) in animals include rabies, measles, poliovirus, herpes simplex, human rhinovirus, influenza and pertussis.

Measles is of particular interest because the live attenuated measles vaccine in common use is extremely effective in generating long-lasting immune responses when given to infants. This might be ideal to protect young people in countries where HIV is widespread.

The recombinant rabies virus vaccine potentially has a number of advantages, since few people are vaccinated against rabies, the attenuated rabies virus infects most human cells but does no damage and it may produce ongoing exposure to HIV antigens in the body. Research in mice has found that a rabies-based HIV vaccine produced HIV-specific neutralising antibodies and cytotoxic T-cells that targeted HIV-infected cells (Schnell).

Recombinant sub-unit vaccines

Recombinant sub-unit vaccines stimulate antibodies to HIV by mimicking proteins on the surface of HIV. A range of HIV proteins has been produced as potential vaccines for HIV. Initially, the main targets for vaccine developers were the viral envelope protein gp120, and its precursor gp160, in the hope that they would prevent HIV entering human cells. More recently, vaccine developers have experimented with other HIV proteins, including regulatory proteins such as Tat, which may modify the course of disease in monkeys.

Envelope proteins

The first HIV vaccine to enter full-scale efficacy testing was the AIDSVAX gp120-based vaccine. This was designed to induce neutralising antibodies in the hope of preventing or aborting infection with HIV.

One AIDSVAX version, based on two different isolates of subtype B viruses, was tested among 5400 people at risk of sexual transmission of HIV in a randomised placebo-controlled trial in the United States, Canada, Puerto Rico and the Netherlands. The trial produced no evidence of protection among the trial volunteers as a whole, although the vaccine did elicit HIV antibodies (rgp120 HIV Vaccine Study Group). A second trial, of an AIDSVAX formulation based on Thai subtype E and subtype B viruses, began in March 1999. This study recruited 2500 injecting drug users in Thailand, but found absolutely no evidence of protection (Pitisutithum).

Modified envelopes

Other strategies for stimulating the immune system to produce antibodies have stemmed from better understanding of the way HIV's proteins interact with the cells they infect. For example, HIV's proteins are often hidden from the immune system by a coating of sugar molecules: removing some of these molecules from the protein's surface may lead to neutralising antibodies that can act against the virus Secondly, there are 'variable loop' regions within the virus's proteins. In these regions, mutations and changes in the protein's structure have no effect on the virus's ability to replicate and cause disease, but they enable it to escape from immune responses directed against those regions by acting as 'decoys'. Studies have shown that removing parts these loops produces stronger antibody responses. For more, see **broadly neutralising antibodies** above.

Regulatory proteins

Several groups of researchers have been investigating the use of HIV proteins other than the envelope proteins in vaccines, such as the regulatory proteins Tat and Nef.

Tat we have looked at above: nef is also of interest, despite the fact that some HIV strains can infect and cause disease without it. If cellular immune responses target cells expressing Nef, they could select for less virulent viruses.

More recently, researchers have reported animal studies using a vaccine consisting of an envelope protein plus a Nef-Tat fusion protein. The combination of these two elements was able to protect monkeys against disease, though not against infection, after challenge with a highly pathogenic simian / human immunodeficiency virus (SHIV). This vaccine is now being evaluated in clinical trials in the United States and Belgium.

Peptide vaccines

Instead of vaccinating with a whole protein, another approach is to use a fragment of a protein, called a peptide, which consists of a few amino acids. A vaccine containing the V3 sequences from several strains of HIV has been used in animals and produced antibodies able to neutralise several laboratory-adapted virus strains. Peptide vaccines have been tested in HIV-positive patients, with some antibody and cellular immune responses against HIV [(Pinto, Kran). Whether these will be translated into protection in HIV-negative people, however, remains to be established.

L inking a peptide to a lipid has also been explored as an HIV vaccine technique. The lipid carries the peptide directly into cell membranes where it can be presented to the immune system with maximum efficiency. A number of preliminary clinical trials of such vaccines have been carried out and a phase II trial using lipopeptides as boosters for canarypox vaccines is planned.

DNA vaccines

DNA vaccines are small pieces of DNA containing genes from HIV, which can be grown in bacteria. After injection, the animal's cells effectively make the vaccine themselves by expressing the HIV genes. Although they work well in mice, it has been more difficult to get DNA vaccines to work in primates, including humans, as it is difficult to get enough DNA into each injection. There are also safety considerations inherent in the design of DNA vaccines, since the genetic material of HIV could effectively result in infection with the virus.

A further problem is that a single mutation in HIV's genetic material can be sufficient to undermine the protection of an HIV vaccine. In one study, in which eight monkeys were vaccinated and challenged with the virus, one monkey became sick and died within six months of initial infection after its virus mutated to be resistant to the vaccine (Barouch). Although a range of DNA vaccines could be used, this would result in even larger doses of DNA being needed. DNA vaccines that trigger the production of cytokines have also been tested. Experiments in monkeys show that this approach works surprisingly well, but this has been less successful in human studies (Boyer).

Replicons

Replicons may be a better way of getting HIV's genes into cells, by using a carrier virus to transport the vaccine genes. Replicons have the same physical properties as viruses, including the ability to enter cells of specific kinds, but they have the advantage of not reproducing after entering the human cell, so there is little or no immune response to the carrier virus. Thus, one replicon system could be used repeatedly in the same person, to deliver a series of different vaccines or gene therapies.

The three leading replicon systems for HIV vaccines are based on Venezuelan equine encephalitis (VEE), Semliki forest virus (SFV), and adeno-associated virus (AAV). All three have shown some success in animal studies. Papillomaviruses have also been developed as the basis for replicons, which appear to offer the possibility of mucosal immunity to HIV antigens following oral immunisation in mice (Zhang). However, it remains to be seen if this can be translated into comparable effects in monkeys or people.

Prime-boost vaccination strategies

A number of trials into prime-boost strategies for HIV vaccination have been attempted. In general, these use two different vaccines, in order to strengthen the immune response to a single vaccine, or to complement an antibody response with a cell-based immune response.

Vaccines - a summary of the issues

So, more than twenty years after the discovery of HIV there is still no preventive vaccine against AIDS. However, while the first vaccine to complete a full-scale clinical trial has so far failed to show any convincing evidence of protection, and despite all the obstacles to developing one, other more credible candidate vaccines are entering trials in increasing numbers. Progress has been made by showing that vaccines can alter the course of HIV-like disease in monkeys and the identification of antibodies that can protect against infection with a wide range of HIV strains.

HIV has focused attention on the need for new vaccine technologies (discussed in the *HIV & AIDS Treatments Directory*) and these in turn raise questions about how an HIV vaccine can be evaluated and, if effective, made available to those who need it.

Preventive vaccines against HIV and AIDS are actively being pursued by governments and inter-governmental agencies, the pharmaceutical industry and non-governmental organisations. Progress towards this important but challenging goal requires a long-term commitment to partnerships across sectors, with the active involvement of communities affected by HIV.

The need for a vaccine

Historically, vaccination is the only strategy that has ever led to the elimination of a viral disease, namely smallpox, in poor countries as well as in wealthy ones, for women and children as well as for adult men. While the biology of HIV is less favourable than smallpox to vaccine development, some experimental vaccines do, to varying degrees, protect animals against related viruses.

An ideal vaccine would be cheap to produce, stable at room temperature, easy to transport and administer without special equipment, completely safe, and would need only one dose to provide complete lifelong protection against all routes of transmission and all variants of HIV. All current vaccine candidates are likely to fall short of these criteria, although even an imperfect vaccine could deliver public health benefits and provide further insights for prevention and treatment strategies.

To achieve this, we need to think in terms of a series of vaccines to be developed and tested, in parallel and then against each other, possibly in combinations, and successively improved over many years. This process will require extended collaborations between countries with the technical resources to develop the vaccines and those with the largest populations affected by HIV. It will require private sector expertise in manufacturing and production of vaccines, underpinned by public financial and legal guarantees where market mechanisms fail to secure the investment to take products forwards. It will need community education and mobilisation to enable evaluation to proceed in an ethically acceptable way, with backing from governments and international institutions.

For the communities worst affected by HIV and AIDS, whose members must be involved in any programme to evaluate preventive vaccines, there are increasingly complex medical and social issues to be addressed. At a community level, any vaccine will need to be evaluated and used in combination with other treatment and prevention strategies. It is essential that this happens in ways that reinforce those other strategies and do not undermine them.

Preventing infection

Firstly, a vaccine might prevent a person becoming infected with HIV (sterilising immunity). Measuring this effect is simple in principle. A population of individuals at risk is recruited into a clinical trial, and a proportion is vaccinated. After follow-up for a number of months or years, the number of new infections in the vaccinated group is compared to the number in a control group. If there are fewer infections in the vaccinated group, this may be evidence for the efficacy of the vaccine.

The prototype for a trial to measure this was the VaxGen Phase III trial discussed below, where the primary endpoint was the number of people who became HIV-positive in the vaccine recipient group compared to the   placebo recipient group.

Delaying illness

Secondly, a vaccine might delay or prevent the progression of illness, despite HIV infection. This effect is likely to depend on a cellular immune response directed against HIV-infected cells. There is evidence from animal studies that such effects can be achieved. In a clinical trial they would be detected using viral load tests, comparing individuals who had received a vaccine and then went on to be infected to others who became infected without first having received the vaccine.

Extracting the true protective effect of a vaccine that delays infection is obviously more difficult. However a statistician working for the US HIV Vaccine Trials Network has argued that an initial trial might still randomise people individually, in a similar design to the AIDSVAX trials, to receive vaccine or placebo. In a population with a 2% risk of HIV infection every year, it should be possible to get answers from a trial that recruited 5,000 people over 12 months and followed them for another four years. This would show if the vaccine did, in fact, have an impact on HIV infection rates - and would be large enough to tell the difference between a vaccine that was 30% effective and one that was 60% effective.

With no protection against infection, this trial design would also make it possible to compare two groups of people with HIV for an average follow-up of around 18 months. This might be long enough to look at some markers of progression (viral load and falling CD4 counts) although this could be obscured by treatment. As follow-up increased, the likelihood of treatment obscuring any effect of the vaccine could become greater (Self). (It might also be reduced, if treatment is driven by CD4 counts, since better control of the virus should lead to deferred treatment.)

If it were possible to show that the need for antiviral treatment was delayed through vaccination, hopefully by years, at least this would provide a clear cost-benefit rationale for providing such a vaccine to populations at risk.

A vaccine in this category might also, in principle, be directed at making HIV disease easier to treat, for example, by specifically blocking the development of drug-resistant viruses. It might also be possible to direct the immune response against specific parts of the virus that are responsible for its virulence, so that viruses which escape from the vaccine-induced response cause less damage than would otherwise be the case.

Blocking transmission

Thirdly, a vaccine might **reduce the chance of onward HIV transmission**. For example, from a mother to her baby, or through sexual transmission. This, like the second effect, would be likely to follow from a reduced viral load seen in vaccinated individuals compared to those who had not been vaccinated.

The greatest benefit from a vaccine would be if it reduced viral load in vaccinees in the period immediately after infection and before antibodies were produced. If so, this should be reflected relatively rapidly in lower rates of new HIV diagnoses over the course of the study, in communities that have received the vaccine compared to those which have not.

The greatest value of a vaccine with this as its main effect would be seen at a population level. The ideal way to test it would therefore be to compare populations in which a vaccine is available with those in which it is not (Self). It would be necessary to ensure a continuing high uptake of HIV testing, which is likely to depend on excellent and expanding access to treatment. The proper comparison would then be between populations, all of which had high levels of access to treatment, some of which were also provided with a vaccine and in which the majority of the HIV-negative population were persuaded to take that vaccine.

The success of a clinical trial based on this principle would depend on identifying and randomising populations which were large enough for most sexual contact to be taking place within them but small enough for the trial to be feasible.

This proposed trial design sets up a number of challenges. Results could vary, as for different STI control strategies, depending on the maturity of the epidemic. The size of the communities compared, the actual level of vaccine coverage achieved, and the extent to which community membership and patterns of sexual mixing remain stable over the period of the study, may all be issues. So, too, is the question of how and from whom consent should be sought for such a study.

Nonetheless, this proposal would eliminate the conflict sometimes perceived between treatment and care, including ARV access, and prevention, including vaccines. It could also strengthen the case for providing HIV/AIDS treatment and care in smaller and more rural communities, where such trials would be most likely to give clear results.

In practice, this would probably need to follow on after a trial which had demonstrated a reduced early viral load in people infected with the virus, and in which lower levels of the virus in semen and/or vaginal fluids can be linked to vaccination.

Regardless of whether such trials can be carried out, this proposal   rightly draws attention to the ultimate test of the value of such a vaccine. This must be whether it reduces the burden both of disease and of its treatment, in   populations where it is made available as compared to those where it is not.

Preventive trials: Phase I, II, III

HIV preventive vaccine trials are generally discussed in terms of three phases, I, II and III.

Phase I involves low-risk volunteers, usually from 20 to 80 in number, who receive a candidate vaccine, or perhaps just a component of such a vaccine, and are monitored for between six months and two years to assess immune response and safety. More than forty different vaccine candidates have now undergone Phase I clinical trials. Most have proven to be at least as safe as any other vaccine and most have induced some immune responses.

Phase II trials would include high-risk volunteers, drawn from populations in which efficacy trials might later be carried out. These look at how to maximise immune response in terms of dosage and methods of administration. They would normally be larger than Phase I trials, possibly running into hundreds of volunteers.

Both Phase I and Phase II trials may be placebo-controlled in order to distinguish adverse effects linked to the vaccine from those which are not. The experience of running trials in high-risk seronegative populations has been that many 'adverse events' are reported, most of which have nothing to do with vaccination.

The aim of a Phase III trial might be to assess whether a candidate vaccine is able to prevent infection, or to prevent disease in the presence of infection, or to prevent onward transmission of the virus. In other words, to discover whether a potential vaccine works. Through giving the vaccine to larger numbers of people, it is also possible to identify rarer side-effects and problems.

In practice, the design of Phase III trials has been dominated by the first objective - preventing HIV infection - although the first such trials also include a follow-up phase aimed at evaluating the second objective - delaying disease. In future trials, the emphasis is likely to shift.

Phase III trials are costly and have an impact on all other aspects of the response to HIV and AIDS. This is because they must recruit populations at high risk of HIV transmission, deliver vaccines and   placebos in combination with other prevention interventions, and evaluate the outcomes.

A 'successful' Phase III trial would be enough to get a vaccine licensed, at least in the country or region where it is carried out, but the real work of getting vaccines into proper use is then only beginning.

By 2003, only one type of vaccine had entered Phase III trials, as described below.

Logistical issues in Phase III trials

The size and length of follow-up for a Phase III (efficacy) trial will depend on:

- the incidence of HIV in the population where the trial is taking place

- the likely efficacy of the vaccine

- volunteer drop-out and non-response rates

- the trial design, and the outcome(s) being assessed (as previously discussed).

If a trial is too small, runs for too short a period, and the vaccine has a limited effect, then it may be inconclusive. Alternatively, if a trial is too big, it could waste resources.

Once a vaccine has been identified which is at least partially effective, it would become necessary to compare that vaccine with other potential vaccines. These trials might be looking for simpler vaccination schedules giving at least the same level of protection, longer duration of protection, and/or reductions in new HIV cases from a lower baseline. All of this implies that trial size and/or duration needs to increase as soon as a partially effective vaccine is identified.

As of June 2006, there were 31 trials taking place of HIV candidate vaccines worldwide. See the IAVI database of AIDS vaccines in human trials for a continuously-updated list at http://www.iavireport.org/specials/OngoingTrialsofPreventiveHIV Vaccines.pdf

- There was one phase III efficacy trial taking place in Thailand. This is the controversial RV144 prime-boost trial using the ALVAC vCP1521 canarypox vector vaccine as prime and the AIDSVAX gp120 envelope clade B/AE subunit vaccine as boost. There are about 7,000 volunteers enrolled. This started in October 2003 and is due to continue till at least 2008.

There were three phase II trials.

- The largest is the STEP trial of the Merck clade B adenovirus-5 trivalent vector vaccine. This will recruit about 3,000 volunteers worldwide. This started in September 2004.

- The second is the HVTN204 prime-boost clades A, B and C trial of a naked DNA vaccine (VRC-HIVDNA016) as prime and the adenovirus VRC-HIVADV014-00-VP vector vaccine as boost. This started in September 2005, is taking place in the USA and Latin America, and will recruit 480 volunteers.

- The third is the IAVI A002 trial of the tgAAC09 clade C adeno-associated virus replicon vaccine, taking place in South Africa, Uganda and Zambia. This started in November 2005 and has so far recruited 78 volunteers in South Africa.

All the others are small phase I trials in low-risk populations.

Mobilising support worldwide

On 18 May 1997, US President Bill Clinton challenged the US research community to find an effective vaccine within the next ten years and set this as a national goal. That year's summit of the G8 countries, held in Denver, also recognised the need for an HIV vaccine; subsequent G8 summits have reiterated this commitment. The Commonwealth Heads of Government Meeting held in Durban, South Africa, in 1999, included a paragraph personally committing the leaders to advancing the response to HIV and AIDS including vaccine development. (For further information, see www.para55.org.)

Such commitments underpin the support for vaccine and microbicide development included in the final statement of the UN General Assembly Special Session on AIDS held in New York in June 2001.

Researchers in the United States, Australia, Britain, Cuba, France, Germany, Japan and South Africa among others have developed vaccine candidates. Clinical trials for HIV vaccines are ongoing or have taken place in the past in the United States, Thailand, various European countries including Britain, France and the Netherlands, Brazil, China, Cuba, Haiti, Kenya, Trinidad, Uganda. Other countries in which trials are planned, or are under serious discussion, some of them with vaccine research programmes, include Argentina, Botswana, Cote d'Ivoire,

Honduras, India, Nigeria, Peru, Russia, South Africa and Tanzania.

The International AIDS Vaccine Initiative

IAVI was constituted in 1995 in the USA as a non-governmental organisation sponsored by various US foundations and donors and is headed by Dr Seth Berkley.

IAVI was founded out of a judgement that the global effort towards a preventive vaccine was in trouble, following a 1994 decision not to proceed with US efficacy trials for gp120 vaccines. It has lobbied the US government, other G8 countries, intergovernmental organisations including the World Bank and UN agencies and entered into working agreements with the European Union, South Africa, India, China, Brazil and other countries. It has equally sought to engage with corporations and community organisations, with formal partnerships agreed between IAVI and agencies in a number of countries including Britain's National AIDS Trust.

One key idea that it has promoted is the creation of a guaranteed and credible market for vaccines, by securing the promise of major loans to buy any proven vaccine on behalf of governments of countries that are in the greatest need. Such loans could be repaid from future savings on humanitarian aid and need not add to the debts of the countries worst affected by HIV.

IAVI funds research specifically directed at vaccines which would be appropriate for countries where the need is greatest and the resources most limited.

By 2001 it had funds and pledges totalling more than US $230 million towards a fundraising target of US $550 million needed to fund vaccine development work plan through to the year 2007, following its *Scientific Blueprint: 2000*. The largest single funder so far has been the Bill and Melinda Gates Foundation. Other major supporters include the Rockefeller, Sloan and Starr Foundations, UNAIDS the World Bank, and a number of governments. These include the UK (through the Department for International Development), Canada, Ireland, the Netherlands, Norway, Sweden and the USA (through USAID).

IAVI publishes a scientific newsletter, *IAVI Report*, and makes its publications freely available through its website, www.iavi.org.

The Global HIV Vaccine Enterprise (GHVE)

The GHVE is a new organisation set up in 2004 after a position paper in *Science* journal argued that an AIDS vaccine is one of the most difficult challenges facing biomedical science today, and while important progress has been made, there is a critical limitation in the way vaccine R&D is currently conducted.

Most of the work is undertaken by small groups of investigators-academic laboratories and biotechnology companies-who typically operate independently of each other, and the scale of their projects is often too small to adequately address major scientific questions. The pace of progress could be increased through greater cooperation and collaboration and more funding targeted to large projects that tackle major questions.

Enterprise members agree to reach consensus on scientific priorities, voluntarily divide responsibility for addressing them and establish joint ventures that pool expertise, infrastructure and resources. They agree to iteratively apply each other's advances so that the best science emerges as quickly as possible and unnecessary duplication is avoided.

The GHVE lists its six aims as

1 Reaching a scientific consensus on the most promising research directions in HIV vaccine science, explicitly noting that vaccines that elicit both cellular and humoral immunity will be necessary.

2 Standardising assays that measure correlates of immune protection.

3   Developing a vaccine manufacturing process that makes consistent batches over time.

4. Supporting greater capacity to mount large clinical trials through on-site manufacturing capacity, enhancing research infrastructure, including trial sites and laboratories, training and supporting qualified staff and educating the public about vaccine trials to help with recruitment of informed study participants.

5. Standardising regulatory systems for clinical trials, especially in developing countries, which often lack expertise and well-defined processes for reviewing and approving clinical trials and assessing results.

6. Agreeing on intellectual property arrangements that balance the need to incentivise and protect individual researchers or companies, and the need to promote greater and more rapid sharing of information among scientists that can lead to potential breakthroughs in HIV vaccine research.

Enterprise members will develop systems for more openly exchanging information as well as share research protocols so that the work of one group is compatible with others. In these ways, the Enterprise is patterned after the Human Genome Project, a scientific alliance that is widely credited with speeding the successful identification of all of the genes in human DNA.

The *Science* paper argued for additional resources, given that total global spending to develop a vaccine is just a fraction of spending to combat the epidemic, and more resources would better position vaccine efforts for success. Enterprise members will mobilise new resources and see that they are targeted to priority areas. The Enterprise received the endorsement of leaders of G8 nations at their summit in 2004, and the G8 pledged to take up the issue of additional resources for vaccine R&D at future summits.

In September 2005 the first Chief Executive of the GHVE was appointed - Dr. Adel Mahmoud, former president of Merck Vaccines.

The AIDS Vaccine Advocacy Coalition (AVAC)

AVAC is a community and consumer based organization, founded in December 1995 to accelerate the ethical development and global delivery of vaccines against HIV/AIDS. It provides independent analysis, policy advocacy, public education and mobilization to enhance AIDS vaccine research and development.

AVAC publishes the aids Vaccine Handbook, a comprehensive (404 page) introduction to AIDS vaccine science, ethics and community advocacy. It can be downloaded from http://www.avac.org/primer2.htm . AVAC also issues reports of various aspects of the development of vaccines and the other new prevention technologies.

In the introduction, Executive Director Mitchell Warren says:

An effective AIDS vaccine remains the world's best chance to contain this relentless epidemic. But the search for an AIDS vaccine must not come at the expense of our immediate response. And it doesn't have to. Testing vaccines requires that we do all the other key things anyway: delivering the best-possible risk-reduction and counselling tools; ensuring confidential, voluntary counselling and testing; providing referral to comprehensive treatment.

The handbook covers:

■   The basics of AIDS vaccine science

■   Clinical trials including being a volunteer; the ethics of trials, including making sure that trials leave communities better rather than worse off; ensuring community participation and readiness; and how to work with trials that 'fail' as in the AIDSVAX trial

■   The experience and ethics of doing vaccine trials with different vulnerable communities

■   Global advocacy and political leadership

■   Personal accounts of involvement with trials.

AVAC has also set up a small-grants fund that will function as a small-scale "emergency fund" to assist needy clinical sites that require immediate help with purchases such as additional medical or lab supplies not covered by grants or contracts for vaccine research.

The Global Alliance for Vaccines and Immunization (GAVI)

GAVI is not an HIV vaccine development organisation, but may become important if an effective vaccine is found. It was founded amid concern that existing financing mechanisms were not enabling vaccination programmes in the developing world to be sustained. Founded in 2000, it is a global alliance of Governments in industrialised and developing countries, UNICEF, WHO, the World Bank, the Bill & Melinda Gates Foundation, non-governmental organizations, vaccine manufacturers from industrialised and developing countries, and public health and research institutions.

GAVI has been financed by ten governments to date -Canada, Denmark, France, Ireland, Luxembourg, the Netherlands, Norway, Sweden, the United Kingdom, and the United States - as well as the European Union, private contributors, and the Bill & Melinda Gates Foundation.

GAVI's aim is to help strengthen health and immunization systems in the developing world, accelerate access to selected vaccines and new vaccine technologies, especially vaccines that are new or underused, and improve injection safety.

It provides multi-year grants to more than 70 of the world's poorest countries to enable them to put on vaccination programmes, especially in children.

Ethical issues in trial design

The general ethical principles that govern all clinical research apply to vaccine trials, and there are a number of international statements on medical ethics that apply. It is fundamental that participation in trials must be voluntary and based on individual informed consent.

The principal difference between preventive vaccine trials and HIV therapeutic trials is that because participants might otherwise have a normal life expectancy and a low level of disability, the level of potentially acceptable risk is much lower.

In the case of HIV preventive vaccines, much of the discussion of ethics of trials has been driven by perceived and actual disparities of power between those at high risk of HIV and those carrying out the research, and between Western countries and multinational companies and communities in developing countries. There is an obvious danger of exploitation, if benefits and risks from research are not evenly shared. There is also a danger that if governments and international agencies are over-protective, the effort will be stalled.

UNAIDS' guidelines

In 1997-99, UNAIDS sponsored a series of consultations leading to the publication of a detailed eighteen-point guidance document in May 2000. The following section outlines and comments on this guidance, which can be read in full on the UNAIDS website (www.unaids.org).

HIV vaccines development (point 1)

UNAIDS begins with the need to develop vaccines and make them available: 'it is imperative that they benefit the population at greatest risk of infection.' It distinguishes between 'investigators', 'host countries' where trials might be held and 'communities' from which volunteers would be drawn, 'donors and international agencies' and 'sponsor countries' acknowledging that vaccines are being developed in public-private partnerships rather than on a purely commercial basis.

Vaccine availability (point 2)

Issues of availability including but not limited to availability in the country and population where a vaccine is tested need to be addressed throughout the process of vaccine development. 'The discussions should include decisions regarding payments, royalties, subsidies, technology and intellectual property, as well as distribution costs, channels and modalities, including vaccination strategies, target populations, and number of doses.'

Capacity building (point 3)

A recurring theme, with the goal of enabling host countries and communities to participate as equal partners in the process.

Research protocols and study populations (point 4)

Any study must be scientifically sound and have the potential to benefit the population recruited into the study. An ethical trial must be capable of answering the questions it sets out to answer, using the most efficient and humane means of addressing scientific uncertainty, e.g. to show whether a candidate vaccine is immunogenic, safe and/or effective. The relevance of this point is greater for populations at high risk in host countries than for populations at low risk in sponsor countries, where exploitation is seen as less of a danger.

Community participation (point 5)

'Community representatives should be involved in an early and sustained manner in the design, development, implementation, and distribution of results of HIV vaccine research.' The guidance identifies categories of interested people who should be consulted in the course of setting up arrangements for community participation, including those eligible to volunteer for a specific study as well as care-givers and people living with HIV.

Scientific and ethical review (point 6)

Host countries must be capable of independent scientific and ethical review of research proposals, an area in which capacity building by agencies independent of vaccine developers may be needed.

Vulnerable populations (point 7)

This refers to the need to recognise and take steps to overcome social factors that may make research participants vulnerable to exploitation. This vulnerability is not solely economic, and may derive from inadequate respect for human rights on a variety of grounds.

Clinical trial phases (point 8)

This breaks with past guidance on international clinical research, which has required that early phase trials should be confined to the country in which a product is first developed. UNAIDS acknowledges that any country may legitimately decide to conduct phase I trials, provided there is sufficiently strong scientific, clinical, and ethical review infrastructure to protect the volunteers. The case for doing this is enhanced when a vaccine candidate is based on isolates of the virus from a particular community, country or region where trials will be carried out.

Potential harms (point 9)

Likely harms need to be identified in research protocols, and fully explained to trial volunteers in the informed consent process, including an explanation of how people will receive treatment and compensation if needed.

'HIV infection acquired during participation in an HIV preventive vaccine trial should not be considered an injury subject to compensation unless it is directly attributable to the vaccine itself, or to direct contamination through research-related activities. In addition to compensation for biological/medical injuries, appropriate consideration should be given to compensation for social or economic harms, e.g. job loss as a result of testing positive following vaccine administration.'

A distinction is made here between the need for compensation for HIV infection and the need for access to treatment and care, which is addressed separately. It would seem better to prevent social or economic harms rather than merely to plan for compensation. This is why 'consideration should also be given to setting up an ombudsperson who can intervene with outside parties, if necessary and requested, on behalf of participants, as well as to providing documentation to participants that they can use to show that their false positive is due to their participation in research.'

Benefits (point 10)

Potential benefits to trial volunteers from participation should be clearly explained to them, without presenting them in such a way as to unduly influence the decision to join a trial.

Control group (point 11)

'As long as there is no known effective HIV preventive vaccine, a placebo control arm should be considered ethically acceptable in a phase III HIV preventive vaccine trial. However, where it is ethically and scientifically acceptable, consideration should be given to the use in the control arm of a vaccine to prevent a relevant condition apart from HIV.' (The examples given are hepatitis B and tetanus.) The guidance might have pointed out that the failure to provide for a blinded control group in any trial involving high-risk volunteers might lead volunteers to assume that a vaccine protects them when it does not and increase their HIV risk, leading to real harm. If volunteers are to take part in a blinded trial they must remain ignorant for the duration of the trial of whether they have received an HIV vaccine, without losing the ability to check their own HIV status.

Informed consent (point 12)

This is a 'strategy and process' arising from a 'process of consultation between community representatives, researchers, sponsor(s) and regulatory bodies.' Individuals must be free to decide for themselves whether to take part, on the basis of 'complete, accurate, and appropriately conveyed and understood information.' Furthermore, 'efforts should be taken to ensure throughout the trial that participants continue to understand and to participate freely as the trial progresses.' Informed consent is needed separately for HIV tests before, during or after the trial.

The guidance observes that in any preventive vaccine trial it must be possible to distinguish the effects of the vaccine from those of natural infection. The costs and feasibility of doing this will vary between different vaccines. Vaccines based on the fullest possible range of viral components may need special and costly provision.

The most obvious test of remaining virus-free is failure to isolate the virus from a blood sample. However, even with a well-equipped laboratory it can still be difficult to isolate HIV from some people who are clearly infected with it, so a negative result on this test may not be convincing. Alternatives like p24 antigen tests (moderately expensive) and PCR tests (more expensive) would not be triggered by most likely vaccines. Some vaccine designers have deliberately excluded the HIV protein gp41 from vaccine systems so that commercially available ELISA tests for antibodies to gp41 may be used for this purpose (Corey, 1996; Yao, 1996).

Informed consent special measures (point 13)

This lists categories of people whose ability to consent freely on their own account may be limited by their social, legal, economic or gender status, for whom additional protective measures may be needed.

Risk-reduction interventions (point 14)

'Appropriate risk-reduction counselling and access to prevention methods should be provided to all vaccine trial participants, with new methods being added as they are discovered and validated.'

One issue, which has much exercised people, is a supposed conflict of interest between trial volunteers, who surely want to stay uninfected at all costs, and researchers 'needing' some people to become infected to prove that others those vaccinated are genuinely protected. In practice, this conflict can be resolved by implementing prevention programmes that in theory and practice reduce the HIV risk of trial volunteers, whether or not they receive a vaccine.

Monitoring informed consent and interventions (point 15)

This needs to be provided for, with plans made before the trial begins.

Care and treatment (point 16)

'Sponsors need to ensure care and treatment for participants who become HIV-infected during the course of the trial.' This does not imply an obligation for sponsors to provide care and treatment for everyone in a community where a trial is taking place, nor for everyone identified as HIV-positive during the course of screening trial volunteers. UNAIDS found during its consultations that there was no consensus as to what level of care and treatment needs to be provided during a vaccine trial. As this issue has been one of the most contentious, it is worth quoting the guidance point in full:

'Care and treatment for HIV/AIDS and its associated complications should be provided to participants in HIV preventive vaccine trials, with the ideal being to provide the best proven therapy, and the minimum to provide the highest level of care attainable in the host country in light of the circumstances listed below. A comprehensive care package should be agreed upon through a host/community/sponsor dialogue which reaches consensus prior to initiation of a trial, taking into consideration the following:

- level of care and treatment available in the sponsor country

- highest level of care available in the host country

- highest level of treatment available in the host country, including the availability of antiretroviral therapy outside the research context in the host country

- availability of infrastructure to provide care and treatment in the context of research

- potential duration and sustainability of care and treatment for the trial participant.

Women (point 17)

This observes that as women including those who are potentially pregnant, are pregnant, or are breastfeeding, should receive future preventive HIV vaccines, women should be included in clinical trials. The implication is that there should not be an absolute exclusion of pregnant or breastfeeding women from the later stages of HIV vaccine trials, although the need to warn women of potential risks to their children as part of the informed consent process is clearly set out.

Children (point 18)

This states, 'children should be included in clinical trials' and discusses the circumstances in which adolescents need to give individual informed consent, noting that the requirement for additional consent by parents or guardians will vary between countries depending on their legal provisions. In the case of breastfed infants, the requirement would be for consent by a parent on behalf of the child, or both parents if required by national legislation.

Trials that 'fail'

It is still possible to get a lot of information from a trial that is a failure in the sense of not showing efficacy and there is an ethical obligation to plan any trial to make the most of that information.

UNAIDS makes the point that the sponsors of a trial in a developing country should always aim to enhance the capacity of the country and community where a trial takes place, to deliver treatment and care and to engage in future research.

It is equally reasonable to expect that a community where a full-scale vaccine trial takes place will gain from the extra effort that is made to deliver effective HIV counselling and prevention to volunteers, and the empowerment of volunteers and those who represent the community through the trial process. Put simply, 'it should be a better place than if the trial hadn't happened.'

It has been argued that Phase III trials should go ahead for HIV vaccines even without strong evidence from Phase II trials that they will work, on account of what can be learned even from a partially effective vaccine. That said, some evidence suggesting that a vaccine will work is very desirable before proceeding to a Phase III trial. Investors would certainly want this, as mass-production of a commercial product should begin before a trial starts, so there would be no question of differences between the vaccine used in the trial and the one subsequently put on the market.

Vaxgen's trials

The leading example of a biotech company developing an HIV preventive vaccine is VaxGen with its *AIDSVAX* products. VaxGen is a company spun-off from Genentech (a biotech company now largely owned by Roche) to develop Genentech's gp120 recombinant vaccine after the US government refusal to support Phase III trials of a prototype in 1994. VaxGen succeeded in raising private funds to run Phase III trials in the USA, Canada, the Netherlands, Puerto Rico and Thailand. It is greatly to their credit that they completed the trials despite many expert opinions to the effect that it would be impossible to recruit or retain volunteers. In fact, trial volunteer retention was higher than predicted in all settings and higher in Thailand than in North America.

The first VaxGen trial

The first VaxGen trial recruited 5,417 volunteers at risk of HIV infection from sexual transmission, around 90% of whom were gay men. One third of the volunteers were randomised in a double-blind trial to receive placebo injections and two thirds a 'bivalent' vaccine based on a genetically engineered version of the gp120 surface protein from two different HIV-1 subtype B isolates.

The protocol for the trial involved seven injections over thirty months (0, 1, 6, 12, 18, 24 and 30 months) with follow-up visits for blood tests two weeks after each injection and six months after the last injection. All volunteers were given prevention advice and counselling.

All volunteers who became HIV-positive during the study are due to be followed up every four months for 24 months. There is no restriction on the treatments HIV-positive volunteers may receive, although treatments are not provided directly as part of the study. Social harms experienced by volunteers, including self-reported risk behaviour, were closely monitored.

5,009 volunteers received at least three of the seven scheduled injections and were included in 'on treatment' analysis which did not, in the event, differ substantially from the 'intent to treat analysis' which included all volunteers for whom an outcome was known.

VaxGen's results: no overall protection

The results of the first phase III HIV vaccine study released in February 2003 showed that Vaxgen's AIDSVAX offered no significant protection against HIV infection in the study population as a whole.

The annual study infection rate 2.7% which was not significantly different between placebo and vaccine recipients. Among all volunteers the level of apparent 'protection' was just 3.8% (p-value = 0.76; confidence interval: -23% to 24%). In other words, it was 95% certain that the **upper limit** for protection was below 25%. The trial had been designed in the hope that if the **lower limit** was above 30%, the vaccine could still be licensed for use in the USA.

The second VaxGen Phase III trial commenced in Thailand during 1999, using a gp120 vaccine based on 'subtype E' (now classified as a 'circulating recombinant form') and subtype B isolates of the virus. This recruited 2,500 volunteers from drug treatment centres around Bangkok, to evaluate protection from direct blood exposure, with an equal number of placebo recipients and vaccine recipients. The annual infection rate was exactly the same in vaccine and placebo recipients: 3.4% a year for both arms, or a vaccine efficacy of exactly zero.

The ongoing VaxGen/ALVAC trial: incrementalists versus serendipists

As we have said above, the AIDSVAX gp120 vaccine continues to be used as the 'boost' in the RV144 phase III trial in combination with the ALVAC vCP1521 canarypox vector as prime. This, the only current phase III trial has attracted fierce criticism form scientists and activists alike. In 2004, 22 researchers wrote to *Science* stating that the US government was wasting its resources on funding a trial of a vaccine combination where there is no evidence that either component works well on its own.

Other researchers said that the addition of the gp120 boost would only muddy the results and make it difficult to establish if the ALVAC vaccine had any immune stimulating effect. "There is no credible scientific justification for the inclusion of gp120 in the trial," said the article's co-author John Moore. "It's an expensive, inert component that complicates any analysis of the final outcome."

The trial's sponsors, NAID, defended the decision to proceed with the trial. NIAID's Margaret Johnston said that, although the results are arguably modest, early studies showed that the combination augments immune responses relative to each vaccine alone, and that the combination vaccine induced CD8 responses in 25%-45% of individuals. However the critics said the enhanced responses seen could be just as well studied in a smaller trial and is was a waste not only of money but of human resources - in the shape of human volunteers who would probably ben excluded from a future vaccine trial.

The central dilemma in AIDS vaccine research seems to be embodied by the RV144 trial. The field is split between researchers who say that vaccine development is incremental and that 'more immune protection than the last one' is sufficient reason for a trial to move ahead. People arguing this point of view say that the only 'failed' vaccine trial is one that produces no information and that even the numerous candidate vaccines that have produced little immune response or, if they have, have yet to show that that translates into efficacy, are part of an immense scientific project that is teaching us huge lessons about virology and immunology.

Researchers sympathetic to the opposite point of view say that, historically, successful vaccines have not been developed incrementally, but have usually come out of the serendipitous success of an often new approach. Like Robert Gallo, they argue that we are at too early a stage in HIV vaccine development to start incrementally developing anything; the incremental stage comes when we have strong candidates that will provide real efficacy. It is a waste of human and financial resources to put on large trials of products that are suspected not to be efficacious and it may be unethical if it provides volunteers with a false sense of security against HIV infection.

Ethical Implications for people with HIV

People with and without HIV, living in the same HIV-affected community, may have very different perspectives on all aspects of life, with major implications for HIV prevention programmes. In particular, gay and bisexual men are both united and divided in responding to AIDS, with one of the major divisions being on the basis of HIV status. It is therefore essential in planning any primary prevention programme, including vaccine research, to consider its impact on people with HIV as well as on those without.

For people with HIV, the call for vaccine research has sometimes been perceived as a kind of abandonment and as a potential diversion of funds away from therapeutic research.

Some of these concerns are realistic: large-scale vaccine trials would certainly be expensive. There can be no absolute guarantee that funding for any particular kind of AIDS research will be maintained, since this depends on political will and judgements, including scientific judgements, of the strength of competing priorities.

Some of the concerns, as has been argued in this chapter, may now be outdated. Insights from preventive vaccine research are likely to be of genuine value to people living with HIV. If therapeutic vaccines prove feasible, these will be of direct value to people with HIV. The line between what is a therapeutic and what is a preventative vaccine is likely to grow ever more blurred over time, as argued by Robin Shattock.

In any case, many people with HIV passionately want to see an end to the epidemic, since they have lost more than anyone else and can see preventive vaccines as a part of the answer.

Since some of the stigma of being HIV-positive arises from fear of infection, a vaccine which offers genuine protection is also a potential remedy for social stigma. Arguably the biggest obstacle to participation in vaccine research is that it means people facing up to the risks that they are running. At a practical level, it means taking an antibody test and acknowledging the possibility of being HIV-positive. How to ensure treatment programmes are in place in resource-poor settings for the not inconsiderable number of people who test positive during screening for a trial remains one of the thorniest issues in trial design, community liaison and funding.

Ethical implications for HIV-negative people

What of those who are HIV-negative and at risk? Many will want to participate, for obvious reasons, but some will not.

It might mean identification as a person at particular risk of HIV, and so being linked to people from whom you would prefer to keep a psychological and social distance. A small-scale interview study of gay men in France who declined to take part in vaccine trials found this to be their dominant problem. This contrasted, however, with Brazilian studies where the dominant reasons for not participating were given as concerns about side-effects and lack of credibility of a vaccine product (Silva).

However, one of the fundamental problems with being HIV-negative and at risk is that being HIV-negative is a 'non-status'. Like virginity, it cannot be aspired to, only lost. Prevention of HIV by methods other than vaccination never succeeds for longer than 'the time being'. For people who are HIV-negative, vaccines offer the possibility of acquiring a status as a 'protected person' which they could work towards for themselves or for others.

There are particular ethical implications for people who volunteer for vaccine trials, many of them common to all trials of new prevention technologies:

- Will participation in the trial provide a false sense of security and/or change behaviour so that people are more rather than less at risk of HIV infection?

- How can we ensure fully informed consent when working with communities of people who may be stigmatised, vulnerable to incentives to take part in unethical trials, illiterate and innumerate or at least not educated about the science of HIV and vaccines?

- How do we ensure the fairest and most comprehensive treatment for those who seroconvert in the course of a trial?

- Some CD8 vaccines will induce the production of antibodies that will mean that vaccine recipients test 'HIV-positive', at least on an ELISA test. How do we educate these people about the meaning of their antibody response, and how do we monitor them in the future for HIV infection?

Securing global access

If a successful vaccine is developed, large-scale investment will be needed to make it available on a global scale. IAVI has made five recommendations to secure that investment and general access, especially if any reliance is placed on private sector involvement in the process. (IAVI, 2000a):

- Effective pricing and global financing mechanisms must be developed to ensure that vaccines are promptly available for use where they are needed.

- Mechanisms must be developed to make reliable estimates of demand for specific vaccines and to ensure creation of production capacity to permit accelerated worldwide access.

- Appropriate delivery systems, policies, and procedures must be developed for adolescents, sexually active adults and other at-risk populations.

- National regulations and international guidelines governing vaccine approval and use must be harmonised.

- To demonstrate global commitment to effective worldwide deployment of important vaccines, immediate efforts should be undertaken . building on existing mechanisms, such as the Global Alliance for Vaccines and Immunization (GAVI) and the Global Fund for Children's Vaccines (GFCV) - to achieve maximum use in developing countries of one or more currently under-utilised non-AIDS vaccines.

Tiered or 'equity' pricing - where prices reflect what countries can afford - will be needed from the moment an HIV vaccine is launched. This implies safeguards, including political support in wealthier countries, against the international trading of cheaper vaccines from developing countries into wealthier countries.

The traditional pattern is that new products are introduced first into wealthy countries, sold at premium prices which enable the manufacturers to recoup their costs in developing the vaccine. Fifteen or more years later, when development costs have been written off and patents have expired, prices can be reduced sufficiently for international agencies to purchase them for use in developing countries. IAVI is saying that this traditional pattern is unacceptable for HIV, and in fact should be unacceptable for any vaccine or treatment.

There are encouraging signs that this thinking is now being adopted by some of the larger companies in the field, in respect of a range of new vaccines that are being developed against diseases that are either confined to countries with limited

resources or present far greater public health problems in those countries than in wealthier, industrialised countries.

Financing refers to the need for both 'push' and 'pull' mechanisms to overcome the perception that there are no profits in making vaccines. Direct public investment in vaccine development by private companies is one form that 'push' mechanisms can take. The French and American governments, and the European Commission, are already doing this. Purchase funds, underwritten by international development agencies such as the World Bank, or by individual governments committing themselves to purchase future vaccines meeting set criteria, are examples of 'pull' mechanisms. Many years ago, the State of California enacted specific legislation limiting liability and guaranteeing purchase of any effective vaccine, and this seems to have helped Californian biotechnology companies (Chiron and Genentech, later VaxGen) take an early lead in this area.

It may never be possible to make an accurate assessment of the demand for any HIV vaccine until it is in widespread use. Nonetheless, it is important to realise that companies will be unlikely to risk large sums of money building manufacturing facilities on a global scale, unless there is some assurance for them that their money will not be wasted.

To produce a potential vaccine on a small scale, to test out an idea in a very few animals, is well within the capability of a well-equipped academic laboratory. However, to produce a vaccine in bulk, to the high industrial standards required by regulatory bodies for any product given to humans, is a very different matter. Expertise in this area is almost entirely located in the pharmaceutical industry, and indeed four large companies produce most of the world's commercial vaccines. These are Merck, Aventis Pasteur, American Home Products (Wyeth Lederle), and GlaxoSmithKline, all of which have had some level of involvement in   HIV vaccine development.

A new and interesting model that is emerging in the UK is represented by Cobra Pharmaceuticals, a company that makes vaccines on behalf of developers, owning some of the delivery technology (in particular, for DNA vaccines) but not seeking to produce or market vaccines for end-users. While they currently make vaccines primarily on a pilot scale, they plan to expand facilities to produce in larger quantities. Such facilities might be developed in public-private partnerships, with public investment to enhance the scale of multi-purpose manufacturing facilities.

Delivery systems to administer vaccines to adults are not widespread. Most vaccines are given to young children, and in many countries it would require new systems of medical records and administrative measures to identify and invite adults or even adolescents to be vaccinated.

There is a need to standardise procedures and criteria across different countries' regulatory agencies. Within Europe, there is now a system which provides both for mutual recognition of decisions to license pharmaceutical products and for Europe-wide registration through the European Medicines Evaluation Agency (EMEA). However, drug regulation is more variable in other countries: South Africa has a professional regulatory agency, but many others do not. A related issue is the absence of any fast-tracking procedure for vaccines, to prioritise those where the safety concerns are minimal and the disease against which they are directed is most serious as a public health problem.

Liability issues may be real. Vaccines are given to people who are well, including young children, often at an age or in circumstances where they may, perhaps coincidentally, be diagnosed with other conditions. In the United States, lawsuits about such cases led most pharmaceutical companies to stop manufacturing vaccines, until legislation was passed setting a ceiling on such liabilities. However, the damage had been done.

As vaccines succeed in eradicating a feared disease, the real adverse effects of the vaccines may match or outweigh the immediate threat to individuals from the disease itself. Public health authorities have not always been effective in dealing with this issue, with an ever-present temptation to deny that these effects occur and to resist compensating those who suffer for a very real public benefit.

The UK government's Policy and Innovation Unit, part of the Cabinet Office, recently published a detailed review of incentives for private investment in meeting global public health needs, with particular reference to HIV, TB and malaria.

An evolving programme

It is unlikely that there will only ever be one vaccine or one clinical trial. The first candidate vaccines will probably have limited efficacy and will certainly be cumbersome to deliver. Most require multiple injections over an extended period. This means that a series of extended clinical trials will prove necessary, over the next fifteen or twenty years.

It has been argued mathematically (Anderson and Garnett) that even a low-efficacy vaccine targeted at high-risk populations could have a major impact on the course of an HIV epidemic, provided that limited effect was long-lasting. Such a vaccine would obviously have to be offered in the context of a wider prevention campaign.

It may be that very different vaccines, eliciting entirely different immune responses, prove equally capable of preventing HIV disease.

It may be that sexual transmission (in the general population, including gay men and injecting drug users) and blood-borne transmission (injecting drug users, healthcare workers and others exposed to blood) ultimately require different vaccines.

If there will be no single magic bullet in the foreseeable future, then it follows:

- that vaccine research must be multidisciplinary and integrated with other prevention research

- that we must find ways to test and later to deploy vaccines in ways that complement and reinforce other prevention methods, and vice versa.

Conclusions

The mobilisation and renewal of effort which has begun at a global level with the launch of the International AIDS Vaccine Initiative needs to be matched and extended at national and community levels.

Vaccine research needs to be constructed as a partnership, including volunteer participants and their communities, researchers, governments and other funding agencies, public research teams and private companies producing vaccines.

The UK and other European governments and institutions could help by clarifying what they want to achieve through vaccine research, and how they propose to advance it. They could work to remove obstacles and create incentives for private sector involvement in vaccine development, following the lead of the US state of California which enacted laws ten years ago, limiting liability for vaccine-related injuries and committing funds for the purchase of any vaccine proven to be effective.

Community leaders and activists can help by informing themselves and those they are working with on the issues surrounding vaccine research and development, and by passing that information to policy makers in government and industry.

There is no certainty that this effort will succeed, although there is good reason to believe that it can. It is, however, completely certain that without sustained efforts now, we could easily be in the very same position in ten years' time.

The experience with hepatitis B, where technically successful vaccines have been on the market for more than two decades, yet new infections continue to occur even in wealthy countries, shows that it takes more than a vaccine to stop an epidemic.

'An ideal HIV vaccine would be oral, inexpensive, safe, and heat stable; it would require only a single dose, last a lifetime, and be effective against all strains of the virus and all routes of exposure. Short of this ideal, practical limitation will constrain the efficacy of any vaccine ... Reaching those at greatest risk for HIV infection promises to be as complex with vaccination as it has been with behavioural interventions. Even a successful vaccine will be only one component of a broad prevention strategy aimed at reducing the number of new infections by diminishing the incidences of exposure to HIV, through reduction of risk behaviour and other means.' (Stryker)

Nonetheless, the impact of demonstrating an effective vaccine, even an imperfect one, would be immensely positive for the global response to AIDS. It would open up a real possibility of working towards the elimination of HIV, rather than the temporary and partial control of it. Money spent on controlling and treating HIV in the meantime would become a supporting investment towards an achievable and finite end, rather than a potentially unending drain on resources. The mobilising and energising effect this could have across the whole range of HIV-related needs should not be underestimated.

Websites

AIDS Vaccine Advocacy Coalition, www.avac.org

Bill and Melinda Gates Foundation, www.gatesfoundation.org

Global Alliance for Vaccines and Immunisation (GAVI),

Global HIV Vaccines Enterprise, http://www.hivvaccineenterprise.org

HIV Vaccine Trials network, www.hvtn.org/

International AIDS Vaccine Initiative, www.iavi.org

IAVI database of AIDS vaccines in human trials, http://www.iavireport.org/specials/OngoingTrialsofPreventiveHIV Vaccines.pdf

International Council of AIDS Service Organisations, www.icaso.org

UNAIDS, www.unaids.org

US National Institutes of Health AIDS Vaccine Research Working Group. www.niaid.nih.gov/daids/vaccine/avrc.htm

WHO-UNAIDS HIV Vaccine Initiative, www.who.int/vaccine_research/diseases/hiv/en/

References

Baba TW et al. Pathogenicity of live, attenuated SIV after mucosal infection of neonatal macaques. Science 267: 1820-1825, 1995

Barouch DH et al. Eventual AIDS vaccine failure in a rhesus monkey by viral escape from cytotoxic T lymphocytes., Nature 415: 335-339, 2002

Boyer JD et al. Vaccination of seronegative volunteers with a human immunodeficiency virus type 1 env/rev DNA vaccine induces antigen-specific proliferation and lymphocyte production of beta-chemokines., J Infect Dis 181: 476-483, 2000

Daniel MD et al. Protective effects of a live attenuated SIV vaccine with a deletion in the nef gene., Science 258: 1938-1941, 1992

Esparza J. Vaccines: State-of-the-art and future directions. 15th International AIDS Conference, Bangkok. Plenary address, abstract ThPl15. 2004.

Gallo RB. The end or the beginning of the drive to an HIV-preventive vaccine: a view from over 20 years. Lancet. 366(9500):1894-8. 2005.

Isaacs R. Impact of pre-existing immunity on the immunogenicity of Ad5-based vaccines., AIDS Vaccine 04, Lausanne, abstract 69, 2004

Kran AMB et al. HLA- and dose-dependent immunogenicity of a peptide-based HIV-1 immunotherapy candidate (Vacc 4x)., AIDS 18: 1875-1883, 2004

Pinto LA et al. HIV-specific immunity following immunization with HIV synthetic envelope peptides in asymptomatic HIV-infected patients., AIDS 13: 335-339, 2002

Pitisutithum P. Efficacy of AIDSVAX B/E vaccines in injecting drug use. Eleventh Conference on Retroviruses and Opportunistic Infections, San Francisco, abstract 107, 2004

rgp120 HIV Vaccine Study Group. Placebo-controlled phase 3 trial of a recombinant glycoprotein 120 vaccine to prevent HIV-1 infection. rgp120 Vaccine Study Group., J Infect Dis 191: 654-665, 2005

Schnell MJ et al. Recombinant rabies virus as potential live-viral vaccines for HIV-1., Proc Natl Acad Sci U S A 97: 3544-3549, 2000

Shearer GM. HIV-specific T cell immunity in exposed-seronegatives. 3rd Conference on Retroviruses and Opportunistic Infections. Abstract no. S42. 1996.

Shiver JW et al. Replication-incompetent adenoviral vaccine vector elicits effective anti-immunodeficiency-virus immunity. Nature 415(6869):272-3.

Stiegler G et al. A potent cross-clade neutralizing human monoclonal antibody against a novel epitope on gp41 of human immunodeficiency virus type 1. AIDS Res Hum Retroviruses 17(18):1757-65. 2001.

Zhang H et al. Human immunodeficiency virus type 1 Gag-specific mucosal immunity after oral immunization with papillomavirus pseudoviruses encoding Gag., J Virol 78: 10249-10257, 2004

Zhu T et al. Breakthrough HIV-1 infection in long-term exposed seronegative individuals. 15th International AIDS Conference, Bangkok. Abstract number: TuOrA1141. 2004.

HIV prevention: which methods work?

Evidence-based HIV prevention

What is evidence-based prevention?

This chapter is intended to provide a practical introduction to the evidence regarding the effectiveness of HIV prevention methods.

After two decades of AIDS and HIV prevention activities, there are increasing demands amongst funders and practitioners for evidence that HIV prevention methods work. The phrase 'evidence-based prevention' has been coined to describe the need for HIV prevention activities to be developed in line with evidence regarding risk factors and outcomes. The notion of an 'evidence-based' approach follows calls in NHS clinical practice for greater standardisation of patient care through the adoption of 'best practice' which is backed up by evidence from sound clinical trials.

The call for evidence-based prevention is only part of a wider demand that health promotion activities, psychotherapy and counselling, and other non-drug-based interventions are subjected to the same kind of scrutiny as drug treatments.

With drug treatments (and surgical procedures, a surprisingly high proportion of which have never been scientifically evaluated) the potential for harming patients with untested treatments is obvious.

But prevention done the wrong way can be harmful too. To take one of the most prominent examples, the COL-1492 study evaluating the use of nonoxynol-9 as a possible microbicide in 765 women in west Africa resulted in frequent users of N-9 having twice the rate of HIV infection as users of a placebo.

Behavioural interventions can have negative results too. In a recent meta-analysis of adherence interventions, for instance (Amico), most interventions were positive or neutral in their effect. But a trial in which 40 participants wrote about an optimistic future in which they would only take one medication a day had a significantly negative effect, with nearly 60% worse adherence in the intervention group.

In the big meta-review cited below (Albarracin), programmes that used threat-inducing arguments to encourage condom use (such as the fear of pregnancy) and normative arguments ('everyone else does it, you should too') had significantly negative effects across participants as a whole, though there were exceptions (for instance, people under 21 responded positively to normative arguments).

It is therefore important scientifically to review the effectiveness of prevention programmes as to do otherwise would not only waste public money but might significantly increase HIV infection.

This chapter reviews:

- The evidence provided by a couple of large meta-reviews of HIV prevention programmes

- The underlying philosophies of HIV prevention, and how and why people change their behaviour

- How and why do we know that HIV prevention efforts have worked, and issues in measuring effectiveness

- Some more research evidence regarding effective interventions.

How do we know HIV prevention efforts have worked?

Effectiveness reviews

In recent years HIV prevention workers, researchers and funders have become increasingly concerned with identifying how best to spend limited funds. This requires a better understanding of which HIV prevention initiatives have been most effective, and which ones are least effective.

A study funded by the UK Health Education Authority (now part of the National Institute for Health and Clinical Excellence) attempted to identify examples of effective interventions, using criteria developed in other health care fields (Oakley). These criteria demanded that studies reporting on the effectiveness of prevention interventions should ideally display the following characteristics:

- A clear definition of aims

- A description of the intervention package and design sufficiently detailed to allow replication

- A randomly allocated control group or matched comparison group*

- Data on numbers of participants recruited to the experimental and control groups

- Baseline (pre-intervention) data for both groups*

- Post-intervention data for both groups*

- Drop-out rates for both groups

- Findings for each outcome measure as defined in the aims of the study.*

However, the review used only four of these characteristics (those marked with an asterisk) when defining studies with a 'sound' methodology. Paradoxically, for a review intended to develop awareness of effective interventions, replicability (point 2) wasn't amongst these criteria!

The study found that just 18 out of 68 outcome evaluations could be described as methodologically 'sound'. Just nine of these studies were conducted with adults in high risk groups. These studies are amongst those discussed in more detail in *What is known about the effectiveness of interventions?* later in this chapter. A number of other studies published since this article appeared are also discussed below.

Another review discusses the question of sound methodology in more detailed terms. A review funded by the US National Institutes of Mental Health and the US Centers for Disease Control proposes a series of standard reporting requirements in HIV and STD prevention behavioural interventions which will allow comparisons between effectiveness studies.

- Describe recruitment and sampling methods: In order for any study to be replicated it is essential that the description of the methodology is as full as possible. It is also important for the reader to be able to judge whether any aspects of the methodology could have biased the results. For example, was the sample a volunteer group or random sampling? How were they selected?

- What proportion of potential participants were recruited into the study?

- What was the refusal rate? What differences exist between participants and non-participants?

- Define the sample size required to produce statistical significance. When a study is designed, statistical methods should be used to define how large a sample will be required in order to detect a certain magnitude of effect on a behavioural or biological outcome. For example, researchers might predict that in order to detect a 20% reduction in syringe sharing, they would need to recruit 100 people into a study in order to be certain that a 20% reduction wasn't due to chance, but to the effects of the intervention. This is called statistical power.

- Was there a control group, and if so, how were people randomised? A control group can guard against the effects of being studied (such as people telling researchers what they think they want to hear)

- Report length of follow-up. This allows readers to judge whether there is evidence of a sustained effect

- Describe the theory of behaviour change and education underlying the intervention. This allows the reader to judge whether the design of the intervention is likely to test the theoretical assumptions underlying the intervention

- Describe the intervention. Too many study reports fail to describe the intervention in sufficient detail. What were the messages communicated to participants? How many sessions/exposures were there?

- Describe outcome measurements used. A more detailed discussion of outcome measures follows later in this chapter

- Report results of mediation analysis. Mediators are the elements of an intervention which mediate between the intervention itself and the behaviour change. "Mediators are generally conceptual variables designed to be addressed by the intervention because they are believed to cause behaviour change, such as perceived social norms, skills, self-efficacy or perceptions of risk. Mediation analysis involves demonstrating that the intervention changed the mediator as well as the behavioural outcome" and that controlling the mediator also affects levels of risk behaviour. If this relationship cannot be proven, then another factor is responsible for behaviour change, and the theoretical relationship between the mediator and the behaviour targeted for intervention is unproven.

References

Oakley A et al. Behavioural interventions for HIV/AIDS prevention, AIDS 9 pp479-486, 1995.

O'Leary A, DiClemente R et al. Reflections on the design and reporting of STD/HIV behavioural intervention research, AIDS Education and Research, 9 Supp A, 1997.

What works?
Two meta-reviews

1. Dolores Albarracin et al, 2005

The largest ever meta-review (study of studies) of HIV prevention interventions (Albarracin) reviewed the effects of 354 HIV prevention interventions and compared their effect with the results for 99 control groups within 33 countries over a 17-year span (though three-quarters of studies were US-based).

Altogether 104,054 people took part in the HIV prevention programmes while another 34,751 were included in control groups (the number in control groups was smaller because many studies compared the effect with matched cohorts or historical controls).

About 45% of participants were men (allowing for a few studies in which gender was not identified); their average age was 26; 34% were white, 47% Afro-American or African and 13% Latino. Only 36% of participants had completed high school.

Many studies did not record which risk groups participants belonged to but 11% were designed specifically for gay men, 15% for injecting drug users, 17% for multiple-partner heterosexuals, 14% for recreational drug users, and 8.5% for sex workers (programmes could target more than one risk group). Fifty-five per cent of participants reported multiple partners.

Of note, very few studies recorded the HIV status of participants, possibly because of a presumption that participants were negative, although in studies where serostatus was recorded, it was 20%.

Baseline condom use was poor - before the interventions 64% of participants 'never or almost never' used condoms, 34% 'sometimes' used them and only 2.3% 'always or almost always' used them. The total proportion of acts of intercourse in which condoms were used was 32.3%.

The size of the meta-review allowed Albarracin and colleagues to calculate the effectiveness of prevention interventions for particular groups of people, both in terms of demographic characteristics like gender, age and race, and in terms of risk category.

It also enabled them to calculate the effectiveness of *specific* kinds of intervention well enough to provide a set of 'decision trees' at the end of the study to help prevention workers decide on the best kind of intervention for a specific group in future.

There was one important limitation to Albarracin's survey. She only used condom use as her primary endpoint. She therefore did not include studies which had other aims, such as abstinence, sexual delay or reduction in the number of partners, nor did she look at the ultimate effect, HIV incidence.

However, the size of the study did allow her to also calculate the effectiveness of programmes on *intervening* effects between the intervention and the condom use.

This is important because it is an aid to theoretical rigour of design. An intervention may be based on one of the theories outlined below and produce a positive result; but without measuring how participants' psychological attitudes have changed, it leaves open the possibility that the change in condom use is due to other factors such as the introduction of treatment. Or it could find out that the intervention did indeed produce the desired psychological effect - but that this change had a negative effect. This was what happened with threat-inducing arguments, where presumably the heightened perception of increased threat ("I will catch HIV unless I use condoms") led to a feeling of helplessness rather than the thing behavioural studies are looking to increase, namely *self-efficacy*.

Self-efficacy is very different from general self-confidence. It is the self-confidence that one can perform a specific task. Neglecting the importance of tying the increased confidence to a task can also result in negative effects. For instance, programmes that taught interpersonal skills such as assertiveness training also had negative effects in some groups. This may be because the increased interpersonal skills were not tied specifically enough to a particular behaviour and may even have been used negatively - as in improving participants' abilities to pick up partners or persuade them not to use condoms.

Albarracin analysed interventions according to the following categories (many studies would use more than one method):

- 'Attitudinal': containing arguments designed to induce a positive attitude about using condoms - 48% of programmes

- 'Normative': containing arguments designed to increase social responsibility or increased perceived peer-group or societal pressure to use condoms - 15% of programmes

- 'Behavioural': containing verbal training or arguments designed to improve participants' condom-using behaviours - 20% of programmes

- 'Behavioural skills': containing training getting participants to practise behavioural skills - 22% of programmes

- 'Threat': containing 'persuasive arguments designed to increase perceptions of threat [of HIV infection or poor sexual health] among recipients' - 47% of programmes

- Most programmes (94%) provided information about HIV

- Twenty-two per cent of programmes distributed condoms to intervention groups and 7% to control groups

- Eighteen per cent of programmes administered an HIV test

- Forty-nine per cent included 'active' interventions such as HIV counselling and testing and behavioural skills training.

- Two-thirds of interventions (where it was recorded) were delivered to groups, 20% to individuals and 8% to both

- Thirty per cent were delivered in clinics, 31% in schools, 21% in community venues such the street, community centres or gay bars, and just 3% consisted of a mass communication.

Results

As stated above, Albarracin's bottom-line finding was that 'active' intervention programmes that required participants to practise a skill or do something else health-enhancing like produced an average 38% increase in occasions of sex in which condoms were used, relative to baseline. Activities include role-playing safer-sex negotiation situations and practising putting on condoms. They also included programmes that involved the taking of an HIV test. Because baseline condom use was 32.3%, this resulted in an absolute increase in condom use of 7.8%.

These are the increases in the proportion of sex acts in which condoms were used. In addition, the baseline proportion of people sometimes using condoms 'at least sometimes' implies that 17% more people would start to use condoms at least sometimes.

'Passive' programmes were ones in which participants merely received a communication such as reading or being taught information, or seeing a video. These produced on average a 13% increase in condom use, relative to baseline, or a 4.2% absolute increase.

Of note, there was also a condom use increase of 8%, relative to baseline, in the control groups. This is probably due to the well-known effect in which inclusion of participants the control group of a study tends to improve their results, not so because of a 'placebo effect' in this case - how can you have a placebo that looks like an intervention? - but because control groups were generally provided with some intervention, such as leaflets, or were on the waiting list for interventions, and were therefore an already motivated group.

The effect of active interventions was therefore to increase condom use by 30% over control groups, and of passive interventions by 5%.

The only exception to this difference between passive and active interventions was in condom provision where - unsurprisingly - simply providing participants with condoms worked better than requiring them to actively ask for them to be provided.

Most types of intervention were effective to some degree, though ones that taught behavioural skills and which induced positive attitudes towards condom use worked best.

The effects observed were strongest for interventions that took place in clinical settings (which, in Albarracin's definition, also included HIV voluntary organisations that offered some sort of clinically-relevant service.) The effects of most types of intervention did not reach significance for interventions conducted in schools or in community settings, though condom provision had a significantly positive effect in community settings.

What may be the most significant single finding of the meta-review was that interventions that increased participants' sense of the threat of HIV or of related outcomes such as STDs or pregnancy had a consistently negative effect, across all categories of recipient.

Put simply, if you frightened people about HIV they used condoms *less*, not more. Remember that nearly half of all programmes included some element of threat arguments.

Normative arguments didn't work either, except with young people under 21. Otherwise, in fact, young people were rather a resistant audience, showing much less tendency to use more condoms after interventions.

Men responded particularly badly to threat arguments (fear) and women to normative arguments (guilt) though both sexes responded equally well to behavioural-skills training.

Africans responded badly to both threats and normative arguments though they did respond well to general training in interpersonal skills as well as specific skills, unlike whites and Latinos. All groups responded well to teaching behavioural skills, not just in condom use but to management skills such as safer-sex negotiation.

High-risk groups (including gay men) generally did not respond as well as low-risk groups, but this may have been a statistical effect whereby groups that already had relatively high levels of condom use did not increase their use as much as groups that initially had low levels. They responded particularly badly to normative and attitudinal arguments. But they responded well to condom provision and condom use training.

Albarracin acknowledges that if she had used sexual abstinence or partner reduction as the outcome measure, threat arguments might be found to work. Scaring people is a legitimate tactic in health promotion if you want to stop people doing something, such as smoking cigarettes or drink-driving. It's much less likely to get people to take positive self-protective steps such as using condoms.

One finding was the striking paucity of trials of programmes for HIV prevention for people with HIV. Seroprevalence data among trial groups was only available in 22 of the 354 trials, "which," comments Albarracin, "severely limited the possibility of analysing the different intervention components." Albarracin was able to show that the higher the HIV prevalence was in groups of participants where it was reported, the more positive the behaviour change which, as she comments, "indicates that HIV-positive people generally increase their condom use," a finding backed up by other studies.

However the lack of statistical power meant that only attitudinal arguments encouraging condom use, fear-inducing arguments about the consequences of not using them, and condom provision could have their effectiveness measured. Fear-inducing arguments and condom provision had a neutral impact. But attitudinal arguments actually had a negative impact on people with HIV: programmes that *didn't* try and get HIV-positive people to have a more favourable attitude towards condoms worked better than ones that did (p=<.001).

Albarracin's finding than just 3% of papers addressed mass-media campaigns also underlines the paucity of research into the effectiveness of this kind of intervention. See **Mass Media Campaigns** below for more on this.

We'll return to Albarracin's meta-review when we look at the theories of behaviour change that underlie the planning of prevention programmes.

2. Wayne Johnson et al., 2002

We take this as an example of a smaller meta-review of HIV prevention interventions targeting a specific population - in this case, gay men. There are so many HIV intervention studies conducted that an attempt to review all meta-reviews - to study the studies of studies - is beyond the scope of this section. However Johnson's is interesting partly because it is about the group that still has the highest HIV incidence in the USA and the UK, and partly because it supports a number of Albarracin's conclusions, but equally interestingly does not support others.

Johnson sifted through 99 HIV prevention studies conducted in the USA to find nine that specifically targeted gay men (and comments on the fact that the highest-incidence group in the USA only had 10% of studies devoted to it). The date of studies ranged from 1989 to 1998 and Hamilton comments that he would have had at least twice the data to work with if he had included later studies. Altogether 2,270 gay men participated in the interventions.

The bottom-line effect of the interventions was a reduction of 26% in instances of unprotected anal sex relative to baseline. Because only 32% of gay men reported unprotected sex before the interventions (a big contrast to Albarracin's populations, where only 32% *did* use condoms) this represents an absolute decrease in unprotected sex acts of 8.5%.

Many of Johnson's findings mirror Albarracin's. He divided up his interventions in a slightly different way thus (with some interventions using a number of methods):

- Training in *interpersonal* skills such as safer-sex negotiation, discloser and communication

- Training in *personal* skills such as self-management, decision-making and stress management

- Programmes designed to enhance *self-esteem* or community pride

- Programmes designed to increase the *social acceptability* of condom use by means such as peer leader endorsement and outreach by peer volunteers (similar to Albarracin's 'normative' studies)

- Programmes designed to enhance *responsibility* by the use of means such as behaviour contracts and agreements.

Like Albarracin, Johnson found that interventions that included interpersonal skills training produced the most clearly favourable effects. Behaviour contracts and responsibility agreements produced the weakest effects.

In contrast to Albarracin, Johnson found that the three interventions that took place in the community worked better that ones that involved small-group training, though these worked too. Two of these were similarly-designed studies which recruited community 'opinion leaders' as disseminators of information and advice about safer sex in gay bars and clubs. See **Community mobilisation** below for more detail on these studies.

The success of these programmes may be culturally-specific, as when the same concept was tried in Glasgow, Scotland it did not work. It may also, be a statistical artefact; the participants in the gay-venue studies had higher levels of unprotected sex, which is concordant with Albarracin's finding that the lower the baseline level of condom use, the greater the improvement interventions tend to produce.

Also in contrast to Albarracin, interventions generally worked better on younger people, and significantly worse in men over 33. Johnson comments that this may also be because older men tended to have baseline higher levels of condom use. It may also be because the majority of interventions that targeted young people in Albarracin's meta-review took place in schools - and it has proved particularly difficult to deliver sex education programmes of proven efficacy in schools, as witnessed recently by the failure of a particularly well-designed programme in Mexican schools (Walker).

One of Johnson's most important findings was to identify significant 'antagonisms' between particular methods. For instance, studies that included personal skills training and self-esteem boosting were effective as long as they did *not* also include arguments for the acceptability of condom use or safer sex. Similarly, programmes for young people worked particularly well if they had low baseline levels of condom use as long as they did *not* include behavioural contracts. This is valuable preliminary work towards finding out what components of an ideal HIV prevention programme work well together, and which don't.

Do Johnson's findings apply to programmes for other risk groups? Well, in the same supplement issue of the *Journal of Acquired Immune Deficiency Syndromes* there are meta-reviews of prevention programmes for safer-sex among drug users (Semaan), for sexually-experienced adolescents (Mullen), and for heterosexual adults (Neumann). Their results are pretty comparable:

- Johnson found a significantly protective effect for interventions with gay men (Odds Ratio 0.69, equivalent to a 26% reduction of instances of unprotected anal sex.)

- Semaan's meta-review of 33 HIV prevention interventions on the sexual risk behaviours of drug users in the USA found a significantly protective effect for this group (Odds Ratio 0.61, equivalent to the proportion of drug users who reduced sexual risk being 12.6% higher in intervention groups than control groups.)

- Mullen's review of 16 behavioural interventions in sexually experienced adolescents found they had a significant effect in reducing instances of unprotected sex (Odds Ratio 0.66) but not in the number of partners (OR 0.89) or STDs (OR 1.18).

- Neumann 's meta-review of 14 behavioral and social interventions for heterosexual adults found statistically significant effects in reducing unprotected sex (Odds Ratio 0.69 and in reducing STD infections (OR 0.74).

HIV prevention programmes show a remarkable consistency of effect across different groups. However there was less information in the above studies than there was in Albarracin's big review as to which methods work best.

Summary

- Averaged over all interventions and all risk groups, HIV prevention programmes show a remarkable consistency of success, with increases in safer sex/condom use in the order of 25%

- 'Active' programmes that get people to practise behavioural skills work about three times better than passive programmes that just deliver information

- Programmes that encourage positive behaviours and develop self-efficacy work better than normative programmes (appeals to social responsibility), though the latter work well for young people

- Programmes that use 'scare tactics' and the threat of AIDS have significantly *negative* effects (except possibly for people with HIV: see below)

- There has been very little randomised controlled research into the efficacy of mass-media HIV prevention initiatives

- Similarly, there has been little into the effect of HIV prevention interventions on people with HIV (but see Positive Prevention below)

- Programmes work best if delivered by experts in clinical settings or by organisations that already offer services to people with HIV.

3. And the UK?

A 2003 meta-review (Ellis) by the Health Development Agency (HDA - now part of NICE, the National Institute for Health and Clinical Excellence) of reviews assessing the effectiveness of interventions in the UK came up with a considerably slimmer body of evidence than the largely US-based meta-reviews above.

It found no research in the UK on which specific modifying factors produced better outcomes: no studies of cost-effectiveness: and no studies of whether theory-based interventions were more effective.

Among its list of 'key evidence gaps', it found:

- Very little review-level evidence relevant to UK gay men

- Very little review-level evidence relevant to UK commercial sex workers

- No review-level evidence relevant to UK African communities

- No review-level evidence about interventions with people with HIV

- And, crucially, very little review-level evidence about the vast majority of interventions. None on condom distribution

schemes, small media (booklets) and community development work.

.and this is not a comprehensive list. So what *did* it find?

- It found that cognitive-behavioural group work interventions that concentrate on role-playing, communication skills and sexual negotiation can be effective for gay men; it also found that community-level interventions involving peers and popular opinion leaders could be effective in influencing gay men's sexual risk behaviour.

- It found that community-level, especially peer-led, interventions can be effective in influencing the sexual risk behaviour of commercial sex workers.

- It found that small group interventions delivered at the community level can be effective in influencing the sexual risk behaviour of black and minority ethnic women.

- And it found that a positive HIV diagnosis positively influenced sexual risk behaviour, but no evidence that a negative one did.

This was the total amount of statistically significant evidence it was able to cull from UK HIV prevention studies.

The HDA was at pains to point out that, for the many different HIV prevention programmes that have been carried out in the UK since the beginning of the epidemic, lack of evidence of effectiveness was not the same as evidence of lack of effectiveness. However, the lack of scientifically rigorous research into HIV prevention in the UK, especially into the difference in effectiveness between methods, does not serve as a good foundation for future programmes.

References

Albarracin D et al. A test of major assumptions about behaviour change: a comprehensive look at the effects of passive and active HIV-prevention interventions since the beginning of the epidemic. *Psychological Bulletin* 131(6), 856-897. 2005.

Ellis S et al. HIV Prevention: a Review of Reviews Assessing the Effectiveness of Interventions to Reduce the Risk of Sexual Transmission. Health Development Agency, 2003. This report may be downloaded from http://www.nice.org.uk/page.aspx?o=502571

Johnson WD et al. HIV Prevention Research for Men who have Sex with Men: a Systematic Review and Meta-analysis. *JAIDS***30**:Supplement 1, S118-S129. 2002.

Mullen PD et al. Meta-analysis of the Effects of Behavioral HIV Prevention Interventions on the Sexual Risk Behavior of Sexually Experienced Adolescents in Controlled Studies in the United States. *JAIDS* 30 Supplement 1:S94-S105. 2002.

Neumann MS et al. Review and Meta-analysis of HIV Prevention Intervention Research for Heterosexual Adult Populations in the United States.

Semaan S et al. A Meta-analysis of the Effect of HIV Prevention Interventions on the Sex Behaviors of Drug Users in the United States. *JAIDS*30 Supplement 1:S73-S93. 2002.

Van Damme L et al. Effectiveness of COL-1492, a nonoxynol-9 vaginal gel, on HIV-1 transmission in female sex workers: a randomised controlled trial. *Lancet* 360:971-977, 2002.

Walker D et al. HIV prevention in Mexican schools: prospective randomised evaluation of intervention. *BMJ* 332:1189-1194. 2006.

The theory and philosophy of HIV prevention

1. Theoretical models of behaviour change

Many of the programmes Albarracin surveyed will have been devised with a particular theory in mind about how people change their behaviour, and programmes that are theory-based have been shown in general to work better. Programmes devised without a consistent theory of behaviour change may offer subtly contradictory or antagonistic messages, as Wayne Johnson tentatively shows.

In another paper (Durantini) from Dolores Albarracin's team at the University of Florida which used the same data as her previous one, experts trained in the theory and technique of at least one method of behaviour change produced better results when they led interventions than did briefly-trained peer educators; the one exception was that peer educators worked at least as well with younger people under 21 as long as the educator was of the same gender and/or ethnicity as the group trained.

The theoretical models discussed here have been developed and tested by researchers working within the fields of medical sociology and psychology to account for the effects of a wide range of health promotion activities. This section discusses the main theoretical models and their relevance to HIV prevention, and relates research literature on HIV prevention to these models.

HIV prevention is always based on a set of assumptions about the ways in which people make decisions about risks, and how they respond to attempts to persuade them to change their behaviour. Sometimes these assumptions are broadly correct, but sometimes researchers have discovered significant problems with such assumptions when they are tested.

The core difference between these theories is that they postulate different *routes* people travel in the process of changing their behaviour. Or, to put it another way, they give different weight to different drivers of behaviour, usually seeing one particular one as primary. These may be divided roughly into theories that see *information* about the health threat to be avoided as the main driver; ones that see the learning of *behavioural and interpersonal skills* as the main driver; and ones that see *social pressure and personal self-efficacy* as the most powerful influences.

This is summarised in a diagram from the Durantini paper:

Reference

Durantini MR et al. Conceptualizing the Influence of Social Agents of Behavior Change: a Meta-Analysis of the Effectiveness of HIV-Prevention Interventionists for Different Groups. *Psychological Bulletin* 132(2) 212-248. 2006.

The health beliefs model

This model (and the similar protection-motivation model) attempt to explain how individuals will take action to avoid ill health. First, individuals must recognise that they are susceptible to a particular condition (at risk), and must perceive that the severity of the condition is such that it is worth avoiding.

They must also perceive that the benefits of avoidance are worth surmounting any barriers to changing their behaviour, and that they have the self-efficacy (in terms of skills, assertiveness etc) to change their behaviour. Cues to action are considered important in assisting all stages of change in this model. A cue for action could be a poster, a face-to-face encounter with an outreach worker or a conversation with a friend.

Rosenstock argues that *programs to deal with a health problem should be based in part on knowledge of how many and which members of a target population feel susceptible to AIDS, believe it to constitute a serious health problem and believe that the threat could be reduced by changing their behaviour at an acceptable psychological cost.*

The attractions of this model are obvious, especially because responses to cues to action at each of the theorised stages are easily measurable by surveys of knowledge and attitudes and of self-reported behaviour.

But the model does not offer much insight into long-term sustenance of behaviour change, and allows sexual and drug-using behaviour to be framed in terms of 'relapse' if it does not conform to the model of behaviour change offered to the target audience. The notion of relapse assumes that behaviour change is a once-and-for-all event rather than an evolution which requires 'sustenance' and support, and does not take into account new situations in which previous learning will be inappropriate. An example might be the decision to abandon condom use in a relationship, which can be more fully explained by the 'reasoned action' model discussed below.

The model does offer some useful tools for questioning assumptions embedded in HIV prevention. For example, it can often come as a surprise to those involved in HIV prevention to discover that members of the target audience consider the consequences of HIV infection to be less serious than other outcomes (such as demonstrating a lack of trust in a partner or a loss of sexual pleasure from condom use). Rosenstock argues that behaviour change is most likely to occur in circumstances where severity and susceptibility are rated highly by individuals, and as Dowsett argues, gay and bisexual men in particular have come to very uneven perceptions of risk as a consequence of their experiences after almost 20 years of warnings about AIDS.

The health beliefs model of individual behaviour change has been widely criticised for its lack of reference to the social and

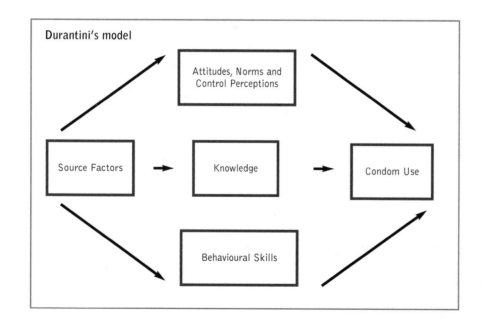

Durantini's model

- Attitudes, Norms and Control Perceptions
- Source Factors
- Knowledge
- Condom Use
- Behavioural Skills

interactive context in which individuals come to judge their susceptibility to risks. In particular, critics have argued that it makes no reference to the pressures from peers or partners which may encourage risky behaviour. This is ironic given the emphasis placed on 'self-efficacy' by some proponents of the model, who have developed educational programmes which focus on the development of skills designed to deal with precisely such pressures. The social learning model discussed immediately below grew out of the Health Beliefs model during the 1970s and 1980s as educators began to appreciate its limitations for explaining how and why people change their behaviour, and the need for concentrating on the development of skills or cognitive techniques.

One earlier meta-analysis (Gerrard) found that there was no association between a person's perceived vulnerability to HIV and the care they took to have safer sex. And, as seen above, interventions that attempted to reinforce the threat of AIDS were generally counter-productive.

Albarracin says:

The health beliefs model and the [similar] *protection motivation theory both suggest that inducing perceptions of threat concerning HIV should increase condom use.Communications designed on this basis typically use highly emotional scare tactics in the hope that negative affect will stimulate condom use. For example.one campaign presented an image of the Grim Reaper as the source of an HIV-prevention message. Other, less extreme communications based on the dame assumptions may describe the consequences of the disease, provide data on infection rates, or conduct a detailed interview about HIV risk behaviour to sensitise participants to risk. As noted, however, these strategies may be counterproductive for proactive target behaviours like condom use.*

However, there are some suggestions that interventions that stress the negative consequences of HIV transmission may work well for one particular audience: people who already have HIV.

Rothman and Salovey (1997) proposed and demonstrated that threatening (*loss-framed*) persuasive messages are effective only when the target behaviour consists of avoiding a risk factor (such as avoiding lung cancer). The same messages, however, are presumably detrimental when one wishes to promote a proactive measure (such as signing on to a smoking cessation course). HIV-positive people may be motivated much more by the negative consequences of infecting others (which can be as severe as criminal prosecution) than the relatively meager reward of behaving responsibly.

Alabarracin found that interventions stressing the threat of HIV transmission at least had a neutral, rather than negative, impact on people who already had HIV in contrast to their negative impact on seronegative people. At the 2006 Retrovirus Conference, Jean Richardson of the University of Southern California demonstrated conclusively that 'loss framed' messages work better in people with HIV than 'gain-framed' ones.

She divided a group of 585 people with HIV (86% males, 74% gay, with men and women represented equally among the heterosexuals) into three groups that received HIV counselling.

The counsellors were asked to fame their messages with a particular slant. The control group talked neutrally with their clients about everyday concerns such as medication adherence. The 'gain frame' counsellors put in positive messages about safer sex into their discourse with clients: you will protect your partner if you use condoms, you'll stay free of STDs, you will feel in control of your behaviour, and so on. The 'loss frame' counsellors gave essentially the same messages the opposite slant: if you *don't* use condoms you will expose your partners to HIV, you are more likely to get STDs, you will feel out of control, and so on.

The findings were very statistically significant. 'Gain framed' messages produced no significant change in behaviour relative to control. But 'loss framed' messages produced a reduction in instances of unprotected sex of 12.5% in people with one regular partner and 38% in people with two or more partners.

Richardson commented that she had 'hoped' there would be no difference in the results of the framing of the messages - possibly because loss-framed messages sound punitive. But it does look as if, when working with people with HIV and *only* with them, the emotional weight of negative messages may work better than positive ones do.

References

Catania J et al. Towards an understanding of risk behaviour: An AIDS risk reduction model, Health Education Quarterly 17, 53-72, 1990.

Dowsett G. Practicing desire: homosexual sex in the era of AIDS, Stanford University Press, 1996.

Richardson J. Prevention in HIV Clinical Settings. 13th Conference on Retroviruses and Opportunistic Infections, Denver, Abstract 165. 2006.

Rosenstock IM et al. The Health belief model and HIV risk behaviour change in Preventing AIDS: theories and models of behavioural interventions DiClemente RJ & Peterson JL (Eds), Plenum Press, New York, 1996. </reference>

Rothman AJ and Salovey P. Shaping perceptions to motivate healthy behaviour: The role of message framing. *Psychological Bulletin* 121(1), 3-19. 1997.

Social-cognitive and information-motivation-behavioural skills models

Bandura's social-cognitive learning theory is a general theory of self-regulatory agency, which proposes that *perceived self-efficacy* lies at the center of human behavior. According to this model, effective self-regulation of behaviour and personal change requires that people believe in their efficacy to control their motivation, thoughts, affective states, and behaviours. In other words, people are unlikely to change unless they want to, believe they can, feel they will, and have the behavioural skills to actually change.

People develop the social and self-regulatory skills required to translate their concerns regarding this information into preventive action (e.g. negotiating safer sex and condom use). This model also proposes that people will require practice and feedback in order to develop self-efficacy in taking preventive action (e.g. learning how to use condoms), and social supports for the desired personal changes will be essential.

The environment in which social learning takes place is created by the interaction between three forces: personal factors such as gender, biological attributes; interactive aspects such as negotiation and the nature of the emotional interaction (is this anonymous sex; what does it mean to refuse to share a needle with a sexual partner?); and social/cultural setting (for example the meanings attached to sex between men).

This model does not offer a strong theoretical explanation for why people choose to change, but as Bandura argues, "the major problem is not teaching people safer sex guidelines, which is easily achievable, but equipping them with skills and self-beliefs that enable them to put the guidelines into action consistently in the face of counteracting pressures".

A refinement of the social-cognitive learning theory is the information-motivation-behavioural skills model (Fisher and Fisher). This also assumes that information, motivation, and behavioural skills underlie behavioral change. The information-motivation- behavioral skills model, however, is a feedback-loop model: it also assumes that the three components exert potentiating effects on each other.

To this extent, the finding by Albarracin that information has positive influences on behavior *only* when accompanied with active, behavioral strategies can be taken as evidence that the confluence of strategies is as important as the selection of each individual approach.

Examples of successful programmes which improved self-efficacy include controlled programmes with gay men and with African-American youth in the US. In both programmes groups identified to be at high risk were taught how to negotiate safer sex in high risk situations through role play with feedback. Both programmes used control groups. In the gay men's programme the control group received no intervention, whilst in the African-American youth programme, the control group received an information-only intervention.

Recipients of the self-efficacy programmes reported lower levels of unprotected sex with partners over extended periods of follow-up, although it is impossible to control for lying in studies with self-reported outcome measures (see below). Nevertheless, especially noteworthy is the fact that the African-American youth study was carried out first in young men and then replicated in young women in another neighbourhood with the same positive outcome (Jemmott).

One programme, not especially with HIV prevention as its main aim, which uses the development of self-efficacy as its core strategy is the Positive Self-Management Programme (PSMP). See the **Self-Management of Life with HIV** section in the **Mental health and quality of life** chapter of the AIDS Reference Manual for more.

References

Bandura A. Social cognitive theory and exercise of control over HIV infection in Preventing AIDS: theories and models of behavioural interventions DiClemente RJ & Peterson JL Eds, Plenum Press, New York, 1994.

Fisher JD and Fisher WA. Theoretical approaches to individual-level change in HIV risk behaviour. In JL Peterson and CC diClemente (eds.), *Handbook of HIV Prevention*, pp 3-55. New York: Springer. ISBN 0-306-46223-0.

Jemmott JB et al. Reductions in HIV risk associated sexual behaviours among black male adolescents: Effects of an AIDS prevention intervention Am J Pub Health 82 pp372-77, 1992.

Jemmott JB et al. Increasing condom use intentions amongst sexually active black adolescent women, Nursing Research 41, pp 273-278, 1992. Kelly JA et al. Behavioural intervention to reduce AIDS risk activities J Consult Clin Psychology 57 pp56-67, 1989

Reasoned action model

The reasoned action model (Fishbein) assumes that most forms of human behaviour are a matter of choice. Thus the most immediate determinant of any given behaviour is an individual's intention whether or not to perform that behaviour. This in turn is influenced by the degree to the person has a positive attitude towards the behaviour, and the degree to which they expect that important others will think that they should perform the behaviour. It therefore combines elements of self-efficacy with elements of social norm-forming. Changing these underlying beliefs about the desirability of an action is what will produce the greatest long-term changes in behaviour. For example, if someone is told not to do something by someone they respect, they are more likely to act on that warning, according to the reasoned action model.

This model is strongly biased towards explaining the success of information giving, and measuring its impact through knowledge and attitudes surveys. It is also strongly biased towards changing subjective beliefs, but doesn't prescribe a particular methodology for doing so.

Research in this area has investigated the cognitive structures which underlie sexual decision-making rather less. There are very few reports of tests of methodologies used to alter beliefs and intentions amongst people at risk of HIV infection, despite the strength of association demonstrated between intention and behaviour in such areas as smoking control, alcoholism treatment, contraceptive behaviour and weight loss.

Albarracin's meta-analysis teased apart the attitudinal and normative parts of the reasoned-action model. It confirmed that programmes that attempted to help participants develop a more positive attitude towards condom use generally worked. However it found that normative arguments only worked in young people under 21.

Albarracin explains this finding thus:

This result does not imply that younger individuals are normatively driven whereas older ones are not. Instead, it appears to suggest that younger individuals do not perceive that making decisions based on social consensus is undesirable, whereas adults are more prone to try to act independently even when they cannot escape being influenced by norms - even if the influence ends up being a reaction against the norms.

One study which has looked at the cognitive structures underlying decision-making about safer sex is research conducted by Australian psychologist Ron Gold. He looked at the underlying justifications which gay men used to explain to themselves why it was permissible to have unprotected sex with partners.

These justifications were overwhelmingly clustered three themes:

- assumptions about partners' HIV status

- feelings of invulnerability

- desire for intimacy.

Another study by the same research team looked at cues which subjects used to judge the HIV status of a partner. Gold interviewed 66 men with an average age of 26 who had reported unprotected sex in the previous six months. Participants were asked to make judgements about the likely HIV status of potential partners based on written descriptions. Gold found that participants were more likely to rate men with attributes of intelligence, well-adjusted personality and a healthy appearance as potentially 'safe' partners, while men rated highly attractive were more likely to be judged 'unsafe'.

Another study which looked at the cognitive basis for sexual decision-making was Sigma Research's review of the rationales underlying unprotected sex. Hickson argues that the strongest influence upon the decision to abandon condom use is assumptions made about self and partner's HIV status.

References

Fishbein M. Using information to change STD-related behaviours in Preventing AIDS: theories and models of behavioural interventions DiClemente RJ & Peterson JL Eds, Plenum Press, New York, 1994.

Gold R et al. On the need to mind the gap: on-line versus off-line cognitions underlying sexual risk-taking, in D Terry et al, The theory of reasoned action: its applications to AIDS preventive behaviour, Pergamon, Oxford, 1993.

Gold R et al. Desire for unprotected intercourse preceding its occurrence: the case of young gay men with an anonymous partner, Int J of STD and AIDS, 4:326-329, 1993.

Gold R et al. Situational factors and thought processes associated with unprotected intercourse in gay men, Psychology and Health 5:259-278, 1991.

Hickson F et al. Perceptions of own and partner's HIV status and unprotected anal intercourse among gay men, Second Conference on Biopsychosocial Aspects of AIDS, 1994.

Stages of behaviour change models

The behaviour-change-stage model (Prochaska) offers an explanation of the stages through which an individual will progress during a change in health behaviour. This model is particularly associated with notions of 'relapse' behaviour, and has been used widely in the treatment of alcoholism and smoking. It divides behaviour change into the following stages:

1. **Pre-contemplation:** lack of awareness of risk or no intention to change risk behaviour

2. **Contemplation:** beginning to consider behaviour change without commitment to do anything immediately

3. **Preparation:** a definite intention to take preventive action in the near future

4. **Action:** modification of behaviour, environment or cognitive experience to overcome the problem

5. **Maintenance:** the stabilisation of the new behaviour and avoidance of relapse.

This model was used as the basis for the US AIDS Community Demonstration Projects, which targeted five at-risk populations in five US cities. Messages were developed from the experiences of community members to model behaviour change steps, and messages were developed to target people considered to be at each of these five stages.

A similar model is the AIDS Risk Reduction Model of Catania, which divides behavioural change into three stages, each with several influencing factors:

1: Recognition and labeling of one's behaviour as high risk

Influences:

- knowledge of sexual activities associated with HIV transmission;

- believing that one is personally susceptible to contracting HIV;

- believing that having AIDS is undesirable;

- social norms and networking.

2: Making a commitment to reduce high-risk sexual contacts and to increase low-risk activities

Influences:

- cost and benefits;

- enjoyment (e.g., will the changes affect my enjoyment of sex?);

- response efficacy (e.g., will the changes successfully reduce my risk of HIV infection?);

- self-efficacy;

- knowledge of the health utility and enjoyability of a sexual practice

- social factors (group norms and social support)

3: Taking action. This stage is broken down into three phases:

- information seeking;

- obtaining remedies;

- enacting solutions.

- Depending on the individual, phases may occur concurrently or phases may be skipped.

Influences

- social networks and problem-solving choices (self-help, informal and formal help);

- prior experiences with problems and solutions;

- level of self-esteem;

- resource requirements of acquiring help;

- ability to communicate verbally with sexual partner;

- sexual partner's beliefs and behaviours.

Both theories, then, attempt to define a sequence of stages that go from behaviour initiation to adoption to maintenance. Successful interventions should be the ones that focus on the particular stage of change the individual is experiencing and facilitate forward progression.

Presumably, knowledge of HIV/AIDS or more general risk perceptions may serve to prompt change when people are not yet performing the behaviour, but may not elicit movement beyond the initial stage. Similarly, inducing favourable attitudes may be important at the very initial stages but not when people are already performing the behaviour and are aware of its outcomes. People who have already adopted the idea of change and begun to perform the behaviour may then need *new* skills to foster complete success.

Albarracin's meta-analysis suggests that, consistent with these theories, behavioural and self-management skills training are more important later than earlier in the change process. On the other hand, contrary to expectation, attitudinal and informational arguments were equally important for both inconsistent and more consistent condom users.

Albarracin comments: "From this point of view, our data suggest that *everything* might be more effective when people have previously engaged in condom use, rather than supporting the specific predictions made by Prochaska and colleagues." In other words: it gets easier the more you practice, but you still need the most basic kind of backup and reinforcement in terms of getting information and keeping attitudes positive if you're not to relapse. People are engaged on a kind of 'Continuous Professional Development' course when it comes to the maintenance of safer sex.

This finding should give some cheer to the developers of mass-media and prevention information campaigns. They imply that although behavioural-skills training is generally a necessary part of an effective HIV-prevention programme, the provision of information, though it does not effect change in itself, can prompt people to *think* about changing and can help them maintain safer behaviour when they have done.

References
Catania JA et al. Towards an Understanding of Risk Behaviour: and AIDS Risk Reduction Model (ARRM). *Health Education Quarterly,* 17, 53-72. 1990.

Prochaska JO et al. In search of how people change: applications to addictive behaviours Am Psychol 47 pp1102-1114, 1992.

Social diffusion model

Innovations are diffused through social networks over time by well-established rules; health-related behaviours are no exception.

A body of social theory called social diffusion theory has studied the diffusion of innovations in fields such agriculture, international development and marketing. More than 4,500 studies have been published on the diffusion of innovations.

Diffusion of innovations theory has been adopted for the study of the adoption of behaviour intended to avoid HIV infection. Diffusion theorists argue that a behaviour or innovation will be adopted if it is judged to have a high degree of utility, and if it is compatible with how individuals already think and act.

However, an innovation will only be considered if it is known about, and one of the major problems facing HIV educators is the difficulty of frank communication about HIV risk and how best to protect oneself and one's partners. The taboo status of much discussion about HIV makes it difficult for individuals to judge the utility of an innovation such as condom use, because frank discussion of condom use is impossible on television.

Diffusion research has also observed that innovations will tend to be adopted in a population according to a distribution that follows an S-shaped curve: that is, few at first, then an increasing proportion, and a few late adopters. Diffusion researchers have been very interested to define the characteristics of who adopts early, and who influences those who adopt an innovation later. They discovered that rates of adoption varied according to the homogeneity of the group, with innovations diffusing more rapidly in groups which were relatively homogenous. 'Change agents' who modelled a new innovation or disseminated information about it were most likely to be successful if they came from that group. The decentralisation of diffusion is also judged to be important. If many different individuals are diffusing an innovation, it is likely to be diffused more quickly.

Two other factors cited as important in the diffusion of innovations have particular relevance to HIV prevention. 'Testability' - opportunities for individuals to experiment with an innovation - and visibility - the knowledge that others are already doing it - are crucial steps in the diffusion process.

One of the earliest successes in reducing HIV incidence comes from Uganda, where HIV incidence went into a sharp decline in the late 1980s. It was accompanied, and probably caused, by an equally sharp reduction, unique among African countries at the time, in the average number of sexual partners people had (see **B is for being faithful and behaviour change** for more on this.)

This decline appears to be evidence that it was not merely the ending of war and the restoring of civil order on the accession of President Yoweri Museveni in 1986, which would involve men returning from the army and militias to their families, which created this change in behaviour patterns.

According to Low-Beer, Stoneburner and colleagues:

Ugandans are relatively more likely to receive AIDS information through friendship and other personal networks than through mass media or other sources, and are significantly more likely to know of a friend or relative with AIDS. Social communication elements, as suggested by these kinds of indicators, may be necessary to bridge the motivational gap between AIDS prevention activities and behavior change sufficient to affect HIV incidence.

In other words, Low-Beer is arguing that the social diffusion model in which there is (a) a wide personal acquaintance with HIV/AIDS in the population and (b) the encouragement and willingness to speak about it and pass knowledge on in informal social networks is the method that has worked best to influence behaviour change. Similar changes now appear to be taking place in other countries, including the highest-prevalence ones such as Zimbabwe.

A wide personal acquaintance with HIV/AIDS is the inevitable consequence of a developing untreated epidemic: the encouragement and willingness to speak about it, however, can be influenced by political leadership and widespread awareness-raising work. Such work was, supporters say, initiated by Museveni when he started his AIDS awareness campaign in 1986, which included his famous 'Zero Grazing' policy, which urged monogamy on all Ugandans.

It is easy to see how this model applies to the development of safer sex and safer drug use in the 1980s, but what does it have to offer HIV prevention workers once the initial lessons have been learnt? It's reasonable to argue that ongoing HIV prevention work is a process of continual innovation as interventions are refined.

Dearing describes how the innovation of bleach as a decontaminant of syringes was successfully diffused in San Francisco in the 1980s. Bleach was adopted because it interfered very little with the process of drug injecting, and because it was viewed as a highly effective decontaminant by drugs workers and by drug injectors. It was successfully diffused by outreach teams which took bleach to the places where injecting drugs users scored drugs or injected. Watters notes that seroprevalence amongst IDUs in San Francisco began to level off after bleach was introduced, whereas other cities which did not adopt the innovation saw a continued rise in prevalence in the following years. Several other projects which relied upon a social diffusion model are discussed under *Community mobilisation* below.

References

Dearing JW et al. Diffusion theory and HIV risk behaviour change in Preventing AIDS: theories and models of behavioural interventions DiClemente RJ & Peterson JL Eds, Plenum Press, New York, 1994.

Low-Beer D, Stoneburner R. Behaviour and communication change in reducing HIV: is Uganda unique? *African Journal of AIDS Research* 2(1): 9-21. 2003.

Watters JK. Epidemiology and prevention of HIV in intravenous drug users in San Francisco 1986-1990, Sixth International Conference on AIDS, Abstract No.FC 106, 1990.

Social/environmental change

The final model assumes that social or environmental changes are necessary in order to change individual behaviour, and that influencing group norms, social policy, sexual mixing patterns and the social and medical infrastructure are the key routes to achieving this change. This model proposes the necessity of working with social groups, not individuals, and underlies such notions as peer education and community mobilisation. But it is also the theoretical underpinning for activism, advocacy and political lobbying.

Friedman and Des Jarlais argue that it is only by reference to social factors that we can understand differences in HIV prevalence amongst different ethnic groups of injecting drug users in the US. Many other examples of social determinants of HIV risk are discussed elsewhere in this volume (see *Understanding the epidemic*), and the social change model is extremely influential in setting the agenda for HIV prevention. However, an over-emphasis on the social/environmental change model can lead to the downgrading of individual behavioural and cognitive techniques which are of proven efficacy.

Probably the best way to use social change models with individuals is to develop 'community pride' programmes which lead to the development of greater self-efficacy and the reduction of isolation among participants. In Wayne Johnson's meta-review, for instance, two of the nine programmes (Choi and Peterson) were for gay men of specific ethnicity: Asians and Pacific Islanders, and African-Americans, respectively.

The Choi workshop consisted of a single three-hour session of group counselling which, among other things, aimed to help gay Asians and Pacific Islanders "develop positive self-identity and mutual social support." Similarly, the Peterson intervention, which consisted of three weekly three-hour sessions, as well as teaching things like self-management, also used "attempts to develop self-identity and social support among African-American MSM."

References

Choi KH et al. The efficacy of brief group counselling in HIV risk reduction among homosexual Asian and Pacific Islander men. *AIDS* 10:81-7. 1996.

Friedman S & Des Jarlais D. Social models for changing health-relevant behaviour, in DIClemente R & Peterson JL (Eds): Preventing AIDS: Theories and methods of behavioural interventions, Plenum Press, New York, 1994.

Peterson JL et al. Evaluation on an HIV risk reduction intervention among African-American homosexual and bisexual men. *AIDS* 10:319-325. 1996.

2. Differing philosophies of HIV prevention

A: Harm reduction or risk elimination?

Since the beginning of the epidemic we have been faced with two competing philosophies about the relationship between acceptable levels of risk and sustainable degrees of behaviour change and public health measures.

One model, that of harm reduction, has sought to demonstrate that the risks of HIV transmission are identifiable and that proven methods of protection against infection exist. These include:

- Avoidance of serodiscordant unprotected sex

- Avoidance of needle-sharing, and provision of sterilised needles and oral substitution drugs such as methadone or buprenorphine

- Use of condoms in penetrative sex, and provision of them

- Screening of the blood supply

- Heat treatment of Factor VIII or provision or safe recombinant clotting factor

- Avoidance of breastfeeding where feasible and necessary

- Adoption of universal precautions in medical settings where invasive procedures take place.

Thus HIV prevention based on a harm reduction philosophy involves substituting less harmful activities for those which pose the greatest risk. For example, the promotion of needle exchanges is a form of risk or harm reduction; it does not eliminate the potentially harmful activity of injecting drugs, but it does offer a means of reducing the risk of HIV infection.

Similarly, the promotion of condoms to gay men for anal sex is seen as preferable to a policy of discouraging gay men from having anal sex altogether. It offers gay men a choice of ways in which to reduce their level of risk, and offers substitutes which are proven to be of lower risk, e.g. oral sex instead of unprotected anal sex. Exactly the same strategy has been employed with workers in the sex industry in many countries.

The majority of debates around the New Prevention Technologies such as pre-exposure prophylaxis, microbicides and mass circumcision are about whether these harm reduction methods actually *will* reduce harm. Indeed, the whole debate about programmes that promote abstinence versus ones that promote condoms hinges on whether, if you take the danger out of sex, you will 'encourage' people to take risks they would otherwise not have done.

Risk elimination

Risk elimination, on the other hand, depends on the belief that protecting both public health and the health of the individual requires the elimination of risk. Risk elimination approaches take two forms:

- The promotion of abstinence over condoms and needle exchanges. This approach questions the efficacy of 'safer sex' as it is commonly conceived, and suggests that injecting drug use is just as harmful as the sharing of injecting equipment.

- The highlighting of very low risks as unacceptable risks.

The previous edition of this Manual argues strongly against risk elimination. But in the real world, things are not so simple, and it is possible to at least make a case that, by providing harm-reduction methods, HIV prevention workers may at times potentially facilitate sexual contacts that would not otherwise have happened.

In one 2005 study from Uganda (Kajubi) researchers from Makerere University randomised 378 young men aged 18-30 from two urban communities near Kampala into two groups.

The intervention group attended a three-hour workshop teaching them about how condoms stopped HIV and STDs, how to put on a condom, strategies for negotiating condom use with partners and talking about barriers to having safer sex. They were then given vouchers to redeem for free condoms provided by young people in their local community.

The control group was just given a general lecture on the HIV situation in Uganda and given the free vouchers but no condom tuition.

The men taught how to use condoms certainly used (a lot) more - 110 per man in the six-month period after the study compared with 13 per man in the control group. However the public health benefit of this was offset by the fact that they had an increased number of partners. In contrast, the control group reduced their partners.

Men taught condom use increased their average number of partners from 2.13 to 2.44 in the six months whereas the control group decreased their number of partners from 2.20 to 2.03. This was highly statistically significant (P = 0.004)

The control group had fewer partners whether regular or casual. In contrast, the intervention group, while reducing their number of casual partners slightly, had considerably more regular partners.

This would not matter if condom use was consistent. But while the amount of unprotected sex the control group had was reduced with both regular and casual partners, the condom group only reduced unprotected sex with all partners slightly - and actually slightly increased the amount of unprotected sex they had with casual partners.

After adjusting for the fact that men in the condom group were on the whole somewhat older and more likely to be married, the researchers calculated that providing the men with condom lessons actually led to them having 48% more unprotected sex than the ones without lessons.

The researchers commented: "Prevention interventions in generalised HIV epidemics need to promote all aspects of sexual risk reduction to slow HIV transmission."

However, it will be noted, Kabuji and colleagues do not therefore propose risk elimination methods instead - such as the probably fruitless task of telling young male Ugandans to be sexually abstinent. They simply advocate for a comprehensive programme of HIV prevention rather than relying on one single intervention.

In other situations, worrying about very low risks can have the paradoxical consequence of inducing fatalism about past sexual practices and reducing adherence to current tried and tested safer sex guidelines, as a 1992 Dutch study showed amongst gay men. Those who became worried that oral sex was risky were most likely to abandon the use of condoms in anal sex, believing themselves to be already exposed to the virus through oral sex.

Another example are the costly and anxiety-provoking 'lookback' exercises that have been conducted by hospitals when a health care professional who has performed exposure-prone procedures has been found to have HIV. These have been done to address public (and professional) anxiety about the tiny risk of infection through an invasive procedure (there have only ever been four documented cases of HIV transmission from a healthcare worker to a patient). However it may be argued that they do more to provoke anxiety than contain it, and draw attention away from the need for universal precautions to be employed in all invasive procedures. This undermines confidence in such precautions, misinforms the public about the risk of HIV infection, and in some cases has resulted in harassment and exposure of the healthcare worker.

These lookbacks have become less frequent since 2001, when the Department of Health altered its guidance so that patient notification only happens where an injury to the infected healthcare worker has happened.

Of course, we have to make allowance for what we do not know and err on the side of caution in predicting the risks of the developing epidemics. Worst-case predictions are intended to be treated as such precisely in order to prevent such scenarios from coming about. However, when such scenarios interfere with demonstrably effective health education, they become almost as dangerous as denial of any risk whatsoever.

A further principle associated with risk reduction is that of minimal disruption. Changes in behaviour are thought to be more sustainable if they involve the least possible change in behaviour required to protect oneself. This is why for many people, cutting down the amount of fat one eats is likely to be a far more realistic, if minimal, form of risk reduction than giving it up altogether. Advice of this sort works with the grain of long established and pleasurable behaviour, rather than against it. Sexual habits are deeply rooted in everyone's lives, and require rather more than will-power to change.

Those who advocate risk elimination argue that the public have the right to be aware of all the risks associated with HIV infection, and to make up their own minds on the basis of such information. Such an argument presupposes:

- That everyone makes up their mind about potential risks on the basis of all the available facts

- That taking steps to reduce certain risks automatically makes it more likely that some people who would previously have avoided that risk will now decide to take it

- That perceptions of risk in the community are all formed by the same factors, leading to an even perception of risk. An example might be sexually transmitted diseases: some people regard these as more disastrous because they have less sex, or because they interfere with an existing relationship, or because the consequences of a sexually transmitted disease might be more

- That the facts are presented neutrally

- That information about AIDS and HIV is not received by people in the light of previous prejudice, misinformation or blaming

- That the information is presented in such a way as to be easily understood

- That everyone is equally capable of acting upon that information to protect themselves

- That there are unlimited resources to present information about even the tiniest theoretical risks. An example of this might be the choice between educating gay men about the dangers of unprotected anal intercourse and the much smaller danger from oral sex.

Realistic risk reduction advice

Following on from the criticisms of risk elimination, it is important that risk reduction advice should be:

- Evidence based. We have already seen evidence above that messages that aim to instil fear of infection may be counter-productive, as they make people feel helpless

- Easily understood by those it is intended to reach

- Implementable. In other words, people have to be willing and able to take the suggested precautions. To suggest that all sex is risky is to invite denial of any risk attached to sexual activity

- Persuasive, not punitive

- Not more disruptive than absolutely necessary.

For further discussion of these issues see *Safer sex* and *Drug use*.

Reference

Kabuji P et al. Increasing Condom Use without Reducing HIV Risk: Results of a Controlled Community Trial in Uganda. *JAIDS* 40(1):77-82. 2005.

B: HIV prevention or sexual health promotion?

The Government's strategy on the promotion of health in England for the 1990s, entitled *The Health of the Nation* (HMSO, 1991), was been the most influential publication in the UK to use the term sexual health promotion. Subsequent strategy documents have emphasised the importance of sexual health promotion, and in 1998 the Department of Health set targets for reducing the number of teenage pregnancies as one of the key planks of sexual health promotion.

The publication in July 2001 of the National Strategy for Sexual Health and HIV, which was subtitled "Better Prevention, Better Services, Better Sexual Health," only set this tendency in stone. The intention had originally been to write a long-overdue HIV strategy for the UK but this was changed to encompass a broader sexual health strategy.

There is a reduced emphasis on HIV prevention compared with the 1980s, despite the fact that the rate of new infections within the UK continues at approximately nearly 3,000 per year.

In this context sexual health promotion covers prevention activity focused on different topics, but mainly referring to contraception and sexually transmitted diseases including HIV infection. This gradual policy shift forced many HIV prevention workers to reorientate their work to fit within this wider framework; to coordinate more closely with other prevention activity; to take a more positive health promotion approach, or simply to use different terminology to ensure continued funding. Being aware of this change in emphasis is all the more important because of the likelihood of HIV-specific funding being removed in the near future and, following the NHS reforms, the new contractual requirements of purchasing authorities.

HIV prevention

Traditionally, prevention is described as being at three levels: primary, secondary and tertiary:

- Primary HIV prevention refers to activity focused on preventing uninfected people becoming infected and on preventing infected people transmitting HIV (e.g. through sex education; condom promotional campaigns; needle exchange schemes)

- Secondary HIV prevention refers to activity aimed at enabling people with HIV to stay well (e.g. HIV antibody testing to allow people to know their status; welfare rights advice; lifestyle behaviour change programmes; anti-discriminatory lobbying)

- Tertiary HIV prevention aims to minimise the effects of ill-health experienced by someone who is symptomatic with HIV disease (e.g. the prophylactic use of drugs and complementary therapies; welfare rights advice to maximise benefits; immuno-supportive educational programmes; disability lobbying).

However, such a distinction of activity has been neither so wide nor so obvious in practice; in general terms HIV prevention has implicitly referred only to primary prevention with the additional recognition that people with HIV are themselves involved in ensuring that they do not pass the infection on and that the primary prevention of other STDs is in itself important secondary HIV prevention for them. In this way, HIV prevention has mainly focused upon elements of sex education (safer sex promotion) irrespective of HIV status.

This division hasn't been helped by the existence of a rival set or categories which defines 'primary prevention' purely as activity focused on preventing uninfected people becoming infected, and 'secondary prevention' as being prevention measures targeted at people who already have HIV. This distinction is still sometimes made in the USA.

However it has been pointed out (not least by people with HIV and their advocates) that HIV prevention whether for people with or without HIV involves the same set of changed behaviours and that some of the same ways of changing them may work. It also implies a hierarchy of importance when it comes to targeting people for prevention programmes - a hierarchy that some advocates for the targeting of people with HIV for prevention activities feel is the wrong way round.

However findings such as the fact that HIV-positive people modify their sexual risk behaviour after diagnosis and there is little evidence that negative people do (see **Counsellingand HIV antibody testing** below), or that people with HIV respond positively to 'loss framed' messages that HIV-negative people find disempowering, may indicate that interventions to help stop people *transmitting* HIV may need to be based on different theories of change and involve different methodology and content than prevention to stop people *acquiring* HIV.

Sexual health promotion

However, both groups of people have the same set of needs if a wider sexual health promotion attitude is taken. If HIV is viewed as just one of a number of acute and chronic conditions that impact on sexual health (albeit one of the most serious and expensive ones), 'positive prevention' may legitimately be seen as a specialised division or primary **sexual health promotion**.

Sexual health promotion can be used to mean a wide variety of things and justify both prescriptive and more liberal approaches.

For example, there have been fears voiced that this term could be used to return to an era of medicalisation as far as the topic of sex is concerned - focusing on disease and the mechanics of sexual behaviour at the expense of sexual pleasure, desire and identity.

This is most obvious in situations where sexual health promotion refers to clinic-based contraception and sexually transmitted disease services. However, this need not be the case even where the focus is on medical services; sexual health promotion can be used to widen the approach of such services to include a social dimension and an example of this is given below (see French & George, 1994).

Advocates of new prevention technologies, however, would counter this by saying that it is precisely medicalised prevention interventions that we badly need; since prevention measures focused on teaching behavioural skills, social responsibility or better communication can only prevent a certain proportion of infections, the most humane, proactive and cost-effective thing to do is to campaign for interventions that do not require people to change their behaviour or psychological attitudes, but prevent HIV infection physically.

Circumcising a heterosexual man, for instance, is safe when done under medical supervision; is a one-off operation; and it may protect him from 65% to 75% of future HIV infections. Side-effects occur, such as loss of sexual pleasure, but they are relatively rare (see **C is also for circumcision** under **developing prevention technologies**). Circumcision may therefore protect the health of this person and of his community better than prevention workshops which offer only 26% efficacy and whose impact tends to wear off over time (in Johnson's meta-analysis, condom-use rates were already becoming lower when they were investigated six months after the end of interventions, in comparison to ones that were evaluated only one or two months after the intervention).

The crucial aspect of sexual health promotion is obviously choice, and making sure that even 'medicalised' interventions are consciously chosen and consented to as part of a person's general determination to reduce the risk to their sexual health.

In the USA, the Centers for Disease Control (CDC) are putting into action a plan to test every adult between 15 and 65 for HIV at least once, in the knowledge that diagnosed people tend to reduce their sexual risk behaviour by at least 50% (and also so that people can be treated before presenting so late that they have AIDS).

However the CDC was also responding to political disapproval of community HIV prevention programmes. On 15 April 2003 they initiated what they called the Serostatus Approach to Fighting the Epidemic (SAFE). This involved a refocusing and reallocation of HIV prevention resources on to people with HIV.

Henceforward, the CDC announced, it would focus on a drive to maximise the number of people tested for HIV. Once people had tested HIV-positive they would be managed by "ongoing case management, medical interventions, and support for other psychosocial stressors."

There is some justification for laying a very strong emphasis on testing as a key element in HIV prevention. According to the CDC's own statistics, there are over 900,000 people with HIV in the USA. About 700,000 know their status. The annual incidence rate is about five per cent a year. But HIV incidence in people infected by people who know their status is less than two per cent (1.73%). Conversely, HIV incidence in partners of HIV-positive people who do *not* know their status is nearly 11% a year (10.79%) (Holtgrave and Anderson).

But HIV prevention for positive people cannot consist solely of testing. There has not been the same effort put into developing prevention advice and programmes for people who *are* diagnosed as part of this screening drive. Exactly a year after the CDC's policy was adopted Terje Anderson, Director of the National Association of People with AIDS (NAPWA), criticised its approach (Anderson). He said the narrow emphasis on testing and individualised counselling was inherently stigmatising:

The lack of any mention of anything that isn't an individual level intervention delivered behind closed doors in a doctor's or social worker's office - the lack of any mention of anything that happens in the community - lays individual responsibility for transmission on each person with HIV, lays no responsibility on their negative partners, makes possible no conversation about the social context that puts people at risk, and treats people with HIV as vectors of infection and not as full people.

In other words, CDC's strategy was to test HIV-positive people, tell them not to pass their infection on, blame them if they did, and possibly treat 'stressors' such as depression and drug use, but not necessarily to provide People Living with HIV with any training in how to minimise the risk of transmission themselves.

So sexual health promotion can be used positively to facilitate discussion about sex and encourage the growth of educational and personal development opportunities (e.g. in youth work, with targeted groups). However, they can also be used in a restrictive, medicalised way to allow only the presentation of biology and treating HIV transmission with preventative medicine as if it was possible to do so in the same way that statins are used to prevent heart disease. There was also an unspoken set of questions about how exactly contact tracing would be performed under the new testing regime.

Sexual health promotion could also refer to activities which enable people who identify collectively to express their own needs. Such community-based activity spans a wide range and can be thought of in terms of the amount of real power people have in determining the allocation of resources to meeting needs. The terms community mobilisation and community development have both been used to describe aspects of this kind of work.

Finally, sexual health promotion can also embrace the role of policy makers and opinion formers in creating a local or national climate which itself promotes sexual health. This can cover anything from liberal or prescriptive mass-media messages, enabling or restrictive legal frameworks or policies and guidelines (e.g. sex education guidelines in schools; age of consent laws; improving the availability of sexually explicit material for 'health' reasons; allowing condom advertising on TV).

References

Anderson T. Expanding the Boundaries of Positive Prevention Programs. Fourth Annual Center for AIDS Prevention Studies Conference, San Francisco. Plenary two. See http://hivinsite.ucsf.edu/InSite?page=cfcaps2004-01&ss=xsl%2Fconf-t2 . 2004.

Department of Health: The Health of the Nation, June 1991, HMSO.

Department of Health: HIV/AIDS and Sexual Health: the Health of the Nation Key Area Handbook, 1992, HMSO.

Department of Health: National Strategy for Sexual Health and HIV, July 2001. May be downloaded from
http://www.dh.gov.uk/assetRoot/04/05/89/45/04058945.pdfHoltgrave DR, Anderson T. Utilizing HIV transmission rates to assist in prioritizing HIV prevention services. *Int J STD AIDS* . 15(12):789-92. 2004.

The limitations of the evidence-based approach

Are randomised, controlled trials appropriate in HIV prevention?

There has been considerable debate amongst health promotion professionals and researchers over what constitutes evidence of effectiveness in health promotion. One of the chief disagreements has arisen over the question of the research methodology that should be used to measure effectiveness. Oakley and colleagues have argued that the gold standard measure for effectiveness is a randomised controlled trial (RCT). However, this view has been criticised as a relic of biomedical research which isn't appropriate for the assessment of behavioural interventions (Fraser).

An obvious parallel can be drawn with HIV treatment research. In a treatment environment where there is just one new drug available and little previous treatment experience, it's easy to recruit and randomise people and judge the effects of the drug, providing you have an agreed endpoint, or outcome measure. But when you have disagreements about the endpoint's validity, even this form of simple study becomes difficult to interpret.

The situation becomes much more difficult when the standard of care has improved greatly, and many drugs can now be combined to treat a disease. It becomes a lot more difficult to find people who have never been exposed to anti-HIV drugs. It's unethical to give people just one drug. It must be added to the standard of care, and the study can't last very long because of the medical and commercial urgency of proving that new drugs work. So we don't know whether the drugs produce long-term changes, or whether the regimens will need to be changed frequently.

Substitute HIV prevention intervention for drugs in this scenario and it's easy to understand why randomised controlled trials are inappropriate in some circumstances (although the circumstances in which they may be appropriate are discussed in *Outcome measures* below).

Researchers are adapting to the new virology and the new treatment environment by designing new sorts of trials and being much more flexible about the kinds of evidence that will be needed to license drugs and develop effective treatment strategies. There is no reason why the HIV prevention field needs to ignore these lessons or to adopt a methodology simply because it is a medical orthodoxy. In reality, one of the big attractions of the randomised controlled trial in a conservative culture may be its capacity to slow down the diffusion of innovations and reduce spending on experimental approaches. It contributes to the rationing of scarce resources, but it may not be the best way of determining how prevention money should be spent.

Stifling innovation

There is also a danger that researchers and practitioners will be unwilling to draw inferences from study results, and will persist in advocating conservative solutions to prevention problems rather than following paths which are plausible. This is exactly what happened in the field of HIV treatment, where some researchers and purchasing authorities have insisted on obtaining evidence from one or several clinical endpoint trials in order to validate particular treatment strategies, rather than being prepared to extrapolate from existing evidence as to which treatment strategies might be biologically plausible.

Yet the history of HIV treatment shows that since the advent of antiretroviral therapy, it is those who have advocated biologically plausible therapy who have tended to get things right. For instance, triple combination therapy was advocated on the basis of biological plausibility over two years before clinical trials proved that it was superior to dual therapy or monotherapy.

Inadequate service provision

This leads us to another danger of the evidence-based approach as it is currently being pioneered. This is the possibility that health authorities will only choose to fund the approaches which are validated by randomised controlled trials or the effectiveness reviews cited above. Lucas has argued that the approaches cited as most effective by such reviews should only be seen as the minimum contents of a package of prevention measures. They should not become a prescription for purchasing.

Nor do such reviews give any guidance on the allocation of resources between different types of programme. This isn't possible without some concomitant analysis of outcome measures. Whilst a programme which increases people's ability to talk about safer sex may have been proven by an RCT, how effective is the intervention at changing infection rates? Ultimately, resource allocation must be judged according to the capacity of different elements of a prevention programme to exert the best possible effect on new infections.

With meta-reviews we are beginning to collect data that can allow us to judge which measures will have the most effect on this outcome. However these reviews of reviews are only as powerful evidentially as the studies whose findings they analyse. While many studies use outcome measure like condom use and unprotected sex acts, fewer use change in partner numbers or STD incidence.

Still fewer use the ultimate endpoint of HIV prevention interventions - change in HIV incidence. This is largely because even in a high-risk population, incidence, at a few per cent a year, is usually too small for anything other than a huge trial to be sufficiently powered to produce a statistically significant result. The same incidence problem has bedevilled studies of the New Prevention Technologies, especially as control groups recruited into the trials often modify their behaviour positively as well.

Currently available effectiveness reviews have another weakness. They don't tell commissioners or providers what sort of agency is best suited to carry out particular types of interventions. Of course, you can make a guess, and evidence is beginning to seep through. For instance, a number of meta-reviews have found that prevention programmes conducted at clinics often have a statistical edge.

But it helps if you understand the models of behaviour change which underlie a particular intervention package. For example, a community mobilisation approach proposed by a local health promotion agency needs to be considered as an example of a social diffusion intervention. What does social diffusion theory in general tell us about the likely nature of the agents best placed to bring about change in a community or group? Is a local health promotion agency best placed to develop this type of programme effectively? Is the community mobilisation approach likely to be the best method of allocating scarce resources, or might other methods of diffusion have a higher contact rate (and a speedier diffusion process)?

In summary, the current limitations of effectiveness reviews suggest the need for better efforts to define the aims and objectives of prevention efforts. A more outcome-focussed set of aims and objectives would allow purchasers and providers to think through the implications of different interventions with more attention to establishing realistic measures of efficacy.

For example, take a town with a large gay population which has a very limited range of prevention activities. This town is not close to any other major gay centre, so it's realistic to use several inter-related outcome measures to measure the overall effectiveness of prevention activities. These might be gonorrhoea reports as short-term indicator, and if possible over the longer-term, HIV incidence in a cohort recruited from the local gay population.

The aim of local prevention activities would be to effect a reduction in both these indicators within a given budget. But what should the package of local prevention activities consist of? To define this package a purchaser could take one of several approaches:

- Fund several different outcomes: number of condoms distributed; number of gay men attending counselling sessions for partners having unprotected sex; number of workshop sessions provided for men having risky sex; number of peer educators/volunteers trained according to the overall aims of the local HIV prevention strategy.

Evaluation of projects funded under this strategy would follow two tracks: process investigation of service delivery, and self-reported behavioural and cognitive changes amongst a sample of gay men recruited from users of these services. Waiting list control groups for some of these interventions could also be required as additional back-up.

This strategy takes account of several different models of the ways in which people change their behaviour, and seeks to deploy these in a mesh of prevention activities to be targeted at the local gay community

- However, it doesn't help purchasers judge where they will get the most value for money. What is the factor leading to most new infections in the locality? Is it unprotected sex in relationships? Is it unprotected sex in saunas and sex clubs? Or are gay men reporting a large number of unprotected contacts whilst using recreational drugs? Whilst these factors can be extrapolated from the research literature, local action research and ethnography will be a vital precursor to funding a cost-effective local strategy. The other vital element during this phase of commissioning is the maintenance of existing levels of service.

Local needs assessment need not reproduce national behavioural data, but it can often give an idea of particular local factors which are facilitating new infections - or more likely, local opportunities for exploiting social networks. For example, a local needs assessment need not investigate what sort of risk-taking activity is going on amongst local men, but it will need to map local gay networks.

Research in commissioning and project design

A conference, *Building Bridges*, held in the mid 1990's indicated the extent to which the processes of effectiveness research, needs assessment, service provision and commissioning remain separated.

A number of issues were identified by presentations at the conference:

- Action research ought to be embedded into HIV prevention activities

- Greater education amongst all involved in project design and management regarding assumptions about behaviour change, risk behaviour and valid outcome measures in relation to the above

- Avoiding hoodwinking of commissioners and providers by researchers

- Avoiding research in the interest of researchers rather than providers or commissioners

- Greater involvement in the research process for those who will be responsible for implementing changes proposed as a consequence of research

- Better dissemination of findings to those stakeholders/ change agents.

All these issues are discussed in the *Building Bridges* conference report, and in particular, in presentations by Graham Hart and by Nicola Woodward.

References

Deverell K (Ed). Building bridges: linking research and primary HIV prevention (Conference report), NAM, 1996.

Fraser, E. How effective are effectiveness reviews? Health Education Journal 1996 55 p 359-362.

Lucas G. Effectiveness reviews, Current HIV Education Research, Spring 1997, HEA.

Oakley A et al. Behavioural interventions for HIV/AIDS prevention, AIDS 9 pp479-486, 1995.

Measuring effectiveness

Outcome measures

Researchers and prevention workers have attempted to assess the effectiveness of interventions by using a number of measures:

- Changes in knowledge and attitudes

- Numbers of persons reached

- Changes in uptake of condoms or injecting equipment

- Changes in reported behaviour amongst a cohort

- Changes in reports of sexually transmitted infections

- Changes in HIV incidence or prevalence in the population

- Changes in HIV incidence or prevalence in a cohort.

This section looks at the value of these measurements, with reference to recent examples from international research, and then goes on to summarise what is known about effective interventions. This list of measurements covers those used in process evaluations and those used in outcome evaluations.

A couple of papers in *AIDS* journal have reviewed what indicators ideally ought to be measured in the evaluation of national HIV prevention programmes, and in the case of the State of California (Page-Shafer), which indicators could and could not be measured.

References

Mertens T et al. Prevention indicators for evaluating the progress of national AIDS programmes. *AIDS* 8(10):1359-69. 1994.Page-Shafer K. Evaluating national HIV prevention indicators: a case study in San Francisco. *AIDS* 14(13): 2015-2026. 2000.

Knowledge and attitudes

Investigation of the effects of HIV prevention campaigns on the knowledge and attitudes of the target population was one of the first measurements of effectiveness to be adopted by researchers. It was considered to be a crucial first step in determining whether or not information about HIV and AIDS had been received and understood by the target population.

During the 1980s knowledge and attitudes surveys carried out in the UK showed wide and rapid dissemination of messages about HIV infection and AIDS, but also showed alarming levels of miscomprehension of these basic messages. These surveys tended to investigate the impact of basic HIV awareness campaigns, and provided useful baseline data.

Such surveys are of limited usefulness today except in situations where new concepts are being introduced to a population. For example, knowledge and attitudes surveys amongst gay and bisexual men in the UK over the past eight to ten years have repeatedly demonstrated high and unvarying levels of knowledge about AIDS, HIV, modes of transmission and safer sex. There is also no automatic relationship between levels of knowledge and behaviour.

Hickson et al note that whilst UK samples of gay men consistently demonstrate very high levels of knowledge about HIV risks, a significant proportion practice unprotected anal intercourse with regular partners.

In some studies an *inverse* relationship has been observed between knowledge and risk behaviour. It is older gay men who are well-educated about HIV risks who are having the most unsafe sex, either because knowledge can be used at the service of rationalising risks (as in decisions to have unprotected sex based on a person's viral load - see **Disclosure, Serosorting and negotiated Safety**) or because people worry less about long-term threats to the health as they get older.

Another form of 'knowledge and attitudes' research which may be more relevant is the evaluation of skills acquisition, although this can be difficult to measure realistically. The skills acquired might be condom use or the ability to raise the topic of safer sex with prospective partners, and skill acquisition must be measured by self-report.

The final form of attitudinal research is investigation of responses to published materials, media campaigns or particular issues identified as important to the design of prevention initiatives. Examples include evaluation of leaflets by focus groups or assessment of comprehension of core messages by questionnaire or focus group.

Such investigations may be necessary in order to establish the acceptability of a certain type of intervention for a target group, or to test an assumption about methods of communication or influence. However, information derived from qualitative evaluations of this sort tends to be much more ambiguous than quantitative data, and contrary to the traditional view that 'you can use statistics to prove anything', it is arguable that you can use qualitative research to prove anything you want it to prove, depending on how you interpret what is said to the researcher. Qualitative research of this nature is better thought of as useful because it teases out and articulates behaviours that can then be the subjects of quantitative research.

Numbers of people reached

Numbers reached by an intervention are a very basic measure of its success, but a high contact rate does not lead automatically to large measurable effects on behaviour or incidence. A project which reaches a relatively small number of people may have a much greater long-term effect on behaviour and incidence, especially if those people are either opinion leaders themselves or the section of a particular community that demonstrates the highest-risk behaviour. Measures of quantity are not very useful unless they are accompanied by measures of quality.

It is also useful to focus on demographic groups such as women or young people if research evidence suggests that these groups are at particular risk of HIV infection. For example, there is some evidence that younger injecting drug users are at greatest risk of HIV infection, and it may be appropriate to set targets for contacts with this group as a surrogate or mediator for an effective intervention to reduce HIV transmission amongst injecting drug users.

However, there is no clear evidence that young gay men are at greater risk of HIV infection than those over 30 (rather the reverse), or that black or Asian men are at intrinsically greater risk purely as a consequence of demographic factors, so a demographic target for this group would be inappropriate as one of the mediators for reduced HIV transmission.

Changes in uptake of condoms or injecting equipment

One way of measuring whether an intervention is working is to look at changes in the uptake of condoms or injecting equipment over time. This form of measurement is relatively easy to carry out, since it only involves monitoring the output of a project. However, there is no guarantee that the output of a project can be related to changes in behaviour or incidence.

For example, whilst a project may experience a 25% increase in demand for condoms over the course of a year, there may be no change in the incidence of gonorrhoea in the locality. This might be due to the fact that individuals are ceasing to obtain condoms from any other source, and relying on a project to provide for their total needs. Or the increase might be explained by an increasing uptake of condoms by those who travel in from other districts and who use sexual health services in other districts. Interventions targeted at gay men carried out by individual London health authorities which are measured locally are a good example of this problem (Kelley). It may even be because the provision of condoms contributes to greater risk behaviour, as seen in the Ugandan study above (Kabuji).

A variant of uptake measurements is the assessment of returns of injecting equipment to syringe exchange projects.

Reference
Kelley P et al. How far will you go? A survey of London gay men's migration and mobility, Gay Men Fighting AIDS, 1997.

Changes in addiction and treatment patterns

There is substantial evidence that addiction to heroin and drug treatment are strong predictors of HIV risk and risk reduction respectively (Rhodes). Measurements of changes in the time that elapses between the onset of addiction and the first demand for treatment, and of changes in drop out rates from treatment programmes are likely to be important indicators of prevention efforts with injecting drug users. However, it is important to be aware that certain types of treatment programme are in themselves likely to be more successful. Programmes which permit long-term maintenance rather than graduated reduction in dosage were most likely to be successful.

Reference
Rhodes T. Risk, behaviour and change, Health Education Authority, 1994.

Changes in self-reported behaviour amongst a cohort or sample

Much of the evidence regarding the effectiveness of HIV prevention measures comes from studies of prospective cohorts. These groups of people are recruited at the beginning of an intervention and followed through the study period to assess changes in behaviour. Such studies are reliant on the self-reported sexual or drug-using behaviour of participants, and also carry the risk that participants will be lost to follow-up, thus biasing the results towards the more co-operative or compliant participants.

However, a range of techniques have been developed by behavioural researchers to reduce these potential biases.

For example, Project Sigma, a UK investigation of gay men's sexual behaviour, used two methods to elicit information about reported sexual behaviour. One was the standard questionnaire method; the other was the process of keeping a sexual diary over the period of a month. Significant discrepancies in self-reporting were noted when the two accounts were compared by researchers (Coxon).

An example of a study in which changes in self-reported behaviour were the measured outcome is the investigation of community diffusion amongst gay men in three small US towns by Kelly et al. This study, described in more detail in *Community mobilisation*, used measures such as frequency of condom use and instances of anal intercourse.

Reference
Coxon T. Between the sheets: gay men's sexual diaries, Cassell, 1995.

Changes in reports of sexually transmitted infections

Gonorrhoea incidence has been used as a surrogate marker for unprotected sex by a wide range of researchers. Gonorrhoea incidence is a very responsive marker of changes in sexual behaviour because of the short incubation period of the infection. Active gonorrhoea is also implicated as one of the factors which increases the risk of HIV transmission, so it is reasonable to assume that a fall in gonorrhoea incidence will influence HIV incidence too. A 1994 study in Tanzania demonstrated a strong association between reduced gonorrhoea incidence and reduced HIV incidence by dividing a district into two and pursuing an aggressive screening and treatment programme for STDs in one area, whilst continuing standard HIV prevention activities in the other (Grosskurth).

Between 1993 and 1995 the US state of Louisiana distributed 21 million free condoms in communities defined as high risk (those with highest HIV prevalence and gonorrhoea incidence). Gonorrhoea reports declined 22% statewide during the programme, and researchers noted a strong association between the highest density of free condom outlets, numbers of condoms distributed and greatest decline in gonorrhoea reports when they assessed trends on a district by district basis (Cohen).

This programme was accompanied by a cohort study (n = 620) which compared changes in self-reported condom use between intervention and non-intervention districts. Condom use rose by 14% in intervention districts and 7% in non-intervention districts. The study was not designed to test either the validity of self-reports (for example by cross-checking with partners), or to distinguish between levels of condom use amongst those with many sexual partners and those with few sexual partners.

Nevertheless, at a population level this study offers proof of the concept that social marketing/free distribution of condoms has a significant impact on sexual health which may contribute to HIV prevention.

However. in recent years studies have started to notice a 'disconnect' between HIV incidence rates and the rates of STDs in gonorrhoea. Increases in STIs in gay men, especially syphilis, has not led to a concomitant increase in HIV infections. This has shaken the assumption that increases in STI rates can be used as surrogate markers or predictors of increases in HIV. In the US, or instance, huge increases in syphilis in gay men have not coincided with equally big increases in HIV. Serosorting may be one reason why an increase in STIs in gay men, especially syphilis, has not led to a concomitant increase in HIV infections.

Conversely, in certain African countries like Zimbabwe, STI rates have gone down while HIV incidence has not, because more HIV infections are now occurring within marriages and fewer within casual encounters. For more on this see **Disclosure, Serosorting and negotiated Safety**.

References

Cohen D et al. Operation Protect: a statewide condom social marketing program Eleventh International Conference on AIDS, Abstract No. ThC4379, 1996.Grosskurth P et al. Impact of improved treatment of sexually transmitted diseases on HIV infection in rural Tanzania: randomised controlled trial, Lancet pp530-536, 1995.

Changes in HIV incidence or prevalence in the population

HIV prevention workers and researchers have often pointed to changes in HIV incidence or prevalence as evidence that HIV prevention efforts are succeeding or failing.

However, one should be very cautious when drawing on such data. For example, it is extremely difficult to tease apart the range of factors which may be responsible for changes in **incidence** over time. The most controversial example is the question of whether changes in HIV incidence amongst gay men during the 1980s were a consequence of changes in behaviour or an inevitable feature of the normal pattern of an epidemic.

Whilst it is clear from international data that early safer sex education coincided with rapid falls in sexually transmitted infections, and that HIV incidence peaked in gay communities in 1983/84, it has been argued that the subsequent decline in HIV incidence may be attributable to a declining number of men in the primary phase of infection capable of transmitting HIV easily to their partners.

According to this model, a slight reduction in the transmission rate at a relatively early stage in the epidemic would have a disproportionate effect on the multiplication rate of the epidemic. For example, if the average number of partners per month amongst a group with 10% HIV incidence per annum fell by 50% (from eight per month to four per month), the chance of encountering an individual recently infected with HIV would fall by a correspondingly greater multiple.

Thus relatively minor and short-term interventions - such as closing bathhouses - may have had a much greater long-term

effect than the widespread adoption of safer sex, providing that they occurred relatively early in the course of the epidemic.

This model also depends on the assumption that infectivity is very high during primary infection (assumed to last for 3-4 months after exposure), and much lower thereafter. One of the justifications for universal testing has been that it will catch a higher proportion of people in primary infection, when they are much more infectious. Estimates of the proportion of HIV infections attributable from someone in primary infection have been as high as 50-60%.

Recent mathematical studies by Professor Roy Anderson's team at Imperial College (Fraser) have suggested that people in primary infection are indeed very infectious - but that in most situations the majority of infections are transmitted by people with chronic, asymptomatic infection, because the time during which people are in this state is in the order of 30-40 times longer, even in the absence of ARV treatment.

An analysis of infections in the Rakai cohort in Uganda showed that people in primary infection were on average 28 times more infectious than people in chronic symptomatic infection. But because the periods of chronic infection was so much longer, it actually contributed a much higher proportion of infections.

Fraser's models indicated that transmission during primary infection accounted for no more than 12% of infections; that transmission on chronic infection accounted for 71%; and that transmission from people with symptomatic AIDS, when viral loads were generally higher, accounted for the other 17%.

The kind of intervention needed therefore depends on the stage of epidemic a particular community has reached. Behaviour-skills training may work better in mature epidemics where the majority of people are in chronic infection: but much more interventionist measures such as early HIV testing including RNA testing may be needed in situations where there is a rapidly proliferating chain of HIV infection happening among a community.

Changes in **prevalence** amongst some segments of the population may indicate that HIV prevention efforts are succeeding in a broad sense, or may give indications of increasing transmission rates. However, it takes a leap of faith to correlate such changes with prevention programmes unless a long time span is being used.

For example, it is reasonable to argue that a fall in HIV prevalence amongst Ugandan women attending antenatal clinics for the birth of their first child suggests that prevention efforts have reduced HIV prevalence in that country, since this group of women are likely to have become sexually active since the beginning of the AIDS epidemic (Asiimwe-Okiror). But a fall in HIV prevalence in the course of one or two years in a much smaller locality cannot be attributed to the efforts of prevention activities in that locality.

For example, a fall in HIV prevalence was noted amongst gay men attending GUM clinics in London by the unlinked anonymised HIV prevalence survey (UA) between 1990 and 1995. However, researchers noted that it would be wrong to assume that this reflected a fall in incidence amongst gay men in the capital. The fall in prevalence could be explained by a change in policy at one of the GUM clinics participating in the survey; diagnosed HIV-positive men were no longer treated in the same GUM clinic sessions as undiagnosed gay men, and would not be routinely tested for HIV as part of the UA survey.

Changes in HIV diagnoses are a similarly unreliable guide to the success of prevention efforts, although presentation for a voluntary HIV test appears to be remarkably responsive to media coverage.

References

Asiimwe-Okiror G. Declines in HIV prevalence in Ugandan pregnant women and its relationship to HIV incidence and risk reduction, Eleventh International Conference on AIDS Abstract No. MoC905, 1996.

Fraser C. Quantifying the Impact of Primary Infection on HIV Transmission and Control. 13th Conference on Retroviruses and Opportunistic Infections, Denver, USA. Abstract 162. 2006.

Koopman J. Core groups cause primary infection to dominate HIV transmission even when more than 90% of virus is excreted during later stages of infection, Eleventh International Conference on AIDS, Abstract No. MoC570, 1996.</reference>

Changes in incidence amongst a cohort

A measure which can give a crude measure of the generalised effect of prevention efforts over time is HIV incidence in a prospective cohort. Two examples of such cohorts are the Sigma gay men's cohort in the UK, and cohorts of injecting drug users recruited by researchers monitoring the success of city-wide needle exchange projects in North America. Data derived from these cohorts demonstrates the strengths and weaknesses of this measure.

The Sigma cohort reported an increase in HIV incidence amongst its sample in 1990-91 following relatively stable incidence since the cohort began testing in 1987. However, it is important to note that the Sigma cohort was a 'decaying' cohort, with a high drop out rate. Such incidence trends become indicative rather than authoritative in cohorts over long periods of time.

Syringe exchange incidence studies have generally demonstrated a decline in incidence. However, a study in Montreal, Canada, demonstrated a greater risk of seroconversion amongst syringe exchange users than non-users during a mean follow-up period of 15 months (33% versus13%) (Bruneau).

However, another study of all needle exchanges in the Canadian city of Vancouver showed that needle exchanges tended to attract those injecting drug users already identified by other studies as those at highest risk - unstable, high frequency injectors with multiple risks including sex work, unprotected sex with other IDUs, polydrug use and high frequency of sharing with strangers. Injecting drug users who used syringe exchanges less frequently (less than once a week) were less likely to share these characteristics (Archibald). These two studies of syringe exchange illustrate the danger of jumping to unwarranted conclusions solely on the basis of incidence data.

References

Archibald C et al. Needle exchange program attracts high risk injection drug users, Eleventh International Conference on AIDS, Abstract No. TuC.320, 1996.

Bruneau J et al. Increased HIV seroprevalence and seroincidence associated with participation in needle exchange program, Eleventh International Conference on AIDS, Abstract No. TuC.323, 1996.

Summary

This review of efficacy measures is intended to highlight the huge difficulties in applying simple measurements to the evaluation of HIV prevention programmes. From the examples cited above, it should be evident that the more robust measures of effectiveness are those which form part of an inter-linked sequence of measurements which test the various assumptions underlying a programme. For example, it would be desirable in assessing the success of a nationwide HIV prevention programme targeted at a gay men to include the following measurements as performance indicators:

- measures of awareness of particular interventions

- measures of understanding of messages

- process efficiency measures of numbers reached

- baseline incidence

- a large cohort to measure changes in incidence over time

- a qualitative research project which looked at the sexual behaviour of cohort seroconverters, such as self-reported reasons for unprotected sex

- proof of concept or mediator studies which tested assumptions such as: increased availability of condoms translates into increased use of condoms by people who would otherwise have engaged in unprotected anal intercourse; or, knowledge of own or partner's HIV status influences condom use.

Can randomised, controlled trials be used in HIV prevention research?

A number of the proof of concept studies identified above appear to demand controlled study. It has been argued in the past that randomised controlled studies in HIV prevention are extremely difficult, particularly if HIV incidence is the outcome measure used. However, there is no reason why studies which examine particular elements of a prevention strategy, and which use carefully chosen outcome measures, should not be conducted successfully.

The major difficulty in using such studies as 'proof of concept' investigations lies not so much in the element of randomisation or the selection of a valid control group, but in the resources needed to mount such studies. Relatively large studies will be needed to draw valid conclusions, and national research networks do not yet exist in the genitourinary setting to mirror those developed by the Medical Research Council for its anti-retroviral studies. Such a network could be developed alongside efforts to establish a national gay men's vaccine cohort (See *Developing prevention technologies: HIV & AIDS vaccines*).

Further reading

Outcome measures are also discussed in:

- Risk, intervention and change, by Tim Rhodes, HEA, 1994.

- Outcomes in HIV prevention by Chris Bonell, HIV Project, 1996 and Using outcomes in HIV prevention: a how-to guide by Chris Bonell and Paul Devlin, HIV Project, 1997.

What is known about the effectiveness of interventions?

Methodology or message: which is more important?

A fundamental confusion often arises in discussions of effectiveness regarding the relative importance of methodologies and messages. Two points need to be made at the outset of this effectiveness review:

- Most controlled research into the effectiveness of methods has concentrated on methodology. Implicit within this has been the assumption that there is a 'core curriculum' of HIV information and skills which need to be taught. There is no discussion in the literature of the detailed content of programmes, so we have no way of comparing whether some programmes proven to be effective actually say contradictory things

- All controlled research which demonstrates effectiveness has relied on the adaptation of the 'core curriculum' of skills and information to the culture and needs of the target group. Nevertheless, similar outcomes have been seen in all controlled studies - the intervention, whatever it is, has a greater impact than doing nothing.

Further investigation of the methodology versus message question is needed in HIV prevention research before it is possible to argue either that 'doing something is better than doing nothing', or that 'doing nothing may sometimes be a better use of resources than doing something'. For example, investigation of the relative impact of campaigns which promote undifferentiated safer sex messages to negative and positive men versus campaigns which promote negotiated safety would be a useful way of testing this question.

Research on the effectiveness of interventions for specific communities

A lack of research on interventions for African communities

This review largely covers interventions with gay men, students and injecting drug users because little or no research has been conducted in the UK on interventions targeted at African communities.

A detailed preliminary evaluation of a number of UK projects targeted at African communities (Maharaj) had been published by the Health and Education Research Unit of the University of London Institute of Education in 1996.

However by 2005, when the Medical Research Council published its own review (Prost) of research among black African communities affected by HIV in the UK and Europe, it could still find no randomised controlled trials on HIV prevention interventions among Africans, though there have been significant surveys of treatment and social needs (Project NASAH), sexual attitudes and lifestyles (the Padare Project) and HIV prevalence and testing (the Mayisha Projects).

The review included 129 studies, of any kind, of which 29 were published in peer-reviewed journals.

Twenty-four of these were descriptive quantitative studies, and five were qualitative studies. A total of 100 'grey literature' publications (mainly reports and online publications) encompassing quantitative and qualitative data were also included.

There were no studies in peer-reviewed journals describing HIV prevention interventions with people of sub-Saharan African origin. However, information on existing interventions was available through 'grey literature', and details of 31 interventions were thus obtained, 22 in the UK and nine in other European countries.

Only one of these actually attempted to measure its own efficacy in terms of public health indicators. This consisted of two King's Fund-financed seminars for 40 people, with four follow-up workshops, offering information and advice on HIV and sexual health to Swahili-speaking young people in Islington. It measured, and found, a significant reduction in the number of unwanted sexual health outcomes (unwanted pregnancies and STIs) among seminar attendees. This is the only prevention study among UK (or European) Africans that had as an outcome measure anything other than a measurement of the pace of the project itself such as leaflets distributed, phone calls made, or clients contacted.

References

Maharaj, K et al. An assessment of HIV prevention interventions with refugees and asylum seekers. Health and Education Research Unit of the University of London Institute of Education, 1996.

Prost, A. A Review of Research among Black African Communities Affected by HIV in the UK and Europe. Medical Research Council, 2005.

Research on interventions for injecting drug users

This section does not attempt to duplicate an excellent and lengthy summary which has already been published by the Health Education Authority, and a book by the same authors:

- Tim Rhodes. *Risk, Intervention and Change: HIV prevention and drug use.* HEA, 80 pages. 1994. ISBN 0-752-10121-8.

- Richard Hartnoll and Tim Rhodes. *AIDS, Drugs and Prevention.* Routledge, 260 pages, 1996. ISBN 0-415-10204-9

Research on interventions with gay and bisexual men

Excellent summaries of psychosocial factors involved in HIV risk reduction and the success of interventions can be found in:

- Ralph DiClemente and John Peterson. *Preventing AIDS: Theories and methods of behavioural interventions,* edited by, Springer, New York, 1994. See especially Chapter Fourteen. ISBN 0-306-44606-5

- Jeffrey A Kelly. *Changing HIV Risk Behavior: Practical Strategies.* The Guilford Press, New York, 195 pages, 1995. ISBN 1-572-30009-4.

What is known about the effectiveness of specific approaches

Mass media campaigns

The success of mass media campaigns in increasing awareness of HIV and risk behaviours have been well reported elsewhere, and research suggests that the content of mass media messages is a crucial determinant of the success of advertising and media campaigns. The UK 'Iceberg and Tombstone' campaign of the 1980s is widely credited with raising public awareness of AIDS at an early enough stage to keep the UK a low-prevalence country relative to the USA and some other European countries - much as its content was criticised at the time. The African 'ABC' campaign that has covered much of an entire continent in roadside posters is also seen as an essential component of prevention activities in the region.

In Switzerland (Lehmann) a booklet about AIDS was mailed to every Swiss household in March 1986. Of the population aged 20-69, to whom the book was sent, 56% read the booklet. For those who read the booklet compared with those who did not the results showed an improvement in knowledge and a better understanding of the risks of specific behaviours and of exposed groups and thus less fear of becoming infected through daily activities. The Swiss campaign was the subject of a number of qualitative and qualitative studies which are still ongoing (Dubois-Arber).

However subsequent, smaller campaigns have not been evaluated properly in terms of actual behavioural change, and most research into mass media campaigns dates from the early days of the epidemic, or at least the pre-HAART era. There has been very little rigorous evaluation of mass media campaigns in the last 10 years. Dolores Albarracin reports that only 3% of the 354 HIV interventions she reviewed were evaluations of the efficacy of mass-media campaigns.

The difficulty with mass-market interventions such as posters, leaflets, websites and social-marketing campaigns is partly due to the problem of finding a satisfactory control group who have not seen the intervention. As a result, a lot of 'research' into the effectiveness of mass-media campaigns stops short of obtaining efficacy evidence and only conducts focus-group-style research into the degree of penetration and recognition of campaigns and qualitative data on whether consumers thought they were effective.

However, it's important to emphasise that absence of evidence as to the effectiveness of mass-market campaigns does not mean evidence of absence.

References

Dubois-Arber F et al. Long term global evaluation of a national AIDS prevention strategy: the case of Switzerland. *AIDS* 13(18), 2571-2582. 1999.

Lehmann P et al. Campaign against AIDS in Switzerland: evaluation of a nationwide educational programme. *BMJ* 295 pp1118-1120, 1987.

Moatti JP et al. Impact on the general public of media campaigns against AIDS: a French evaluation, *Health Policy* 21 pp233-247, 1992.

Small media

Small media refers to interventions such as leaflets, posters and advertising in small circulation or community publications.

The primary evaluative tools which have been used to assess the impact of these interventions have been investigations of numbers who have seen the leaflet or advert, its comprehensibility and its relevance to the target audience. Small media interventions may be measured for other impacts if they are part of a specific campaign with a defined set of aims and objectives. An example of this might be a leaflet or advertising campaign which seeks to introduce messages about 'negotiated safety' or assumptions about HIV status. It would be possible to measure the impact compared with baseline in awareness of the ideas communicated in the leaflets or adverts, but would it be possible to correlate this awareness with changes in behaviour? Is this a reasonable expectation?

If an intervention's aims and objectives are correlated with a particular set of assumptions about how behaviour changes in response to informational cues (see *Models of behaviour change* above), some researchers argue that it is reasonable to assume that changes in behaviour have occurred in response to informational interventions. However, research needs to be designed in such a way as to prove that it was exposure to the leaflet or poster which was an essential component of the intervention, rather than other factors such as participation in the study which influenced behaviour.

An Australian study has shown that small media in the form of posters have little or no impact on behaviour amongst those already exposed to a message by other means. Men who had reported unprotected sex were randomised either to a cognitive behavioural intervention, to receive copies once a month of posters judged by the researchers to be good examples of gay men's safer sex promotion, or to a control group which received no intervention.

Participants were asked to record their reactions to the material, and also their sexual behaviour during the follow-up period. Those randomised to the poster group reported that they found the posters attractive and that the posters put across the safer sex message effectively, yet reported little or no change in levels of unprotected sex during the follow-up period in comparison with the no-intervention control group. In contrast, the cognitive intervention group reported a much lower rate of unprotected sex (Gold).

Such findings are problematic because of the resources allocated to the development of small media interventions. They are seen as the core of AIDS education because they are low-budget and because they can slot into many other programmes of work, such as outreach or peer education.

- An effective small media intervention is likely to have the following characteristics:

- Cultural sensitivity to the idioms and styles of the target audience

- Visual impact, attractiveness

- Tailored to the educational level of the target audience

- The target audience has repeated exposures to the intervention.

Given these characteristics, it is amazing how many small media interventions in the HIV prevention field ignore fundamental rules of marketing and advertising, and how rarely professionals in the fields of copywriting and marketing are employed to develop such materials. This is not a consequence of budgetary restrictions, by and large, but of a failure to appreciate that health communications are no different from other forms of marketing or PR. This is not an argument for turning HIV prevention over to advertising agencies, but for allowing the finished product to be created by communications professionals rather than a committee.

References
Gold R: AIDS education: has it gone wrong? National AIDS Bulletin, March 1996.

Counselling and HIV antibody testing

Evidence of the effectiveness of HIV antibody testing and counselling in altering behaviour is contradictory. A major review published in 1991 concluded that no reliable, controlled data existed to confirm the value of HIV testing as a prevention measure.

This was the case, at least, where the result of the test was a negative one. HIV testing *has* been found to have a significant

impact on the risk behaviour of people who test positive - see **positive prevention** below.

Only amongst heterosexual couples was there any clear evidence that counselling and testing had any impact on the practice of safer sex. Amongst injecting drug users in contact with methadone maintenance programmes, HIV testing and counselling were associated with reductions in needle sharing, but there were no differences between those who tested positive or negative, suggesting that knowledge of HIV status was not the critical factor in encouraging safer behaviour (Higgins).

Amongst gay men there is no strong evidence that knowledge of HIV status in itself predisposes to safer sexual behaviour, although this has been inferred from a number of studies (Kippax).

All studies which have reported on the effects of testing and counselling have been uncontrolled, and it has been suggested that the self-selecting nature of such studies may bias the results, because those who come forward for testing may be more motivated to change their behaviour. However, testing may speed the process of behaviour change in the view of some commentators, and may act as a reinforcer of intentions regarding behaviour change, particularly if the practice of HIV testing receives social or peer support (Cohen).

It is important to tease apart the impact of the knowledge of serostatus from the impact of any pre- or post-test counselling.

In the latter case, even if testing was proven to have a significant impact on subsequent behaviour, it is still questionable whether a successful counselling intervention that reinforced the general impact of serostatus could be replicated by others. This is due to the subjective nature of the counselling encounter, which relies on the skills of the counsellor, the information content of the counselling session and the number of 'doses'.

Sigma Research has shown wide variation in the content of counselling sessions and in their impact on individuals in the South-East of England, and there may be variations even within a counselling team. Recent research at the Chelsea and Westminster GUM clinic in London showed that significant divergences existed amongst both counsellors and clinicians regarding definitions of high, low and medium risk sex acts.

There is no guarantee that counselling interventions, even if they are standardised, will be received in similar ways by all clients. Critics of the Health Beliefs and Reasoned Action models of behaviour change have pointed out that social and peer pressures may act against 'rational' assessment of information provided by counsellors, and that using HIV testing as a means of changing people's behaviour presupposes that people will act on the risk reduction information they are given (Beardsell).

References
Beardsell S et al. Should wider HIV testing be encouraged on the grounds of HIV prevention? AIDS Care 6:1,1994

Cohen M. Changing to safer sex: personality, logic and habit, in Aggleton P et al Eds: AIDS: Responses, interventions and care Falmer Press, London, 1991.

Higgins DL et al. Evidence for the effects of HIV antibody testing and counselling on risk behaviours, JAMA 226 pp2419-2429, 1991.

Peer education

Peer education has been one of the most important methods by which information about HIV and behaviour change has been transmitted. Peer education models have been especially common amongst students, ethnic minorities and gay men. However, it is difficult to separate peer education from other components of HIV prevention activity in research reports. See *Community mobilisation* and *Group cognitive interventions* below for further discussion of the role of peer education.

Workshops

There is little or no evaluation of workshops as an intervention despite the increasing frequency with which they are offered. It is also difficult to define whether workshops constitute a group cognitive intervention (attempting to reframe people's thinking about their sexual behaviour), a behavioural intervention (attempting to offer techniques for avoiding situations, negotiating condom use etc) or whether they are a purely informational intervention. Most workshop programmes appear to offer a combination of these approaches, and any evaluation needs to make clear the balance of aims and objectives, and to define outcomes suitable for measuring each of these objectives.

An informal insight in the role of workshops within community mobilisation was offered by Tom Coates, a researcher on the US-based Men's Network research project, at the Berlin AIDS conference in 1993. Coates observed that whilst exposure to safer sex messages through events such as parties and discos was associated with a reduction in unprotected sex, workshops organised by the group tended only to attract those who had a high commitment to safer sex at baseline. In other words, they may be a technique for maintaining safer behaviour, but may be a less attractive change agent for those who are having risky unprotected sex (Coates). However, it is also worth considering ways in which workshops have been marketed to the target audience when their success is being evaluated. Are the organisers using methods likely to recruit people who are most likely to demonstrate post-intervention changes in behaviour, or are they preaching to the converted? Evaluation of any workshop programme should include pre-testing of the recruitment materials to ensure that they will attract people at higher risk of HIV infection or of having unprotected sex.

References

Coates T et al. Prevention in developed countries, Abtsract No. RT-08, Ninth International Conference on AIDS, 1993.

Outreach work

Outreach work has developed in a number of settings thought to expose individuals to high risk of HIV infection. These include public sex environments (PSEs), commercial sex premises (saunas, massage parlours) and gay clubs. Outreach work has also occurred on the streets amongst injecting drug users, homeless youth and commercial sex workers.

The attraction of outreach work is that it can bring individuals into contact with services and messages they might not have received otherwise (e.g. Bleach and teach in San Francisco, see *Social diffusion* below). It also reaches people at earlier stages in their drug using careers, although there is no clear evidence that it is a superior method for reaching men who are just becoming homosexually active.

Outreach work is highly labour intensive when professionalised, and difficult to regulate when performed by volunteers. There is a considerable literature on outreach projects with injecting drug users (e.g. Rhodes 1991), which have been evaluated more thoroughly than work in cottages and cruising areas (PSEs). Rhodes et al found that existing outreach methods among injecting drug users had a number of limitations:

- They only reached those who were relatively easy to reach 'hard to reach' drug users

- Outreach tends to target individuals rather than the social networks in which they use drugs or have sex, despite the fact that community-wide norms influence behaviours

- Drug users had a variety of other needs which took precedence over receiving advice about HIV risk. They wanted housing, money and treatment.

Nevertheless, Rhodes concluded that outreach had an important role to play in HIV prevention work with injecting drug users, a view endorsed by the Department of Health and NHS Executive in its 1997 guidance on purchasing effective treatment and care for drug misusers. However, the guidance also recommended that providers should collect data including statistics on 'the effect of contact', without a clear discussion of how purchasers might judge when the aims and objectives of an outreach project were either realistic or being met effectively in terms of behaviour

change. Specific outcome measures for assessing behaviour change and project efficacy amongst IDUs are discussed in *Risk behaviour: injecting drug users* below.

Outreach work with gay and bisexual men in public sex environments has been one of the preferred models of intervention with this group, based on a number of assumptions:

- A significant population of hard to reach gay and bisexual men exists who can only be reached through such settings, and who will otherwise remain uninformed about HIV risks

- Cottages and cruising areas are a significant locus of unsafe sexual activity.

Evidence from research in the UK tends to contradict both these assumptions. Many cruising areas are heavily used by gay men who also frequent the commercial gay scene, as the Sigma Research Pride surveys have demonstrated. Weatherburn has also shown that men who do not use the commercial gay scene with a high degree of frequency and who may not identify as gay, nevertheless have a high level of knowledge about HIV. Other researchers have shown that unprotected sex is less likely to occur in cottages than at home.

However, research by GMFA on the sexual behaviour and condom use of men using London's largest cruising area indicates that:

- A large proportion of men who use that location to meet sex partners will have anal sex with those partners, either on the Heath or later, at home

- Condoms distributed by GMFA were used on the Heath

- A large proportion of men did not bring condoms to the Heath

- A large proportion of those who did bring condoms did not bring lubricant, or brought condoms which may be unsuitable for anal sex.

- The population reached on the Heath was not disproportionately different from that identified by another GMFA survey (Kelley, 1997) as regular users of the commercial gay scene.

This research suggests that outreach which concentrates on face to face contacts will be less cost-effective than outreach targeted at sites where a high volume of sexual contacts takes place, and where many opportunities exist to supply appropriate condoms and lubricant.

References

Kelley P, et al: How far will you go?, GMFA, 1997.

Rhodes T, et al: Hard to reach or out of reach: an evaluation of an innovative model of HIV outreach education, Tufnell Press, London, 1991.

Rhodes T, et al: Out of the agency and onto the streets: a review of HIV outreach health education in Europe and the United States , ISDD, 1991.

Rhodes T: Outreach work with drug users: principles and practice, Council of Europe, 1996.

Weatherburn P, et al: No aggregate change in homosexual HIV risk behaviour change among gay men attending the Gay Pride festivals, 1993-1996, AIDS 10 pp771-774, 1996.

Weatherburn P, et al: Behaviourally bisexual men, HEA, 1996.

Group cognitive/skills interventions

A number of group cognitive interventions have been tested in well-controlled studies. They draw from different models of behaviour change, but all involve the development of skills and cognitive frameworks to help people sustain safer behaviour. Some methods are more labour intensive than others, and some could be adapted to other media. All have been proven to work with particular populations.

The first is a 12 session AIDS risk reduction programme targeted at gay men during the late 1980s in the US state of

Mississippi. The programme recruited 104 men at high risk for HIV infection and randomised them into two groups: immediate intervention versus a four-month delay. The delay group served as a short-term control group.

Baseline data showed that participants in both groups used condoms in approximately 23% of all instances of anal intercourse. However, the study report does not differentiate between anal intercourse with regular partners and casual partners.

Programme participants were then exposed to a series of workshops on safer sex, assertiveness training, how to deal with risky sexual situations, how to avoid sex when intoxicated, how to raise the topic of safer sex and how to deal with safer sex within relationships.

Four months after the intervention participants had used condoms in 66% of all instances of anal intercourse, whilst members of the control group had used condoms in just 19% of all instances of anal intercourse. This rate of condom use was sustained during over two years of follow-up, and 60% of subjects completely refrained from unprotected anal intercourse during the follow-up period (Kelly).

Despite the short period of controlled study, it is reasonable to argue that this intervention had a significant effect on behaviour, but it raises the question of whether or not the success of the intervention was dose-related i.e. would a similar effect have been seen with six or even one workshop instead of twelve?

A US study shows that such methods can be translated to other population groups. A study of 197 African-American and Hispanic women with sexual histories suggesting HIV risk were invited to participate in a programme based at a Milwaukee primary health care clinic. They were randomised to two groups. One received a five session HIV risk reduction programme led by female group leaders. Women in the control group attended five sessions on unrelated health topics.

The HIV risk reduction programme included skills training in condom use, sexual assertiveness, examination of the circumstances which triggered risky behaviour for individuals and peer support for efforts to change behaviour. All skills training was developed with the assistance of a focus group to ensure that it was culturally appropriate.

Three months after the conclusion of the programme women in the intervention group reported condom use in 56% of sexual encounters involving vaginal intercourse. This was up from baseline of 26%. The number who used condoms at any time during the preceding three months rose from 43% to 66%. Participants also reported using condoms with a larger proportion of their male partners than at baseline. In contrast no changes in any of these variables were reported in the control group. Moreover, the women in the intervention group tended to have a more complete understanding of HIV risks, to have a more accurate personal estimation of their risk, and to view themselves as more personally vulnerable to HIV infection (Kelly 1992).

The study evaluation also looked at the quality of the skills developed by women to see whether the skills training component might have contributed to behaviour change. After three months women who had received skills training were rated by blinded evaluators as significantly more effective in resisting pressure to have sex without a condom, and in persuading a partner to postpone sex until a condom could be obtained.

Another US study piloted an intervention aimed at pregnant women that used a novel measure of efficacy: the use of credit cards which could be redeemed at local pharmacies to obtain condoms or spermicide. The programme enrolled 206 young single pregnant women in Akron and randomised them to one of three groups: HIV prevention, general health promotion and no intervention.

Women in the HIV prevention group were exposed to four small group sessions of 1 to 2 hours, which began after the fourteenth week of pregnancy. The group sessions focussed on the development of a sound 'health action' plan. To enhance cross-group consistency, sessions were built around the use of culturally relevant health videos. The thematic content of the health promotion and HIV prevention was linked, but specific content differed. For example, if participants were invited to focus on activities which might have a negative impact on the foetus, the health promotion group would be directed to discuss the impact of smoking and drinking, whilst the HIV groups would look at mother-to-baby transmission of HIV. Skills development included negotiation and assertiveness skills, role playing, problem solving and aversive conditioning (imagining adverse consequences of behaviour).

All study participants were also given credit cards that could be used only at local pharmacies to obtain either condoms or spermicide. The uptake of condoms and spermicide was used to measure the impact of the workshops. Interestingly there was no significant difference in the uptake of condoms or spermicide between the HIV prevention and health promotion groups, but there was a difference in behaviour: women in the HIV prevention group were more likely to use condoms or spermicide with their partners, and had a stronger intention to do so, after three and six months of follow up. However, the benefits obtained from the HIV prevention intervention were only moderately greater than those obtained from the health promotion group (Hobfoll). Both groups did better on all scores (HIV-related knowledge, safer sex intentions and behaviours, discussion of HIV risk with partners and condom usage) than the no-intervention control group.

This study would tend to suggest that free condom availability needs to be supported by educational activity and skills training if it is to be translated into safer behaviour.

A number of other US programmes have also provided controlled evidence of the effectiveness of multiple session workshop programmes focussing on the development of knowledge and skills. These include a study of HIV prevention workshops with homeless youth in hostel accommodation (Rotheram-Borus), which demonstrated that the level of change was proportional to the 'dose', with the greatest reductions in unprotected sex amongst those who attended 15 or more sessions during a period of three weeks' residence in a hostel (sessions lasted less than an hour).

Several studies discussed above (see *Social learning* in *Understanding behaviour change* above) also provide evidence of the success and replicability of the skills-based workshop approach (Jemmott). On the other hand, several randomised, controlled studies of group skills interventions show no advantage to participation in such programmes.

A programme for 102 Los Angeles youths with an average age of 12 showed no significant change in 19 of 21 attitudes and opinions about sexual behaviour and condom use. Researchers speculated that the intervention was too short (eight one hour sessions) and that the use of teenage mothers who achieved a good rapport with students may not have discouraged students from early sexual intercourse, but instead glamorised teen pregnancy (Kirby).

Another skills-based intervention which included the use of a comic book, videotape and a group skills curriculum showed no difference in levels of condom use between the intervention group and control group at six months (Gillmore), but researchers suggested that the null result may be attributable to the fact that the sample group were recruited from juvenile detention centres, and may have had no opportunity to practice the skills learnt during the workshops!

The research literature leaves unanswered the question of how many workshops might be adequate in order to sustain behaviour change. Unfortunately, no evaluation exists of the workshop programme developed by Gay Men Fighting AIDS in the UK, which contains many of the elements described above. The Sex Day format has been delivered to several thousand men in the UK since its inception in 1992, but no research evidence has been collected on the behavioural effects of this one-session intervention. It has been argued that a controlled trial of such an intervention would be impossible because it would be difficult to distinguish the effects of the intervention from those of other

HIV prevention activities. However, as the studies above show, this problem does not seem to have arisen for researchers looking at other high-risk populations.

References

Gillmore MR, et al. Effects of a skills-based intervention to encourage condom use among high risk heterosexually active adolescents, AIDS Education and Prevention 9, Supp A, 1997.

Hobfoll SE, et al. Reducing inner city women's risk activities: a study of single, pregnant women, Health Psychology 13:5 pp397-403, 1994.

Kelly J, et a. Behavioural interventions to reduce AIDS risk activities, Journal of Consulting and Clinical Psychology 57:1 pp60-67, 1989.

Kelly J, et al: HIV/AIDS prevention groups for high risk inner city women: intervention outcomes and effects on risk behaviour, paper to American Public Health Association, Nov 1992.

Kirby D, et al: An impact evaluation of Project SNAPP: an AIDS and pregnancy prevention middle school programme, AIDS Education and Prevention 9, SuppA, 1997.

Individual cognitive interventions

The cognitive interventions discussed above all rely on group formats for their delivery. This makes them labour intensive and unsuitable for large population interventions. However, a number of research teams have reported individual cognitive interventions which have proved effective.

Ron Gold reported a randomised controlled study using individual diaries to encourage men to examine their intentions and self-justifications regarding unprotected anal intercourse. Gay men were randomised to three groups and asked to keep a sexual diary for 16 weeks and send in completed pages each week. After four weeks men were randomised to one of three groups: a control group who received no intervention, a group who received safer sex posters with the request to evaluate their impact and effectiveness, and a group who were asked to fill in a questionnaire.

The questionnaire group were asked to reflect upon a recent occasion when they had engaged in unprotected anal intercourse, and were given a list of possible self-justifications for having unsafe sex. They were asked to indicate the extent to which each of these self-justifications had been on their mind at the moment they had decided to engage in unprotected anal intercourse. They were then asked to select the self-justifications that had been in their mind most strongly at the time; to indicate how reasonable each of these seemed to them now, looking back on it, an to briefly justify these responses. The men were thus asked to reflect on their thinking in the heat of the moment, and to justify it in the cold light of day.

A significant difference in sexual behaviour emerged by the end of the study period. Whilst there was no significant difference between the three groups in the numbers who had unprotected anal intercourse at least once, there was a significant difference between the self-justifications group and the others in terms of the amount of unprotected anal intercourse that took place during the 16 week study. 42% of the control group and 41% of the poster group had unprotected anal intercourse more than once, whereas only 17% of the self-justifications group had anal intercourse more than once.

Gold argues that the technique may exhibit a greater effect when individuals have unprotected sex after engaging in an examination of why they had unprotected sex. He comments: "Presumably their first post-intervention slip-up provoked and disturbed the men; their perception that they had done it again concentrated their mind on the problem. At that point they really began to absorb the lessons of the intervention."

References

Gold R, et al: AIDS education: has it gone wrong? National AIDS Bulletin March, 1995.

Community mobilisation

Community mobilisation is a term akin to community development, but it is used here to distinguish it from community development methods used in other health areas because it has a specific history in the HIV field.

Community mobilisation has been studied in several well-controlled trials in the United States. The most famous example is the Kelly study of opinion leaders, a randomised, controlled trial conducted amongst gay men in paired towns in four US states. The study tested the argument of social diffusion theorists, that if 15-20% of a population adopts an innovation, then it will be conveyed through natural social networking to cause community wide change. Many historians of safer sex have argued that this is how safer sex came to be adopted by gay men during the mid-1980s.

The study utilised 'opinion leaders' who were identified as the people most likely to influence their peers. Opinion leaders were identified by asking bartenders to nominate people they considered to be most liked and trusted by patrons. The opinion leaders selected were then invited to attend group sessions at which they were trained in ways of delivering HIV risk reduction messages to their peers. These methods included endorsing the benefits and timeliness of risk behaviour change, recommending strategies for implementing change and correcting risk misperceptions amongst their friends. The men were then invited to initiate twenty conversations amongst their friends over the following weeks.

The study was carried out in four states, with two cities in each state compared, one serving as a control and one as an intervention site. Three months and again six months later, surveys of all men entering bars in the intervention cities and control cities were carried out. The response rate was 85%, and unprotected anal intercourse in the intervention cities declined from 33% at baseline to under 25% at nine months, a reduction of 28%. No change was found in the control group.

The reported incidence of unprotected insertive anal sex fell from 27% to 18% over the same time period in the intervention cities, but the incidence of unprotected receptive anal sex fell more slowly. There was no change in the control cities.

When researchers analysed the results to determine the factors accounting for the changes in behaviour they had observed, they found that men who spent the most time in bars had the highest levels of risk behaviour at baseline. But they also showed the greatest reduction in such behaviour following intervention. Since most peer conversations probably took place in bars, the researchers hypothesised that there was a dose response effect. This was corroborated by men's own reports: those who reported being engaged in the greatest number of risk reduction conversations also reported the greatest reduction in risk behaviour.

Another US project, similar to Gay Men Fighting AIDS and a number of other UK projects in its design, was the Mpowerment project. This was tested by US National Institutes of Mental Health researchers in two West Coast cities, Santa Barbara, California, and Eugene, Oregon, in 1992.

Eugene received the intervention first whilst Santa Barbara served as control, and longitudinal cohorts of gay men aged 18 to 29 were recruited and assessed before and after by mail-back survey.

The project tested the hypothesis that involvement with the process of peer education would have an effect on risk behaviour. By allowing the community to take responsibility for behaviour change efforts, it was hoped to foster a deeper and longer lasting effect than one achieved by professionals.

A core group of 15 self-selected volunteers was recruited and given a brief to design the project, with advice from local academics, public health professionals and AIDS service organisations. The project developed several arms: peer outreach conducted by volunteers in bars, community events and events organised by the group itself. This outreach work also served to recruit other peer educators in a rolling programme of recruitment.

The group also organised a storefront drop-in centre and small group sessions focussing on safer sex information and skill development. The latter were attended by 170 young men in the town (estimated to represent at least 15% of the local gay population).

One year after the intervention a 26% reduction was reported in the number of individuals who reported any instance of unprotected anal intercourse. This included a 45% reduction in respondents reporting any unprotected anal intercourse with non-primary partners and a 24% reduction in those reporting an unprotected anal intercourse with primary partners. In contrast there was no change in these variables in the control city (Kegeles).

A study amongst injecting drugs users provides evidence that such methods need not be confined to gay men. The US National Institutes of Drug Abuse has studied the use of peer educators amongst injecting drug users, and concluded that a project employing volunteer drug users as peer educators and community development facilitators not only reduced the sharing of injecting equipment, but led to fall in HIV incidence in Chicago (Wiebel). However, this is the only controlled study amongst IDUs.

A problem with all of these examples of community mobilisation is the difficulty we have in judging the relationship contexts in which unprotected sex was taking place in these studies. Whilst the Mpowerment study did ask questions about unprotected sex with regular partners, the Kelly studies did not, and critics of the community mobilisation approach have argued that such interventions are only likely to have an effect on those having unprotected sex with casual partners. Those in regular partnerships may see themselves as immune from such messages and may need to be targeted specifically. However, these criticisms ignore the fact that all studies of community mobilisation have been studies of a methodology, not a message. In order to prove that community mobilisation is an inappropriate way to target men in relationships, it is necessary to design a study which looks at the diffusion of messages about unprotected sex in relationships. This has not yet happened.

Clearly these studies do not answer all the questions which might arise about the distribution of resources in a community mobilisation type project, but they do suggest that the level of contacts achieved need not be analogous to the total population of a district. However, the Kelly studies suggest that dosage and exposure were important elements in the success of the project.

Both studies support the need for knowledge of local sexual and social networks, and sensitivity to the customs and idiom of the local community. The selection of local informants is a crucial first stage in a community mobilisation project: if this goes wrong the project could veer off course.

There is also a danger that culturally specific problems could arise in replicating community mobilisation-type efforts in other countries. Evidence of this was supplied at a recent meeting of the British Psychological Society by Graham Hart, who reported on a study being conducted by the Medical Research Council's Medical Sociology Unit in Edinburgh and Glasgow, intended to replicate some elements of the Kelly and Kegeles studies (Williamson).

Among men who reported speakingwith peer educators 49% reported thinking about their sexualbehaviour and 26% reported changing their sexual behaviour. Lead researcher Lisa Williamson said that the study "appears to be an effective interventiontool in terms of the uptake of sexual health services, but isless effective in achieving actual sexual behaviour change amonghomosexual men."

Hart reported that local informants were none too keen on the idea of encouraging popular local figures to discuss intimate details of people's sex lives, because their popularity tended to be proportional to their store of local gossip! Many people would be unwilling to discuss intimate sexual matters with such popular but indiscreet figures.

Nevertheless, such evidence does suggest that the general concept of community mobilisation has a valuable contribution to make to HIV prevention activities. However, design and evaluation of future projects should proceed with an awareness of the limitations of current evidence, and should seek to add to the body of research knowledge about community mobilisation strategies. For example, is it adequate to reach 15-20% of the population to diffuse a message, and how would you measure this? What is the best balance of activities within community mobilisation?

References

Kegeles S, et a. The Mpowerment project: a community level HIV prevention intervention for young gay and bisexual men, Am J Public Health, in press, 1997.

Kelly JA, et al. HIV risk behaviour reduction following intervention with key opinion leaders of the population: an experimental analysis, Am J Public Health 81 pp168-171, 1991.

Kelly JA, et al. Community AIDS/HIV risk reduction: the effects of endorsements by popular people in three cities, Am J Public Health, 82 pp1483-1489, 1992.

Williamson, LM. The Gay Men's Task Force: the impact of peer education on the sexual health behaviour of homosexual men in Glasgow.

Social marketing

Social marketing is an approach which seeks to promote an innovation of social utility by using a variety of methods, including free distribution, promotion of the innovation and subsidised sale of the innovation.

Social marketing has had two huge successes in the AIDS epidemic: condom distribution and needle exchange. Needle exchange is discussed in detail above, as is condom distribution.

No research in the UK has yet been designed which is able to evaluate the impact of condom distribution on sexual behaviour, but social marketing theory suggests that well planned free condom distribution will have a number of impacts:

- Maintains the visibility of condoms in settings where people meet sexual partners

- Models condom use and the acceptability of carrying condoms

- Allows individuals to initiate conversations about condom use

- Provides appropriate condoms and lubricants

- Makes condoms easily available at times of day when people are likely to meet sexual partners

- Reduces the cost of condom use, and makes them available free

- Puts condoms into the hands of people who might not otherwise buy them, and who might choose to have sex on the spur of the moment.

Social marketing of condoms should also be backed up by media promotion which highlights each of these characteristics in ways designed to appeal to the target audience. A model example is a feature article published by the gay men's weekly *Boyz*, which interviewed men in the street about carrying condoms, and whether they had ever missed out on sex as a result of failing to carry condoms. The article modelled the acceptability and desirability of carrying condoms, and of ensuring that they were not out of date or damaged. Purchasing of condom distribution should include a plan for media coverage and promotion, and purchasers should ensure that agencies are resourced to deliver such editorial coverage among the target group media as a key part of their role.

Internet interventions

With the success of gay cruising sites like Gaydar and Gay.com, the Internet has become the meeting-place of choice for many gay men, offering as it does, initial anonymity and safety and a chance to get to know prospective partners before meeting them in person.

Researchers in London (Bolding) have found that by 2003 the proportion of gay men in the city who had met partners online had increased to over 50%, and 75% of HIV-positive men had done so. See **D is for disclosure, serosorting and negotiated safety** for more on the internet and its potential role in disclosure and serosorting.

In an article in Positive Nation by this writer in the same year, Sigma Research's Ford Hickson said: "The internet has led to increases in the number of men who have sex with men, and the number of partners they have, and the proportion who have anal sex, protected and unprotected."

The internet therefore offers an ideal place in which both to survey gay men about their sexual habits, and the inline survey has become such an important research tool that for last year's Gay Men's Sex Survey, Sigma Research abandoned their long-established practice of researchers interrogating gay men about their sex lives at gay festivals and for the first time distributed the survey only in two forms, as booklets in gay venues and as an online questionnaire.

The internet also has considerable power, potentially at least, to offer prevention interventions. The question is, what should these look like? The internet is much more than a set of pages on a computer screen. It is a tool for people to conduct their own sexual health research; a 'safe space' for people to explore sexual fantasies and fears; an intimate, dialogue-based meeting place; and the biggest lonely hearts column and porn magazine ever.

In the Positive Nation article, Mark Watson, European Director of Gay.com, said that the internet's interactive nature was its greatest strength, but one that HIV prevention organisations had not yet fully exploited.

Gaymen's encounters are in real time. The Internet is a 4D area and we have 2D prevention campaigns. Click on the Terrence Higgins Trust's gay men's prevention resources links and you'll get poster pdfs. The internet enables people to meet where they don't feel they will encounter social disapproval if they talk about fucking without condoms. That discussion is not about 'deliberate infection.' It's about guys discussing condom use - and being HIV-positive - in a place where it doesn't feel unsexy to do so.

The internet offers various possibilities for prevention interventions:

Banner ads with click-throughs to sexual health information sites and HIV and STD testing services.

- Example: InSPOT (www.inspot.org), a peer STD partner-notification site whereby people diagnosed with an STD can anonymously notify people they've met online

Social-marketing sites that aim to give positive messages about HIV prevention

- Examples: HIV Stops With Me (www.hivstopswithme.org), a site, backed by a poster campaign, featuring interviews with HIV-positive people about their life stories, relationships and safer sex strategies. Tagline: "Positive People Preventing HIV"

Moderated sexual health chatrooms

- Example: the Terrence Higgins Trust now run a 'Health Info' chatroom within the Gaydar chatrooms, only visible to people whose Gaydar profile locates them in England and Wales: HIV Scotland run a 'Scottish Netreach' site for people there.

HIV and sexual health information sites for people with specific needs such as drug users, ethnic minorities, youth, etc.

- Example: www.tweaker.org, an information and resource site, also offering a discussion board, for gay men who use methamphetamine (crystal meth)

Moderated or unmoderated internet discussion boards on sexual health and HIV

- Examples: numerous contact sites, such as Gay.com, offer discussion boards on various subjects such as health, relationships, HIV, coming out and lifestyle.

Contact and cruising sites specifically for people who with to find a partner of the same HIV status or who are specifically seeking protected sex

- Examples: there are a number of contact sites specifically for people with HIV in the USA, but only a few in the UK, such as the Positive Nation personal ads. In the USA www.safesexcity.com offers a site for gay men who specifically pledge to maintain safer sex.

Active interventions where sexual health workers engage people seeking unsafe sex or 'PnP' (sex, usually unsafe, with recreational drugs)

- This is a controversial intervention, as this kind of unsolicited contact can annoy internet users and, if the health worker is pretending to be a prospective contact, would be considered unethical by many people. It has been found useful in certain populations such as Spanish-speaking sites for gay men in the USA.

Does all this internet activity help people maintain sexual health? InSPOT is one of a number of sites run by the US consultancy ISIS (Internet Sexuality Information Services - www.isis-inc.org) a not-for-profit organisation that aims to help sexual health providers develop innovative ways of reaching people and offering online help. ISIS developed a syphilis testing campaign (www.stdtest.org) that offered theatre and book coupons in return for getting a test, and banner ads on cruising sites. The banner ads got 32,000 hits in two months on gay.com and 5,000 redeemed their test coupons.

In terms of information provision and discussion, unsolicited messaging via email or chat messages does not usually work. In a 2001 survey of people (of all sexualities) who completed an online survey of sexual risk behaviour (Bull) most indicated they would visit a websitefor STD/HIV prevention information (61%), but fewer would openan E-mail (45%) or chat (30%) about the topic.

One of the most promising ways of using the internet is by using discussion boards to help people provide each other with mutual support and information, thus mobilising a 'virtual community' - something that works for classic car collectors or Star Trek fans, so it should work for people worried about HIV too.

The potential pitfalls of this approach include the internet's well-known tendency to encourage abuse ('flaming') and contributors posting inaccurate or harmful information. For this reason discussion boards need to be tightly moderated - which considerably increases their cost. Marginalised communities like African immigrants with unsettled residency status are also less likely to have the ability to access the internet in privacy which such interventions need.

References

Bolding G. Sex with casual partners among London MSM: is the Internet more risky? 15th International AIDS Conference, Bangkok. Abstract WePeC6053. 2004.

Bull SS et al. Barriers to STD/HIV prevention on the Internet. *Health Education Research* 16(6): 661-670. 2001.

Cairns G. Cybersafersex - Catching HIV in the Net. *Positive Nation* 106: 38-9. 2004.

What interventions can be recommended?

A number of conclusions can be drawn from the evidence discussed in this chapter and in other effectiveness reviews.

Community mobilisation methods have been proven to work

Research evidence clearly demonstrates that community-based education efforts which rely on diffusion techniques and the development of skills lead to behaviour change. There are also sound theoretical reasons (see *Social diffusion* above) for assuming that well-planned and carefully managed community mobilisation interventions which are sensitive to the values and the diversity of a community will be successful in reducing the incidence of HIV infection, although no study has yet been designed to test this assumption.

There is a dose-response in HIV prevention activities

A variety of intervention studies provide evidence that greater exposure to HIV prevention messages, skills building and community norms which promote safer behaviour will be more effective than one-off or occasional interventions. This requires the development of a sequence of activities which are co-ordinated to achieve an adequate level of exposure amongst members of the target group, not one-off interventions.

Intervention techniques are adaptable to different communities and risk situations

The medium is not the message. Many of the interventions described in this chapter can be adapted to different communities and to communicate different types of messages. There is no reason why techniques already successfully deployed amongst gay men, African-American youth and injecting drug users should not work with other groups, provided that they are culturally sensitive. Nor is there any reason to abandon tried and tested methods simply because HIV prevention messages are becoming more complex.

Interventions must have a sound basis in research on risk and behavioural change

Much HIV prevention work taking place now is based on a mish-mash of theories about behaviour change and HIV risk factors. All the interventions discussed in this chapter have one thing in common: a clearly thought-out rationale based on a set of research findings about HIV risk and the way that human behaviour can be influenced.

A variety of tools exist for measuring the success of prevention activities: use them

Using a combination of outcome measures may be the best way of evaluating the effectiveness of a programme of interventions. Unless very sound evidence exists of the relationship between one variable and HIV incidence, the value of a project should not be assessed on the basis of changes in one variable alone. HIV prevention needs to develop performance indicators which measure quality hand in hand with quantity of activity.

Interventions should challenge reasoning, not just risk perception

Many of the interventions discussed contained cognitive components designed to make people think about the ways they rationalise risky activities. This is not proof in itself that reasoning needs to be foregrounded in future activities, but it does suggest a potentially useful avenue for research and project development.

How can we get best value for money in HIV prevention now?

It depends which population is being targeted. Amongst gay men, community mobilisation coupled with more interventionist counselling techniques in STD clinics might yield the best returns, together with a continued emphasis on condom distribution. Face-to-face outreach work does not appear cost-effective in comparison with media work and free condom distribution, particularly in large population centres. Research which can

identify the reasons for seroconversions, and which can clarify the future role of GUM clinics in HIV prevention is urgently needed, and would be a good investment.

Amongst African communities, diffusion of safer sex messages is likely to be best accomplished by community organisations and community organisers, but the measurement of outcomes is hampered by fact that it will be difficult to judge whether HIV infections have been avoided as a consequence of HIV prevention activities in the UK or in African countries. However, recent evidence gathered by a variety of research projects suggests that there are big variations between African communities in levels of knowledge about HIV, and an investment is needed in action research which can point the way towards more extensive activities.

Amongst injecting drugs users, an investment in treatment and maintenance of injecting drug users together with the continuation of syringe exchange programmes is likely to keep HIV incidence low.

Needs assessment and evaluation: further reading

This chapter does not offer detailed guidance on population needs assessment or evaluation methodologies because a wealth of literature now exists on this subject. Amongst the best sources of information are:

Rhodes T. Risk intervention and change: HIV prevention and drug use, Health Education Authority, 1994.

Scott P. Purchasing HIV Prevention: a No-Nonsense Guide for Use with Gay and Bisexual Men, Health Education Authority, London, 1995.

Scott P, and Warwick I, with Durbin H. A Pilot Needs Assessment and Evaluation Training Project, The HIV Project, London, 1996.

Scott P. Moving Targets: An assessment of the needs of gay man and of bisexual men in relation to HIV prevention in Enfield and Haringey, a report published by Enfield and Haringey Health Authority, London, 1996.

Warwick I, Orr K and Whitty G. Local HIV prevention needs assessment for gay and bisexual men: a review and recommendations for action, Health Education Authority, 1995.

Weatherburn P, et al. Behaviourally bisexual men in the UK: identifying needs for HIV prevention, Health Education Authority, 1996.

Woodhead D, Warwick I and Whitty G: Developing Local HIV Prevention Assessments with Gay and Bisexual Men, Health Education Authority, London, 1995.

Further sources of information

This review is not an exhaustive discussion of all evaluated interventions in HIV prevention. It raises a number of issues about research into such interventions, and highlights particularly successful interventions. For further information about research in each of these areas, you can go to:

- EppiCentre (Evidence for Policy and Practice Information and Co-ordinating, University of London Institute of Education) (020 7612 6393; health@ioe.ac). Website: http://eppi.ioe.ac.uk/ . In July 2004 the EPPI Centre conducted a systematic review of research relevant to the development and implementation of effective and appropriate interventions among gay men in the UK. This can be downloaded from the website.

Charges apply to individuals outside the North Thames region for EppiCentre services.

- A useful summary of research evidence from the US is available at http://www.AIDSCAP. Copies of a twenty page review of current data can be downloaded, along with factsheets (somewhat rudimentary and US biased in their data analysis).

- A review article, *Prevention of HIV infection*, by Kyung-Hee Choi and Thomas J. Coates, was published in AIDS, 1994, 8:1371-1389. It includes discussion of interventions in developing countries

- A book, *Preventing AIDS: Theories and methods of behavioural interventions* by Ralph DiClemente and John Peterson (Plenum Press, New York, 1994) provides a useful and detailed overview of interventions reported up to 1994, although its focus is largely confined to US populations

- A supplement to the journal *AIDS Education and Prevention* (volume 9, number 1), on effectiveness of behavioural interventions, was published in 1997

- A review, *AIDS prevention strategies that work: a review of National Institutes of Mental Health-sponsored research*, was published in 1996 by the Office on AIDS and the US National Institutes of Mental Health.

Positive prevention

The idea that HIV-positive people should be the principal target for HIV prevention programmes is not a new one. After all, Positive People form 50% of the people present at any HIV transmission event and yet are a minority of the population. So programmes directed at them will have a disproportionate effect.

Positive Prevention encompasses two ideas: HIV prevention *targeted* at people with HIV, and HIV prevention *led* by people with HIV.

Targeting evidence-based HIV prevention and sexual harm reduction programmes at people with HIV makes sense:

- on an economic level because an HIV-positive person is involved in every HIV transmission event,

- on a legal level because people with HIV are at risk of prosecution for transmission,

- on a human rights level because people with HIV have demonstrably greater sexual and mental health needs.

The idea of positive-*led* prevention comes from the scientific evidence that, once diagnosed, people with HIV do take steps to reduce the risk of infecting others.

the uninfected. In a recent paper, the International HIV/AIDS Alliance suggested why:

"Most prevention strategies to date have been targeted at uninfected people to prevent them from becoming infected with HIV. Historically, there has been a reluctance to work on HIV/STI prevention with people with HIV because of perceptions that the concept of prevention for people already infected is inherently contradictory.

"There have also been justifiable concerns about victimising an already stigmatised group. In addition, there has been a reluctance to acknowledge that people with HIV have sex, and also to get to grips with the complex ethical issues surrounding people with HIV's responsibilities towards others."

'Positive Prevention' is therefore potentially an extremely effective tool against HIV, but not always one that has a positive effect on *people* with HIV.

The paper that contains the quote above was drafted by the AIDS Alliance in 2002. It proposes a very wide definition of what 'positive prevention' is, dividing the activity into 17 different strategies thus:

3.1 Individually focused health promotion	3.2 Sealing up, targeting and improving service and commodity delivery	3.3 Community mobilisation	3.4 Advocacy, policy change and community awareness
Strategy 1: Promoting voluntary councelling and testing	Strategy 5: Ensuring availability of voluntary testing	Strategy 9: Facilitating post-test clubs and other peer support groups	Strategy 14: Involving people with HIV in decision-making for Positive Prevention
Strategy 2: Providing post-test and ongoing councelling for positive people	Strategy 6: Provoding antiretroviral treatment for Positive Prevention	Strategy 10: Implementing focused communication campaigns	Strategy 15: Advocacy for Positive Prevention
Strategy 3: Encouraging beneficial disclosure and ethical partner notification	Strategy 7: Reducing stigma and integrating Positive Prevention into treatment centres	Strategy 11: Training people with HIV as peer outreach workers	Strategy 16: Legal reviews and legislative reform
Strategy 4: Providing councelling for sero-discordant couples	Strategy 8: Providing services for preventing mother-to-child transmission	Strategy 12: Reinforcing Positive Prevention through home-based care	Strategy 17: Advocacy for access to treatment
		Strategy 13: Addressing HIV-related gender-based violence in Positive Prevention	

Since, as discussed above, it is easier to support and reinforce an existing behaviour than to completely change it, HIV prevention strategies should be advised from the 'bottom up' by what people with HIV and their partners already do. They should be tailored to help people sustain behaviour that supports good sexual health and relationships, and to address barriers to adopting those behaviours (such as fear of disclosure, depression or substance abuse).

One 1999 paper (King-Spooner) comments:

"Preventive interventions with positive individuals are likely to have a greater impact on the epidemic, for an equivalent input of cost, time, resources, than preventative interventions focused on negative individuals. A change in the risky behaviour of an HIV-positive person will, on average, and in almost all affected populations, have a much bigger impact on the spread of the virus than an equivalent change in the behaviour of an HIV-negative person."

Yet throughout the history of the epidemic far fewer prevention resources have been directed at people living with HIV than at

What's interesting about this grid of 17 strategies is that it doesn't in any way make any recommendations as to the content or methodology of any of the strategies it recommends. How is voluntary counselling and testing to be promoted, and how voluntary is voluntary? What kind of counselling works best? How does one encourage beneficial disclosure and reduce stigma? What kind of peer support works best and how can it promote safer sex practices? What content should focused communication campaigns have? And, if you involve people with HIV in positive prevention, what will they say they want?

In other words, with Positive prevention we are back revisiting the HIV prevention versus sexual health promotion debate. Should positive prevention be a public health endeavour aimed at helping or coercing, by whatever means work best, people with HIV to keep their virus to themselves? Or should it be positive-*led* promotion, a way of helping people with HIV as a shared-interest community develop sexual health strategies and HIV prevention strategies that work best for them?

We have already mentioned above under **Counsellingand HIV antibody testing** that one version of 'positive prevention' is the medicalised one currently being spearheaded by the Centres for the Disease Control in the USA which aims to divert funds away from HIV intervention programmes targeting the whole community, or vulnerable communities, and instead use them to get more people tested for HIV and to offer them intensive support - though they are rather vaguer about post-test support.

Responding to political disapproval of community HIV prevention programmes, on 15 April 2003 the US Centers for Disease Control initiated what they called the Serostatus Approach to Fighting the Epidemic (SAFE). This involved a refocusing and reallocation of HIV prevention resources on to people with HIV. Henceforward, the CDC announced, it would focus on a drive to maximise the number of people tested for HIV - some papers, indeed recommended universal testing for all adults. Once people had tested HIV-positive they would be managed by "ongoing case management, medical interventions, and support for other psychosocial stressors."

There is some justification for laying a very strong emphasis on testing as a key element in HIV prevention. According to the CDC's own statistics, there are over 900,000 people with HIV in the USA. About 700,000 know their status. The annual incidence (new infection) rate is about five per cent a year. But if you just count those infected by people who know their status, it is less than two per cent (1.73%). Conversely, HIV incidence in partners of HIV+ people who do *not* know their status is nearly 11% a year (10.79%) (Holtgrave and Anderson).

The figures above detailing reduction in incidence after testing tell us nothing about whether people with HIV actually modify their behaviour to reduce the chance of infecting others post-testing. And they tell us even less about how to support them in making any behaviour change, if they do.

Testing people with HIV will obviously bring down infection rates in itself because many will be start taking antiretrovirals. A study of gay men in San Francisco (Porco) calculated that the average HIV infectivity of the population declined by 60% after the introduction of HAART.

However other studies have found that this did not result in immediate declines in incidence, but rather increases (Katz); HIV incidence doubled from 2.1% a year to 4.2% a year in San Francisco between 1995 and 1999. Mathematical modelling (Law) has calculated that it would only take a 30% increase in serodiscordant unprotected sex to counterbalance a 50% decline in infectiousness.

This underlines the importance of testing, because it suggests that if incidence in the partners of tested HIV-positive people is indeed less than a sixth of that in the partners of untested people, then a large proportion of HIV must be transmitted by untested people or those infected since their last test.

This has led, in the USA at least, to calls for universal HIV testing -with two surveys (Sanders, Paltiel) showing this would be cost-effective - and more recently with a change of heart in prevention activists leading to the decision to allow the sale of over-the-counter HIV tests. It is more doubtful if universal testing in the UK would be cost-effective, as we still only have a third of the USA's HIV prevalence. And prevention experts and public bodies alike in the UK do not seem to be ready for self testing.

However the decrease in incidence from tested partners cannot be due entirely to reduced infectiousness due to their taking HAART . No more than 74% of the tested US HIV-positive population is taking HAART (McNaghten) of which no more than 80% are virally suppressed at any one time. Therefore, at best, one would expect incidence in the partners of tested HIV-positive to be about 40% of those with untested partners. Instead it is about 16% of that figure. In other words the reduction in HIV infectivity accounts for less than half of the reduction in incidence.

So what positive-led prevention should do is to answer the following three questions:

- How did those tested people managed to reduce the number of people they infected post-testing?

- What behaviour changes did they make to achieve this?

- And what could be done better to support them in those behaviour changes?

Why positive prevention may look very different

It's an interesting question as to why, when it seems such an obvious idea, the development of interventions for people with HIV has been such a relatively neglected idea.

As we said above in the discussion on 'primary and secondary prevention' (under **HIV prevention or sexual health promotion?**), people with HIV have fundamentally the same need for interventions that can help them attain and maintain better sexual health as people without HIV.

However, the motives for maintaining safer sex, and therefore the kind of psychological reinforcement that best supports it, may also be very different.

In November 2000 a CHAPS campaign, "In Two Minds", depicted the rationalisations gay men may make to give themselves 'permission' to have unprotected sex. The head is depicted giving the reason *for* safer sex; the groin giving the rationalisation against it. All but one picture were of models depicting HIV-negative men. The THT wanted to include an HIV-positive man in the campaign, but ran into difficulties deciding what it should depict him thinking.

An extract from a *Positive Nation* piece that discussed this campaign is worth featuring because it depicts how different the decision processes are that HIV-positive people make, and the difficulty of fitting them into a 'One size fits all' campaign. The problem they had was that the HIV-negative men had a clear and identical motive (rationalised away differently) for avoiding HIV, namely fear of infection. But what was the positive man's motive?

Jack Summerside of CHAPS told Positive Nation: "In the first draft of the advert, he was saying '*What if he trusts me to protect him?*'' The team did not think this would work because they did not believe that HIV-positive men, realistically, were motivated by pure altruism. So if positive men aren't scared of infection, what are they scared of? Research provides the answer: Isolation, ostracism, and being unwanted.

"So in the end we reverted to a line we'd tried out earlier. '*I'll get a hard time if he finds out I've got HIV and didn't use a condom.*'"

The difficulty of finding a wording that fitted with the rest of the campaign typifies the problem of attempting to skirt round the fact that in many ways negative and positive gay men are totally different 'interest communities'. They are united by their gay identity and by personal bonds. But the motives for maintaining sexual safety are utterly different.

The THT are to be praised for including a positive image in this campaign (though more than one might have been better). But the difficulty of finding a wording that fitted with the rest of the campaign typifies the problem of attempting to skirt round the fact that in many ways negative and positive gay men are totally different 'interest communities'.

They are united by their gay identity and by personal bonds. But the motives for maintaining sexual safety are utterly different.

If one looks at HIV prevention from the theoretical viewpoint of the Health Beliefs Model, the activity is about reinforcing and reminding people that unpleasant emotions are a consequence of HIV transmission. In this case HIV-negative people are motivated by an emotion - fear - that is caused by contemplating an existential and unvarying *physical* phenomenon - death and disease.

In contrast, HIV-positive people are motivated by an emotion - shame - that is caused by contemplating a contingent and variable *social* phenomenon - stigma and isolation. Campaigns and prevention interventions may run into problems - not least, that of reinforcing stigma - when they try to reinforce this emotion in the same way.

The findings from the Albarracin meta-review that 'threat' messages were not as counterproductive when used to frame prevention messages for people with HIV, as they were for people without, and Jean Richardson's finding that 'loss framed' messages work better for people with HIV, give some credence to this idea.

The other reason positive prevention may look very different is that, historically, the steps people with HIV and especially gay men have taken to contain their infection may look at the time very different from what health-promotion experts are recommending.

The best example of this is the controversy about 'barebacking'.

'Barebacking' originally signified a transgressive, eroticised seeking out and adoption of unprotected sex by gay men as a rebellion against the norms of HIV prevention messages. As well as involving the sexual charge of doing socially proscribed acts, it has also involved an eroticisation of HIV and HIV transmission themselves, with language terms evolving such as 'bugchaser' and 'giftgiver' for men who seek - or who *fantasise* about seeking - to respectively receive and transmit HIV.

These may be seen as attempts to conquer the extreme anxiety of AIDS by controlling it via eroticisation; similarly, sado-masochism may be seen as a way of controlling anxieties about humiliation and inadequacy. Or they can be seen as an extreme version of compensation for the all-pervasive shadow of HIV stigma - defiantly making 'cool' and sexy what is deemed by society to be most sinful and depraved.

Unsurprisingly 'barebacking' created a media furore, with documentary films like *The Gift* (Louise Hogarth, 2002) exploring this apparently self-destructive gay subculture. But what barebacking *was* and what it *did* may have been two different things. Because it involved a way whereby HIV-positive men attempted to make the deeply unsexy (HIV and disease) sexy and thereby conquer their own internalised stigma, it seems to have become in part a *code* for "I'm HIV-positive", if for no other reason that the next question to a barebacker seeking sex in a chatroom is usually "are you poz?"

In other words, it usually involved disclosure: disclosure not as an act of pure altruism or social responsibility, but disclosure in the service of sex, and therefore motivated much more powerfully than pure altruism could be.

In a 2003 paper (Race) entitled "Re-evaluation of Risk among Gay Men", Kane Race of the National Centre in HIV Social Research at the University of New South Wales comments:

It is unknown at this stage whether barebacking has had a positive or negative effect on new HIV infections. While there are sporadic reports that some HIV-negative gay men make sense of some of the unprotected anal intercourse in which they engage in terms of barebacking, the phenomenon tends to be associated with HIV-positive men. Thus, the effect may be to increase, rather than decrease, the degree of seroconcordance in the total number of sexual encounters. Barebacking may have the effect of partner sorting in a manner analogous to negotiated safety. Unlike HIV-negative men, HIV-positive men require only one HIV test to adequately ascertain their HIV status, thus this possible prevention ethic need not occur in the context of a regular relationship.

What this implies is that people with HIV often do seek to reduce the risk of passing on their infection to others, but may do so in ways that are contrary to received public health opinion or run ahead of it and are also extremely difficult to imagine promoting.

An example is serosorting - the restriction of unprotected sex to people with the same HIV status. Although this may be starting to contribute significantly to apparent reductions in HIV incidence in some US cities (Truong), public health workers are not yet ready to promote it as an HIV prevention measure, as it looks uncomfortably like promoting unprotected sex.

In a recent article in the *Bay Area Reporter* (Bajko) Jeff McConnell, an HIV prevention researcher, said: "If you are talking to a guy who uses condoms all the time and has a perfect record, you wouldn't want to counsel him on serosorting.but if you are counselling an individual who cannot use condoms consistently or refuses to use them, you do want to talk to them about serosorting." But co-researcher Dr Robert Grant said: "I think that it may be deemed inappropriate for public health messages to recommend one type of partnership over another."

The way to square this circle, of course, is to provide the kind of HIV prevention that doesn't involve *telling* people to do anything. Positive prevention may have to involve detaching HIV prevention form the idea of 'health promotion' altogether, making it something much more like a combination of community mobilisation and self-efficacy training.

What works in Positive Prevention?

Two meta-reviews of HIV prevention interventions specifically directed at people with HIV have come out in the first few months of 2006, finally amending the dearth of review-level research in the area - although they still concentrate entirely on US studies.

In the first, Nicole Crepaz of the Centers for Disease Control sifted through 310 studies of prevention programmes for people with HIV and filtered out all but the 12 whose standard of evidence stood up to the most rigorous scientific scrutiny. In total 4,052 people with HIV participated in these 12 programmes.

Crepaz concluded that HIV-positive people responded at least as well as HIV-negative people, and possibly better, to prevention interventions. She found a significant reduction of sexual risk incidents in participants in the 12 programmes (Odds Ratio 0.57), and a reduction in the amount of STIs (Odds Ratio 0.21, though only a minority of programmes measured this). Programmes designed to reduce needle-sharing in drug users also produced significant improvements in risk behaviour (OR 0.47).

By comparing one study with another, Crepaz found that the most effective interventions were ones that:

- Specifically taught people how to negotiate condom use and safer sex as their main focus

- Also included help for other aspects of living with HIV, such as disclosing your status, medication adherence and maintaining self-esteem

- Were intensive, that is which involved at least 10 sessions delivered over at least three months

- Were delivered in a clinical setting or at a voluntary organisation that already provided services to people with HIV, rather than in outreach or community settings

- Were at least partly delivered by professional counsellors

- And were at least partly delivered on a one-to-one basis.

Crepaz found that the least effective programmes were those which simply delivered information on transmission risk and condom effectiveness.

In the second meta-review, Blair T Johnson of the University of Connecticut analysed 15 studies, some of them ones that Crepaz also analysed. Some of the studies were split into different more than one different intervention (including the 'gain frame' and 'loss frame' trial by Jean Richardson cited above) so Johnson was able to study a total of 19 different interventions.

Programmes used varied techniques such as group therapy, support, role-plays, videos, telephone support and one-to-one counselling and lasted from 18 days to 45 weeks.

Johnson found that, on average, they produced an overall increase in condom use of 16% overall relative to baseline - not as good as Albarracin's 'active' programmes, but as good as or better than her 'passive' ones. Johnson, like Albarracin, used this measure of effectiveness as it was the one used most frequently as the measure of success.

However Johnson found no change whatsoever in the number of partners people had after intervention. Only seven out of the 19 programmes measured if the number of partners changed, however, and Johnson suggests that this may have been confounded by people doing things not measured by researchers instead of reducing partners, such as serosorting. The most effective, a 2000 programme directed at HIV-positive teenagers in Los Angeles, increased their condom use by 82% compared with a control group. However some were unsuccessful, and the only non-US programme, directed at HIV-positive people in Tanzania, actually reduced condom use by 25%. Johnson found that programmes that worked had three characteristics.

Firstly, they tended to be directed at younger people. Programmes where the average age of participants was 20 worked five times better than ones directed at 40-year-olds. Johnson hypothesised that older people tend more often to be in long-term relationships where sexual habits are harder to shift, and says that better interventions for long-term couples where one partner has HIV need to be devised.

Secondly, the ones that worked were either motivational or taught people behavioural skills, and programmes which did both worked even better. 'Motivational' was the word Johnson used for programmes that provided things that improved participants' overall quality of life such as increased social support or self-confidence.

Programmes that provided information on HIV risk alone had no effect; ones that added in either motivation or behavioural skills increased condom use by 12%; and ones providing all three things increased it by 33%.

Thirdly, and disappointingly, programmes directed at gay men didn't work, by and large and, conversely, ones that excluded gay men were effective, increasing condom use by 42%.

However Johnson doesn't see this as evidence that gay men are uniquely deaf to safer-sex advice and support. He points out that not one single programme directed at gay men provided both ingredients proven to be necessary - they either provided greater social support or taught behavioural skills but not one did both.

Johnson criticises the lack of scientific research into ways of helping HIV-positive people maintain safer sex and reduce HIV transmission. He comments:

Perhaps the most surprising finding of this work is that more than two decades into the epidemic, there have been so few randomly-controlled trials of interventions that focus in people living with HIV, though there have been literally hundreds of studies conducted with uninfected populations. There is an urgent need for research in this area.

References

Bajko Matthew S. Few Health Officials Ready to Promote Serosorting. *Bay Area Reporter* 08 May 2006.

Crepaz N et al. Do prevention interventions reduce HIV risk behaviours among people living with HIV? A meta-analytic review of controlled trials. *AIDS* 20:143-157. 2006.

Holtgrave DR, Anderson T. Utilizing HIV transmission rates to assist in prioritizing HIV prevention services. *Int J STD AIDS*. 15(12):789-92. 2004.

International HIV/AIDS Alliance. Positive Prevention: Draft background paper. July 2003. May be downloaded from http://www.aidsalliance.org/sw9438.asp

Johnson BT et al. Sexual risk reduction for persons living with HIV: Research synthesis of randomised controlled trials, 1993 to 2004. *JAIDS* 41(5): 642-650. 2006.

Katz MH. Impact of Highly Active Antiretroviral Treatment on HIV Seroincidence among Men Who Have Sex with Men: San Francisco.*American Journal of Public Health* 92(3):

King-Spooner S. HIV prevention and the positive population. *Int J STD AIDS* 10(3):141-50. 1999.

Law MG. Modelling the effect of combination antiretroviral treatments on HIV incidence. *AIDS* 15(10) 1287-1294. 2001.

McNaghten AD. Gender disparity in HIV treatment and AIDS opportunistic illnesses (OI). Int Conf AIDS, Bangkok, July 2004. Abstract MoOrC1032.

Paltiel DA et al. Expanded screening for HIV in the United States -- An analysis of cost-effectiveness. *N Engl J Med* 352:586-95. 2005.

Porco TC et al. Decline in HIV infectivity following the introduction of highly active antiretroviral therapy. *AIDS* 18(1):81-8. 2004.

Race KD. Revaluation of Risk among Gay Men. *Social Research,* Issues Paper No. 1. National Centre in HIV Social Research, University of New South Wales. August 2003.

Sanders GD et al. Cost-effectiveness of screening for HIV in the era of highly active antiretroviral therapy. *N Engl J Med* 352:570-85. 2005.

Truong HM et al. Increases in "Serosorting" May Prevent Further Expansion of the HIV Epidemic among MSM in San Francisco. 11th Conference on Retroviruses and Opportunistic Infections, San Francisco. Abstract 843. 2004.

Drug use and harm reduction

Why do people use drugs?

People who use drugs do so for a number of different reasons including; for enjoyment, for fun, for excitement, because they are curious, to escape, to relax, to give them more confidence, to stay awake, to go to sleep, out of habit, because they are dependent, to help them cope with life, to manage physical and/or mental health problems, because their friends do, to experiment, to enhance a good experience or because they are bored. Every individual will use drugs for their individual reason or combination of reasons.

If you include legal drugs such as alcohol, cigarettes and caffeine (found in tea, coffee, chocolate), it is possible to see that we are all more likely than not to use drugs at some time in our lives.

With the popularity of so-called 'recreational drugs' such as Ecstasy, more and more young people will be experiencing illicit drug use even if they do not see themselves as drug users. Only the minority of drug users will ever feel they have a problem with their drug use, and not all of these will approach specialist services.

Drug groups

Drugs tend to be classified according to their effects into three main groups.

Stimulants

The physical effects of these drugs included an over-stimulation of the nervous system creating energised muscles, increased heart rate, increased blood pressure and decreased appetite. A stimulant can cause heart, blood vessel and seizure problems, particularly if large amounts are used or if the user is extra sensitive.

A moderate dose of the stronger stimulants can make one feel more confident, outgoing, eager to perform, euphoric and excited. Larger doses or prolonged use of the stronger stimulants can cause anxiety, paranoia and mental confusion.

Drugs in this group include; Caffeine, Nicotine, Amphetamine, Cocaine / Crack, Anabolic Steroids, Amyl Nitrates and Ecstasy.

Depressants

The physical effects of these drugs include slowed heart rate and respiration, decreased muscular coordination and energy and a dulling of the senses. Downers can cause constipation, nausea and sexual dysfunction.

Initially, small doses can act like stimulants because they lower inhibitions, but as more is taken the overall depressants effect begins to dominate, dulling the mind and slowing the body. Downers can also induce euphoria, or a sense of well-being.

Solvents and Gases can cause dizziness, slurred speech, unsteady gait, and drowsiness. Solvents can be quite toxic to lung, brain, liver and kidney tissues, and some can lower blood pressure, causing the user to faint or lose balance. With small amounts of solvents, impulsiveness, excitement and irritability are common.

Drugs in this group include; Alcohol, Solvents, Gases, GHB, Barbiturates, Benzodiazepines, Opiates (Heroin, Morphine, Methadone, Narcotic Analgesics), Ketamine and Rohypnol.

Hallucinogens

These drugs can distort perceptions to induce delusions or hallucinations. The physical effects can cause nausea and dizziness. Marijuana increases appetite and makes the eyes bloodshot. LSD raises the blood pressure and causes sweating. Drugs that alter perceptual function overload or distort messages to and from the brain stem, the sensory switchboard for the mind, so that many physical stimuli, particularly visual ones, are intensified or distorted. Imaginary messages can also be created by the brain. Drugs in this group include; LSD, Magic Mushrooms, Cannabis / Grass / Skunk and Ecstasy

Factors which influence the effects of drugs

There are a number of factors which influence the experience that an individual will have when taking drugs, therefore not everybody who takes a substance will have the same experience.

Drug factors

The effects of drugs will depend on a number of factors including which substance is taken, whether it is a stimulant, depressant or a hallucinogenic drug, as well as the amount of each drug taken. The purity of illicit drugs is unknown, and so the user will never know how much of the active ingredient is in what they are taking. The overall effect of each substance will also vary according to what other drugs it is taken with, both illicit drugs and prescribed drugs. The method of use and the period of time over which the substance is used will also impact on the effects of the drugs on the individual.

Individual factors

Individual factors will also influence the effects of the drugs. These included their state of mind when they take drugs (how the user is feeling), their state of health and their expectation regarding what will happen. If the individual is low in mood and feeling unwell they are less likely to have a positive experience when taking substances than if they are in a positive state of mind and feel physically well. In addition, if the individual thinks they have taken one substance, but have actually taken another substance then they will not experience the effect that they are expecting. For example, with Ecstasy users may expect to experience the effects of taking a stimulant drugs, but if the tablet actually contains a depressant, such as ketamine, they will experience a different effect. Knowledge and experience will also have an effect - somebody who has taken the substance before will know what to expect. Other issues include weight, sex and age, which can impact on the size of the drug effect on the individual.

Situational factors

Situational factors will also have an impact on the drug experience. Where the person is when they take the drugs and who they are with can be important. If a person takes a drug at a party with friends they may have a positive experience, however, if they then lose their friends and the party gets raided by the police, for example, then they are much more likely to experience negative effects, such as paranoia and anxiety. What the individual has to do next is also important - if they are able to go home and relax then they are less likely to experience any negative effects than say for example, they had to go to work or to a family gathering. Atmosphere and situation are therefore important factors in the drug experience. How often the user uses the drug is also important, as frequent use can have an impact on the user's physical health, such as weakening the immune system and leaving them feeling run down, which may make the drug use more difficult to tolerate. Regular use can also leave the user feeling tired, depressed or anxious as a result of regular 'come downs' which may mean the individual is not able to recover fully before they use again, thereby increasing the chance of a negative experience.

Potential problems of drug use

It is worth noting that many individuals who take drugs do not experience any problems at all. This may depend on the individual's level of use, social support and financial situation. However, potentiall problems could include:

Lifestyle

Regular or frequent drug use can lead to problems at school, college or work particularly if it effects the individual's concentration or attendance. Regular drug use can leave the individual feeling irritable or tired and drug users may find that they have problems with relationships with friends, family members or partners. Conflicts can be caused as a result of their drug use if other people do not approve of their use, and these can include conflicts with authority due to the illegal nature of much drug use. Regular use can lead to financial problems, and this may have a knock on effect on the individual's ability to pay bills or rent.

Physical health

An individuals' physical health can be affected as a result of the drugs used, the method of drug use (such as injecting) as well as due to accidents whilst on drugs. When under the influence of drugs individuals may engage in more risk taking behaviour and this can lead to accidents, for example drink driving.

Mental health

An individuals' mental health can be affected as a result of drug use. The 'come down' effect can leave many users having mood changes - they may feel depressed, anxious or even have suicidal thoughts following a period of drug use. Some individuals may also have these feelings when they have taken certain substances, and may also feel paranoid or have disturbing thoughts when on substances. Regular drug use can lead to individuals losing their self-confidence without drugs which can lead to a psychological dependency.

Legal issues

As a result of the illegal nature of many drugs, users risk being arrested for possession and possibly dealing offences. Many 'recreational users' may find themselves facing a dealing charge simply from 'sorting out' supplies for their friends for the weekend. An arrest for drug-related offences can result in a criminal record and possibly prison, which can have an impact on the individual's future regarding work and travel. Other offences can include those committed when the individual is under the influence of drugs, such as drink driving, as well as offences that may be committed to support a drug habit.

How people use drugs

People who use drugs may do so at a number of different levels. This will affect their ability to make decisions about their drug use and possible risky behaviour.

Experimental

Experimental drug use generally includes people who may try a substance once or twice but after that do not use it again. Many individuals may experiment with one or two substances at some point in their lives.

Recreational

People may use drugs at a recreational level. At this level they will use them infrequently and often only on particular occasions or at certain social events, such as when going out clubbing. Recreational users are not that likely to be injecting, but this is not an absolute rule.

Dependent

This can be either physical dependency, where the person would experience withdrawal symptoms when they stop using, or psychological dependency when they feel unable to stop using

People who use drugs from the opiate family (i.e. heroin, methadone) or the benzodiazepine family (i.e. valium or temazepam) may become physically dependent if they use daily for 1-2 weeks, although this varies between individuals. Physical dependency means they will have withdrawal symptoms if they stop using, and is typically associated with depressant drugs such as heroin, methadone, benzodiazepines, alcohol and nicotine.

Many people experience psychological dependency on a number of different drugs including those already mentioned but also stimulants (i.e. cocaine, speed, crack) and even cannabis or caffeine. This type of dependency can be very hard to break. Many users will therefore have to deal with cravings (a desire to use) brought on by their physical and psychological dependency.

Some drug users do not want to or are unable to stop and may look to drug maintenance programmes or controlled drug use as a way of better managing their drug use. With controlled use individuals move from chaotic dependent use to using in a very structured and organised way. Some agencies offer support to help people make this transition and this can help individuals reduce the problems associated with drug use and enable them to make clearer choices about safer drug use.

In addition to dependency on drugs, some people experience a psychological dependency on injecting, known as needle fixation. This may make it very difficult to stop injecting.

How drugs get to the brain

By mouth

When someone takes a drug orally it passes through the oesophagus and stomach lining to the small intestine where it is absorbed into the tiny blood vessels (capillaries) lining the stomach, and diffuse into the bloodstream. Drugs taken this way have to pass through mouth enzymes and stomach acids before they can get to the brain, so the effects are delayed. It takes 20-30 minutes to take effect, especially after a meal when it may take longer. Drugs in liquid form, such as alcohol, tablets, such as ecstasy and benzodiazepines and powders, such as amphetamines can be taken this way.

By sniffing

Drugs taken this way are absorbed by the tiny blood vessels enmeshed in the mucous membrane lining the nasal passages. The effects are usually more intense and occur more quickly than with the oral route. It takes about 3-5 minutes for the drug to take effect. Drugs taken this way can include cocaine, amphetamines, MDMA powder and crushed tablets.

By contact

Drugs taken this way are absorbed through the skin, tongue or anus. Drugs to treat addiction to nicotine are applied to the skin in saturated adhesive patches where they release measured quantities of the drug over a period of time. Drugs taken through the skin, such as nicotine patches, or tongue, such as LSD, can take about 5-10 minutes to take effect. When suppositories are used, the drug travels into the body via the anal blood vessels and this can take 10-15 minutes to take effect.

By injection

Drugs may be injected into the bloodstream intravenously (IV), into a muscle mass (IM) or under the skin (subcutaneous or skin popping). Injection is a quick and potent way to absorb a drug. It takes 15-30 seconds to take effect if taken IV or 3-5 minutes when taken IM and 'skin-popping'. Injection is the most dangerous method, and exposes the body to many potential health problems, such as hepatitis, abscesses, septicaemia and HIV. Drugs such as heroin, crushed tablets, such as Valium or temazepam, and sometime amphetamines can be taken this way.

By smoking

When an individual smokes, the vaporised drug enters the lungs and is rapidly absorbed through the tiny blood vessels lining the air sacs of the bronchi. From the lungs, the drug-laden blood is pumped back to the heart and then directly to the body and brain, acting more quickly than any other method. It takes approx. 7-10 seconds for the drug to take effect. Drugs taken this way include nicotine and cannabis, in the form of a cigarette or joint. Cannabis and crack cocaine can also be smoked in a bong or pipe.

Why people inject drugs

People inject drugs for their own individual reasons, but there are some common themes:

- By injecting a drug, the effect will be more intense and immediate than if smoked or taken orally.

- A smaller amount of the drug is needed to get the same effect when injecting, and therefore, at first, it will work out cheaper to inject than to smoke.

- There is a 'thrill' associated with the process of injecting (needle fixation).

- Some people find that injecting makes them feel less nauseous than smoking.

Injecting a drug is more risky than smoking or swallowing the drug as there is the likelihood of sharing injecting equipment, with the associated risk of HIV and many other infections. There is also a greater risk of overdosing.

The importance of safer injecting

HIV and other blood-borne viruses can be transmitted via unsafe injecting practices. This includes through sharing injecting equipment, including water, spoons, filters, but the most important risk comes from sharing needles and syringes.

Safer injecting will:

- Protect you from HIV / AIDS.

- Protect you from other infections such as hepatitis.

- Help protect you from dirty hits.

- Help protect you from other damage when you inject yourself, such as abscesses, septicaemia or collapsed veins.

The essentials of safer injecting

- Get hold of new needles. Find out how to get them free from needle exchanges.

- Use them when you inject. Work out in advance how to make sure you have enough needles to see you through so you never have to share them with anyone else.

- Learn how to clean your works. This is important for those times and situations when you can't get hold of new needles. However, it is important to remember that it is best not to share at all.

Unsafe injecting

Again, people share injecting equipment for a number of individual reasons which may relate to the moment, or to broader issues. However, there are common themes:

- A drug user may inject unsafely if he or she does not have the correct information about safer injecting.

- If the drug user does not have easy access to sterile injecting equipment ('works') at the moment of using drugs, he or she will be much more likely to share.

- If a drug user is withdrawing from a drug and feeling sick, he or she will be much more likely to take risks and share injecting equipment.

If users are given clear information about how to inject safely, where to obtain new injecting equipment and methods of cleaning works, the client may be enabled to act on that information. However, information alone does not routinely result in behaviour change and clients who may usually inject safely may nevertheless in particular circumstances put themselves at risk.

Therefore, in educating drug users, there should be discussion of strategies for coping with difficult situations when a client might feel inclined to share works. For example, individuals who always intend to use sterile needles, but who often end up in their dealer's house without injecting equipment (and consequently share needles) may be encouraged to use a dealer who has clean 'works' at their house or to develop a routine of visiting a chemist or needle exchange on the way to the dealer.

Access to new needles will differ throughout the country. Many needle exchanges are run as part of community drug agencies, or sometimes HIV teams. There are other needle exchanges that do not run from a fixed project base. These may be the only local exchange facility or an extension of a project based service. These schemes may run in a number of different ways:

- Satellite schemes: a needle exchange is brought into a host agency for regular sessions. This could be in a probation office, a youth club, community centre or GP practice.

- Mobile schemes: A needle-exchange which operates from a van or bus visiting fixed places on a regular basis.

- Delivery schemes: Some outreach teams run delivery services for all or some groups of users.

- Dealer-based schemes: some outreach workers deliver needles and syringes to dealers who give out sterile equipment to their customers.

Disposal of used works

Access to disposal facilities will vary throughout the country. Sharps bins will be available through needle exchanges and drug services. One thing to remember is that sharps bins should not be overfilled or this could lead to spikes piercing the plastic. Bins should only be filled two-thirds full.

With larger syringes, separate the barrel and the plunger, and take the needle out. Then put the needle inside the barrel, replace the plunger, and push it until the needle bends and jams. Then bag the works and dispose of it in a bin. This should not be done with small syringes, because the needle can stick through the barrel.

Understanding injection drug use and harm reduction

Research into risk behaviour has primarily focused on individual risk factors rather than social risk factors such as membership of networks of drug users or the size of equipment-sharing customs of these networks. This section looks at the main risk factors identified by individual behavioural and social/network research.

Levels of equipment sharing

Levels of equipment sharing appear to be strongly influenced by situational factors. The most important of these is the availability of clean injecting equipment (Stimson 1989). There is a clear correlation between the availability of clean injecting equipment, the levels of sharing and the prevalence of HIV amongst drug users. Dependent drug users may be more prone when they are withdrawing (Gossop 1993).

However, close social relationships may also encourage sharing. For example, women in Glasgow did not tend to see sharing with sexual partners as a risk activity, but as a reciprocal act no different from any other form of sharing which takes place in a close relationship (Barnard 1993).

Numerous recent studies have also shown higher levels of needle sharing amongst younger injectors who have begun using drugs since the advent of needle exchange and HIV prevention. However, younger injectors were not necessarily at greater risk of HIV infection unless they were sharing with older, more experienced injectors (Friedman 1990).

These findings suggest that ethnographic research which maps the social networks and sites in which drug injecting takes place are likely to be an important part of local HIV prevention work with injecting drug users.

Prisons provide an important social context for equipment sharing. Prisons may enhance HIV risk by blocking access to sterile injecting equipment and by encouraging the sharing of injecting equipment. Access to materials such as bleach or detergent which can be used to clean injecting equipment may also be highly restricted. Prison may also promote a switch from non-injecting drug use to injection drug use due to reduced opportunities for drug use. In addition, with random drug testing taking place in prisons some people may switch from using cannabis which can stay in the body for up to 30 days to drugs such as heroin, which only stays in the body for 2-4 days, to avoid detection (Stark et al. 1999).

Sexual behaviour of injecting drug users

Levels of condom use among drug injectors and their sexual partners are similar to those reported in other studies of heterosexual behaviour. For example, 68% of IDUs reported that they never used condoms with primary partners during a six month period (Rhodes et al. 1999), although rates of condom usage with casual partners were higher.

References

Barnard M et al: Needle sharing in context: patterns of sharing amongst women and men injectors and HIV risks, Addiction 88: 805-812, 1993.

Friedman SR et al: AIDS and the social relations of intravenous drug users, Millbank Quarterly, 86 (S1), 1990.

Gossop M et al: Severity of heroin dependence and HIV risk: sharing injecting equipment, AIDS Care 5: 159-168, 1993.

Gostin L et al: Prevention of HIV/AIDS and other blood borne diseases amongst injection drug users: a national survey on the regulation of syringes and needles, JAMA 277(1): 53-62, 1997.

Maden A et al: Drug dependence in prison, BMJ 302: 880, 1991.

Power K et al: Intravenous drug use and HIV transmission amongst inmates in Scottish prisons, British J Addiction 83: 649-653, 1992.

Rhodes T et al. Drug injecting, rapid HIV spread and the risk environment: implications for assessment and response. AIDS 13 Supp A S259-270, 1999.

Stark, C et al (eds). Illegal Drug use in the United Kingdom; Prevention, treatment and enforcement. Ashgate Publishing Ltd. 1999.

Stimson G et al: Syringe exchange programmes for injecting drug users, AIDS 5: 253-260, 1989.

Harm reduction

What is harm reduction?

It is a philosophy that recognises that some people will use drugs regardless. It is a damage limitation strategy. Harm reduction does not condone drug-taking but simply acknowledges that it takes place; and therefore the pragmatic response is to provide information and advice about minimising risks.

Needle exchanges came about as a harm reduction strategy. In the UK, needle exchanges and harm reduction have been overwhelming successes. In many parts of the UK, where there is a well developed range of services offering prescribed drugs and needle exchange, the HIV prevalence rate among injecting drug users is between 1-2%. Its effectiveness in the UK can be seen by comparison with New York which had no needle exchange and where 70% of drug users are HIV-positive (Parsons et al. 1997).

This highlights the need for drug and HIV agencies to be familiar with harm reduction strategies for preventing HIV infection among drug users.

Why harm reduction?

Most injecting drug use is both illegal and socially driven underground. A whole body of research exists which shows that punitive or coercive attempts to try to 'stamp out' drug use don't succeed. What's worse is that they drive drug use even further underground and make HIV prevention services inaccessible to the majority of drug users.

If our primary aim is the reduction of HIV transmission and the provision of quality services to drug users with HIV or AIDS, then it is essential to adopt an approach that recognises the difficulties of accessing drug users and the dangers of alienating them.

It is important to begin with advice and with services that drug users will themselves value. It is important to give minimum necessary advice about risk and harm reduction rather than maximal advice requiring drug users to make total changes to their lives in a short space of time, as this will alienate clients and drive them away from services.

- Harm reduction focuses on giving advice about;

- not sharing injecting equipment.

- cleaning injecting equipment for those situations where there is no option but sharing.

- safer sex.

- using all drugs via all methods.

- the wider health context of safer injecting.

- preventing and dealing with an overdose.

- referral to accessible services.

- implementing harm reduction techniques in the real world.

If users are looking for services to help them give up drug use then clearly it is important to provide speedy and reliable referrals to these and to ensure that they are as user-friendly as possible.

The Harm Reduction approach has been implemented for all drug users. Following the death of Leah Betts in 1995 and other high-profile ecstasy deaths organisations such as the Dance International Network and other user groups have been established to give advice to clubbers about taking all drugs safely. Traditionally drug services in the UK were set up for primarily heroin- using clients; however, in recent years services have been developed to meet the changing face of drug use within the UK.

Services are now established for clients who use cocaine / crack primarily, as well as other non- opiate drug users, such as Ecstasy and other so called 'recreational drugs', who in the past were not able to access support (Stark et al. 1999).

Safer sex

It should be remembered that all drug users are also sexually active and may, like the rest of the population, be heterosexual, gay, bisexual or lesbian. People under the influence of any substances, including alcohol, may engage in more risky behaviour, including engaging in unsafe sex. Due to the potential prevalence of HIV infection among injecting drug users they are also likely to be particularly at risk from HIV through unsafe sex and this issue should not be overlooked.

Implementing harm reduction techniques in the real world

For many people risk reduction can be complicated by other factors. Someone's social and economic situation will strongly affect their ability to take on information and change their behaviour. In some cases practical help with benefits and housing may be the most effective harm reduction strategy as this may create the setting for someone to use the information they have learned about safer drug use.

Unexpected barriers may appear which cause people to be at risk. Someone may get sterile injecting equipment but drop it when they see the police coming towards them. Also people's emotional state and mental health may affect their ability to implement harm reduction strategies. Someone who is very upset may take a risk they would otherwise avoid. Finally, if someone has consumed a large amount of drugs or alcohol this may restrict their ability to act more safely.

It is vital to acknowledge the realities of people's lives and accept that change is a process, not a one-off event. If small changes are noted they need to be positively reinforced and built upon.

Policy and practice

Since the 1960s heroin users have been offered drug treatment programmes based on heroin substitutes such as physeptone, DF118, diamorphine and, most commonly, oral methadone, and more recently lofexidine and buprenorphine. There are different views as to the role and value of drug treatment programmes. Some people believe that heroin substitutes should only be employed to support drug users to stop using heroin: an abstinence policy. Others believe that heroin substitutes can also be used to help people control their drug use through maintenance programmes: a harm reduction policy.

Since the advent of HIV infection a stronger harm reduction approach has been promoted. The Advisory Council on the Misuse of Drugs (ACMD) in their first AIDS and Drug Misuse Report (1989) argued that preventing the spread of HIV infection should take precedence over attempts to reduce drug taking, as HIV posed a greater threat to the individual and society.

The second ACMD report on *AIDS and Drug Misuse* (1991) stressed the role of prescribing as a harm reduction tool. This was again reinforced in the Department of Health's advice to doctors in their report: *Drug Misuse and Dependence: Guidelines on Clinical Management* (1991).

However, despite a shift in policy towards harm reduction over the last ten years, practice remains divided between abstinence and harm reduction policies and will vary from area to area and from project to project. On one side are those who still take an abstinence approach to prescribing, offering reduction programmes to those who wish to stop using drugs. On the other side are those offering low threshold schemes where as many users as possible are promoted to enter drug maintenance programmes to encourage them into services and away from daily injecting.

Within these two extremes can be found a whole spectrum of various practices and policies. It is important to recognise that even where very experimental harm reduction drug prescribing is offered to users, some will still wish to stop using. Prescribing is generally far more available than ten years ago and is increasingly accepted as a valuable tool in preventing the spread of HIV infection among injecting drug users and reducing other drug related harm.

Drug treatment programmes are usually undertaken by drug dependency units (DDUs), community drug teams (CDTs) or street drug agencies. DDUs will have their own medical team. CDTs and street agencies may have their own medical staff or work in conjunction with general practitioners. Some GPs may also prescribe without support from drug agencies.

Finally, some private doctors prescribe to drug users. They will usually tend to be more harm reduction orientated or liberal in their prescribing and offer options such as injectable alternatives to street heroin which are less available on the NHS.

In May 2003 the 56th World Health Assembly endorsed the WHO Global Health Sector Strategy (GHSS) for HIV/AIDS 2003-2007. The Strategy lists the core components of a health sector response to HIV/AIDS, including "promoting harm reduction among injecting drug users, such as wide access to sterile injecting equipment, and drug dependence treatment and outreach services to help reduce frequency of injecting drug use". There is ample evidence that harm reduction programmes work in both developing and developed countries, and can prevent, stabilise and reverse AIDS epidemics among injecting drug users (Deveau et al, 2006).

Harm reduction has been surrounded by controversy since the mid 1980s when needle exchanges and substitution treatments were first introduced in Western Europe. Globally drug users receive little or no sympathy from the general population, and too often the issues of drug use, HIV and harm reduction strategies are entangled in political, religious and moral debates to the detriment of prevention and care efforts. Attitudes on how to tackle drug use differ greatly, but all governments promote drug use prevention through supply and demand reduction techniques. In many countries the main barriers to effectively scaling up harm reduction interventions remain repressive laws and policies that increase HIV transmission among and from injecting drug users. Some politically conservative countries do not agree with some elements of harm reduction on the principle that providing clean equipment or methadone substitute encourages drug abuse. They believe that needle exchange services are a waste of money and only promote injecting drug use, when the message should be abstinence from drugs. Substitution drug treatment is a difficult concept for many to accept; critics argue that this prolongs drug addiction or provides users with drugs to sell on the street to fund further drug use.

Although outreach work is the most accepted form of harm reduction, some believe it makes life easier for drug users, by teaching them safer methods of injecting, and is overall a waste of resources.

The International Harm Reduction Development Program (IHRD) is an organisation that works to reduce HIV and other harms related to injecting drug use. It presses for policies that reduce stigmatisation of illicit drug users and protect their human rights. It has supported more than 200 programs in Central and Eastern Europe, the former Soviet Union, and Asia, bases its activities on the philosophy that people unable or unwilling to abstain from drug use can make positive changes to protect their health and the health of others. Since 2001, IHRD has prioritised advocacy to expand availability of needle exchange, opiate substitution treatment, and treatment for HIV; to reform discriminatory policies and practices; and to increase the political participation of people who use drugs and those living with HIV.

Substitution Therapy

A report by the WHO in March 2005 reviewed many global studies and concluded that substitution treatment is a 'critical component' of prevention policy, significantly reducing opioid dependency and HIV infection rates (WHO, 2005). The WHO's essential drugs list includes medicines that are required to meet a minimum standard of health care in all countries and drugs are only added to the list if a committee of experts concludes they are the most effective drug for a priority health condition. Adding methadone and buprenorphine to this list emphasise the important roles they play in helping active drug users benefit from HIV treatment and any delay is detrimental to the coverage and quality of treatment for opiate addicted persons, including those living with HIV/AIDS.

Drug substitution treatment has proven effective in rehabilitating and stabilising IDUs, and in reducing HIV infection rates (Keen et al, 2003). Researchers from the University of Philadelphia monitored 152 injecting users receiving methadone maintenance treatment and 103 injecting users on no treatment over a period of 18 months, all of whom were HIV-negative at the beginning of the study. The results showed that over the 18 months, only 3.5% of those on treatment became infected with HIV, as opposed to 22% not on treatment (Metzger et al, 1993)

Another study in Amsterdam followed a group of 582 IDU's on methadone maintenance treatment for an average of three years. The HIV infection rate was 6.0 per 100 person-years among those who continued injecting throughout the treatment, and 0.2 per 100 person-years in those who stopped injecting while on treatment. These results indicate that oral methadone treatment is critical in stopping drug users injecting, though a small minority will later revert to high-risk behaviour (Langendam et al, 2000) In addition, studies have also found a decline in crime rates and commercial sex work when IDUs no longer have to find ways to fund their expensive addictions (Gossop et al, 2005)

Despite WHO recommendation that substitution therapy is an essential component of harm reduction programmes for injecting drug users this guidance continues to be ignored throughout Eastern Europe and Central Asia due to a suspicion of substitute therapy merely perpetuates drug dependency. It is not available in Albania, Armenia, Azerbaijan, Belarus, Kazakhstan, Russia, Tajikistan, Turkmenistan and Uzbekistan. Even where substitution therapy programmes do exist, entry criteria and practices affect the ability of drug users to access treatment. Any illicit drug use alongside substitution therapy may result in termination of the therapy, and patients often have no control over the methadone doses they receive, which can be particularly problematic in those receiving efavirenz-based antiretroviral therapy, which can reduce methadone levels by 50%. The duration of substitution therapy also needs to be adequate to ensure treatment effectiveness; programmes that give only six months inevitably perpetuate a cycle of drug dependence because drug users don't have long enough to address the psychosocial factors underlying their drug use. This places HIV treatment beyond the reach of hundreds of thousands of injecting drug users who form the core group of the HIV epidemic in some areas.

The absence of available stimulant substitution treatment produces a set of challenges for engaging stimulant into HIV prevention programmes.

Heroin Prescriptions

Canada, Germany, Netherlands, Spain and Switzerland provides injecting drug users with access to a prescription of heroin of known quality, purity and potency, obtained from health services or other legal channels. This represents an essential component for retaining opiate-dependent drug users in any kind of treatment and is an essential component of HIV prevention, treatment and care. However, there is strong opposition to heroin prescribing in many countries.

Needle Exchanges

The lack of a clean needle is not going to deter a drug user from injecting. However, access to clean needles can draw them into programmes and can protect users from infection long enough to provide them with ongoing opportunities to use services such as methadone substitution therapy. Needle exchange programmes (NEPs) have reduced HIV transmission rates among IDU's in areas where they have been established. One of the most definitive studies of NEPs was carried out in 1997, focusing on 81 cities worldwide. It found that HIV infection rates increased by 5.9% per year in the 52 cities without NEPs, and decreased by 5.8% per year in the 29 cities that did provide NEPs (Hurley et al, 1997) An eleven-year study of HIV among IDU's in New York found that HIV prevalence rates fell from 54% to 13% following the introduction of NEPs (Jarlais et al, 2005). The World Health Organisation (2004) reviewed the effectiveness of NEPs in many countries; the results produced convincing evidence that NEPs significantly reduced HIV infection, and no evidence that they encourage drug use (WHO, 2004a).

The inappropriate disposal of needles and syringes is often cited as a fundamental reason why communities reject needle and syringe exchange programmes. Therefore sharp bins or containers placed in toilets or other localities out of the view of the general public may be one way to address this.

Safe injecting rooms

Safe injecting rooms are a safe spaces for injection with medical personal on hand to provide first aid in the event of an overdose. Whilst they are still a controversial harm reduction intervention, countries including Australia, Canada and Switzerland have introduced them and have shown that they can save thousands of lives.

Prisons

In health terms, prison may be the most dangerous environment that most drug users will ever encounter; yet injecting drug users are disproportionately over represented in such institutions (Deveau et al, 2006). By December 2000, nineteen prisons in three countries, Germany, Spain and Switzerland, had needle and syringe exchange programmes. These programmes have begun to demonstrate the feasibility and efficacy of harm reduction, medical treatment and health promotion efforts in prisons without any reported unintended negative consequences (Dolan et al, 2003). More recently, needle and syringe exchange programmes have been implemented in 53 prisons in 6 countries (Belarus, Germany, Kyrgyzstan, Moldova, Spain and Switzerland,) (Lines et al, 2004). Whilst this can be an effective way of addressing the spread of HIV in prisons it remains a contentious issue in many countries.

Outreach Projects

Community-based outreach prevention focuses on promoting a change in high-risk behaviour. Educating users about HIV prevention, helping them to get into rehabilitation programmes, and tackling the issues of IDU's and sexual transmission, are all part of outreach prevention (UNAIDS, 2006) A recent report from the WHO reviewed data from over 40 studies on outreach prevention; it concluded that outreach prevention methods significantly reduce high-risk behaviour in IDU's and are successful in directing them to rehabilitation services (WHO, 2004b).

Many countries, including projects in Thailand, Vietnam and Kenya use former drug users as outreach workers as they know where to find other drug users and can refer them into services. Whilst this is an inexpensive way of reaching this population they are not always entirely reliable and can be a challenge to work with. Utilising these workers, without providing appropriate training may be exposing them to temptation and the ongoing health and well-being of these community-based workers needs to be monitored. Whilst a Kenyan outreach project reported a decline in injecting, from 94% to 85% and in needle sharing, from 41% to 15%, it can be a challenge to get the drug users to accept them as many deny injecting. Many also refuse HIV testing and accessing health prevention as it can be seen as a diversion from getting money to support their addiction. Project need to put more emphasis on mobile services which are more accessible in the hopes that that will increase client participation (Deveau et al, 2006).

Voluntary Testing

Voluntary testing may be particularly important for prevention efforts as many drug users may not protect themselves because they assume that they are already infected. The flip side of this however, is that an increase in alcohol and drug use often results when people learn that they are HIV-positive, so testing services need to be closely linked with HIV care and counselling services.

References

Deveau C et al. Prevention of HIV/AIDS among drug users as a vulnerable population. The 2006 HIV/AIDS Implementers Meeting of the President's Emergency Plan for AIDS Relief, Durban, South Africa, abstract 89, 2006.

Dolan K, Rutter S, and Wodak AD (2003). Prison based syringe exchange programs: A review of international research and development. Addiction, 98: p. 153-158.

Gossop M, et al (2005, 1st September), 'Reductions in criminal convictions after addiction treatment: 5-year follow up' (http://www.ncbi.nlm.nih.gov/entrez/query.fcgi?cmd=Retrieve&db=PubMed&list_uids=16102373&dopt=Abstract), Drug Alcohol Depend; 79(3).

Hurley SF, et al (1997, 21th June), 'Effectiveness of needle-exchange programmes for prevention of HIV infection' (http://www.ncbi.nlm.nih.gov/entrez/query.fcgi?db=pubmed&list_uids=9269214&cmd=Retrieve&indexed=google), The Lancet; 349(9068):1797-800.

Jarlais D, et al (2005, 19th October), 'Reductions in hepatitis C virus and HIV infections among injecting drug users in New York City, 1990 - 2001 (http://www.ncbi.nlm.nih.gov/entrez/query.fcgi?cmd=Retrieve&db=PubMed&list_uids=16251819&dopt=Abstract)', AIDS2005; 19(3).

Keen J, et al (2003, June), 'Does methadone maintenance treatment based on the new national guidelines work in a primary care setting? (http://www.pubmedcentral.nih.gov/articlerender.fcgi?artid=1314620)', British Journal of General Practice; 53(491).

Langendam MW, et al (2000, April), 'Methadone maintenance and cessation of injecting drug use: results from the Amsterdam Cohort Study' (http://cat.inist.fr/?aModele=afficheN&cpsidt=1367323), Addiction; 95(4).

Lines R, Jürgens R, Stöver H, Laticevschi D and Nelles J (2004). Prison Needle Exchange: A Review of International Evidence and Experience, Canadian HIV//AIDS Legal Network, Montreal. Available at www.aidslaw.ca cited 8 December 2004.

Metzger DS, et al (1993, 6th September), 'HIV seroconversion among intravenous drug users in and out-of-treatment: an 18-month prospective follow up (http://www.ncbi.nlm.nih.gov/entrez/query.fcgi?db=pubmed&cmd=Retrieve&dopt=AbstractPlus&list_uids=8340896&query_hl=7&itool=pubmed_docsum)', J Acquir Immune Defic Syndr; 6(9).

UNAIDS. (2006). '2006 Report on the global aids epidemic'.

WHO/UNODC/UNAIDS position paper. Substitution maintenance therapy in the management of opioid dependence and HIV/AIDS prevention. 2004

http://www.who.int/substance_abuse/publications/en/PositionPaper_English.pdf

World Health Organisation, 'Effectiveness of sterile needle and syringe programming in reducing HIV/AIDS among injecting drug users (http://www.who.int/hiv/pub/idu/en/)'. 2004a.

World Health Organisation. Effectiveness of Community Based Outreach in Preventing HIV / AIDS among Injecting drug users. 2004b.

World Health Organisation. 'Effectiveness of drug dependence treatment in preventing HIV among injecting drug users (http://www.who.int/hiv/pub/idu/en/)'. (2005, March)

Attitudes towards addiction

Addiction is defined as physical or psychological dependence on a substance. Addicts are often written off by society as people unable to change their behaviour by definition, and viewed as people whose behaviour is contagious; addicts are simultaneously victims and pushers of drugs in the eyes of some, and such views have led to punitive and frequently dismissive attitudes towards the health of drug users and their capacity for change. For example, even when the risk of hepatitis B infection through the sharing of syringes was well-known, pharmacists in Edinburgh during the early 1980s resisted supplying clean syringes on the grounds that this would encourage drug use.

Fortunately such responses are rare in the UK today, but attitudes towards the treatment of injecting drug use remain punitive. There are frequent complaints from addicts about the unwillingness of doctors to prescribe methadone, for instance, and a widespread unwillingness to consider the supply of purified heroin as a maintenance option and as an early 'stabilisation' stage in the reduction of drug use. Addicts also complain of widespread 'addictophobia' amongst healthcare professionals, leading to poor standards of care and a lack of understanding or compassion.

Drug users are still negatively portrayed in the media and by society in general. The high correlation between drug use and crime results in the label of all drug users being criminals and as a result known drug users may be banned from local shops as they are assumed to be shoplifters and may find themselves being picked up more frequently by the police. Should drug users be victims of crime they get very little police and / or public support, for example, a drug user who sells sex to fund their drug use who may be attacked or raped.

Within wider society, drug users may find they become discriminated against within their community, and parents who are drug users may find that social services become more involved due to the believe that drug users can't be good parents.

Since the 1970s there has been an increasing tendency to view the phenomenon of addiction as a medical or psychological problem which requires treatment and to which some individuals are more predisposed than others. This view has arisen largely as a result of research which has sought to disprove the notion that addiction is the result of an incorrect moral choice. Researchers claim to have located biochemical characteristics and brain structures which predispose some people to addiction to heroin and alcohol, whilst others claim that alcoholism is an inherited behaviour. Research which has sought to locate the roots of addiction in biochemical processes or psychological events in childhood has tended to draw attention away from the social construction of addiction: why some communities are more vulnerable to addiction than others, the economics of illicit drug use and what addiction and drug use symbolise to those who use drugs.

In recent years the government has increased funding for services for drug users through the criminal justice system. There are extensive Arrest Referral Schemes throughout the UK, where drug workers see users in police stations with the aim of moving them into treatment. Drug Treatment and Testing Orders have increased, with drug users being offered the opportunity to attend a treatment programme rather than receiving a custodial sentence. The problem is that demand for treatment outweighs the supply and in many areas the waiting list for accessing services is long. This makes it difficult for people to get into treatment when they are motivated to address their drug use.

High rates of injecting drug use are concentrated amongst economically deprived communities in the developed world, and injecting drug users are more likely to be men than women, especially in Mediterranean countries and amongst ethnic minorities in the USA. Addicts become addicts not only because drugs meet a need at the point addiction begins, but also because social forces dictate that some people will need drugs more than others, come into contact with drugs more than others, and have fewer options for escaping addiction than others. Many addicts say that injecting drug use was a way of beating boredom, of escaping the limiting horizons of an economically deprived life, poor educational opportunities, unemployment and poverty.

Some addicts describe injecting drug use as a rite of passage, a graduation into the drug culture which gives the individual status and mystique amongst his or her peers. This process is said to be very widespread in southern European countries irrespective of economic status. Despite this identity little sense of community around their shared behaviour exists amongst injecting drug users. Many users will have strong bonds only with a very small group of other users, and not with a wider, invisible community of users. This lack of identification has made community-based responses by injecting drug users rare; most responses have been led by former users now working in the drugs field.

References & further reading: drug users and drug addiction

Genser SG et al. Sex for crack as an AIDS risk behaviour: an ethnographic study, VIII International AIDS Conference, Amsterdam, abstract WeC 1032, 1992.

Gossop, M. Living with Drugs. Ashgate Publishing Ltd. 1996.

Kim AA et al. Increased risk of HIV and sexually transmitted disease transmission among gay or bisexual men who use Viagra, San Francisco 2000-2001, AIDS 16(10): 1425-1428, 2002

Lindsay MK et al. Crack cocaine: a risk factor for HIV, Obstet Gynecol 80(6): 981-984, 1992.

Murji, K. Policing Drugs. Ashgate Publishing Ltd. 1998.

Parsons et al. Over a decade of syringe exchange; results from 1997 UK survey. The Centre for research on drugs and health behaviour. www.harmreduction.org/research 1997

Patterson TP et al. HIV-positive methamphetamine users: Social and behavioural outcomes of binge use, XIV International AIDS Conference, Barcelona, abstract E11681, 2002.

Piaseczna MA et al. Predictors of HIV seroconversion among young men who have sex with men in Canada, XIV International AIDS Conference, Barcelona, abstract MoPeC3450, 2002.

Rhodes T et al. Drug injecting, rapid HIV spread and the risk environment: implications for assessment and response. AIDS 13 Supp A S259-270, 1999.

Riley SC et al. Patterns of recreational drug use at dance events in Edinburgh, Scotland, Addiction 96(7): 1035-1047, 2001.

Riehman K. Injecting drug use and AIDS in developing countries: determinants and issues for policy consideration. World Bank (available from http://www.worldbank.org/aids-econ/confront/backgrnd/riehman/index.htm)

Schoenfisch S et al. Risk of HIV infection and behavioural changes associated with crack cocaine use in prenatal patients, IX International AIDS Conference, Berlin, abstract PoC 15-2920, 1993.

Sherr L et al. Viagra use and sexual risk among HIV-positive and HIV-negative gay men in London. XIII International AIDS Conference, Durban, abstract WePpD1409, 2000.

Stark, C et al (eds). Illegal Drug use in the United Kingdom; Prevention, treatment and enforcement. Ashgate. 1999.

Sterk C. Cocaine and seropositivity, Lancet 8593: 1052-1053, 1988.

Drugs and the law

Introduction

For the very latest information on the legality, popularity and adverse effects of recreational drugs, visit Drugscope, the UK's leading drugs charity and centre of expertise on drugs at www.drugscope.org.uk or the governments drug information agency at www.talktofrank.com.

Drugs in the UK are controlled by two laws: the Medicines Act (1968) and the Misuse of Drugs Act (1971). The Medicines Act bans the non-medical use of certain drugs. The Misuse of Drugs Act places banned drugs in different classes. The penalties for offences involving a drug depend on the class it is in. Class A

drugs carry the highest penalties, Class C the lowest. First offenders that are charged with possessing drugs for their own use may get off with only a caution or a fine. However, even a caution means a criminal record.

Regular offenders, people selling drugs, or drug smugglers, can be sentenced to life imprisonment for trafficking.

It is an offence to allow anyone on your premises to produce, give away or sell illegal drugs. It's an offence even to offer to supply the drug free of charge. So if a parent knows that their child is sharing drugs with a friend in their house and does nothing to stop it, the parent has committed an offence.

Services for drug users

Introduction

This section is intended to give the reader an understanding of drugs services in the United Kingdom. It's intended to allow someone approaching work with drug users for the first time to have an understanding of how policy has been developed, and equally importantly, how this policy has been integrated at a local level in the development of new projects and in the refocusing of more traditional services.

This chapter also seeks to highlight key issues for those reviewing or rethinking their services in the light of HIV infection. This chapter cannot and should not replace the process of needs assessment, and it is vital to recognise that each area will have its own distinct drug scenes and cultures.

The development of drug services

In order to understand the current position concerning the provision of drug services, it is necessary to provide a brief overview of the development of services in Britain.

The 1980s in Britain was an era in which the recorded prevalence and spread of drug use increased among most sectors of the population. In the last five years of the decade, the Home Office Notifications of new drug users (Misuse of Drugs Act, Class 1) increased by 46% (from 12,424 to 26,954) and the number of re-notifications has also continued to increase. However, these statistics perhaps represent as little as 10% of the overall number of long-term users. The Home Office has now discontinued its notification system for new drug users.

The Advisory Committee on the Misuse of Drugs (ACMD) was established in 1981 to advise central government on developing responses to drug use. In 1982 in their Treatment and Rehabilitation Report, the ACMD recommended the development of Drug Advisory Committees to coordinate local services both within the voluntary and statutory sectors. The ACMD first report, AIDS and Drug Misuse (1989) stated that 'the spread of HIV is a greater danger to individual and public than drug misuse'. This promoted a shift towards harm reduction policies. It became a priority to draw as many drug users into services in order to prevent the spread of HIV infection and minimise drug related harm.

With the Criminal Justice Act (1991) community agencies were encouraged to consider offering community sentence options for drug users. It is the Probation Service's role to promote these developments and drug treatment services, including residential rehabilitation projects now offer alternatives to custody or parole packages for drug using offenders.

The Children Act (1989) has implications for those working with drug users with children or younger drug users and this provides an alternative route to funding through social services.

Funding of drugs services

Services for drug users are provided across the voluntary, statutory and private sectors and funding will vary according to the provider's status.

The NHS and Community Care Act (1990) introduced an internal market into health and social care. Primary Care Trusts (PCT's) were given the resources and the responsibility for purchasing services to meet the health needs of their population. In practice, needs far outstripped the available budget and difficult decisions have to be made about choices and priorities. The role of regional Health Authorities (RHA) also changed to an advisory role and to monitoring the development of the purchaser/provider split.

While the NHS traditionally has been the largest statutory provider of drug services, other statutory agencies such as Social Services, the Probation Service, and the Youth Service have become increasingly active in providing or funding drug services. In particular, Social Services (within the framework of the Community Care legislation and the Children Act) and the Probation Service (within the framework of the Criminal Justice Act) provide top-up funding for residential rehabilitation projects. Social Services also had new responsibilities under the Act and were required to produce a Community Care Plan, outlining social care provision.

The voluntary sector tends to have a more eclectic funding base and draws money from the commercial and charitable sectors but also receives money from health and local authorities and central government. Many services are increasingly seeking to generate income, and a number of drug training agencies receive significant percentages of their finance from this source.

The coexistence of different approaches

Direct services for people who use drugs have been developed from a number of traditions and beliefs. Many services have been developed by concerned local people in the voluntary sector, or following bursts of central government monies.

The development of district drug advisory committees and the implementation of the NHS and Community Care Act sought to promote a better understanding of what services where required and also clarity in how these services were provided.

National Treatment Agency

The National Treatment Agency (NTA) is a special health authority, created by the Government in 2001 to ensure that there is more treatment, better treatment and fairer treatment available to all those who need it.

Their overall purpose is to:

- double the number of people in effective, well-managed treatment from 100,000 in 1998 to 200,000 in 2008.

- increase the proportion of people who successfully complete or, if appropriate, continue treatment.

This is the first time an organisation has been established to oversee the development of drug treatment services at a national level. Parallel structures have been established with the Scottish Executive (www.drugmisuse.isdscotland.org) and the Welsh (www.wales.gov.uk) and Northern Ireland Assemblies. (www.healthpromotionagency.org.uk)

The NTA exists to serve the needs of drug treatment service users, their unpaid carers and the communities in which they live. They work in partnership with service providers, commissioners of treatment services and communities to improve the quality and effectiveness of treatment.

Around four million people in England and Wales use at least one illicit drug each year, and around one million people use at least one of the most dangerous drugs (such as heroin and crack). For most people this will be a passing phase and they will not continue to take drugs or require any special treatment in order to deal with it. A minority of approximately 250-300,000 will, however, develop serious drug problems, typically involving heroin and/or cocaine.

While the numbers of people with serious drug problems may be small, drug misuse affects everyone. Providing drug misusers with well-managed, effective treatment is the most successful way of tackling all of these harms. But giving up and staying off drugs is difficult. Most drug misusers relapse and need to return to treatment a number of times before getting their habit under control. However, around 50% of those who do complete a comprehensive treatment programme are still drug-free after five years. Drug misuse causes economic and social decline in some of our most deprived communities. Drug treatment helps to reduce the demand for drugs. It can also enable drug misusers to reintegrate into society and become economically and socially active citizens. Treatment for drug misuse can help to reduce the offending rates of drug misusers who commit crimes to fund their habit. For every £1 that is spent on drug treatment, society gets £3 worth of benefit from reductions in offending.

Drug treatment gives clients the opportunity to improve their health, rebuild relationships and return to education or employment. Drug misuse causes around 1,350 premature deaths each year in England and getting into treatment reduces the chances of someone overdosing. Injecting drugs can contribute directly to the spread HIV and hepatitis. Getting good advice and information from a service can help to reduce risky behaviour as well as provide vaccinations against hepatitis B and treatment for HIV and Hepatitis.

UK drugs strategy

A new government 10-year plan was announced by the Drugs Co-ordinator in April 1998 and a new prison service drug strategy was announced in May 1998. The Government's drugs strategy, updated in 2002, aims to give direction and coherence to separate government initiatives related to drug misuse. This strategy sets the context in which the NTA works to tackle the harms associated with problematic drug misuse. The NTA is responsible for the treatment aim, and is actively involved in all other areas of the strategy.

The national strategy has four aims:

- To help young people resist drug use in order to achieve their full potential in society.

- To stifle the availability of illegal drugs on our streets.

- To protect our communities from drug-related anti-social and criminal behaviour.

- To enable people with drug problems to overcome them and live healthy, crime-free lives.

Improving the commissioning of drug treatment services

Approximately £450 million was spent on drug treatment in England in 2003/04. The aim of the NTA is to ensure that money is spent to best effect, on treatment that really works and that meets the needs of local people. Drug action teams (DAT's) are responsible for using central government and local funding to pay for (or commission) treatment from NHS and voluntary sector organisations.

The NTA's nine regional teams provide guidance and support to DAT's on how to spend this money. This includes ensuring that DAT's are able to provide drug misusers with a full range of services. For example, all DAT's should be able to provide drug misusers' with access to advice and information, needle exchanges, counselling, community based prescribing, inpatient detoxification and residential rehabilitation.

DAT's are local consortiums that bring together representatives of all the local agencies involved in tackling the misuse of drugs, including primary care trusts, local authority, police, probation. There are 149 DAT's in England covering all local authorities.

Promoting best practice in drug treatment

NTA believes that treatment should be based on evidence rather than unfounded theory. They provide a summary of existing research, carried out by studies and test new approaches to treatment in order to identify what works, and then publish the findings and recommendations. Service users and their unpaid carers have a vital role to play in improving services, and the NTA actively promote their involvement at local, regional and national level. In order to ensure equally high standards of treatment across the country, they have developed a set of basic standards that all services should meet. This is the first time that a national standard will have been set for drug treatment.

Improving the performance of drug treatment services and staff

As well as providing information and guidance to drug treatment workers to help them improve their performance, the NTA also work with the key organisations and colleges to improve training for new and existing staff. For example, the Royal College of General Practitioners and the Royal College of Psychiatrists to increase the level of tuition on drug misuse in standard doctor's training.

They also work in partnership with other parts of the health service, including public health and social services, as well as criminal justice agencies including the probation and prison services. These partnerships are vital because drug misusers come into regular contact with these services. By working with these services drug misusers can be provided with appropriate support and treatment.

Prevention work with those who do not use drugs

Education and prevention work seeks to prevent anyone (especially young people) from beginning to use drugs. The belief is that we must work with young people now to try to reduce the level of drug use in the future.

The present Government have placed a great deal of emphasis on this approach, funding a number of Home Office Drugs Prevention Teams to promote drugs education and prevention work in areas of high drug prevalence. Originally it was felt that those engaging in education and prevention work should focus exclusively on prevention.

More recently it has been recognised that education and prevention work should acknowledge and work with the fact that many young people may be experimenting with drug use.

The quality of education and prevention work varies considerably. It ranges from simplistic and probably ineffective 'just say no' messages and scare tactics to more sophisticated attempts to allow young people to reflect on the potential risks and problems associated with both illicit and legal drug use.

Education and prevention work may be undertaken by specialist drugs education and prevention teams, health promotion departments, youth clubs or youth workers, or schools. It may also be part of the work of a agency which offers direct services to drug users. The Home Office or your local health promotion department should be able to advise you on your local services.

Local drug services can be found on the governments' website www.talktofrank.com or through drugscope www.drugscope.co.uk

A map of service provision

Three levels of drug services exist ranging from the general to the highly specialised:

- Services for a wide range of drug users.

- Specialised services: drug dependency treatment and HIV services.

- Rehabilitation and in-patient detoxification.

A person has to want help to address their drug use or otherwise the treatment will not have a successful outcome. This is a key issue that will impact on the success of any government initiative to direct individuals into treatment as a result of involvement with the criminal justice system.

What kind of help an individual wants will also influence which type of drug service they access. Not all drug users will see their drug use as problematic or want to achieve abstinence. Many users, particularly more recreational users may want information and advice on harm reduction, and this will influence the service they may choose to access.

Individuals will also differ in terms of what they perceive to be their biggest problem and/or need. Many drug users may feel that they need support around issues such as financial, benefits, work, legal, housing, social, welfare, physical, mental, emotional, sexual health etc, rather than their drug use per se, which they may not consider to be a problem or their biggest problem.

The background of drug workers can also vary hugely, from those who are trained social workers, counsellors and nurses, through to ex-users who have no professional qualifications. This may

impact on the philosophy of the agency and the services that are offered. In inner city areas drug and alcohol projects tend to be separate, but in other areas one agency may provide a service for both drug and alcohol-using clients.

List of services for drug users

Needle exchanges

These may exist as separate projects which encompass wider harm reduction and primary health care services for injecting drug users or may be attached to other services, such as CDT's or street agencies.

They will often require users to give minimal information and are usually happy for people to register under false names. They will usually offer far more than just a needle exchange and will often have a primary health care nurse who can advise users about safer injecting practice and look at problems that may have arisen from injecting. These are usually very friendly projects which are not there to push users into stopping but to promote harm reduction techniques.

In addition, a number of districts have developed pharmacy-based exchanges where chemists are organised to give injecting equipment to injecting drug users. Pharmacy schemes may allow drug users to get sterile equipment with greater anonymity but it does reduce access to the harm reduction and primary health care services. Even where there is no formal scheme many chemists will sell needles and syringes and some drug users may prefer the anonymity of a commercial transaction. Pharmacies involved in the needle exchange scheme will usually display a yellow sticker, with red and green arrows, on their door so that they can be identified.

A further variation of this service is mobile or delivery service. In both these cases the needle exchange goes to the users either through satellite clinics in local areas, in buses or vans or through delivery services.

Any area may have one or more of the above schemes. In some areas it may be necessary to run a range of outlets to offer the widest access to service users. In addition, some areas have developed fixed injecting equipment disposal sites in areas where discarded injecting equipment has been a problem.

Community drug teams (CDTs) and street agencies

These services will usually be based in the community and will be outpatient or non-residential projects. Clients can usually refer themselves directly to these services. Some services have open access sessions, or 'drop-ins' where no appointment is needed. Others work by appointments only

Projects often describe their services as offering 'advice, information and referral'. This usually covers health education advice about drugs and their effects, access to community-based prescribing services, drugs counselling, complementary therapies, group work, satellite services and referral on to other specialist drug teams. Some agencies will also offer broader housing and welfare rights advice to drug users in addition.

Most services will have access to a nurse, if only part-time. The nurse will offer HIV testing, Hep C testing, Hep B vaccinations, wound dressing, safer injecting advice and onward referral as necessary.

CDTs or street agencies will offer services to users of all types of drugs. Traditionally these were set up to work with the less chaotic end of drug use, e.g. recreational drug users, and with non-injecting heroin users, however, there tends to be less of a clear distinction now. Increased demand has meant that many CDTs work in a 'shared-care' agreement with clients GPs. The doctor will prescribe according to the recommendations of the drug worker, who will also provide key working or counselling.

Street agencies and CDTs have traditionally been run in the non-statutory sector, however more recently CDTs are also being funded by greater number of local and health authority based teams.

Alcohol services

In inner city areas there tends to be a separate service for alcohol users, although in outer city or more rural areas one agency will provide a service for both drug and alcohol users. Most alcohol services seem to be provided by the voluntary sector.

Alcohol services will offer a range of services including key-working / counselling, community alcohol detox, referral to residential detox and rehabilitation, relapse prevention support. Some services may also offer a range of support groups which clients can access, such as harm reduction or relapse prevention groups. The ethos of the agencies can vary, but tend to provide services for patients who want to reduce the harm associated with their drinking as well as for those who wish to achieve abstinence.

Alcohol services are often not as knowledgeable around HIV issues, mainly due to the lack of a direct link between alcohol use and the risk of possible infection. However, as increased alcohol use is a well-established risk for newly diagnosed patients, they may be seeing lots of HIV-positive clients without realising it because the client does not disclose. Therefore it is important for alcohol services to have some knowledge and information around HIV and the issues affecting positive individuals.

Self-help groups

In addition to services provided for people with drug-related problems, there is a range of self help organisations. The largest of these are the 'Twelve Step' family of self-help groups (i.e. Narcotics Anonymous, Alcoholics Anonymous, Cocaine Anonymous, Families Anonymous, etc.). These support and encourage people to become and stay drug free through attending support groups on a regular basis. They are self-run groups, by ex- users for ex- and current users.

In addition, local areas may run other self-help groups for users or their families. A large number of independent family support groups are coordinated through the national charity, AdFam.

The other significant area of self-help support is the range of groups for people with HIV. These may be available to all people with HIV or designed for particular affected groups, such as drug users.

General practitioners (GPs)

Outside specialist drugs agencies, GPs remain the other key primary provider of services. Many GPs have played a central role in prescribing heroin substitutes (such as methadone) to heroin users. With the Department of Health's report, *Drug Misuse and Dependence: Guidelines on Clinical Management* (1991), this role has been strongly reinforced. GPs may prescribe independently to drug users or increasingly work collaboratively with street agencies or CDT's. This may take the form of a shared contract of care or of specific joint working as a result of

the drugs agency responding to the non-medical needs of the client.

Specialised services: drug dependency treatment and HIV services

These services are for drug users who may have more acute drug problems or require some type of specialist intervention. They may be hospital or community based but again will largely be outpatient or non-residential services. Clients may still be able to self-refer but in some cases a professional referral may be required.

Drug Dependency Units (DDUs)

Drug Dependency Units are usually led by a consultant psychiatrist specialising in drug or substance misuse and will be staffed by one or more of the following professions - social workers, psychiatric and general nurses, counsellors and clinical psychologists.

DDUs were established within the NHS in the 1960s in order to respond to the growing number of opiate users, and are predominately run by the NHS. They continue to provide services mainly to opiate users and traditionally they were the service that prescribed methadone. In establishing DDUs, the Government intended to draw prescribing away from GPs into specialist units. However, as drug prevalence increased over the next 30 years this became less realistic and in the light of recent moves towards community care, less desirable.

Increasingly DDUs will be one of a range of prescribers in any areas, with community agencies and now GPs also actively involved. In many areas DDUs are becoming specialised, seeking to use their skills to work with the most problematic drug users or those requiring the specialist skills of the multi-disciplinary team e.g. drug users with mental health problems, poly-drug users, pregnant women etc, those that cannot be managed by the GP. In these cases the DDUs are likely to leave the bulk of prescribing to community agencies and GPs. However, in some areas, particularly those with relatively low drug prevalence, DDUs may be the main or only prescriber. Some areas may not have a DDU but may have a consultant psychiatrist with some responsibility for drug misuse.

Most services will have a full time nurse, who can offer HIV & Hepatitis testing, Hepatitis B vaccinations, wound dressing and onward referral as necessary, for example to the tissue viability nurse. They can have very long waiting lists depending on the area, up to one year.

HIV teams

With HIV prevalence among injecting drug users highest in London and Scotland, a range of services have been developed for drug users with HIV infection in these areas. These services may be dedicated teams or consist of workers based within DDUs, HIV outpatient clinics, HIV day centres or social services teams. These post holders will have a specific remit for HIV care and should not be confused with HIV counsellors employed to undertake harm reduction work or HIV antibody pre-test counselling.

Finally, a range of varied services is provided to drug users by HIV service organisations throughout the country. There is an extensive listing of all organisations throughout the UK offering HIV and AIDS-related services in the *UK AIDS Directory*. However, with a decrease in funding to HIV organisations, some of these services are not as prevalent as they used to be.

Rehabilitation and inpatient detoxification

Services at this level are for drug users who may require interventions that cannot be undertaken in the community or that require longer term support. These services may be hospital-based or in residential communities. Clients generally need to be assessed for community care funding by their local social services substance misuse team and generally need to be referred there by professionals.

Inpatient detoxification units

Some drug users require detoxification on an inpatient or residential setting. These projects offer a range of detoxification packages which may include some level of therapeutic support, either individually or in group-setting. These projects are largely focused towards the needs of alcohol and /or opiate users but are increasingly considering the needs of other types of drug users, such as crack cocaine users. Inpatient detoxification centres may be run within the NHS or by the voluntary or private sectors. They may be run through community-based residential projects or in hospitals. The location may affect the range and diversity of the services available.

The programme is generally between 2-4 weeks and as the focus is to become drug-free medical interventions are the priority. A small number of units allow people on drug treatment programmes to stabilise their use. There tends to be quite a long waiting list due to the fact that demand greatly outweighs supply.

Residential rehabilitation projects

Some drug users require longer-term therapeutic support to tackle their drug problems. A number of projects, widely known as 'rehabs', have been set up in the voluntary sector providing a wide range of different types of residential support. These are based on many different philosophies and stays vary usually from 3 -6 months and offer a combination of individual key-working / counselling and groups. Some services provide longer support in the form of supported housing to assist clients to re-integrate into mainstream society, after they have completed the treatment programme.

Rehabilitation projects cater for between 6-35 clients, can be mixed or single sex, city- or countryside-based. Some rehabs specialise in providing services to particular client groups such as younger users, women or parents with children. The majority of users will enter rehabs drug-free, having completed an inpatient or community detoxification programme. These services will usually require individuals to have an assessment for community care funding to pay for their treatment.

'Rehabs' tend to be holistic in approach and will support clients around a wide range of issues as well as their drug use, such as education programmes, support around legal, social and family issues.

Access to rehabs is a postcode lottery to some degree, with different boroughs or areas having a different attitude towards funding rehabs. Some boroughs or areas may only fund certain rehabs, meaning that the client may not be able to choose which one they want to go to. The time taken to get into rehab can vary,

but tends to be a minimum of three months, generally longer, again as demand far outweighs supply.

Day programmes

Day programmes are very similar to residential rehabs' in terms of treatment and support offered, however clients live in the community whilst attending. This can have both advantages and disadvantages. Clients are not in a protected environment whilst in treatment as they have to continue to live in the community and face the risks of relapse whilst attending the programme. However, this can help them develop coping skills by managing high-risk situations whilst in treatment, getting the support they need to manage 'real life'.

The advantages of a day care programme is that clients who have family or for other reasons cannot go away for a period of time can still access treatment. In addition, it is cheaper for the funder to send people to a day programme than sending them to a residential rehab. Clients tend to attend day programmes between 9am -5pm Monday-Friday and programmes are usually funded for twelve weeks.

Hospices or residential projects for drug users with HIV

In major centres of high HIV prevalence among injecting drug users, a small number of dedicated residential, respite and hospice projects, such as Mildmay Hospital in London, exist and can provide support for drug users. People are usually referred via community or outpatient services. These units run either within the voluntary or health sector.

Training and development

Training is provided both through the voluntary and statutory sectors. Trainers may be attached to drug teams, part of broader training teams (e.g. within Social Services) or in a small number of cases be dedicated drugs or drugs and HIV training units. In addition, there are a number of freelance trainers operating in the private sector.

A number of agencies or individuals offer consultancy or management services to drugs agencies. These may be freelance staff or be part of training or direct drugs agencies. A number of large charities exist to develop and manage drugs projects which may include some of these services within the infrastructure.

Making services accessible to drug users

The need for accessibility

There has always been a pressing need to engage drug users in services to reduce the possible harm or risks associated with drug using. The advent of HIV has heightened this need and has been reflected in the shift towards harm reduction policies. When abstinence was the dominant philosophy it was often argued that drug users would come to services when they were ready to stop using. HIV underlined the inadequacies of this approach.

Whether people are attempting to set up new services or re-profile existing ones, it is crucial to ensure that projects are viewed as approachable and accessible to potential clients.

Social, economic and legal factors may prevent people from accessing services. Often the user's lifestyle may require support to manage and may actively obstruct them from accessing services.

The location of services may influence the user's decision whether to attend the project or not. A team based in a psychiatric hospital may be viewed as less accessible than a team based in a shop front on a high street. In addition more obvious factors such as access to public transport and disabled access also will also affect this choice. A project's location in terms of the local community will also influence accessibility. A team based in a major drug using area may be attractive, and a team's location in relation to local ethnic communities may also help or impinge on access due to stigma or drug use and discrimination faced by drug users.

The range and style of services will also affect access. Users may feel happy attending only projects with a particular philosophy (e.g. 'Twelve Step' programme). Alternatively users may be clear from personal experience that only a certain type of service will work for them (e.g. residential services).

Users may prefer to use a project that can offer them support in a wide range of areas such as health care, welfare, benefits and housing advice etc, rather than one that exclusively focuses on their drug use. Others will judge a project by its style or friendliness and in particular this may affect the 'word on the street' about a project.

The structure of services may also affect a user's ability to engage. Appointments systems may prove an obstruction to a user whose lifestyle is very unstructured. Asking people with drug dependence to spend all day being assessed when they need to be out raising money and buying drugs is a strategy likely to fail. The needs of parents and the employed also have to be considered.

Waiting times and ability to respond to a crisis is important as users may be influenced by a team's ability to respond quickly. Many users approach services at a point of crisis. If they are put on a three-month waiting list when they approach services they may have dropped out by the time the crisis has eased. The quality of services affects the 'word on the street' about a project. A team that responds slowly, is able to offer a limited range of services and is viewed as judgmental is likely to struggle to access clients.

The drug user's self-esteem may be low and they may have poor self confidence; the client may find it difficult to consider change or feel confident enough to enter services. Accessible services need to develop strategies for coping with the consequences of low self-esteem.

Planning services for HIV-positive drug users

Workers or teams seeking to attract or engage this population will have to consider the following factors that exclude drug users with HIV infection from services:

Drug users often do not view HIV as their primary problem and therefore find traditional HIV services unresponsive. Drug users may view their drug use, homelessness, or legal problems as their most immediate concern. Among the most excluded section of drug users, drug use, homelessness, legal complications, financial difficulties, social and psychological problems may all combine to suppress the client's self - esteem. Users may view drug services as inaccessible if it runs an appointment only service or if the potential client wishes to continue using illicit drugs if the service follows an abstinence-based philosophy.

Where drug users with HIV infection do initially engage with services they often drop out because of the large number of agencies they have to attend to access services. So communication between services is important to facilitate engagement.

Drug users with HIV infection are largely invisible and not accessible via traditional services alone. The illegal nature of the community compounds this problem. The increased urgency of the need to reach drug users in the last ten years is reflected in a proliferation of outreach workers and teams largely funded from dedicated HIV money. Outreach services aim to access 'hard to reach groups' such as people from ethnic or cultural communities, the homeless, cocaine users, or younger users. Many CDT's or street agencies use outreach workers as a way to draw users into projects or to take services out to them.

Many agencies have developed a number of strategies and techniques to engage 'hard to reach' clients. These include:

Satellite services

In areas of high drug use, other agencies may also provide frontline services to drug users. This may be services such as the Probation Service, Social Services, the Youth Service (both in the statutory and voluntary sectors), Homeless Services and counselling services for young people. Some of these services employ specialist drug workers, or the local drug service may send a worker to this service for specialist support.

What they can do will depend on the agency, at a minimum they can offer information and advice and referral on to appropriate services.

Mobile schemes

In order to reach users who may not be able to travel to a project base it may be more appropriate to take services out through the use of a van or bus. Through the establishment of regular and known stops users may be encouraged into services. This is particularly useful in rural areas or in areas where a lack of public transport makes an area isolated (e.g. housing estates.)

Delivery schemes

Again, in order to take services out to those who may not otherwise attend a project, a phone number (usually a mobile one) is advertised. Users are invited to ring to request an outreach worker to deliver needles and syringes or condoms. This type of scheme is labour intensive and is best used to gradually draw people into a project-based service or to reach well defined hard-to-reach groups.

Detached work

This style of outreach was largely developed within the youth service but has been adapted to drugs work. Users are targeted through street dealer scenes, key meeting places or using arenas. Again this method is labour intensive but allows outreach workers the opportunity to intervene in areas with a street drug or prostitution scene.

Paraphernalia

'Wraps' with project and harm reduction advice printed on them were developed by the Drug Advice and Information Service in Brighton and they allow the project to reach users who do not come into the service. Lighters and matchboxes are a regular part of social interaction and are used as part of preparing some drugs for injection. Most smokers know how matches and lighters are inadvertently passed from one person to another. When developed by the Healthy Options Team in East London it was felt better to make no mention of drugs on the matchboxes or lighters, as this might put the user at risk from the police. Instead, project information was given. In all such techniques, careful piloting with service users is needed.

It should also be remembered that with the exception of needles and syringes it is illegal to supply paraphernalia, such as citric acid (used to prepare heroin for injection) or sterile water. However, the local Crown Prosecution Service may agree to overlook this if they feel it is in the public interest.

Dealer-based schemes

This type of scheme recognises that dealers are better placed to see large numbers of drug users and pass on equipment and information than outreach workers. The dealer may need to have the benefits of the scheme 'sold' to them (e.g. being viewed as more convenient than rival dealers), or to be offered other incentives. Care will need to be taken not to increase the dealer's risk of getting arrested as this would ensure no future dealer compliance. It may also be wise to liaise with the police to get their backing for such a venture.

Peer-led initiatives

These techniques are more appropriate to areas where the drugs scene happens behind closed doors. Outreach workers ask clients to introduce them to other users, or to bring new users into the service from which new contacts are made. The workers aim to keep finding new users to act as the introduction to the next user group. The outreach worker may need to consider the benefits or rewards for the drug user who provides the contacts, and giving money or goods such as cigarettes may be options.

The fact that users attending services come into regular contact with their peers can be used to pass on messages regarding safer drug use. The user who attends the service can be given information and clean drug paraphernalia which they can pass on to other users.

Peer education

In this technique users are offered training on a range of drugs and HIV-related issues. At the end of their course they are sent back into their using community and alongside their drug-using or -dealing they become peer educators and volunteer outreach workers. It is advisable to offer regular contact to allow the volunteer outreach worker to seek support, advice and information updates.

Benefits of user involvement

Drugs users have not had a strong history of involvement in the services provided to them, but with the promotion of quality assurance initiatives this is changing. Some agencies have sought to establish services from a user perspective, working with the active participation of the using community.

Working with a community approach proved highly successful in spreading risk reduction messages and techniques not only in the gay communities but also in more loosely organised networks of gay and bisexual men that are more nearly akin to the networks that exist amongst drug users.

Adapting this model to work with drug users is problematic due to the illegal nature of the community, and may require a complete shift of emphasis in service delivery. This remains daunting to many agencies, as accepting a model of community development also allows for drug users to have a far greater say in, and responsibility for, their social and health care. However, this is in line with the case management approach promoted within community care legislation.

Where a community development approach has been undertaken with drug users, a greater ownership and support of the community-orientated project improves access, opens avenues of advertising through user networks and improves client retention. This approach can be highly effective in either reaching wide sections of the drug using community or in targeting specific populations.

It is also cost effective as user involvement in their development ensures the relevance of and accessibility of new campaigns and services. Where a sense of community has been developed among users, clients may see this as motive enough to become involved in supporting the delivery of services.

Within the gay communities the role of community members as professionals has acted as a validation of the community and helped make sure that some of its values (such as safer sex rather than abstinence from sex) are adopted by HIV services. This remains problematic in drug services as many agencies expect workers who have been drug users to have been drug-free for at least two years. To operate a community development model may require these employment policies to be rethought.

A community development approach offers the opportunity to include and involve drug users in their services. Limited existing evidence shows that drug users may be motivated to respond to this approach with significant benefit to drug agencies. However, it requires a commitment to rethink service delivery from a user perspective and to include clients as equals within the development process. It is important to consider issues of personal safety as poor planning could put workers in danger. Plus, if users feel put at risk by outreach workers then they are unlikely to be receptive.

Outreach work must be based on needs assessment, solid preparation and careful development. Without clear aims and objectives outreach is unlikely to be successful and could prove a waste of resources. However, it does offer the opportunity to reach out to drug users who would otherwise remain out of touch with services.

Evaluating and monitoring drug services

Evaluation and monitoring remain essential tools in assessing the effectiveness and quality of services, and it is the responsibility of NTA to monitor the quality of services provided.

Services now need to set objectives on an annual basis which are agreed and monitored within the framework of service agreements with purchasing authorities. This allows quantitative data collection to be set in context, with agencies working to sustain or increase activity levels. Qualitative data systems to monitor waiting times, client retention rates, success rates and behaviour change among clients all add to the depth of evaluation of services. Increasingly, consumer evaluation is being seen as an essential tool in monitoring quality. It may, for the first time, force some agencies to listen to the comments of drug users. Complaints procedures are now being seen as a positive opportunity to engage consumers' comments on services. This has led to a stronger emphasis on both formal and informal complaints procedures. In addition to formal evaluation techniques, some projects are seeking to promote greater user consultation at a less formal level through comments boxes.

Resources

Leaflets

The following organisations can provide leaflets, posters and training courses on a wide range of drug and alcohol-related issues.

www.lifeline.org.uk

www.hit.org.uk

www.drugscope.org.uk

Poster

Overdose Aid (Drugscope, Waterbridge House, 32-34 Loman Street, London SE1 0EE, 020 7928 1211)

Books and reports

The Centre for Research on Drugs and Health Behaviour (Charing Cross and Westminster Medical School, 200 Seagrove Road, London SW6 1RQ, 020 8846 6565) has conducted extensive research on needle exchanges, HIV infection and outreach work in the UK.

Drugscope has an extensive library and publishes a bimonthly magazine Druglink (see above under Poster).

Counselling drug users about HIV and AIDS by Geraldine Mulleady (Blackwell Scientific, £15.99, 1992) is an excellent and detailed guide to counselling drug users.

The Alcohol and Drug Wildcard: Substance Use and Psychiatric Problems in People With HIV (Ucsf Aids Health Project Monograph Series, No. 2)

Joan E. Zweben
(http://www.amazon.co.uk/exec/obidos/search-handle-url/index=books-uk&field-author=zweben,%20joan%20e./026-2514221-2930846)

Patt Denning
(http://www.amazon.co.uk/exec/obidos/search-handle-url/index=books-uk&field-author=denning,%20patt/026-2514221-2930846)

A to Z of drugs

Acid

see LSD

Alcohol

Alcohol comes in many forms, from beer and wine to spirits. It is a controlled but legalised drug in the sense that it is available only through certain licensed outlets and to persons over 18 years of age. Alcohol is a major contributor towards ill-health and disease in the UK, and leads to greater loss of life than any of the other drugs discussed in this section. Alcoholism is a widespread problem in the UK

Alcohol has a depressant effect; it relaxes the central nervous system and leads to a pleasant and uninhibited feeling. Most people feel merry and relaxed after a couple of drinks, but greater alcohol use can lead to poor co-ordination, exaggerated emotional reactions and eventually unconsciousness. Large amounts of alcohol may lead to coma and death.

Long-term consumption of large quantities of alcohol can lead to liver damage, heart disease and brain damage. Alcoholics frequently have poor nutrition and consequent poor health.

There is no evidence that moderate drinking is harmful, and many people find that a few drinks help to relieve feelings of stress or anxiety. Moderate drinking is also linked to a reduced risk of heart disease, although it is unclear why.

Small amounts of alcohol, especially before a meal, can help to increase appetite which can be valuable when someone is at risk of weight loss.

The government recently changed their advice on safer drinking. The recommended consumption has increased from 14 to 21 units per week for women and from 21 -28 units for men. However, the advice is that women should only drink 2-3 units per day and men 3-4 units per day. This advice comes about to address the issue of binge drinking which recognises that drinking all units in 1 or 2 sessions per week can be more detrimental to health than drinking a small amount every day. (http://www.alcoholconcern.org.uk/). However, heavy drinking can affect your immune system and may slow down recovery from infections. People who drink heavily often tend to neglect their diets.

Alcohol can react badly with some medicines, so it is best to check with the pharmacist or doctor when prescribed new medications to find out whether it is safe to drink alcohol with them. There is a particular problem with some treatments for tuberculosis (rifampicin and rifabutin) and the antibiotic metronidazole and related drugs. However, there is no direct incompatibility between alcohol and any of the current antiretrovirals (see section later on drug interactions).

The adverse consequences of heavy alcohol consumption on the HIV-infected patient as it relates to disease progression are poorly understood and to date existing studies have failed to find an association between alcohol use, progression to AIDS or infectiousness.

However a 2005 study of monkeys given large doses of alcohol - the equivalent of four pints of beer a day over a seven-week period - found that rates of viral replication and viral load increased by 1.9 logs (nearly 89-fold). However although CD4 counts initially declined faster in monkeys given alcohol than the control animals, the difference in CD4 cells was not significant by the end of the study (Kumar, 2005), Another study by Bagby (2006) suggests that heavy drinking can accelerate time to AIDS among rhesus macaques infected with simian immunodeficiency virus (SIV), The monkeys were exposed to alcohol for four days a week at levels designed to simulate 'binge' drinking, and compared with a control group. The monkeys receiving alcohol had higher viral loads in the blood in the early months after being infected with the virus, which is associated with more rapid disease progression. As SIV infection in rhesus macaques is so similar to what happens in HIV-infected humans, they conclude that it is important to reduce alcohol use in HIV-positive individuals as the speed of progression of AIDS for alcohol users is in part affected by past and current drinking very early on in the disease. It is known that each episode of alcohol intoxication can suppress multiple elements of immune function in humans and this suppression can be largely responsible for the increased incidence of infections such as pneumonia. However, chronic alcohol consumption can also stimulate the immune system, leading to diseases like hepatitis. Bagby's (2006) research suggests that both effects are involved: immunosuppression could increase the incidence of opportunistic infections, and immune stimulation could activate cells infected with the virus, causing more cells to become infected.

Another study by Poonia (2006) carried out on monkeys has found that long-term alcohol consumption can affect the turnover of immune system cells in the intestine, and the depletion of these cells by simian immunodeficiency virus (SIV). They found that monkeys given alcohol had lower levels of effector memory CD8 T-cells in the intestine, which are responsible for the rapid identification and killing of cells infected with organisms the body has already encountered. They also showed a depletion of central memory CD4 T-cells in the intestines after infection and had higher levels of SIV in the intestine, lymph nodes and spleen. The investigators conclude that alcohol increases the number of the major target cells for SIV in the intestine, and that this allows replication to be enhanced. They provide some evidence that alcohol could inhibit the turnover of T-cells, resulting in the altered proportions of the different cell types. Although studies have not examined any similar effects of alcohol and HIV on immune cells in humans, these results suggest that long-term intake of large amounts of alcohol may affect the activity of the immune system during early HIV infection. This, in turn, may cause higher viral loads by increasing HIV replication.

Reference

Bagby GJ et al. *Chronic binge ethanol consumption accelerates progression of simian immunodeficiency virus disease.* Alcoholism: Clinical and Experimental Research 30 (10): 1-10, 2006.

Kumar R et al. Increased viral replication in simian immunodeficiency virus/simian HIV-infected macaques with self-administering model of chronic alcohol consumption. J Acquir Immune Defic Syndr 39: 386-390, 2005. Poonia B et al. *Intestinal lymphocyte subsets and turnover are affected by chronic alcohol consumption: implications for SIV / HIV infection.* J Acquir Immune Defic Syndr 41: 537-547, 2006.

Amphetamines/speed

Often known as speed, whizz, billy or uppers. See also **Crystal Meth.**

Amphetamines are stimulants normally taken by mouth or snorted up the nose. Amphetamines usually come in powder form, although tablets may also be encountered. It is sold in 'wraps' of one gram, and the price has remained fairly stable at around £10 a gram for many years. Speed is usually cut with other forms of powder such as ascorbic acid, icing sugar, cornflour and talc.

Amphetamines can also be injected. It is important to be aware that HIV can be transmitted through sharing needles and syringes used to inject speed in just the same way as with heroin. The frequency of injecting speed seems to vary widely from one part of the country to another.

Most amphetamines come in the form of amphetamine sulphate powder. Amphetamines are treated as Class B drugs under the Misuse of Drugs Acts unless they are prepared for injection, in which case they are classified as Class A drugs.

Amphetamines cause the heartbeat to speed up, appetite to diminish, the pupils to widen and mood to improve. Users experience a rush of confidence and energy which can last for three to four hours before they begin to 'come down'. Feelings of anxiety and restlessness begin to take over at this point. Grinding of the teeth is a common side-effect of amphetamine use. Repeated use of amphetamines leads to tolerance and can lead to more exaggerated feelings of anxiety, paranoia and panic. Long-term heavy use may result in mental disturbances which become more pronounced with time.

Amphetamines postpone the need for food and rest but don't eliminate these needs altogether. This means that regular users can begin to suffer from poor diet and weight loss. In turn this affects resistance to infection, so HIV-positive users need to be especially wary of over-taxing the body with repeated amphetamine use.

The effect of speed use on diet and sleep means that women who are regular users of the drug may experience irregular periods. Speed also affects unborn children, leading to low birth weight, although it is not thought to lead to birth defects.

Crystal meth - see below - is a form of amphetamine which gives a longer-lasting and more intense 'high'. Although there is little evidence that 'regular' speed users have faster progression to AIDS, crystal meth has been found to increase the rate of HIV replication and accelerate HIV- related dementia.

Amyl/butyl nitrites

see Poppers.

Anabolic steroids

Anabolic steroids are hormones which are commonly used as drugs to build muscle. In the human body their effect is to enhance masculine characteristics. Bodybuilders and, increasingly, regular gym-goers, use anabolic steroids to build lean muscle mass and body mass, usually in cycles of four weeks on, followed by time off.

People, mostly men, with HIV are sometimes prescribed testosterone hormone replacement therapy, because some men with HIV are hypogonadal (have low natural production of testosterone). When given by a nurse or doctor, the dose and frequency of this type of anabolic steroid use does not necessarily cause the same kind of hazards to health as the unregulated use of non-prescription steroids bought in the gym or on the black market and self-administered.

All steroids can elevate liver enzymes but levels usually return to normal once the cycle is stopped. Long-term heavy use may increase the risk of developing liver cancer. The injectable, water-based suspension of testosterone, commonly used by bodybuilders, is highly toxic to the liver, and can encourage the development of acne, male pattern baldness, testicular atrophy (shrinkage) and impotence. Steroids also affect the hormonal and reproductive system in men, lowering the production of testosterone, which in turn reduces sperm production. These steroids tend to be used because large gains in muscle mass are seen in very short periods of time. Methandrostenolone (Dianabol) shares this side-effect profile in both its oral and injectable forms. Testosterone enanthate and testosterone propionate are also toxic. Testosterone cypionate causes severe disturbances in the production of the body's own testosterone and high levels of water retention have been reported anecdotally.

Rare side-effects of steroid usage include stomach pain, insomnia, and high blood pressure. In men, side-effects include enlarged prostate (causing difficulty with urination) and breast development.

Women run the risk of developing male characteristics such as growth of facial and body hair, deepening of the voice and decrease in breast size, all of which appear to be irreversible. These characteristics may be passed on to a female foetus if the woman is pregnant while taking the drugs. Women report increased sex drive and menstrual irregularities and the clitoris may become enlarged.

Counterfeit steroids are common, and may contain impurities which can in turn result in infections or abscesses. Incorrect selection of an injection site may lead to the disruption of a major nerve, with consequent paralysis or pain in the area served by that nerve.

Steroids are usually supplied in liquid capsules and injected so there is increasing concern about the chances of HIV transmission through sharing needles to inject steroids. Needle-sharing appears to be a common practice amongst anabolic steroid users, but it is dangerous for exactly the same reason that sharing needles for injecting recreational drugs is dangerous, because of the risk of blood-borne infections. As with other injected drugs, clean needles and syringes should be used. Recent surveys have found that up to a third of needles exchanged at UK needle exchange programmes are from users of anabolic steroids.

Anabolic steroids are Prescription Only drugs under the Medicines Act. They can only be sold by a pharmacist on the presentation of a doctor's prescription. Anabolic steroids are also class C drugs under the Misuse of Drugs Act (1971). It is not an offence to possess anabolic steroids for personal use, unless they are counterfeit. It is an offence to supply them.

Barbiturates

Also known as barbs, downers, and names related to colours and trade names e.g. blues, reds, sekkies etc.

Barbiturates are used medically to calm people down and as sleeping pills. Most barbiturates come in powdered form and are sold in coloured capsules. They are usually taken by mouth, occasionally with alcohol, although some users inject the powder inside the capsule.

Barbiturates depress the central nervous system in the same way as alcohol and the effects will last for three to six hours, depending on the dose. Larger doses can make the user clumsy, which can lead to accidents. Happiness, misery and mental confusion are all possible as a result of use.

Large doses can produce unconsciousness and eventually breathing failure and death. Death from overdose is a real danger as the amount which can cause an overdose is very near the normal dose, and gets progressively narrower with use, as users develop tolerance. The chances of an overdose occurring are far greater if alcohol is taken at the same time.

Long-term users are likely to develop a tolerance to and dependence on barbiturates. The dependence is both physical and mental. The effects of withdrawing from a high dose can include irritability, nervousness, sleeplessness, faintness, sickness, twitching, delirium and convulsions. Sudden withdrawal from high doses of barbiturates can result in death. The risks associated with barbiturate use are increased if the drug is injected. Infections due to drug injecting and a build-up of undissolved tablet in the skin tissue may occur. Injecting sedatives is possibly the most dangerous form of drug use.

Heavy users are especially liable to bronchitis and pneumonia (because the cough reflex is suppressed), hypothermia (because the peripheral blood vessels dilate, but the drug blocks normal responses to cold). Prolonged regular use of barbiturates in the later stages of pregnancy can result in withdrawal symptoms in new-born babies.

Barbiturates are Prescription Only drugs under the Medicines Act (1968). This means they can only be sold from a pharmacy in accordance with a doctor's prescription. Barbiturates are also controlled as class B drugs under the Misuse of Drugs Act (http://www.drugscope.org.uk/druginfo/drugsearch/ds_results.asp?file=%5cwip%5cl1%5cl%5cl%5cdrug%20laws.html) (1971). Doctors can still prescribe them and patients take them but unauthorised possession or supply is an offence.

Benzodiazepines

see tranquillisers

Buprenorphine

Buprenorphine (trade name Subutex) is an opioid drug that is similar to heroin. It is prescribed as a substitute to heroin, in the same way as methadone, and can help to reduce the withdrawal symptoms and cravings associated with stopping heroin use. It is sometimes preferred to methadone, as it is reported that some people feel more 'clear headed' with buprenorphine than methadone. Also, some people have argued that buprenorphine is easier to detox from and more difficult to overdose with than methadone.

Cannabis

Also known as marijuana, blow, dope, puff, grass, weed, hash, wacky baccy, spliff, skunk.

Cannabis is the most widely used illicit drug in the UK. The supply and possession of cannabis is illegal in the UK and is likely to remain so for the foreseeable future. Cannabis was downgraded from a Class B drug to a Class C drug in January 2004. Supplying the drug carries the risk of a prison sentence of up to fourteen years, whilst possession for any reason could result in a two-year sentence. Similarly, growing cannabis at home for your own use could also lead to a prison sentence. In practice, the police often just issue a caution to people caught in possession of the drug, and it is possible that only persistent offenders are likely to find themselves in court.

Cannabis comes in two forms: cannabis resin (hashish) and marijuana, the dried leaves of *Cannabis sativa*. Cannabis is sold as blocks of compressed resin by the eighth or quarter of an ounce; marijuana is sold as dried leaves. Marijuana, or grass or weed as it is generally known, varies in strength; a variety called 'skunk' is now widely available in the UK. It contains much more THC, the active ingredient which causes the hallucinogenic properties, than other forms of grass.

Cannabis can be smoked, usually with tobacco, eaten, drunk as a tea or snorted as a snuff. The drug affects the central nervous system, and as a result, users may experience relief from pain, feel light-headed, relaxed, or sleepy. The drug can also stimulate appetite; inducing the so-called 'munchies'. In 1996, a clinical trial in San Francisco found that people with HIV wasting disease who used cannabis were more likely to put on weight. The drug is also widely used to relieve insomnia and the symptoms of anxiety and stress. It is also used by people with multiple sclerosis as a muscle relaxant. However, cannabis is also known to impair co-ordination, can cause nausea and vomiting, as well as anxiety and paranoia, which in long-term use may become chronic.

The effects of cannabis tend to depend on the pre-existing mood of the user, the amount used and the situation in which it is used. The most common, and also the most sought-after effects, are talkativeness, cheerfulness, relaxation and greater appreciation of sound and colour. Cannabis reduces individuals' abilities to do complicated tasks and can affect the short-term memory.

Because people can't concentrate as well, it is dangerous to drive or work machinery soon after using the drug. A driver under the influence of cannabis may be just as much of a danger as a driver under the influence of alcohol.

Smoking cannabis is likely to harm an unborn child in just the same way as smoking tobacco, but there is no evidence that it exaggerates these effects.

Medical marijuana

Cannabis has been widely promoted as a medication in its own right, particularly as an appetite stimulant and as pain relief, and cases of elderly patients with conditions such as multiple sclerosis arrested for growing or possessing cannabis have occasionally hit the headlines. It has been used informally by people with HIV for the same reasons since the beginning of the epidemic and in San Francisco a 'medical marijuana' dispensary was operated by AIDS-dissident group ACT-UP SF.

To assess the extent of cannabis use, researchers from the Chelsea and Westminster Hospital asked patients attending the hospital's HIV clinic to complete an anonymous questionnaire about their use of cannabis and the effects of the drug on their HIV-related symptoms.

"Despite the fact that cannabis is still illegal, its use for medical purposes appears to be quite widespread," they write. "A large number of patients reported that cannabis improved symptom control."

In total, 523 patients completed the questionnaire. Of these, 143 (27%) reported ever using cannabis to improve their symptoms. The majority (71%) only smoked cannabis, with 2% eating and drinking it and the rest combining eating, drinking and smoking the drug. Most patients (55%) took cannabis daily.

When asked why they took cannabis, 54% of the patients replied "to treat symptoms," and 20% using it to "reduce symptom frequency." Sixty-six per cent used cannabis to "relieve anxiety" and 52% to "relieve depression."

However, 85% said that they used cannabis to "aid relaxation" and 43% "for a high." It is not clear from the study to what extent these proportions overlapped.

Patients using cannabis reported significant improvements in symptoms. The greatest improvement was seen in appetite. Seventy-eight per cent of the cannabis users reported a lack of appetite, but 97% of these experienced an improvement after using the drug (p < 0.001).

Forty-five per cent of the cannabis users reported pain, but the drug improved this in 94%. This included muscle pain (94%), nerve pain (90%), tingling (85%) and headache (65%).

Statistically significant improvements were also reported for nausea (93%), anxiety (93%) and depression (86%), as well as numbness (72%), weight loss (69%), tremor (66%), constipation (50%), tiredness (40%) and diarrhoea (36%).

However, 47% of the cannabis users reported memory loss after taking the drug (p = 0.043).

Cannabis and mental health

Cannabis, however, has also been associated with the development of psychosis, especially in young users, leading to demands that the drug be re-classified. Chronic loss of memory and shortened attention span have been observed in long-term users of the drug, in some cases even after they have ceased, and there is evidence that long-term users can develop psychological dependency on the drug. Chronic use of cannabis has also been associated with the onset or long-term worsening of certain mental illnesses, most notably depression and psychosis and there is growing evidence of a link particularly in young people who start smoking strong forms of skunk at an early age.

A recent study in the British Medical Journal (Henquet), for example, found that young people who started smoking cannabis between the ages of 14 to 20 were 67% more likely than non-users to develop psychotic illnesses four years after they started smoking. This association was much stronger in young people who had already been assessed as being vulnerable to psychosis.

A longitudinal New Zealand study (Arseneault) which followed 1,000 people born in 1977 for 25 years found that young people who had started using cannabis by the age of 15 were 4.5 times

as likely to develop schizophrenia in adulthood, while people who were heavy cannabis users before the age of 18 were six times more likely.

References

Arseneault L. Cannabis use in adolescence and risk for adult psychosis: longitudinal prospective study. BMJ 325: 1212-1213. 2002.

Henquet C et al. Prospective cohort study of cannabis use, predisposition for psychosis, and psychotic symptoms in young people. BMJ 330(7481):11-15. 2005.

Woolridge E et al. Cannabis use in HIV for pain and other medical symptoms. J Pain Symptom Manage 29: 358-367, 2005.

Cocaine

Also known as Charlie, snow, coke, powder. See also **Crack** below.

Cocaine is a stimulant made from the leaves of the South American coca shrub. It comes in the form of a white powder, and normally costs in the region of £50 a gram. Cocaine use is becoming increasingly widespread throughout the UK, as is crack cocaine. It is a Class A drug under the Misuse of Drugs Act (1971). Dealing carries a maximum life prison sentence and unlimited fine, and possession can mean up to seven years in prison and a fine of £5,000.

In common with most other street drugs, users are rarely sold a pure form of cocaine. The drug is often cut with other cheaper drugs such as amphetamines (speed), talc or detergents which can be poisonous or cause irritation, leading to infection, particularly if injected.

Usually snorted into the nose, it provides a feeling of excitement, exhilaration and self-confidence lasting for about 15-30 minutes. Cocaine can also be rubbed into the gums, onto the teeth and into the anus or vagina before penetrative sex. Cocaine and crack can also be made into a solution for injection. Users will frequently take repeated doses to maintain the high and as a result over a few hours anxiety, agitation and paranoia can develop, as well as tolerance for the drug, leading to the need for higher doses. Due to the short acting nature of cocaine, people who inject risk doing considerable damage to their veins due to the need to inject more frequently. Users are often tempted to step up the dose because of the feelings of physical and mental well-being produced by the drug.

After stopping use, users will feel tired, sleepy and depressed, which reinforces the temptation to repeat the dose.

With regular use, increasingly unpleasant effects develop which generally persuade people to 'give it a break'. Happiness is replaced by an uncomfortable state of restlessness, excitability, sickness, sleeplessness and weight loss. With continued use this may change to a persecuted state of mind. Regular users may seem nervous, excitable and suspicious. Confused exhaustion due to lack of sleep is common. All these effects generally clear up once the drug is stopped.

Repeated sniffing damages the nose membranes and may damage the structure separating the nostrils. The effect of cocaine use on diet and sleep means that women who are regular users of the drug may experience irregular periods. Cocaine also affects unborn children in several ways (www.marchofdimes.com/professionals)

- It may be linked to spontaneous abortion.

- Cocaine is expelled from the mother's body far more quickly than from the foetus.

- Women who use cocaine during pregnancy are more likely to deliver prematurely.

- Frequent users of cocaine are more likely to suffer a difficult delivery.

- The babies of cocaine users are more likely to be of low birth weight.

- Babies of women who use cocaine during pregnancy are much more likely to die after birth than babies of non-users, probably due to low birth weight and premature delivery.

- Children of cocaine users are likely to display jittery and disturbed behaviour during the first year of life, but there is no clear evidence that children of cocaine users will be less intelligent, have more severe behavioural problems or suffer retarded growth in later years.

All these apply to the babies of crack cocaine users too.

There is increasing evidence that sharing snorting equipment may permit the transmission of hepatitis C virus. Rubbing cocaine into the gums, vagina, or anus can cause ulceration, which could increase transmission of HIV or other sexually transmitted infections. Sharing injecting equipment also presents a risk for transmission of HIV, hepatitis viruses, and other blood-borne infections (www.nida.nih.gov/ResearchReports/Cocaine).

Crack

Also known as rocks or freebase cocaine. See also *Cocaine*.

Crack is a cheaper variant of cocaine and is becoming more widely used in the UK. Crack is an illegal Class A drug: dealing carries a maximum life prison sentence and unlimited fine, and possession can mean up to seven years in prison and a fine of £5,000.

Crack is sold in the form of small rocks, which are smoked either in cigarettes or in a pipe. Historically, crack has been associated with poor urban populations, but in fact is used by people from a wide social spectrum.

Crack is a very efficient way of delivering cocaine to the brain, and the initial rush is very strong. The pleasurable high followed by unpleasant side-effects encourages repeated compulsive use, which can easily lead to dependency.

Crack users are more likely to have problems with their drug use than those snorting cocaine and run into problems much earlier in their drug use.

Crack use has been associated with a high incidence of STIs, and crack use may increase the risk of oral transmission of HIV due to burns and ulcers in the mouth caused by crack smoking. Crack can also be injected, and some users prefer 'snowballs', where heroin and crack are taken together.

There is evidence that crack/cocaine may accelerate HIV replication. In 2002 scientists exposing HIV-implanted mice to the equivalent of a dose of smoked crack cocaine daily for 10-12 days found that the proportion of CD4 and CD8 cells that had become infected with HIV was 38.8%, compared with 15.5% in control animals. The cocaine-treated mice had a threefold greater decline in CD4 counts and in their CD4:CD8 ratio, and a 40-fold increase in viral load.

Reference

Roth MD et al. Cocaine enhances human immunodeficiency virus replication in a model of severe combined immunodeficient mice implanted with human peripheral blood leukocytes. J Infect Dis 185: 701-705, 2002.

Crystal meth

Also known as methamphetamine, tina, crystal meths, krank, tweak, ice, yaba

Methamphetamine was originally manufactured by the Nazis to help keep their troops awake for days at a time. It has been popular with gay men on the West Coast of North America for the last decade, and, as Yaba, is now more popular than heroin in Thailand. As the use of crystal meth has moved across the US to the East Coast, there are concerns that it is now being targeted at Europe and the UK. There have been recent reports that crystal meth is being used by UK gay men, mainly at private parties. At the moment it is unclear how easily available crystal meth is and how widely it is being used.

A derivative of synthetic amphetamines, it can be manufactured far more quickly and easily than traditional forms of amphetamine. The main ingredients, which include salt, household cleaning products, distilled cold medicines and lithium from camera batteries can be bought legally and the drug can be made at home. However, it can come in pill form, as powder to be snorted or injected, or in its crystal form 'ice', smoked in a pipe. In the UK, reports suggest that crystal meth is available in a number of different forms including paste, crystals and possibly suspended as a solution.

Crystal meth brings on a feeling of exhilaration and a sharpening of focus, which leads to intense feelings of sexual power which can result in marathon sex for hours on end. Several recent studies have linked the use of crystal meth with increased sexual risk-taking, especially when combined with *Viagra* (see also *Viagra* below). It has been reported in the States that crystal meth has been a factor in almost half of new HIV infections amongst gay men.

Smoking crystal meth results in body temperature rises and rapid cardiac and respiratory rates developing as the blood pressure increases.

The effects and dependence potential of crystal meth are similar to that of amphetamine misuse, although since it is more potent, the dangers involved are greater with an increased chance of overdose. Overuse can bring on paranoia, short term memory loss, wild rages and mood swings as well as damage to the immune system. Although it does not appear to be physically addictive, psychological dependence for the drug does occur.

Overdosing can lead to severe convulsions followed by circulatory and respiratory collapse, coma and death. Some people have died after taking small doses.

Crystal meth is used widely and is particularly popular amongst urban gay men. At times hysterically blamed for rising levels of unprotected sex and HIV infection in gay men, especially in US cities. A study by Bolding (2006) into the sexual behaviour of gay men in London found that approximately 10% of gay men in London have used methamphetamine (http://www.aidsmap.com/en/docs/2F1E4CD0-8E53-40C5-B580-3AB8E8820C77.asp). It was used by 13% of HIV-positive men in the previous year and 8% of HIV-negative men. However most men were infrequent users of the drug; of those who were HIV-positive 9% said that they had used the drug once or twice in the previous twelve months, 3% said they used it once or twice a month, but less than 1% said they used on a weekly basis. Higher rates of use were found amongst gay men living in London, with 7% reporting use of the drug at least once during the last year with 20% of HIV-positive men saying they had used it at least once during the previous twelve months. The highest level of methamphetamine use was found amongst HIV-positive men with multiple sexual partners. The findings are broadly in line with that of the 2005 National Gay Men's Sex Survey which found that a little over 6% of gay men in London reported use of the drug in the previous year, although higher levels of use were seen amongst HIV-positive men (http://www.aidsmap.com/en/news/0EF82EBE-0D65-4B30-ACF1-FE1225555A1D.asp).

At the 12th Retrovirus Conference in February 2005, Grant Colfax of the San Francisco Department of Public Health said that poppers, cocaine and crystal meth were the biggest single contributory factor to continued HIV transmission between gay men. Colfax told the conference that using crystal raised the risk of unsafe sex two to three times, and the risk of HIV infection by

60%. A Californian study involving 68 gay men seeking treatment for methamphetamine dependence revealed that 61% were HIV-positive, and that these men were more likely to have injected the drug, to have had a sexually transmitted infection, to have had a larger number of sexual partners and to have had unprotected anal sex.

However, the association between methamphetamine use and HIV risk behaviours was not clear-cut as 90% of men also reported using cocaine, ketamine and ecstasy and men who use these drugs were also twice as likely to report unsafe sex (Bolding, 2006). HIV-negative gay men who use methamphetamine are twice as likely as men who do not use it to become infected with HIV (Plankey, 2006). However, the use of poppers (amyl nitrate), which is legally available and common on the gay scenes in industrialised countries, lead to a similar increase in the risk of becoming infected with HIV. Buchacz (2005) also found that gay men who use methamphetamine were more likely to report unprotected anal sex and were three times more likely to test positive for HIV than non- users. Even when the use of other recreational drugs, alcohol and poppers was controlled they still found a strong association between methamphetamine use and recent infection with HIV (odds ratio 2.5).

Receptive unprotected anal sex raised the risk of infection by nearly 300%. But because taking drugs during sex was more common than getting penetrated without condoms, the "attributable fraction" of HIV cases due to drug use (that is, the contribution drug use made to HIV transmission) was 29%, beating unprotected receptive anal sex by one per cent.

On the surface, Colfax admitted, it was puzzling that using a drug was even more risky than directly indulging in the sexual behaviour most likely to transmit HIV.

However, all sorts of factors could come together to make users of coke and crystal particularly vulnerable. Pain was dulled, so injuries for HIV to pass through could be more common. Other drug users were already more likely to be HIV-positive, and also less likely to remember to take HIV medication, and therefore more infectious. And users might simply not be able to remember what they'd done.

In addition, he said, drugs suppressed the immune system, and poppers caused increased blood flow to the anal region. All of these factors made transmission more likely.

Colfax said that a number of studies have shown that drug use in gay men was two to three times higher than in straight men of comparable age, and two to three times as high again in HIV-positive gay men.

Interestingly, and in contrast with findings about other HIV risks, young white gay men were particularly at risk. In one study of young men under 25 in seven US cities, half of all white men said they had used crystal, four in ten cocaine and one in eight crack. In contrast, only one in six young black men had used crystal meth, one in eight coke and one in 20 crack. "So much for urban stereotypes," commented Colfax.

He then looked at what could be done to help gay men stop using. One study of group support had shown no effect, but it may simply have been too intense. (It was a three-times-weekly Narcotics Anonymous-type meeting.) Behavioural therapy produced modest reductions. More typical one-to-one counselling reduced the number of unsafe-sex episodes by three-quarters, but didn't stop men using drugs. (It may have just helped them feel good enough about themselves to use condoms.)

One of the most promising approaches, he said, was a New York incentive scheme that gave users substantial rewards in the form of department store vouchers if they produced consecutive urine tests free of drugs. But this was obviously only appropriate for the 25% or so of crystal and coke users who are dependent, rather than recreational weekend users.

He also looked at substitution therapy, or giving another drug to stop drug use - nicotine patches for smokers, Antabuse for alcoholics, methadone for heroin addicts.

No substitute drug had worked so far for "uppers" like coke or crystal, he said, but there was a trial in heterosexuals with problem crystal use of a drug called bupropion. This raises the levels of dopamine, the brain chemical over-stimulated by coke and meth. Dopamine crashes during comedown, tempting users to have another tweak. Results were yet to come out and, as with methadone, some people feared substitution therapy would have no influence on sexual-risk behaviour, or even increase it.

Finally, Colfax said, although he didn't have time to comment, there was probably no substitute for a strong community response, and he praised community campaigns to make crystal less 'sexy'.

It can be argued that methamphetamine is a new and serious challenge to both HIV treatment and prevention (Urbina, 2004). The viral loads of HIV-positive people who used methamphetamine are significantly higher than those of individuals who do not take the drug (Ellis, 2003). Stimulant drugs, such as methamphetamine, can increase viral load by dysregulating inflammatory cytokine production. Current users of the drug had higher viral loads than either past users or the drug or patients who had never used the drug, a finding that is consistent with earlier laboratory studies. However, as viral load was comparable in patients not taking HAART, regardless of methamphetamine use, they believe that poorer adherence to anti-HIV treatment regimens explains the higher viral loads.

In 2005 (Chang) US scientists used magnetic resonance imaging to determine the level of neurotransmitters in the brain which are markers of healthy neurones. They found lower levels of the neurotransmitter Nacetylaspartate in the basal ganglia, cells which control the co-ordination of movement. These cells are also the ones most frequently damaged by HIV itself. The investigators speculate that the additive effect of HIV and methamphetamine may be related to the drug's effect on the neurotransmitter dopamine. Methamphetamine causes the release of massive amounts of dopamine from the ends of neurones, notably in the basal ganglia. This release of dopamine often causes the ends of the neurones to shrivel and eventually die back. The researchers hypothesise that this release of dopamine can also stimulate HIV replication and worsen the damage caused by the drug. A study involving FIV, the feline equivalent of HIV, found that methamphetamine increases the ability of FIV to multiply and mutate 15-fold suggesting that the neurotoxic effects of methamphetamine and HIV could increase the risks and severity of HIV-associated dementia.

For more on interactions between crystal meth and HIV drugs, see **drug interactions** below.

References

Bolding G et al. *Use of crystal methamphetamine among gay men in London.* Addiction 101 (online edition), 2006.

Buchacz K et.al. *Amphetamine use is associated with increased HIV incidence among men who have sex with men in San Francisco.* AIDS 19: 1423 - 1424, 2005

Chang L et al. Additive effects of HIV and chronic methamphetamine use of brain metabolite abnormalities. *Am J Psychiatry* 162: 361-369, 2005.

Colfax G. The Epidemiology of Substance Use and Sexual Risk Behavior among Men Who Have Sex with Men: Implications for HIV Prevention Interventions. 12th Conference on Retroviruses and Opportunistic Infections. Boston, 2005. Paper no. 55.

Plankey MW et al. *The relationship of methamphetamine and popper use with HIV seroconversion among MSM in the multicenter AIDS cohort study.* Sixteenth International AIDS Conference, Toronto, abstract THPE712, 2006.

Urbina A et al. *Crystal methamphetamine, its analogues, and HIV infection: medical and psychiatric aspects of a new epidemic.* Clinical Infectious Diseases 38 (on-line edition). 2004.

Ecstasy

Also known as E, doves, MDMA, MDA, X.

One of the most widely used illicit drugs in the UK, E is now the most popular party drug on the club scene. It is an amphetamine-based drug which has mildly hallucinogenic effects. It is commonly used at nightclubs and raves because it can greatly enhance mood, energy levels, feelings of empathy with others, perception of colour and music. In the UK, ecstasy is an illegal Class A drug. Dealing carries a maximum life prison sentence and unlimited fine, and possession up to seven years in prison and a £5,000 fine.

The drug is sold in tablet form and can be bought for between £2 - £5. MDMA powder can sometimes also be bought for approx. £20-40 a gram. After about 30 to 45 minutes the drug gives an intense high, which may last for several hours. Because the body becomes tolerant of the drug, people may end up taking larger quantities to induce similar feelings of euphoria.

As with all recreational drugs, it is difficult to know what the ecstasy tablet you are using really contains. The doses found in street drugs are not controlled, and the ecstasy pill you buy might contain much larger quantities of the drug. Often ecstasy will have been cut with other substances which could be poisonous, or with other drugs, usually amphetamines or LSD, but occasionally heroin.

In the short-term, ecstasy can cause dehydration, headache, chills, eye twitching, jaw clenching, blurred vision, nausea and vomiting, and like many drugs taken to get high, is commonly accompanied by a low period or come-down. Long-term use has been linked to poor mental health, depression, psychotic episodes and memory problems.

People can have an allergic reaction to the drug, which can be fatal (though deaths related to ecstasy are very rare relative to the extent of its consumption). The drug has also been associated with heart and lung problems, dramatic increases in body temperature, kidney failure, and liver damage. The potential liver toxicities of ecstasy and other recreational drugs are of particular concern to people with HIV as liver damage can make you very ill in its own right, and stop the body from processing anti-HIV drugs properly.

Ecstasy has been linked to unsafe sex by a number of studies of sexual behaviour amongst gay men. Some ecstasy users may argue that since the drug relaxes blood vessels, making erections difficult to maintain, unsafe sexual practices are being reduced by the drug. However, this does not prevent an ecstasy user being the receptive partner. Furthermore, the anti-impotency drug *Viagra,* which became more widely available in the UK in 1998, is being combined with ecstasy to enhance the atmosphere of sexual risk-taking that is occurring amongst club-going gay men in the UK.

People who are taking prescribed medication such as *Prozac* or other selective serotonin reuptake inhibitors should avoid ecstasy, since interactions between the two drugs can have unpleasant effects. Ecstasy is commonly combined with LSD, speed and/or ketamine in a sequence designed to extend and deepen the experience. LSD tends to add visual intensity but can also lead to feelings of paranoia, disorientation and distress if taken in a high dose (see LSD) or in an already unsettled state of mind.

Speed tends to lengthen the duration of the effect, and some forms of E have a high content of MDA, a chemical which is on the amphetamine end of the hallucinogen-amphetamine scale. Ketamine (see below) can cause radical disorientation and a feeling of being cut off from the surrounding world, but can also intensify the visual/hallucinogenic experience. People coming down from E may take sleeping tablets, tranquillisers or Prozac to help them chill out and to assist sleep. Some people report feelings of depression some days after use, perhaps because the drug disrupts the long-term balance of serotonin, a brain chemical which influences mood.

There have been concerns expressed that long-term ecstasy use cause brain damage, based on research carried out in animals and tests in small numbers of humans. So far this research has produced conflicting results.

Women with a history of genitourinary tract infection should use with caution, since women who use it seem to suffer from GU infections more frequently than others. Nothing is known about the effects of the drug on the unborn child.

People taking protease inhibitors, particularly ones boosted with ritonavir, need to be especially careful taking ecstasy and certain other drugs including GHB and *Viagra* because ritonavir can increase the levels of drug in the body dangerously. MDMA levels in patients taking ritonavir reach three to ten times those seen in other people.

In October 1996 Londoner Philip Kay died after taking 2.5 ecstasy tablets: the inquest found that he had levels of the drug in his body equivalent to taking 22 tablets. He had started taking full-dose ritonavir a few weeks earlier.

Refrences

For an account of Philip Kay's death by his partner Jim Lumb, see http://www.ecstasy.org/experiences/trip66.html

GHB

Also known as GBH, Liquid ecstasy, GBL, BDO.

GHB (gammahydroxybutyrate) has recently become popular on the club scene, with users enjoying an alcohol-like high with positive sexual effects.

Originally used as a general anaesthetic, it was also used by body builders in the 1980s because of its ability to stimulate growth hormone. GHB affects the release of dopamine in the brain, causing effects ranging from relaxation to sleep at low doses. At higher doses, the drug lowers blood pressure and in some cases people find breathing difficult. Overdosing can lead to a loss of consciousness and coma. It is not recommended that asthmatics or those with any form of respiratory or low blood pressure disorders take this drug.

The drug is usually sold in small 30 ml plastic containers (approx. £15) and consumed in capfuls. A small capful can make you feel uninhibited, exhilarated, relaxed and feeling good with the effects lasting as long as a day, although it is difficult to give a clear 'safe' dose, as the concentration of the liquid will vary.

Bigger doses can lead to disorientation, nausea, a numbing of the muscles or muscle spasms and vomiting. Users need to be careful as there is only a small difference between a desirable dose and an overdose.

Boosted protease inhibitors significantly increase the levels of GHB in the system, and there have been many anecdotal and at least one confirmed case of GHB overdose in patients taking PIs.

Reference

Harrington RD et al. Life-threatening interactions between HIV-1 protease inhibitors and the illicit drugs MDMA and gamma hydroxybutyrate. Arch Intern Med 159: 2221-2224, 1999.

Heroin

Also known as smack, junk, H, skag, dikes (for diconal), amps (injectable ampoules).

See *Opiates.*

Ketamine

Also known as K, Special K

Ketamine is a dissociative anaesthetic which makes people feel detached from their immediate environment; it can also turn muscles rigid so that the user is frozen until the drug wears off. Users say that they experience their bodies very differently whilst on ketamine, perhaps one of the reasons that it is frequently combined with ecstasy and LSD. Ketamine is largely used on the club scene.

Ketamine is a prescription-only medicine and is not illegal to possess. However, you can be prosecuted under the Medicines Act for selling the drug without a license. Ketamine comes as a liquid, a white powder or pill, which can be swallowed, snorted or injected. The drug begins to take effect after about twenty minutes when taken orally, and usually starts very gradually. The body heats up and the user begins to notice an altered sense of their body when moving about. Some users report intense hallucinogenic effects in the mind's eye; others report difficulty in moving, and may freeze completely.

The psychological effect of ketamine may be to plunge the user into what is often called a 'K-hole', a place from which it's difficult to return or for others to reach until the drug wears off. For this reason it is important that ketamine users be looked after by others whilst in this state, since they may not be able to look after themselves or communicate that they are having difficulties such as violent overheating, difficulty in swallowing or choking, all of which can occur on ketamine.

Eating or drinking in the hours before taking ketamine could lead to vomiting, as with any anaesthetic.

The effects of long-term ketamine use may include memory loss and mental disturbances. Several deaths from ketamine use have been reported in the UK.

Khat

Also know as Khat, quat, qat, qaadka, chat,

Khat is a stimulant with similar effects to amphetamine. It comes from a leafy green plant of the same name. Used mostly in Africa, Khat is getting more common in Europe, particularly in immigrant communities.

It is chewed over a number of hours and a small bunch of leaves costs around £4. Chewing it can make people feel more alert and talkative. Although it is a stimulant, many users report a feeling of calm if chewed over a few hours. Some describe it as being 'blissed out'. It can also suppress the appetite.

Khat can make a user psychologically dependent so when they stop using it they feel depressed. If you use it a lot, you may develop insomnia, heart problems and sexual problems like impotence

It can give you feelings of anxiety and aggression with some people finding that it makes them irritable, in some cases very angry and even violent. There is some evidence to suggest that it can make pre-existing mental health problems worse.

Khat is not an illegal drug in the UK. It can be used or traded without penalty, however it is an illegal substance in many other countries like the US.

LSD

Also known as acid, trips, microdots.

LSD is a chemical - lysergic acid diethylamide - sold in the form of tablets or tiny pieces of blotting paper impregnated with the drug. These 'blotters' are often printed with a pattern to distinguish them from other brands of LSD. It is a Class A drug.

LSD begins to take effect 30 to 60 minutes after it is taken, and the trip begins to intensify, lasting for six to eight hours. The effect will then begin to fade, although the length of the trip depends on the strength of the LSD; a trip can quite easily last longer if a large quantity is used.

LSD has an extremely dramatic effect on all the senses in most people. Once again the effects are dose related. Users report visual effects such as intensified colours, distorted shapes and sizes, and movement in stationary objects. Perceptions will change and these will depend on the mood of the user, the setting in which the drug is taken and the company in which the user takes the drug. Sometimes the trip will be extremely euphoric, but on other occasions it might be terrifying.

Individuals who haven't used the drug before would be well advised to start with a half or even a quarter of a tab in order to become accustomed to the extraordinary effects of the drug, which can be intensely frightening for the uninitiated.

Individuals are able to influence the progress of the trip, as are companions of the drug user, so if an individual appears to be having a bad trip it is very important that companions look after the user, and guide them to a safe place, mentally and physically. Friendly reassurance and physical contact are very helpful in this state.

LSD can cause 'flashbacks', short-lived, vivid re-experiences of part of a previous trip long after the drug's effect has ceased. Other psychological reactions can include the worsening of mental illness in people with underlying mental conditions.

LSD is not thought to affect the immune system, although many people report feelings of exhaustion after a trip. The drug is not thought to affect unborn children.

Magic Mushrooms

Also known as magic's, mushies, liberty cap, psilocybe semilanceata, psilocybin, shrooms

Magic Mushrooms are mushrooms which grow in the wild that produce similar effects to LSD when you eat them. There are two main types; the most common form is a species called psilocybe, the other more potent variety is amanita muscaria. There are deadly poisonous species of amanitas.

After picking, they are both either eaten raw or dried out and stored. Most people take between 1-5 grams. They are free if you know where to find them or up to £5 for a handful.

The effects for both mushrooms can take between 30 minutes to two hours to happen. The strongest part of the trip takes 4-10 hours and the after-effects usually last a further 2-6 hours. The more you take, the longer your trip could last. The effects include a distortion of colour, sound and objects. They can speed up and slow down time and movement and can make a user feel more emotionally sensitive, with some people reporting that they feel more creative and enlightened.

Up until 18 July 2005, freshly-picked magic mushrooms were not a controlled drug under UK law, though drying them for later use was illegal. The Drugs Act 2005 removed this anomaly and they are now a class A drug - though this has been criticised as a disproportionate response.

Nicotine

The negative consequences of smoking tobacco on health are well documented and well known.

Crothers et al (2005) in a large prospective observational cohort of HIV-positive male veterans found that smokers on potent antiretroviral therapy were twice as likely to die than non-smokers, and more likely to suffer from increased respiratory symptoms, chronic obstructive pulmonary disease (COPD), and bacterial pneumonia.

An American study (http://www.aidsmpa.com/en/news/CA194F69-8234-4EEA-81AF-E2FE2C2A0412.asp) (Feldman et al, 2006) found that even when taking anti-HIV treatment, HIV-positive women smokers were 36% more likely than HIV-positive women non-smokers to develop an AIDS-defining illness. They also found that smokers had a 53% increased risk of dying compared to non-smokers. The CD4 cell count of smokers was also lower over time than non-smokers. The smokers were more likely to be current or former users of illegal drugs, have hepatitis C virus and to have a previous history of AIDS. However, even after they took these factors into account they still found that smokers did less well on HIV treatment than non-smokers. Smokers were less likely to take their HIV treatment properly, so the researchers restricted their analysis to the women who took at least 95% of their doses. Once again, they found smokers were more likely to develop new AIDS-defining illness or die than non-smokers. They concluded that HIV treatment is not as beneficial for smokers than non-smokers.

A meta-analysis of studies of smoking and HIV acquisition and of progression to AIDS (Furber) found that five of six papers looking at smoking and the risk of acquiring HIV infection found that smoking tobacco was an independent risk factor. In these studies smokers had an adjusted odds ratio of between 1.6 to 3.5 of infection with HIV, "a magnitude of public health significance", according to the investigators. However nine out of ten papers looking at the link between smoking and progression to AIDS found no such link.

References

Feldman JG et al. *Association of cigarette smoking with HIV prognosis among women in the HAART era.* Am J Public Health 96(6): 1060-1065, 2006.

Furber AS et al. *Is smoking tobacco an independent risk factor for HIV infection and progression to AIDS?* Sexually Transmitted Infections 83: 41 - 46, 2007.Crothers K et al. *The impact of cigarette smoking on mortality, quality of life, and comorbid illness among HIV-positive veterans.* Journal of General Internal Medicine 20 (12), 1142-1145, 2005.

Opiates

Includes heroin, methadone, Diconal, morphine, dipapanone, pethidine, codeine, Distalgesic (dextropropoxyphene), Temgesic (buprenorphine). Also known as smack, junk, H, skag, dikes (for Diconal), amps (injectable ampoules).

Opiates are drugs made from the opium poppy. Opium is the dried 'milk' of the poppy. It contains morphine and codeine, both effective painkillers and from morphine it is not difficult to produce heroin. In pure form heroin is a white powder and twice as strong as morphine. A number of man-made opioids are also manufactured as painkillers, such as methadone, Morphine Sulfate and Oxymorphone Numorphon. They can be injected, smoked or sniffed.

When taken, opiates depress the nervous system and have a euphoric effect. Many people report a feeling of drowsiness, warmth, well-being and contentment. These pleasurable feelings are associated with the fact that opiates induce relaxed detachment from the impact of pain and anxiety and from desires for food and sex etc, yet at the same time as the person remains fully aware.

Injection of opiates into the veins intensifies these effects and makes them almost instantaneous, producing a short-lived burst of pleasurable sensation ('rush'). Injection under the skin or into the muscle gives a slower and more intense effect than intravenous injection. When smoked, the effects of heroin can be

expected to come on about as quickly as intravenous injection, but to be much less intense as the available dose is used over a period of time rather than injected all at once.

Tolerance develops to opiates so that someone in search of frequently repeated euphoria must increase the dose and/or change their method of administration. However, there comes a point when no further increase in dose can restore the positive effects of the drug and it is taken just to feel 'normal'.

Intravenous injection maximises the effects of a given amount of heroin and produces a much more intense immediate experience, so as tolerance develops (and perhaps as money runs short) there may be a tendency to move from sniffing or smoking heroin to injection.

Since (unlike barbiturates) tolerance also develops to the respiratory depressant effects of opiates, gradual escalation of dose does not in itself lead to risk of death through overdose. However, fatal overdoses can happen when opiate users take their usual dose after a break during which tolerance has faded.

After as little as several weeks on high and frequent doses, sudden withdrawal results in a variable degree of discomfort generally comparable to a bout of flu. The effects start 8 to 24 hours after the last 'fix' and include aches, tremor, sweating and chills, sneezing and yawning, muscular spasms. They generally fade in seven to ten days but feelings of weakness, loss of well-being and sleep disturbance can last for several months. Abrupt opiate withdrawal is rarely life threatening and is considerably less dangerous than withdrawal from alcohol or barbiturates.

Physical dependence is not as significant as the strong psychological dependence developed by some long-term users. Dependence of any kind is not inevitable and some people use heroin on an occasional basis. The physiological effects of long-term opiate use are rarely serious in themselves. They include respiratory complaints, constipation and irregular periods. At higher doses chronic sedation can occur, but at lower doses users can function normally.

However the consequences of injecting opiates and of a drug-using lifestyle can be serious. Among regular injectors, there is commonly physical damage associated with poor hygiene and the injection of contaminants. Contaminants contribute to respiratory disease, skin lesions, tetanus (with injection under the skin) and other complications depending on the agent used and the individual's sensitivity. Decreased appetite and apathy can contribute to disease caused by poor nutrition, self-neglect and bad housing. Repeated heroin sniffing may damage structures in the nose.

On the other hand, because opiates in themselves are relatively safe drugs, addicts in receipt of opiates on prescription and who maintain a stable, hygienic lifestyle can be virtually indistinguishable from non-drug users, and suffer no serious physical damage. However as opiates are the most commonly injected drugs of misuse in Britain, those users who do inject face a high risk of becoming infected with HIV if they share needles.

Methadone is a form of opiate usually supplied on prescription to addicts as an alternative to injecting. It is usually taken as a liquid, although it is available in ampules. In order to withdraw from opiate use addicts may gradually reduce their dose of methadone over a long period of time in order to reduce physical and psychological dependence on the drug. Opiate use during pregnancy may result in smaller babies, who suffer severe withdrawal symptoms after birth.

Poppers

Also known as amyl, butyl, isobutyl nitrite (collectively known as alkyl nitrites).

Amyl nitrite in the past was used medically to ease the chest pain caused by angina pectoris. When inhaled the drug causes the dilation of blood vessels, allowing more blood to reach the heart. The drug also causes a rush of blood to the brain, a speeded-up heartbeat, the relaxation of muscle tissue and an intense high lasting just a few minutes. It is for these reasons that sniffing amyl nitrite and a related compound, butyl nitrite, became popular amongst gay men both in gay clubs and during sex.

The drug is used to intensify pleasure whilst dancing and whilst having sex. Sniffing poppers also relaxes the anal sphincter muscle, allowing anal intercourse to take place more easily. Use of poppers is not just restricted to gay men, however; a recent UK survey found that 20% of 16 year-olds claimed to have used nitrites, and it is frequently used on the club scene.

After-effects of sniffing poppers may include headaches, skin rashes, weakness, sinus pain, burns if the liquid comes into contact with the skin, and nausea. People with a history of heart trouble or anaemia should avoid using the drug, as should those with breathing problems, or glaucoma. In extreme cases excessive use of poppers can lead to methaemoglobulinemia, in which the lips and skin take on a blue tinge, and vomiting, shock and unconsciousness may follow. Deaths have been reported as a consequence of this condition.

Amyl nitrite is very rarely used in medicine these days but is controlled under the Medicines Act (1968). Possession is not illegal but supply can be an offence. The sale of poppers without a prescription was found to be illegal following a prosecution brought by the Royal Pharmaceutical Society against several sex shops which sold poppers. However, the law has not yet changed, although a recent European Union directive and a decision of the Medicines Control Agency (who administers the Medicines Act) means that any substance on sale with a psychoactive or mood-altering effect could be classed as a medicine and so be controlled under the Medicines Act.

Poppers may have long-term carcinogenic effects, according to studies in animals, but some researchers have suggested that poppers are excreted from the body very quickly after use. Any long-term carcinogenic effect in humans remains to be established.

Poppers should not be combined with the anti-impotence drug *Viagra* since this can lead to loss of blood pressure and could potentially be fatal.

Tranquillisers

Also known as benzodiazepines, *Valium, Ativan, Librium, temazepam*

Most tranquillisers are prescribed for anxiety and sleeping problems, and suppress mental activity and alertness. They are widely prescribed in the UK. Tolerance develops after two weeks when used as sleeping pills and four months when used against anxiety, but if use continues after tolerance develops it is possible that the user has become psychologically dependent.

Withdrawal effects upon ceasing tranquilliser use after long periods are common, and range from mild to severe. These include: insomnia; anxiety; heightened sensitivity to light, touch, noise and sound; irritability; nausea; vomiting and tremors. In extreme cases convulsions and fits occur which may be life-threatening.

Tranquillisers are often employed by drug users as a means of blunting the effects of anxiety, such as when supplies of a normal drug are unavailable or when coming down from a trip. In non-anxious people they do not produce pleasurable feelings, with the exception of *Valium*, which may produce mild euphoric feelings. Large quantities of benzodiazepines mixed with alcohol may be dangerous.

Withdrawal symptoms seem particularly noticeable with shorter-acting benzodiazepines such as lorazepam and temazepam. Regular high dose benzodiazepine use in late pregnancy can sometimes result in withdrawal effects in the new-born baby.

Viagra

Viagra (sildenafil citrate is a treatment for impotence that has become increasingly common as a recreational drug, particularly amongst gay men who want to counteract the impotence side-effect of ecstasy. Several studies have linked Viagra use to increased risk of unprotected sex and STIs, although is it unclear whether this is because Viagra enables men to have more partners or increases the length of sexual exposure. It is also possible that these men simply added Viagra to their risk-taking repertoire.

The most common side-effects of Viagra are headaches, facial flushing, indigestion, nasal congestion and transient disturbance of colour vision. In the clinical trials, 30% of participants reported a side-effect but only 2% stopped taking the drug due to side-effects.

Viagra should not be taken in conjunction with 'poppers' or nitrates (e.g. amyl nitrate) or with drugs used to treat angina. If nitrates and Viagra are taken together, blood pressure may fall to dangerously low levels.

HIV & drug users: A different clinical picture

In the UK less than 3% of new HIV infections were attributed to injecting drug use in both 2000 and 2001. Drug users with a history of IVDU are highly likely to be co-infected with hepatitis B and C viruses, anywhere between 40 -100% depending on location (Brettle 2001) However, recent research has shown that 30% of IDUs share needles and 60% share of other paraphernalia (www.nta.nhs.uk/programme/docs/Harmreductiondraftscopingpaper.pdf)

This has lead to an increase in Hepatitis C, especially amongst younger drug users, and suggests a risk of an increase of HIV amongst drug users.

Illegal drug use and alcohol use can impact on HIV-positive people in many ways.

Clinical issues - medical conditions

The clinical picture of HIV in drug using populations is significantly different from HIV in other populations. For example, there are almost no cases of Kaposi's Sarcoma in male IDUs who are HIV-positive but there is a five-fold risk of death from bacterial infections in HIV-positive drug users vs. HIV-positive non-drug users. IDUs seem to be more susceptible of bacterial pneumonia as a result of HIV infection. This condition and pulmonary tuberculosis, also common in the drug users, have both AIDS defining illnesses.

A database was established to look at particular manifestations of HIV in drug users. Many of the most common diseases are bacterial infections, pulmonary tuberculosis, sexually transmitted diseases, hepatitis, and malignancies other than KS and lymphomas. When IDUs develop pneumonias, it is more often bacterial pneumonia, which requires a different course of treatment, or TB-related, rather not PCP.

Certain malignancies, not considered AIDS-defining but definitely life - threatening, are also occurring mostly in IDUs. These include lung cancer and cancers of the GI tract. In HIV-positive women, cervical diseases and superimposed HPV infection are important clinical conditions that must not be underestimated. Cervical cancer was added as an AIDS defining illness in 1993.

Some medical problems / symptoms will be as a result of the drug use and some due to the HIV. Alcohol / illicit drug use can precipitate or exacerbate medical conditions and result in an overlapping of symptoms. Certainly fever, infection and diarrhoea are quite common in drug users. Symptoms of HIV such as weight loss, diarrhoea, and fever may be caused either by drug use or withdrawal. Consequently, the clinical manifestations of HIV can be combined with, masked by, or mimicked by the effects of drugs and alcohol.

Often so-called behavioural problems associated with 'problem drinkers and drug users' are misdiagnosed disorders associated with brain lesions or central and peripheral nervous system toxicities. It is absolutely imperative that clinicians look beyond stereotypes and prejudices when treating drug addicts and recognise coexistent, parallel pathophysiology that may be occurring (Selwin 1996).

Pain management is another important issue to consider when treating heroin users, as they will need more narcotic, not less. Dosages that are considered dangerous for other people, may be required for drug users, because of their capacity and tolerance for narcotics. Former addicts and recovering addicts may also need slightly higher doses of pain medications. Just because a person may have a history of drug addiction doesn't mean that they shouldn't be given pain medication when they need it (Selwin 1996).

Hepatitis

It is estimated that between 15-40% of alcoholics are hepatitis C positive (http://www.alcoholconcern.org.uk/). It is reported that between 50 - 80% of IDUs are hepatitis C positive and 20% are hepatitis B positive. Rates of hepatitis C in Crack users and amongst people who snort drugs (cocaine, amphetamines) are increasing due to sharing of, for example, bank notes, for snorting or pipes for smoking crack.

Hepatitis, delta-hepatitis (which can accompany hepatitis B) and hepatitis C show serologic abnormalities in the presence of HIV. Whilst they don't become more active or severe in people with HIV, HIV-positive drug users are more likely to carry hepatitis longer and thus remain infectious for a longer period of time. (Selwin 1996)

Co-infection of HIV and hepatitis can result in a more complex medical picture. It can accelerate the time course to cirrhosis. Alcohol can even in modest amounts be a major risk factor for the development of HCV infection-related cirrhosis.

Whilst hepatitis B vaccination programmes are being offered in a number of drug services, take up is not high enough, resulting in an increased risk of rates. However, prognosis of hepatitis B has not been shown to be adversely affected by co-infection with HIV.

Hepatitis C appears to have a more accelerated course to fibrosis, cirrhosis and hepatic failure in HIV-positive individuals. Some researchers believe that hepatitis C may accelerate HIV progression. The hepatotoxicity of many antiretroviral medications complicates the treatment of HIV in hepatitis C carriers.

Pancreatitis

Pancreatitis is an inflammation of the pancreas, which can result as a consequence of chronic alcohol use and also an adverse effect of several HIV medications. (ddI & ddC)

Peripheral neuropathy

Peripheral neuropathy describes damage to the peripheral nervous system, the vast communications network that transmits information from the brain and spinal cord (the central nervous system) to every other part of the body. Peripheral neuropathy occurs most frequently in people who smoke, are over age 40, and have difficulty controlling their blood sugar levels. It can be caused as a consequence of chronic alcohol use, HIV medications (ddI, ddC, d4T) and HIV infection.

Dementia

Dementia is a progressive brain dysfunction, leads to a gradually increasing restriction of daily activities. Heavy alcohol use can have an adverse effect on the Central Nervous System. It exacerbates the detrimental effect of HIV infection on the brain and complicates the course of HIV-associated dementia. Both alcohol-related dementia and HIV dementia are associated with frontal lobe pathology and neuronal loss.

Liver damage

Alcohol and Illicit drug use can put extra strain on the liver, leading to liver damage. Any drug can cause potential liver toxicity's which are a concern to people with HIV as liver damage in itself can make people ill and it can stop the body from processing anti-HIV drugs properly.

Cardiomyopathy

Cardiomyopathy is a serious disease in which the heart muscle becomes inflamed and doesn't work as well as it should. There may be multiple causes including viral infections. Alcohol, cocaine and HIV infection may have additive or synergistic effects, and HIV infection and alcohol or cocaine independently can increase the risk of cardiomyopathy.

Bacterial pneumonia

Bacterial pneumonia is an infection that causes irritation, swelling, and congestion in the lungs. Alcohol and HIV infection may have additive or synergistic effects, and both HIV infection and alcohol independently can increase the risk of bacterial pneumonia. When IDUs develop pneumonia, it is more often bacterial pneumonia or TB related, rather than PCP.

Bacterial infections caused by encapsulated organisms such as *S. pneumoniae* and *H. influenza*, especially pneumonia are common in HIV infected IDUs.

Cardiovascular Disease

HIV-positive patients have signs of damage to the lining of blood vessels and that the damage was more pronounced in the patients who had higher viral loads, particularly injection drug users (Solages, 2006). Reduced flexibility of blood vessels in response to blood flow is the earliest detectable sign of the development of cardiovascular disease. This reduced flexibility, called 'endothelial dysfunction', is caused by the failure of cells lining blood vessels to stimulate the vessels to widen when blood flow increases. They found that current injection drug use had a significant association with artery dilation in the HIV-positive patients. HIV viral load emerged as being significantly associated with endothelial dysfunction and concluded that the effects of intravenous drug use on endothelial function may be caused by higher viral loads in the injecting drug users, possibly due to reduced adherence to their anti-HIV medication.

Reference

Alcabes P, Friedland G. Injection drug use and HIV infection. Clin Inf Dis. 20: 1467-1479. 1995.

Celetano DD et al. Self-reported ART in IDUs. JAMA 280: 544-546, 1998.

Chaisson, et al. Race, sex, drug use and progression of HIV disease. NEJM 333: 751-756, 1995.

Floris-Moore, et al. Gender and Hospitalisation Patterns Among HIV-Infected Drug Users Before and After the Availability of Highly Active Antiretroviral Therapy Journal of Acquired Immune Deficiency Syndromes (http://www.lwwonline.com/article.asp?issn=1525-4135&vol=34&iss=3&page=331) 2004.

Mannheimer SB, et al. Use of antiretroviral therapy by drug users with HIV infection. JAMA. 281(8): 699 [discussion 700-701], 1999.

Michaels SH, et al. Letter. JAMA. 281(8): 699-700, 1999.

O'Connor PG, et al. Medical progress: medical care for injection-drug users with HIV infection. NEJM. 331(7): 450-459, 1994.

Selwin, P. HIV and Drug Users: A Different Clinical Picture. Being Alive Newsletter, 1996.

Selwyn PA, et al. Clinical manifestations and predictors of disease progression in drug users with HIV infection. NEJM. 327(24): 1697-1703, 1992.

Solages A et al. *Endothelial function in HIV-infected persons.* Clin Infect Dis 42: 1325-1332, 2006.

Strathdee SA, et al. Barriers to use of free ART in IDUs. JAMA. 280: 547-549, 1998.

Clinical - psychiatric conditions

Depression

There is a strong link between HIV and depression. Some of these symptoms may be induced by HIV disease itself or by HIV medications.

In addition, many recreational drugs can both cause depression or anxiety and be used as 'self-medication' by people suffering from them.

Drug-related depression can be caused by alcohol or alcohol withdrawal, amphetamines, cocaine, ecstasy, crystal, cannabis and ketamine. There is a lack of adequate scientific data about the relationship between depression and recreational drug use, however, there is significant understanding based on clinical experience.

The drug ecstasy affects the serotonin system, the same neurotransmitters that are affected by antidepressants. There is growing evidence to suggest that ecstasy may have very long-term effects that may ultimately bring on depression and anxiety problems. For some individuals, it may not take much ecstasy use for this to occur.

Depression may lead an individual to seek relief in the use of alcohol or other recreational drugs. In turn, these drugs may cause or exacerbate depression. If antidepressants are used with recreational drugs, it will decrease the users chances of getting better. It is therefore important for users to seek help in reducing drug use as well as getting direct treatment for the depression.

Individuals who have experienced physical and sexual assaults may be more susceptible to use alcohol and / or illicit drug use as a way of coping, and this can have a detrimental effect on the health of people who are HIV-positive. The role of trauma in HIV is only just starting to be explored. However, if sexual abuse is the route of transmission of HIV this can make it more difficult for an individual to come to terms with their diagnosis.

Psychosis

Psychosis is defined as a state of mental illness in which the subject has lost insight into their own thought processes. Whereas people suffering normal or 'neurotic' depression or anxiety will be only too well aware that they have a problem, psychotics attribute symptoms to influences outside themselves. Psychosis is most commonly caused by schizophrenia, but is also seen in severe bipolar illness (manic-depression).

For links between cannabis and psychosis, see under cannabis above; other hallucinogens like LSD can also precipitate psychosis, especially in young people and those with a predisposition to it.

References

Markowitz JC et al. Treating depression in HIV-positive patients. AIDS 8(4): 403-412, 1994.

Markowitz JC et al. Treatment of depressive symptoms in human immunodeficiency virus-positive patients. Archives of General Psychiatry 55: 452-457, 1998.

Vincent E et al. Impact of HAART-related side-effects on unsafe sexual behaviours in HIV-infected injecting drug users: 7-year follow-up. AIDS 18: 1321-1325, 2004.

Yang Y et al. Hepatitis C and neuropsychological function in treatment-naive HIV-1-infected subjects - A5097s baseline analysis. Eleventh Conference on Retroviruses and Opportunistic Infections, San Francisco, abstract 26, 2004.

Yun LWH et al. Antidepressant treatment improves adherence to antiretroviral therapy among depressed HIV-infected patients. J Acquired Immune Defic Syndr 38: 432-438, 2005.

Immunological issues

There is now some evidence that using certain recreational drugs can cause significant damage to the immune system and affect HIV disease progression, although it is not possible to distinguish the effects of the drugs themselves from their consequences, including sleep deprivation, poor nutrition and disturbances in adherence to HAART

A 2001 study found that weekly use of either hallucinogens (e.g. ecstasy, LSD) or cocaine strongly and independently predicted death in a cohort of 370 HIV-positive men in a San Francisco cohort: statistically, they were than two and half times more likely to die than men who did not use recreational drugs. Use of hallucinogens was also associated with a faster progression to AIDS (Vittinghof 2001).

Regular drug users report more frequent bouts of colds, flu and unexplainable viruses when they're taking drugs (and placing great stress on their bodies) than when they're giving themselves a break. This suggests that damage to the immune system is short term rather than long term. Alcohol and illicit drugs are thought to temporarily reduce the action of your body's natural killer cells, which are the cells needed to attack infections. It is also likely to have an affect on T-cell / CD4 count if only in the short term.

Whilst the immune system is lowered, opportunistic infections may be more likely, but there is no firm evidence. If these opportunistic infections are serious enough, they could pose a long-term problem for your body's immune system. However, there is mixed evidence regarding whether use of drugs will speed up the progression of HIV.

In injectors, impurities and bacteria are injected directly into the blood stream, combined with poor diet and so on may be as harmful for the immune system as much as the drugs used.

See also under **cocaine** above.

Reference

Vittinghoff E et al. Cofactors for HIV disease progression in a cohort of homosexual and bisexual men. J Acquir Immune Defic Syndr 27(3): 308-314, 2001.

Behavioural issues

Risk-taking behaviour

Being under the influence of drugs or alcohol may increase risk-taking behaviour.

Sex

For a lot of people, drugs and sex go together. Drug users might trade sex for drugs. Some people think that sexual activity is more enjoyable when they are using drugs.

Drug use, including alcohol, increases the chance that people will not protect themselves during sexual activity or will engage in high-risk sexual activities. Someone who is trading sex for drugs might find it difficult to set limits on what they are willing to do. Anyone using drugs is less likely to remember about using protection, or to care about it, thereby increasing their risk of contracting and transmitting HIV (AIDS.org Fact Sheet: Drug Use and HIV).

For the link between unprotected sex and crystal meth (methamphetamine), see under **crystal meth** above.

Drugs

Being under the influence of alcohol or drugs also increases the likelihood of using other drugs which can have an effect on the immune system, as well as the users' ability to make informed choices. It has been shown that alcohol and other substance use can increase the likelihood of injecting, sharing needles and other drug use paraphernalia such as injecting equipment or sharing pipes or bank notes when snorting. This places individuals at a risk of transmission and/or re-infection of blood-borne viruses such as Hepatitis B&C and a risk of re-infection with other strains of HIV including drug resistant strains which can have an impact on treatment options (www.thebody.com/cdc/factdrug.html).

Lifestyle

Drug use, whether occasional / recreational or dependent can have an impact on the users lifestyle. During periods of drug use, an individual's lifestyle can become more chaotic, due to a change in patterns of behaviour, such as being away from home and this can have an impact on adherence.

Good nutrition helps keep your immune system strong, enabling you to better fight disease. A healthy diet improves quality of life. However, drug use may also interrupt eating patterns, leading to ill health and can affect medication absorption if it needs to be taken with or after food. Good nutrition helps the body process the many medications taken by people with HIV.

Weight loss, wasting, and malnutrition continue to be common problems in HIV, despite more effective antiretroviral medications, and can contribute to HIV disease progression. Diet (and exercise) may help with symptoms such as diarrhoea, nausea, and fatigue, and with fat redistribution and metabolic abnormalities such as high blood sugar, cholesterol, and triglycerides (www.tufts.edu/med/nutrition-infection/hiv/health.html).

Smoking tends to go hand in hand with other drug use, including drinking and so-called 'recreational drug' use. People with HIV disease are more likely to smoke than HIV-negative people. Smoking can interfere with normal lung function in healthy people. In people with HIV, smoking weakens the immune system and can make it more difficult to fight off HIV-related infections, especially infections relating to the lungs. Having HIV increases the risk of chronic lung disease. This is a risk for smoking marijuana as well as tobacco. Smoking can interfere with processing of medications by the liver and people with HIV who smoke are more likely to suffer complications from HIV medication than those who don't. It can also worsen liver problems like hepatitis.

Smoking increases the risk of some long-term side-effects of HIV disease and treatment. These include osteoporosis (weak bones that can lead to fractures). HIV treatment slightly increases the risk of heart attack, but smoking is the major controllable risk factor for heart attacks or strokes.

People with HIV disease who smoke are more likely to develop several opportunistic infections related to HIV, including thrush, oral hairy leukoplakia (whitish mouth sores), bacterial pneumonia and pneumocystis pneumonia (PCP).

For women, smoking can increase the risk and severity of infection with human papillomavirus (HPV). This increases the risk of cervical disease.
(http://www.thebody.com/nmai/smoking.html)

Medication compliance

Alcohol / illicit drug use is a risk factor for poorer compliance as use can make adherence more difficult, which may lead to viral resistance and reduce effectiveness of treatment. This includes missed doses as well as not taking medication on time (http://www.aidsmap.com/prediction non-adherent patients).

Medication interactions

A number of anti-retroviral drugs interact with methadone and illicit drugs which can make both more or less potent. An opiate drug user may be unwilling to take any medication if they find that they experience opiate withdrawals due to interactions. It is therefore important that the HIV team and drug service communicates in order to ensure that methadone dose can be increased or decreased according to the anti-retroviral drugs that are being prescribed. All drug users need to be informed of the possible interactions between their prescribed drugs and any recreational drugs that they use so that they can be given appropriate harm reduction advice. It is therefore important that HIV healthcare professionals ask patients about any drugs that they use and create an environment where patients feel they can disclose drug use without any fear of discrimination. (see section on drug interactions later and under **ecstasy** and **GHB** above.)

Access to medical care

Alcohol problems have been shown to be significantly associated with a delay for men in presenting to services for HIV. A similar pattern has also been observed with users of other drugs. Drug users also tend to be poor attenders' to their HIV clinic, which can be the result of past experiences within the medical setting.

Assumptions and judgements are made about alcohol and drug misusers, especially IV drug users. They can experience a lack of sympathy to general medical ailments as professionals may believe that the user 'brought it on themselves and if didn't use drugs, they won't have the problem'. Some professionals may hold attitudes regarding the individuals' lifestyle and therefore believe that if the user has contracted HIV and another blood borne virus then it *'serves them right'*. Receptionists, doctors, nurses and A&E staff may therefore discriminate against drug / alcohol users. In addition, many dentists refuse to treat drug users due to fears around Hepatitis C transmission, or discriminate against people who are HIV or Hepatitis C positive.

Most medical practitioners receive very little training on illicit drug use and don't feel very knowledgeable around drug-related issues or very confident working with drug users. As with the general population, they get their messages from the media and are susceptible to the same images as the rest of the population. Some may be fearful of being manipulated or may have had a bad experience with a drug user in the past and this influences their attitudes to all drug users. In addition, a lack of understanding of drug user and their difficulties may lead them to become frustrated by a lack of behaviour change amongst users.

The structure of the health service can also make it difficult for some drug users to access services. For example an individual's chaotic lifestyle can make it difficult for them to keep appointment times. If the appointment is early in the morning dependent drug users may not be able to attend as they may need to get score drugs to prevent withdrawals. Furthermore, clinic times generally do not fit in with a drug user's lifestyle, and often they may not be able to make it to the clinic before it shuts. The hospital or clinic might be some distance away and they may not be able to afford to get there. Also, long waiting times in clinics or A&E may mean that many drug users can't wait to be seen because they will need to go out use again.

Referral to specialist care has long waiting lists. As many drug users may be homeless or in unstable accommodation they may not find out that they have an appointment or the appointment may be so far in the future that they have forgotten about it when they are due to attend.

The ability to provide an array of social services, along with comprehensive medical care is a crucial, inseparable component in successfully providing treatment for HIV-positive alcohol and drug users. This is a population that has been disenfranchised and marginalised. Providing a warm and non-judgmental medical team is key. If clinicians are going to provide care for them they must first accept their life style, which for most may not be abstinence. Whether individuals are using drugs intravenously or not, they should still be able to receive treatments.

Adherence to medication

Problems with adherence to HAART have also been found in studies on recreational drug and alcohol users, which can affect T-cell counts and viral loads.

Halikitis et al. (2002) found that 51.9% of gay and bisexual men missed one dose of their medicines in the two-month period prior to assessment and 47.5% missed one dose in the last two weeks. Substance users reported more doses missed than non-drug users. Individuals who used club drugs were less adherent than those reporting no substance use and less adherent than those individuals who abused drugs other than club drugs. Reasons given for missing medication included being under the influence (56%), forgot (54%), busy with other things (53%), fell asleep (42%), being away from home (41%) and change in routine (40%). The researchers concluded that club drug use impacted adherence to HAART and needs to be addressed.

Lucas et al. (2001) studied 764 HIV-1 infected patients found that active drug users were more likely to report non-adherence to medication and to have smaller median reductions in HIV-1 RNA from baseline and smaller median increases in CD4 counts from baseline than patients who were non-users and former drug users. The reasons for these effects are unclear, however they may relate to psychological and social problems stemming from drug use.

It has been found that HIV-positive injecting drug users fail to derive the same virological benefit from HAART as either HIV-positive former intravenous drug users or people with HIV who have never injected drugs (Palepu et al. 2003). They compared the proportion of current IV drug users who achieved two successive viral load results below 500 copies/ml after starting HAART. Data on CD4 cell count and HIV viral load were obtained for 578 patients and participants were asked to complete a questionnaire concerning their demographic details and drug-taking risk behaviour. To establish levels of adherence, investigators obtained information on the number of prescriptions being refilled. Current IV drug use was reported by 78 (13%) of patients, a further 96 (17%) said they had used IV drugs and 404 (70%) said they had never used IV drugs.

Adherence was worst in current IV drug users (77%), followed by former users (81.5%) and people who had never used drugs (91.6%). Univariate analysis found that current and former drug users were less likely to achieve an undetectable viral load. They also had a higher baseline viral load (170,000 copies/ml versus 120,000 copies/ml) and receiving fewer months of therapy (14.5 versus 39). The investigators acknowledge that using prescription refill as a measure is unsatisfactory as patients in their study could by obtaining medication but then failing to take it. However, they conclude that when other prognostic variables were controlled for, current IV drug users were less likely to achieve a virological response to HAART. High adherence, longer duration of therapy, lower baseline viral load and NNRTI-based therapy were associated with "superior virological outcome for former and non-injection drug users."

Those users who have a lack of organisation in their personal lives which can occur due to drug use at any level may need help developing a structure to which they can tailor their regimen. Interventions should help minimise or cope with the negative side-effects of HAART, and emphasis the positive aspects of the regime. This can be difficult as many patients may not disclose their drug use to their HIV centre for fear of discrimination or because they don't see themselves as being a drug user.

However, HIV-positive individuals on HAART who use alcohol or recreational drugs are in great need of adherence enhancing interventions to reduce their risk of developing drug resistant virus. This would include looking at the individual's lifestyle, and identifying the times or activities that lead to poorer adherence and giving advice as appropriate. For example, advice may be specifically around ways of adhering at the weekend, when going out clubbing, such as forward planning if the person does not always go home and addressing concerns around drug interactions which may be contributing to the individuals' non-adherence.

The data regarding adherence problems to HAART medication and alcohol and recreational drugs are not always consistent. For example, Saunders et al (2001) studied 78 subjects with varying use of alcohol and recreational drugs (heavy users, moderate users, non-users). In this small sample they found no relationship between alcohol and recreational drug use and adherence problems. The heavy users had reported few problems with adherence but this may have been due to motivation to exaggerate actual compliance.

There have been studies that suggest that HIV-positive drug users who continue to inject heroin may develop AIDS faster than those who use other drugs or give up drugs (Ronald et al, 1994)). However, a pre-HAART review of the literature, conducted in 1994, concluded that "there appears to be little convincing evidence that active drug injection is detrimental to the outcome of HIV infection" (Phillips et al. 1994). However, injecting drug use has been associated with the more rapid evolution of drug resistance, suggesting that active injecting may have implications for the long-term effectiveness of HAART (Carneiro 1999).

References

Carneiro M et al. The effect of drug-injection behaviour on genetic evolution of HIV-1. Journal of Infectious Diseases 180(4): 1025-1032, 1999.

Halkitis P.N., Kutnick A.H., Borkowski T., Parsons J.T. Adherence to HIV medications and club drug use among gay and bisexual men. 2002 XIV International AIDS Conference 2002.

Lucas G.M., Cheever L.W., Chaisson R.E., Moore R.D. Detrimental effects of continued illicit drug use on the treatment of HIV-1 infection. JAIDS 27: 251-259, 2001.

Palepu A et al. Impaired virologic response to highly active antiretroviral therapy associated with ongoing injection drug use. JAIDS 32: 522 - 526, 2003.

Phillips AN et al. Active drug injecting and progression of HIV infection. AIDS 8(3): 385-386, 1994.

Ronald PJM et al. Continued drug use and other cofactors for progression to AIDS among injecting drug users. AIDS 8: 339-343, 1994.

Saunders D.S., Lancee W.J., Rourke S.B. The effect of alcohol and drug use on HAART adherence. Source: http://www.pulsus.com/cahr/abs/abs222.htm.%20oral%20presentation.%202001.

Swanson & Cooper. Dangerous Liaison: Club Drug Use and HIV/AIDS. http://www.thebody.com 2002

Access to ARVs for drug users

At the XVI International AIDS Conference in Toronto in 2006 it was reported that countries facing HIV epidemics among injecting drug users routinely exclude them from HIV treatment, leaving millions vulnerable to disease and potentially fueling the world's fastest-growing HIV/AIDS epidemics. This is despite having lower CD4 counts and higher viral loads (Mocroft et al, 1999). The consequences may be particularly severe in Russia, China, and other countries of Asia, Eastern Europe, and Central Asia where injecting drug users account for the largest share of those diagnosed with HIV.

At the end of 2004, there were 36 156 former/current injecting drug users with access to antiretroviral therapy in 45 developing and transitional countries, of whom 30 000 were in Brazil. This means that only some 6000 injecting drug users from the other

44 countries are receiving antiretroviral therapy. The coverage of antiretroviral therapy was 13.89% (3 668 389 people in need of ART out of 509 690 people estimated in receipt of antiretroviral therapy) However, in spite of the important contribution to the spread of the epidemic made by unsafe injecting practices (e.g. 74% of HIV cases in Eastern Europe and Central Asia are attributed to injecting drug use), injecting drug users represent 7% of the people on antiretroviral therapy (Aceijas, et al. 2005). For example, in Malaysia, there are approx. 15,000 drug users interned in rehabilitation centers, including a significant proportion who are HIV-positive. More than 75% of all HIV infections are estimated to be among injecting drug users, only 12% of those receiving ARV are drug users.

This is often a result of misconceptions held by health care providers regarding active drug use and their adherence to drug regimes that result in hesitancy to offer antiretroviral therapy to active drug users. Yet scientific evidence shows that when properly engaged by an experienced health care provider and adequate support, HIV-positive injecting drug users have clinical outcomes equivalent to those of HIV-positive people who do not use drugs (Paredes et al. 2000).

International organisations, including the World Health Organisation and the International AIDS Society as well as national bodies, including the Brazilian Ministry of Health, the British HIV Association, the Spanish AIDS Study and the United States Department of Health and Human Services recommend no physician should refuse effective therapy to a patient who wants it, including active drug users.

References

Aceijas, C., Oppenheimer, E., Stimson, G.V & Hickman, M. (Paper in preparation). Antiretroviral treatment for injecting drug users in developing and transitional countries.

Mocroft A, Madge S, Johnson AM, et al (1999). A comparison of exposure groups in the EuroSIDA study: starting highly active antiretroviral therapy (HAART), response to HAART, and survival. Journal of Acquired Immune Deficiency Syndromes, 22(4):369-378.

Paredes R, Mocroft A, Ole K, et al (2000). Predictors of virologic success and ensuing failure in HIV-positive patients starting highly active anteretroviral therapy in Europe: Results from the EuroSIDA study. Archives of Internal Medicine; 160(8):1123-1132.

Interactions with ART

Introduction

Anyone who has studied the official information sheets that detail the approved uses of each protease inhibitor will be aware that these drugs can have significant interactions with other prescribed drugs. In some cases this information has been derived from clinical tests in which people took both drugs and were studied through blood tests. But these well-studied interactions are the minority. More often, drug companies' researchers decide which interactions are likely based on the way their drug is metabolised.

Even for some prescribed drugs which are used by substantial numbers of people with HIV, such as the heroin-substitute methadone used in drug treatment programmes, surprisingly little reliable research on interactions with anti-HIV drugs has been conducted. Most of the guidelines on possible interactions are 'informed guesswork' based on the way the drugs in question are metabolised by liver enzymes.

But while there is quite a lot of information about these interactions, it is much harder to find reliable advice about

possible problems if they are taken with illegal drugs. Interactions can impact on effectiveness of prescribed drugs by impacting on the speed that drugs are metabolised, thereby increase side-effects and decrease / increase potency of both prescribed and street drugs.

All the information that exists comes from the same process of 'informed guesswork', where predictions are made by drug company researchers, who 'guess' how the drug is metabolised, and from anecdotal information reported by users. However, it is made more complicated still by several additional problems of reporting from experiences.

- on rare occasions, deaths have been reported even after people have taken only a single ecstasy tablet and no other drugs that could cause interactions.

- researchers often aren't sure how some illegal drugs are processed in the body.

- any available information may relate to the pure form of the drug, such as the chemical MDMA (ecstasy), but 'street' drugs are rarely pure (an ecstasy tablet may well contain MDE or MDA rather than MDMA). For example, if a drug interaction led to a three-fold increase in blood levels of MDMA, the effect might be barely noticeable to someone who took an E containing very little MDMA, but very substantial for someone who took an E that consisted of pure MDMA. Purity of the street drug is unknown so the size of the interaction effect can vary differently for e.g. 1 ecstasy pill depending on what's in it. The same applies to all street drugs.

- research on these issues is sometimes hampered because the government and drug companies are anxious not to be seen as 'condoning' illegal drug use.

Several of these issues were relevant to the ritonavir/ecstasy case, which came to the fore in autumn 1996 when a London club-goer, Philip Kay, died after taking ecstasy. An autopsy found that he had unusually high levels of ecstasy in his blood, which may be at least partially explained by the fact that he was also taking ritonavir. For more information see under **Ecstasy** above.

No formal interaction studies had taken place, although knowledge of the metabolism of the two drugs made it likely that ritonavir would boost ecstasy levels two to three-fold. Philip Kay's partner is sure that he took no more than 2.5 ecstasy tablets, yet at post-mortem he had blood levels of MDMA equivalent to taking 22 tablets - nearly a ten-fold increase. One possibility is that these particular Es contained unusually high amounts of MDMA.

Alternatively, if Kay was naturally a poor metaboliser of MDMA on account of his genetic make-up, that too could have had a bearing on the case. However, Abbott Laboratories has subsequently suggested that abnormally high peak levels of ritonavir during the early weeks of therapy may cause elevations in ecstasy levels if it is taken at this time.

Since then, hospitals have reported other cases due to adverse reactions to ecstasy among people taking protease inhibitors. However, ecstasy is not the only illegal drug that might interact dangerously with prescription drugs, and ritonavir isn't the only anti-HIV drug that may interact with illegal drugs.

Some medications can speed up how quickly the liver clears other medications from the body. When this happens the second medication is cleared faster from the body and this could result in there not being enough medication in the body to work properly. In the case of HIV, inducer drugs can cause some HIV medications to be removed form the bloodstream too quickly and this can lead to viral resistance.

Protease inhibitors are by far the most likely of the anti-HIV drugs to have interactions with recreational drugs in the liver. One key enzyme involved is called cytochrome P450 2D6 (CYP2D6), which is significantly inhibited by ritonavir. What results is a log-jam. It's rather like rush hour at the tube stations- if all the ticket barriers are open, everyone can get through easily. If half are closed, then more people are competing for fewer gates and a build-up begins. In the body, ritonavir closes some of these gates in the liver. When chemicals in MDMA are trying to get through, they are impeded. This could lead to a large build up in the body. Other drugs affected are: speed, anabolic steroids, *Diazepam* (valium), *Rohypnol* (flunitrazepam), *Prozac* (fluoxetine), *Lustral* (sertraline), *Viagra* (sindenafil), GBH and methadone.

It is thought that other protease inhibitors do not inhibit the action of enzymes involved in breaking down recreational drugs to the same extent as ritonavir.

It is possible that the non-nucleoside reverse transcriptase inhibitor (NNRTI) delavirdine, which also inhibits the 3A4 enzyme, could increase levels of some recreational drugs. Another NNRTI, nevirapine has the opposite effect as it induces 3A4 so could lead to reduced levels of any recreational drugs that are metabolised by that enzyme.

General harm reduction advice

Taking combination therapies can be complicated, mixing it with drug and alcohol use can make it more complicated. No one knows how the drugs will interact for certain and mixing prescribed and illegal drugs can increase possible problems and risks.

It is important to discuss any illegal drug use with your prescribing doctor, as other treatment options may be better.

In the first six weeks of a new combination an individual is more vulnerable and there is increased risk. For example, during the first six weeks of ritonavir treatment, the levels of it in the blood are at their highest, so this is when it is most likely that an increase in negative effects will occur. It is therefore best to start with a small dose of any illicit drugs and wait before taking any more. It is best not to mix too many substances and remember that less is more. Any alcohol or drug taking that results in vomiting and/or diarrhoea may have reduced the effectiveness of HIV drugs as it may not have been absorbed. Therefore moderation is the key.

Taking larger amounts or repeated doses can exaggerate the negative effects of both the HIV drugs and the illegal drugs. If possible, let someone know what you've taken, both prescribed and otherwise.

It is important to get plenty of rest before you take drugs. It is important to consider your general mental and physical health as if your depressed or run down, the comedown will be harder to take.

Australian activists have produced guidelines on safer use of party drugs for people with CD4 counts below 400. They advise club-goers not to drink plain water, but rather to dissolve in the water a sachet of oral rehydration salts (such as *Dioralyte* or *Rapolyte*, usually intended to replace lost salts and sugars in people with diarrhoea). Two days before the event, double your dose of acyclovir (if you take it) and start taking co-trimoxazole (one twice a day), folic or folinic acid (once a day) and fluconazole (one twice a day). At the club, take 800mg of acyclovir. Afterwards, take another 800mg of acyclovir and more oral rehydration salts. Carry on taking the other medications for two days after the event.

It is best to wait for as long as possible after taking antiretroviral medication before starting illicit drug use, although it is very important that all HIV medication continues to be taken as prescribed. Skipping treatment will not protect from the negative effects of mixing them with other drugs. The levels of HIV drugs in the individuals system may decrease, but their effects on the liver will remain the same, and so will the potential for a bad reaction. Skipping medication will make it easier for resistance to emerge as it will lower the body's level of the anti-retroviral and increases the change of HIV beating it, thereby increasing viral load.

All mood- and consciousness-altering drugs can have an impact on people's ability to adhere to their medication schedule, leading to non-compliance with treatment regime. This can be because the individual goes out at weekends and does not go home in time to take the medications, or they may miss doses due to changes in sleeping patterns or because they feel too unwell after illicit drug or alcohol use. It is therefore important that people planning to use any substances develop strategies to help them take their medication at the right time and in the right way. For example, it is important for users to plan ahead so that they take enough drugs with them if there is a chance they won't go home after a night out or think about ways of remembering to take medication if routine is changed. A double dose should not be taken if a dose is missed.

Some HIV drugs, such as the protease inhibitor indinavir, have been linked to dehydration, which, coupled with the dehydrating effects of alcohol and stimulants can lead to complications like kidney stones. It is therefore important that the user drink plenty of fluids to avoid dehydration.

Beginning treatment is a serious commitment and therefore it is important that before starting you are sure that you are ready for it and are prepared to make any necessary adjustments in lifestyle to ensure adequate adherence.

The following section provides information on known drug interactions between antiretroviral medications and illicit drugs.

More information on drug interactions and safer drug use is available on the following websites.

www.hiv-druginteractions.org

www.thebody.com

www.aidsmap.com

Drug interactions

Alcohol interactions

Occasional and light use of alcohol is not known to interact with other HIV medications. However, chronic, heavy use of alcohol can be destructive to the liver, which can be dangerous because of the way that drugs are broken down. It can increase the risk of drug toxicity's such as liver damage. Drugs will stay in the system longer, which is likely to cause overdoses and worse side-effects. Some drugs (HIV and otherwise) should not be mixed with alcohol, and so it is important to check.

The enzymes involved in breaking alcohol down are different to those inhibited by ritonavir. However, there might well be some unpleasant side-effects when the alcohol and protease inhibitors interact in the bloodstream, for example drinking alcohol when on a protease inhibitor is likely to increase the potency of the alcohol. Alcohol itself has side-effects, and mixed with tablets that also have side-effects can make these. Alcohol makes the user dehydrated, as does the protease inhibitor indinavir, so if the two are used together there is an increased risk of kidney stones.

If taking the nucleoside reverse transcriptase inhibitor (NRTI) ddI (didanosine) alcohol should be avoided as it can increase the risk of pancreatitits (intense stomach pain that feels like it's going all the way through to your back), which has been fatal to some patients.

Research findings are mixed and the impact of alcohol on HIV disease progression is complex. Any negative observed effect may be due to the impact of alcohol on individual behaviour, including compliance, rather than a direct immunological effect of alcohol. For example, excessive alcohol use can make adherence more difficult. Alcohol use at risky levels is more prevalent among HIV- infected patients and a HIV diagnosis may increase a client's alcohol use.

Current advice is that anyone living with hepatitis C should abstain from alcohol, if possible, or keep consumption to an absolute minimum, in order to protect the liver from chronic damage (cirrhosis). People who have alcohol-related liver damage (especially those with hepatitis C) may however suffer more severe side-effects from some HIV-related medication, especially protease inhibitors.

Amphetamine interactions

The protease inhibitor ritonavir is predicted to increase amphetamine levels in the blood by a factor of 2-3. The other protease inhibitors should have less of an impact, but this is not always the case. This can lead to increased anxiety, manic behaviour, shortness of breath, racing heartbeat, greater dehydration etc. It is therefore best to start with a much lower dose and it is important to take extra care if injecting.

Anabolic steroid interactions

If anabolic steroids are mixed with anti-retroviral drugs (particularly PI's) the result could be a 2-3-fold build-up of steroids in the blood. This would lead to an excess in testosterone which will accentuate an undesirable side-effects, and may lead to increased anger, mood swings, liver and kidney damage, as well as hair loss.

There has been controversy over the effects of anabolic steroids on the immune system. Some experts have argued that steroids are immunosuppressive, but the only study to look at immune status in HIV-positive men receiving anabolic steroid treatment for wasting showed no detrimental effect on CD4 or CD8 levels. Excess testosterone is known to elevate LDL (bad) cholesterol, so those at risk for heart disease or other effects of protease inhibitor -related lipodystrophy should use anabolic steroids with caution.

Buprenorphine

Bruce (2006) reported three cases, which appear to demonstrate that Atazanavir (Reyataz), boosted by low dose ritonavir (Norvir) interacts with the opiate substitute, buprenorphine. In all three cases the patients were also taking drugs from the nucleoside/nucleotide reverse transcriptase inhibitor class, but existing pharmacokinetic knowledge did not provide any reason for the doctors to expect an interaction between any of these antiretrovirals and buprenorphine. Patients taking the standard atazanavir/ritonavir dose of 300mg/100mg once a day in combination with two other anti-HIV drugs, with doses of buprenorphine ranging from 8mg to 14mg a day reported sleepiness, reduced mental function and feeling "doped out". Doctors believe that the interaction occurred because both atazanavir/ritonavir and buprenorphine are processed by the body in the same way, through the liver enzyme CYP3A4.

Cannabis interactions

It is not known how cannabis reacts with anti-HIV drugs. A small American study found that cannabis use did not impact on the effectiveness of the protease inhibitor indinavir, even though the drugs use the same mechanism to pass through the body. However, protease inhibitors may increase THC levels (the active ingredient in marijuana) so smaller doses may have greater effects (i.e. getting stoned quicker)

There is no clear evidence that smoking cannabis in itself affects immunity, but smoking certainly does. If the drug is smoked, long-term use is known to cause many smoking-related respiratory and cardiovascular diseases such as asthma, bronchitis, emphysema and heart disease. This may be of particular concern to people with HIV who have suffered lung damage from TB, or to those with increased lipids from anti-HIV medication, as this may increase the risk of heart attack.

Smoking depletes the body's store of antioxidant nutrients, which can lower resistance to infection. Low levels of the antioxidant nutrients appear as symptoms of HIV infection emerge. Heavy smokers with HIV are especially vulnerable to the development of *Pneumocystis* Pneumonia (PCP). There is also evidence that smoking cannabis can cause cancers of the mouth, throat and lungs.

Cocaine & crack interactions

Cocaine is not metabolised by the body in the same way as anti-HIV drugs so there does not appear to be cause for concern about interactions between them. However, test-tube studies suggest that cocaine alters the functioning of the immune system in several ways, making immune cells more vulnerable to HIV, potentially accelerating immune damage (Nair 2000). In addition, cocaine doubled the speed at which the virus reproduced (up to 20 times), suggesting that HIV disease may progress faster in regular cocaine users (Nair 2000). Mice infected with HIV and then exposed to cocaine for 10 to 12 days had HIV levels 200 to 300-fold higher than counterparts not exposed to cocaine (Roth 2002) and had far fewer CD4 T-cells than mice not given the drug.

However, studies looking at regular cocaine use and disease progression in gay men have produced conflicting results, due to multitude of other social factors (access to healthcare, lifestyle factors). One study found no association, whilst another found that weekly cocaine use was associated with a greater risk of death. Because drug use may be an indicator of other social issues which may have a negative effect on health such as poor access to health care, or other health problems these types of studies can be difficult to interpret.

The use of crack cocaine use was independently associated with progression to clinical AIDS in a prospective cohort study of 222 HIV-positive women and 302 HIV-positive men who attended a hospital-affiliated methadone maintenance programme (Webber 1999).

Most HIV medications, particularly protease inhibitors and non-nucleosides, can slow down how the liver clears other drugs from the body often resulting in increased levels in the bloodstream. In the case of cocaine, which is a short acting drug, this could lead to very high levels in the body, which could lead to overdose, heart attacks and strokes.

Cocaine use may worsen sinus problems, which are frequent in people with HIV. Cocaine produces a shorter high so users need to use more frequently, which if they inject results in an increased risk of contracting and / or transmitting HIV.

Long-term cocaine use can lead to problems with attention and concentration, memory loss and decreased speed in processing information, which can lead to missing antiretroviral doses and ultimately to drug resistance.

Ecstasy interactions

The effects of ecstasy on the immune system and on HIV disease progression are uncertain. There is no definitive evidence that ecstasy affects the immune system, but any drug which affects nutrients in the body may affect resistance to infection. However, there have been reports from some research which suggests that a single dose of ecstasy (100mg) can cause a dramatic fall in the level of T-cells (Swanson & Cooper 2002).

Combined with ritonavir, ecstasy has caused death even when ecstasy is used in normal doses. This is because ritonavir acts to slow down the liver enzyme that breaks it down so it makes the dose 3-10 times stronger, boosting the amount of ecstasy in the blood stream by between 200% and 300%. Ecstasy use could be dangerous with other protease inhibitors and NNRTIs, especially delavirdine, as they are metabolised using a similar process so there is a risk that ecstasy could interact dangerously with them as well. Possible effects could be increased edginess, more teeth grinding, palpitations, joint stiffness, dehydration and a greater chance of liver and kidney damage.

Other drugs that should be avoided whilst on ecstasy, due to interactions, are MAO inhibitors and other sympathomimetics e.g. certain asthma medications (beta-2 antagonists), ephedrine, pseudoephedrine (decongestants) and phenylpropanolamine (diet pills).

GHB interactions

Levels of the recreational drug commonly known as GHB (gamma hydroxybuytrate) may be increased to life-threatening levels if it is taken alongside a protease inhibitor. In a report from Seattle a 29 year-old man receiving treatment with ritonavir and saquinavir became unconscious after taking half a teaspoonful of GHB. He had taken a previous half teaspoonful of GHB and two ecstasy tablets in the preceding 24 hours. The man had not experienced adverse reactions to GHB or ecstasy prior to protease inhibitor treatment. Reporting doctors suggested that ritonavir and saquinavir slowed down metabolism of both drugs and caused the near-fatal reaction.

It is now suggested that GHB used with HAART it could lead to a 2-3 fold build up in blood. The possible symptoms of GHB overdose include vomiting, breathing problems, seizures, stupor and coma, and the dose normally associated with severe distress is greater than 50mg/kg of body weight. In this case the dose has been estimated at less than 10mg/kg body weight (Harrington 1999).

Heroin interactions

There is no clear research on whether heroin and antiretroviral drugs interacts. Some anecdotal reports have suggested that HIV drugs may cause heroin to be metabolised more quickly, resulting in less hit, less buzz and more withdrawal symptoms. However, due to the lack of research it is important that heroin users take care after they have been prescribed a new antiretroviral regime.

Ketamine interactions

When combined with ritonavir can lead to chemical hepatitis, an unpleasant inflammation of the liver resulting in jaundice. Known examples of this have eventually gone away, but damage to the liver is not recommended for HIV-positive people. PIs, particularly ritonavir and sabuinavir, and the NNRTI delavirdine may increase levels of ketamine in the bloodstream, possibly leading to increased heart rate, increased BP or difficulty breathing. This is not certain though.

Methadone interactions

Taking methadone with prescribed drugs, including anti-HIV drugs can have a number of different effects. Some doctors are taking a cautious approach to antiretroviral treatment among people who are also taking drugs such as anti-depressants, stimulants or opiates, possibly admitting them to hospital for observation when treatment is first started.

Drugs which are likely to decrease methadone levels.

Of the NNRTI anti-HIV drugs, nevirapine is likely to decrease methadone levels. A study in Dublin reported that nevirapine reduced methadone levels by 46% within two to three weeks of commencing the drug. Patients began to report opiate withdrawal symptoms 8-10 days after starting, however it is not recommended that methadone dosage be increased at the same time as starting nevirapine. Instead, it may be better to monitor withdrawal symptoms and increase the methadone dose if withdrawal does begin to occur (Clarke 2000).

The NNRTI efavirenz reduces exposure to methadone by about 60% within 24 hours of commencing (Marzolini et al. 2000). This occurs because efavirenz speeds up, or induces, the metabolism of methadone. However, dosage adjustment should not take place immediately because the neurological side-effects of efavirenz may be mistaken for opiate withdrawal. As with nevirapine, close monitoring for withdrawal is recommended. Gradual dose increases of methadone are advised if symptoms of withdrawal occur.

The nucleoside reverse transcriptase inhibitor (NRTI) stavudine (d4T) has been shown to reduce methadone levels by about 25%. Again, an individual should be monitored for withdrawal symptoms, and dose of methadone increased if necessary.

Drugs which are likely to increase methadone levels

On the basis of the liver metabolism if both saquinavir and methadone are taken together then levels of both drugs might increase and so dose reductions may be necessary.

Of the NNRTI anti-HIV drugs, delavirdine is likely to substantially increase levels of methadone, so dose reductions may be necessary.

Merck is currently conducting a formal study of indinavir and methadone. The company suggests that on the basis of their liver metabolism, levels of both drugs might increase and so dose reductions may be necessary.

No effect on methadone level

There has been very little research into interactions between methadone and other nucleoside analogues such as ddI (didanosine), ddC (zalcitabine) and 3TC (lamivudine), although no problems have been reported with combining these drugs.

Drugs with mixed / contradictory effects

Ritonavir has been shown to increase the potency of methadone when studied in the test tube but in real life it seems to have the opposite effect.

Effect of methadone on HAART medication

Methadone maintenance affects the metabolism of numerous antiviral medications commonly prescribed in HIV-positive individuals including NRTIs such as zidovidine, stavudine, didanosine and abacavir as well as NNRTIs such as efaverinz and nevirapine.

Levels of ddI (didanosine) in the blood of methadone users were only 60% of those observed in ddI users not receiving methadone. Methadone delayed the absorption of ddI, which could be a problem because the drug is not stable and the part of the ddI that does not get absorbed quickly can be damaged by stomach acid and, possibly, digestive enzymes. A larger dose may be needed.

Methadone has been found to increase AZT levels twofold. Very high levels of AZT in your system can mimic the early symptoms of opiate withdrawal. Reducing methadone dosages does not make the side-effects of AZT less severe.

Other drugs used by people with HIV

Other drugs often used by people with HIV, such as ketoconazole and itraconazole, which are used to treat fungal infections, may increase the level of methadone.

Rifampicin, which is used to treat TB dramatically reduces levels of methadone, so patients may need to have their methadone increased about three-fold if they are to avoid symptoms of withdrawal. It is important to educate these patients about the interaction; if they were to stop taking rifampicin while still taking three times the normal methadone dose, they could die from methadone overdose. Rifabutin, which is also used to treat TB, may also reduce levels of methadone.

The antidepressants amitriptyline (*Elavil*), fluvoxamine (*Lucox*), the anti-anxiety medication diazepam (*Valium*) and similar drugs such as xanax or halcion can all make methadone more potent.

Ciprofloxacin, which is used to treat gonorrhoea and sometimes urinary tract infections, has been shown to increase levels of methadone in the blood.

It is important that clients are educated about all these interactions because they may be buying methadone over and above their prescription and need to know the potential affects.

Those on methadone maintenance have a slower progression to AIDS than those who are not on a maintenance programme and continually relapse as street drugs can increase progression of HIV. It is also probably best for HIV-positive people who are on Methadone to detox slowly as withdrawal itself is stressful to the body, and this may increase HIV replication and disease progression.

Methamphetamine interactions

Australian doctors have reported what they believe to be a fatal interaction between ritonavir and methamphetamine, which is a popular recreational drug amongst gay men, especially in North America and Australia. A 49 year old Melbourne man taking the anti-HIV drugs ritonavir (400 mg bid), soft gel saquinavir (400 mg bid) and stavudine (d4T) was found dead the morning after injecting methamphetamine and sniffing amyl nitrate. A toxicology analysis showed that the dead man had methamphetamine levels of 0.5 mg/l in his blood, a level seen in many people who have died of methamphetamine overdose. Methamphetamine is metabolised by the liver enzyme cytochrome p450 CYP2D6, which is inhibited by ritonavir. The protease inhibitor could have slowed the metabolism of methamphetamine, thus causing the overdose. However, as this is the first report of a potentially harmful interaction since the introduction of protease inhibitors leading some to suggest that methamphetamine may not be responsible. Amyl nitrate use could also have contributed to the overdose, because it is metabolised to nitric oxide, another cytochrome p450 inhibitor (Hales et al, 2000).Ellis et al (2003) downplayed the possibility that a drug interaction between methamphetamine and protease inhibitors might be responsible for the viral load difference they found in their research stating that no consistent reports of altered drug metabolism exist. However pharmaceutical companies failure to investigate interactions between pharmaceutical products and illicit drugs prevents researchers from gaining a clear understanding of potential interactions.

Popper interactions

The long-term effects of poppers have been a matter of considerable controversy. In the early days it was found that there was a statistical correlation between use of poppers in HIV-positive men and Kaposi's Sarcoma, which is a malignant tumor (http://www.nlm.nih.gov/medlineplus/ency/article/001310.htm) of the connective tissue. However in recent years it has been found that there is a link between the herpes virus (HHV8) and KS. It is thought more likely that this virus, which is transmitted through anal sex causes KS. However, poppers have been used to enhance anal sex, hence perhaps the relationship.

Several studies which have compared HIV-negative and HIV-positive gay men who used poppers have shown that only those with HIV suffered any immune damage or progression to AIDS, thereby showing that use can be more dangerous for HIV-positive individuals. Studies in mice have shown that inhalation of poppers does suppress the immune system and may reduce the CD4+ and CD8+ T cell populations.

Amyl nitrate is metabolised to nitric oxide, which is a cytochrome p450 inhibitor, which is inhibited by ritonavir. Therefore, ritonavir may slow the metabolism of Amyl Nitrates, and increase the risk of overdose.

If Amyl nitrate and Viagra used together can cause dangerous hypotension, which is abnormally low blood pressure, because of the way the two drugs interact. Therefore it is important that these drugs are not mixed.

Tranquilliser interactions

Protease inhibitors may block the breakdown of certain sedatives, leading to increased blood levels of these drugs, especially Diazepam (Valium), with ritonavir having the largest negative effect. This can lead to drowsiness, disorientation, convulsions and coma.

Viagra interactions

Protease inhibitors and NNRTIs are metabolised by the P450 3A4 enzyme in the liver, which also processes *Viagra*. Consequently, anti-HIV drugs and *Viagra* may produce high levels of *Viagra* in the blood and worsen side-effects. Preliminary data on interactions between anti-HIV drugs and *Viagra*, confirmed these suspicions and two months later, the first report of the death of a man who took *Viagra* whilst taking protease inhibitors (in this case ritonavir plus saquinavir) appeared in the medical journal (Hall 1999)

Of the five protease inhibitors, saquinavir has the least effect on the CYP3A4 metabolic pathway and ritonavir has the greatest effect. Tests conducted by Pfizer found levels of saquinavir and ritonavir were not affected by *Viagra*. In contrast, saquinavir doubled the total concentration of *Viagra* in the blood, and ritonavir increased the maximum concentration of *Viagra* four-fold.

Side-effects of interaction may include headaches, facial flushing and redness, visual disturbance, abnormal changes in blood pressure and chest pain. Also, it could cause priapism, which is an abnormally prolonged erection, which may need medical treatment.

Therefore, for people taking ritonavir, it is recommended that *Viagra* should not be used at all given the potential health risks. However, if the two drugs are co-administered, the dose of *Viagra* should not exceed 25mg every 48 hours. Caution is also advised for patients taking any NNRTIs.

Other drugs which are also metabolised by the 3A4 pathway (such as ketoconazole, itraconazole and erythromycin) should be used with caution when taking *Viagra,* and it is recommended that the dose of *Viagra* is similarly reduced. Furthermore, people on these medications which are metabolised by 3A4 should not take two doses of *Viagra* within one 48-hour period.

There is in vitro evidence that the NNRTI nevirapine may lower blood levels of *Viagra* and reduce its effectiveness. Research to date suggests that *Viagra* will not affect the level of nevirapine in the blood.

Amyl nitrate and *Viagra* used together can cause dangerous hypotension, which is abnormally low blood pressure because of the way the two drugs interact. Therefore it is best that these two drugs are not use together.

References

Bruce RD et al. *Three case reports of a clinical pharmacokinetic interaction with buprenorphine and atazanavir plus ritonavir.* AIDS 20: 783 - 784, 2006.

Carneiro M et al. The effect of drug-injection behaviour on genetic evolution of HIV-1. Journal of Infectious Diseases 180(4): 1025-1032, 1999.

Clarke S et al. Managing methadone and non-nucleoside reverse transcriptase inhibitors: guidelines for clinical practice. Seventh Conference on Retroviruses and Opportunistic Infections, San Francisco, abstract 88, 2000.

Ellis RJ et al. *Increased human immunodeficiency virus loads in active methamphetamine users are explained by reduced effectiveness of antiretroviral therapy.* Journal of Infectious Diseases 188 (on-line edition). 2003.

Gavrilin MA et al. Methamphetamine enhances cell-associated feline immunodeficiency virus replication in astrocytes. Journal of NeuroVirology: 8: 240-249, 2002.

Hales G et al. Possible fatal interaction between protease inhibitors and methamphetamine. Antiviral Therapy 5 (1): 19, 2000.

Hall M. Interaction between sildenafil and HIV-1 combination therapy. Lancet 353: 2071-2072, 1999.

Harrington RD et al. Life-threatening interactions between HIV-1 protease inhibitors and the illicit drugs MDMA and gamma hydroxybuytrate. Archives of Internal Medicine 159(18): 2221-2224, 1999.

Hsyu PH et al. Pharmacokinetic and pharmacodynamic interactions between nelfinavir and methadone. Seventh Conference on Retroviruses and Opportunistic Infections, San Francisco, abstract 87, 2000.

Marzolini C (http://www.ncbi.nlm.nih.gov/entrez/query.fcgi?db=pubmed&cmd=search&term=%22marzolini+c%22%5bauthor%5d) et al, Efavirenz decreases methadone blood concentrations. AIDS 14(9): 1291-1292, 2000.

Nair MPN et al. Cocaine differentially modulates chemokine production by mononuclear cells from normal donors and human immunodeficiency virus type 1-infected patients. Clinical and Diagnostic Laboratory Immunology 7(1): 96-100, 2000.

Nandwani R et al. Possible interaction between sildenafil and HIV combination therapy. Lancet 353: 9155, 840, 1999.

Phillips AN et al. Active drug injecting and progression of HIV infection. AIDS 8(3): 385-386, 1994.

Ronald PJM et al. Continued drug use and other cofactors for progression to AIDS among injecting drug users. AIDS 8: 339-343, 1994.

Roth MD, et al. Cocaine enhances human immunodeficiency virus replication in a model of severe combined immunodeficient mice implanted with human peripheral blood leukocytes. Journal of Infectious Diseases 185: 701-705, 2002.

Swanson & Cooper. Dangerous Liaison: Club Drug Use and HIV/AIDS (http://www.thebody.com), 2002

Vittinghoff E et al. Cofactors for HIV disease progression in a cohort of homosexual and bisexual men. J Acquir Immune Defic Syndr 27(3): 308-314, 2001.

Webber MP et al. A prospective study of HIV disease progression in female and male drug users. AIDS 13(2): 257-262, 1999.

Drug users, drug addiction and HIV

Social policy and the epidemic

Drug use can fuel the spread of HIV in several ways. Injection drugs, like heroin, can transmit HIV through use of shared needles or equipment. Non-injection drugs like ecstasy, amphetamines, Viagra, poppers, crystal meth and crack are associated with increased sexual risk-taking behaviours, by impairing judgement, possibly creating strong sexual rushes and/or enabling the user to have more sex for longer.

Drug addiction has been heavily concentrated amongst disadvantaged populations in the US and Europe, particularly in neighbourhoods with high levels of unemployment amongst male youth. In the United States it has been especially concentrated amongst people of colour, while in Europe it has been most concentrated amongst white working-class youth. Ethnic minorities in Europe have been less prone to high levels of injecting drug use than their US counterparts, although this seems to be changing particularly with the increase prevalence of crack cocaine.

Drug addiction is an economically driven social problem with dependent drug users more likely to be poor and socially marginal. However, it should also be noted that a significant number of heroin addicts maintain drug habits whilst working in full-time jobs and raising families. In addition, 'recreational drug use' in the UK has escalated hugely in the past 15 years with 25.4% of 15-29 year-olds reporting that they had used drugs in 2002 (National Statistics, Regional Trends 2002). Thereby increasingly, drug users are people of all ages, social backgrounds and ethnic groups.

There are many debates about the best way of tackling drug use. The UK government joins with other countries in trying to stop the supply of drugs to this country. For example, several million pounds have been given to assist the Pakistan government to eradicate opium poppy fields and help farmers grow other non-drug crops. There are problems with this strategy, however as drugs are often grown in inaccessible areas where the government does not have control of the country and that even when crops are eradicated, production may merely shift elsewhere. Also the prices that farmers get for their alternative, legal crops are nothing like as much for drugs like opium and coca (which is made into cocaine) (World Drug Report 2005, United Nations Office for drugs and crime).

One of the major effects of the increase in drug addiction was a correspondent increase in crime as addicts sought ways of financing their habits It was concern about crime together with the concern of parents and families of users which led to pressure for increasingly punitive policies towards drug addiction during the 1980s in the US, especially amongst some black community leaders. By the mid-1980s, American politicians were firmly committed to a War on Drugs and there was an escalation of traditionally punitive US attitudes towards drug and alcohol use, which continue in the present day.

These policies in the US were to play a major role in sustaining the spread of HIV amongst drug users and the virus had already saturated drug using populations in New York and New Jersey by the time the first cases of AIDS were detected in 1982-83. It was not until 1993 in San Francisco and 1994 in Los Angeles that needle-exchange programmes were approved by city governments, and such schemes were still illegal in ten US states in 1994. Opponents of needle exchange argued that it would promote drug use and maintain addicts on drugs rather than encouraging treatment and rehabilitation.

Many states and municipalities in the United States have acted to improve access to sterile syringes. However, there are still major obstacles to obtaining sterile syringes in the United States as the possession, distribution, and sale of syringes remain a criminal offence in much of the country, and the federal government prohibits the use of its funds for needle exchange programs. In 1999, needle exchange programs exchanged 19 million sterile syringes, which clearly demonstrates the need for the service. Since Connecticut reformed their drug paraphernalia and prescription laws to allow pharmacy sales in 1992, needle sharing among injecting drug users dropped by 40%. By June 2000, 36% of US HIV cases reported to the Centre for Disease Control and Prevention had occurred among injecting drug users, their sexual partners, and children. It was only in 2000 that New York, New Hampshire, and Rhode Island joined the majority of states in allowing pharmacy sales of sterile syringes. People from ethnic minority groups continue to be disproportionately affected by HIV. Among African Americans and Latino's aged 25 to 44 50% of the deaths are caused by injections with contaminated needles. (http://www.drugpolicy.org/reducingharm/needleexchan/).

Similar attitudes determined which cities would be worst affected in the UK. In 1982 pharmacists in Edinburgh decided not to sell clean needles or syringes to injecting drug users as a drug control measure. Police also operated a policy of confiscating injecting equipment from drug users. The effect was to encourage the sharing of injecting equipment at the point when HIV was beginning to enter the drug-using population in Edinburgh. In contrast, Liverpool City Council pursued a policy of drugs education and outreach which resulted in one of the lowest levels of HIV infection amongst drug users in the UK.

In 1986 the British government agreed to a pilot programme testing needle exchanges as an HIV prevention measure. This policy has subsequently been vindicated by the low rates of infection amongst drug users in the UK compared with other European countries (and it is arguable that real rates of infection in the UK have been much lower than seroprevalence figures suggest, because of the migration of large numbers of Southern European drug users to London after having been infected in their countries of origin).

Treatment programme which have concentrated on providing methadone as maintenance treatment as a step towards treatment and abstinence have undoubtedly encouraged contact between drugs services and drug users which do not exist in countries such as Italy, Spain, Portugal and France where treatment options for addicts are more limited and more punitive and methadone is rarely available.

In France the sale of syringes was illegal until 1987; in some areas local governments subsequently pursued punitive policies against drug users, fuelling the spread of HIV. Punitive policies against drug use in some countries also served to shift drug production and consequently consumption to other countries. For example injecting drug use increased in Spain from the late 1970s as a consequence of tougher policies in France, which pushed heroin manufacture over the border.

New drugs and the spread of HIV

Club drugs, or recreational drugs, as they are sometimes called, have only recently been associated with increased high-risk sexual behaviours which, in turn, may cause higher incidence of HIV/AIDS. The most significant new drugs of the past twenty years have been crack, ecstasy, crystal meth and Viagra. Crack played a significant role in spreading HIV in the inner cities of the United States, whereas ecstasy has played a more ambiguous role in North America, Europe and Australasia. More recently, crystal meth and Viagra are playing a significant role in the spread of the HIV epidemic amongst gay scene attendees in North America and Europe.

Crack is a highly addictive derivative of cocaine (see the *A-Z of drugs*), and has become widely available in inner city areas in the US and Europe. Some researchers attribute the spread of HIV amongst women in the US to the practice of trading sex for drugs. Users are reported to trade sex for the next hit of crack in what are known as crack houses, locations where dealers sell the drug to addicts and make pipes available to smoke the drug. Crack houses often appear to bring uninfected women into contact with HIV-positive injecting drug users acting as dealers.

Crack appears to play a significant role in the spread of HIV in the United States because of its role in encouraging high rates of partner change in communities where HIV is already prevalent. A high incidence of other sexually transmitted infections amongst crack users compounds this problem by increasing the chances of transmission. Researchers in Florida found that women who used crack were more likely to be black, to have had more than five sexual partners per month, and that women were more likely to have exchanged sex for money and to have more than five sex partners per month after initiating crack use (Schoenfisch et al. 1993). It has also been noted that crack use may increase the risk of oral transmission of HIV due to burns and sores in the mouth caused by crack smoking, and because at least one study has shown that the sex sold by male and female crack addicts is predominantly oral sex. Sharing crack pipes is also contributing to the spread of Hepatitis C. It has also been noted that prostitution by crack users has led many non-crack users to seek out crack using prostitutes because they offer cheaper sexual services (Genser et al. 1992).

Crack is now prevalent in the UK, chiefly in larger cities, and it seems that the links between crack use and HIV which have appeared in the US will be replicated in the UK. A recent study, looking at the prevalence of recreational drug use in a group of club-goers in Scotland, found that crack use was less than 5%, compared with 80% use of ecstasy and amphetamines. (Riley et al. 2001). However, police figures from 2002 show that the numbers of those arrested for trafficking and possession of crack in Britain have risen by more than 200% since 1999.

Ecstasy has been linked to unsafe sex by a number of studies of sexual behaviour amongst gay men. This suggests a possible link between ecstasy use and the increase in risk behaviour which could lead to HIV infection.   An American study of 169 gay and bisexual men who were mostly club goers, published in July 2000, found that men who used ecstasy were more likely to have unsafe sex than men who drank or used other drugs. Overall, 57% of the men reported having had unprotected sex at least once during the past year- with the odds being higher among those who used ecstasy frequently (Klitzman et al. 2002).

Drugs such as MDMA have become increasingly popular within a significant drug-using subset. A large probability telephone sample of urban men who have sex with men (MSMs) taken at four large American cities found a 52% prevalence of recreational drug use (Stall et al 2001). A separate study in New York City found that 13.7% of a sample of MSMs reported using MDMA within the past six months, using it an average of 6.24 times in that period. Compared with non-users, MDMA users were found to have more male partners, have more one-night stands with men, and have more unprotected anal sex with men. (Klitzman et al. 2002). There was clearly an association between club drug use and high-risk sexual behaviours.

Although there have been no further recent studies on the link between Ecstasy and unsafe sexual practices, the use of ecstasy amongst gay men in the UK has not declined. In 2001, twice as many people suffered from ecstasy-related deaths (40 vs. 20) than in 2000 (Stall et al. 1999). Some ecstasy users argue that since the drug relaxes blood vessels, making erections difficult to maintain, unsafe sexual practices are being reduced by the drug. However, this does not prevent an ecstasy user being the receptive partner. Furthermore, the anti-impotency drug Viagra, which became more widely available in the UK since 1998, is being combined with ecstasy and other drugs increasing the possibility of sexual risk-taking amongst club-going gay men in the UK.

Since HIV-positive men are more likely to suffer from sexual dysfunction than their HIV-negative counterparts, many HIV-positive men receive prescribed *Viagra* from their clinicians. However, *Viagra* is easily available through illicit sources, either on the internet or through adverts in the gay and club-scene press, and increasing numbers of men are using it recreationally.

A study presented at the 13th International AIDS Conference in July 2000 in Durban, conducted quite soon after the licensing of Viagra, among both HIV-positive and HIV-negative gay men using one of five central London gyms found that 15% of all men had ever used *Viagra* (Sherr et al. 2000). The overwhelming majority (83%) had used it recreationally, without prescription and 63% had combined it with other recreational drugs. HIV-negative men were found to be more likely to report serodiscordant unprotected anal intercourse (UAI) in the previous three months, while actually taking the drug, than those who had never taken it (4.0% v 3.8%). Rates of serodiscordant UAI in the previous three months among the HIV-positive men who were taking the drug were barely different to those recorded among HIV-positive men who had never taken the drug (4.0% v 3.8%). The authors concluded that both HIV-positive and HIV-negative men may have added *Viagra* to their risk-taking repertoire, rather than *Viagra* causing the increase in risk behaviour.

A more recent study from San Francisco (Kim et al. 2002) found similar incidences of unprescribed Viagra use, high rates of STIs, and use of *Viagra* with other recreational drugs. Worryingly, 17% of *Viagra* users had combined the drug with poppers (amyl/butyl nitrate) which can lead to dangerously low blood pressure, stroke, heart attack or death. The authors were unable to differentiate whether these MSM were experiencing higher rates of STIs and unprotected sex because *Viagra* enables men to have more partners, *Viagra* increases the length of sexual exposure, or that these men simply added *Viagra* to their risk-taking repertoire.

References

Genser SG et al. Sex for crack as an AIDS risk behaviour: an ethnographic study. VIII International AIDS Conference, Amsterdam, abstract WeC 1032, 1992.

Kim AA et al. Increased risk of HIV and sexually transmitted disease transmission among gay or bisexual men who use Viagra, San Francisco 2000-2001, AIDS 16(10): 1425-1428, 2002.

Klitzman RL, Greenberg JD, Pollack LM, Dolezal C. MDMA ("Ecstasy") use, and its association with high-risk behaviours, mental health, and other factors among gay/bisexual men in New York City. Alcohol and Drug Dependence 66: 115-125, 2002.

Riley SC et al. Patterns of recreational drug use at dance events in Edinburgh, Scotland, Addiction 96(7): 1035-1047, 2001.

Schoenfisch S et al. Risk of HIV infection and behavioural changes associated with crack cocaine use in prenatal patients, IX International AIDS Conference, Berlin, abstract PoC 15-2920, 1993.

Sherr L et al. Viagra use and sexual risk among HIV-positive and HIV-negative gay men in London. XIII International AIDS Conference, Durban, abstract WePpD1409, 2000.

Stall R, Paul JP, Greenwood G, Pollack LM et al. Alcohol use, drug use and alcohol-related problems among men who have sex with men: The Urban Men's Health Study. Addiction 96: 1589-1601, 2001.

International responses to drug users

Injection drug use accounts for only five per cent to ten per cent of cumulative HIV infections globally, but in some parts of the world it is the major mode of HIV transmission and incidence continues to rise. For more information, see the **HIV epidemiology** chapter.

In any country with unsafe drug-injecting practises, a fresh outbreak of HIV is liable to occur at any time. Worst affected are the Russian Federation, Ukraine, and the Baltic states (Estonia, Latvia, and Lithuania), but HIV continues to spread in Belarus, Moldova and Kazakhstan, while more recent epidemics are now evident in Kyrgyzstan and Uzbekistan. In the Russian Federation, a new outbreak of HIV among injecting drug users (IDUs) in the Moscow region in 1999, resulted in the reporting of more than three times as many new cases in that year as in all the previous years combined. It is now estimated that around 860,000 people aged 15-49 are living with HIV in the Russian Federation, although reporting of HIV cases is at best patchy in many areas. The epidemic in Eastern Europe is driven by injecting drug use, and the criminalisation of this practise makes it difficult to gain an accurate picture of the proportion of drug users who are HIV-positive. In some cities, such as Svetlogorsk in Belarus, HIV prevalence among IDUs rose to more than 55% within one year of identifying HIV among the city's IDU population. It is estimated that in China, Malaysia, and Vietnam at least half of HIV infections are associated with drug injection.

HIV epidemics among IDUs are distinguished from those of other populations by their potential for rapid spread of the virus within the IVDU community and outward into the general population. In Bangkok, New York and Odessa, experience has shown that once HIV prevalence reaches a threshold of about 10%, it can surpass 40 - 50% within one to four years. Most of these infections result from sharing or reusing contaminated equipment (mainly needles and syringes) or from injecting tainted drug preparations.

Adolescence is also the time many young people are at risk of experimenting with drugs, and many of the new infections worldwide result from the sharing of drug use paraphernalia by young people (http://www.aacap.org/publications/factsfam/teendrug.htm). Young people often do not have the skills or the incentives to avoid starting doing drugs. Once they have started, many quickly progress from inhaling or snorting to injecting, which dramatically increases their risk of infection. In the Russian Federation, there were 3,008 reported new HIV infections among injecting drug users aged 10 to 19 in 1999. By 2000, that number had more than tripled to 9,612. In Thailand, 80% of women and girls admitted to drug treatment centres during 1999-2000 were under 25. Everywhere in the world, drug use is also associated with heightened sexual transmission of HIV.

Repressive laws and policies as well as punitive policing are the most common responses to drug use and drug users in many countries. A number of countries have recently passed legislation partly inspired by the "zero-tolerance" approach that dominates current US drug policy. In general, official policy in many countries continues to be guided by international conventions on drug use that emphasise drug interdiction and drug user incarceration approaches. Police harassment of drug users is also widespread. It is reported that, in some countries, particularly in Eastern Europe and Central & South East Asia, police round up young people suspected of drug use to search for signs of injecting or force them to be tested for HIV. Those who test positive have their drug use and HIV status registered.

These and other human rights abuses are compounded by the failure to provide needed services to drug users. In many countries, the few official drug treatment programs that do exist often share the punitive approach to drug users that characterises official drug policy, hence many drug users do not access the treatment that is available. Counselling, peer support, and other approaches that address the psychosocial needs of people trying to deal with their addiction are rarely used. Substitution treatment is unavailable in many countries, and illegal in some, despite the overwhelming international evidence that points to the efficacy of harm reduction approaches in reducing the individual and social harms associated with drug use, especially HIV/AIDS and other diseases.

In the UK, for example, with efforts to reduce the supply of and demand for illicit drugs there are also policies and programmes in place which attempt to decrease the adverse health, social and economic consequences of drug use. However, developing harm reduction in many countries brings a number of challenges, especially in those with hostile policies together with negative social attitudes toward drug users and people with HIV/AIDS which inhibits the expansion of harm reduction services to the requisite scale.

Fair and accurate reporting plays a vital role in raising public awareness of and shaping national and international responses to drug use and HIV/AIDS. However, many news stories continue to portray drugs users and people with HIV/AIDS only in terms of the threat they pose to others. All too often, drug users and their families are merely represented as silent objects of law enforcement or drug control campaigns, or not included in media coverage at all.

The spread of injecting and drug use in developing countries

One of the most powerful factors governing the spread of HIV in developing countries is the globalisation of the heroin and cocaine trade, and the unintentional impact of policies to combat that trade.

Heroin trade

In the 1960s the major source of heroin was the Golden Triangle region of South East Asia. Until the 1970s opium was gathered here for shipment to Europe, where it was refined into heroin. This practice ensured that opium was the drug most readily available in SE Asia, and minimised the practice of injecting drug use. However, in the late 1970s heroin factories in Europe began to close down due to law enforcement, and it became safer to refine the drug at the site of production. Cheap heroin soon became easily available in SE Asia, and injecting drug use began to spread along heroin supply routes into Burma, Vietnam, Thailand, southern provinces of China and northern India as injectable quality heroin became more readily available and users developed tolerance to the smoked form of the drug.

New trends in the marketing of illicit drugs have had a major impact on the development of the epidemic. Organised crime syndicates moved into the heroin trade in the 1970s as it became clear that very large profits could be extracted from drug dealing. A flood of new heroin began to enter Europe and America following the fall of the Shah of Iran in 1979, leading to a further increase in heroin addiction. Heroin also begun to spread to African countries, especially Nigeria, as drug trafficking onto Europe and North America began increasingly using West Africa as a relay point.

The route of heroin smuggled into the West crosses through a number of Eastern European countries, and its path is marked by a high concentration of IDUs, and a high HIV prevalence amongst this group even though the HIV epidemics are still young and have so far spared some cities and sub-populations.

The World Drug Report 2005
(http://www.unodc.org/unodc/world_drug_report.html) (UNODC)
states that global illicit opium poppy cultivation increased by
16% in 2004 due entirely to increased cultivation in
Afghanistan. Afghanistan is a high yield area (32kg/ha) and
cultivation increased from 80,000 ha in 2003 to 131,000 ha in
2004 with every province now growing it. Despite this, global
opium poppy cultivation is still less than it was in the early
nineties. Declines were recorded in 2004 in Laos and Myanmar
both low opium yield areas (13kg/ha). The main source of street
heroin in the UK is the Golden Crescent
(http://www.drugscope.org.uk/druginfo/drugsearch/ds_results.asp
?file=1_crescent.html) countries of South West Asia, mainly
Afghanistan, Iran and Pakistan. In June 2005 75% of Europe's
and 95% of the UK's heroin came from Afghanistan, with
UK-based Turkish groups behind 70% of heroin in the UK
(Druglink 2005).

The opium situation in Afghanistan as of August 2005
(http://www.unodc.org/unodc/opium_situation_in_afghanistan.ht
ml) indicates a reduction in the cultivation of poppy by 21%
(autumn 2005), however due to a good growing season the yield
of opium by hectare increased from 32kg per hectare in 2004 to
39kg in 2005; as a result total potential production of opium
decreased by only 2% (World Drug Report 2005, United Nations
Office for drugs and crime).

Cocaine trade

In South America the major drug product is cocaine. Intensive
policing of cocaine supplies has led to shortages, and
subsequently to price increases. When prices rise, more people
may be tempted to inject a drug in order to get maximum value
for money.

The heart of the international cocaine trade is located in the
Andean region of South America. Virtually all of the world's
cocaine base, the intermediate product used to manufacture
cocaine hydrochloride (cocaine HCl), is produced in Peru,
Bolivia, or Colombia. Cocaine base production in Peru and
Bolivia in 1995 represented about 90% of the world's cocaine
base; the remaining 10% was produced in Colombia. Colombian
traffickers were dependent on Peruvian and Bolivian sources for
two-thirds of their cocaine base. Each year, hundreds of tons of
cocaine base were imported by aircraft from Peru and Bolivia.

In 1997, Bolivia's Government implemented the Dignity Plan,
which has all but eliminated illicit cocaine cultivation in the
Chapare jungle. Bolivia's potential cocaine production decreased
from 240 metric tons in 1995 to 70 metric tons in 1999.
Additionally, laboratory analysis indicates that the purity of
Bolivian cocaine has dropped significantly while local base prices
have risen, an indication of reduced availability. Much of
Bolivia's cocaine is now believed to be either consumed in Brazil
or shipped through Brazil to Europe.

In Peru, cocaine production decreased from an estimated 460
metric tons in 1995, to 175 metric tons in 1999. This was in
part due to Peru's air interdiction program, which shut down the
cocaine "airbridge" between Bolivia, Peru and Colombia. This
resulted in a drop in coca prices, taking the profitability out of
coca cultivation. Since 2000 replanting has started again in
previously abandoned fields causing speculation that coca leaf
cultivation may be on the rise. In addition, since 1995 net coca
cultivation in Colombia has more than doubled from 50,000
hectares in 1995 to 136,200 hectares in 2000.

Africa has also attracted the cocaine syndicates' attention.
Nigerian trafficking groups are moving significant amounts of
cocaine from South America to all parts of Africa. Because of
the Nigerian role in the global movement of drugs, West Africa
has become an important transit area for cocaine bound for
destinations throughout Africa. Ghana seized more cocaine than
Jamaica--over a quarter of a metric ton in the first nine months
of 1996 alone--twenty times more than Ghanaian authorities had

seized in all of 1995. Cocaine has also continued to enter South
Africa in important quantities for consumption in the country
and for shipment to other destinations in Africa and Europe.
South African enforcement authorities are establishing working
links with their Brazilian counterparts to help break up the
Nigerian trafficking groups responsible for most of the cocaine
flow into southern Africa.

Current global trends in drug use

There are many different recreational drugs available and the
popularity of each varies around of the world, as does the
popularity of injecting. The estimate global illicit drugs trade
turnover is US $322 billion per year (Wodak, 2006)

It is estimated that in 2004, 4% of the worldwide population
used cannabis, 1% used amphetamine type stimulants, cocaine,
or opiates. These data also give an indication of frequency of
drug use: 200 million people (4.9%) used drugs annually, 110
million people (2.7%) monthly, and 25 million people (0.6%)
more than once a month (Aceijas et al, 2005).

Roughly one tenth of HIV infections are a result of needle
sharing and it is estimated that there are 13.2 million IDU's
worldwide (Needle et al, 2000) with around 80% living in
developing and transitional countries (Aceijas et al, 2005). This
breaks down to an estimated:

- 8.8 million in Eastern and Central Europe, South and
  South-East Asia

- 1.4 million in North America

- 1 million in Latin America

The use of opiates has been increasing worldwide with more than
two-thirds of the countries in the world reporting increases.
Opiate use is highest in developing nations and nations in
transition, while use in developed nations is stable or declining.
One possible reason for the increase in use worldwide is that
production of opium has increased dramatically. Opium and
opiate drugs are most widely used in Asia. Opiate use is much
lower in North America, Central America, South America, and
Europe than it is in Asia. However, there is still enough use to
consider opium a problem drug in those regions. Africa has the
lowest overall use of opium (Carmen 2004)

Cannabis remains the most widespread drug in use worldwide.
The United Nations World Drug Report estimates that cannabis
is the most widely abused substance in all parts of the world,
with around 141 million people using it. The use of cannabis is
increasing overall, but in some regions, notably North America,
Russia, China, and parts of Asia, use has stabilised or decreased
in recent years. Cannabis will probably remain the most widely
used drug because the crop is easily grown in many different
climates and requires no processing for use as drugs. The major
growers of cannabis and major suppliers for the world market
are Morocco, South Africa, Nigeria, Afghanistan, Pakistan,
Mexico, Colombia, and Jamaica. Another trend in cannabis
growing in developed nations is hydroponics and other indoor
growing techniques. Improved cannabis growing techniques result
in a plant with a much higher concentration of
tetrahydrocannabinol, the active ingredient in marijuana and
other cannabis drugs. As a result, the drugs from these crops are
more powerful.

Throughout the 1990s, the use of amphetamine-type stimulants
(ATS) increased dramatically worldwide. The main regions of use
of ATS are in North America, Western Europe, and Asia. By the
end of the 1990s, ATS use had stabilised or declined in North
America and Western Europe. By contrast, use has continued to
increase in Asia. Asia is the leading region for use and

manufacture of ATS, and the potential for spreading the problem to other regions continues (Carmen 2004).

Worldwide, cocaine use has been reported in more than two-thirds of all countries. Although the use of cocaine is declining in North America, the rate of use still leads the world. In Western Europe, cocaine use has continued to rise since 1980. The lowest rates of cocaine use are found in Asia. Law-enforcement efforts have brought down the rate of production in cocaine-producing nations in recent years. Cocaine use is highest in the United States, but use is also high in other countries throughout the Americas and Europe. In general, rates of cocaine use are higher in more affluent countries. The use of amphetamine-type stimulants is highest in Europe and significant in selected other countries in the Americas. African countries generally show more amphetamine-type stimulant use than use of opium and cocaine, where use is low. Cocaine use in Spain has overtaken the United States and left Britain and Ireland behind, with the proportion of people who use the drug rising to more than one in 40. "Spain occupies the top place in the world," the report said, citing United Nations figures on cocaine use around the globe. The reason for such a high rate in Spain is that much of Europe's cocaine is unloaded on to Spanish beaches (El Pais Newspaper, Sept 2005)

Around 25% of all injecting drug users live in South and South-east Asia, and a further 18% in East Asia. Each of China and India is home to more than a million IDU's. The world's highest rates of HIV infection amongst IDU's are found in Asia. By 1999, drug-dependent individuals comprised about 77% of HIV infections in Malaysia and 69% in China, and 66% of AIDS cases in Viet Nam. A further 24% of injecting drug users are found in Eastern Europe and Central Asia. There are around 2 million in Russia, 397,000 in Ukraine and 174,000 in Kazakhstan. IDU's account for 82% of all HIV/AIDS cases in Central Europe and Former Soviet Union states. North America and Latin America respectively account for 10.6% and 7.6% of injecting drug users. There are around 1.3 million in the USA, 800,000 in Brazil and 153,000 in Canada. Around 9.4% of IDU's live in Western Europe, where populations above 200,000 exist in Germany, Italy and Spain (Aceijas et al, 2005).

During the last decade of the 20th century the number of countries reporting injecting drug use rose from 80 to 134 and the proportion of countries with HIV outbreaks among injecting drug users rose from 65% to 84% (Needle et al, 2000). At least 41 countries have HIV prevalence rates above 5% among injecting drug users. HIV prevalence rates above 20% have been recorded at sites in 25 of these countries, and above 50% in 15 of them (Aceijas et al, 2005). Explosive growth is one characteristic of injecting drug use-related HIV epidemics and in several well documented instances, HIV seroprevalence among injecting drug users rose from 1%-2% to 60%-70% in a few years (Grassley et al, 2003).

Recent estimates indicate that at least 10% of all new infections in the world - a figure that rises to 30% when Africa is excluded - can be attributed to injecting drug use; this was about 4 million at the end of 2005, yet many of these drug users are unable to access anti-HIV treatment (UNAIDS, 2002), The worst affected areas for infection through contaminated needle use are Central and Eastern Europe of which Estonia, the Russian Federation and Ukraine appear to have the largest and most widespread epidemics, Central Asia, most of Southern Asia, North Africa, Iran, Pakistan, Nepal, and parts of Latin America (Needle et al, 2000). According to the United Nations Office on Drugs and Crime (UNODC), in Eastern Europe, 60% of injecting drug users are under the age of 26. The recent, dramatic rise in HIV prevalence in South and Southeast Asia is substantially related to injecting drug use (Rhodes et al, 1999). In South and Southeast Asia, including China, Indonesia, Myanmar and Viet Nam, the age at which people begin injecting drug use is reducing with young people being especially susceptible. In countries that have little or no harm reduction services such as needle and syringe programmes are not widely available and drug substitution treatment is illegal with law enforcement still represents the main response in dealing with drug use. This is a public health problem that not only affects people who inject

drugs, but also their sexual partners, their children and the wider community. In some countries, infection through needle sharing is the dominant transmission route. In Russia for example 80% of HIV-positive people were infected in this way (UNAIDS, 2002)

Injecting drug use is becoming a problem in Africa, which is increasingly being used for the trafficking of heroin and cocaine. Studies indicate that drug use is becoming an increasing problem in coastal countries such as Nigeria, Mauritius, Kenya, Tanzania and South Africa (UNODC, 2001). In South Africa injection drug users come from all racial groups and use a wide range of drugs including heroin, methamphetamine, cocaine and even MDMA (Parry et al, 2006). In Kenya the prevalence rate of opiate abuse is 0.1%, giving an estimated 30,000 injection drug users and the problem is growing. Although Kenya has an HIV prevalence of 8%, the potential HIV prevalence amongst IDU's is over 50% UNODC, 2001). The percentage of IDU's sharing syringes within the past six months ranges from 11% in Nigeria to 27% in Kenya (UNODC, 2001). Several small studies suggest that the HIV prevalence in these populations ranges between 8.9% in Nigeria, to 19.4% in South Africa, 29-31% in Tanzania and between 22.9% to 50% in Kenya (UNODC, 2001). In all countries services for drug users are very rare.

A recent study by the Health Protection Agency (2006) suggests that HIV prevalence amongst IDU's in England and Wales is at its highest level since 1992.

The latest figures from the HPA's Unlinked Anonymous Prevalence Monitoring Programme (UAPMP), which provides data to the end of 2005, show that one in 62 IDU's were found to be infected with HIV in 2005, which is equivalent to a national IDU HIV prevalence rate of 1.6%. The highest prevalence was in London where 4% were infected with HIV and elsewhere in England and Wales prevalence was 1%.

Between 1998 and 2003 only 118 new infections in total were attributed to IDU's, in 2004, 131 were attributed to IDU and it is likely that this has increased to an estimated 182 in 2005. Previous reports from the HPA suggest that between 30% and 50% of IDU's are unaware that they are HIV-positive. Since surveillance began in 1982, 76,850 new HIV diagnosis had been made by the end of December 2005 of these, 5.7% were probably acquired through IDU. HIV prevalence amongst IDU's in England and Wales reached a peak of 5.9% in 1990, 1.6% in 1992 and a low of 0.6% in 1996. The report found evidence of a recent increase in risky injecting practices and evidence of an increase in the injecting of crack-cocaine. As far back as 1998 the UK's national drug strategy changed its focus from harm-reduction and the reduction of blood-borne viruses to wider social harms, in particular drug-related crime. This shift in the focus of policy and service provision may well have hindered the promotion of harm reduction measures in response to evolving patterns of drug use and risk behaviours.

An underestimated route of HIV transmission is the use of cocaine, particularly crack-cocaine. Around 13.4 million people use cocaine worldwide, with most use in North America (6.5 million) (Deveau et al, 2006). HIV prevalence among crack-cocaine drug users is lower than amongst IDU's, but studies are now revealing that infection rates are on the rise. The risk is blood can be passed from mouth to mouth if smoking equipment is shared. A study in Canada found that 37% of the 550 enrolled drug users reported sharing smoking equipment every time they took the drug. The programme supplied clean crack-smoking apparatus for 12 months and sharing fell to 13%. The study highlighted that sufficient harm reduction strategies have to be introduced, as more evidence reveals the extent of this overlooked route of HIV transmission.

In spite of laws and governmental measures, such as intensive policing, imprisonment and, in some countries the 'war on drugs', illegal drug use is on the increase. This approach drives many drug users underground, away from social support services, including health services, making contact, providing HIV education and prevention as well as and health care difficult. Yet experience has shown that HIV epidemics among injecting drug users can be halted, if injecting drug users are appropriately supported through a comprehensive harm reduction approach. There is an urgent need to place and maintain pressure on governments to repeal repressive laws and policies towards injecting drug users to adequately support financially harm reduction programmes.

There is a need for more research to be carried out on injecting drug users regarding HIV infection and other health issues. For example, in no country in North Africa and the Middle East, are injecting drug users included as a study group in surveillance systems, which is disastrous in terms of early detection of a HIV epidemic outbreak.

References

Aceijas, C., Stimson, G.V., Hickman, M. & Rhodes, T. Global overview of injecting drug use and HIV infection among injecting drug users, *AIDS*, 18:2295-2303. 2004.

Carmen, A et al. Global overview of injecting drug use and HIV infection among injecting drug users. On behalf of the UN Reference Group on HIV/AIDS Prevention and Care among IDU in Developing and Transitional Countries, 2004.

Deveau C et al. *Prevention of HIV/AIDS among drug users as a vulnerable population.* The 2006 HIV/AIDS Implementers Meeting of the President's Emergency Plan for AIDS Relief, Durban, South Africa, abstract 89, 2006.

Grassly NC, Lowndes CM, Rhodes T. Modelling emerging HIV epidemics: the role of injection drug use and sexual transmission in the Russian Federation, China, and India. *International Journal of Drug Policy*, 14:25-43. 2003.

Health Protection Agency. *Evidence of a continuing increase in the HIV prevalence among injecting drug users in England and Wales* CDR Weekly 16 (11), 2006.

Needle R et al. The Global Research Network on HIV Prevention in Drug Using Populations (GRN) 1998- 2000: trends in the epidemiology, ethnography, and prevention of HIV/AIDS in injecting drug users. In: *2000 Global*

Research Network Meeting on HIV Prevention in Drug Using Populations, Third Annual Meeting Report, 5-7 July, Durban, South Africa. Washington, DC, National Institute on Drug Abuse. 2000.

Needle R et al. *Injection drug use in sub-Saharan Africa: emergence of an under-recognized HIV transmission risk.* The 2006 HIV/AIDS Implementers Meeting of the President's Emergency Plan for AIDS Relief, Durban, South Africa, Abstract 121, 2006.

Parry C et al. *HIV and drug use among injection drug users (IDU's), commercial sex workers (CSWs) and men who have sex with men (MSM) in South Africa.* The 2006 HIV/AIDS Implementers Meeting of the President's Emergency Plan for AIDS Relief, Durban, South Africa, Abstract 126, 2006.

Rhodes T, Ball A, Stimson GV et al. HIV infection associated with drug injecting in the newly independent states, Eastern Europe: the social and economic context of epidemics. *Addiction* 94:1323-1336. 1999.

UNAIDS. *Report of the Global HIV/AIDS Epidemic*, Geneva, Switzerland. 2002.

World Drug Report, UNODC. (2001). *Assistance to country responses on HIV/AIDS associated with injecting drug use by the UN and other agencies*, Report for the Interagency Task Team on injecting drug use.

Yongwanitchit K et al (2006). Bangkok Metropolitan Administration (BMA) outreach program to reduce HIV risks for injecting drug users. The 2006 HIV/AIDS Implementers Meeting of the President's Emergency Plan for AIDS Relief, Durban, South Africa, Abstract 93, 2006.

The economic impact of drug production

The growing and processing of drugs usually takes place in developing nations or nations in transition. For developing nations, drug production may form the basis of the country's economy. Drug growing and processing usually employs a large percentage of the population and may be a major source of income. The money from growing and processing drugs boosts local economies, even though most of the profits do not directly benefit the growers and production workers.

The economic impact of coca production is significant. In 1999 Colombia produced 520 metric tons of coca worth an estimated $494 million. Peru produced 305 metric tons of coca worth an estimated $134 million. Bolivia produced 70 metric tons of coca worth an estimated $63 million.

The huge economic impact of drug production on source countries makes elimination of this production a major problem. In poor nations, people usually consider the money-making

opportunities worth the risks. Many times, the risks are lessened through corrupt governments that make profits from the illicit drug production. Some countries simply lack the resources or manpower to combat illicit drug growing and production.

The Opening up of Eastern Europe and the Russian Federation

The opening up of the countries of Eastern Europe and the Russian Federation to the West offers opportunities for such countries to learn from and participate in the debates and research which have shaped drug policy-making and programming in Western Europe, North America, Australia and, increasingly, parts of Asia. However, these cannot merely be replicated as that would be to ignore the particularities of history, culture and society as well as the characteristics of drug use and drug users in countries of the region.

In Poland, the Ukraine and Belarus there is now a growing understanding amongst academics and policy makers of the implications of the emerging twin epidemics of injecting drug use and HIV infection. Experience in other parts of the world has demonstrated that injecting drug use practices are both locally specific and very diverse. Yet there remains both a lack of basic information regarding injecting drug use practices, and a need to develop local capacity to collect and analyse such data.

There is a need for basic information on the context in which drug injecting takes place. This includes such information as what are the social profiles of those involved, what is the nature of the sub-culture and norms surrounding drug injecting, where does injecting take place and what health or other services are accessible and trusted.

Developments in democracy and governance in the region may make such a process particularly appropriate and timely for those countries as it can build on existing efforts to increase institutional capacity, decentralise decision-making, democratise political systems and promote citizen and community participation. Such a development framework also allows the conceptual focus to widen beyond the individual to an understanding that HIV infection is as much to do with the social contexts as it is with an individual's behaviour. Work on injecting drug use and HIV must be placed in the contexts of poverty, gender, social disaffection and hypocrisy (Rhodes 1999).

References

Rhodes T et al. Drug injecting, rapid HIV spread and the risk environment: implications for assessment and response. AIDS 13 Supp A S259-270, 1999.

Russian Federation

The countries of the former USSR present some of the most dramatic trends in the worldwide HIV/AIDS epidemic. Fuelled by injecting drug use, the epidemic unfolds against a complicated backdrop of economic crisis, rapid social change, increased poverty and unemployment, growing prostitution and changes in sexual norms. Previously characterised by very low prevalence rates, the region now faces an extremely steep increase in the number of new infections, up from 420,000 at end-1999 to at least 700,000 one year later. In 2000 alone, more new infections were registered in the Russian Federation than in all previous years combined. Some might consider Russia's HIV problems modest in comparison with southern Africa, with prevalence hovering around 1%, compared with 30-35% in some parts of southern Africa. However, Russia is already suffering net population decline and HIV is beginning to show signs of moving beyond the predominantly male injecting drug user population.

The total number of drug users had risen 900% in the decade ending in early 2004 (Pravda, 2004), which has been traced in part to the increased availability of cheap heroin trafficked through central Asia and across the former Soviet states from Afghanistan and Turkey (Dehne et al, 1999). There is some evidence to suggest that the aftermath of the events of September 11, 2001 in Afghanistan and central Asia has not stemmed the flow of heroin through the region and may even exacerbate it in the long run (Lubin et al, 2002).

Drug use is the main cause of HIV's spread in Russia (http://www.avert.org/ecstatee.htm), where around 2% of adults have injected narcotics, Estimates of the number of active drug users in Russia in February 2004 ranged from 1 to 4 million, although it is believed the high end of that range reflected the reality. In 2004, officials predicted that Russia could have over 35 million drug users by 2014 (Pravda, 2004). At the same time the Commonwealth of Independent States, which includes twelve former Soviet states, predicted that in 2010 the twelve countries would have 25 million drug users of whom 10 million would be living with HIV/AIDS (NewsInfo, 2004) the vast majority in Russia. Kozlov (2006) showed that both heroin and psychostimulant drugs such as amphetamines are being injected. Most individuals reported sharing injecting equipment, with 79% sharing needles.

As in many parts of the world the exchange of sex for drugs and the use of sex work to support drug habits provide important links between injection drug use and commercial sex. Estimates in 2003 suggest that some 40% of sex workers in Moscow were regular injectors of heroin (Webster, 2003) and between 15-50% of women injection drug users engage in sex work with some regularity. The median number of sexual partners in the previous six months reported by women who sold sex was five. Overall, the investigators noted that

The dominant drug of choice overall in Russia remains injected heroin, but homemade preparations of ephedrine, including methamphetamine in a liquid form known as *vint* (meaning "screw") are also widely injected (Rhodes et al, 2004). Use of powdered or refined heroin builds on a longer tradition of consumption of home-produced opiates of various kinds. Mini-laboratories exist in virtually every neighbourhood, and Russian methods of producing opiates carry a particular risk - the use of human blood in the production process. Blood is used to neutralise toxins present in the opiate liquid derived from poppy straw because acetic anhydride, the chemical used in larger laboratories, is too expensive. On average, one glass of liquid will require 5ml of blood, virtually guaranteeing that HIV could be transmitted.

The reliance on drug preparations made in the home also established a tradition of group injecting. One person will provide some of the ingredients, one will provide the cooker and filtersor other equipment, and so on, and the overall process is much cheaper when carried out in groups than by individuals (Grund, 2001). Group situations such as this lead frequently to the collective use of injecting equipment in Russia(Rhodes et al, 2003) and is associated with high risk of transmission of HIV. In 2004 studies indicated between 36 - 82% of drug users shared needles depending on the city (Rhodes et al, 2004). The sharing of injecting equipment is also common because syringes of any sort are in very short supply. All syringes now have to be imported into the former Soviet Union, but supply is dependent on the availability of foreign currency to pay for the goods. Drug dealers will offer injections from ready loaded syringes, or will squirt a prepared dose from a larger syringe, which may have been used for prior injecting and contaminated with HIV-infected blood, into another syringe.

Researchers have also recorded frequent use of practices that entail squirting drug preparations from one user's syringe into another by "front-loading" (into a syringe from which the needle has been removed) or "back-loading" (into a syringe from which the plunger has been removed), both of which increase the risk of infectious disease transmission.

Studies in Russian cities conducted between 1997 and 2002 found a wide range of HIV prevalence rates among IDUs ranging from 0% - 65% (UNDP 2004; Rhodes*et al*. 2004). Although

only 52% of registered infections are among IDUs, the Russian Federal AIDS Centre has estimated that in 2002 over 90% of actual infections are among IDUs (Rhodes *et al*. 2004). A large part of this increase is among sex workers (many of whom are also IDUs and/or are sexual partners of IDUs): One study estimated that 80% of HIV-positive women were involved in both injecting drug use and sex work (Smolskaya et al. 2000 quoted in Rhodes et al. 2004). Young people throughout the region are particularly and increasingly vulnerable. HIV is concentrated largely among 18- to 30 year-olds, the average HIV-infected IDU is 24 years old, with up to 5% of young people in Moscow being HIV-positive (Burrows and Sarang 2005).

By 2002, an estimated 93% of persons registered by the government as HIV-positive since the beginning of the epidemic were injection drug users (CEEHRN, 2002) In contrast, in 2002 an estimated 12% of new HIV transmission was sexual-that figure climbed to 17.5% in the first half of 2003-indicating the foothold that the epidemic is gaining in the general population (UNDP, 2004). Whilst infection rates may have reached saturation levels in at least some of the currently affected drug user populations, new outbreaks could still emerge (Rhodes et al, 2004).

HIV prevention efforts are being crippled by religious dogmatism and extremely repressive attitudes towards injecting drug use. In addition there is hostility towards non-governmental organisations perceived to be influenced by the west. Punitive laws against drug use make harm reduction programmes involving needle exchange, supply of sterile injecting equipment and substitution therapy difficult if not impossible, For example, the Humanitarian Action in St Petersburg explained how in-service training of police officers had dispelled the widespread belief that outreach workers were distributing drugs and led to an end to harassment. Lars Kalling, the UN Special Envoy for HIV/AIDS in Eastern Europe, told the conference that 700,000 new infections could be averted between now and 2015 if governments in the region establish effective prevention programmes. However, political resistance to harm reduction programmes in the region remains entrenched, despite growing fears that Russia is facing a profound demographic crisis that will result in a shrinking population.

In 2003, Russia's entire HIV prevention budget was just $1 million, and funding for harm reduction fell by 29% between 2002 and 2005 (Wolfe, 2005). Foreign donors have helped to support outreach programmes and needle exchanges in some regions, but they are few and far between. In 2006, President Putin increased the federal budget for HIV and AIDS programmes, and promised to do more to tackle the epidemic. This however has coincided with increased hostility towards non-governmental organisations and increased criticism of "foreign" ideas such as condom promotion and harm reduction. Moral objections to homosexuality, drug use and commercial sex continue to remain a hindrance to HIV prevention in Russia (Alcorn, 2006) with substitution treatment remaining illegal (Niedowski, 2006)

Needle exchanges

In 2004, there were an estimated 75 syringe exchange programs across the Russian Federation, of which 42 were run by government institutions and 33 by NGOs (Rhodes et al, 2004). 56 of the 89 regions report having at least one functioning syringe exchange (HRW, 2004a) In June 2006 this had reduced to just 60 needle exchanges, which is fewer than there were in 2002 and none are in Moscow. It is also legal in Russia to purchase syringes at a drug store, which service as the most important source of syringes for most drug users.

The range of services provided at syringe exchange points can make the utilisation of these services a more promising avenue for HIV prevention than the purchase of syringes in drug stores. Significant reductions in risky behaviour, including sharing of syringes, linked to participation in syringe exchange programs have been demonstrated repeatedly in Russia (Rhodes et al, 2004) ''but such results have generally not been associated with drug store purchases of syringes.

Police harassment is one of the most important factors that exacerbate risky behaviour among drug users. In a 2002 study of drug use in five Russian cities, 44% of drug users said they had been stopped by the police in the month prior to being interviewed, and two third of these said that their injecting equipment had been confiscated by the police (Rhodes et al, 2003). Over 40% added that they rarely carried syringes for fear of encountering the police with them. Drug users who had been arrested or detained by the police for drug-related offences were over four times more likely than other users to have shared syringes in the previous four weeks. Some drug users also avoid the drug stores because police frequently targeted people buying syringes at such locations (Trubnikov, 2003).

Harm reduction programs, particularly needle exchange, have had unclear legal status in Russia. The 1996 Criminal Code of the Russian Federation defined as crimes the manufacture, acquisition, keeping, carriage, sending, or sale of illegal narcotics (article 228) and the "inclining to consumption" of illegal drugs (article 230), interpreted by most observers to refer both to consumption and to inducing another person to consume illicit drugs. The 1998 Federal Law on Drugs and Psychotropic Substances similarly defines crimes related to the manufacture, use, and sale of illicit drugs and does not address harm reduction activities explicitly. Expert observers noted in recent years that the lack of explicit treatment of harm reduction activities in the law has enabled law enforcement officials to interpret the law as prohibiting activities such as syringe exchange and particularly to charge that harm reduction activities can have the effect of promoting drug use (Butler, 2003).

In December 2003, article 230 of the Criminal Code on consumption of illicit drugs was amended. It added that the given article does not cover promotion of use of relevant tools and equipment necessary for use. This amendment was hailed by some observers as a breakthrough for legal protection of harm reduction services. The new regulations were meant to be in place by March 2004, however since late 2003 an edict was issued saying that programs that "exchange disposable syringes for drug abusers" constitute "open promotion of illegal drugs" and suggesting that regional authorities should consider whether there were grounds for invoking criminal law against operators of these services. It also suggested that authorities in countries such as the Netherlands, Switzerland, and Canada had disavowed harm reduction and particularly syringe exchange programs as erroneous policy leading to promotion of drug use, a patently untrue statement. There was a swift international reaction to this letter, denouncing the analysis and defending the HIV prevention record of syringe exchange services (HRW, 2004b).

In February 2004 another public statement stated that the SDCC would not ban syringe exchange programs, but sought to license them and ensure that they are carried out in government health facilities. Syringe exchange services are seen to serve both a prevention and a treatment function, which some observers have taken to mean that he was suggesting HIV testing of drug users who seek sterile syringes at exchange services meaning that users of syringe exchange services should not be able to keep their anonymity. The statement also stated that syringes should not be exchanged in mobile units such as buses, a measure that would hit NGOs especially hard as they run mobile units.

A Ministry of Health statement in February 2004 expressed general support for HIV prevention activities among persons at risk of HIV/AIDS but did not address needle exchange specifically. Dr. Alexander Golyusov, director of the HIV/AIDS unit in the Ministry of Health in February 2004 stated that no decision had been taken to shut down or curtail needle exchange. He said the ministry saw it as very important to work respectfully with drug users on HIV prevention, to treat them with humanity in order to bring more benefits. However, the main point of schemes is seen by the authorities as not in giving away needles, but working with people to change their mentality and understanding as giving away needles without consultation is seen as only bringing harm.

Prisons

Being in prison or other state detention is an important risk factor for HIV in Russia as a very high percentage of drug users will find themselves in state custody at some time in their lives. Injection drug use is reportedly widespread; between 22 - 65% (Rhodes et al, 2004). HIV prevention services such as provision of sterile syringes or disinfectant materials are virtually absent (Holley, 2004). Official statistics indicate that from 1996 to 2003, HIV prevalence in Russian prisons rose more than thirty-fold from less than one per 1000 inmates to 42.1 per 1000 inmates (Roshchupkin, 2003). According to a 2002 report, about 34,000 HIV-positive persons-over 15% of the persons officially counted as HIV-positive in the country-were in state custody, of which the large majority found out about their HIV status in prison (Rhodes et al, 2004).

Outreach

The SDCC asserted that drug users and former drug users should not be permitted to work in HIV prevention services for injection drug users. This runs counter to the conclusion of UNAIDS and HIV service providers all over the world that peer-led education can be most effective for HIV prevention among drug users and other marginalised persons (Amirkhanian, et al, 1999).

Possession

The State Duma's December 2003 amendment of the Criminal Code was also hailed as an opportunity to revise the criminal drug possession laws in Russia, which have historically defined harsh penalties for very small levels of individual possession of narcotics. In the late 1990s, Russia reduced by a factor of fifty the amount of heroin and other drugs the possession of which would entail mandatory imprisonment. Activists noted that the main motivation for the 2003 changes may have been to reduce the severe overcrowding of prisons. The Duma's amendments expressed the view that individual possession of "less than ten average doses" should not be a criminal offence. The SDCC circulated a proposal that would have defined the minimum dose for criminal possession of heroin at 0.0001 grams, a dose smaller than in any other country that defines legal minimum amounts for criminal prosecution. It also recommended corresponding minimum doses of cannabis and methamphetamines.

Substitute therapy

Substitution therapy such as methadone maintenance therapy is illegal in Russia, and the 2003 amendments to the drug law did not change this despite it being available in most of the other former Soviet states for some years (CEEHRN, 2002). The Ministry of Health state that they are concerned by first-hand accounts from drug users that methadone is more addictive or "harder to get off" than heroin and that other countries' experiences have been "contradictory." Despite growing pressure from the international public health community Russia's chief public health official has reported that methadone substitution therapy will not made available in the near future. The concern is that if the right of free-of-charge distribution of methadone is given to NGOs, it will not be always possible to control exact observance of legislation. They also argue that even if methadone is implemented in [state] clinics, there are chances that the medical personnel will plunder the drug or drug users will trade in surpluses of methadone.

The refusal of Russia to legalise methadone and support substitution therapy has been widely criticised by international experts. The Open Society Institute has noted that in criminalizing use of methadone, Russia is denying itself one of the potentially most effective tools at its disposal to stem HIV transmission (Malinowska - Sempruch, et al, 2003). In particular in 2006 Russia received strong criticism from 49 leading drug treatment and HIV researchers and other experts from around the world issued a letter of concern over a highly influential anti-methadone article published in the *Russian Medical Newspaper (Meditsinskaya Gazeta)*.

The article assembled numerous inaccuracies, misstatements of fact and even references to non-existent scientific studies in order to attack the use of methadone as a substitution therapy; included the claim that substitution therapy is contrary to the 1961 UN Convention on Narcotic Drugs. In fact the convention does not address methadone substitution therapy because it was not used at the time; it's only use in 1961 was as a painkiller. The article claimed that methadone substitution therapy is ineffective, creates a new body of drug addicts and causes harmful long-term side-effects, yet no references are provided by the Russian authors to support these claims. It also claimed that advocates of methadone substitution therapy are advancing the economic interests of methadone manufacturers. This is inaccurate as methadone costs pennies to produce and is a generic product manufactured by many companies. Finally, it claimed that recent WHO guidance on substitution therapy runs counter to all previous UN conventions and decisions. In fact, the 2004 position paper was endorsed by UNODC, the drug control body of the UN, and reflected policies already practiced throughout the European Union, China, India, the United States, Canada and Australia.

Antiretroviral therapy

Due to fears about poor adherence, virtually no current injecting drug users in Russia receive treatment with antiretroviral therapy. Indeed, only 5,000 individuals in the whole of Russia received antiretroviral therapy in 2005, but there are hopes that treatment programmes will increase this figure to over 30,000 during 2007. Long (2006) stated that the current policy of only providing antiretroviral therapy to individuals who do not inject drugs does not make any public health, or economic sense. Using a mathematical model assessing the public health benefits and economic cost of a number of HIV treatment strategies they calculated that treating both IDU's and non IDU's was the strategy that would prevent the most new HIV infections over a 20 year period. They found that it would cost only $300 more per year per life-year gained than the most conservative strategy, which provided treatment only to patients who did not inject drugs.

References

Alcorn K, "Russian HIV prevention mired in moralism and xenophobia (http://www.nam.org.uk/en/news/0626DB82-0C78-4A83-A7D6-9AC3A8A7E2F2.asp)" Aidsmap news, 22 May 2006

Amirkhanian, Y.A., Kelly, J.A., Kabakshieva, E., McAuliffe, T.L., & Vassileva, S. (1999) "Evaluation of a social network HIV prevention intervention program for young men who have sex with men in Russia and Bulgaria," AIDS Education and Prevention, vol. 15, no. 3, pp. 205-207

Burrows and Sarang. Mixed Signals: Responses to HIV/AIDS in the Russian Federation, 2005.

Butler, W.E. (2003). "HIV/AIDS and Drug Misuse in Russia: Harm Reduction Programmes and the Russian Legal System," London, Family Health International, p. 11-13;

Central and Eastern European Harm Reduction Network (CEEHRN). (2002) "Injecting Drug Users, HIV/AIDS Treatment and Primary Care in Central and Eastern Europe and the Former Soviet Union" (report of a survey), Vilnius.

Dehne, K.L., Grund, J-P,C., Khodakevich, L. & Kobyshcha, Y. (1999). "The HIV/AIDS Epidemic among Drug Injectors in Eastern Europe: Patterns, Trends and Determinants," Journal of Drug Issues 29 (4),

Grund, J-P. (2001) "A Candle Lit from Both Sides: The HIV Epidemic in Russia," in Karen NcElrath, ed. HIV and AIDS: A Global View (Westport, Connecticut: Greenwood Press, 2001). Excerpt available at http://johnranard.com/fire_within/candle_text_body.html.

Human Rights Watch (2004a). Interview with Dr. Alexander Golyusov, director, HIV/AIDS Unit, Ministry of Health, Moscow, February 26.

Human Rights Watch. (2004b) Interview with Lev Levinson, director, New Drug Policy Project, Moscow, February 24.

Kozlov AP et al (2006) HIV incidence and factors associated with HIV acquisition among injection drug users in St Petersburg, Russia. AIDS 20: 901 - 906, 2006.

Long EF et al (2006) Effectiveness and cost-effectiveness of strategies to expand antiretroviral therapy in St Petersburg, Russia. AIDS 20: 2207 - 2215, 2006.

Lubin, N., Klaits, A. Barsegian, I. (2002). "Narcotics interdiction in Afghanistan and Central Asia: Challenges for international assistance" (report to the Open Society Institute).

Malinowska-Sempruch, K., Hoover, J. & Alexandrova, A. (2003) "Unintended Consequences: Drug Policies Fuel the HIV Epidemic in Russia and Ukraine," New York: Open Society Institute, p. 6.

Mikhailov, A.G. (2003). State Drug Control Committee of Russia, letter no. 509, November 19, 2003, made available in English by the New Drug Policy Project, Moscow.

News Info. Ru. (2004). CIS 2010: 25 million drug addicts, 10 million of them living with HIV," available at http://www.tpaa.net/articles/reg_010504_cis_drugs.html.

Niedowski E, "Russia resists needle swap", Baltimore Sun, 9 June 2006

Pravda. (2004)."Sad tally, Russia counts more than 4 million addicts," February 20, 2004 [online], available at http://newsfromrussia.com/main/2004/02/20/52421.html.

Rhodes, T., Mikhailova, L., Sarang, A., Lowndes, C.M., Rylkov, A., Khutorskoy, M. & Renton, A. (2003). "Situational factors influencing drug injecting, risk reduction and syringe exchange in Togliatti City, Russian Federation: A qualitative study of micro risk environment," Social Science and Medicine vol. 57, p. 40.

Rhodes, T., Sarang, A., Bobrik, A., Bobkov, E. and Platt, L. (2004) "HIV transmission and HIV prevention associated with injecting drug use in the Russian Federation," International Journal of Drug Policy, vol. 15, no. 1, pp. 2.

Roshchupkin, G. (2003). "HIV/AIDS Prevention in Prisons in Russia," in T. Lokshina, ed. Situation of Prisoners in Contemporary Russia (Moscow: Moscow Helsinki Group, 2003), p. 213; UNDP, Reversing the Epidemic, p.33.

Stachowiak, J. & Beyrer, C. (2002). "HIV Follows Heroin Trafficking Routes," John Hopkins Bloomberg School of Public Health, October 14, 2002 [online] http://www.eurasianet.org/health.security/presentations/hiv_trafficking.shtml.

Trubnikov, M.N., Khodakevich, L.N., Barkov, D.A. & Blagovo, D.V. "Sources of injecting equipment for drug users in Moscow, Russia," International ....

Webster, P. (2003). "HIV/AIDS explosion in Russia triggers research boom," Lancet, vol. 361 p. 2133.

Eastern Europe

In the Newly Independent States in Eastern Europe (NIS) a rapid spread of drug use and drug injecting has occurred since 1990, paralleled by major social dislocation and change. Shifts to private economic production have occurred in the context of sharp declines in gross domestic product and have led to dramatic unemployment, increased income differentials and poverty, and the rapid expansion of criminal economies. Further suggestions of the link between social conditions and ill-health are indicated by the parallel increases in alcohol consumption and morbidity (Rhodes et al. 1999). Since this time there is overwhelming evidence confirms that there has been a massive increase in the trafficking, production and distribution of injectable drugs.

Changes in drug supply, including price and availability, linked to changing international patterns of drug production and trafficking, itself linked to the opening up of borders between Eastern and Western Europe, lead to an increase in drug use. Evidence also suggests that rising drug consumption is also manifesting itself as an increase in drug injecting and the sharing of injection equipment.

According to recent estimates there are currently between 2.3 and 4 million injecting drug users in the region and the number of users is growing. These trends are exacerbating a range of devastating drug-related harms such as HIV/AIDS (Rhodes et al. 1999).

Unauthorised possession of needles and syringes is illegal in many countries in the region. Lack of access to clean injection equipment therefore forces many users to share, which puts them at risk of contracting HIV. Many users of illegal drugs refuse to visit health care professionals for fear of contact with state agencies or the police. Consequently, they lack knowledge about the health risks of injecting drug use in general, and their own health situation in particular. In many countries, deteriorating health care systems struggle to provide the public with even the most basic information on HIV/AIDS. Bearing a double stigma, HIV-positive drug injectors face even more discrimination in accessing treatment and care.

Poland

From 1985 to 31 July 1996 there were 4166 reported cases of HIV infection in Poland, at least 2802 of these were illicit drug users. A study of injecting drug users (IDU) attending two detoxification centres in Warsaw found 46% to be infected with HIV (Rhodes 1999).

Belarus

Belarus has had a sharp increase in registered cases of HIV infection since June 1996, mostly among injecting drug users, particularly in Svetlogorsk. According to the police in Svetlogorsk, most young people below the age of 17 years have experimented with drug injecting. It is estimated that 4,000 -7,000 injecting drug users live in Svetlogorsk. Before June 1996 nearly all HIV test results from Svetlogorsk were negative. In June of the same year, 6 of 33 (18%) IDU-tested HIV-positive. In July 173 of 333 (50%) tested HIV-positive. By October 482 cases of HIV infection were registered, mostly among IDU. These figures indicate an extremely rapid spread of HIV (Rhodes 1999).

Ukraine

Ukraine is experiencing an extensive and rapidly expanding HIV epidemic, with around 1.4% of Ukrainian adults living with HIV at the end of 2005; the highest rate in Europe (Deveau et al, 2006).Most infections are among injecting drug users, however, as in other countries it is rapidly spreading from these people to their sexual partners and onwards to the rest of the population. In 2003, Ukraine had 45 needle exchanges, reaching about only 10% of injecting drug users. Most of these were funded by foreign donors such as the Open Society Institute. A national survey in 2004 found that only 20% of drug injectors reported avoiding non-sterile injecting equipment and practised safe sex.

Ukraine's national AIDS law, recognised as a model in the region, incorporates human rights protections for people living with HIV/AIDS. These include specific provisions that bar refusal of medical care based on HIV status, and guarantee access to appropriate medication, the right to HIV/AIDS information as well as confidentiality of HIV test results. Its national law and policy support syringe exchange and opiate-substitution therapy, which the World Health Organisation and UNAIDS have endorsed as essential to strategies aimed at HIV prevention and care for drug users (CEEHRN, 2002). However, Human Rights Watch found that abusive practices, problematic regulations, and a failure to implement crucial provisions of national AIDS policies render these protections meaningless for most Ukrainians living with or at highest risk of HIV. Healthcare workers' discriminatory practices toward people they know or suspect to be HIV-positive exists. They frequently refuse to treat such people and routinely disclose confidential information about HIV status therefore many people do not seek HIV testing out of fear that their status, if HIV-positive, could be revealed.

Police abuse, sometimes amounting to torture, keeps drug users away from needles exchange. The criminalisation of even trace amounts of drugs means drug users are easy targets for police seeking to fulfil arrest quotas. Police extort money and information from drug users, sometimes using the mere possession of syringes as an excuse to harass or arrest them and outreach workers providing services to them. However, proposed changes in Ukraine's drug laws to criminalise possession of smaller amounts of drugs than are currently prohibited threaten to exacerbate these abuses.

Substitution therapy, in the form of Buprenorphine reaches only a fraction of the drug users in need of it. According to the World Health Organisation, at least 60,000 drug users need substitution therapy but, to date, only 200 treatment slots are available. The use of the cheaper alternative, methadone was blocked by the national drug control authority due to fears of diversion of methadone supplies from clinics and pharmacies. Drug treatment clinics are required to officially register drug users who are referred to them for treatment, and to share this information with law enforcement agencies. This practice keeps many drug users from seeking healthcare or drug treatment services. The lack of ongoing investment in services targeted at drug users is likely to hamper comprehensive efforts to contain the extensive epidemic among injecting drug users. This relates to the highly-stigmatised nature of injecting drug use and the massive discrimination experienced by those who engage or are associated with it. Furthermore, active injecting drug users are not considered capable of adhering to antiretroviral therapy and are excluded from treatment.

References

Central and Eastern European Harm Reduction Network (CEEHRN). (2002) "Injecting Drug Users, HIV/AIDS Treatment and Primary Care in Central and Eastern Europe and the Former Soviet Union" (report of a survey), Vilnius.

Deveau C et al. *Prevention of HIV/AIDS among drug users as a vulnerable population.* The 2006 HIV/AIDS Implementers Meeting of the President's Emergency Plan for AIDS Relief, Durban, South Africa, abstract 89, 2006.

Drug use in Asia

In Asia, economic, social and political instability is similarly paving the way for increases in drug production, injecting drug use, sex work and cross border migration - all recognised factors in the spread of HIV. Shifts in trade, transportation and communication networks across Asia are also facilitating the spread of drug injecting, needle-sharing and consequently, of HIV (Suwanwela & Poshyachinda 1986). Drug use lies behind the bulk of the HIV/AIDS epidemics in China, Malaysia and Vietnam, accounting for a respective 69%, 77 and 66% of infections in these countries, estimates indicate (Kin, 1995). In Myanmar an estimated 1 in 3 injecting drug users were HIV-infected in 2004 and In Jakarta, Indonesia, HIV prevalence as high as 48% has been found in injecting drug users in rehabilitation centres (UNAIDS, 2006). Vietnam has an HIV epidemic largely spread through injection drug users. Needle sharing is commonplace, with HIV infections as high as 40% among the drug-injecting populations in some cities (Chau, 2006).

In Thailand infection rates among injecting drug users have remained extremely high, at 35-50%, and are still rising in some areas (UNDP, 2004) HIV prevention for injecting drug users and their sexual partners has not been a priority in Thailand even though this route of transmission plays a significant role in the spread of HIV (HRW, 2004) The official "war on drugs" has resulted in the incarceration of large numbers of IDU's, hastening the spread of HIV in prisons where risk behaviors continue but prevention services and drug treatment are often unavailable. In 2004 Prime Minister Thaksin said that the government saw the need to treat drug users as patients, not criminals, and proposed plans to reduce transmission among this group. However, the schemes, which included free needle distribution and methadone treatments, have yet to emerge. Needles are available at pharmacies but these pharmacies are watched by the police who quickly arrest drug users often in a brutal and violent manner. As a result of this and a heavy-handed government operation to crackdown on drug trafficking in 2003, drug use has been driven underground, making it more difficult for prevention campaigns to target this group (HRW, 2004). In recent years, funding for HIV prevention has fallen by two thirds and public concern has dwindled. Methamphetamine became a widely used drug in SE Asia around 1998, particularly in Thailand where it is known as 'Yaba'. In 2001 use had reached epidemic proportions, with Thai authorities estimating that over 2.5 million people were regular users (Poshyachinda 1992).

Despite this, in many Asian countries, it was still poorly addressed in the national HIV/AIDS plan of most affected Asian countries with India, Malaysia, Myanmar and Nepal only gave "inadequate" attention to the drug use issue in their AIDS plans (Kin 1995). Moreover, HIV/AIDS was not addressed in the national drug plan of affected countries, such as China, Malaysia, Myanmar and Nepal. Indeed, only Vietnam addressed the issue in its national drug plan.

In countries that promise a mandatory death penalty for drug importation and trafficking it is no surprise that harm reduction for current drug users is a rather political topic. While it is not unlawful to carry syringes and needles in nearly all countries, the police still arrest people for the possession of injecting equipment in India, Malaysia, Myanmar and Nepal. Only one affected country, Vietnam, has a needle and syringe exchange available, although India and Nepal have limited programmes (Poshyachinda 1993). Pharmacies are open late at night to provide drug users with a place to get clean needles, however many feel they cannot go there without fear of prosecution, thereby limiting the accessible of these services.

Policy-makers are also currently against substitution therapy in all countries except Thailand, Vietnam and Hong Kong, although some, such as India and Nepal, are considering it. Hong Kong, which has an extensive number of methadone clinics, has only a low HIV infection rate (Poshyachinda 1993). Most countries in this region, including India, Malaysia, Nepal and Myanmar have treatment which is abstinence-oriented, with a 1961 convention on narcotics, which calls for drugs only to be used for certain purposes such as medical reasons, still influencing many countries.

The UNAIDS Report in 2006 on the Global AIDS Epidemic found that in recent years rates have continued to increase and HIV infections have begun to migrate from high-risk populations to the general population. Failure to target populations at high risk of HIV exposure, such as injecting drug users has resulted in a full-fledged epidemic in recent years that is growing despite increased funding from local governments and the international community.

References

Chau LTM. *Community-based outreach for high-risk injection drug using populations in an emergency plan country: Vietnam 2004-2005.* The 2006 HIV/AIDS Implementers Meeting of the President's Emergency Plan for AIDS Relief, Durban, South Africa, Abstract 127, 2006.

Human Rights Watch, 'Not enough graves: the war on drugs, HIV/AIDS, and violations of human rights' (http://www.hrw.org/campaigns/aids/2004/thai.htm), Vol. 16 No. 8 (C). 2004

Kin F. Injecting drug use among heroin users in Malaysia: Summary of research findings. Report of the WHO Drug Injecting Project Planning Meeting, Phase II. Bangkok, Thailand. September 11-15, 1995.

Poshyachinda V. Drug injecting and Hiv infection among the population of drug abusers in Asia. Bulletin on Narcotics. XLV(1): 77-90, 1993.

Poshyachinda V. Drugs and AIDS in South-east Asia. Forsenic Science International. 62: 15-28. 1992.

Poshyachinda V. Drug injecting and Hiv infection among the population of drug abusers in Asia. Bulletin on Narcotics. XLV(1): 77-90, 1993.

Suwanwela C. and Poshyachinda V. Drug abuse in Asia. Bulletin on Narcotics XXXVIII (1&2): 41-53. 1986.

UNAIDS. Report on the Global AIDS Epidemic. 2006

UNDP (2004), 'Thailand's Response to HIV/AIDS' (http://www.undp.or.th/HIVReport.htm)

China

According to Chinese law drug users must be rehabilitated and consequently the country has adopted compulsory measures as the main approach, with drug users being sent to compulsory rehabilitation centres (CRCs). Because of the zero tolerance attitude to drug use, the government has been slow to implement HIV/AIDS prevention and control measures for IDU's (Deveau et al, 2006).

In 2000 there were 860,000 registered drug users in China, but unofficial estimates put the number of drug users closer to six or seven million. The popularity of injecting drugs has increased over time, and many studies are now showing no less than 50% of drug users are injecting, and in many reports the figure rises to over 80%. The sharing of needles and syringes is a common practice, with frequently 60% or more of users sharing. Injecting equipment is reported to be easily accessible and relatively cheap from either medical clinics or pharmacies in most urban centres, although it is unclear what the availability is in more rural areas (UNAIDS, 2006).

The use of contaminated needles in injecting drugs provides the most common HIV transmission route in China. Needle-sharing accounted for half of the 62,000 reported HIV cases in 2002 (China's Ministry of Health and the United Nations Theme Group on HIV/AIDS in China). Injecting drug use accelerated after China began reforming its economic system in 1979, an effort that opened the country's doors to foreign trade, travel, and investments. Heroin and opium entered the country from the "golden triangle"; the poppy-growing border area of Myanmar,

Laos, and Thailand. Heroin use steadily spread from the border area along trafficking routes in western China and to prosperous eastern provinces. Today, more than one million injecting drug users are registered with China's Public Security Bureau, although some estimates place the actual total at around three million (China's Country Coordinating Mechanism, 2004).

At one surveillance site in Xinjiang, 84% of injecting drug users had HIV. In the border town of Ruili in Yunnan, the province that reported the first HIV case among drug users in 1989, around 80% of drug users were infected. Infection rates at other surveillance sites in the most affected provinces range from 12 - 75% (Geneva: UNAIDS, 2002).

Activities aimed at educating injecting drug users about HIV transmission currently take place at detoxification centres run by the Public Security Bureau at several pilot sites or by international NGOs. The government hopes to expand outreach to 60% of drug users within five years through 210 additional outreach centres (China's Country Coordinating Mechanism, 2002)In 2005, only nine methadone clinics operated in seven southern and western provinces, serving roughly 1,800 drug users (Thompson 2005). Methadone is generally provided at no cost to the user either by the government or by a nongovernmental organisation (NGO) operating the facility. In five years, the government hopes to have 190 clinics jointly operated by the Public Security Bureau, the health bureau, the Food and Drug Administration, and NGOs. These clinics are expected to provide treatment to more than 50,000 drug users, which is still below the estimated demand.

Recently the Chinese government has shown a change in its attitude towards preventing HIV transmission among injecting drug users. In March 2004 a pilot programme began providing methadone treatment for IDU's, and a study found the rates of heroin use, intravenous injection and crime related to drug use had decreased. Clean needle exchange programmes were also set up at around 50 sites in several provinces during 2004 and have since expanded. China's response to HIV is improving, but coverage is still too patchy to have a substantial impact. However, the policies promoting the arrest and incarceration of drug users have made drug users reluctant to access HIV prevention services (Deveau et al, 2006).

The policy environment for harm reduction in China has been liberalised, allowing local authorities to embark on needle-exchange programs. Similar programs will increasingly be implemented in the six other provinces where HIV infection among drug users is most prevalent. The Yunnan law also requires that individuals and entities such as clinics and companies maintain the confidentiality of a person's HIV status. Other provisions relate to the officials' responsibilities to carry out and enforce the directives. The legislation stipulates punishments, including fines for government and health officials and doctors who ignore the AIDS law, fail to perform HIV/AIDS surveillance, refuse to treat patients with HIV and AIDS, disclose patients' personal details, or distribute antiretroviral medicine without approval (Order of the People's Government of Yunnan Province 2004).

However, effective implementation of harm-reduction programs requires the active participation of relevant local communities, including mayors, the court system, and public security officials. Implementing these programs is not simple as some officials oppose public health approaches that seem to condone or support illegal activity. To these officials, needle-exchange programs and condom distribution may appear to be at odds with the bid to legally crack down on drug dealers and drug users.

References

A Joint Assessment of HIV/AIDS Prevention, Treatment and Care in China (2004), State Council HIV/AIDS Working Committee Office and UN Theme Group on HIV/AIDS in China

China's Ministry of Health and the United Nations Theme Group on HIV/AIDS in China, "Joint Assessment Report on HIV/AIDS Prevention and Control in China: June 17, 2003," accessed online at www.youandaids.org/unfiles/joint_assessment_exec_summary_china.doc, on Aug. 3, 2004.

China's Country Coordinating Mechanism, "Reducing HIV transmission among and from vulnerable groups and alleviating its impact in seven provinces in China," Round

4 HIVAIDS Proposal to the Global Fund to Fight AIDS, Tuberculosis and Malaria, accessed online at www.theglobalfund.org/search/portfolio.aspx?countryID=CHN#HIV/AIDS, on Aug. 3, 2004.

China's Country Coordinating Mechanism, Round 4 HIV/AIDS Proposal.

Deveau C et al. *Prevention of HIV/AIDS among drug users as a vulnerable population.* The 2006 HIV/AIDS Implementers Meeting of the President's Emergency Plan for AIDS Relief, Durban, South Africa, abstract 89, 2006.

Order of the People's Government of Yunnan Province No. 121, articles 22 and 23.

Thompson. Injecting Drug Use Fuelling Spread of HIV in China, 2005.

UN Theme Group on HIV/AIDS in China, "HIV/AIDS: China's Titanic Peril-2001 Update of the AIDS Situation and Needs Assessment Report" (Geneva: UNAIDS, 2002): 16.

UNAIDS. Report on the Global AIDS Epidemic. 2006

Xia, M et al. Risk factors for HIV infection among drug users in Yunnan Province, China: association with intravenous drug use and protective effect of boiling reusable needles and syringes."AIDS 8: 1701-1706, 1994.

Central Asian Republics

The Central Asian republics, close to the main production areas of opium in Afghanistan, minor opium producers themselves, and main corridors for drug trafficking to Russia and Europe, have experienced very large increases in illicit drug use including injecting drug use in recent years. According to UNDCP, opiate use prevalence may be approaching 1% of the population older than 15 years. In Temirtau in Kazakhstan, a city of 200,000, at least 3,000 of the 32,000 young people between 15 and 29 years are believed to be injecting drug users. The very big and growing populations of primarily young drug injectors in the Central Asian republics are at high and immediate risk of HIV infection. As in Russia heroin is gradually replacing home made opiates as the most commonly injected drug (Rhodes 1999).

In response to the first outbreak of HIV among injecting drug users in Central Asia, occurring in 1997 in Temirtau, Kazakhstan, local authorities adopted, on a pilot basis, legislation and regulations, which enabled the establishment of a pilot project on harm reduction the same year. In 1998 a series of rapid assessments and responses on HIV and injecting drug use were implemented in five cities in Kazakhstan, Kyrgyzstan and Uzbekistan. Subsequently, pilot projects in terms of so-called harm reduction trust points have been set up in all five countries, providing needle exchange, counselling, access to anonymous and confidential HIV and STI testing, condoms and information materials. (Rhodes 1999).

The governmental rehabilitation and detoxification programmes are largely insufficient for the number of drug addicts, and have little, if anything to offer other than punitive approaches. Injecting drug users remain strongly stigmatised, considered criminals by the public, a stigma which is reinforced by governmental campaigns against drug trafficking, which tend to blur the difference between drug addiction and drug trafficking. Consequently, the specialised STI, HIV/AIDS and narcological institutes are still largely unable to establish contact and credibility with vulnerable groups such as injecting drug users.

The pilot projects have clearly demonstrated their relevance and the high demand for such services, yet at the same time the shortcomings. In Kazakhstan more than 70% of the clients request access to drug treatment, but the existing capacity is grossly inadequate and the cost of the services well beyond what drug users can afford. According to the national Kyrgyz AIDS centres, the existing services, while providing services for three to four times as many clients as initially envisaged, only reach about two per cents of the IDU population. In countries like Uzbekistan, where services are new, few drug users seek them of fear of being arrested by the police. In this case, outreach by volunteers, often former drug users themselves, has been the only option. (Rhodes 1999).

Injecting drug use is also fuelling the epidemic in Iran: when tested, 15% of men injecting drugs in Tehran were found to be HIV-positive. Approximately one half of the prison inmate population is incarcerated for drug-related charges and one in five injection drug users have reported sharing needles in prison.

Reference
Deveau C et al. *Prevention of HIV/AIDS among drug users as a vulnerable population.* The 2006 HIV/AIDS Implementers Meeting of the President's Emergency Plan for AIDS Relief, Durban, South Africa, abstract 89, 2006.

Rhodes T et al. Drug injecting, rapid HIV spread and the risk environment: implications for assessment and response. AIDS 13 Supp A S259-270, 1999.

India, Pakistan & Bangladesh

In 2000 it was estimated that there were over 400,000 IDUs in India (Deany 2000). IVDU related HIV infections make up only about 6-20% of all HIV infections nationwide. However, while the states of Manipur, Mizoram, and Nagaland account for less than 1% of the total population in the country, they contribute nearly 16% of the total number of HIV-positive individuals. Around the early 1990s the prevalence of HIV/AIDS among IDUs zoomed from 0 - 60% in areas such as Manipur and drug users were routinely ostracised and arrested (Sarkar et al. 1995).

Transmission through injecting drug use is still a major driving factor in the spread of HIV in India, particularly in the north-eastern states such as Manipur. It is also a major problem in urban areas outside the north, such as Mumbai, Kolkata and Chennai (Panda, 2002). Nationally, HIV prevalence among injecting drug users appears to have declined slightly in recent years, from 13% in 2003 to 10% in 2005 (NACO, 2006). The Indian government's approach to drug use is based around law-enforcement and prosecution, rather than harm reduction (Charles & Bewley-Taylor, 2005), with very little done in terms of treating drug users or helping them to stop using drugs. These tough regulations on drug users make it hard to reach this group with HIV messages. In the 1990s former Intravenous Drug Users (IDUs), started to meet in secret, to support each other. This was probably the start of a self-help movement and currently there are over 50 Self-Help Groups (SHG's) for the youth. Several organisations, including the Care Foundation and the Manipur Network of Positive People, are battling Manipur's biggest twin threat - drugs and HIV/AIDS. In 1991, the Social Awareness Service Organisation (SASO), a NGO, started providing drug users with clean-use techniques, by making available syringes for individual use, counselling and medication in an effort to curtail the spread of HIV/AIDS among this user community in the state. Now, drug users can visit drop-in centres at any NGO and get new syringes, pick up vials of distilled water, get free tea, watch TV or play carom. (Rhodes 1999).

There was no history of IDU in Pakistan until after the Afghan war, when drugs flowed from Afghanistan to Pakistan for export. This has produced a rapid increase in availability of heroin. There are an estimated three million drug users in Pakistan. However, these estimates are from the early 1990s and are likely to be understated. In the past, it was believed that injection drug use was uncommon, but recent evidence from Karachi, Pakistan's largest city, suggests that about 20-25% of drug users inject their drug. There is little official recognition of injection drug use, and no official surveillance of HIV in this group (McCormick 1995). In Pakistan as many as 25% of injection drug users in Karachi tested HIV-positive in 2004 yet only one year earlier, the same community reported a single case of HIV infection (UNAIDS, 2006).

In Bangladesh, rates of HIV among injecting drug users increased from 1.7% in 2001 to 4.9% in 2005. A large proportion of injecting drug users (as many as 1 in 5 in some regions) report buying sex and fewer than 1 in 10 consistently used a condom during commercial sex (UNAIDS, 2006).

Reference
Charles M., Bewley-Taylor D. (2005), 'Briefing Paper 10; Drug policy in India - compounding harm?' (http://www.internationaldrugpolicy.net/publications.htm), The Berkley Foundation Drug Policy Programme

Deany. HIV and Injecting Drug Use: A New Challenge to Sustainable Human Development UNDP HIV and Development Programme: UNDP Asia-Pacific Regional Programme on HIV and Development, 2000

McCormick J. A general description of HIV and intravenous drug use (and needle use) in Karachi, Pakistan. Report of the WHO Drug Injecting Project Planning Meeting, Phase II. Bangkok, Thailand. September 11-15, 1995.

Panda S. (2002), 'The HIV/AIDS epidemic in India: an overview', in Panda S., Chatterjee A. and Abdul-Quader A.S. (Eds.), 'The epidemic and the response in India', p.20

Rhodes T. Outreach work with drug users: principles and practices. Council of Europe Press, 1996. (Also available in Russian).

Rhodes T et al. Drug injecting, rapid HIV spread and the risk environment: implications for assessment and response. AIDS 13 Supp A S259-270, 1999.

Sarkar S. Drug Injecting in Manipur, India. Report of the WHO Drug Injecting Project Planning Meeting, Phase II. Bangkok, Thailand. September 11-15, 1995.

UNAIDS. Report on the Global AIDS Epidemic. 2006

Africa

Although longitudinal studies are lacking, the evidence from secondary data sources suggests a growing problem of drug misuse in many sub-Saharan African countries. Many cities are trafficking routes for cannabis, heroin, cocaine, and other psychotropic substances (Day 1992). The spill-over effects are reflected in the reported increase in the misuse of heroin and cocaine in many countries, with anecdotal reports of the injecting of these substances from some of these countries (United Nations Drug Control Programme [UNDCP] 1994). Trends in drug misuse in sub-Saharan Africa indicate the potential diffusion of injecting drug use with major and severe implications for the future transmission of HIV and other blood-borne diseases. To date, drug policy control efforts have focused on supply reduction (reducing the availability of drugs) and demand reduction (reducing the use of drugs). Harm reduction interventions, which focus on reducing harmful consequences of drug use, have become established in many developed countries but have yet to be developed systematically in sub-Saharan Africa.

In recent years cannabis use has increased extensively with the typical cannabis user being young (age 10 to 30 years) and male. Use has been reported among students, farmers, soldiers, street children, and civil servants (Ohaeri and Odejide 1991; Ekpo et al. 1995). Substances such as stimulants are obtained from licit and illicit sources, are widely used in sub-Saharan Africa (Baasher 1989) and have been reported from Burkina Faso, Chad, Gabon, Ghana, Mali, Senegal, and South Africa (United Nations Economic and Social Council 1994). The stimulants are usually smuggled into African countries where they are consumed mainly by adolescents (predominantly students) and unskilled labourers, such as drivers and farmers, for the purpose of keeping awake or alert to study or work.

The misuse of barbiturates is more limited, having been reported from Cote D'Ivoire, Mali, Mauritius, and Tanzania (United Nations Economic and Social Council 1994). Ineffective pharmacy control systems, as well as poor prescribing protocols for health professionals, have been partly blamed for the latter (Asuni and Pela 1986). There is widespread use of khat (catha edulis) in the eastern countries of Somalia, Kenya, and Ethiopia where its use is legal and in Eritrea and Tanzania where it is an illegal substance. Khat is reported to be used by students to improve their academic performance, by truck drivers to keep themselves awake, and by labourers to supply the extra vigor and energy they need to work. The trafficking in, and the use of, Mandrax (methaqualone) is a major concern in the southern and eastern countries of Zambia, South Africa, Swaziland, Namibia, Mauritius, Kenya, Uganda, and Tanzania (UNDCP 1994). Synthetic narcotic analgesics (e.g. Wellcanol) are well-known misused substances in South Africa, Sudan, and Tanzania. The sniffing of glues and petrol is found among street children and juveniles in Kenya, Tanzania, Sudan, Somalia, Swaziland, and Zambia (UNDCP 1994).

In the early 1980s, West Africa became an important trans-shipment route for heroin from south-east Asia en route to Europe and North America, and for cocaine from South America, initially involving Nigeria and then Cote D'Ivoire, Mali, Ghana, and Senegal. Since then, the use of heroin has been increasing in almost all of the countries in the continent, particularly those hitherto recognised as drug trafficking transit

zones (e.g., Nigeria, Liberia, Cote D'Ivoire, Senegal, Chad, Ghana, Kenya, South Africa, and Mauritius) (Day 1992). Similarly, cocaine use is reported as a problem in Nigeria, Ghana, Mali, South Africa, Tanzania, and Uganda and as a limited but growing problem in Cote D'Ivoire, Gabon, Kenya, Mauritius, and Senegal (United Nations Economic and Social Council 1994).

A recent multisource review in 1995 indicated that drug injecting had been reported in Cote D'Ivoire, Nigeria, Gabon, Ghana, Mauritius, Senegal, South Africa, Tanzania, Uganda, and Zambia (Stimson and Adelekan 1996). Wellcanol is reported to be injected in South Africa, Tanzania and Uganda.

The increasing presence of drug trafficking routes, the ineffective supply control strategies, the increased availability of heroin and cocaine, and the reduction in prices of heroin and cocaine (Olukoya 1995) in many sub-Saharan African countries indicate a real potential for the rapid diffusion of injecting practices in this region. Given the current profile of HIV infection in Africa, the introduction of high-risk injecting practices would bring further huge personal, community, and national costs.

The development of harm reduction programmes are difficult due to logistic problems such as access to populations, both physically because of poor access to the media, poor transport and communications, and because of low educational levels (Stimson and Adelekan 1996; Wodak et al.1993).

The healthcare system in many countries is generally characterised by an insufficient allocation of resources for service development, a lack of qualified personnel, and poorly developed information gathering systems. As a result the majority of African people do not have easy and ready access to good quality and affordable health services.

Drug misuse is still highly criminalised, and users can receive a lengthy prison sentence for the possession or use of a small quantity of illegal substances. The emphasis on criminalisation further prevents accessibility of the already marginalised drug-dependent individuals to the limited services available. Needle exchanges for drug users can also be difficult to set up when some medical centres still do not have access to regular clean needles.

A recent study which looked at 63 female sex workers who are heroin injectors in Dar es Salaam, Tanzania have found evidence of a new needle sharing practice they call 'flashblood', which is the term used to describe drawing blood back in a syringe until the barrel is full, and then passing the syringe to a female companion who injects the blood. By injecting the syringe about 4 cc's of blood, women believe that they can avert symptoms associated with heroin withdrawal because the first injector's blood is thought to have 'some heroin in it.' Female sex workers began the flashblood practice amongst themselves in the last couple of months in an altruistic attempt to help their impoverished and more desperate associates. Male injectors interviewed are still unaware of this practice (McCurdy, 2005).

During 2003, one kete of high quality, mostly pure white heroin cost US$0.50. One kete was all many injectors needed to get high. Now the price of heroin has increased to US$1 per kete, and the heroin is reportedly adulterated. By the summer of 2005, most injectors claimed they need two kete to get high.

Women most affected by the increase in cost and decline in quality of heroin are those who are in poor health as the result of chronic heroin abuse. Because of their appearance and obvious poor health, these women are unable to attract enough clients to support their habits.

Female sex workers in Dar es Salaam will agree to forgo the condom at the clients' request if they are desperate for money. Many Tanzanian men prefer not to use condoms and routinely ask female sex workers not to use them. Female heroin injectors who are desperate, like the women who accept 'flashblood', are the most likely to agree to forgo condoms. The practice of flashblood is an exaggeration of the practice of needle sharing which magnifies HIV transmission risk. If the first injector is

HIV or HCV infected, the amount of virus directly transmitted into the bloodstream by the second injector could be quite large.

Injection drug use has emerged in East Africa in the last five to six years, and it is spreading rapidly throughout the region (Beckerleg 2004; Beckerleg & Hundt 2004; McCurdy 2005). If the practice of 'flashblood' spreads from Dar es Salaam to other cities in East Africa, its impact on the rate of HIV and HCV transmission could be substantial. Heroin injection now appears to be occurring in most large towns of Kenya and Tanzania. A study of 336 heroin users in Nairobi, Kenya found that 44.9% were, or had been, injectors [UNIDCP, 1997]. Of 101 current injectors, 52.5% were HIV- positive. This compares with a 13.5% prevalence rate among heroin users who had never injected.

South Africa is by far the largest market for illicit drugs entering Southern Africa. Its relative affluence within the region makes it a tempting 'emerging market' in its own right. The country's geography, porous borders and international trade links with Asia, Latin America, Western Europe and North America have made it an attractive drug transit country. Drug trafficking and abuse have escalated in recent years, with the point of escalation traceable to the liberalisation of most aspects of society in the years immediately surrounding the country's first democratic elections in 1994. South Africa is a society in transition. Drug use correlates strongly with the pressures placed upon social capital by rapid modernisation and the decline in traditional social relationships and forms of family structure.

Among the non-White population, social injustice and the weakened family bonds which resulted from decades of apartheid policies have created an environment in which temporary escape from the harsh reality of everyday life is often sought through the consumption of psychoactive substances. Among the White population, anecdotal evidence also supports a connection between increased substance abuse and both increased availability of drugs and the psychological consequences of adjusting to life in the "new" South Africa. The use of "club drugs" (principally ecstasy and LSD, but including a wide range of substances) has grown dramatically in this community since the early 1990s, in part due to active interaction with the youth cultures of industrialised nations. While amphetamine-type stimulants, notably ecstasy, are mainly imported from Europe to satisfy domestic demand in the club scene, there is also evidence of local manufacturing of these substances. A study in Botswana (Weiser, 2006) found that heavy and problem alcohol consumption is associated with HIV sexual risk behaviours in both men and women. They were significantly more likely to have unprotected sex with a non-monogamous partner, have multiple sexual partners, or buy or sell sex than individuals who did not drink. This suggests that HIV prevention initiatives to be integrated into programmes targeting alcohol abuse. Furthermore, alcohol's deep-seated cultural and social meanings, related to social status, gender identity, and family and communal structures in Botswana and elsewhere in Africa needs to be addressed if HIV preventions is to have any success.

References

Abiodun OA, Adelekan ML et al. Pattern of substance abuse among secondary school students in ilorin, Northern Nigeria. West African Journal of Medicine 13(2): 91-97. 1994.

Adelekan ML. Self-reported drug use among secondary school students in the Nigerian. State of Ogun. Bulletin on Narcotics 41(1 and 2): 109-116. 1989.

Adelekan ML and Adeniran RA. Rehabilitation and follow-up issues in drug abusers managed at the Neuropsychiatric Hospital, Abeokuta, Nigeria. West African Journal of Medicine 10(1): 354-360. 1991.

Adelekan ML et al. Monitoring trends in substance use through a repeat cross-sectional survey in a Nigerian university. Drugs: Education, Prevention and Policy 3(3): 239-247, 1996.

Adelekan M and Stimson GV. Problems and prospects of implementing harm reduction for HIV and injecting drug use in high-risk sub-Saharan African countries. Forthcoming in Journal of Drug Issues, special issue on AIDS and Drug Use, 1996.

Asuni T and Pela OA. 1986 Drug abuse in Africa. Bulletin on Narcotics 38(1 and 2): 55-60.

Beckerleg S. How 'Cool' is heroin injection at the Kenya coast. Drugs: Education, Prevention & Policy (11)1, 67-78, 2004.

Beckerleg S and Hundt GL. The characteristics and recent growth of heroin injecting in a Kenyan coastal town. Addiction Research & Theory (12)1: 41-54, 2004.

Day G. 1992 Geographical, economical and political situation in West Africa: Significance of drug trafficking and abuse. In Drug control in Africa: Experiences from a seminar for West African countries, Padova: ARFI, 1992

Eide AH and Acuda SW. Drug use among secondary school students in Zimbabwe. Addiction 90(11): 1517-1527, 1995

Ekpo M et al. Lagos "area boys and girls" in rehabilitation: Their substance use and psychosocial profiles. East African Medical Journal 72(5): 311-316. European Centre for the Epidemiological Monitoring of AIDS, 1995

McCurdy SA et al. The emerging heroin epidemic in Dar es Salaam , Tanzania : Youth hangouts, maghetto and injecting practices. AIDS Care 17 (Supplement 1): S65-76, 2005.

McCurdy S et al. 'Flashblood' and HIV risk among IDUs in Tanzania.

afaids@eforums.healthdev.org. 2005.

Ohaeri JU and Odejide AO. Admissions for drug and alcohol-related problems in Nigerian psychiatric care facilities in one year. Drug and Alcohol Dependence 31: 101-109. 1991.

Olukoya SA. Worrisome development: Hard drug consumption is gaining ground in Nigeria. Newswatch 21-22, 1995

Stimson G & Choopanya K: Global Perspectives on Drug Injecting. Drug Injecting and HIV Infection, 1998.

Stimson GV and Adelekan M L. The diffusion of drug injecting in developing countries. International Journal of Drug Policy 7(4): 246-256. 1996.

United Nations International Drug Control Programme (1997). World Drug Report. Oxford, Oxford University Press.Meursing, K., and N. Morojele. Use of alcohol among high school students in Lesotho. British Journal of Addiction 84(11): 1337-1342, 1989.

United Nations Drug Control Programme 1994 Report of the expert forum on demand reduction in east and southern Africa. Nairobi, Kenya, November 1-5, 1994.

United Nations International Drug Control Programme. United Nations Economic and Social Council 1994 Examination of the world situation with respect to drug abuse, including illicit demand, illicit trafficking and supply. Commission on Narcotic Drugs, E/CN.7/1994/4.

Weiser SD et al. A population-based study on alcohol and high-risk sexual behaviours in Botswana. PloS Medicine 3: 1940 - 1948, 2006.

Wodak A et al. An evolving public health crisis: HIV infection among injecting drug users in developing countries. In Psychoactive Drugs and Harm Reduction: From Faith to Science, eds. N. Heather, A. Wodak, E. Nadelman, and P. O'Hare, 280-294, 1993.

Australia

Harm reduction is taken much more seriously in Australia (http://www.avert.org/ausstatg.htm), where federal funding enables a wide range of outlets - including drug treatment centres, hospitals, health centres, chemists and vending machines - to distribute many millions of clean needles each year. These and other harm reduction services have been supported since the 1980s, and have been highly effective at controlling HIV. According to official estimates, the $100 million spent on needle exchanges by state and federal governments between 1990 and 2000 prevented around 25,000 HIV infections, and reduced health spending by around $1.8 billion (in US dollars) (Deveau et al, 2006).

Reference

Deveau C et al. Prevention of HIV/AIDS among drug users as a vulnerable population. The 2006 HIV/AIDS Implementers Meeting of the President's Emergency Plan for AIDS Relief, Durban, South Africa, abstract 89, 2006.

United States

According to a 1996 study an estimated 2.4 million Americans have used heroin at some time in their lives and nearly 216,000 of them reported using it within the month preceding the survey, with injecting being most common method of taking it (Deveau et al, 2006). Other drugs such as crystal methamphetamine, favoured by the gay community, and steroids, used by body-builders - also carry the risks of injecting without the stigma of heroin use. The prevalence of drug use in America shows clearly that the potential for HIV transmission amongst American IDU's is very high. In 2004, some 34% of women and 21% of men who were diagnosed with HIV were injecting drug users who were assumed to have been infected as a result of their drug use (Deveau et al, 2006).

Needle exchange schemes are often unpopular - even criminalised - in much of America. Many states have 'drug paraphernalia' laws that make it a crime to possess or distribute needles or syringes, and five U.S. states impose a total ban on sales of syringes in pharmacies without a prescription. The US is the only country that provides no federal funding for needle exchange services and federal policies do not permit support of clean needle exchange programmes. This is an intervention that has repeatedly been demonstrated to be a cost-effective way to reduce HIV transmission but which religious and social conservatives see as "enabling" drug use. This is despite experts believe that an expansion of needle exchange services helped to reverse an extensive HIV epidemic among drug users in New York City during the 1990s. As a result needle exchange schemes have been opened and closed as the political climate has shifted. One significant development came in September 2004 when Arnold Schwarzenegger, Governor of California, signed legislation permitting the sale of sterile syringes without a prescription - something not previously possible in California. As of May 2006, there were 185 needle exchange schemes operating in 36 states, as well as Washington D.C., Puerto Rico, and Native American Lands. This is fewer schemes than in Scotland, where the population is around sixty times smaller.

In a political climate where religious conservatives, more obsessed about the "sin" than what happens to the "sinner," have great influence over US policy, it is unlikely that political policies will change, at least for the next few years. The United States also refuses to fund needle exchanges in other countries and the federal government is using its economic power to try to export this view to the rest of the world - recently America tried unsuccessfully to pressure the United Nations Office on Drugs and Crime to remove all support for harm reduction programs (Deveau et al, 2006).

In 2004 IDUs accounted for 17% of all AIDS cases amongst African Americans. Injecting drug use is the second leading cause of HIV infection in African American women and the third leading cause of HIV infection in African American men. HIV rates amongst black IDU's were particularly fuelled by the rise in crack cocaine use seen within the community in the mid 1980. Positive trends can also been in the overall statistics on AIDS in African Americans. Despite HIV continuing to disproportionately affect the black population, the overall number of infections being recorded has actually been dropping by around 5% every year since 2001. CDC officials are uncertain as to why this drop has occurred, but some have suggested it may partially be due to a new needle exchange programme implemented in New York that has caused a massive decline in the number of injecting drug users being infected with HIV (Black AIDS Institute, 2006).

References

Deveau C et al. *Prevention of HIV/AIDS among drug users as a vulnerable population.* The 2006 HIV/AIDS Implementers Meeting of the President's Emergency Plan for AIDS Relief, Durban, South Africa, abstract 89, 2006.

The black AIDS Institute 'AIDS in blackface: 25 years of an Epidemic. (http://www.blackaids.org)' June 2006.

UNAIDS. Report on the Global AIDS Epidemic. 2006

Latin America

Drug use is increasingly common in many Latin America countries, which in part may be due to the recent shift from dictatorships to democracies. In Argentina, Brazil, Uruguay and Paraguay (UNAIDS, 2006).injecting drug use has been a major driving factor behind the spread of HIV, with cocaine and heroin being the most commonly injected drugs. The proportion of HIV cases attributed to IDUs in the Southern cone countries of Chile, Argentina, Uruguay, and Paraguay at 30% (Perez-Gomez 1995).

In Brazil drug injectors have become the second largest HIV transmission category in Brazil, making up more than one-quarter of all AIDS cases reported by 1991 (Lima et al 1992). Harm reduction programmes have been implemented in Brazil, which have contributed to declining HIV prevalence rates in several cities (Hacker & Friedman, 2005). For example, the city of Santos saw a 20% decline in HIV prevalence among

IDU's between 1998 and 2000. The total number of needle exchanges in Brazil increased from 12 in 1998 to 40 by the end of 2000, with around 150,000 syringes exchanged between 1999 and 2000 (Okie, 2006). Clean needles are available in prisons, which has contributed to 76% of Brazil's injecting drug users reported no sharing of needles and syringes (Berkman, et al, 2005). Access to treatment is also widespread, with 30,000 IDU's receiving ARVs at the end of 2005 (Okie, 2006)

In Argentina, drug injectors are the second largest category of HIV transmission in Argentina. The proportion of AIDS cases attributed to injecting drug use has increased, rising from 11.3% in 1987 to 39% in 1991 (Perez-Gomez 1995). Some harm reduction activities have also been carried out in Argentinean cities, however Argentina lacks harm reduction programmes at national, state and local level (Frasca, 2005) This is despite a severe HIV epidemic among injecting drug users: one study carried out in Buenos Aires found a HIV prevalence rate of 44% among this group (UNAIDS, 2006)

In countries, such as Bolivia, Peru and Ecuador, the spread of HIV through injecting drug use has been limited in scope. In the past Columbia did not have a history of injecting drug use, however since then there has been an increase in injection drug use of locally produced heroin. (Perez-Gomez 1995). In Chile, data are scarce, and in Venezuela the role of injecting drug use in the HIV epidemic is negligible. However, the availability of heroin is increasing in these countries, which may lead to a change in the situation in coming years (Frasca, 2005). Many countries face severe restrictions in carrying out harm reductions programmes due to restrictive laws and a lack of political support.

In several Southern Cone countries, 'pasta base' or 'paco' - a form of cocaine, which is smoked - has become extremely popular in recent years, both among poorer populations and the middle-classes.Although the rise in popularity of pasta base has generally had negative health implications, there is evidence to suggest that some drug users have started smoking cocaine in this form instead of injecting it. This may be reducing the level of needle-sharing in the region, thereby reducing the number of people becoming infected with HIV through injecting drug use (UNAIDS, 2006).

Whilst some impressive prevention campaigns in the region have been carried out through outreach work these are only small-scale and most countries still need to expand harm-reduction programmes for injecting drug users (Bonfman et al, 2002). For the most part, governments have neglected high infection rates among vulnerable groups, and rising rates among the general population.

References

Berkman A, Garica J et al. (2005) "A Critical Analysis of the Brazilian Response to HIV/AIDS: Lessons Learned for Controlling and Mitigating the Epidemic in Developing Countries (http://www.ncbi.nlm.nih.gov/entrez/query.fcgi?cmd=Retrieve&db=PubMed&list_uids=15933232)", American Journal of Public Health 95(7).

Bronfman, M. N. et al. (2002), Mobile populations and HIV/AIDS in Central America and Mexico: research for action, AIDS (http://www.aidsonline.com): Volume 16 Supplement 3 December 2002 pp S42-S49

Frasca T. (2005), "AIDS in Latin America", Palgrave/Macmillan, p.135

Hacker MA, Friedman SR (2005), 'The role of "long-term" and "new" injectors in a declining HIV/AIDS epidemic in Rio de Janeiro, Brazil', Substance Use & Misuse. 2005;40(1):99-123.

Lima ES et al. Injecting-drug users and the spread of HIV in Brazil. AIDS and Public Policy Journal. 7(3): 170-174, 1992.

Okie S. (May 2006), 'Fighting HIV - lessons from Brazil' (http://content.nejm.org/cgi/content/short/354/19/1977), The New England Journal of Medicine 354;19

Perez-Gomez, A. "Drug injecting in Bogota, Columbia." Report of the WHO Drug Injecting Project Planning Meeting, Phase II. Bangkok, Thailand. September 11-15, 1995.

UNAIDS. 'UNAIDS fact sheet: Latin America' (http://www.unaids.org/en/Regions_Countries/Regions/LatinAmerica.asp) . 2006.

Conclusions

The spread of HIV among IDUs highlights many development issues. It is notable that some of the countries and communities most at risk from HIV and injecting drug use are often some of the least developed. Drug use and HIV affect the most vulnerable and marginalised groups within communities, from slum populations in New Delhi and hill tribes in Northern Thailand, to disadvantaged young people in Central and Eastern Europe. When IDUs are women, the stigma and vulnerability they face is even worse.

Communities in remote areas, which are marginalised and have little control over their economic and social development, are natural habitats for the cultivation, trafficking and consumption of drugs. Production leads to economic dependence on drug traffickers rather than to social and economic development. Increased drug use also leads to increased health problems in producer countries, especially where the use and sharing of needles for injecting drugs facilitates the spread of HIV (Ahmed 1988). Risk behaviours leading to HIV transmission through shared needles and syringes are closely linked to development problems such as poverty and lack of sustainable livelihoods, exploitation, inadequate education and political repression. The exact nature of the links between risk behaviours and specific development problems remains unclear but exploring these links may make a significant contribution to increasing understanding of both development and the epidemic (Deany 2000).

Injecting drug use poses an enormous threat to sustainable human development. In some countries the scale of injecting drug use creates a potentially massive group of susceptible individuals for the further spread of HIV as once HIV enters the injecting population, countries can expect large and sustained HIV epidemics.

Drug use often provokes moralistic or judgmental attitudes and responses. Perceiving (and treating) drug users as a 'species apart' may reinforce a sense of moral superiority, but it is unproductive and indefensible. Potentially, anyone could become a drug user or find themselves the parent, partner, child, sibling, colleague or friend of a user. Stigmatising and marginalising injecting drug users are likely to leave them alienated, fearful, and out of touch with the support and services they may most need.

Legal and ethical factors are also creating challenges to the enabling environment. For example, the illegal nature of drug use can lead young people to hide their drug consumption, preferring to inject rather than risk detection through the smell of smoking. This is despite the risk that injecting poses for HIV transmission through clandestine sharing of injecting equipment (Hart 1989).

Countries experiencing these epidemics may lack the capacity to develop policy and programmatic responses which deal appropriately with drug use. Where responses are developed, they mainly target the long-term goals of eradication of drug supply and drug use, rather than the more pressing problem of HIV transmission. The relationship between drug use and HIV transmission differs between countries and changes to policies and programmes must therefore be developed separately through a process of ongoing analysis, policy dialogue and monitoring of responses.

There is a growing body of knowledge and experience in the development and implementation of effective HIV prevention responses among IDUs and an increased willingness on the part of my countries to try to these in order to try to prevent or limit a HIV epidemic tried. These include drug and HIV/AIDS policy reform, methods for involving affected communities in developing responses, outreach and peer education, needle and syringe exchange, and drug substitution programmes to decrease injecting.

Despite recent expansion of responses, within individual countries, these tend to be several years behind the pace and scale of the actual epidemic. This appears to be the result of a range of factors closely linked to development and including:

- The current policy environment, making it difficult for community-based programmes to prevent HIV among injecting drug users.

- Lack of policy dialogue between sectors of government responsible for responses to HIV and drug use.

- Economic, social and political dislocation, leading to increases in drug injecting, needle sharing and, consequently, HIV.

- Low community capacity, in terms of skills, resources and experience to respond to HIV among IDUs.

- Injecting drug users, especially women, being demonised for their drug use, rather than supported, placing them at particular risk of both human rights abuses and HIV infection.

- Donor agencies and countries alike failing to recognise the long-term threat to development posed by HIV and injecting drug use.

The challenge is to find new ways to build the capacity of communities to understand and respond more effectively to this emerging development problem. At the same time, donors, governments and the international community need to be persuaded to make HIV prevention among injecting drug users a much more urgent global priority, as well as a local reality.

References

Deany. HIV and Injecting Drug Use: A New Challenge to Sustainable Human Development UNDP HIV and Development Programme: UNDP Asia-Pacific Regional Programme on HIV and Development. 2000.

Hepatitis co-infection

Hepatitis is a word derived from ancient Greek. It means inflammation of the liver. The causes of liver inflammation are many and varied and include heavy alcohol or recreational drug use, the toxic effects of various medications and certain viral infections.

A number of viruses can cause the liver to become inflamed. However, the viruses that are responsible for most cases of inflammatory liver disease worldwide belong to a group called the hepatitis viruses. They are labelled with letters ranging from A to G, in order of discovery. The first three viruses to be identified, therefore, were named hepatitis A, hepatitis B and hepatitis C. These are commonly abbreviated as HAV, HBV and HCV.

This chapter is exclusively concerned with viral hepatitis, with a particular focus on hepatitis B and C and the implications of co-infection with HIV. Hepatitis B and C are transmitted from person to person in similar ways to HIV. As a result, many people infected with HIV are also co-infected with either HBV or HCV or both. Such co-infection is a cause for concern because it can complicate the treatment of HIV and may reduce the effectiveness of highly active antiretroviral treatment (HAART).

Treatments are available for some forms of viral hepatitis, while others types can only be left to resolve naturally. For a complete discussion of current therapeutic options for HIV-HCV and HIV-HBV co-infected individuals, see the *HIV & AIDS Treatments Directory*.

The toxic effects of HAART on the liver may be exacerbated by the presence of any one of the hepatitis viruses. That's why it is important for HIV-positive people to avoid co-infection. There are vaccines available that can prevent HAV and HBV infection.

BHIVA guidelines recommend that HIV-positive people who are not already co-infected or who do not have natural immunity receive vaccinations against hepatitis A and B.

The hepatitis viruses are grouped together because they are all implicated in inflammatory liver disease. However, the genetic make-up, transmission routes and disease course of the infections they cause differ greatly. Hepatitis A infection, for example, is acute and self-limiting, like flu. In contrast, hepatitis C infection, like HIV infection, is a chronic infection that causes mild initial symptoms or none but can go on to cause accumulating and sometimes lethal damage. Hepatitis B infection, meanwhile, has an obvious acute phase that is often self-limiting, but may become established as a chronic infection. In addition, HBV infection has the characteristic, when chronic, of 'flaring up' intermittently, in a similar way to some other viral infections, such as herpes.

The damage the hepatitis viruses cause can be classified as either **cytopathic** or **immunopathic**. Cytopathic means the virus causes damage directly, by injuring the cells that it infects. Hepatitis A does this. Immunopathic means that it is the response of the body's immune system to the viruses that causes the damage; chronic hepatitis B causes damage this way, which explains its sometimes unpredictable course. In the case of hepatitis C, both mechanisms may be involved.

Doctors also divide liver failure into two types: **cytolytic** (the classic kind, where liver cells rupture and die) and **cholestatic** (where, because of swelling, the liver's tubes and ducts get blocked, causing waste products to build up).

Liver function tests

Liver function tests are blood tests that are used to assess how well the liver is functioning. There are a number of markers in the blood that can be measured to help gauge the state of the liver. We describe here some of the most common and most significant tests. It is important to stress that no one set of test results is diagnostic of liver disease. The results of a variety of tests over a period of time are needed before a diagnosis can be made and course of treatment (if necessary) prescribed.

In addition to blood tests, a procedure known as a liver biopsy may be carried out. This involves taking a sample of someone's liver and examining it under a microscope. This procedure is described in more detail below.

Blood tests

The most important liver function tests are the blood tests for **ALT (alanine aminotransferase)** and **AST (aspartate aminotransferase).** These are enzymes that are stored in liver cells and are released into the blood stream when those cells become inflamed or destroyed, causing ALT and AST levels to rise dramatically. ALT and AST tests do not identify what the cause of the damage is or whether it is ongoing or temporary. Rather, they suggest, but do not prove, ongoing liver inflammation.

ALT and AST should routinely be monitored in people with HIV, whether or not they have viral hepatitis. ALT is specific to liver cells, whereas AST isn't, being present in red blood cells and cardiac and skeletal muscle as well as the liver. Normal levels of both ALT and AST are less than 40 IUs (international units) per litre. Over 200 is evidence of severe toxicity, and scores in the thousands of liver failure. You may also hear ALT/AST tests expressed in terms of multiples of the 'upper limit of normal', i.e. multiples of 40 IUs/litre. The ratio of ALT to AST in the blood can sometimes help differentiate between the causes of liver damage.

Alkaline phosphatase, another enzyme, is produced by the bile ducts. High levels are usually indicative of obstruction of the bile ducts, though levels may also be high in kidney and intestinal disease. Normal levels are 30-130 IU per litre.

Gamma Glutamic Transpeptidase (GGT) is an enzyme present in a number of body tissues. It is found in high concentrations in the liver and the bile ducts. It is often measured to confirm that raised alkaline phosphatase levels are indeed caused by liver disease. Elevated levels of GGT may also indicate liver damage caused by alcohol or certain medications.

Bilirubin is a waste product, resulting from the breakdown of old red blood cells. It is responsible for the yellow coloration of bruises and the brown of faeces. Jaundice, with its characteristic yellowing of the skin, results from an excess of bilirubin in the blood and tissues. Dark amber urine is another sign of elevated levels of bilirubin.

There are two types of this enzyme: **unconjugated** bilirubin is fat-soluble, and an excess of it indicates cytolytic liver disease and cirrhosis; **conjugated** bilirubin is water-soluble, and excess indicates cholestatic disease.

Normal blood levels of bilirubin are around 17 micromols per litre, though higher levels do not necessarily suggest liver damage. However, high levels of bilirubin (more than twice the 'normal' level) combined with ALT levels over four times normal *is* indicative of possible liver failure.

Elevated levels of the protein **alpha-feta protein (AFP or a-FP)** are common in people with chronic hepatitis. But at very high levels, it is indicative of liver or testicular cancer, so it is important to keep an eye on it. Pregnant women are also tested for AFP, as elevated levels may suggest foetal abnormality.

Albumin is a substance made in large quantities by the liver to regulate the body's fluid balance. It acts like a sponge, mopping up surplus fluid. If the liver cannot make enough albumin the result is ascites, an accumulation of fluid in the abdomen which is a sign of end-stage liver failure. This means the liver has 'decompensated'; that is, it has come to the end of its reserves. Normal levels of albumin are 35-51 grams per decilitre.

Prothrombin time is the time taken for blood to clot when mixed with a reagent in a test tube. It is normally 10-15 seconds; longer than this indicates the liver is failing to make enough clotting factors.

Biopsy

A liver biopsy is a surgical procedure in which a long needle is inserted into the abdomen and a sliver of the organ is removed. The liver sample is examined microscopically to determine whether the liver is damaged and, if so, the extent and type of damage.

Fibrosis is the development of hard tissue in the liver as a result of inflammation. It is reversible if the inflammation is reduced or prevented.

Cirrhosis is a scarring of the liver that causes loss of liver function. Generally speaking, damage caused by cirrhosis is irreversible. However, in rare instances, liver tissue can recover from cirrhosis, although how this happens and why is not well understood. This phenomenon can make the distinction between severe fibrosis and mild cirrhosis a little less clear.

The liver is a large organ; it can cope with some damage, with functioning parts working harder to compensate for loss of function elsewhere. However, unless the cause of the damage is removed or ameliorated, the damage may become progressive, leading, ultimately, to total liver failure.

An **ultra-sound scan (USS)** is a non-invasive procedure which is used to detect liver tumours in people with pre-existing liver cirrhosis. Cirrhosis cannot be detected on an USS. A special camera is moved over the stomach and pictures are taken of the internal organs. These pictures are not high definition and need to be interpreted by a specialist.   Someone with cirrhosis will be recommended to have a scan every six months.

Recent advances in non-invasive procedures for assessing liver injury include the **Fibroscan,** This is a modified ultrasound probe which, held against the skin, detects the degree of stiffness in liver tissue. A French study (De Lédinghen) found that it was efficient in detecting high-grade fibrosis and cirrhosis in patients with HIV.

Another kind of test uses microscopic air bubbles injected into a vein. An ultrasound probe is then used to see if they make it freely through the blood vessels in the liver. Fibrosis blocks the blood vessels and the bubbles get trapped.

Hepatitis A

The Hepatitis A virus (HAV) causes an acute, self-limiting infection. The usual pattern of the disease is to be infected, show symptoms and then to recover naturally. HAV belongs to the Picornaviridae family of viruses, which also includes polioviruses, Coxsackie viruses and many of the viruses that cause the common cold.

HAV infection is fairly uncommon in the UK, with around 1,000 to 1,100 cases being reported annually since 2000. The number of cases has declined dramatically since hitting a peak of over 7,000 cases in the early 1990s. HAV infection is less common than both HBV infection and HCV infection. However, HAV infection accounts for two-thirds of UK reports of acute hepatitis, because it is the most likely kind to cause symptoms.

Hepatitis A is very common in much of the developing world. It is also three times as common in Mediterranean countries and used to be four times more common in the USA, though vaccination has brought the annual number of cases there down to near-UK levels.

About one in five adults in the UK and one in three in the US show signs of having been infected with hepatitis A at some point in their lives. This compares to over 90% of adults in Africa, most middle-eastern countries and much of south and south-east Asia. Seven in 10 children in developing countries show signs of infection, compared with only one in 50 in the UK.

There are about 1.4 million cases of hepatitis A reported a year globally, and that is estimated to be about a tenth of the true total. Travellers who are not immune to hepatitis A, either through vaccination or previous infection, are 100 times more likely to get hepatitis A than typhoid abroad, and 1,000 times more likely to get it than cholera. The proportion of hepatitis A cases that were acquired through foreign travel increased from one in 16 in 1990 to one in seven in 1998. Non-immune travellers should get themselves vaccinated for hepatitis A - see **Treatment** below. Other people at higher risk of hepatitis A include gay men and injecting drug users.

Symptoms

HAV infection has a wide range of symptoms, including nausea, vomiting, fatigue and jaundice. Occasionally, these symptoms are severe and recuperation can take a few months. However, some people experience few or no symptoms. Hepatitis A does not become a chronic condition and the infection does not last in the body for more than a couple of months. Very, very rarely, HAV infection can cause liver failure and death.

After someone is infected with hepatitis A, there is an incubation period of about three to four weeks (sometimes two, sometimes as long as six) before they start to feel ill. However, they are infectious from one to two weeks after catching hepatitis A. Therefore, it is unwise for anyone who has been in contact with someone with hepatitis A to assume that, because they themselves have no symptoms, they are neither infected nor infectious.

The first symptoms are usually fatigue and weakness, usually followed by loss of appetite and nausea, which may sometimes be quite severe. Food, especially fatty food, will feel quite indigestible. Vomiting is not uncommon. Some people develop a fever, though this is not always the case. About one-in-four to one-in-six people with hepatitis A require hospitalisation for a short while. This is often because they get dehydrated through vomiting, so rehydration is necessary. Extreme thirst is a common symptom of HAV infection.

In the first few days after symptoms show themselves, hepatitis A can feel like a particularly nasty intestinal illness. But a week to 10 days after the first symptoms show, people usually develop jaundice - an unmistakable sign of hepatitis caused by the build-up of bilirubin (see above). As well as accumulating in the skin and the whites of the eyes, causing the yellow discoloration typical of jaundice, bilirubin also becomes concentrated in sweat, which can cause severe itching and a difference in body odour. Urine becomes dark orange or brown, as the body attempts to get rid of the excess bilirubin. Meanwhile, stools (faeces) turn pale and float, because liver inflammation inhibits the production of bile and the digestion of fat.

Once jaundice develops, people start to become less infectious, though they are still somewhat infectious up to a week after it disappears. Thereafter, symptoms slowly ease. Most people start to feel well again about six weeks after first noticing symptoms. However, about 15% of people with HAV infection develop 'relapsing' symptoms, where they can get ill again and even develop jaundice for short periods over the following six to nine months.

About 20% of adults infected with HAV don't get jaundice. Hepatitis A in **children** is very different. Most children under six only get mild symptoms, and only one in 10 will get jaundice. Only half of 6-14 year olds infected with HAV get jaundice.

Co-infections

In general, hepatitis A is no more dangerous to people with HIV than those without. However, one study found that co-infection of HIV and HAV leads to higher and longer-lasting levels of hepatitis A virus circulating in the blood (Ida 2002). Although the duration of symptoms was unaffected by HIV status, HIV-infected patients exhibited HAV in the blood for a median of 53 days, compared with 22 days amongst HIV-negative individuals. The amount of hepatitis A in the blood was significantly higher among those with HIV, regardless of HIV viral load or CD4 count.

Hepatitis A is **much more dangerous** to people who have pre-existing liver damage due to hepatitis B or C, or other causes, such as alcohol-induced cirrhosis, because the liver's capacity for recovery is reduced. For this reason, people with hepatitis C or chronic hepatitis B should get vaccinated for hepatitis A.

Transmission

HAV is transmitted by the faecal-oral route. The faeces of someone with HAV are infectious and, if ingested, will cause the infection to be passed on. Commonly, this happens in countries where untreated sewage is discharged into the water supply or where uncooked foods that have been washed in contaminated water are eaten. Another route of transmission is through consuming undercooked food, particularly shellfish. As most tropical and middle-eastern countries have far higher rates of hepatitis A than the UK, travellers should get vaccinated before going abroad.

HAV-infected persons are infectious for only a relatively brief period of time. However, many sexual practices facilitate faecal-oral transmission of HAV, and non-apparent faecal contamination is not unusual during anal sex. **Rimming** is an obvious risk for HAV transmission. Using condoms for anal sex does not prevent HAV transmission. Clusters of HAV infection have, on occasion, been traced to public-sex venues in the UK and Europe.

The risks of sexual transmission of HAV, particularly among gay men, can be greatly reduced by scrupulous hygiene: the hands and genitals (and any sex toys that are used) should be washed thoroughly before and after sex, and rimming should be avoided.

Only about six-in-ten hepatitis A infections can be traced to another person. When a child gets hepatitis A, they don't tend to develop symptoms; so, unless there is an obvious source of infection, it is often assumed that they got it from another child. However, workers in child-care centres are one group who display higher rates of HAV infection than the population as a whole. It's thought that this may be due to poor hygiene - when changing nappies, for example.

Hepatitis A can be spread both through transfusion of blood products and from mother to baby in the womb, but this is very rare.

Tests

Exposure is usually confirmed by an HAV antibody test. There are two types of antibody tests, each of which tells us something different.

A positive immunoglobulin M (**IgM**) test means that you currently have active hepatitis A, or have had it very recently. IgM levels become undetectable in the blood a few months after infection.

A positive immunoglobulin G (**IgG**) test means either that you have hepatitis A now, have had it in the past and are now immune to it, or have had a vaccination against it that has 'taken' successfully.

It is also possible to perform a viral load (PCR) test for HAV, but, as HAV infection is usually obvious, this is rarely done.

Treatment

People with HAV infection are usually advised to rest in bed and take plenty of fluids until the symptoms have passed. Occasionally, immunoglobulin may be given to people who have not been vaccinated but are thought to have been infected with HAV.

When someone has acute hepatitis, their liver's ability to process drugs and medicines will be limited, so additional medicines are generally not prescribed and certain classes   of drugs, such as tranquillisers, are to be avoided altogether.

However, people who take anti-HIV medication should not stop taking it if they get symptoms of HAV infection. Their HIV clinician may want to monitor the level of drugs in their body and temporarily lower the dose if liver function is not as efficient as usual.

Is there a vaccine?

Yes. Hepatitis A vaccination is safe, effective and strongly to be recommended to people with HIV, though appears most effective if administered when a person's CD4 count is above 500 (Smith 2002). People with HIV should receive two doses of the vaccine six to 12 months apart (BHIVA 2004a).

The hepatitis A vaccinations that are currently available are *Havrix* and *Vaqta*, along with the combined HAV/HBV vaccine *Twinrix*.

People at high risk of getting hepatitis A, including gay men, injecting drug users, people intending to travel to the developing world and people who work with young children, should be vaccinated.

In the USA, 11 states recommend hepatitis A vaccination for all children.

For the fullest protection, adults receive two vaccine shots spaced at six-month intervals, and children receive three. However, studies in travellers have shown that a single shot, ideally (but not essentially) administered at least four weeks before travel, offers a significant degree of protection.

Hepatitis A vaccination is currently being offered to gay men as part of the B Safe Campaign (www.hepbsafe.com).

The immunity conferred by the hepatitis A vaccine lasts about 15 years; a booster shot is then recommended.

Before the invention of HAV vaccines, people were offered shots of immunoglobulin antibodies (immune serum globulin or ISG) as a preventative. This is still offered to people at very high risk of exposure, such as members of a household where someone has hepatitis A, because it acts faster than the HAV vaccine.

Hepatitis B

Isolated in 1965, hepatitis B (HBV) is classified as a hepadnavirus. Hepatitis B infection is generally immunopathic: the damage that occurs in the bodies of infected patients is primarily caused by their own immune response to the presence of the virus, rather than the pathogen itself. In the case of HBV, the damage mainly happens in the liver; this is known as autoimmune hepatitis. However, when HBV is highly active and replicating in large numbers, it may cause damage to cells on its own and so work cytopathically as well.

Knowledge of HBV has changed significantly in the past decade, and people who were told they had 'natural immunity' to hepatitis B in the past may not have it. Anyone in this situation should be re-tested in case they are infectious or have undetected chronic HBV.

Disease progression

In the period immediately following exposure to hepatitis B the majority of adults develop an acute illness, with symptoms ranging from influenza to severe jaundice (yellow skin and eyes). This illness is debilitating in just under half of those infected. A

tiny minority develop fulminant infection, which means that the patient's liver is overwhelmed. This can be fatal.

Most adults infected with HBV - estimated at over 90% - recover spontaneously. There is a high level of circulating virus in the acute phase and so people are often highly infectious to others during this time. This is a non-specific, debilitating illness in about 20% of people, involving fatigue, loss of appetite and nausea and sometimes depression. About a third of those infected get characteristic hepatitis symptoms like jaundice.

Five to ten per cent of people infected with HBV and 95% of children infected as infants suffer chronic detectable infection. Some of these people eventually get rid of HBV, usually within the first two years of infection. The longer HBV is present, however, the more difficult it is to clear. Persons in this group suffer from varying degrees of illness associated with **chronic hepatitis B.**

There are three broad categories of chronic infection, although individuals may not necessarily fit comfortably in any one category;

- Healthy carriers do not manifest symptoms. HBV persists, but is not accompanied by liver inflammation. The immune system appears not to react too violently to HBV, despite the presence of high levels of virus - a state known as immunotolerance. They remain infectious to other people.

- Periodically symptomatic persons experience episodes of active liver inflammation caused by a process called immunoelimination. The immune system appears to stop tolerating the presence of HBV and symptomatic liver disease follows, as the immune system attacks infected liver cells. It is not known exactly why this occurs. Sometimes, the active episodes end and the person returns to an immunotolerant state like healthy carriers; at other times, it becomes progressive liver disease. Levels of the virus increase when people have active immunoelimination episodes and so they become more infectious.

- About 25% of people with chronic HBV infection go on to develop progressive liver disease, which is characterised by ongoing liver inflammation. It seems that people who are most at risk of progression to this phase have immune systems that continue to try to eliminate HBV, but fail to do so. The immune system attacks infected liver cells in a vain attempt to clear the virus, causing serious injury in the process. This can develop into cirrhosis and, for a small minority, liver cancer.

As with all forms of chronic hepatitis, there is a risk of cirrhosis developing. Chronic hepatitis B also significantly increases a person's risk of hepatocellular carcinoma (HCC) or liver cancer. Currently, it is thought that about five to 15% of chronic HBV patients will progress to HCC. The majority of people with HCC already have cirrhosis, but over a third do not. The liver should routinely be monitored for tumours in people with chronic HBV. It remains unclear whether or not HBV co-infection hastens the progress of HIV infection.

What this all means is that only about two per cent of people who catch hepatitis B will eventually die from it - although that translates as many millions of people worldwide, because it is such a common disease.

How common is hepatitis B?

Around 2,500 cases of hepatitis B are reported in the UK a year, of which around 1,500 are acute cases. But, as only a third of people get anything other than very mild symptoms, the true figure is probably considerably larger: the Health Protection Agency's estimate is about 7,700.

The uncertainty is reflected in two US surveys: one in 1998 put the number of new hepatitis B cases a year at 10,500; the other, in 2001, put it at 100,000.

It is estimated that the proportion of the UK population that has ever had hepatitis B is around one in thirty, or about two million people. Gay men are five times more likely to catch hepatitis B than the general population - about one in six has caught it.

The prevalence of chronic hepatitis B in the UK is estimated to be 0.2 to 0.3% of the population, or about 180,000 people. Since 20 to 30% of these will go on to develop cirrhosis and liver failure, it can be seen that hepatitis B is a considerable public health problem.

Globally, HBV infection is an even bigger health problem. About 350 million people in the world currently have either acute or chronic hepatitis B infection, or about six per cent of the world's population. The World Health Organisation estimates that hepatitis B causes one million deaths a year worldwide.

Transmission routes

The hepatitis B virus can enter the body through mucous membranes. This is usually when semen, vaginal fluid or the blood of an infected individual gets into the mouth, eyes, penis (inside the urethra), rectum or vagina of an uninfected person.

The virus can also enter the bloodstream via needles or through cuts or wounds. Hepatitis B cannot be contracted through unbroken skin. No research to date has proven transmission from the saliva of an infected individual.

Hepatitis B is easily passed on among intravenous drug users: it can be spread via the sharing of spoons, filters and other paraphernalia, as well as hypodermic needles and syringes.

Sharing any piece of equipment that is likely to break the skin and have blood, semen or vaginal fluid on it on it is a risk for transmission of hepatitis B. A small percentage of people with hepatitis B may have been infected by practices that can lead to the drawing of blood, including tattooing, piercing and shaving.

Hepatitis B can be found in infectious quantities in blood, semen and vaginal fluid. It is therefore transmissible by any unprotected sexual contact which involves the combination of body fluids between partners. Oral sex with ejaculation is a risk factor for HBV transmission. Sexual practices which involve blood-to-blood contact or breaking of the skin also constitute a risk. No research to date has established direct evidence of HBV transmission from wet kisses.

Hepatitis B was a major concern for people with haemophilia prior to the heat-treating of blood products in the mid-1980s (UKHCDO 2004). It is still possible that people could be infected with hepatitis B from blood transfusions if the blood is not screened for the virus. However, all blood collected now in Britain is screened for hepatitis B.

Vertical transmission is a common route, especially in Asia and north Africa. Children born with hepatitis B are much more likely to develop chronic HBV than people contracting the virus by other routes.

Occupational transmission

The risk of exposure in healthcare settings from needle stick injuries is higher for hepatitis B than either HIV or hepatitis C. All health workers providing patient care in the UK should be vaccinated against HBV and some employers insist upon it. The transmission rate has been found to vary between 6 and 30% (1 in 17 to 1 in 3). The rate for HIV is between 0.2 and 0.4%, or between 1 in 500 and 1 in 250 (University of Virginia 2001).

Tests for HBV

There are a number of tests for hepatitis B that try to ascertain if someone is immune, a chronic carrier or has never had the disease. The results for some of these tests can be confusing to experienced liver doctors, never mind patients.

The history of testing for HBV has been of a series of certainties that have gradually been eroded by the finding of new exceptions to received wisdom. People who were believed to have recovered from acute HBV have later been shown to have a chronic infection. Some who were thought to be immune and no longer infectious have been shown to have passed on the virus. Others who had been believed to have cleared the virus have been found to have low levels of it circulating in the blood.

Classifying someone as either recovered, immune or no longer infectious has become a difficult task that may be produce the right result in the majority of cases, but, inevitably, the wrong one in others. Co-infection with HIV only makes the picture more complex.

Antibody and antigen tests

The tests done initially are usually antigen and antibody tests. **Antigens** are fragments of viral protein which appear at different times during hepatitis B infection. **Antibodies** are proteins made by immune cells that react with viral antigens and confer a degree of immunity.

There are three antigens that can be tested for: the surface or 's' antigen, the core or 'c' antigen and the 'e' antigen, which is another protein in the core of the viral particle. These are abbreviated to HBsAg, HBcAg and HBeAg, with 'HB' standing for Hepatitis B and 'Ag' for Antigen.

These three antigens may provoke the immune system to make an antibody, which can also be tested for. These antibody tests are labelled anti-HBs, anti-HBc and anti-HBe tests (or, confusingly, HBsAb, HBcAb and HbeAb). The immune system produces antibodies to the antigens at different stages of the disease.

Seven different tests are performed whose combined results can usually show whether you've got acute or chronic hepatitis B, how active it is, or whether you've recovered.

- **Hepatitis B surface antigen (HBsAg)** If you test positive for this, it means you either have acute or chronic infection, which may be active or inactive, but you haven't recovered.

- **HBsAg antibody (Anti-HBs)** If you test positive for this, it usually means (except in 'occult infection', see below) that you have recovered completely from hepatitis B and are now immune to it.

- **Hepatitis B core antigen (HBcAg)** A positive test for this means you've caught hepatitis B at some time - whether or not you have recovered from it.

- **HBc antibody (Anti-HBc)** A positive test for this means you're in the acute phase of the infection, not the chronic one.

- **Hepatitis B E antigen (HBeAg)** This is the most sensitive test for disease where the virus is actively reproducing, whether in the chronic or acute phase. In the chronic phase, a positive HBeAg test is an indicator that liver fibrosis is occurring.

- **HBe antibody (Anti-HBe)** Usually positive *except* during particularly active chronic infection, or if you've completely recovered.

- There is also a **DNA (PCR) test** for hepatitis B, which is positive during early acute infection and active chronic infection.

Antibodies can also be lost from the body after a period of time, and with HBV it seems quite possible to have some of the HBV antibodies without others, in what seem to be quite illogical ways. They can also be present or lacking in ways that are confusing to liver doctors, so do not be surprised if results are difficult to interpret.

All other combinations require expert interpretation and often repetition of these tests, alongside others to try and understand the situation. This may be immediately after the first set of tests, to act as a means of confirming the results, or they may become part of a yearly monitoring routine.

Presence of the virus

When there is uncertainty over the result of antigen and antibody tests, the HBV-DNA test is used to detect and quantify the presence of HBV virus in the blood. This test can be a good idea in people with HIV in any event, because HIV may impact on the presence of antibodies, either affecting the immune system's production of them or causing the antibodies to be lost more quickly.

A positive HBV-DNA result indicates that the virus is present and active and that the person is definitely infected. The sensitivity of the HBV-DNA test varies, with newer ones being much more sensitive and older ones much less so. It is worth asking how low a level of the virus can be detected by the test being used. The HBV-PCR test is a sensitive indicator of the presence of the virus in the blood, but less accurate in determining the level of circulating virus and so less useful at staging the disease. This test can show low levels of the virus circulating that are not detected by older HBV-DNA tests. The newer HBV-DNA tests are almost as sensitive as the PCR test with limits of detection as low as 100-200 copies/ml.

The 'e' antigen test was previously used as a marker for infectivity, in the belief that when the immune system had produced antibodies to this antigen and the antigen had disappeared, the person had achieved immunity. This is true for many people and can be a way of assessing if treatment has worked and made someone immune.

However, there is a mutation of the hepatitis B virus that means it does not produce the 'e' antigen at all, in which case tests for it are inevitably negative despite ongoing infection. In people with this mutant form of HBV, no 'e' antibody will be produced either. As antibodies may later be lost by a person anyway, someone who tests negative on both 'e' antigen and antibody has either recovered and developed natural immunity from the usual HBV infection or has the mutant form and is suffering chronic HBV.

This means that anti-HBV testing does not work in all cases, but is still useful for many in determining the stage and resolution of the infection.

Occult infection

A patient is said to have occult, or hidden, hepatitis B infection if they test positive for hepatitis B DNA and are positive for hepatitis B anticore but do not have the usual markers of hepatitis B infection: hepatitis B surface antigen and hepatitis B antibodies.

Three studies published in 2007 suggested that only about half the HIV patients attending US HIV clinics were being monitored for the presence of hepatitis B infection. They also found that anything between one in four and one in 10 patients who had hepatitis B may have occult infection.

Although having the occult version of infection did not appear to be associated with liver damage, hepatitis B is an unpredictable virus that can reappear and 'flare up' at any time, so closer monitoring is clearly warranted.

In the first study, from Cincinnati, Ohio (Shire), 909 patients from the city's University HIV Clinic were picked at random. They were not already known to have hepatitis B, but when given viral load tests for the virus, 43 of them (4.7% or one in 21) turned out to have it.

Out of these, 12 (28%) did not have a positive result to the surface antigen test (HBsAg). The patients who were HBsAG-positive had elevated liver enzyme levels. This indicates that liver damage due to hepatitis B was ongoing; that if they'd been monitored properly this would have been found out earlier; and that they should probably have been receiving treatment. However, patients who were not positive for HBsAG did not have elevated liver enzyme levels. Whether such infection might turn into episodes of active liver inflammation, especially if a person's immune status changes, is unknown.

The fact that patients are not being properly monitored for hepatitis B was underlined by another study from Texas (Jain). This found that, out of 155 people with HIV who started HIV combination therapy between 1999 and 2003, only one in six had a viral load test for hepatitis B before starting HIV therapy and only a third had a hepatitis B check in the year after starting therapy. Hepatitis B monitoring improved over time, but even in the latest year studied (2003) only just over half of patients had a hepatitis B check. This is despite US guidelines that say every HIV patient should be monitored for HBV co-infection. This study's authors comment that "improved physician adherence to these guidelines is needed."

The third study, from the Penn Center for AIDS Research in Philadelphia (Lo Rey), underlined the findings of the other two. Out of 179 randomly selected HIV patients who were negative on the HBsAg test, 17 (or nearly one in 10) had a positive hepatitis B viral load test, i.e. had 'occult' infection. These patients were also positive for antibodies to hepatitis B's surface antigen (anti-HBs) - which should mean they've had hepatitis B, but have got rid of it.

"The presence of anti-HBs does not rule out occult hepatitis B," say the researchers. "Future studies should examine the long-term clinical implications of occult hepatitis B in HIV-infected patients."

Signs of active liver disease

The standard liver function tests mentioned in the section on **Hepatitis A** above are also used to help define whether the person has liver damage.

Genotypes of HBV

Different types of the same virus are known as **genotypes**. Six different genotypes have been identified for HBV and are labelled alphabetically from A to G.

The test to define an individual's genotype is rarely done for hepatitis B and usually only for research purposes, because the results currently have no impact on treatment recommendations. The different genotypes probably affect how likely the disease is to become chronic, how aggressive it is and how it responds to treatment. But more research is needed before specific recommendations can be made.

Genotypes A and D are prevalent in Europe and the USA, while genotype E seems to be restricted to Africa and F is prevalent in Central and South America. Genotypes B and C are common in East Asia. Genotype G was found in both France and the US. The mutant form of HBV that causes the virus not to produce the 'e' antigen (HBeAg) may occur with each genotype but is more thought to be more frequent in genotypes B and D than genotype A.

Treatment

The purpose of treatment will vary, depending on a person's situation. It may be to improve the state of a person's liver, reduce the level of circulating virus, increase production of antibodies to the 'e' antigen or all three of these.

Acute HBV

Treatment in acute hepatitis B has not been shown to be effective.

The only qualification to this is in the case of newborn babies of mothers with HIV and HBV. Although this may not be classically defined as 'acute infection', there is an increased risk of developing chronic infection. Such babies should receive Hepatitis B Immunoglobulin at birth and have a course of the vaccine to try to avoid chronic infection (BHIVA 2004a).

Chronic HBV

There are a number of treatments for chronic HBV, including interferon and six nucleoside analogue drugs, three of which are also used to treat HIV.

Because some (or even most) of these treatments are active against HIV as well, this complicates matters in HIV co-infection. If the person is not on anti-HIV therapy, it is very important not to expose them to an anti-HIV drug on its own and provoke HIV to develop resistance to that drug, as this will make treating HIV much harder.

Hepatitis B can also develop resistance to some drugs, and so a management strategy for both conditions together is vital. If a drug is active against one virus but resisted by the second virus, removing the drug is probably a bad idea, and the rest of the treatment should be changed to take account of this.

An individual's circumstances will impact on the choice of therapy, but, generally, people not taking any HIV medication should avoid the drugs that have an effect on HIV. People already on HIV combination therapy should try to ensure that this combination includes drugs that are active against HBV as well.

Interferon is a subcutaneous injection, the classic form of which is called alpha-interferon. It is taken for four to six months. There is no recommended dose for the UK, but US guidelines propose five million units daily or ten million three times per week for at least 16 weeks (Lok 2001). European guidelines merely note that treatment is more effective at higher doses (EASL 2003).

The use of alpha-interferon is likely to be superseded by the use of pegylated interferon, which is a longer lasting form of interferon and only needs to be injected once a week. Results from the use of alpha-interferon are poor, being successful in fewer than a third of cases, regardless of which marker of treatment success is used. It also produces many uncomfortable side-effects. Furthermore, it tends to reduce the level of a person's CD4 cells, which may make it a less attractive option for someone who is not taking HIV treatment. HBV does not seem to develop resistance against interferon.

Lamivudine (3TC, *Epivir* - also branded as *Zeffix* when used as an anti-hepatitis B drug) comes in tablet form. The dose for HBV is lower than that required for HIV and so it should not be used at the lower dose in people not on HIV treatment, as it is likely to lead to HIV resistance to lamivudine. If a person's HIV has already become resistant to lamivudine, it may still be used against hepatitis B, though HBV can develop its own resistance to lamivudine. It should not be used alone in people not already on HIV therapy.

Emtricitabine (FTC, *Emtriva*) is similar to lamivudine and also comes as a tablet. It seems to work for longer but is cross-resistant with lamivudine. This means that once HBV has become resistant to lamivudine it will also be resistant to emtricitabine and vice versa. They should not be used together. Emtricitabine is also effective against HIV, and for this reason should not be used alone in people not already on HIV therapy.

Adefovir (*Hepsera*) is a tablet that was tried as an anti-HIV drug but was not very successful. It does however work well against hepatitis B. At the level prescribed for HBV, it was presumed to have no effect on HIV - but see below. It works against HBV that is resistant to lamivudine and, presumably, emtricitabine as well.

Tenofovir (*Viread*) is a tablet taken once a day. It is also active against HIV and so should not be used alone in people who are not on anti-HIV therapy. It seems to be effective against HBV that is resistant to lamivudine.

Tenofovir and emtricitabine are also co-formulated as *Truvada* and Epivir is co-formulated with abacavir as *Kivexa*.

Entecavir (*Baraclude*) was approved in 2005. It is a nucleoside analogue drug. The recommended dose of entecavir for chronic hepatitis B virus infection in nucleoside analogue treatment-naive adults and adolescents 16 years of age and older is 0.5mg once a day. For patients with a history of detectable hepatitis B viral loads while receiving 3TC or known 3TC resistance mutations, the recommended dose is 1mg once a day. The higher dose must be taken at least two hours before or two hours after a meal.

Telbivudine (*Tyzeka; Sebivo* in the USA) was approved in 2007. Another nucleoside analogue, it is taken as a single daily dose of 600 mg per day. Phase II studies showed that telbivudine is associated with significantly greater HBV suppression than lamivudine over the first year of treatment and beyond, with 60% of patients who are HBeAg-positive achieving complete HBV viral suppression versus 40% on lamivudine.

Recent problems with hepatitis B drugs and HIV

A study presented at the 14th CROI Conference in 2007 (McMahon) found that, contrary to expectation, entecavir was active against HIV as well as hepatitis B and that patients taking it as their only therapy might develop the M184V resistance mutation in HIV, which also confers resistance to lamivudine and emtricitabine.

Presenter Dr Chloe Thio from Johns Hopkins University reported on three cases in which HIV/HBV co-infected patients not receiving antiretroviral therapy experienced at least a 1-log decline in HIV viral load after starting entecavir for hepatitis B treatment. HIV RNA levels later rebounded in two of these individuals.

To explore this effect, Dr Thio and colleagues performed a laboratory analysis in which HIV-infected CD4 cells were exposed to increasing concentrations of antiviral drugs. To assess the emergence of resistance mutations, they obtained and cloned HIV isolates from the patient described in the first case report at several time points while on entecavir monotherapy. In addition, they used PCR testing to determine whether HIV replication was affected by exposure to entecavir.

They found that entecavir potently inhibited HIV replication with a 50% inhibitory concentration (IC50) between 0.1 and 1 nM, which is below the plasma concentration typically achieved with a normal dose of entecavir for hepatitis B treatment. PCR tests showed that entecavir inhibited the activity of the HIV reverse transcriptase enzyme, thereby slowing viral replication.

The analysis of the HIV samples from the co-infected patient showed that the M184V mutation accumulated over time. At baseline, none of the HIV clones harboured the mutation, compared with 61% at four months and 96% at six months after starting entecavir.

The researchers concluded that entecavir is a potent - but partial - inhibitor of HIV replication in vivo and in vitro, and that it can select for the M184V mutation, which confers high-level resistance to entecavir.

As adefovir is also a partial inhibitor of HIV at the doses given to supporess hepatitis B, this would also be the case with this drug.

Dr Thio and colleagues concluded that these results have important implications for the treatment of hepatitis B in HIV-positive individuals. "Entecavir should not be used in HIV/HBV co-infected individuals not on a fully suppressive HIV regimen without careful consideration of other options," they wrote.

After these case reports came to light in the month preceding the Retrovirus conference, Health Canada issued warning about the use of entecavir alone in HIV/HBV co-infected patients.

In addition, the US Food and Drug Administration and Bristol-Myers Squibb notified healthcare providers that the entecavir product label is being revised to reflect the new information. The label originally stated that "entecavir has no clinically relevant HIV activity."

Bristol-Myers Squibb's recent letter to health professionals says: "Healthcare professionals are advised that when considering therapy with *Baraclude* in an HIV/HBV co-infected patient not receiving HAART, the risk of developing HIV resistance cannot be excluded, based on current information."

As noted, there are few antiviral agents active against HBV but not HIV. With entecavir out of the picture, only the most recently approved anti-HBV drug - telbivudine - remains. Given the latest entecavir results, it should be carefully tested for even minor anti-HIV activity, using the most sensitive assays.

Another option is to treat HIV/HBV co-infected patients with multiple anti-HBV drugs, thus slowing the emergence of resistance to a single agent. Finally, reconsideration could be given to starting such individuals on antiretroviral therapy along with anti-HBV therapy, with regular monitoring for

hepatotoxicity, since patients who require hepatitis B treatment may have advanced liver disease.

For HIV, combining drugs to prevent viral resistance and ensure effective suppression of the virus has been very successful. It is very possible this approach will be used with HBV to overcome issues of resistance in the future.

Is there a vaccine?

Yes. Hepatitis B vaccination is safe and recommended in people with HIV. The *Recombinax HB, HBVaxPro* and *Engerix-B* vaccinations (the latter also combined with the hepatitis A vaccine as *Twinrix*) are available.

In people with HIV, vaccination appears most effective if administered when the CD4 count is above 500 (BHIVA 2004a). It is given as four injections over a 12-month period, with three in the first two months and another after a year. A more rapid approach, with three injections in a month and another after a year, has not been evaluated in people with HIV.

The vaccine appears to be somewhat less effective in people with HIV, with a higher proportion needing a booster dose or a repeat of the whole vaccination cycle in order to achieve full immunisation (Smith 2002). Protective antibodies produced after vaccination disappear over time, and this seems to happen more quickly in people co-infected with HIV (Rey 2000). Annual checks to ensure that the immune system maintains an effective level of protective antibodies are recommended (BHIVA 2004a).

People at high risk of getting hepatitis B include gay men, injecting drug users, medical workers and people intending to travel to the developing world.

In most developed countries there is universal hepatitis B vaccination for children - for instance, the USA adopted universal hepatitis B vaccination in children in 1991.

Interestingly, one of the exceptions is the UK (another is the Netherlands). The justification for this was that the UK was an exceptionally low-prevalence country, but with rates among immigrants and people of Asian ethnic background increasing, this is no longer the case, and the Foundation for Liver Research has been campaigning for universal child vaccination.

Gay men in the UK have been targeted by the B Safe campaign, but it is still estimated that only 50 per cent of gay men susceptible to hepatitis B have had the vaccination.

The immunity conferred by the hepatitis B vaccine lasts about 15 years and people should get a booster shot about every ten years to ensure continued immunity.

HBV vaccination can be obtained through GPs. If you do not wish to discuss with your GP those aspects of your lifestyle which may put you at risk of HBV infection, you may obtain the vaccination through a GUM clinic or through a local drugs project.

Nurses and health care workers should be offered the vaccination as part of routine occupational health procedures.

Hepatitis C

Only explicitly identified in 1989, hepatitis C (HCV) is classified as a flavivirus. Prior to being isolated, it was known to exist and was usually described as non-A, non-B hepatitis or 'serum hepatitis', as it was known to be transmitted through blood and blood products.

The virus replication process is quite error-prone and so results in a very high level of mutation. HCV also exists in at least six different genotypes, each with very different degrees of persistence and pathogenicity.

Hepatitis C is the most common type of viral hepatitis in the UK, affecting almost every adult with haemophilia, a majority of IDUs and an increasing number of gay men. It is also a significant problem worldwide and a major concern for people with HIV.

In the UK, as in many other countries, the prevalence of hepatitis C infection is uncertain, because this is a disease which more often than not causes no symptoms at first, and which may only start causing them decades later. The Department of Health estimates that about 0.5% of the general population in England has been infected with hepatitis C. Since the early 1990s, the number of people diagnosed each year with HCV infection has increased significantly, from under 1,000 to over 9,000.

Some people clear the virus in the acute stage: this means that around 0.4% of the general population in England (200,000 people) may have chronic hepatitis C infection - or more than three times as many people as have HIV. Other estimates put the number as high as 400,000. However, up to the end of 2003 only 38,000 laboratory reports of HIV infection had been received, so over three-quarters of people in Britain with the virus do not know they have it.

This puts the UK at the low-prevalence end of global hepatitis C infection. Worldwide the number of people with chronic hepatitis C has been estimated at 170 million (about half the number with chronic hepatitis B), although some estimates are as high at 400 million. The highest prevalence rates appear to be in Asia and Africa. In some countries, such as Egypt, it is estimated that up to 22% of the population has hepatitis C.

In the USA, HCV antibody surveillance has shown that prevalence of chronic hepatitis C in the general population is about 1.3%, with a prevalence of four per cent in people in their 40s (Armstrong). A 2002 study found that HCV prevalence in a cohort of military veterans in New York was 10.6%. In Europe, the infection rate is at its lowest in the north of the continent, with prevalence rates generally rising in the south and east.

Rates of co-infection with HIV vary in Britain, with the largest HIV clinic suggesting that nearly 12% of people with HIV are co-infected with hepatitis C. In parts of the world, such as Russia, where the predominant mode of HIV transmission is through injecting drug use, hepatitis C co-infection rates are as high as 80% (Lioznov). About 25 to 35% of the US HIV-positive population has hepatitis C. In Europe, data from the EuroSIDA cohort of European people with HIV indicate that 33% were co-infected with HCV, and among injecting drug users the rate increased to over 75% (Stubbe).

Disease progression

HCV is a highly variable disease with major differences in how aggressive it is, what symptoms it causes and how it responds to treatment. HCV is a long-lasting disease and, once established as chronic, it appears to remain in the body for life. Although generally a slow-acting condition, usually taking decades to cause cirrhosis and liver failure in some people, it can significantly damage the liver within a few years in others. Some people experience almost no symptoms, while others are significantly incapacitated. Fatigue, abdominal pain and nausea are the most common symptoms, but there are many others, not all of which are confined to the liver.

Hepatitis C is both immunopathic and cytopathic. Cytopathic means the virus causes damage directly, by injuring the cells that it infects while immunopathic means that it is the response of the body's immune system to the viruses that causes the damage. It is because HCV causes both mechanisms of injury to cells that the symptoms are so varied. HCV is described as being hepatotropic and lymphatotropic, meaning that it inhabits both the liver and the lymphatic system.

People with HCV have a higher likelihood of getting Hepatocellular Carcinoma (HCC), better known as liver cancer, and are possibly at greater risk of non-Hodgkin's lymphoma. It remains uncertain if hepatitis C affects the progression of HIV - but HIV infection certainly accelerates the progression of hepatitis C, with co-infected people with low CD4 counts progressing to cirrhosis about three times faster than mono-infected people.

Less than a third of people suffer an acute phase at the time of infection, with symptoms usually including jaundice and fatigue, but less severely than in HBV infection. About 15% of people clear the hepatitis C virus spontaneously, but the majority of people suffer from chronic infection, most experiencing no noticeable symptoms at the time of infection.

Of the 85% who develop chronic infection, around five to ten per cent become asymptomatic carriers with no progression, similar to occult hepatitis B infection. Around 65 to 70% will develop a stable chronic infection with little or slow progression to liver fibrosis, but with periodically raised liver enzyme levels. About 20 to 30% will develop progressive chronic hepatitis leading to cirrhosis, and 1.5% will develop liver cancer (Alter). About 60% of people with chronic hepatitis C have raised ALT levels (see **liver function tests** above) at any one time (Armstrong).

However, the figures that have appeared are based upon current cross-sections of patients rather than long term follow-up of infected patients, so may be misleading. It is not really known what proportion of HCV patients will eventually go on to experience the various symptoms associated with liver disease. Some analyses conclude that progression occurs across the whole HCV-positive population at differing speeds (Dienstag) and suggest that HCV can cause other life-threatening conditions. Precise breakdowns of proportions progressing to various types and stages of disease are still a matter of conjecture.

On the other hand, we may also be underestimating the proportion of people who clear the virus spontaneously in acute infection. This may be because most people at risk of hepatitis C are not monitored closely enough to identify acute infections. In one closely-monitored patient group, the cohort of gay men with HIV at London's Chelsea and Westminster Hospital, 24% of those who acquired hepatitis C through sexual transmission spontaneously cleared their infection (Gilleece).

Certain factors have been identified as speeding up the progression to fibrosis and cirrhosis (including HIV infection with a low CD4 count) and others that were originally thought likely have been shown not to. A number of others remain unproven or only hinted at by research data.

Factors related to the virus

- Duration of infection: the risk of liver disease increases with time. There is no time point beyond which one can say 'If I haven't got liver disease now, I never will'.

- Genotype: it seems that the different genotypes may affect the course of the disease in people. For example, genotype 3 appears to be the easiest for the body to clear, but may progress to fibrosis faster, and genotype 4 may be harder for the body to clear than the other major genotypes. This is, however, a complex area and past assertions about some genotypes being more virulent were later refuted, so this may change again.

- Viral load: unlike in HIV infection, a high viral load prior to treatment does not predict a faster or more severe disease progression and may be entirely unrelated.

Factors related to the person

- Age at infection: contracting hepatitis C after age 40 has been associated with greater risk of progression in some studies.

- Alcohol consumption: a greatly increased risk of cirrhosis is associated with sustained alcohol consumption of greater than 40g (five units or two pints of most lagers) each day. One study found a fifteen-fold greater rate of progression to fibrosis in people who drank more than this amount compared with people who drank no alcohol at all. It may be that there is no safe limit for alcohol consumption if you have hepatitis C (or indeed chronic hepatitis B).

- An individual's genetic make-up.

- HIV infection and a low CD4 count: a CD4 count of less than 200 is associated with an increased risk of cirrhosis. Those with higher CD4 counts were at no greater risk than their HIV-negative counterparts, suggesting that immune suppression facilitates liver disease.

- Other hepatitis viruses: co-infection with hepatitis A or hepatitis B increases the risk of liver disease.

- Gender: men seem to progress faster to liver disease.

All of these effects only show themselves across a population, and so, while a young woman with a healthy lifestyle will be unlikely to quickly develop serious liver disease, there is no guarantee.

Most of these factors are also beyond the control of a person; no one can change their age or genetic make up, for example. Reducing alcohol consumption and avoiding other hepatitis infections are the only things that are truly within the control of a person. How someone responds to this is up to the individual, and whilst not drinking alcohol may be fine for one person, it may remove a significant social support structure for others. People with HCV may also chose to drink fully aware of the consequences for their health, just as smokers are almost always aware of the likely impact on their future health of smoking.

Transmission

Hepatitis C has a number of routes of transmission. Transmission by injection is the most common route, but infections of HCV through sex are a particular issue for gay men with HIV. Co-infection with HIV has also been shown to increase the infectivity of people with hepatitis C.

Injecting drug use

Hepatitis C is easily passed on in situations of intravenous drug use. HCV is spread via the sharing of spoons, filters and other paraphernalia, as well as hypodermic needles and syringes.

Overall, HCV infection rates among intravenous drug users (IDUs) are extremely high, varying between 60% and 77% in studies in the UK. In 2000, the Department of Health estimated that one-third of IDUs attending GUM clinics in England and Wales were infected with HCV, of whom only 40% were aware of their infection. The prevalence of HCV among injecting drug users varied by region, the highest numbers being in London and the North-West.

One in 12 IDUs who began injecting in the past three years were HCV-positive. IDUs who had been in prison were almost twice as likely to have been infected with HCV than those who had not.

Sexual transmission

HCV can be and is transmitted sexually. But sexual transmission seems to happen most frequently between men who have sex with men and are HIV-positive. Sexual transmission among heterosexuals who do not have HIV appears extremely unlikely by comparison (Marincovich 2003).

The amount of circulating hepatitis C in the blood stream is significantly increased in people with HIV (Eyster 1994) and this may mean they are more infectious in sexual situations. The impact of HIV on the immune system may also mean that people with HIV are more likely to contract HCV sexually from someone infected, and it may be the combination of these two factors that leads to the noticeably higher rate of sexual transmission rates amongst HIV-positive gay men.

Outbreaks of acute HCV have been seen in London and Paris among gay men attending HIV clinics, and sex seems to be the route of transmission. Researchers from Naples found that HCV infection was almost three times higher in those who were HIV-positive compared to HIV-negative controls (15.1% versus 5.2%; P = 0.005). Significantly, 18.7% of those who had regular heterosexual or gay sex with an HIV-positive partner were HCV-positive, compared with only 1.6% for the partners of HIV-negative controls (Filippini 2001).

Abresica (2002) in Italy found that 20% of women who had been infected with HIV by HIV/HCV co-infected partners were also infected with HCV, leading the co-authors to conclude: "It's probable that HIV and its related opportunistic infections of the female genital tract could strongly facilitate HCV sexual transmission." However, other retrospective studies have found little or no sexual transmission of HCV among heterosexual couples where one had HIV.

Research suggests also that sexual practices which involve contact with blood are associated with hepatitis C transmission. These include unprotected anal sex, sex during menstruation and fisting.

Occupational exposure

As with hepatitis B and HIV, there is the risk of exposure in healthcare settings from needle stick injuries. The transmission rate has been found to vary between 0.4 and 2% (between 1 in 250 and 1 in 50). The rate for HIV is between 0.2 and 0.4%, or between 1 in 500 and 1 in 250 (University of Virginia 2001).

Vertical transmission

Estimates of the rate of mother-to-baby transmission of HCV range from 0% to 36%, but the risk of transmission appears to be increased in mothers who are co-infected with HCV and HIV. This may be due to the generally higher HCV viral load in co-infected people.

Most transmission is known to occur around the time of delivery, and planned Caesarean section, before the rupture of membranes, lowers transmission rates compared to emergency Caesarean or vaginal delivery. Breastfeeding is not considered to be a route of transmission and, in the United States, the Centers for Disease Control (CDC) do not consider bottle feeding of uninfected infants to be necessary. Bleeding or cracked nipples are a theoretical route of transmission.

Household contact:

Sharing any piece of equipment that is likely to get blood on it, such as a razor or toothbrush, is a definite but small risk for transmission of hepatitis C.

Intra-mucosally: sharing rolled-up notes or other equipment to snort cocaine

According to a large scale American survey of over 500,000 blood donors, risks of exposure to HCV were associated with intra-nasal cocaine use. The results of this survey do not amount to proof of intra-nasal transmission in themselves, but rather a correlation (Conty-Cantilena 1996). A study from the Royal Free Hospital in north London also supported the idea that this is a route of transmission (Danta 2003).

Blood transfusions and blood products

The very high rates of HCV infection in haemophiliacs, particularly those treated prior to the introduction of donor and blood screening and sterilisation in 1986, reflect the ease of transmission via this route (UKHCDO 2004). A small number of people have also contracted HCV from blood transfusions and organ transplants. The Skipton Fund has been set up to provide a two-stage financial payment to people infected with HCV in the UK from medical treatment.

Vaccination programmes and traditional acupuncture

It is now known that large numbers of people were infected with HCV by 'shared needle' vaccination programmes, particularly in Southern Europe, Asia and Africa. It has been particularly blamed as the reason for the huge number of infections in Egypt. Acupuncture may have also spread the virus in Asia prior to the introduction of sterilisation techniques

Cosmetics and tattoos

A small percentage of the HCV-positive population have been infected by cosmetic contact. Practices that can lead to the drawing of blood, including tattooing, piercing and shaving, are assumed to be responsible.

Tests for HCV

Exposure to HCV, though not chronic infection, is shown by an HCV antibody test. As some people naturally clear the virus from their body, chronic infection is only diagnosed in people who test positive to a PCR test. The PCR test is similar to a viral load test for HIV in that it detects that the virus is present in the blood. It may also be called an HCV RNA test. Antibodies to HCV do not mean someone is immune to HCV in future, even if they have naturally cleared the virus or have been successfully treated.

HIV can cause the antibodies to HCV to disappear in some people, a factor which may have caused some people with HIV to have tested negative for HCV in the past. If hepatitis C infection is suspected - because someone has jaundice or their liver function tests suggest inflammation - then the HCV PCR test should be carried out (BHIVA 2004b).

The standard liver function tests mentioned at the start of this chapter are also used to help define whether a person has liver damage.

The genotype test for HCV is an important one for people who are going to have treatment. There are six major genotypes of the virus (with others that are only found in specific parts of the world), which are labelled numerically from one to six. Some genotypes are further divided into subtypes such as 1a and 1b. Genotype 1 is the most common in the United States, accounting for more than 75% of all infections. Genotype 3 is the most frequent on the Indian subcontinent. Most infections in Egypt are genotype 4, whilst genotype 5 is usually only found in southern Africa. Genotype 6 is found in south-east Asia.

In the UK, it is thought that about two-thirds of HCV-infected people have genotype 1, most of the rest being 2 or 3. Genotypes 2 and 3 respond better to current therapy than genotypes 1 and 4. Much less is known about the response to treatment of genotypes 5 and 6.

Treatment

Treatments are dependent on a number of factors. The results of biopsies and liver function tests, along with how a person is feeling, are used to decide whether treatment is recommended or not. Since many people can live for decades without symptoms or significant liver damage, treatment is not always recommended to people - or wanted by them.

The current standard-of-care treatment is pegylated interferon and ribavirin. Pegylated interferon is a once-a-week injection and ribavirin a tablet taken twice a day. It is an arduous treatment, usually causing many side-effects that can significantly debilitate people. Almost all the side-effects disappear when treatment stops, but a few can be permanent.

This is a treatment that is taken for a set period of time and either cures people of HCV or fails to do so. If the treatment has little or no impact on the level of hepatitis C in the bloodstream after twelve weeks, it is stopped. If it does significantly reduce the level of virus, preferably to a level below detection, treatment continues to the end of the course.

The length of time a person takes treatment currently depends on the particular HCV genotype they have and also upon whether they have HIV co-infection. People who do not have HIV and those with genotypes 2 and 3 require treatment for 24 weeks, while those with other genotypes generally take treatment for 48 weeks.

Some people respond to the medication while they are taking it, but the virus is not completely eradicated from their system, reappearing in the bloodstream once the treatment programme has finished. This is often described as a *partial response*. People for whom the treatment cures them of HCV are described as *sustained responders*, because their response to medication is sustained beyond the period of treatment. Three-quarters of people with HCV genotypes 2 and 3 are cured by pegylated Interferon and ribavirin, and just over half of those with genotype 1.

In people co-infected with HIV, treatment can be more important, because removing HCV from the system may reduce the load on a liver that may have to deal with metabolising HIV therapies as well. Current expert opinion is that period of treatment of pegylated Interferon and ribavirin should be extended for people with HIV: those with Genotypes 2 and 3 should take treatment for 48 weeks, while those with the other genotypes should have 72 weeks of treatment. This opinion arises from the poorer results seen in people with HIV and HCV who took the treatment for the standard lengths of time. Extending treatment to 72 weeks has produced diminishing returns as people find it hard to tolerate for that length of time.

In the largest trial of pegylated interferon and ribavirin in co-infected people so far conducted, the APRICOT trial (Torriani 2004), the sustained response rate overall was 40% after 48 weeks of treatment. But there was a big difference between genotypes 2 and 3, where 62% of patients responded, and genotype 1, where only 29% had a sustained response.

This difference was even more pronounced in a smaller study, ACTG 5071 (Chung), which only found a sustained response rate of 14% but 73% in genotype 2 and 3.

Higher rates of sustained response have been found in those recently infected with HCV, with 60% of the Chelsea and Westminster cohort of gay men with HIV who caught HCV achieving a sustained viral response (Gilleece). However, this is poor compared to mono-infected people, where SVR rates of 90 to 98% have been seen in people treated during acute infection.

Response to therapy at 12 weeks predicts whether or not a person will achieve a sustained virological response six months after treatment is completed. If an individual has failed to achieve a reduction in their HCV viral load of at least 100-fold (2 logs) by this time, many experts recommend discontinuing HCV therapy given the high incidence of side-effects and the low likelihood of achieving a sustained response. For those with cirrhosis or liver failure, transplantation is a viable option if the person's HIV prognosis is good. For a complete discussion of current therapeutic options for HIV-HCV co-infected individuals, see the *HIV & AIDS Treatments Directory*.

Future treatments and vaccines

A large number of different drugs with different modes of action are being developed to treat hepatitis C infection. These include 'improved' versions of interferon (examples are *Albuferon*, *Infergen* and lambda and tau-interferon) and of ribavirin (taribavirin and levovirin).

Existing anti-inflammatory drugs are being looked at to see if they can control the immune-modulated damage caused by hepatitis C and delay or prevent fibrosis. Examples include thalidomide, etanercept, thymosin and mycophenolate.

HCV protease and integrase inhibitors are also currently being tested in trials. Boehringer Ingelheim has a serine-protease inhibitor called BILN-2061 in phase II trials, while Vertex Pharmaceuticals recently presented the first clinical data on its HCV protease inhibitor, called VX-950, and Schering-Plough received fast-track approval for their compound SCH 503034. Experimental nucleoside analogues include valopicitabine (NM-283) and isatoribine (ANA245).

A number of other drug targets are being investigated. Preventative and therapeutic vaccines for hepatitis C are also being developed, although these are in the early stages of development and are hampered by the difficulty of stimulating an immune response against all the many variant forms of HCV (Houghton 2003)

As some of these drugs are in reasonably late-stage clinical trials, many people with hepatitis C who are not progressing rapidly to fibrosis or are not in acute infection are weighing up the pros and cons of taking a hard-to-tolerate treatment now against waiting two to three years for anti-HCV therapies that may be considerably more potent and/or easy to take.

However, many of the experimental drugs are virustatic rather than virucidal drugs; this means that they will work like anti-HIV drugs, in that they will slow down or prevent viral replication instead of effecting a permanent cure. Because of this, the use of interferon in conjunction with these new agents is likely to be the gold standard of treatment for some years to come.

For more on current and future hepatitis C treatment options, see the *HIV & AIDS Treatments Directory*.

The hepatitis C treatment lottery

People co-infected with hepatitis C and HIV are even more likely to suffer from multiple socio-economic disadvantages than people with HIV. These vary from a double stigma against both diseases to poor physical and mental health, as well as the social marginalisation experienced by injecting drug users.

One study found a 57.3% prevalence of depression among HIV-infected patients and a 69.8% prevalence of depression among patients co-infected with HIV and hepatitis C (HCV), compared with an estimated five to ten per cent prevalence in the general adult population of primary care patients (Hooshyar). Substance abuse, which affects an estimated 8.3% of the general US population aged 12 and over, affected 28.8% of HIV-infected patients in the study, and 47.9% of HIV/HCV-infected patients.

What this adds up to is that the already rather poor success rates for current HCV treatment are further exacerbated by the fact that only a small proportion of people who are eligible for hepatitis C treatment end up getting it, even where it is available.

This is partly due to factors to do with the patients: people who are current injecting drug users may have neither the stability of lifestyle to adhere to a year's worth of interferon therapy nor the mental stability to tolerate some of its neuropsychological side-effects.

However, there is a lot of evidence that physicians' perceptions of such patients' ability to tolerate and adhere to an expensive and partially-effective treatment are at least as influential as any other factors. Current injecting drug use is often used as a blanket exclusion criterion for people with hepatitis C, regardless of any other assessment of the patient's ability to adhere to treatment, as is current psychiatric treatment. This can result in a tiny proportion of patients who might benefit from hepatitis C treatment actually ending up being cured.

In one typical example from New York (Burger), of 528 HIV/HCV co-infected persons at one clinic, only 193 (37%) were referred for treatment. Of these, 107 (55%) were considered suitable candidates according to criteria that included persons with controlled substance use, stable psychiatric illnesses and anaemia responsive to growth factors.

During the evaluation process, 32 of those selected for treatment subsequently became ineligible due to inconsistent follow-up. Twenty declined treatment, and 16 deferred treatment, with seven remaining under evaluation. Twenty-four were ineligible because of repeatedly missing their initial appointment, seven because of active psychiatric illness, 21 because of uncontrolled substance abuse, 37 due to medical reasons, and six because their hepatitis C infection had spontaneously resolved. Among the 252 patients with detectable viral load who had *not* been referred, 58 were found to be eligible for treatment; while 19 of these were previously treated, a substantial number of patients refused evaluation.

In short, out of 528 patients, only 165 (31%) were eligible for treatment under the clinic's criteria; only 107 (20%) were actually referred for treatment; and only 32 (six per cent) actually started taking a treatment that, in a patient group with predominantly genotype 1 infection, stood about a 30% chance of success. Similar 'ultimate cure' rates of about two per cent have been found from other studies in both Europe and America.

There is, in short, a huge need not only for cheaper, more tolerable and effective hepatitis C treatment, but also for criteria that make it more easily accessible and usable by the patients who need it most.

Multiple co-infections

There have been suggestions that people with HCV who become infected with hepatitis A were at risk of fulminant hepatitis and possible death (Vento et al 1998). However, a larger follow-up study showed no deaths from acute hepatitis A infection in those with HCV (Mele et al. 1998). None of the people in the studies had HIV as well, so beyond highlighting the importance of being vaccinated, it is difficult to give any recommendations.

For people with HIV and hepatitis C, contracting hepatitis B is obviously not a good thing. In practice, there has not been much evidence to suggest that HBV illness is worse or the chance of liver failure increases in people who already have HCV. Little research has focused on people with multiple hepatitis viruses and no recommendations have come from the studies that have been done.

It seems that other factors, such as alcohol consumption, have a greater influence on the chances of developing liver cancer. Therefore, the prognosis for patients with multiple viruses is probably worse, but maybe not dramatically so.

Conclusion

Hepatitis C is a complex condition and is linked to a number of other medical disorders, some of which are serious, as well as to multiple socio-economic stressors. Because the full picture is still emerging, it is not yet possible to give a complete list of symptoms, their likelihood of appearance in individual persons, the possible factors influencing their occurrence and the overall impact of HCV infection on quality of life and longevity. HIV co-infection complicates this even more.

Hepatitis D

Hepatitis D, once called the 'delta agent', is an issue for people with hepatitis B. HDV only infects people who already have hepatitis B and exacerbates the condition.

Transmission

Either people are infected with both at the same time or contract hepatitis D after having already got hepatitis B. It is often diagnosed when someone with chronic HBV suddenly becomes significantly worse or the acute infection of HBV is particularly severe. It has similar routes of transmission to hepatitis A and is endemic around the Mediterranean.

Tests

Exposure is usually confirmed by an antibody test.

Treatment

Treatment is normally bed rest and taking plenty of fluids until the symptoms have passed. The treatments for hepatitis B are used with people who have both viruses.

Is there a vaccine?

No. Although there is no vaccine specific for HDV, successful vaccination against hepatitis B prevents infection with HDV.

Hepatitis E

Hepatitis E was once classified as a member of the Calciviridae family but has since been reclassified into its own family called simply 'HEV-like viruses'. It has some structural similarities to the rubella virus.

HEV is especially severe for pregnant women, in whom it can cause fulminant hepatitis and lead to death of the foetus in up to a fifth of infected women. It has been also been known to cause fulminant hepatitis in a few other cases.

Transmission

Like hepatitis A, HEV is transmitted via the faecal-oral route. This means that the faeces of someone with HEV are infectious and if another person ingests this faecal matter, they contract the disease. Commonly, this happens in countries where untreated sewage is discharged straight into rivers that also supply drinking water or where uncooked foods that have been washed in contaminated water are consumed.

HEV-infected persons are infectious for only a relatively brief period of time.

However, many sexual practices facilitate faecal-oral transmission of HEV, and inapparent faecal contamination is not unusual during anal sex. Rimming is an obvious risk for HEV.

Tests

Hepatitis E can be diagnosed by an antibody test, and a PCR test, which shows presence of the virus, is also available.

Treatment

Similar to that for Hepatitis A. The infection usually resolves itself within a few weeks or months. Bed rest and drinking plenty of fluids is the usual recommendation for someone with HEV.

Is there a vaccine?

Not yet. One is being trialled by the US army in Nepal but is not yet commercially available. The hope is that if it proves effective it will become available in 2007.

Epidemiology

Although cases have been identified all over the world, it is found more frequently in Asia, north Africa and Mexico and is the commonest form of hepatitis in India. In the western world, it is generally considered to be a disease which affects travellers to developing countries.

Hepatitis F

Hepatitis F is a hypothetical virus. In the 1990s, several laboratories claimed to have identified hepatitis F. Before any of these claims could be substantiated, another virus affecting the liver was found and named Hepatitis G. When the claim for hepatitis F was discounted it would have been too confusing to re-designate HGV as hepatitis F. So HFV remains unassigned.

Hepatitis G

Hepatitis G is a virus that may not even cause hepatitis.

HGV was discovered in the mid-1990s at the same time as GBV-C, and they are believed to be different strains of the same virus. It is sometimes designated HGV/GBV-C. It is a flavivirus like HCV and was originally found in a person with liver disease, which may be why it was believed to be a hepatitis virus.

It is uncertain whether HGV really does cause hepatitis or what impact it has on other infections. Some studies have found it to slow the progression of HIV while others have found no impact. No study has proven it to be the cause of liver damage yet or indeed that it causes any health problems. It is commonly found in people who already have HIV, HBV and HCV, probably because of the similarity of transmission routes, as well as in the general population.

Transmission routes

It is transmitted by blood and blood products, sexual activity and from mother to child at birth. Since it does not appear to cause any disease, it is not tested for in blood donors.

Tests

Testing for a virus that does not seem to cause any illness is generally confined to research purposes. Blood can be tested for antibodies and a PCR test can show the presence of the virus.

Treatment

Since it does not appear to cause illness, there is no treatment, although interferon was used at one point to try to eradicate the virus from the body.

Liver disease

Patients with chronic hepatitis will be significantly more susceptible to cirrhosis and liver cancer than the general population; and these two conditions evoke the most apprehension.

Cirrhosis

Patients with cirrhotic livers may start to experience symptoms caused by the inability of blood to flow freely through the organ; as a result blood is diverted around the liver, which can cause a number of secondary symptoms.

Patients will also experience symptoms related to the deterioration in effective function of the liver. They include:

- Ascites, which leads to the swelling of the abdomen, caused by the accumulation of fluid.

- Varices are distended blood vessels around the stomach and gullet which enlarge because the blood is trying to find a way around the scarred liver. These blood vessels can bleed into the stomach, which necessitates immediate treatment.

The symptoms are vomiting up blood and/or passing black faeces.

- Circulatory changes. Because a cirrhotic liver doesn't break down certain blood chemicals as efficiently, blood vessels can become blocked, leading to the heart having to work harder and the dilation of blood vessels

- Encephalopathy. Patients may experience impaired mental function because the liver is not breaking down waste products in the blood as efficiently as it should or because blood is bypassing the liver. Laxatives are sometimes used to treat this.

- Liver failure may develop as a result of long-term progression via cirrhosis or as a result of fulminant hepatitis, which is characterised by the overwhelming of liver cells by pathogens and toxins, resulting in widespread necrosis (cell inflammation and death). It is treated by a transplant.

- Liver transplants currently have a high success rate. Survival rates for five years after the operation are around 80%.

Liver cancer

The exact mechanism through which the hepatitis viruses cause cancer is the subject of considerable scientific speculation. Hepatocellular carcinoma (HCC) is a particularly nasty form of cancer which can sometimes be treated by liver transplantation.

HIV co-infection is not a reason by itself to prevent a transplant and a number of successful liver transplants have already been performed in Britain on people co-infected with HIV. In the majority of people, HCC comes after they have developed cirrhosis. However, a number of people have developed liver cancer without having cirrhosis first.

Complementary therapies

Silymarin or milk thistle is the most common alternative medication used by persons with hepatitis. It has been used to treat all forms of liver disease for over 2000 years. However, its effects have never been properly evaluated in controlled trials.

The widespread use of herbal products can pose serious health risks. Many alternative therapies are associated with significant liver toxicity. Agents to avoid include: chaparral leaf, valerian, skullcap, misteltoe, germander, Jin Bu Huan, and pyrrolizidine alkaloids.

For more on complementary approaches, see *Directory of Complementary Therapies in HIV & AIDS*.

References

Abrescia N et al. Sexual transmission of HCV in sexually infected HIV women. Fourteenth International AIDS Conference, Barcelona, abstract C11013, 2002.

Alter H. Patterns of hepatitis C infection. Presented at the 37th Annual Meeting of the Infectious Diseases Society of America; Philadelphia, Pa; November 18-21, 1999. Session 70, S111.

Armstrong GL et al. The Prevalence of Hepatitis C Virus Infection in the United States, 1999 through 2002. Ann Int Med 144(10): 705-714. 2006.

BHIVA Guidelines : HIV and Chronic Hepatitis: Co-Infection with HIV and Hepatitis B Virus Infection, 2004(a). Available at www.bhiva.org/guidelines/2004/HBV/index.html

BHIVA guidelines for treatment and management of HIV and Hepatitis C coinfection, 2004(b) available at www.bhiva.org/guidelines/2004/HCV/index.html

Burger S. Limited success of hepatitis C treatment in an inner city population with Human Immunodeficiency Virus coinfection. XVI International AIDS Conference, Toronto. Abstract CDB0345. 2006.

Chung R et al. Peginterferon alfa-2a plus ribavirin versus interferon alfa-2a plus ribavirin for chronic hepatitis C in HIV-coinfected persons. NEJM 351: 451-459, 2004.

Conty-Cantilena C et al. Routes of infection, viremia, and liver disease in blood donors found to have hepatitis C virus infection. New England Journal of Medicine 334: 169, 1996.

Danta M, Brown D, Jacobs M et al. Epidemiology of acute HCV infection in a London cohort of HIV-positive homosexual males. 54th Annual Meeting of the American Association for the Study of Liver Diseases, Boston, Massachusetts, abstract 561, 2003.

De Lédinghen V et al. Diagnosis of hepatic fibrosis and cirrhosis by transient elastography in HIV/hepatitis C virus-coinfected patients. J Acquir Immune Defic Syndr 41: 175-179, 2006.

Department of Health. Hepatitis C: essential information for professionals and guidance on testing. 2004. See www.dh.gov.uk/en/Publicationsandstatistics/Publications/PublicationsPolicyAndGuidance/DH_4097933

Dienstag J. Gastroenterology 112, No 2: 651-655, 1997.

EASL International Consensus Conference on Hepatitis B Journal of Hepatology, S3-S25, 2003.

Eyster ME et al. Increasing hepatitis C virus RNA levels in hemophiliacs: relationship to human immunodeficiency virus infection and liver disease. Multicenter Hemophilia Cohort Study Blood; 84(4): 1020-1023, 1994.

Filippini P et al. Does HIV Infection Favor the Sexual Transmission of Hepatitis C? Sexually Transmitted Diseases, 28(12): 725-729, 2001.

Gibb D et al. Early report: Mother-to-child transmission of hepatitis C virus: evidence for preventable peripartum transmission. Lancet 356: 904-907, 2000.

Gilleece YC et al. Is the treatment of acute hepatitis C in HIV-positive individuals effective? Eleventh Annual Conference of the British HIV Association, abstract O26, Dublin, April 20 - 23rd, 2005.

Hooshyar D. Depression High Among HIV-Positive Patients: Rates Are More than Five Times Greater. AIDS Alert 19(3): 34, 2004.

Ida S et al. Influence of human immunodeficiency virus type 1 infection on acute hepatitis A virus infection. Clinical Infectious Diseases, 34: 379-385, 2002.

Jain MK et al. Do HIV care providers appropriately manage hepatitis B in coinfected patients treated with antiretroviral therapy? Clin Inf Dis 44: 996-1000, 2007.

Lioznov D et al.HIV Disease Burden in St. Petersburg, Russia. 11th Conference on Retroviruses and Opportunistic Infections, abstract 868. 2004.

Lo Rey V et al. Prevalence, risk factors and outcomes for occult hepatitis B infection among HIV-infected patients. JAIDS 44(3): 315-320. 2007.

Lok, ASF and Mcmahon, BJ. Chronic Hepatitis B, Hepatology 34: 1225-1241, 2001.

McMahon M et al. The anti-hepatitis B drug entecavir inhibits HIV-1 replication and selects HIV-1 variants resistant to antiretroviral drugs. Fourteenth Conference on Retroviruses and Opportunistic Infections, Los Angeles, abstract 136LB, 2007.

Mele et al. Hepatitis associated with hepatitis A superinfection in patients with chronic hepatitis C (http://content.nejm.org/cgi/content/short/338/24/1771) New England Journal of Medicine 338: 1771-1773, Jun 11, 1998.

Rey D, Krantz V, Partisani M et al. Increasing the number of hepatitis B injections augments anti-HBs response rate in HIV-infected patients. Effect on viral load. Vaccine 18: 1161-1165, 1998.

Shire NJ et al. The prevalence and significance of occult hepatitis B virus in a prospective cohort of HIV-infected patients. JAIDS 44(3): 309-314. 2007.

Smith PT et al. Comparison of the efficacy of Hepatitis A and Hepatitis B vaccination in HIV infected patients. XIV International AIDS Conference, Barcelona, abstract B3156, 2002.

Stubbe et al. Infection with GB Virus C in Patients with Chronic Liver Disease. Journal of Medical Virology 51: 175-18, 1997.

Torriani et al. Peginterferon Alfa-2a plus Ribavirin for Chronic Hepatitis C Virus Infection in HIV-Infected Patients New England Journal of Medicine 351: 438-450, 2004.

UKHCDO The impact of HIV on mortality rates in the complete UK haemophilia population. AIDS 18: 525-533, 2004.

University of Virginia (2001) see www.healthsystem.virginia.edu/internet/epinet/estimates.cfm

Vento et al. Fulminant hepatitis associated with hepatitis A virus superinfection in patients with chronic hepatitis C. New England Journal of Medicine 338: 286-290, 1998.

TB and HIV

Introduction

This year marks the 125th anniversary of the discovery of Mycobacterium tuberculosis (TB). In 1882, Robert Koch identified the bacterium while studying a sputum smear through a microscope. TB disease, however, has been a known scourge since the time of the Pharaohs, and has claimed many lives throughout history, including those of Franz Kafka, George Orwell and Eleanor Roosevelt.

During Europe's industrial revolution in the 1800s, TB was a leading killer, particularly among disadvantaged people living in cramped quarters with poor access to light, nutrition and clean water. Then came increased economic prosperity, public health improvements, widespread vaccination programmes, antibiotic treatments and, finally, isoniazid preventive therapy (IPT). Each of these helped make TB very much less prevalent in the industrialised world between 1940 and 1980.

This mid-twentieth century success may have led to complacency among public health experts and pharmaceutical researchers. Well into the 1980s, many thought TB could be completely eradicated, as smallpox had been, but with the onset of HIV and AIDS and the breakdown of health care systems, there was a worldwide resurgence of the deadly disease. TB takes two million lives a year, 99% of which are in the developing world. Today, TB is as much a threat as it was in the pre-antibiotic era.

Because tuberculosis continues to be a disease of the poor, striking where HIV is rife, there has usually been little outcry from its sufferers. The pharmaceutical industry has paid only scant attention and apparently sees little market incentive to develop new treatments. It may be because people have lived and died with TB since the beginning of human evolution that there has never been an urgent public and medical response, as there was when HIV was first identified in the 1980s.

Catalysed by the growing threat of multi-drug resistant (MDR) and extensively drug-resistant (XDR) TB, however, HIV and TB activists are belatedly joining forces to demand better TB control through integrated services and research into improved and novel TB technologies such as vaccines, diagnostics and drugs.

Tuberculosis - the facts

Transmission

Mycobacterium tuberculosis, the tuberculosis bacterium, is contagious and spread mainly through the air, in the same way as the common cold. Close contact with people who have infectious TB creates ideal conditions for its spread. Tuberculosis is not transmitted through a person's clothes, bed linen, cooking utensils or dishes.

Symptoms

Active TB infection is characterised by a persistent cough lasting for more than two weeks, shortness of breath, chest pain, night sweats, weight loss and fever. Greenish or yellow sputum or sputum containing blood are also symptoms of TB. Pulmonary tuberculosis can easily be confused with other diseases of the respiratory system.

Latent and active TB infection

Only one in ten people infected with *M. tuberculosis* will progress to the disease state, as a healthy immune system keeps the infection dormant. This is known as latent TB infection (LTBI). HIV has begun to affect the rate of active infections, however, because people with HIV are more vulnerable to infection. When people have weakened immune systems, latent bacteria in their lungs can begin to multiply and become an active TB infection, which can migrate to other parts of the body, such as the brain, kidneys or spine. This is known as disseminated or extra-pulmonary TB.

TB is a preventable and curable disease, but, if left untreated, all forms of TB are deadly. On average, a person with untreated pulmonary TB will infect ten to fifteen other people each year.

TB/HIV

It is imperative that people living with HIV and TB are identified at the earliest possible stage, because the risk of the TB becoming active increases by ten per cent per year in those with HIV. This represents a 50% greater risk than for those who are HIV-negative (WHO 2007a). People living with HIV and untreated TB have a 90% mortality rate (WHO 2007a) within a few months of TB infection. This makes TB a leading cause of death in people with HIV worldwide. The chances of developing

TB rise six-fold during the year following seroconversion and continue to increase as the CD4 count progressively declines. The majority of TB/HIV co-infection cases are in sub-Saharan Africa, where HIV has fanned the resurgence of TB. Some African countries have HIV/TB co-infection rates of 70%.

The dual epidemics of HIV and TB feed off each other: HIV is the highest risk factor for the transformation of latent into active TB, while TB fuels the progress of HIV infection in the body. TB progresses faster in people with HIV and presents earlier than other opportunistic infections. If diagnosed in time, though, TB in those with HIV is treatable with a variety of antibiotics, and this treatment can prolong life by at least two years.

However, the last new antibiotic class (the rifamycins) to be approved was discovered over 40 years ago. Over time, some strains of the TB bacterium have acquired resistance to one or more of the antibiotics used to treat the disease. These strains are known as multi-drug resistant TB (MDR-TB) and extensively-drug resistant TB (XDR-TB). These resistant strains are much more difficult and expensive to treat and are often fatal.

New tools for the diagnosis and treatment of TB are urgently needed. Diagnosis of TB in people with HIV cannot rely on standard microscopy alone - a more sensitive test is needed. Similarly, new TB drugs must address the interactions between TB drugs and the commonly used HIV treatment drugs. At present, these interactions (particularly those between protease inhibitors and the rifamycins) and the liver toxicity that HIV treatments can cause make treating TB and HIV at the same time somewhat problematic. In the past, TB and HIV have been treated separately, despite the overlapping nature of their epidemics. In some countries, such as Russia, a long-standing TB treatment establishment has found it difficult to integrate their services with a new HIV treatment service. More recently, there have been moves towards the integration of TB and HIV services, in an attempt to achieve significant gains in the control of both TB and HIV. New initiatives include offering counselling and voluntary HIV testing to TB patients, while actively screening HIV-positive patients for TB. Research shows that TB patients are more willing to accept HIV testing than the general population - so it is hoped that TB treatment programmes can become significant conduits for antiretroviral treatment.

The epidemiology of TB

Global

Some 8-10 million new cases of tuberculosis appear each year. A third of the world's population, two billion people, are infected with TB. The proportion is similar among the world's 40 million people living with HIV - a third of them have TB (WHO 2007a) - but the impact on them is disproportionately severe.

In 2004, according to WHO estimates, 80% of new TB cases occurred in Africa, South East Asia and the Western Pacific. People living with HIV accounted for 741,000 of those new TB infections. Deaths from TB were in keeping with the annual

average of almost two million per year, and there were 425,000 documented cases of MDR-TB in new or previously treated TB patients. Though most regions are seeing a decline in TB incidence of around 0.6% a year, *global* incidence is rising at 1%, due to 4% increases in Africa and eastern Europe.

Nine of the world's 22 high-TB burden African countries have HIV prevalence rates of at least four per cent. HIV, along with weak health systems, insufficient health staffing and human resources, and limited links between TB and HIV control, fuel the TB epidemic. Most worrying is the limited availability of drug resistance data from those regions, due to sub-standard laboratories.

The United Kingdom

Tuberculosis infection rates have risen steadily in England and Wales since the late 1980s (Rose 2002). The largest observed increase from the previous year was seen in 2005: overall, UK case numbers increased 11%, from 7,321 cases reported in 2004 to 8,113 in 2005 (14.7 per 100,000 population). The number of pulmonary cases increased by 7% and the number of extra-pulmonary by 17% (HPA 2006a).

Most of the UK's TB cases occur in large cities, with London accounting for most of these, at 43% of all reported cases in 2005 - 46.3 per 100,000 (HPA 2006b). This meets the WHO definition of a high tuberculosis incidence region. This rate is comparable to the average rate of TB incidence across all 53 countries of the WHO European region - which includes the former Soviet Union and Central Asia (Ditiu 2006).

The incidence of tuberculosis in the UK-born population remains low and is in slow but steady decline. However, TB in the UK's foreign-born population is on the rise, and reflects an increase in TB rates in migrants from high-TB-burdened regions such as Africa and South Asia. Indian, Pakistani, and Bangladeshi immigrants accounted for the highest number of *cases* - 2414 in 2005 - while the highest *rates* occurred in African immigrants - 399 per 100,000 (HPA 2006c). Only 22% of these foreign-born cases had arrived during the previous two years. This suggests that those immigrants with TB didn't necessarily acquire it in their country of origin. TB rates among UK-born ethnic minorities also continue to grow compared to the UK-born white population, either due to travel or to close contact with other infectious cases within the UK.

Those worst affected by tuberculosis are people who live in poverty and who also have other afflictions, such as homelessness, mental illness and/or injecting drug use. These are often incompatible with routine TB treatment, and can lead to an increased risk of MDR-TB and onward transmission. According to a 2004 TB and housing study, nearly one in 50 homeless people in London had TB - 25 times the national average (London Regional Public Health Group 2004).

Europe

In Central Europe and other established market economy regions, TB incidence represented only 1.7% of the global total in 2003. Even so, many countries in Europe have experienced a levelling off of TB rates, which were previously declining, that began in the 1980s. This was due to increased poverty, immigration and HIV - and to the failure to maintain the necessary public health infrastructure for TB control (Stop TB Partnership 2006-a).

In Europe, in 2005, an estimated 4.7% of those with TB were HIV-positive (Ditiu 2006). The proportion of HIV/TB co-infection is highest in Portugal and Spain, but has increased significantly in Estonia and Latvia. In other countries of the Balkans and Eastern Europe, HIV/TB co-infection levels remain below one per cent (Ditiu 2006).

Eastern Europe and Central Asia, however - the former Soviet countries - are experiencing a MDR-TB crisis. Patients in some of these regions are ten times more likely to have MDR-TB than are patients in the rest of the world, according to the WHO. Drug-resistant strains are stronger than in other regions, and are often resistant to first-line drugs and to some second-line drugs.

Prisons in the former Soviet Union have been a hotbed for the spread of both TB and MDR-TB, due to overcrowding, inadequate ventilation and malnutrition. TB incidence rates among prisoners are 50 times and mortality rates more than 28 times those in the general population. TB has spread through the region by piggybacking off the HIV epidemic since the 1990s, particularly among injecting drug users. An estimated 50-90% of all HIV cases in Eastern Europe and Central Asia are in intravenous drug users 2006b).

The resurgence of TB in Europe is attributed not just to HIV, however, but also to economic decline, for instance in the collapse of the Soviet Union and civil unrest in the Balkans and the Caucasus. Years of neglect have left many countries with out of date and ineffective, vertical TB control practices. Moreover, there is a lack of coordination between TB and HIV/AIDS control programmes and no clear strategy to address the IDU situation in the region.

Global targets

The devastation caused by TB in the context of the HIV pandemic, especially in sub-Saharan Africa and the former USSR, along with the spread of MDR-TB in large cities in the industrialised nations in the 1990s, motivated the World Health Organisation's global scale-up of TB control. In 1991, the World Health Assembly (WHA) declared TB a global health emergency and set targets of detecting 70% of the world's smear-positive TB cases and curing 85% of them by 2000 (WHO 1991c).

Additionally, WHO declared TB a global emergency in 1993 and in 1994-1995 launched DOTS, (Directly Observed Therapy, short course), a five-element strategy for diagnosis and treatment, which was adopted by countries in encouraging numbers. Nevertheless, progress in case detection was slow, and global targets were delayed to 2005, when, because of the African and Eastern European epidemics, these goals went unmet and are still substantially below the target.

The Stop TB Partnership, established to address the constraints of DOTS, put forth new goals in its Global Plan to Stop TB 2006-2015, calling for the halving of TB prevalence and deaths by 2015 compared with 1990 levels. The Plan serves to stimulate research and development into new tools such as diagnostics, drugs and vaccines. This is in line with the Millennium Development Goals (MDGs) to have halted and begun to reverse the incidence of TB by 2015.

The Partnership's ultimate goal is the elimination of TB as a public health problem by 2050. But critics say that the growing problems of MDR-TB and XDR-TB and the lack of collective political will from either the G8 or the high TB-burdened countries make this goal unrealistic. For example, a 2006 report by the US Treatment Action Group found that a mere $400 million was spent globally on new tools (diagnostics, vaccines and drugs) and operational research in 2005 (Feuer 2006). Compare this to the Global Plan's call for $9 billion to be spent on new tools research between 2006-2015.

Universal access

There has been a growing demand from the TB and HIV communities for universal access to integrated TB and HIV prevention, treatment, care and support. A groundswell of voices was prompted by the cluster of deaths from XDR-TB in 2005 in South Africa - the highest rates recorded thus far.

Specifically, the community emphasises the need for:

- Immediate and visible commitments to halt the spread of XDR-TB;

- Immediate financing to control for MDR and XDR-TB, and to accelerate the development of appropriate diagnostics and drugs;

- An increased investment in basic TB control programmes as the key to preventing the further spread of TB;

- The delivery of TB and HIV care and treatment in the context of fully functioning primary health care systems;

- A substantial investment of additional resources in accelerated research and development of new diagnostic, prevention and treatment technologies;

- The most vulnerable populations to be provided with TB and HIV services and to redress the social injustices that fuel the dual epidemics.

Diagnostics

Tests that detect TB bacteria

Sputum smear microscopy is the most widely used technique for diagnosing tuberculosis. This inexpensive and widely used method examines three sputum samples under a microscope over at least two days to assess whether they contain TB mycobacteria.

However, this method does not identify the majority of HIV-related TB cases. Many people with active TB do not have sufficient TB mycobacteria in their lungs for the sputum smear to detect the infection. This especially applies to those who are co-infected with HIV, who often have extra-pulmonary TB. In these cases, TB infection spreads out from the lungs into other tissues, leaving the sputum sample with too few bacteria to diagnose.

TB in children also goes undetected by sputum microscopy, because they are often unable to produce enough sputum for a reliable sample. In summary, this assay, which dates back to the 19th century, only detects around half of all TB cases.

A more sensitive method, even among HIV-infected people, is the culture test, which consists of incubating a sputum sample over a few weeks to see whether it contains live mycobacteria. A setback to the culture diagnostic is that it requires three to eight weeks to be sure no bacteria are present - time that patients and doctors faced with life or death decisions cannot afford to wait. Other tests, which use liquid media, can grow the bacteria more quickly - in twelve days or so. While these tests have far greater sensitivity, they are expensive and technically demanding. Neither test is available in resource-poor settings where the TB/HIV burden is high.

Despite the time and cost restraints of the different methods of culturing TB, such methods have another advantage in addition to their better diagnostic rates. This is that the results provide a drug-susceptibility profile, allowing the detection of drug resistance. Hence the push to implement liquid culture tests as a tool to detect and treat for first-line drug resistance. And on the horizon there are DNA amplification tests that may be able to identify drug resistance in minutes.

Additional methods of TB detection

In addition to tests that detect for TB bacteria there are two other methods for identifying TB infection: clinical examination based on symptoms and a measure of immune response to TB.

Clinical examination plus a symptom questionnaire is a useful initial screening step to TB detection, as many individuals with a cough that has lasted longer than three weeks turn out to have pulmonary TB.

The tuberculin skin test (TST), also called the Mantoux test, is an immune response test. TST is used to observe the skin's response to an injection of a mycobacterium-isolated protein, a **purified protein derivative** (PPD). A marked swelling (induration) in the skin will arise within two to three days if the person is infected with TB. A large induration indicates active TB infection.

However, those with HIV are much less likely to be reactive to PPD, and those who have been vaccinated with the bacille Calmette-Guérin (BCG) vaccination - which is most people in the world - often present false positives.

In PPD positive individuals, additional tests such as chest X-rays are needed to verify whether active disease is present. Unfortunately, the chest X-ray is equally variable in its ability to detect TB in those with HIV, because their TB bacteria are usually disseminated throughout the body.

Research

Because two-thirds of HIV-associated TB cases are either sputum smear-negative or extra-pulmonary, there is an urgent need for research into novel and improved tools to hasten the accurate diagnosis of these cases and those of MDR-TB and paediatric TB. The need for better diagnostics is even more pressing given the fact that tuberculosis is, for the most part, a curable disease.

As with TB treatment, the last few years have witnessed the creation of public-private partnerships, such as the Foundation for Innovative Diagnostics, to expedite research in TB diagnostics. However, basic science challenges persist as researchers struggle to understand the tuberculosis bacilli, to distinguish between latent and active TB and to identify markers that predict conversion from latent to active TB.

Currently, there are four diagnostics products that are poised to go or have gone into the demonstration phase - large-scale field studies. These include culture-based MDR assays, and one that can detect rifampicin resistance from sputum specimens without the need for culture, so that results are available in as little as two days, rather than several weeks. There are eight more products at different stages of development. Full availability, though, is anticipated to take at least five more years.

Treatment

Tuberculosis has been a curable disease since the discovery of combination antibiotic therapy in the 1950s. After screening for the bacteria, if patients are infected they should be given either prophylactic treatment to thwart the development of the disease, or a combination of antibiotic drugs if they already have an active infection. Effective treatment will be life extending, will quickly render the TB patient non-contagious and so subsequently prevent the further spread of the disease.

Antiretrovirals (ARVs) reduce the risk of active TB infection in those with HIV, but not enough to obviate the need for TB treatment. The medical management of HIV-related tuberculosis is complex. Challenges include overlapping side-effects, drug interactions, a high pill burden and poor drug absorption. However the biggest potential problem is Immune Response Inflammatory Syndrome (IRIS), in which sometimes-lethal manifestations of TB infection reappear in patients starting

ARVs because the immune system suddenly starts responding to the bacterium it was previously too weak to fight. For this reason, the question of whether to start TB and HIV treatment together or to delay HIV treatment until after the first phase of TB treatment requires fine judgement (see below for more), and it is recommended that the patient seeks an experienced health provider with expertise in treating both diseases.

First-line therapy

Curative treatment can take six to eight months for first-line therapy, and requires four drugs - rifampicin (R), isoniazid (H), pyrazinamide (Z), and ethambutol (E) - to be taken daily for two months. A continuation phase follows, with either four months of rifampicin/isoniazid (RH) or six months of ethambutol/isoniazid (EH). For convenience, treatment is available in combination tablets; the pill burden for this first-line treatment can be as high as eleven pills a day. Some ARVs are contraindicated with TB medications, particularly rifamycins taken with nevirapine (a first-line ARV) or ritonavir-boosted protease inhibitors (a standard in second-line ARV regimens). When taken with ARVs, rifamycins can lower ARV concentrations and promote drug resistance or toxicity. Rifampicin can also reduce the effectiveness of the contraceptive pill. WHO recommends treating for TB before starting on ARVs if the patient's CD4 count is above 350, in order to avoid harmful drug interactions. However, if patients have low CD4 counts (and the majority presenting for HIV and TB treatment in resource-poor settings do), then treatment for TB and HIV should start together. A South African study presented at the 2007 CROI meeting (Lawn 2007) found that mortality in patients with TB and HIV who did not receive ARV treatment was 50% in three months and the benefits of co-treatment far outweighed the risks, with deaths from TB in those not receiving ARVs more than 30 times more common than deaths due to IRIS in those who did receive ARVs.

Second-line therapy

TB strains that are resistant to both rifampicin (R) and isoniazid (H) are considered multi-drug resistant. These strains arise from inadequate supplies or improper use of first-line therapy, and require second-line drugs to treat and cure. The two most important drug classes used to treat MDR-TB, the aminoglycosides and fluoroquinolones, are less effective than first-line drugs, and must be taken for at least 18-24 months. They are highly toxic, often require hospitalisation, and are extremely expensive, sometimes as much as 300 times more expensive than a treatment course for ordinary TB.

Adherence

In order to ensure treatment success, medication must be taken until all the mycobacteria are dead. The patient's symptoms may be alleviated within two-three weeks of starting treatment, and they may need encouragement to see the treatment through to the end, in order to prevent drug resistance developing and/or further spread of the bacteria.

The WHO recommends DOTS - Directly Observed Treatment, short course - to ensure adherence and thorough treatment. This strategy has the patient take his/her pills in the presence of a health care worker or a community volunteer who can supervise the therapy. Although DOTS cures 95% of TB cases, critics say that the DOTS model puts considerable strain on patients, who often have to travel a long distance every day for several months to receive treatment. An alternative approach that is gaining popularity is to encourage the patients to take responsibility for their own treatment through education and counselling. This is similar to the flexible approaches adopted for other chronic diseases.

Immune reconstitution syndrome

IRIS presents as a temporary exacerbation of TB symptoms, or as radiographic manifestations of TB, after HIV treatment with ARVs is initiated. This mysterious phenomenon, which can be lethal, is thought to be the result of immune reconstitution as a consequence of effective antiretroviral therapy while still in the presence of high levels of TB. In one South African study (Lawn 2005), 23% of patients starting ARVs and TB treatment together showed some evidence of IRIS; rates observed elsewhere have varied from eight per cent to 45%. Symptoms may be treated with nonsteroidal or steroidal anti-inflammatory agents, of which the most frequently used is prednisolone.

Prophylactic therapy

After ruling out the presence of active TB, isoniazid preventive therapy (IPT) can be helpful in preventing its onset in people with HIV infection, reducing risk by up to 62% in those who test PPD positive and by 36% overall. Benefits from IPT may wane, however, after one to two years in high TB prevalence settings (Chaisson 2007). IPT is helpful when people still have robust immunity and their TB is likely to be latent, but not after they have already developed active TB.

The risk that drug resistance will develop from the use of IPT appears to be very low. For patients who have pre-existing isoniazid-resistant latent TB infection, rifampin may be substituted as preventive therapy. There's no evidence of increased toxicity when taking both IPT and ARVs. No preventive therapy has been shown to be effective for MDR- or XDR-TB, but new agents are currently being screened (Chaisson 2007).

Research

TB presents challenges today that were unforeseeable 40 years ago when the last class of antibiotics (rifamycins) was discovered. Improved and novel drugs are needed: firstly, to decrease the pill burden on patients; secondly, that can be taken concurrently with ARVs without risk of side-effects; and thirdly, to treat MDR-TB and paediatric TB.

The resurgence of worldwide TB on the back of the HIV pandemic has sparked a renewed commitment to look for more efficient drugs to combat the disease. The beginning of the millennium saw the creation of public-private partnerships, such as the Global Alliance for TB Drug Development, which hoped to accelerate research. There are currently 30 drugs targeting TB in development, of which six are in clinical trials. Two

fluoroquinolone drugs, moxifoxacin and gatifloxacin, are in late-stage clinical trials, and researchers are hoping they may be able to shorten the course of TB therapy to two months. Both are already market-approved and sold worldwide as broad-spectrum antibiotics.

Other drugs such as diarylquinolone (TMC207) and nitroimidazole are still in early-phase testing; they hold promise for use in first-line and MDR-TB treatment. Optimism around these candidates is tempered by the fact that these new agents need to be effective and safe enough to be added to the standard four-drug therapy, which achieves cure rates of 95% - a tall order. It's anticipated that the next approved drug won't be available for at least five years.

Nutrition

New research demonstrates that nutrition is a vital component in the management of TB. If a patient is underweight or does not experience significant weight gain while on treatment, the relapse rate of TB is much higher than it is in well-nourished TB patients (Khan 2006).

Generally, the body needs extra energy to control TB. A varied diet will ensure the patient gets all the nutrients the body needs. Alcohol should be avoided; it's high in calories but offers no nutrients. It's also hard on the liver, especially when taken alongside isoniazid, pyrazinamide, or rifampicin.

It is best to choose foods high in protein, such as meat, poultry, fish, milk, and dried beans, peas and lentils. (When taking isoniazid, some cheeses and fish may cause itchy skin, headaches and light-headedness.) The following nutrients are also recommended: vitamin B6 pyridoxine, vitamin A, vitamin C, iron, protein and calcium.

Vaccines

BCG

The bacille Calmette-Guérin (BCG) vaccine, named for its discoverers Albert Calmette and Camille Guérin in 1921, is one of the globe's most widely administered vaccines, with roughly 100 million doses given to children each year (Treatment Action Group 2006). It is created from a strain of weakened bovine tuberculosis and given to newborns to induce an immune response against meningitis and disseminated TB, not primary infection. Although efficacy rates vary between zero and 75%, depending on geography, any protective effect of BCG typically diminishes within 10-15 years or during adolescence, and does not prevent the reactivation of latent pulmonary infection.

In low-TB prevalence settings, such as the USA, BCG vaccination is not standard practice. Also, children known to have HIV should not be BCG vaccinated.

Research

Improved TB vaccines are seen as a key to global TB control, but even with advances in mycobacterial immunology and genomics stimulating research into the discovery of new TB vaccines, it is unlikely that one will be available for routine use in the near future. Questions remain - for instance, regarding host immunity to TB and the identification of TB genes and antigens. This absence of basic science knowledge is considered a paradoxical result of the BCG vaccine's effectiveness: there was a lack of investment in new research because BCG was considered an appropriate response to the epidemic.

Because a third of the world is infected with TB, in order to control the disease a therapeutic vaccine that would work against latent TB is essential. This means that a successful strategy would not focus on neonates or the use of BCG alone, but would require post-exposure vaccines that could be taken concurrently with TB medication to reduce the duration of treatment.

Currently, there are four vaccines in early phase research, including recombinant BCG vaccines, a recombinant protein and a heat-killed *M. vaccae* and a vaccinia virus - the latter two vaccines are being studied as possible post-exposure vaccines.

Drug-resistant TB

Multi-drug resistant tuberculosis (MDR-TB)

Drug-resistant TB is a form of TB that does not respond to one of the standard treatments using first-line drugs. Multi-drug resistant (MDR) TB is defined as TB strains that are resistant to first-line drugs rifampin and isoniazid. MDR-TB is a serious global health problem threatening TB control everywhere, but particularly in Eastern Europe, Central Asia and increasingly in Africa. Because of globalisation, wealthy countries are not impervious to MDR-TB's reach.

According to the latest estimates, ten per cent of all new TB infections are resistant to at least one anti-TB drug. Each year, 420,000 new cases of MDR-TB, with 116,000 deaths, are detected (Zignol 2006). Mortality rates among MDR-TB cases are nearly 50%. WHO estimates that less than two per cent of the world's annual MDR-TB cases are treated according to WHO guidelines (Stop TB Partnership 2006), meaning that MDR-TB is a death sentence for many people.

By far the highest rates of MDR-TB are seen in Russia and the former Soviet countries, where over six per cent of newly diagnosed TB is MDR, with a maximum of 14% in Kazakhstan and Estonia. In few other countries of the world does MDR as a proportion of newly-diagnosed TB form more than 3% of cases: exceptions are China, Iran, Myanmar, Mozambique, Côte d'Ivoire, Peru and Ecuador (Ditiu).

Similarly, Russia and some former Soviet countries see the highest rates of MDR-TB amongst previously treated patients, due to suboptimal therapy. Countries of the world where more than 40% of previously treated patients have MDR-TB include Russia, Kazakhstan, Uzbekistan and Lithuania but also include Iran and Oman. Countries where 20-40% of previously-treated patients have MDR-TB range from China and Thailand through Egypt to Mexico and even include Italy; sub-Saharan Africa has relatively low rates of MDR-TB in previously treated patients, only because treatment is less available or because HIV co-infected patients die too soon for MDR-TB to become established.

There are two origins of MDR-TB: transmission from one person to another and, more commonly, when a person's own TB develops resistance because of suboptimal treatment. This can happen in various ways: when patients are not properly supported to complete their regimens; when patients are prescribed the wrong treatment, the wrong dose, or prescribed treatment for too short a period of time; when the drug supply is inconsistent; or when the drugs are of poor quality. Summarily, drug resistance arises in places with poor TB control programmes. But even in the best of circumstances there's a risk of resistance developing, because the 40 year-old anti-TB drugs are losing their potency.

Diagnostics

Diagnosing MDR-TB requires even more sophisticated technology than is needed for drug-sensitive TB. The only way to diagnose drug-resistant TB is to culture the bacteria, but many labs, particularly in resource-poor settings, don't have the necessary equipment or the trained personnel.

Treatment

Second-line TB drugs used to treat MDR-TB must be taken for at least 18- 24 months, are an estimated 100 times more expensive than first-line therapy and are less effective. The treatments are toxic, causing a range of serous side-effects including hepatitis, depression, hallucinations and dizziness. Often the patient needs to be hospitalised in isolation for long periods of time. Moreover, supplies of second-line drugs can be erratic.

Research

Researchers are pursuing treatment that requires fewer months on therapy in a bid to boost adherence and consequently prevent future drug resistance developing. They're also pursuing drugs that act in new ways against TB, to avoid cross-resistance, and others that won't interfere with ARVs.

Extensively drug-resistant tuberculosis (XDR-TB)

XDR-TB has emerged worldwide as a threat to public health and TB control, raising concerns of a future epidemic of untreatable TB.

XDR-TB occurs when resistance to second-line drugs develops. This is MDR-TB plus resistance to the fluoroquinolone drugs and resistance to at least one of the injectable drugs - amikacin, kanamycin and capreomycin.

XDR-TB cases have been confirmed worldwide, including all G8 countries. The exact distribution is unknown and it's not certain, though it's likely, whether XDR-TB is more common in countries with MDR-TB, or whether it is a sporadic phenomenon linked to suboptimal treatment anywhere. In March of 2006, the problem of XDR was first defined by the Centers for Disease Control (CDC) and the World Health Organization (WHO). They found that two per cent of MDR-TB isolates were XDR; an additional survey showed that in some places perhaps as many as 19% of MDR-TB cases were in fact XDR-TB (Wright 2006). It is estimated that each year there are some 27,000 cases of XDR-TB, with 16,000 deaths (Zignol 2006). XDR-TB has been around for years; it's only since the ramping up of drug-resistance surveillance worldwide that cases are being reported in greater numbers.

As with MDR-TB, there are two causes of XDR-TB: transmission from one person to another, and, more commonly, a person's own MDR-TB developing further resistance because of suboptimal treatment. And, again as with MDR-TB, this can happen for a number of reasons: when patients are not properly supported to complete their regimens; when patients are prescribed the wrong treatment, the wrong dose, or prescribed treatment for too short a period of time; when the drug supply is inconsistent; or when the drugs are of poor quality.

As with drug-sensitive TB, 90% of people infected with XDR-TB never develop the disease. People with HIV infection are more likely to fall ill, but overall, the chances of being infected with XDR-TB are even lower than they are for drug-susceptible TB, because cases of XDR-TB are more rare. For people with HIV, ARV treatments are likely to reduce the risk of XDR-TB, as they do for drug-sensitive TB.

A person diagnosed with drug-sensitive TB can avoid getting XDR-TB by following their prescribed drug regimen exactly. No doses should be missed, especially in intermittent treatment, where drugs are to be taken every other day. Treatment should always be taken through to the end. If a patient is suffering from side-effects, it is best to inform their health worker to find a solution.

Because XDR-TB is resistant to first- and second-line drugs, it is extremely difficult to treat, and consequently has high mortality rates; however, in countries with good TB control programmes, 50-60% cure rates are possible. Successful treatment of XDR-TB requires that all six classes of second-line drugs are available to clinicians with expertise in XDR-TB treatment.

XDR-TB has exposed weaknesses in the globe's TB control programmes, which lack laboratory capacity to monitor drug resistance. To evaluate for drug resistance, bacteria needs to be cultivated and tested in a laboratory, which can take 6-16 weeks. Most African countries cannot carry out first- or second-line resistance testing in order to diagnose and treat XDR-TB properly. Consequently, WHO is currently developing a strategic plan to scale up laboratory monitoring; however, there is still a need for the development of international standards for drug-sensitivity testing.

Infection control

Another fault-line exposed by XDR-TB is the lack of infection control in most developing countries. There is a need for adequate control, such as proper ventilation and minimizing contact with other patients, particularly those with HIV, in every health facility that sees TB patients or those suspected to have TB. All national TB programmes should follow International Standards for TB Care. (see www.who.int/tb/publications/2006/istc/en/index)

In 2005, in Kwazulu-Natal, South Africa, the largest outbreak in the history of XDR-TB infection, which killed 52 out of the 53 individuals, raised issues of enforced quarantine and coercive treatment. Public health discourse posits that this will not result in a useful response from the general public. Instead, an effective management system must be put in place for drug-resistant disease. However, the WHO points out that there are rare circumstances in which quarantine must be enforced. See WHO guidance on human rights and involuntary detention for XDR-TB control at www.who.int/tb/xdr/involuntary_treatment/en/index.

Research

Research is imperative to controlling XDR-TB. Improved rapid diagnostics and new drugs to replace the long course of toxic medications for XDR-TB are in the pipeline. It is unlikely that the BCG vaccine works against XDR-TB; therefore a new vaccine is urgently needed.

Growing alarm at XDR-TB's global reach is a wake-up call for greater support for basic TB and HIV care, prevention and control. XDR-TB also underlines the need for better management of MDR-TB, as the majority of XDR-TB is likely to be found in those countries that have high levels of MDR-TB.

References

Chaisson R. *TB prevention for HIV patients: priorities and ongoing research efforts.* Available at http://www.stoptb.org/wg/tb_hiv/assets/documents/Chaisson_CROI2007.ppt.

Ditiu L. *Tuberculosis: a global problem.* Presentation to the Stop TB Partnership, Milan, 23 March 2006.

Feuer et al. *Tuberculosis research & development: a critical analysis, October 2006.* Available at http://www.aidsinfonyc.org/tag/tbhiv/tbrandd2.html#toc

Health Protection Agency - a. *Tuberculosis rates by site of disease (pulmonary vs. extra-pulmonary), England, Wales and Northern Ireland, 2000 - 2005* see http://www.hpa.org.uk/infections/topics_az/tb/epidemiology/figures/figure11.htm

Health Protection Agency-b. *Tuberculosis case reports and rates (per 100,000 population) by region/country, England, Wales and Northern Ireland, 2000 - 2005, 2006.* Available at http://www.hpa.org.uk/infections/topics_az/tb/epidemiology/table15.htm

Health Protection Agency-c. *Focus on tuberculosis, annual surveillance report 2006-England, Wales and Northern Ireland.* 14-21, 2006.

Khan A et al. *Lack of weight gain and relapse risk in a large tuberculosis treatment trial.* American Journal of Respiratory and Critical Care Medicine, 18 May 2006

Lawn S et al. *Immune reconstitution disease associated with mycobacterial infections in HIV-infected individuals receiving antiretrovirals.* Lancet Infectious Diseases 5(6):361-373. 2005.

Lawn S et al. *Early mortality among patients with HIV-associated TB in Africa: implications for the time to initiate ART.* Fourteenth Conference on Retroviruses and Opportunistic Infections, Los Angeles, abstract 81, 2007.

London Regional Public Health Group et al. *TB and housing-meeting the needs of homeless & 'hard to treat' TB patients in London 2004.* Available at http://www.crisis.org.uk/page.builder/researchbank.html

Rose AM, Gatto AJ, Watson JM. *Recent increases in tuberculosis notifications in England and Wales - real or artefact?* J Public Health Med;24:136-7, 2002.

Stop TB Partnership-a. *The Global Plan to Stop TB 2006-2015:* 106, 2006.

Stop TB Partnership-b. *The Global Plan to Stop TB 2006-2015: 91,* 2006.

Stop TB Partnership. *The global plan to stop TB 2006-2015.* Geneva, World Health Organization, 2006 (WHO/HTM/STB/2006.35); http://www.stoptb.org/globalplan/

Treatment Action Group. *What's in the Pipeline: New HIV Drugs, Vaccines, Microbicides, HCV and TB Therapies in Clinical Trials.* August 2006. See http://www.aidsinfonyc.org/tag/tagline/pipeline2006.pdf

World Health Organization-a. *Tuberculosis: Frequently asked questions about TB and HIV,* 2007. Available at http://www.who.int/tb/hiv/faq/en/index.html

World Health Organization-b. *WHO Report 2006: global tuberculosis control, surveillance, planning, financing.* Geneva, WHO (WHO/HTM/TB/2006.362).

World Health Organization-c. *44th* World Health Assembly: Resolution and decision resolution WHA 44.8. Geneva, World Health Organization, 1991.

Wright A et al. *Emergence of Mycobacterium tuberculosis with extensive resistance to second-line drugs - worldwide, 2000-2004.* Morbidity and Mortality Weekly Report 55(11):301-5, 2006.

Zignol M, Hosseini MS, Wright A, Weezenbeek CL, Nunn P, Watt CJ, Williams BG, Dye C. *Global incidence of multidrug-resistant tuberculosis.* J Infect Dis 194:479-85, 2006.

HIV and Black African Communities in the UK

An Overview

There are estimated to be more than 15,750 African people living with diagnosed infection in the UK.[1] In addition several thousand more African people living in the UK have undiagnosed HIV infection since studies have shown that roughly 2/3 of African people in the UK have never tested for HIV.[2] In 2004, the prevalence of previously undiagnosed HIV infection remained highest among heterosexuals born in sub-Saharan Africa (3.8%, 190/4973), in comparison, the prevalence of previously undiagnosed HIV infection was 0.2% (140/59,508) among heterosexuals born in the UK.[3]

African people with HIV have significant ongoing difficulties in the following areas: income, immigration status, housing and living conditions, and access to training, skills and job opportunities. Difficulties in meeting these basic needs clearly lead to reduced quality of life. They have significant and ongoing difficulties associated with anxiety and depression, their ability to sleep, their self-confidence and their personal relationships.[4]

Social exclusion is undoubtedly exacerbated by factors associated with migration. It is likely that a significant proportion of African people with HIV in the UK are (or have been in the past) refugees or asylum seekers, a group already significantly socially excluded.[5] Exclusion associated with being HIV-positive may be significantly compounded by pre-existing social exclusion and social need associated with being an African refugee or asylum seeker.[6]

In order to survive and thrive, refugees and asylum seekers needs to draw on their own personal resources (their ability to work for example) and need to draw on a supportive social environment in their host country. This environment is created first by the support of expatriate communities in the host country as well as in their home country and second by the provision of supportive enabling legislation, policy and services by the host country. African people with HIV are likely to have all of these resources particularly curtailed.[7]

Despite a relatively long history of the epidemic in sub Saharan Africa, HIV remains significantly stigmatised among African communities in the UK and globally.[8,9] Expatriate, diasporic and global African networks play an important role in the survival of African migrants in the UK.[10] However the disclosure of an HIV-positive identity often leads to the withdrawal of vital community support. Thus, African people with HIV in the UK are less able to disclose to and draw support from their family and expatriate communities. Stigma at a community level leads to difficulties in even the most intimate relationships. Sigma Research found that 15% of African people living with HIV had not disclosed their status to their partners and only a third of respondents had disclosed their HIV status to their children or their families.[11] A London study of HIV-positive gay men (mostly white) and black African heterosexual men and women showed that there are striking differences, by ethnicity, in the extent to which people told their family, friends and partners that they have HIV. African men and women in particular may require support in disclosing their HIV status.[12]

The policy of dispersing asylum seekers away from large urban environments often means that those living with HIV are moved away from specialist HIV treatment and care centres as well as being moved to a setting where support and contact within expatriate groups is unlikely. Home Office changes to immigration policy and the recent decision by the Law Lords on May 5th 2005 also mean that a person with HIV who is on treatment will be unlikely to be granted leave to remain on medical grounds under humanitarian protection provisions.[13] If that person is granted discretionary leave to remain it will only be for three years.

In addition to this, changes made earlier this year to the provision of NHS services for overseas visitors impose strict limitations on access to hospital care for non-residents and those whose asylum applications have failed. Broadly speaking, this means that while short term visitors, including students, and failed asylum seekers will be allowed to access HIV testing and other STI screening, long-term treatment for infection will not be provided unless it is paid for privately or via Accident & Emergency.[14]

In short, the current social, legal and policy environment in the UK is not geared towards maximising the health and productivity of African people with HIV.

References

1   A Complex Picture - HIV and other Sexually Transmitted Infections in the United Kingdom: Health Protection Agency, November 2006

2   HIV testing and high risk sexual behaviour among London's migrant African communities: a participatory research study. Sex Transm Infect. 78: 241-245, 2002.

3   A Complex Picture - HIV and other Sexually Transmitted Infections in the United Kingdom: Health Protection Agency, November 2006

4   Project Nasah : an investigation into the HIV treatment information and other needs of African people with HIV resident in England. Sigma Research, 2003

5   All Party Parliamentary Group on AIDS (2003). Migration and HIV: Improving Lives in Britain. An Inquiry into the Impact of the UK, Nationality and Immigration System on People Living with HIV.

6   Refugee Council (2004b), Hungry and homeless: the impact of the withdrawal of state support on asylum seekers, refugee communities and the voluntary sector, London, Refugee Council.

7   Supporting People with HIV: Research into the housing and related support needs of people with HIV in Nottingham City, Sigma Research, March 2006

8   Bhatt C (1995) Primary & secondary HIV prevention issues for African communities. London, HIV Project & New River Health Promotion Department (out of print).

9   Goldin CS. Stigmatization and AIDS - critical issues in public health. Social Science & Medicine, 39(9): 1359-1366, 1994.

10 Outsider status: stigma and discrimination experienced by Gay men and African people with HIV.   Sigma Research, 2004

11 Project Nasah : an investigation into the HIV treatment information and other needs of African people with HIV resident in England. Sigma Research, 2003

12 Disclosing your HIV status: the role of ethnicity among people living with HIV in London, City University, Jonathan Elford, 2006

13 N v. Secretary of State for the Home Department, Int J Refugee Law.2005; 17: 593-629

14 New Developments in Sexual Health and HIV/AIDS Policy, Government response to the Health Select Committee's Third Report of Session 2004-2005

Social and demographic characteristics of the UK Black African population

Black Africans constituted 0.8% of the total population and 10.5% of the ethnic minority population in the 2001 Census - making them the fifth largest ethnic minority group in the UK.[1]

Black Africans were also the fastest growing ethnic minority group, having more than doubled in size between 1991 and 2001.[2]

The Black African grouping is one of the most diverse in terms of country of origin with 34% born in the UK, 16% in Nigeria, 10% in Ghana, 4% in Zimbabwe, 3% in Uganda and the remainder in other African states.[3]

There has been a long history of small-scale migration from Sub-Saharan African nations with Somali sailors settling in Britain in the late nineteenth century and Black African communities forming in the major British seaports. Unsurprisingly in such heterogeneous group, there were a range of factors driving migration. In the post-independence period the number of people travelling to Britain for education and technical training increased as the demand for skills and education could not be met locally. This continues to be a driving force in migration today but economic pressures and political persecution also drive people to travel to Britain. From the 1960s onwards, political instability in various African nations including Kenya, Uganda and Malawi has contributed to increased migration to Britain. More recent conflicts such as those in Rwanda, Sudan and the Democratic Republic of Congo have also led to migration from Africa.[4]

Black Africans are often highly qualified academically but they suffer high levels of unemployment. According to the 2001 census, 27% of Africans had 'higher level qualifications' compared to just 14% in the whole population. However, in 2001/2, around one in seven Black African men was unemployed (15%) compared with 5% of white British men.[5]

Black Africans recorded the lowest proportion of self-employment (as a percentage of all in employment), compared to other ethnic groups, at 6.7% (in 2001/2).

Nigerians and Ghanaians form the two largest communities within the Black African group. Nigerians in the UK are mainly from the Yoruba and Ibo tribes. Most Ghanaians in the UK are from the Ashanti, Fanti, Ga or Ewe tribes.

However, significant numbers have arrived from Somalia, Uganda, Ethiopia, Zimbabwe and the Democratic Republic of Congo in recent years, seeking asylum.

Somalia was the third most frequent country of origin for people seeking asylum in the UK in the second quarter of 2004.[6]

Somalia has existed without a government for more than 15 years, since the former Somali President, Mohammed Siad Barre, was ousted in the civil war of 1991. Since then, the country has experienced a refugee crisis due to complex inter ethnic rivalries, clan warfare and famine.[7]

Zimbabwe was the fourth most frequent country of origin for people seeking asylum in the UK in the second quarter of 2004. The country is currently going through tremendous economic crisis, severe food shortages and violent land reform.[8]

Black Africans speak English and/or African tribal languages from their place of origin, such as Yoruba (Nigeria) and Twi (Ghana). However, those communities which are more recently established in the UK and/or have come to the UK seeking asylum may have lower levels of fluency in English.[9]

A mix of religions is practised within the community, varying by country. According to the 2001 Census, 69% of Black Africans are Christian and 20% Muslim. Only two per cent had no religion. Muslim Black Africans are mainly from North and West Africa, particularly Somalia and Nigeria. For all communities, places of worship were a focus of social gatherings and networking, particularly the Ugandan, Nigerian and Ghanaian communities. For these communities, the church is the focus of a range of activities including social and educational events. Among the predominately Somali community, places of worship themselves were not used for non-religions activities, but the occasion of worship was used for meeting outside and in nearby cafes.[10]

Around three quarters (78%) of Black Africans live in London.

Black Africans form more than 10% of the population of Southwark, Newham, Lambeth and Hackney.

There are large Somali communities in London (particularly Haringay and Hackney) and Manchester, but Cardiff has the oldest and the largest British-born Somali population in the UK.[11]

Africans also reside in growing numbers in the following areas

The North

- Newcastle
- Liverpool
- Manchester
- Leeds
- Bradford
- Sheffield
- Doncaster

Midlands

- Nottingham
- Wolverhampton
- Coventry
- Birmingham
- Stoke-on-Trent

Hertfordshire

- St. Albans
- Milton Keynes

Bedfordshire

- Luton

The West

- Bristol
- Oxford
- Swindon

The South

- Brighton & Hove
- Reading
- Slough
- Southampton

East

- Cambridge
- Southend-on-Sea
- Essex

The Black African community in the UK has a younger age profile than that of Black Caribbean, with 30% aged under 16 years (compared with 20% of Black Caribbean) and 2% aged 65 years and over (compared with 11% of Black Caribbean).[12]

Almost half of Black African households include dependent children (48%), which is lower than the figures for South Asian households, but higher than for other ethnic minority groups.

The lowest proportion of children in workless households is in the Indian communities, at only 8.8%. 28.8% of Black Caribbean children live in workless households, compared to 14.1% of white children. The ethnic group with the highest proportion of children in workless households is the Black African group, at 40.6%.[13]

The African identity tends to vary across generations, similar to other ethnic groups:[14]

- Older generations, and those forced to leave their family and friends, attach a great deal of importance to their African backgrounds, often have very strong ties with their hometowns and may regard themselves as temporary residents despite having lived in the UK for many years.

- The younger generation are generally much more integrated into London/British culture. They tend to describe themselves as 'British-born Nigerian', 'British-born African' and so on, and they may feel they have more in common with other British young people than with their parents' culture.

Men and women were considered by community representatives to have different experiences of migration, access to services, employment, education, family roles, and adapting to life in the UK[15]:

- in some cases, women are thought to have gained greater independence and economic freedom with increased employment and education opportunities and access to welfare benefits. There is a view that women find it easier to obtain employment then men, partly due to the greater discrimination experienced by men; and partly due to the types of jobs available to people without qualifications being in occupations associated with women, for example low paid care or cleaning based occupations which men were not used to having to accept.

- On the other hand women are more isolated and have less access to employment due to family responsibilities (particularly Somali women), language barriers or lack of qualifications. There was a concern that employed women carry a double burden of responsibility as chief carer and wage earner.

- whilst there is evidence of men with highly skilled jobs, there were also reports that men found it very hard to find employment, which reflected their skills, or enabled them to support their families. As a consequence men suffer from loss of status and depression or had to juggle several different full and part-time jobs.

References

1 Focus on People and Migration, Office for National Statistics, 2004

2 The Growth and Decline of Cities and Regions and Minority Ethnic Groups in Britain, Ruth Lupton et al, CASE-Brookings Census Brief, November 2004

3 People Living in Britain, The Black African Group, Commission for Racial Equality, 2007

4 Ibid

5 Office for National Statistics. Census, April 2001.

6 Ethnic Research Network, Twenty interesting facts about the Black African Community in the UK, Winter 2005

7, 8, 9, 10, 11 bid

12 Engaging marginalized communities: Communication Guide, The National Centre for Languages, Frequently asked questions

13 Rising workless households threaten child poverty aim, Paul Bivand, Centre for Economic and Social Inclusion, Labour Market Analysis: Working Brief, September 2005

14 Ethnic Research Network, Twenty interesting facts about the Black African Community in the UK, Winter 2005

15 Needs and Gaps within services to Asylum Seekers and Refugees, Refugee/Asylum Seeker Core Group, South London and Maudsley Trust, April 24, 2001

Epidemiology of HIV infection the UK amongst Black Africans in the UK

The global HIV pandemic continues to worsen particularly in African countries with strong links to the UK. At the end of 2005 - according to revised UN estimates over 38.6 million people were living with HIV.[1] Two-thirds of them are Commonwealth citizens. 8 out of 19 Commonwealth countries in sub-Saharan Africa have HIV/AIDS adult prevalence rates above 10%.[2] Significantly, while Black Africans made up 0.8% of the population in the 2001 census, in 2005 they accounted for two thirds of all new cases reported, however more of these cases are now being contracted within the UK. The number of reports of HIV-infected black Africans who contracted their infection in the UK increased from 43 in 2000 to 182 in 2005.[3]

There are over 3500 HIV diagnoses per year among black Africans (approx 22 000 total)

- Almost two thirds are women

- About one third have been in the UK less than two years

- 90% acquired heterosexually, majority in Africa

- 7% through sex between men (Sigma)

- around 100 children (<15 years) 97% infected through mother to child transmission

- >10% present late (with AIDS symptoms)

- TB most important AIDS defining illness

Since 1999, there have been more diagnoses in heterosexual men and women each year than MSM. Most heterosexual infections diagnosed in the UK were probably acquired in Africa. This accounts consistently for about 75% of new diagnoses in heterosexual men and women each year.[4] Infections acquired in the UK consistently accounts for about 10% of new diagnoses in each year. As the overall numbers rise, so do the numbers in each of these categories.

Ethnicity information became better reported in 2000 due to a change in surveillance methods. There is a marked difference between the "MSM epidemic" and the "heterosexual epidemic" in the UK. Between 2000 and 2003, the four years where ethnicity has been reported - over 85% of MSM are white, over 70% of heterosexual men are black African and over 80% of heterosexual women are black African. The proportion of HIV infections diagnosed in the UK among black Africans has increased from 24% (376 of 1598) in 1996 to 58% (3323 of 5732) of all newly reported HIV infections in the UK, for which ethnicity was recorded, in 2003; these continue to be diagnoses of infections that were predominately acquired abroad.[5]

New diagnoses in the UK from an exposure to HIV in Africa show complex trends over time. Early influences from Eastern Africa include many infections from Uganda. More recently infections from South East Africa have become more influential, with infections from Zimbabwe continuing at high levels. Diagnoses of infections acquired in other regions of Africa continue to rise more gradually.[6]

Many heterosexuals are diagnosed late in the course of their infection - particularly men. A CD4 count of 200 is considered to be AIDS defining in the USA. Although this is not part of the UK definition of AIDS a CD4 count of this level is indication of later stage immunosuppression and the threshold by which antiretroviral therapy should have been started.[7] Heterosexual men are consistently diagnosed at a later stage of infection (around half at a CD4 count of 200 or less) than heterosexual women who in turn are consistently diagnosed at a later stage of infection than men who have sex with men.

After the introduction of HAART (Highly Active Antiretroviral therapy), the majority of AIDS cases diagnosed were in those recently diagnosed with HIV, i.e. individuals diagnosed late in the course of HIV disease. In heterosexual men and women AIDS diagnoses are increasing. (TB plays a large part in these figures). According to the HPA report *A Complex Picture* (2006): "*Two in five (40%) black or ethnic minority (BME) adults were diagnosed late and they were seven times more likely to die within a year of their HIV diagnosis than those with higher CD4 counts (3% compared to 0.4%).*"

It is not possible to measure the numbers who are currently living with diagnosed HIV in the UK from the new diagnoses figures, although it is estimated that around 15,750 Africans living with diagnosed HIV currently reside in the UK - 21% undiagnosed.[8] The mobility and age of those most affected and the long duration of HIV infection mean that people may have left the country or may have died and not been reported.

Every year a survey to measure the numbers currently living with HIV is carried out (SOPHID = Survey of Prevalent HIV Infections Diagnosed) and gives the best estimate of the current picture. SOPHID figures show that the numbers living with diagnosed HIV in England, Wales and Northern Ireland have more than tripled between 1996 and 2005. Breaking down the numbers from the SOPHID survey by ethnicity. White ethnicities make up the largest numbers of individuals living with HIV (50% of the total in 2005) and black African ethnicities are the second most affected group (39% of the total in 2005) The proportion and numbers of black Africans among the total living with HIV has increased.

In total there were thought to be about 63,500 adults living with HIV at the end of 2005 with a third (20,100) who remained unaware of their infection.[9] There are likely to be more than 4000 African men and women in the UK who are unaware of their HIV infection.

References

1 UNAIDS/WHO AIDS Epidemic Update: December 2006

2 AIDS in the Commonwealth, Commonwealth Secretariat, United Nations Statistics Division, 2005

3 A Complex Picture, Health Protection Agency, 2006

4 Ibid

5 A Complex Picture, Health Protection Agency, 2006

6 Africans and HIV in the UK: An epidemiological perspective May 2006, Health Protection Agency

7 BHIVA guidelines for TB/HIV infection - February 2005

8 A Complex Picture, Health Protection Agency, 2006

9 Ibid

Socio-economic issues for Africans living with HIV

Studies have found that many HIV-positive black Africans faced major social issues related to immigration, housing, employment, and income. As a result, HIV was only one of many issues and it was not necessarily the most important. Treatment issues were a lower priority than practical day-to-day living concerns, such as housing and having enough money to buy food and clothing. The largest differential between African and white British people with HIV was the extent to which [basic] practical needs were problematic[1]. Being a woman, especially a mother, and being a migrant were at least as important as HIV status in shaping the lives of HIV-positive African women in London[2].

The NASAH and PADARE project both showed that the respondents were well qualified, with almost all respondents having some qualifications and about one-half with college or university education. However, the numbers in employment were low (less than 20%), with almost one-half unemployed and registered for benefits. Most respondents in both studies thus had limited access to economic resources, and poverty characterised their lives, despite their high educational levels.[3] This trend was also noted among African women with HIV in London. Similarly, the SHIBAH project found that fewer than 20% of respondents were employed for over 10 hours per week.[4] The Access All Areas study findings were similar, with 80% of respondents educated to degree level or above, but only 22% in some form of employment or voluntary work.[5]

Compared to other people with HIV in the UK Black African people living with HIV in the UK are:[6]

- Ten times more likely to experience problems getting enough money to live on

- seven times more likely to report problems with their living conditions

- three times more likely to report problems with discrimination

- and twice as likely to report problems with getting about (mobility) and personal relationships

Both the Nasah and PADARE projects clearly conveyed that the main problem for Africans living with HIV was 'getting enough money to live on'. Similarly, Project Nasah's second briefing sheet on the needs of African people living with HIV reports that 'poverty dominates the lives of Africans living with HIV in England': having enough money to live on was cited as a major concern by 77% of respondents. Increasing access to employment must be a high priority area for interventions with Africans living with HIV.

Many HIV-positive migrants may be of working age and well educated but unable to find work because of their immigration status. In London, the NASAH and PADARE studies have demonstrated that less than 20% of black Africans living with HIV are employed, despite being well qualified. Similarly, only one fifth of the 124 respondents in the SHIBAH study were in paid employment. Since July 2002, asylum seekers are not allowed to work until they are granted either refugee or humanitarian status.[7] When destitute, they are entirely dependent on NASS for financial support. However, many African migrants would prefer to support themselves and use their skills rather than rather than being supported.[8]

'Routes into Work', rub by Positive Futures, enabled 29% of its clients to find employment. However, only 6% of African men found employment as a result of the intervention. Positive Futures deduced that African clients did not see the immediate benefits from such services because of immigration problems and institutionalised racism in the job market.[9]

References

1 Project Nasah, Sigma Research, Weatherburn et al. 2003

2 My Heart is Loaded, African women with HIV surviving in London, Dr Jane Anderson Centre for Infectious Diseases, Barts and The London, 2005

3 Chinouya, M. and Davidson, O. (2003).The PADARE project: Assessing the health related knowledge, attitudes and behaviours of HIV-positive African Accessing Services In North Central London. African HIV Policy Network: London.

4 Health First: Chinouya, M., Ssanyu-Sseruma, W., Kwok, A. (2005). The SHIBAH Report: A Study of Sexual Health Issues Affecting Black Africans Living with HIV in Lambeth, Southwark, and Lewisham. Health First: London.

5 Positive Futures. (2002). Access All Areas: A Study of the Accessibility of Positive Futures Services for people from Black and Ethnic Minorities. London.

6 Project Nasah, Sigma Research, Weatherburn et al. 2003

7 The Nationality, Immigration and Asylum Act 2002: changes to the asylum system in the UK, Refugee Council, December 2002.

8 Chinouya, M., Reynolds, R. (2001). HIV Prevention and African Communities Living in England: A Framework for Action. National AIDS Trust: London.

9 Positive Futures. (2002). Access All Areas: A Study of the Accessibility of Positive Futures Services for people from Black and Ethnic Minorities. London.

Stigma and discrimination

Fear of discrimination may have a more detrimental effect on the health and well being of HIV-positive people in the UK than actual discrimination.[1] However, research suggests that one in 10 HIV-positive people in the UK have experienced prejudice and discrimination from neighbours, and for African people with HIV the figure is higher.[2]

Black African people in the UK are rendered significantly less powerful than other groups by a range of factors. Social and institutional racism are compounded by anti-asylum discourses and practices (these include media representations, legislation, political processes and policy), which collectively demonise African people as a potential threat. Central to these discourses and practices is the notion that Black African people have the capacity to spread disease and to drain state resources. These notions find strength in the fact that an HIV epidemic exists in Africa and that a significant proportion of African people entering the UK are HIV-positive.[3]

African people with HIV find themselves stigmatised not only within broader British society (for being Black, African, an asylum seeker and having HIV), but also within African populations in the UK, not only because they are suspected of being promiscuous, or a bad parent, or gay, but also because they are a 'Black African with HIV in Britain'. This is seen as living proof that the overarching racism and xenophobia are 'justified', and in the eyes of fellow Africans, those with HIV are portrayed as denigrating the reputation of the entire community. Africans describe that the most painful form of rejection came from their own family and friends. Stigma classically works in this way, making a powerless community turn on itself rather than trying to gain power.[4]

Black African people with HIV have great disincentives to be open about HIV in society at large, but even more so among their own African networks because such a disclosure will result in almost certain rejection from what is sometimes a sole source of support. Therefore, many feel that they must keep their HIV status a secret. The problem is that this causes severe personal stress and often means that they cannot access social (and sometimes clinical) services. Thus, such stigma has a direct, highly detrimental effect on the health of African people with HIV.[5]

Many black African communities regularly describe discriminatory practices in NHS and social service settings.[6] Such practices served as a further disincentive to access the services needed by Black African people living with HIV.

Finally, African people with HIV find the area of work highly problematic. Those who are not legally allowed to work are open to the exploitative practices of the illegal labor market. The presence of a chronic or acute illness such as HIV can only increase their vulnerability. Those who can work are deterred from doing so because they do not feel free to disclose their HIV status to employers. This is because first, they feel powerless to resist the possible discrimination that might result, and second because they feel that they have little control of that information once it is revealed. In closed migrant groups, control of such information is paramount. As a consequence many do not seek work, or else they seek illegal or menial work for which they are overqualified because it does not demand disclosure.[7]

References

1 Sick with worry: Prejudice haunts people with HIV, The Guardian, Raekha Prasad, Wednesday November 28, 2001

2 Prejudice, Discrimination and HIV - A Report, Terrence Higgins Trust, Policy Campaigns and Research Division, November 2001

3 Outsider status: stigma and discrimination experienced by gay men and African people with HIV, Dodds, Catherine et al, Sigma Research, 2004

4,5 ibid

6 Elford J et al. *Discrimination experienced by people living with HIV*. HIV Med 7 (supplement 1), abstract P93, 2006.

7 Outsider status: stigma and discrimination experienced by gay men and African people with HIV, Dodds, Catherine et al, Sigma Research, 2004

Testing

An unlinked and anonymous seroprevalence survey undertaken among heterosexual attendees at seven GUM clinics in London in 1999 and 2000 found that one in 16 woman and one in 33 men born in sub-Saharan Africa were infected with HIV. Thirty-nine per cent of those that were HIV-positive remained undiagnosed after the visit.

Similarly, Mayisha II found that two-thirds of black Africans living with HIV in England were undiagnosed. High levels of undiagnosed HIV infection and, frequently, late diagnosis following longstanding HIV infection, make a powerful case for interventions emphasising the benefits of early testing.

Fear of stigma and discrimination are preventing Africans in the United Kingdom from testing for HIV, according to the finding from Mayisha II.[1] Although investigators found that a high proportion of individuals participating in the study were willing to undergo anonymous oral HIV testing, they also established that almost half of all individuals had never had an HIV test, and that a significant number of individuals participating in the study had undiagnosed HIV infection.

In interviews researchers asked individuals about their attitudes to HIV and reasons for not having an HIV test.[2] Some individuals said that they feared a positive HIV test would jeopardise their right to remain in the UK. HIV was frequently associated with "immorality" and sexual "misbehaviour" and there was a fear of rejection, retribution or reprisals from family members or the wider community. A study on 'pathways to HIV testing' found that only 28% of black Africans surveyed thought they might be HIV-positive before diagnosis (versus 41% of white patients), indicating that black Africans often do not suspect their status.

Encouraging innovative approaches to VCT promotion is a priority for primary and secondary HIV prevention interventions with black African communities.[3] African adults residing in the UK often present with a different clinical spectrum to non- Africans: co-infection with Tuberculosis and late presentation to HIV services, often at the onset of symptoms from AIDS-related illnesses, are frequent. Moreover, African adults often discover their status at a more advanced stage of disease progression and with lower CD4 counts at diagnosis. These factors put considerable incentive on developing interventions encouraging early testing.[4]

Research shows that poor access to services and strained relationships with healthcare providers are factors that lead many Africans in the UK to present late for HIV care.[5] While many positive Africans are diagnosed in Genitourinary Medicine (GUM) clinics, a sizeable proportion also learn their status as hospital in-patients following an AIDS related illness: Project

Nasah, a survey of 435 HIV-positive Africans showed that, while the majority of respondents had been diagnosed in GUM clinics, 38% were diagnosed as hospital in-patients, and 5% through general practice. One study suggests that black African patients see general practitioners as an important source of information on HIV/AIDS, highlighting the potential for making information about VCT or VCT services themselves more readily available through primary care.[6]

References

1 MAYISHA II Collaborative Group (2005). Mayisha II Main Study Report: Assessing the feasibility and acceptability of community based prevalence surveys of HIV among black Africans in England. Health Protection Agency Centre for Infections: London.

2 Elam G et al. *Barriers to voluntary confidential HIV testing among African men and women in England: results from the Mayisha II community-based survey of sexual attitudes and lifestyles among Africans in England*. HIV Med 7 (supplement 1), abstract 028, 2006.

3 Del Amo, J. et al. (1996b). Spectrum of disease in Africans with AIDS in London. AIDS 10(13): 1563-1569.

4 Ibid

5 Erwin, J., Morgan, M., Britten, N., Gray, K., Peters, B. (2002). Pathways to HIV testing and care by black African and white patients in London. Sexually Transmitted Infections 78(1): 37-39.

6 McMunn A., Mwanje, R., Pozniak, A.L. (1997). Issues facing Africans in London with HIV infection. Genitourinary Medicine 73(3): 157-158.

Disclosure

Stigma and discrimination obstruct disclosure and discourage people from accessing healthcare, social care, or applying for work, thereby contributing to the social exclusion of people living with HIV. African respondents interviewed by Sigma research reported numerous experiences of racism and discrimination while living in the UK; stigmatising attitudes from doctors and healthcare staff, and HIV-related stigma within black African communities. Fear of stigma can lead to persons living with HIV refraining from disclosing their status to sexual partners, children, friends, and to the broader community. It also can lead people to conceal their needs for social and emotional support, and delaying access to medical treatments. In the broader community stigma is compounded by immediate social networks and within the family.[1]

Many HIV-positive people feel unable to access community and social support groups because of the fear of disclosing their HIV status. For many Africans living with HIV it might be difficult to manage disclosure if they live in very close-knit communities, and may feel that they lack control over 'who knows' their HIV status. Stigma may thus lead some persons to isolate themselves from potential support networks for fear of unintentional disclosure. Black Africans testing for HIV at a London hospital were found to be twice more likely than white people to be worried about future discrimination if they tested positive, and four times more likely to be worried about meeting someone they knew at the clinic. Concern with stigma and discrimination explains why many positive African resolve to keep their serostatus secret.

Black Africans are significantly less likely than white patients to disclose their HIV status to family and friends. Africans are concerned that the 'social cost' of knowing one's status, whether intentional or not, can be larger because of the potential loss of inclusion from both the majority population and from the smaller ethnic communities. Some studies show that positive Africans are more likely to disclose their status to close friends and to their GPs than to family.[2] A recent study of white gay man and Black African heterosexuals in London showed striking differences, by ethnicity, in the extent to which people told their family, friends and partners that they have HIV. African men and women in particular may require support in disclosing their HIV status.[3]

References

■ Sigma Research (2004). Outsider status - Stigma and discrimination experienced by Gay men and African people with HIV, London, Sigma

■ McMunn, A, Mwanje, R., Paine K, Pozniak, A.L. (1998). Health service utilization in London's African migrant communities: implications for HIV prevention.AIDS Care 10(4): 453-462.

■ HIV and AIDS in African communities: A framework for better prevention and care, Department of Health, African HIV Policy Network, National AIDS Trust, 20 December 2004

Prevention

Sexual attitudes, knowledge and behaviour of HIV-positive Africans

To date there are no estimates of HIV prevalence linked to sexual behaviour in a community sample of Africans in the UK. What we know primarily comes from four reports, including the Padare study and the Shibah report, and the largest sample from Mayisha I and II.

The PADARE study surveyed 214 black Africans with HIV in London, the majority of who were born in Zimbabwe, Uganda, Zambia and Congo. Only 3% were born in the UK.

The Sexual Health Issues of Black Africans with HIV (SHIBAH) Project consisted of a survey of 124 HIV-positive black Africans in Lambeth, Southwark and Lewisham and in-depth interviews with 20 survey respondents.

Mayisha I and II: **Mayisha I** surveyed 748 migrants from five sub-SaharanAfrican communities (Congo, Kenya, Uganda, Zambia, Zimbabwe)resident in London.[1] The information collected included data on demographic characteristics, utilisation ofsexual health services, HIV testing history, sexual behaviour,and attitudes. **Mayisha II** included a survey of sexual attitudes and lifestyles of 1,500 Black African men and women aged 16 years and over recruited from social and commercial venues in London, Luton and the West Midlands using a brief, validated, self-completion questionnaire.

Studies on sexual behaviour among ethnic minority groups in the UK found that many black Africans had low self-perceived risk, and, consequently, low condom use.

Similarly, in the SHIBAH survey, 56% of black Africans living with HIV 'always' used condoms, 33% 'sometimes', and 10% 'never'. PADARE, SHIBAH, and Mayisha I found relatively low levels of sexual health knowledge among black Africans surveyed in London. The PADARE study, in particular, revealed important knowledge gaps: 16% of the participants felt they could be cured of HIV in the UK, while 8% thought an undetectable viral load meant they could not pass on the infection to anyone else. In Mayisha I, over 90% of the men and women surveyed strongly agreed with the statement 'I think I could convince a new sexual partner to use a condom, even if they did not want to use one'. In both Mayisha I and PADARE, a majority of participants reported the intention to use condoms with new partners, but few actually did: while the majority of 214 positive black African respondents in PADARE had had sex in the last four weeks, 40% reported using a condom only on some or on no occasions, and 29% had had unprotected sex. In Mayisha II, only 49.2% of men and 38.7% of women who answered the question about condom use reported using a condom the last time they had sex. These findings indicate relatively low condom use, which is related to the acceptability of condoms and their conflicting link to protection and promiscuity. The condom is seen as a symbol of protection among black Africans in the UK. Yet there is evidence that the use of condoms is still perceived by many as indicating a lack of trust between partners. In Mayisha II for example, the majority of respondents felt that condom use was not appropriate or necessary in long-term relationships, and implied partner distrust.

Levels of condom use and confidence in communicating with partners about sexual health must be understood within the broader context of relationships, and as linked to issues of trust, fidelity, and the desire for children.[2] Serial monogamy is 'the expected pattern among Africans women', who view multiple partnering as 'physically and emotionally risky'. The majority of black African respondents in the study thought that sexual relationships should be based on fidelity, trust, and stable partnerships. Trust and faithfulness are also seen as key values by the respondents of Mayisha II, views that are often underpinned by strong religious beliefs.

References

1   Fenton, K. A., Chinouya M, Davidson, O., Copas .A., MAYISHA study team. (2002). HIV testing and high risk sexual behaviour London's migrant African communities: a participatory research study. Sexually Transmitted Infections 78: 241-245.

2   Elam, G., Fenton, K., Johnson, A., Nazroo, J., & Ritchie, J. (1999). Exploring ethnicity and sexual health: A qualitative study of sexual attitudes and lifestyles of five ethnic minority communities in Camden & Islington. London: University College London.

Relationships

The PADARE study showed that casual relationships are frequent among young black Africans in the UK, with 22% of both men and women reporting that their most recent partner was a casual one. PADARE also found that black Africans had partners among people of Caribbean origin, whites, and other black British people. Recent evidence shows that heterosexual HIV transmission is occurring within the UK among people infected in West Africa.[1] However, more research needs to be carried out in order to better understand patterns of sexual mixing and the potential risk of HIV transmission, both within black African groups and between different ethnic groups.

Several interventions in the UK have sought to empower black African men and women to negotiate safer sex with their partners. However, HIV-related stigma remains a major barrier to open discussions about sexual health. As noted in PADARE and Mayisha II, emotions and the desire to seem 'trustworthy' play an important role in sexual decision-making, and sometimes override concerns about health. In some contexts, the 'imperatives' of relationships take precedence over awareness of the benefits of HIV testing.

There were also fears that questioning a partner's HIV status in the context of a new relationship might be interpreted as distrust. Respondents often assumed that a partner's potential risk was easily identified, and that risk could be avoided by carefully choosing one's partners. This was linked to notions of 'safe' and 'unsafe' identities; studies show that a partner's potential risk could be 'weighed up' by considering their previous sexual history, marital status, and cultural or educational background. However sex in relationships often preceded discussions about previous sexual history, and partners tended to reduce their use of condoms as the duration and intimacy of relationships increased.

A joint report from the National AIDS Trust, the African HIV Policy Network, and the Department of Health highlights the 'predominance of traditional attitudes towards sexual relationships and behaviours' among African communities in the UK.[2] Culturally patterned attitudes towards sexual behaviour may create gender role prescriptions that limit women's agency in negotiating safer sex, foster expectations of monogamy and fidelity, and raise issues of secrecy around sex or particular sexual practices.[3] The ways in which people learn about sex are culturally mediated: In many African families, sexual matters are seldom discussed between parents and children, and that, instead, other relatives or peers may be more active in giving information about sex and sexual health. Interventions with people of sub-Saharan African origin living with HIV therefore need to take into account culturally defined attitudes towards sexual behaviour and sex education.

In Mayisha II sexual health was seen by respondents as an important issue, with around two-fifths of men and women having ever attended a sexual health clinic. Half of female respondents and 43% of the men reported that they had ever had a voluntary confidential HIV test - the majority of which were within the past five years. Respondents' accounts indicated the importance of community outreach work and HIV awareness raising events as key factors in motivating them to take a voluntary HIV test, but fear of stigmatisation or deportation and expectations of HIV as a 'death sentence' continue to deter others from taking the test. Feelings about condom use were mixed. Around half of those that responded had used a condom the last time they had sex, but respondents tended to agree that condom use was not appropriate or necessary in long term relationships - condom use implying lack of trust in such situations.

References

1   Dougan, S., Patel, B., Tosswill, J.H., Sinka, K. (2005). Diagnoses of HIV-1 and HIV-2 in England, Wales, and Northern Ireland associated with West Africa. Sexually Transmitted Infections 81: 338-341.

2   Department of Health, African HIV Policy Network, National AIDS Trust. (2004). HIV and AIDS in African Communities: A Framework for Better Prevention and Care. London.

3   Chinouya Mudari, M., O'Brien, M. (2005). AIDS and African Childhood in London. The Paradox of African Traditions and Modern concerns on Childhood. London.

Prevention for African communities nationally

In 1997, the Department of Health (DoH), through Enfield & Haringey Health Authority, commissioned several HIV primary prevention interventions in England and Wales to address known and undiagnosed HIV infection in relatively recently arrived African populations. In October 2001, the DoH entrusted the African HIV Policy Network, an African led organisation, with the management of the project (www.ahpn.org). The National African HIV Prevention Programme, or NAHIP as it has come to be known, commenced formally with the appointment of Project Manager. An advisory group made up of professionals from health promotion, research, policy, community groups, epidemiology, behavioural science and the DoH assists in the strategic management of the programme.

In June 2003 NAHIP began developing a multi-agency collaborative health promotion network to deliver national HIV interventions. Voluntary organisations with experience in HIV prevention and health promotion with African communities were asked to submit statements of interest in order to form a working partnership with NAHIP. Ten organisations were recruited

through a selection process overseen by the NAHIP Advisory group and have since been working together to produce a range of resources to be used in HIV prevention campaigns. For further information and to download resources visit the NAHIP website: www.nahip.org.uk.

A key HIV prevention resource produced by NAHIP was the 'Doing it well' handbook.   The handbook provides a framework on how to conduct individual, group and community level health promotion interventions with and for African communities in England.   Other projects implemented by NAHIP include an Audit of HIV Resources Targeting Africans in the UK, and skills and training course, for those involved in HIV prevention, anti-stigma initiatives as well as care and support.[1]

Reference

1   National African HIV Prevention Programme: Pulle, S., Lubega, J., Davidson, O. & Chinouya, M. (2005). Doing It Well: A good practice guide for choosing and implementing community-based HIV prevention interventions with African communities in England. London.

African HIV Framework

In response to the increase in reported HIV prevalence amongst African populations, the Department of Health (DoH), National AIDS Trust (NAT) and the AHPN developed a Framework for Better Prevention and Care for African Communities (2001), which was then later published in 2005. The African Framework supported the National Sexual Health and HIV Strategy, the Commissioning Toolkit and the White Paper, Choosing Health. The African Framework was also a response to the DoH's National Sexual Health and HIV Strategy, which calls for a national strategic approach to the response to HIV.

The work also came out of a growing sense among African HIV community organizations that a national approach to HIV prevention and care was critically important. Until now, there has been very little that defines and describes the national issues in relation to HIV prevention and care needs for African communities. There is a growing body of excellent local work, or work focusing on specific subpopulations, but the ability for us all to look at the pertinent needs and issues across England was hampered by an absence of strategy. The Department of Health has committed itself to producing a second edition of the Framework, taking account of further research and the input of African communities and providers by the end of 2006.

Diagnosis and treatment

Both the NASAH and PADARE surveys showed that over one-half of participants had been diagnosed in the UK less than 3 years ago. Whilst there is evidence that black Africans present later with HIV, this may be attributable to their not being in the UK rather than to problems accessing health care in the UK. Diagnosis in the UK may not be their first diagnosis. Sigma Research found that 21% of respondents were probably first diagnosed with HIV prior to residence in the UK, although reports identify a lower figure of 7% among black African women.[1] Additionally, three-quarters of Africans newly diagnosed with HIV in London visited their GP in the two years before their HIV was detected, often with symptoms suggestive of HIV infection.

Investigators from 15 HIV treatment centres in London conducted a survey between 2004 and early 2006 involving 236 Africans who had been recently diagnosed with HIV. They were asked about their use of primary care in the two years before their HIV diagnosis.

HIV testing was mentioned to 16% of individuals by their GP. A GP mentioning an HIV test was a powerful incentive for testing, with 55% of individuals recommended a test attending for one. What's more, 56% of all individuals said that they would have attended for an HIV test if their GP had told them that they were at risk of the infection.[2]

A previous HIV test was reported by a third of individuals, and a third of these said that this test had been in the UK. The investigators calculated that 20% of Africans recently diagnosed with HIV had been infected with the virus since their arrival in the UK.

Reactions to diagnosis were largely similar to those reported for other groups of HIV-positive people, with an initial period of shock often followed by confusion, social withdrawal and depression. However, the NASAH study found that major depression was more common among African than white people with HIV, a finding possibly related to the often difficult socio-economic circumstances of the former. African women frequently reported anxiety and uncertainty. Despite major depression being more common among African than white people with HIV, with HIV. Black Africans were almost three times less likely to be referred to a specialist mental health unit in London.[3] Individuals of African origin have also been shown to be less likely to be referred by health advisors for psychological assessment, in part because they do not discuss their HIV-related distress unless questions are asked. There is evidence that an HIV diagnosis is particularly stressful for those African people in the UK who have uncertain immigration status. It is also clear from the research evidence that many had experienced AIDS in Africa where treatment availability has been limited and the death rate remains high.[4] For the many Africans who have experienced HIV in Africa, or indeed for those whose immigration status was not clear, positive test results represented a death sentence. As a result, they view their immigration status and continued residence in the UK as a matter of life and death. Respondents in all studies showed that they were active participants in the management of their health.

In all the above studies, between two-thirds and three-quarters had taken anti-HIV treatment at some point. Other methods used to manage health included nutrition, religion and use of complementary therapies.

Reference

1   Weatherburn, P., Ssanyu-Seruma, W. & Hickson, F. (2003) Project NASAH: An investigation into the HIV treatment, information and other needs of African people with HIV resident in England. Sigma Research, NAM Publications, National AIDS Trust and African HIV Policy Network.

2   Burns F et al. *Could primary care be doing more?* HIV Med 7 (Supplement 1), abstract 029, 2006.

3   Are we meeting the psychological needs of Black African HIV-positive individuals in London? Controlled study of referrals to a psychological medicine unit, AIDS Care. 2001 Aug;13(4):413-9

4   The psychosocial and health care needs of HIV-positive people in the United Kingdom: a review, G Green and R Smith, Department of Health and Human Sciences, University of Essex, Colchester, UK

Treatment

Project *Nasah* recruited over 400 black Africans with HIV in the UK to investigate their HIV treatment information and other needs. A total of 435 people were interviewed for the study, their age and sex being representative of the demographics of the African HIV community in the UK. Interviewees were recruited by African interviewers through peer networks in London, Greater Manchester, West Yorkshire and Oxfordshire.

Anti-HIV therapy was currently being taken by 73% of the sample, with people reporting that they were unemployed, off sick or retired most likely to report use of HAART.

Eight times as many HIV-positive Africans living in the UK have problems with knowledge about their HIV treatments than HIV-positive white British, but are nevertheless just as likely to adhere to treatment. Although 36% reported problems with adherence in *Nasah*, this was comparable to the 31% of the *What do you need?* sample, largely made up of gay men.

Although the majority of people interviewed in the *Nasah* study said that they had had no problems obtaining HIV treatment information in the last year, 27% did report difficulties and this figure is eight times greater than the white British sample in *What do you need?* 36% said that they were dissatisfied with their knowledge of treatments. One in seven Africans said they did not know enough about the medication they were taking currently, and 32% indicated that they felt unsure that they knew all they should.   A recent HIV diagnosis may explain the larger proportion of Africans who reported difficulties or said they needed to know more about treatments.

Areas of knowledge felt to be most lacking were:

- Lipodystrophy (63% not satisfied or unsure they knew enough)

- Clinical trials (65%)

- Side-effects of treatment (38%)

- Illnesses related to HIV (37%)

- Resistance (38%)

- Looking after children (37%)

- Pregnancy and HIV (35%)

Treatment information interventions

Talking with medical staff was overwhelmingly judged by Africans to be the method that had been most important to them in finding out about anti-HIV treatments - 63% reported it to be the most important method, compared to 11% who cited talking to other people with HIV, and 6% who reported talking to workers from HIV organisations as the most important method.

Forty one per cent said that they always understood what medical staff told them, and 56% said that they 'usually' understood. Three per cent never understood what they were told, and 16% of current treatment takers never told their clinician that they had missed doses although the relationship with medical staff emerged clearly as the most important source of information for Africans. Oral sources had been thought to be the most important source of treatment information, but *Nasah* found that over 90% had read treatment newsletters or leaflets in the past year, 86% had found them an important learning tool and 74% wanted to access them in the future.

In addition, nearly two-third of the sample reported wanting to read more about treatments. Nor did stigma or fear of disclosure of health status appear to deter people from having HIV information in their homes, with 86% saying that they took HIV treatment information home with them from the clinic and 27% reporting a subscription to an HIV treatments newsletter.

Immigration and migration and HIV for African communities

The relatively rapid rise in HIV infections in the UK comes at a time when the Government is under increasing public pressure to reduce the number of asylum seekers and migrants coming into the country, on the grounds that they are overburdening the education, health and social welfare infrastructure.[1]

References
1   Migration, public health and compulsory screening for TB and HIV, IPPR, Richard Coker, November 2003

What is a refugee?

- An asylum seeker is someone who has submitted a claim for asylum and is awaiting a decision from the home office

- A refugee is someone who has been accepted to stay in the UK under the Geneva Convention and given leave to remain in the UK for four years. After that period an individual can apply for settled status. They can also request reunion with a spouse and any children less than 18 years of age. Under the terms of the 1951 Geneva Convention, a refugee is defined as any person who "owing to well-founded fear of being persecuted for reasons of race, religion, nationality, membership of a particular social group or political opinion, is outside the country of his nationality and is unable or, owing to such fear, is unwilling to return to it."

- Someone who is given indefinite leave to remain in the UK is given permanent residence in Britain indefinitely. Family reunion is only permitted if the individual is able to support their family and will not rely on public funding to do so.

The belief that most asylum seekers come to Britain for welfare benefits is at odds with the fact that many are highly skilled and previously enjoyed a high standard of living.[1] Many pay the equivalent of several thousand pounds to a trafficker to reach a place of potential asylum. The skills of health professionals, teachers, and other workers could benefit Britain, but it is difficult for their experience and qualifications to be recognised. Much social research has shown that black African people are among the most highly educated social groups in the UK.

Some Africans moved to the UK for the purpose of career development or study, and many others have done so as a result of persecution, illness, civil conflict, insecurity, genocide and poverty. So for many there is no real option to return 'home' and most describe their existence in the UK as one of necessity rather than choice.

There is evidence of fear that an HIV-positive status would be detrimental to asylum application[2]. A particularly vulnerable migrant group affected by HIV are those who have been forced to leave their country of origin. According to the British Medical Association, 'Health care for asylum seekers in Britain is patchy, belated and often inappropriate'[3]. There are problems with access to health care, including difficulty in finding a GP, problems related to not speaking English, lack of cultural sensitivity, high levels of mental health difficulties, and disrupted social support. More specifically, asylum seekers may have witnessed or experienced physical and/or sexual violence. As such many Africans may find it difficult to establish working relationships with service providers, as their belief in the world as a safe place has been shattered and trusting relationships are therefore very difficult to form. Adherence to treatment may thus be threatened.

References
1   Asylum seekers and refugees in Britain: What brings asylum seekers to the United Kingdom? Angela Burnett, *senior medical examiner* and Michael Peel, *senior*

medical examiner Medical Foundation for the Care of Victims of Torture, BMJ. 2001 February 24; 322(7284): 485-488.

2   Atrill R, Kinniburgh J, Power L. Social Exclusion and HIV. London, Terrence Higgins Trust 2001.

3   Asylum seekers and health: A British Medical Association and Medical Foundation for the Care of the Victims of Torture dossier October 2001

Treatment tourism

There is little evidence that migrants come to the UK specifically to seek treatment for HIV/AIDS, which the media has termed 'treatment tourism'. The Terrence Higgins Trust and the George House Trust examined the records of 60 recent service users from three agencies in South London, Manchester and the West Midlands, and noted that only 13 of 60 migrants had sought asylum, while 12 had come to study.[1] The most common time span between entry and diagnosis was ten to twelve months, and 75% of migrants waited more than 9 months after entry to test. The most common reason given for testing was the onset of symptomatic HIV, with many falling severely ill before diagnosis. As many migrants do not suspect their status, it appears extremely unlikely that they arrive in Europe with a view to seeking medical treatment for HIV/AIDS. A recent study demonstrated a correlation between HIV presentation in the UK, migration, and political upheaval in African countries: an increase in the number of persons presenting with HIV during or following periods of political conflict was demonstrable for Ugandans, Congolese, Rwandans, Somalians, and Ethiopians.[2]

On the other hand, few people from countries with high HIV prevalence and low levels of conflict, such as Botswana, presented in the UK. This confirms the link between political conflict, migration and HIV. It also goes some way to show that 'health tourism', i.e. relocation for the purpose of gaining access to HIV services, is not the driving force behind recent African migration to the UK.

1   *Footnote from witness:* "Recent Migrants using HIV Services in England", Terrence Higgins Trust and George House Trust, 2003.

2   Forsyth, S., Burns, F., French, P. (2005). Conflict and changing patterns of migration from Africa: the impact on HIV services in London, UK. AIDS 19: 635-637.

Migration policy and HIV

Section 55

Although the National Strategy for HIV and Sexual Health and HIV (NSSHH) identifies asylum seekers as 'a group at special risk' in need of information and advice on sexual health, at a broad level asylum seekers face a number of barriers when accessing health care. Difficulties in accessing health care attributable to asylum seeker status are in part related to the regulations imposed under Section 55 of the Immigration and Asylum Act enforced as from 8 January 2003[1]. This Section denies the right to claim asylum to individuals who do not apply 'as soon as is practicably possible' - a regulation which has the potential to leave asylum seekers destitute, which is a particularly dangerous position for those who are HIV-positive[2]. All those who manage to claim asylum within the stated time are transferred to 'induction centres' for up to a week. From these centres, which are under the management of the National Asylum Support Service (NASS), they are sent to either a known address or to detention centres, whilst their claims are processed.

The government has announced a reversal of its policy of denying asylum seekers practical support unless they make their claim as 'soon as is reasonably practicable'. The decision comes after the government lost its appeal against High Court rulings in the cases of three asylum seekers in May 2004. The appellants argued that Section 55 breached asylum seekers human rights. The Government is currently considering an appeal to the House of Lords[3].

References

1 The Exclusion of Failed Asylum Seekers from Free NHS Care; A Policy Analysis and Impact Assessment, Robert Harris, International Health BSc Dissertation, April 2005

2 H. Weston, NAZ Project, unpublished report.

3 Destitution by design: Withdrawal of support from in-country asylum applicants: An impact assessment for London, Greater London Authoruty, February 2004

Detention

The British Medical Association expressed concerns that conditions in detention centres were inappropriate for the long-term health needs of asylum seekers and refugees.[1] The All-Party Parliamentary Group on AIDS (APPGA) received evidence that conditions inside NASS-run centres were inappropriate for those living with HIV. There were no specialist HIV services. Detention could actively prevent individuals from adhering to their HAART regimes. For instance, some antiretroviral drugs should be taken with food, but administration of drugs in detention centres was not necessarily in conjunction with meals, so individuals were prevented from adhering to their HAART regimes. They had little privacy for storing and taking complex medication, and levels of financial support could prevent the purchase of appropriate healthy food or transport to HIV treatment and care clinics. The APPG recommended that 'the government should not place individuals with HIV in detention or removal centres for immigration purposes, where it is not possible to provide suitable Medical care. Detention can undermine efforts to maintain good health'.[2]

References

1 Safe from harm? Health and social care for vulnerable refugees and asylum seekers, Refugee Council conferences Supported by the King's Fund and the Social Care Institute for Excellence Regent's College, London , 1 November 2006

2 APPGA, Migration and HIV: Improving Lives in Britain. An Inquiry into the Impact of the UK Nationality and Immigration System on People Living with HIV, July 2003

Dispersal programme

The HIV-positive asylum seeker faces further barriers to receiving appropriate health care as a result of the Home Office policy of dispersal, introduced in April 2000.

Asylum seekers may be dispersed to parts of the country with a low prevalence (from London and southeast England to locations around the United Kingdom) of HIV, little experience of managing HIV infection, a lack of infrastructure, and no appropriate community-based support services in place. More than 100,000 asylum seekers to date have been dispersed, many of who are from regions with HIV epidemics. It is not known how many HIV- positive seekers have been affected by this policy.[1] Asylum seekers may receive only 48 hours notice, and they face immediate cessation of income, housing and legal benefits if they decline dispersal or return to London.

Of the potential barriers to safe dispersal of HIV-infected asylum seekers, it is of particular concern that dispersal is done at short notice and frequently without appropriate transfer of medical information.[2] Inappropriate dispersal of an HIV infected patient could lead to HIV resistance, onward transmission of HIV infection and avoidable morbidity and mortality for the asylum seeker.

- An article published in the British Medical Journal in 2004 further highlighted the issue of dispersal of HIV-positive asylum seekers by providing the findings of a national survey of UK healthcare providers. The research aimed at finding out the experiences and opinions of doctors working in genitourinarymedicine in relation to the dispersalof HIV-positive asylum seekers. The main findings of the study were that most doctors who treat HIV-positive asylum seekers haveunsuccessfully contested dispersal and that

doctors believe that dispersalis disruptive, may compromise HIV care, and may lead to increasedtransmission.

- In 2006, the National AIDS Trust published a report on the dispersal of asylum seekers living with HIV.[3]

- In December 2005, NASS introduced a new policy on the dispersal of asylum seekers with healthcare needs. The new policy states that a delay must be considered when dispersing HIV-positive asylum seekers, and that the treating clinician must be satisfied that continuing treatment has been organised in the patient's destination area. It also states that the provider of accommodation in the destination area has an obligation to ensure that HIV-positive asylum seekers are registered with a GP.[4]

References

1 Asylum policy sparks HIV concern, BBC News, Friday, 6 August, 2004

2 Creighton S, Sethi G, Edwards SG et al. British Medical Journal (08.07.04) Vol. 29; No. 7461: P. 322- 323 - Monday, August 16, 2004.

3 See NAT, (2006) Dispersal of Asylum Seekers with HIV, London

4 UNGASS 2006: HAS THE UK GOVERNMENT KEPT THE PROMISE? AIDS Rights Project, MARCH 2006

Leave to Remain and HIV

The fact that someone is HIV-positive or has AIDS is not in itself a basis for refusing that application. A person is entitled to apply for leave to remain on grounds unrelated to their HIV-positive status. However, there may be cases where a person has no other grounds to remain in the UK, but wishes to seek discretionary leave to remain on the basis that they will not receive adequate medical treatment in their home country.

Such applications in the past may have been bolstered by reference to the European Convention on Human Rights, article 3 of which provides that "no one shall be subjected to torture or to inhuman or degrading treatment or punishment". In this context, reference is often made to the decision of the European Court of Human Rights in the case D v United Kingdom (1997) 24 EHRR 423. In that case, D was serving a period of imprisonment in the UK for a drug related offence. While he was in prison, he was diagnosed as being HIV-positive and suffering from AIDS. After his release, the government proposed to return him to his home country, St Kitts. The European Court noted that D was very close to death, that the care available for him in St Kitts would be inadequate, and that his removal would expose him to a real risk of dying under most distressing circumstances. It would, therefore, potentially amount to inhuman treatment under article 3, meaning that the UK government could not return him to St Kitts as intended.[1]

However, the House of Lords overturned this decision with the recent outcome of N v Secretary of State for the Home Department [2005] UKHL 31. Essentially, the facts of the case are this: N arrived in the UK in 1998 from Uganda, seeking asylum. She was diagnosed as being HIV-positive with a CD4 count of 10 very soon afterwards. Following treatment, her condition is now stable (according to one of the judges, she now has a CD4 count of 414). However, her claim for asylum has been rejected and the Home Secretary proposes to deport her back to Uganda, where it is accepted she would be likely to die within a year or two for lack of medication and proper care.

The Court of Appeal (upholding the Immigration Appeal Tribunal's decision to overturn an earlier decision by the adjudicator) held that deportation would not violate N's rights under article 3 of the European Convention on Human Rights (the right to be free from torture or inhuman or degrading treatment).[2] The House of Lords has now upheld that decision. It is likely that N and the thousands like her will face removal and a significant reduction in life expectancy.

References

1 African HIV Policy Network, Newsletter, Summer 2005, Issue 7

2 http://www.publications.parliament.uk/pa/ld200405/ldjudgmt/jd050505/home-1.htm

Entitlement to health care

Prior to April 2004, NHS treatment of all kinds was available free of charge to anyone who could show that they had been in the UK for more than 12 months. It was also available free to anyone currently applying for asylum or for leave to remain. This situation ensured that anyone who was clearly a long stay resident of the UK, no matter how they became so, would receive the health treatment they needed. The regulations governing NHS charging, and a number of key exemptions to them, were enshrined in the NHS Act 1977 and the NHS (Charges to Overseas Visitors) Regulations 1989. The exemptions included universal free treatment for a range of conditions on public health grounds. These included TB and all sexually transmitted infections except for HIV. For HIV, you had to wait 12 months to access free NHS services.

However, in response to media and political agitation about "treatment tourism" and the cost to the NHS of people allegedly flying in to the UK for the sole or primary purpose of exploiting the UK health system, new restrictions were imposed on all hospital services from April 2004. These new regulations mean that treatment for HIV (or for anything else not specially mentioned in the 1989 Amendment) would never be provided without charge for certain categories of people. This was despite the lack of any research showing the existence or extent of "treatment tourism" in HIV. Most migrants were unlikely to be aware of their status until they had been in the UK for more than nine months[1].

New NHS charging regulations were introduced in April 2004 after consultation. Amongst other changes, some genuinely beneficial (students, for instance, can now access NHS services without charge provided their course is of at least six months duration) the twelve-month rule was removed. This change means that long stay visitors, anyone in the UK without documentation, and anyone refused asylum or leave to remain, but not removed from the UK, are liable to be charged for any NHS services other than those provided in an emergency (usually interpreted as those available at A&E departments) or those outlined in the 1989 exemptions.

It is clear that these changes to the regulations are already causing hardship. It is also beginning to be clear in the case of HIV that, while they may result in a small short term cost reduction to local NHS budgets, in the longer term they are highly likely to have a negative effect in all three major areas - the public purse, the public health and individual health.

In light of the impact the Department of Health has introduced an easement clause. The easement clause means that any treatment and care, including for HIV and other conditions, that is started prior to any decision on asylum application continues to be provided as a free NHS service even if the asylum status changes and until the treatment ends or the person leaves the country. It does not meet the needs of those who are diagnosed after the failure of their asylum claim (or those here permanently but without documentation).[2]

References

1 Charging Manifesto
http://www.ahpn.org/downloads/campaigns/charging_campaign_manifesto1.doc

2 House of Commons Health Committee New Developments inSexual Health and HIV/AIDS Policy: Third Report of Session 2004-05 *Volume I*

Mandatory screening for asylum seekers with HIV

In January 2003, the Cabinet Office, in collaboration with the Department of Health and the Home Office, launched a closed inquiry into "imported infections", examining the impact of some serious communicable diseases on public health in the UK, with particular focus on individuals coming from abroad. The main implication for the HIV sector would be that the Government was considering whether or not to require an HIV test from individuals coming into the UK: students, work-permit holders and asylum seekers in particular[1].

It is inappropriate to routinely screen all asylum applicants for HIV. Mandatory screening is against World Health Organisation guidelines for implementing HIV/AIDS counselling (1993). The 45th World Health Assembly noted that "there is no public health rationale for any measures that limit the rights of the individual, notably measures establishing mandatory screening." It is important to offer confidential voluntary counselling and testing and support those at risk[2]. Separately, some researchers and clinicians have grown impatient with the VCT approach and advocate routinised HIV testing during hospital visits as a remedy to the problem of late diagnosis. Some have argued that HIV testing 'should be widely accepted, without conventional voluntary counselling and testing'. Conversely, other researchers feel that the routinisation of testing would lower quality standards for VCT by side stepping appropriate counselling[3]. Migrants' groups and HIV specialists, in particular, have argued that mandatory testing would entrench the existing stigmatisation of HIV-positive people and act as a further deterrent to accessing services. These views against mandatory testing were collated in a report from the All Party Parliamentary Group on AIDS (UK). The report concluded that the government should foster policies that encourage VCT.[4]

References

1 AHPN Quarterly Newsletter, Issue 4, Vol 3, Autumn 2004

2 Angela Burnett, Asylum seekers and refugees in Britain The health of survivors of torture and organised violence BMJ 2001;322:606-609 (10 March)

3 Manavi, K., Welsby, P. (2005). HIV Testing no longer needs special status. British Medical Journal 13:133-176.

4 All Party Parliamentary Group on AIDS (2003). Migration and HIV: Improving Lives in Britain. An Inquiry into the Impact of the UK Nationality and Immigration System on People Living with HIV.

Prosecution of HIV transmission

The first three men who were convicted for committing Grievous Bodily Harm (GBH) in England for transmitting HIV to female sexual partners, were all of Black African origin, and were either seeking asylum or had refugee status. These cases raise a range of issues for African people living with HIV in the UK.

In October 2003, a London judge disallowed evidence about two complainants' knowledge of Mohammed Dica's diagnosis, because he deemed their consent irrelevant. Mr. Dica was convicted and given an eight-year prison sentence, but the conviction was quashed in March by the Appeal Court. At his third retrial in March 2005, Mr. Dica was convicted on one count of recklessly inflicting grievous bodily harm contrary to Section 20 of the *OAPA 1861*. He was ordered to serve out the remainder of his four and a half year sentence on that conviction.

In January 2004, Kouassi Adaye pled guilty to charges including GBH relating to the transmission of HIV to a woman in

Liverpool. Despite not being tested at the time of transmission, the judge said Mr. Adaye should have known his status as, one week before he had sex with the complainant, his wife telephoned from South Africa to say that she was positive[1].

In November 2003, Feston Konzani was charged with 5 counts of inflicting grievous bodily harm with intent, in Middlesbrough. He was convicted on three counts of reckless transmission and sentenced to a total of ten years imprisonment. Feston was a Malawian asylum seeker.

These men have been variously described in local and national press coverage as 'terrorists', 'assassins', and 'monsters'. While many of us may not dispute that the actions attributed to them are immoral, there are important questions to be raised about the purpose of using the criminal law in such instances. If criminalisation contributes to the environment of fear and blame that drives the epidemic, is it an effective means of addressing HIV transmission?[2]

African people with diagnosed HIV have strong opinions regarding the issue of criminalisation, as noted in *Outsider Status*, a report on stigma and discrimination experienced by people living with HIV. Many questioned why responsibility for transmission was not considered to be shared between both partners. Large proportions were also upset by sensational press coverage that spread misinformation about HIV, while appearing to indict all HIV-positive Black African migrants in the UK. Some challenged the criminal justice system's exclusive selection of Black African male migrants for the development of this case law, while also raising questions about the strength of evidence for and against the defendants. A small proportion of African research participants argued that non-disclosure of positive status before unprotected sex should result in prosecution, but the majority of respondents argued that the negative impacts far outweighed any possible good that could come from such convictions[3].

Criminalisation of HIV transmission is of key importance to all African people living with HIV in the UK. The African HIV community is already discussing the issues raised by these cases.

References

1 HIV in the courts: the best course of action? Catherine Dodds, Research Fellow, Sigma Research, University of Portsmouth, AHPN Quarterly Newsletter, Issue 4, Vol 3, Autumn 2004

2 AHPN's Position Paper on the Criminalisation of HIV Transmission, November 2005

3 Sigma Research (2004). Outsider status - Stigma and discrimination experienced by Gay men and African people with HIV. London, Sigma

Gender

Women are now the fastest growing group of newly diagnosed HIV-positive people in the UK, with a significant percentage of them being from minority ethnic communities, mainly black African. In 1992, women made up 12% of people living with HIV and AIDS in the UK. By 1998, the proportion had grown to 35%. An overwhelming majority of those women were black African (at least 80%) and had been infected from a male partner.

Violence against women is a common method of exposure to HIV. It is estimated that over 50% of women refugee and asylum seekers in the UK, the majority of whom come from Africa, are fleeing rape - mostly perpetrated by soldiers, police or agents of the state. The intersection of HIV epidemiology with gender and race may expose black African women to multiple stigma and discrimination because of their race and their presumed or actual status.[1]

The finding from a qualitative study of African women entitled " My Heart is loaded" found that:[2]

- A majority of the women interviewed had already experienced at least one profoundly traumatic life event including rape, murder of partners and family members and various other forms of persecution. In addition to direct experience of HIV related death and ill health in close relatives or friends or child from HIV.

- The lives of most African women are heavily influenced by their capacity to become pregnant and give birth. However this raises additional problems for those who are HIV-positive. Most of the women in this study stressed the importance of motherhood as a source of identity and legitimacy.

- Mothers are traditionally seen as the moral guardians of society. This meant that many of these HIV-positive women were afraid of being stigmatised for not living up to these social expectations.

- Guilt was often especially debilitating among those who were compelled to leave children behind in Africa. Changing circumstances meant that these children often had to be passed between carers and attempts to bring them to the UK were usually difficult and often unsuccessful.

- Many of the women said that the lack of a male partner was one of the most difficult things they had to face. They wanted to be in an intimate relationship but perceived the obstacles to achieving this to be very great. For many, the lack of friends and of a partner resulted in physical and emotional isolation that was very difficult to bear.

Findings from a Project NASAH and the PADARE project found access to health care services was poor. Very few studies have explored the needs of older women living with HIV/AIDS. The SHIBAH report glimpsed the emerging difficulties of women approaching the menopause, and recommended further research amongst this group, in particular the interactions between gender, ageing, HIV and sexual health.

References

1 Womens Resource Centre, *CEDAW Shadow Report:* Statistics about women in the UK (2006)

2 [My Heart is Loaded, African women with HIV surviving in London, Dr Jane Anderson Centre for Infectious Diseases, Barts and The London, 2005

Gender violence

Victimisation in women who are HIV-positive or at risk for HIV has been documented. Over one-third of women with HIV in London reported a history of sexual and physical abuse. There was some evidence that among black African women in the UK those who revealed their positive status were more vulnerable to physical abuse.

Pregnancy

The majority of pregnant women with HIV in England come from overseas, mostly from sub-Saharan Africa. Concerns such as immigration and housing may be uppermost in their minds.[1] Studies have found experiences of poverty, poor housing and racism amongst pregnant asylum seekers. The poverty experienced when living on £30 per week, in relation to HIV, places babies of HIV-positive mothers at higher risk of infection because, when the mothers cannot afford formula milk, they will occasionally resort to breast-feeding. In recent years, however, there has been a substantial improvement in uptake of voluntary confidential antenatal HIV testing among black African women in the UK, resulting in a significant reduction in the number of children infected with HIV through mother to child transmission. Nevertheless, there remains a critical lack of interventions focusing on the needs of children and youths whose lives are affected by HIV, either by being positive themselves, or through having positive parents.[2]

A major impact of HIV for African women in London is related to their capacity to become pregnant and give birth, as motherhood is an important source of identity and legitimacy. In most cultures, motherhood is an important part of women's identity. A number of studies provide evidence that HIV status is not the major influence in reproductive decision-making for many women.[3]

A study of 40 HIV-positive women in London showed that 18% were planning a pregnancy and 30% were still undecided. Women were found to be unsure, at times uninformed, and to desire information about interventions. Anxiety levels were high especially among Black African women, regarding antiretroviral treatments and breastfeeding avoidance.[4]

References

1 Recommended Standards for NHS HIV Care, MedFash, 2003

2 The psychosocial and health care needs of HIV-positive people in the United Kingdom: a review, G Green and R Smith, HIV Medicine, Volume 5 Issue s1 Page 4 - May 2004

3 Ibid

4 Ibid

Children and families

There were over 1100 under 19s known to be infected with HIV living in the UK. The number of affected children, defined as those living in a family where one or more member is HIV infected, is unknown.[1] Over the last decade, the number of women infected with the virus has quadrupled leading us to presume that there are at least 15-20,000 children affected by HIV in the UK.

A disproportionate number of children affected by HIV in the UK are asylum-seeking children whose parents were born in sub-Saharan Africa. Resources are likely to be limited. A high proportion live in one-parent families. Seventy per cent live in lone-parent-headed households, usually without extended family support, and may be separated from at least one parent and siblings.

Other than reproductive issues, the literature on the psychosocial impact of HIV-positive parenting is dominated by the issue of disclosure. This includes disclosure of the parent's HIV status to children and disclosure of a child's HIV status. In both these scenarios, many difficulties are associated with disclosing to children, particularly in cultural settings where the stigma of HIV is high, for example among some black African communities. The literature identifies the following reasons for non-disclosure:[2]

- concerns about discrimination and stigma;

- fears that children may 'tell' indiscriminately;

- negative associations of HIV;

- cultural differences;

- concerns that children are too young and that disclosure may affect their development and well-being;

- the fact that telling is awkward;

- the belief that health is not sufficiently compromised and may not be in the future;

- the fact that disclosure is low on the list of priorities.

A study of 13 families with HIV-infected children attending a South London clinic (where 77% of the families were of African origin) found that parents thought that their child had a partial understanding of their illness and understood clinic visits and treatments. All considered that disclosure should wait until the child was old enough not to tell other people indiscriminately. Parents viewed disclosure as inevitable, but to be delayed as long as possible. They felt it should take place prior to teenage years, before the child became sexually active. Parents reported avoiding the subject as much as possible.[3]

Lack of childcare is also a considerable burden for women living with HIV, and can constitute an important barrier for parents to access healthcare, social services, and employment. HIV prevention strategies must include childcare facilities so as to create an enabling environment for women to access services.[4]

There is wide variability in the cultural ethnic and social composition of children and families living with HIV in the UK. Tensions may emerge between African traditions and modern UK concerns about childhood. The notion of children as people with rights does not fit well with more traditional cultural positions that emphasise parental rights. Balancing the two is a challenge for professionals working with African families in the UK. See the *Children and adolescents* chapter for further details.

References

1 The UK Collaborative Group for HIV and STI Surveillance. A Complex Picture. HIV and other Sexually Transmitted Infections in the United Kingdom: 2006. Health Protection Agency, Centre for Infections. London, November 2006.

2 Ibid

3 Waugh S. Parental views on disclosure of diagnosis to their HIV-positive children. AIDS Care 2003; 15: 169-176.

4 Flowers, P., Davis, M., Hart, G., Rosengarten, M., Frankis, J. and Imrie, J. (2005a) Diagnosis, Stigma and Identity among HIV-positive Black African living in the UK.

Black African men

African men are less likely than women to access HIV prevention services and are 'less visible in settings where HIV prevention was likely to be discussed. African men perceive HIV prevention gatherings as being primarily focused on women's needs, children, relationships and contraception.

Gender roles tend to change upon migration: where men are the 'traditional' decision makers regarding children and the family, the socio-economic difficulties they face as a result of migration often leads to a renegotiation of their roles as husbands, fathers and brothers. This in turn might affect their sexual decision-making among couples, but also responsibility-sharing within families, as well as individual men's sexual risk behaviour[1]. HIV prevention interventions must take into account the changing roles and needs of African men, particularly younger men, and involve them in the design of interventions.

References

1 Chinouya, M., Reynolds, R. (2001). HIV Prevention and African Communities Living in England: A Framework for Action. National AIDS Trust: London.

Black African men who have sex with men

Very little is known about the sexual health and HIV prevention needs of black gay and bisexual men. Twenty per cent of African men interviewed for the PADARE Project said they had had sex with other men in the year prior to interview, which would indicate that African MSM constitute a small but significant portion of the African community in the UK. Moreover, recent evidence suggests that black and ethnic minority MSM are highly affected by HIV/AIDS:

- An estimated 500,000 homosexually active men live in the UK, of which approximately half are exclusively gay, with London home to over 12,000 black behaviourally homosexual men.[1]

- A review of ethnicity data from two national HIV/AIDS surveillance and unlinked anonymous data from 14 clinics showed that Black African men who had sex with men accounted for 12% of new diagnosis.[2]

- a recent study using UK National HIV prevalence data estimates that 7% of black and ethnic minority MSM living in the UK were diagnosed with HIV, compared with 3% of white MSM in 2002.[3]

- According the HPA report a complex picture BME men accounted for 10% of MSM accessing care in 2005 (1935/18 642). Of these 1935 BME men, the majority (48%; 921/1935) were of other/mixed ethnicity, with 20% (387) black Caribbean and 13% (253) black African.[4]

- 6% of black African men infected through sex between men (»SOPHID 2002: Individuals of black-African ethnic origin)

Furthermore, a study by Sigma Research using self-reported data showed that 18% of black gay and bisexual men were living with diagnosed HIV in the UK in 2004, compared with 10% of white gay/bisexual men. HIV prevention is hampered by the fact that black MSM shoulder discrimination both from the black African community and the gay community at large.[5] An African gay man told the investigators of Mayisha II study about the tensions that his sexuality caused, and how he was denounced as an "abomination" in his church when the pastor became aware of his sexuality.

Some interventions have sought to involve black MSM as peer educators in raising HIV awareness, and dedicated support groups. However more research is critically required to understand the sexual health needs of black African/ Caribbean MSM and the best ways to reach them with prevention interventions. HIV prevention interventions therefore need to take into account the needs of African men and encourage them to manage interventions. There is little or no action being taken to address the needs of African gay men, and there are few African led organizations that include African gay men in their interventions.

The UK has seen several community development and social support initiatives for various groups of Black gay and bisexual men.

Interventions:

- The main focus of the Big Up @ GMFA group includes building Black gay communities, providing targeted interventions for the sexual and mental well-being of African and Caribbean men who have sex with men, and challenging homophobia and racism.

- In November 2002 Terrence Higgins Trust launched the Black Gay Equality Campaign, a series of four posters depicting family members who had learnt or were learning to accept a gay family member. The campaign was launched at the annual Black Gay Community Awards held in London.

- Club Afreaka is a monthly nightclub for African MSM. It opened its doors at the Black Cap in Camden Town on 10th July 2003 and is now at the G-Lounge. (Gay men's venues).

- Tumaini (a conference style/social event) was held on 20th November 2004, was an interactive event that brought together gay men of African descent

- The Black connection is a monthly group where Black gay and bisexual men come together to meet, talk, socialise and share experiences about their lives in a supportive and attitude free environment.

References

1 Two Years of Working with Black Gay Men, Simon Nelson, Terrence Higgins Trust, 2003

2 Epidemiology of HIV among black and minority ethnic men who have sex with men in...
Dougan et al. *Sex Transm Infect.*2005; 81: 345-350

3 Dougan, S., Elford, J. Rice, B., Brown, A.E., Sinka, K., Evans. B.G., Gill, O.N., Fenton, K. (2005). Epidemiology of HIV among black and ethnic minority ethnic men who have sex with men in England and Wales. Sexually Transmitted Infections 81: 345-350.

4 A Complex Picture. HIV and other Sexually Transmitted Infections. in the United Kingdom: Health Protection Agency, 2006

5 Redefining community, restoring identity: The role of social class, ethnicity and migration in the lives of gay men in London, *2003*

Psychosocial needs of Black African people living with HIV

Studies that have explored the psychological concerns of sexual health clinic attendees from Black African groups in London show that contrast to the higher levels of subjective psychological distress reported by African clinic attendees (26%) and a significant proportion who said they would like to see a psychologist (36%), no referrals to psychology services were made. This evidence substantiates existing arguments concerning a general reluctance to refer black people to 'talking therapies'.

Research has raised questions about the cultural appropriateness of HIV counseling services for black Africans in the UK, especially as the uptake of counseling and psychological support services by African patients is low. This has been explained by the fact that talking to a stranger about family issues might not be culturally appropriate, but also because of practitioners' lack of cultural competency.[1,2] Studies have shown that black Africans talked about not 'being able to listen' to what was being said about HIV care during post-diagnosis counselling because of the impact of grief.

Reports also indicate that for black African people the fear of stigma leads to a lack of disclosure, and in turn lack of disclosure seems to be linked to a lack of social support and social isolation. Many describe a distinct lack of social support and report a lack of opportunity to talk about their HIV status and that the fear of meeting people from the community is a barrier to using self-help groups. Thus, because status disclosure is difficult, social isolation and lack of social support are exacerbated. Weatherburn et al. found a lack of social support in practical areas such as doing household chores, mobility and getting enough money to live on. Almost half of those living with children had difficulties looking after them. Although problems with practical needs were the experience of a minority of HIV-positive people, the impact could be considerable.[3]

Relationship problems were experienced by nearly one-third of respondents, although whether problems would have emerged regardless of HIV status was unclear. Sexual problems were also experienced.

References

1   Flowers, P., Davis, M., Hart, G., Rosengarten, M., Frankis, J. and Imrie, J. (2005a) Diagnosis, Stigma and Identity among HIV-positive Black African living in the UK.

2   Ohen, L., Hunte, S. and Wallace, C. (2004). Who provides Social Advice to HIV-positive clients. Lambeth Primary Care Trust, London.

3   Malanda, S, Meadows, J., Catalan, J. (2001) Are we meeting the psychological needs of Black African HIV-positive individuals in London? Controlled Study of referrals to a psychological medicine unit. AIDS Care 13 (4): 413-419.

Faith

Active involvement with a religious group has been linked to increased social support and a sense of belonging as well as spiritual support among older HIV-infected adults. The majority of respondents in all studies stated that religion was important, and religious faith was found to be a major source of support for African women in coping with their difficulties.[1]

Faith is significant in managing daily life with an positive HIV diagnosis, however the church also represents a threatening space marked by lack of confidentiality, and the generation of stigma. Faith leaders have limited capacity in dealing with HIV-related issues within their congregations. Faith leaders are willing to work in partnership with statutory agencies, but need their capacity to be developed to support those who were living with HIV.

References

1   My Heart is Loaded, African women with HIV surviving in London, Dr Jane Anderson Centre for Infectious Diseases, Barts and The London, 2005

Need for further research

Of primary importance is greater research into the epidemiological and demographic features of the Black African HIV epidemic in England, particularly as the dispersal system forces many new and vulnerable people out of London where much HIV health prevention and care activity is located.

- Large social mapping of Black African communities in order to identify the setting and methodologies for accessing Black African communities

- The demographic distribution of HIV amongst Black African communities in England

- Pan-London behavioural surveillance.

Health services and health prevention interventions

- Understanding barriers to use of sexual health services

- Evaluation of HIV prevention initiatives

- Development of research tools to reflect Black African community experience.

- African patients' experience of HAART needs further exploration to inform future secondary prevention interventions.

Epidemiology and monitoring

- Research that explores and identifies the sexual health and HIV prevention needs of black gay and bisexual men.

- much remains unknown about the epidemiological and demographic features of the African HIV epidemic, and this becomes more urgent as the dispersal system forces many new and vulnerable people out of London.

- Sexual behaviour - there is a critical need for a better understanding of the sexual behaviours and attitudes of Africans with or at risk of HIV, in the context of cultural practices and beliefs, relationships, gender disparity, and economic status.

- Gender specific research - there is an urgent need for more understanding of attitudes, beliefs and practices surrounding breastfeeding, pregnancy and termination, experiences of antenatal testing, male approaches to condom use, experiences and behaviours of African men, sexual negotiation and masculinity.

- Specific sub-populations - more information is needed on asylum seekers and visitors, the role of drugs and alcohol, African men who have sex with men and African sex workers.

- Health services and prevention interventions - patterns of service use by African communities, evaluation of HIV prevention interventions, the development of research tools to reflect African community experience.

- There is a significant lack of rigorous qualitative and quantitative research on the social care needs of African people living with HIV in the UK. The needs of African people with HIV are influenced by policy and practices which are far broader than those pertaining to HIV, health or social care, falling instead, within the remit of broader social exclusion policy and interventions. Research undertaken solely from the perspective of HIV prevention, treatment information need or clinical service need (as the majority of past research has done so) cannot hope to capture the ways in which social care and health need among this group necessitates interventions on more levels that we are used to considering.

- Tackling HIV related discrimination among primary health care staff continues to be highlighted by the Department of Health as an urgent priority. Rather than undertaking yet another investigation of the experiences of people living with HIV in health care settings, a new approach is most certainly required. Comparative evaluations of existing HIV training programmes for health care staff could contribute to the development of a best-practice evidence base. Such work should also include an examination of the impact of PEPSE training among front-line Accident and Emergency staff in those PCTs that make such preventive treatment accessible.

In September 2001 the African HIV Research Forum was launched. Its main aim is to bring together individuals and organisations to focus on all aspects of HIV research relating to the various African communities within the United Kingdom www.ahrf.org.uk.

Women and HIV

Women living with HIV represent around half of the total global population living with the virus. For these women HIV presents a number of specific challenges and difficulties relating both to their sex and gender. It is the intention of this chapter to present some of these challenges and difficulties and to acknowledge those problems unique to women. This chapter also aims to discuss specific concerns for HIV-positive women living with HIV.

Women and HIV - a growing challenge

In recent years it has been recognised that the epidemiology of HIV and AIDS (i.e. the nature of the epidemic) is becoming increasingly feminised. The 2006 UNAIDS Update on the AIDS Epidemic[1] presents international information about the number of people affected by HIV, how these infections are distributed world-wide and also how different areas of the worlds face different challenges in trying to stop the spread of HIV.

Women and HIV - epidemiological information

Worldwide, women account for almost 50% of the people living with HIV. Women face a double burden with HIV, not only are they often disproportionately represented in terms of numbers but they also carry much of the burden of caring for other people who are positive. The table below lists the proportion of people living with HIV who are also women: it can be seen from the table below that areas with higher proportions of women in their HIV-positive population generally correspond with areas of higher prevalence. (See Epidemiology Chapter)

Proportion of people living with HIV who are women

Area	Percentage
sub-Saharan Africa	59
Caribbean	50
Middle East and North Africa	48
Oceania	47
Latin America	31
Eastern Europe and Central Asia	30
South and South-East Easia	29
East Asia	29
Western and Central Europe	28
North America	26
Global	48

Sub-Saharan Africa, in keeping with its devastating challenge from HIV and AIDS also faces the largest challenge in terms of the proportion of women living with the virus. For every ten adult men living with HIV in that area there are about 14 adult women who are infected. Women in this region are described as bearing a 'disproportionate part of the burden of HIV' since, not only do they make up the majority of the positive population but they also are most likely to be carers for other positive people. In many areas prevalence data is conveniently collected by testing rates of HIV infection in pregnant women attending clinics. In **Zimbabwe**[2] 2004 data showed the prevalence of HIV in Harare, the capital, as having fallen from 30% in 2000 to 24% in 2006. However, despite this apparent decline in prevalence the life expectancy in this country has fallen to 37 years for men and only 34 years for women. In **South Africa**[3] prevalence of HIV in young people (aged 15-25 years) was shown to be 4.8% in

young men and 17% in young women - a fourfold difference. This increased risk for young women is reflected in other Sub Saharan countries. However, delaying sexual activity only appears to delay one's infection with HIV in **Lesotho**[4] where recent surveys display starkly an increasing risk for women as they grow older with less than 10% of women testing positive at aged 18-19, 30% at aged 22 but almost 40% by the age of 24. In **Uganda**, prevalence rates for women are almost 8% compared to 5% for men while in **Ghana**[5] women were nearly three times as likely to be HIV-positive if they were married compared to if they had never been married.

While much of women's disproportionate HIV burden in Africa appears to be fuelled by heterosexual transmissions, other areas reflect different epidemiological patterns. In **China**[6], for example, almost half (44%) of people living with HIV are believed to have acquired their infection through injecting drug use, however, in 2005 it was estimated that around 50% of infections occurred through unprotected sex and the proportion of women infected has risen from 25% of the total of people living with HIV in 2002 to 39% in 2004, reflecting a shift from the most at risk populations to the population at large. In **India and Cambodia**, meanwhile, there are large proportions of women who have become infected through intercourse with a regular partner who themselves were infected through paid sex and in Thailand one third of new infections in 2005 were in married women who were probably infected by their spouses. Meanwhile, in Viet Nam, most positive people have acquired their virus through intravenous drug use and sex work.

In **Eastern Europe and Central Asia** young people aged 15-24 years make up the majority of infections. In **Russia**[7], in 2005, women accounted for over 40% of newly reported HIV infections, reflecting a shift from an epidemic fuelled by intravenous drug use to an increase in the importance of unprotected sex as a transmission route. In the Caribbean, although the total populations are small there is still an adult prevalence rate in the region's countries between 1-4%. Again, the epidemic in the **Caribbean** is largely heterosexual and women are jeopardised by the gender inequalities which lead to them being economically dependent on men and at increased risk of being infected via sex work (either as workers or through regular partners).

In Latin America, where in many countries including **Argentina, Paraguay and Peru**, the population most affected by HIV has been men who have sex with men, the proportion of women affected is increasing. In **Argentina**[8], for example, the ratio of men to women has changed from 15:1 in 1998 to 3:1 in 2005, while in **Chile** increasing numbers of women are becoming HIV-positive through male partners who themselves became positive through sex with other men.

In North America, Western and Central Europe women account for a smaller, yet still substantial, proportion of people living with HIV. In the **United States of America**[9] the proportion of women in people newly diagnosed has increased from 15% before 1995 to 27% in 2004, three quarters of whom were infected during unprotected sex (e.g. with male injecting drug users, through sex work and men who had sex with other men.) The epidemic in the United States of America disproportionately affects ethnic and racial minorities with 70% of new diagnoses between 2001-2004 among African American and Hispanics who together account for only 26% of the population. These ethnic differences are compounded by gender inequalities as starkly reflected in figures for the African American community which show that the rate of new diagnosis for African American men was seven times higher than that for white men while the rate for African American women is 21 times higher than for white women.

Ethnic and gender inequalities are evidenced again in **Canada**[10,11] where aboriginal people accounted for 9% of new infections while comprising only 3.3% on the population. This may be related to rates of intravenous drug in this population where the proportion of female injecting drug users is relatively high.

In the Middle East and North Africa, although most infections have to date been in men there is an increasing proportion of women affected yet in Oceania the picture is different again with young women (aged 15-29) in **Papua New Guinea**[12] experiencing prevalence rates almost twice as high as those for men of the same age.

In **Australia and NewZealand** the epidemic mainly focuses on unprotected sex between men. However, ethnic and gender inequalities similar to those in Canada and America are evidenced in the fact that Australia's Indigenous women are eighteen times more likely to HIV-positive than non-Indigenous women and three times more likely than non-Indigenous men[13].

In **Western and Central Europe** the proportion of women affected has been increasing as the proportion of heterosexual transmissions has grown. These heterosexual transmissions, as is the case in Canada, are most often acquired in areas of high prevalence. In the **UK**[14], while women account for around 30% of all HIV infections via sexual contact or IV drug use since the start of the epidemic, in recent years the proportion of women testing positive has increased and is currently around 40% of the total of new infections each year.

Thus, women are becoming increasingly burdened by the HIV and AIDS epidemic. The next section explores the biological, social and economic factors which influence the particular vulnerability of women.

References

1   UNAIDS, 2006, *Report on the global AIDS epidemic*, Geneva, UNAIDS

2   Mahomva A et al, 2006, HIV Prevalence and trends from data in Zimbabwe, 1997-2004, *Sexually Transmitted Infections*, 82(2)

3   Shisana O et al, 2005, *South African National HIV Prevalence, HIV Incidence, Behaviour and Communication Surveys*, Pretoria, Human Sciences Research Council. Available at http://www.hrsc.ac.za/media/2005/11/20051130_1.html

4   NAC and UNAIDS, 2006, *Lesotho 2005 UNGASS country report: status of the national response to the 2001 Declaration of Commitment on HIV and AIDS, January 2003-December 2005*, Maseru, Government of Lesotho

5   Ghana Statistical Service, Noguchi Memorial Institute for Medical Research, ORC, Macro, 2004, *Ghana Demographic and Health Survey2003*, Calverton, Ghana Statistical Service, Noguchi Memorial Institute for Medical Research, ORC, Macro

6   Ministry of Health China, UNAIDS, WHO, 2006, *2005 update on the HIV and AIDS epidemic and response in China*, Beijing, Ministry of Health, China, UNAIDS, WHO

7   Pokrovskiy, 2006, *The HIV and AIDS epidemic in Russia: trends, lessons and key challenges and opportunities for scaling up the response*, Side presentation to XVI International AIDS Conference, 13-18 August, Toronto

8   National AIDS Programme, 2005, *Epidemiological surveillance report*, December, Buenos Aires

9   US Centers for Disease Control and Prevention, 2006, *A Glance at the HIV and AIDS epidemic*, April, Atlanta, Centres for Disease Control and Prevention, available at http://www.cdc.gov.hiv.resources/factsheets/At-a-glance.htm

10 Boulos D et al, 2006, Estimates of HIV prevalence and incidence in Canada, 2005, Canada Communicable Disease Report 2006, 32(15), available at http://www.phac-aspc.gc.ca/media/nr-rp/2006/20060731-hiv-vih_e.html

11 Public Health Agency of Canada, 2006, *HIV and AIDS among Aboriginal peoples in Canada: a continuing concern - HIV and AIDS epidemic update August 2006*, Ottawa, Public Health Agency of Canada available at: http://phac-aspc.gc.ca/publicat/epui-aepi/epi-06/index.html

12 National AIDS Council Secretariat Papua New Guinea, 2006, *Monitoring the Declaration of Commitment on HIV and AIDS: January 2004-December 2005*, Port Moresby, National AIDS Council Secretariat Papua New Guinea

13 Wright M et al, 2005, Fulfilling Prophecy? Sexually transmitted infections and HIV in Indigenous people in Western Australia, *Medical Journal of Australia*, 183(3):124-128

14 HPA, 2006, A Complex Picture, HIV and other Sexually Transmitted Infections in the UK, 2006, HPA (Health Protection Agency) available at: http://www.hpa.org.uk/publications/2006/hiv_sti_2006/contents.htm

Confronting the crisis: women and HIV

In 2004 UNAIDS/UNFPA/UNIFEM published a global report called *Confronting the Crisis*[1] which explored the HIV epidemic and its impact on women. This substantial piece of work acknowledged the changing nature of the epidemic and its increasing impact on women worldwide. It brought together up-to-date information and thinking about how to respond to this crisis and some of the key messages from the report are outlined below.

This crisis is twofold and involves both the prevention of HIV infection in women and also ensuring access to treatment and care of HIV-positive women.

The vulnerability of women

At the XV1 World AIDS Conference increased coverage was given to those aspects of the HIV epidemic which relate to women. This increased focus on women is highly welcomed and the topic was explored at a High Level Session on Leadership entitled: *Time to Deliver for Women and Girls*. At this session Peter Piot, at that time Executive Director for the Joint United Nations Programme on HIV and AIDS (UNAIDS), made a keynote address which listed and discussed multi-factorial influences which together need to be addressed to slow the increasing HIV burden faced by women[2].

Women are traditionally seen as being vulnerable to HIV infection through two mechanisms: biological vulnerability and social vulnerability.

Biological vulnerability[3]

The biological make up of women's bodies make them more vulnerable to HIV infection. During penetrative vaginal sex the area of mucosal surface exposed to sexual fluids is much greater than the comparable area exposed in a man. This greater surface area coupled with the fact that sperm is a more efficient carrier of HIV than vaginal fluids means that it is around more risky for an HIV-negative woman to have vaginal sex with an HIV-positive man than vice versa (although this can be affected by a partner's infectivity or the presence of other Sexually Transmitted Infections (STIs). Young women are anatomically more vulnerable to infection.

The mucosal surface of the vagina can, at times, be damaged during sexual intercourse. These microlesions may allow greater entry to the virus. The risk from this sort of damage is increased in young women and during coerced sex.

Women also have an increased risk of becoming infected if they have a STI which results in irritation to the vagina (e.g. genital herpes and syphilis). In studies in the United States of America[4] additional factors appear to be associated with increased risk of heterosexual transmission including alcohol use, a history of childhood sexual abuse, current domestic abuse and the use of crack/cocaine.

In addition to their physical properties women are more likely than men to attend hospital and require blood transfusions due to procedures associated with pregnancy and childbirth. Before donated blood products were routinely screened for HIV (and other viruses) this could also increase women's vulnerability.

While biological vulnerability is important this can be mitigated against by the use of male and female condoms and, potentially microbicides (see below.) However, the social and cultural factors which may limit women's ability to deploy these prevention methods compound women's vulnerability. *Confronting the Crisis* suggested that gender inequalities account for the disproportionate burden faced by women. This was echoed by Peter Piot in Toronto who suggested that the epidemic in women was mostly a reflection of power relationships and is only slightly accounted for by biology.

Social and cultural vulnerability

The social and cultural position of women in societies worldwide increases their vulnerability to HIV infection. Inequalities within sexual relationships as well as socio-economic and cultural aspects of their lives impact on the opportunities for them to prevent HIV infection. These two aspects of vulnerability are outlined below.

Sexual vulnerability

The position of women in respect of their sexual lives remains unequal, both in the developing and developed worlds. *Confronting the Crisis* discusses three key factors which contribute to Sub-Saharan women's vulnerability within relationships:

- The culture of silence surrounding sexuality

- Unequal sexual relationships

- Violence against women in relationships.

Although these factors in *Confronting the Crisis* were related directly to Sub-Saharan Africa it is possible to understand their impact in other communities.

The culture of silence

The culture of silence surrounding sexuality makes it difficult for women both to access relevant information about their sexual health and sex lives and to negotiate their sexual relationships[5, 6]. This cultural silence can also extend to knowledge about HIV and AIDS. For example, in one Zambian study less than a quarter of the women asked believed that, even if a woman knew her husband had multiple partners, she would be able to refuse to have sex with him, and only 11% of the women believed she had a right to ask him to use a condom.

This culture of silence means that women are not expected to discuss or make decisions about their sexual lives. Therefore raising the idea of condom use in this context can be very challenging especially when considered alongside other barriers to condom use such as the lack of physical intimacy and loss of spontaneity. Insistence on condom use may also lead to suspicions of infidelity or lack of commitment by a partner.

This culture of silence could be seen as a reflection of power relationships where men are hold power over women. This ultimately can lead to a situation where 'sex' for women is seen purely in terms of penetrative intercourse with a man and therefore women's needs are reduced to just that. This also makes it hard to express desires for other sorts of sexual activity and marginalises lesbian or bisexual women.[7]

Many prevention messages have focussed on the ABC of safer sex, namely 'Abstinence, Being Faithful and using a Condom. Clearly, for many women these ABC's are not within their control.

Unequal sexual relationships

Commercial sex work is covered in a section below.

Women's first sexual experiences are most likely to be with older men which immediately increases their risk as the man is likely to be more sexually experienced. In addition, in many countries women are married in their teens as a way of reducing poverty, as mentioned above in some areas being married is in itself a risk factor for HIV. An Indian study found that some of the contributing factors to this risk were that condoms were seldom used and the women involved found it difficult to discuss their sex lives. Also, if men did suggest using condoms the women suspected they had been unfaithful.

Traditional views of male sexuality mean that promiscuity in men is seen as more acceptable than promiscuity in women who are expected to remain virgins until they marry. Thus women often have less experience in negotiating sexual relations and less accurate information. In some cultures women may engage in anal sex to maintain their virginity. Some surveys report as many as 25% of women as having had anal sex as part of an ongoing heterosexual relationship. Again this carries the additional risks of cuts and abrasions which increase the risk of transmission.

In a further Indian study of a group of 400 women it was found that 25% of the group had STIs and 14% were HIV-positive: 93% of these women were married and 91% had never had sex with anyone but their husbands.

However, it is not only within established relationships that women are vulnerable. In some areas poverty and lack of opportunity can lead to girls and women exchanging sex for food or other necessities. In Southern African countries a 'sugar daddy' is an older man who exchanges sometimes money and other privileges to girls, often to help them support their family in the absence of parents.

Violence against women

It is increasingly recognised that there is a link between violence against women and HIV and AIDS. HIV-positive women are more likely than the general population to have experienced violence and that experience of violence is a risk factor for HIV. The incidence of violence against women is alarmingly high. The fact sheet *Stop Violence against Women, Fight AIDS*[8] reports that in Ethiopia, Bangladesh and India 59%, 50% and 40% of women respectively had experienced sexual violence by an intimate partner. Violence against women is pandemic. It has been reported that almost half of all women in the UK will experience violence in the form of domestic abuse, stalking or sexual assault[9], in addition, a recent UK survey reported by EVAW (End Violence Against Women) reports that 42% of young people aged 16-20 years know girls who have been hit by their boyfriend while 40% of young people know girls who have been forced or pressurised to have sex.[10]

Violence against women often occurs in areas of conflict. It has been reported that in the genocide in Rwanda in 1994 approximately a quarter of a million women experienced sexual violence - many of these women became HIV-positive.

Violence is an important factor in HIV:[11]

- coerced sex can cause abrasions which will increase the risk of HIV transmission

- Experience of violence or fear of violence means that many women are unable to choose when, where and with whom they will have sex.

Socio-economic and cultural vulnerability

The position of women in society increases their vulnerability to HIV. The unequal distribution of economic resources means that women tend to be less economically independent and therefore less in control of making decisions. For example, a woman may be unable to try to persuade a partner to use a condom for financial as well as personal safety reasons. In some areas it is not possible for women to own land and property. If a woman controls their own land and property they are able to retain more control over their household. At the XVI AIDS Conference in Toronto Geeta Rao Gupta, from the International Center for Research on Women, spoke eloquently about how this can impact on women's vulnerability.[12] Land and property do not only provide safety and shelter but they also can act as capital and have been shown to increase women's control over their households and give them the freedom to avoid abusive or unsatisfactory relationships. Geeta Rao Gupta also discussed research which showed that women who owned property were much less likely to experience violence than those who did not (7% versus 40%).

Another economic factor which impacts on women is that in many areas men travel and stay away from home in order to find work. This is often a particular problem for women in rural areas, whose husbands may become infected through commercial sex transactions - and in turn infect their wives.

The lower status of women in societies means that at times access to education is prioritised for male children. Lack of access to education can lead to illiteracy which can reduce people's access to information and services (including HIV prevention information); lack of education will also limit one's career opportunities. Of the 771 million adults in the world who are illiterate, around two-thirds are women.[13] Some areas in particular have extremely low literacy rates: in South and West Asia, sub-Saharan Africa and the Arab States around two-thirds of adult men and only half of adult women are considered to be literate, in addition sub-Saharan Africa has the lowest rate of youth literacy of all regions. It is reasonable to assume that these rates of illiteracy are fuelling the HIV epidemic in general and contributing greatly to the epidemic in women in particular.

Lack of opportunity to access and understand information about HIV can lead to situations where women do not know how to protect themselves, for example, in studies reported in *Confronting the Crisis*, in Vietnam almost half of all young women surveyed believed they could get HIV from a mosquito bite while in Cambodia 30% of young women believed that HIV could be contracted by supernatural means and nearly 35% believed a healthy looking person could not be infected. This situation is described as a 'cause of great concern'.

Many of the positive women in the world are living in areas where access to anti-retroviral treatment (ART) is limited, in sub-Saharan Africa, for example, only approximately 3% of individuals requiring ART actually received it in 2003. However, it is not only the availability of ART which impacts on women's access to treatment; in some areas the treatment of men is prioritised over women. Therefore, if women are not economically independent they may be unable to access treatment on their own behalf. For example, a survey with Zambian women revealed how families on limited budgets chose to pay for treatment only for men in the household and also how property rights - where property of a man who dies passes to his family not to his wife - mean that widows can often be left with no means of support.

Thus, in areas where health services and family planning are not free and easily available women will not be able to access health care or contraception.

Another feature of women's unequal status in the world is that of their role in providing care for people infected. The burden of care in HIV lies with women who, in fulfilling their traditional gendered role, may neglect their own health needs.

There are also some particular cultural practices which increase women's risks:

- **Female genital mutilation - infibulation:** This can increase vulnerability due to the likelihood of bleeding during intercourse. Infibulation is illegal in many areas therefore women undergoing this procedure may be at risk from poor procedures and blood transfusion. The United Nations Family and Population Agency estimates that two million young women undergo this operation each year, largely in Africa.

- **Drying agents:** In some areas of Africa it is the custom to use agents such as herbs to dry or tighten the vagina to increase male pleasure. This may cause cuts and abrasions which increase the risk of HIV transmissibility.

- **Virginity as healing:** Some traditional healers perpetuate the myth that by having sex with a virgin an HIV-positive man may become HIV-negative. This increases the vulnerability of young women.

The section above has given an overview of the factors which influence the HIV epidemic in women. The next section discusses particular issues for female sex workers.

References and further reading

1   UNFPA, UNAIDS and UNIFEM: Women and HIV/AIDS: Confronting the Crisis. ISBN 0-89714-708-1. 2004. See http://www.unfpa.org/publications/detail.cfm?ID=190 . See also UNAIDS Fact Sheet - Women and AIDS - A Growing Challenge

2   Piot P, Keynote Address to the High Level Debate on Leadership: Time to Deliver for Women and Girls, Toronto, August 2006, available at: http://www.kaisernetwork.org/health_cast/player.cfm?id=2727

3   Engender Health, Women's Vulnerability and Risk, part 3 of papers, available at http://www.engenderhealth.org/res/onc/hiv/transmission/hiv3p6.html, 2004

4   NIAID, National Institute of Allergy and Infections Diseases, *HIV Infection in Women - Fact Sheet*, available at http://ww.niaid.nih.gov/factsheets/womenhiv.htm, May 2006

5   Simoni J, Walters K and Nero D, Safer Sex Among HIV-positive women: the role of relationships, *Sex Roles*, Vol. 42, No. 7/8, p 691-708, 2000

6   Wilson T, Sexual and Reproductive Behaviour of Women with HIV Infection, *Clinical Obstetrics and Gynaecology*, Vol. 44, No. 2, p 289-299, 2001

7   Segal L, Sexualities, in Woodward K (ed), 1997, *Identity and Difference*, London, Sage, 1997

8   Global Coalition of Women and AIDS, Factsheet: Stop violence against women fight AIDS, UNAIDS, available at http://www.womenandaids.unaids.org/themes/docs/UNAIDS%20VAW%20Brief.pdf

9   Walby & Allen, Domestic Violence, Sexual Assault and Stalking: Findings from the British Crime Survey, Department of Health, 2004

10 End Violence against Women, A UK Poll of 16-20 Year Olds, ICM, 2006 available at http://amnesty.org.uk/uploads/documents/doc_17400.pdf

11 Gielen AC, McDonell KA, Wu AW, O'Campo P and Faden R. Quality of life among women living with HIV: the importance of violence, social support and self-care behaviours, Social Science and Medicine 52: 315-322, 2001.

12 Gupta G R, Women, HIV and Poverty: Understanding the Nexus for Effective Change, International Centre for Research on Women, Washington, August 2006, available at http://www.icrw.org/docs/speeches/8-15-06-toronto-womenhivpoverty.pdf

13 UNESCO Institute of Statistics, 2006 available at http://www.uis.unesco.org

Female sex workers

UNAIDS' 2006 Report on the Global AIDS Epidemic describes four key populations who are 'at risk and neglected' namely: sex workers, men who have sex with men, infecting drug users and prisoners. For the purposes of this chapter it was therefore felt to be important to include some information about female sex workers, their experience within the epidemic and potential processes through which they can work safely and healthily.

A 2002 report on sex workers by UNAIDS[1] estimated that the total number of people engaged in sex work could number in the tens of millions worldwide. The majority of sex workers are female and most of them are young. In eastern Europe and central Asia it is estimated that 80% of sex workers are under 25 years of age and that those who inject drugs may be even younger. Many of these workers lack experience and information about HIV and what services are available to help them. In a 2003 African study on 33% of the sex workers surveyed knew that they were at risk of HIV infection if they had unprotected sex.

The legal status and associated with sex work differs from county to country. In the UK sex work in itself is not illegal but soliciting and procuring, living off of the earnings or running a brothel is. This leaves working women unprotected by legislation.

Sex workers encounter particular factors which may make them more vulnerable to, and at risk of HIV infection which UNAIDS lists as follows:

- Stigmatisation and marginalisation

- Limited economic options, in particular for women

- Limited access to health, social and legal services

- Limited access to information and prevention means

- Gender-related differences and inequalities

- Sexual exploitation and trafficking

- Harmful, or a lack of protective, legislation and policies

- Exposure to risks associated with lifestyle (e.g. violence, substance use, mobility).

In addition to these factors sex workers are rarely involved in forums where policy initiatives are being discussed so their voices are not heard.

The marginalisation and stigmatisation of sex workers at times has also been associated with HIV, sex workers have been seen as 'vectors of transmission' for spreading the virus while little moral outrage has been directed towards the clients of sex workers in whose hands lies the means of preventing HIV transmission by practicing safer sex. The clients of both female and male sex workers are mostly men. Some countries (e.g. Thailand, Dominican Republic) have introduced 100% condom use policies in brothels and other sex establishments which have appeared to reduce transmission rates. However, this policy is not foolproof and many men will still look elsewhere to find a woman whose situation means she will allow him to have unprotected sex with her.

Other means of reducing HIV transmission via commercial sex has been to introduce licensing of sex workers based on their attendance for sexual health services and potentially HIV testing. Such schemes allow access to health care and information for sex workers but rely on sensitive and quality staffing who are willing to treat clients with dignity or people will not attend.

Compulsory testing of sex workers has also been proposed in some areas as a prevention mechanism, however, this does nothing to protect the workers themselves from infection, compounds the stigmatisation of positive women (as male sex workers tend not to be subject to such licensing arrangements) and, it could be argued, fundamentally restricts human rights whereby only one person in a sexual relationship is required to be subject to medical testing.

As well as these ethical arguments there are practical problems with such schemes, Firstly, if a sex worker is given a licence to practice the customer may request unprotected sex and also, given that positive people are able to have healthy and active sex lives such restrictions are restrictions on positive people working in the sex industry appear not to be grounded in safer sex messages.

In the UK no such schemes are currently in force but there are regular political debates about how best to 'manage' the sex industry. Sex workers' organisations and advocates have lobbied for decriminalisation of such work which would reduce some of the stigma associated and render workers better protected in law. This would also enable women to operate from legitimate establishments thereby protecting themselves from increased risk of violence and exploitation which go with working on the streets. However, decriminalisation remains very controversial.

HIV and AIDS and sex work sit within a wider framework of poverty and gender inequality and, from this perspective UNAIDS (2002) suggests that the following processes may be successful in preventing HIV and caring for those affected:

- Promotion of safer sexual behaviour among sex workers, clients and institutions or groups associated with sex workers such as police and partners. This would involve condom availability and negotiation skills.

- Promotion and availability of STI prevention and care services

- Outreach work that includes health, social and legal services

- Peer education among sex workers, clients and associated groups

- Advocacy for policy and law reform at national and local levels, including respect of human rights.

Sex worker activism

Despite the structural inequalities and discrimination faced by sex workers, many prevention and care campaigns have been initiated from within this population itself. A snapshot of some of the initiatives designed and implemented by workers is presented here to remind us that stereotypical portrayals of this group of women serve only to misrepresent and further stigmatise them.

India

In Sonagachi, Calcutta, India, female sex workers reacted to what they saw as discrimination and started the Durbar Mahila Samanaya Committee (DMSC) - which roughly translates into Indomitable Women's Solidarity Committee - to represent the 60,000 sex workers in West Bengal.[2] Their work was initiated by a peer education project in which the sex workers themselves worked as peer educators who visited each tenement and distributed free condoms. Other sex workers were invited to educational sessions about HIV infections and given access to medical treatment and testing. Clients were also invited to learn about safer sex and a male peer educator was employed to work with the men.

The solidarity and strength of the DMSC has allowed representatives to be involved in policy making and has also empowered the working women to refuse to practices unsafe sex. This has resulted in a significant reduction in the frequency of women having unprotected commercial sex.

Bangladesh

Dhaka, the capital city of Bangladesh, hosts over 10,000 sex workers. Activists (either present or former sex workers) from Durjoy Nari Shango[3], an organisation for female sex workers which has the following objectives:

- Promoting unity

- Prevention of HIV/AIDS

- Building self-esteem

- Skills training to promote alternative methods of income generation.

- Addressing essential needs (shelter/sanitation/education and health care for children of sex workers)

- Establishing social, legal and human rights.

The primary focus of the group is to improve the lives of sex workers' children. Children are often stigmatised and, like their mothers, will not receive equal quality of education or medical treatment. Durjoy's objective is to help integrate the children in the great community by enrolling more children into the public school system and providing education classes at the centre.

Set up in 1998, the organisation now has over 2,500 members who benefit from safer sex education, skills training and drop-in centres. Women work together to monitor each other's whereabouts and to assist if individuals are at risk of violence. The organisation has also made formal presentations and, as well as benefiting from the practical support and activities, women involved have the opportunity to build self-esteem.

Durjoy Nari Shango was awarded a Red Ribbon Award (which celebrates community leadership and action on AIDS) by the XVIth International AIDS Conference.

References

1 UNAIDS Technical Update 2002, Sex work and HIV and AIDS, Geneva UNAIDS

2 See: www.positivenation.co.uk/issue85_6/features/feature6/feature6_1.htm and http://www.walnet.org/pdf/ADVOCACY.PDF

3 See: www.synergyaids.com/documents/Submodulebrothel.pdf and www.redribbonaward.org/content.php?pg=community&event=conference&document=dailyjournal&day=5

Resource

Network of Sex Work Projects - an informal alliance of sex workers and organizations that provide services to sex workers formed as the Network of Sex Work Projects. See www.nswp.org.

In particular see Overs, Cheryl and Longo, Paulo: *Making Sex Work Safe*, Network of Sex Work Projects. 1997.

Prevention

As discussed above, the vulnerability of women to HIV infection can be considered in terms of their biological, sexual and socio-economic and cultural experiences. In order to prevent further catastrophic spread of the virus through the female population government and policy makers have a huge challenge.

Confronting the Crisis summarised principles for prevention strategies which are known to work:

- Challenging the social norms and values that contribute to the lower social status of women and girls and condone violence against them.

- Increasing the self-confidence and self-esteem of girls.

- Strengthening the legal and policy frameworks that support women's rights to economic independence including the right to own and inherit land and property.

- Ensuring access to health services and education, in particular life-skills and sexuality education for both boys and girls.

- Empowering women and girls economically.

These principles emphasise the wider determinants which influence women's ability to remain HIV free and thus acknowledge that this will not be solved by provision of safer sex information alone. In his Keynote address to the XVI World AIDS Conference Peter Piot raised additional areas for discussion. As referred to earlier, the ABC (Abstinence, Be Faithful and use a Condom) approach to prevention is inappropriate for women as none of these are primarily under their control, it is still the case that many HIV policy and programmes do not involve women in their design, it is also the case that work needs to be done with men and boys in alerting them to the way in which traditional gender roles and their behaviours are fuelling the epidemic.

While the principles of prevention strategies outlined above may seem most relevant to the developing world a strong argument could be made for their importance within the UK. Social norms about male and female sexuality continue to portray these as different, with different moral values attached, and women tend to earn less than men and be more likely to be carers of children and other dependant family members. While some areas are encouraging sexual health awareness education for young people via projects such as the SHARE initiative in Scotland[1], a comprehensive prevention programme for women remains elusive.

Traditional prevention campaigns have either been targeted at gay men or a population level behaviour change approach. While recently there have been initiatives promoting testing within the African community there is little in the way of general messages for women. One of the difficulties in developing such an approach is that knowledge about what might work is limited. It has been suggested that, since most women are infected by men, a way forward might be to target initiatives at men (for example IV Drug Users or gay and bisexual men who have sex with women). However, this would not reach all vulnerable women could be seen as placing women as 'victims' in the epidemic by not allowing them the means to protect themselves.

Developing an effective prevention campaign for women is a complex issue. It seems unlikely that prevention messages for 'heterosexuals' will not be effective as this term embraces a diversity of groups and does not distinguish between women and men and therefore cannot be specific about risks.

Most women in Britain who know they have HIV were unaware that they were at risk when they became infected. Often, HIV-positive women report that they knew the risks associated with HIV, but did not know that this risk was related to them. So, despite the challenges, it is important that something is done to address this area or women will continue to consider themselves at low risk for HIV.

Although both female and male condoms protect both partners from the risk of HIV and other STIs neither can be used by a woman without the co-operation of her partner. One way to address this gap in the means of protection may be through the development of microbicides which potentially could supply a woman controlled prevention method.

Microbicides

A microbicide is 'any product which can kill or prevent infection from one or more microbes that can be transmitted during sexual intercourse[2]. A microbicide would be used in the form of a gel, sponge or lubricant and the aim is to develop an agent that will not only prevent transmission of HIV and other STIs but also act as a contraceptive. Further information about microbicides is included in the *Prevention* section of this Manual.

Microbicide development has been discussed at major conferences for many years and as yet there is no immediate short-term likelihood for an effective microbicide to be available on the open market. However, there are several different approaches being researched at the moment. Scientists developing such agents are faced with a complexity of need wherein some applications (e.g. tenofovir gel which is in Phase 2 testing) will protect only against HIV and not other STIs while others may be required to protect against infection but to allow for conception.

It is not envisaged at the moment that microbicides would be as effective at preventing HIV transmission as condoms. Condom use however, as discussed elsewhere, can face several barriers and if a microbicide was discreet and easy to use a woman could protect herself (potentially before or after sex) without the involvement or agreement of her partner. However, according to projections presented at the Microbicides 2002 Conference by Dr. Charlotte Church, of the London School of Tropical Medicine, if a microbicide that was 60% effective reaches the market, and was used consistently by 30% of women at risk, it could prevent 3.7 million infections. The cost of developing microbicides is huge and activists campaign for more funding to be put into this field.

References and Resources

1 For information on the SHARE programme please contact Healthy Respect at NHS Lothian on 0131-536 9000.

2 Weeks M, Mosack K, Abbott M, Sylla L, Valders B and Prince M. American Sexually Transmitted Diseases Association, Microbicide Acceptability Among High Risk Urban U.S. Women: Experiences and Perceptions of Sexually Transmitted HIV Prevention, 2004.

See also:

- ACT-UP New York: Women, AIDS and Activism, South End Press, 1990.
- Gorna, Robin: Vamps Virgins and Victims: How can women fight AIDS? Cassell, 1996. See especially chapters eight and nine.
- National AIDS Trust. HIV Prevention Factsheet, 2005
- UNAIDS: Gender and HIV/AIDS: Taking stock of research and programmes is an extensive discussion of research evidence regarding gender and HIV. A selection of links to other material on Women and HIV can be found in the Links section on www.aidsmap.com .

Women rising to the challenge

In many areas women have been at the forefront of leading the fight against HIV and AIDS. Many community-based organisations have been developed and implemented by positive women themselves. The enterprise, energy and commitment of these women in the face of the challenges listed above are tremendous. Unfortunately there is not space within this chapter to describe even a fraction of the work that has been done, however, it is hoped that the few projects are presented will serve as examples of how women activists are leading the process of change.

Some of the work that women have done is on a small scale local level in response to need. For example, in San Francisco, Jane - an 'older woman living with HIV' - recognised that there was no organisation that addressed the needs of older positive women in her area. She took up this challenge and started a support group in her local area. Other individual women have instigated political lobbying and pressure groups to encourage governments to adopt appropriate HIV and AIDS policy. For example, in Uganda the National Community of women Living with AIDS[1] (NACWOLA), which provides services to over 40,000 women in Uganda, was founded by Beatrice Were, a positive woman who has recently received an award for defending human rights. In addition to this role, Beatrice also co-ordinates ActionAid International and advocates for the rights of positive people in her country.

Women have been instrumental in leading the fight through developing initiatives in peer education which can help influence traditional communities by using language and people relevant to their needs to address issues around HIV and AIDS including safer sex but also care of AIDS orphans. One such internationally recognised initiative is the Stepping Stones programme[2].

Many of the modern heroines of HIV were represented at the XVI World AIDS Conference in Toronto which saw increased coverage of gender issues and increased inclusion of positive women on the programme. One of the co-organisers of the conference was the International Community of Women Living with HIV and AIDS (ICW)[3]. ICW is an international network run for and by HIV-positive women that promotes all positive women's voices and advocates for changes that improve their lives. It was founded in Amsterdam in 1992 to respond to the desperate lack of support and information to HIV-positive women worldwide. ICW works towards ensuring that all HIV-positive women will:

- Have a respected and meaningful involvement at all political levels; local, national, regional, and international, where decisions that affect their lives are being made;

- Have full access to care and treatment; and

- Enjoy the full rights, particularly sexual, reproductive, legal, financial and general health rights; irrespective of our sexuality, culture, age, religion, social or economic status/class and race.

ICW was represented on the Conference High Level Session on Leadership: Time to deliver for women and girls, which developed 5 actions to confront the challenge of HIV in women which are summarised below:

Action 1: Increase funding for AIDS programmes for women, and adapt existing strategies to ensure they are gender integrated.

Action 2: increase meaningful participation of women where AIDS policies are decided, strategies forged and funds allocated.

Action 3: increase access for all women to services as well as prevention options women can initiate themselves, notably microbicides and female condoms. Invest in young people's development and understanding of the gender dimension of the pandemic and provide them with the necessary access to reproductive and sexual health and rights and HIV and AIDS information, education and services.

Action 4: Ensure the rights of women are fully reflected in legislation that protects women against violence, upholds their right to own and inherit property and upholds their right to access sexual and reproductive health services.

Action 5: Empower women by scaling up efforts to secure women's livelihoods, enhance their socio-economic status and better equip them to live health lives in a world with HIV and AIDS.

A full version of these calls to action is available at: www.aids2006.org/admin/images/upload/1261.pdf

It is clear then that, despite the challenges faced by HIV-positive women, they continue to respond with dignity and bravery, it is also clear that at last the international community is beginning not only to recognise this but to start engaging with positive women and listening to their voices. Within the UK, most HIV agencies offer women the opportunity to meet with peers either in a formal or informal setting.

References and further reading

1 See http://hrw.org/english/docs/2006/10/26/uganda14405.htm

2 See http://www.steppingstonesfeedback.org

3 See www.icw.org

Living with HIV

For women, living with HIV requires adjustments and decision-making in relation to one's health, motherhood, one's own mortality and relationships not just with sexual partners but with other friends and family[1]. There are also particular considerations for women and antiretroviral therapy. This section aims to highlight some of these concerns and will cover the following areas:

- Specific health concerns for positive women

- Cervical screening

- Menopause

- Treatment in women
  Introduction
  Side-effects
  Adherence

- Stigma and disclosure

- Sex and relationships
  Contraception and prevention of STIs
  Disclosing your HIV status to a sexual partner

- Pregnancy
  Introduction
  HIV testing in pregnancy
  Conception
  Infertility treatment
  Considerations for pregnant women
  ART treatment in pregnancy
  Drug levels and side-effects in pregnancy
  Single dose nevirapine

- Care of infants born to positive mothers
  Treatment
  Testing
  Breastfeeding

Specific health concerns for positive women

In general terms the signs and symptoms of HIV and AIDS in women and men are similar. However, there are some particular differences and concerns for women: some studies have found that the incidence of some HIV related illnesses are different in men than in women; for example, **Kaposi's sarcoma** appears to be more common in gay men while **herpes simplex virus** appears more likely to produce complications in women. One American study appeared to show that positive women are more likely than positive men to develop **bacterial pneumonia** although the authors of the study speculated that this might be due to factors such as access or use of health care services. **Anaemia** (reduced levels of red blood cells) also appears to be more common in HIV-positive women than positive men.

However, in terms of women-specific concerns, it does appear to be the case that HIV-positive women experience gynaecological problems more frequently and more severely than negative women. These are summarised below[2,3].

- HIV-positive women experience more **vaginal thrush** than negative women and this tends to be more persistent. There are, however, effective oral medications to treat thrush. The presence of any infection as well as causing ill-health to women can increase the risk of vertical and sexual transmission.

- **Human Papilloma Virus (HPV)** infection which can cause genital warts and is linked with cervical cancer occurs more frequently in HIV-positive women as do precancerous changes in the cervix (opening to the womb) called cervical dysplasia. For this reason positive women are recommended to have cervical smear tests performed once a year.

- **Pelvic inflammatory disease (PID)** also seems to be more common in HIV-positive women and more severe.

- HIV-positive women also report more **menstrual problems** than negative women (e.g. heavier or lighter bleeding, irregular or lack of periods). There is some evidence to suggest that menstrual irregularities are associated with lower CD4 counts. If a woman notices any changes to her period this should be reported to her doctor as it may be a sign of HIV disease progression.

- A recent study suggested that HIV-positive women were not, however, at increased risk of severe menstrual problems and suggested that, given the common occurrence of menstrual irregularities in negative women it may be the case that positive women mistakenly attribute these to their HIV status.

Cervical screening

Due to the increased risk of cervical dysplasia mentioned above HIV-positive women are recommended to have cervical smear (PAP) tests performed more regularly than the general population. The current UK recommendation for routine screening is once every twelve months.

Cervical cancer and precancerous changes in the cervix have been known to be linked to HIV and related immunosuppression for many years. In 1993 invasive cervical cancer was listed as an AIDS defining illness. Positive women who experience precancerous changes in the cervix may be at increased risk of this rapidly progressing to cervical cancer.

Early cervical cancer is usually asymptomatic (shows no symptoms); later symptoms can include bleeding after intercourse, watery/bloodstained vaginal discharge or a foul smelling vaginal discharge. If a positive woman experiences any of these symptoms she should attend her doctor/family planning clinic for investigation.

Fortunately precancerous and cancerous changes can be readily detected through a smear test. If any abnormalities are detected she will normally be offered a repeat test and be referred for gynaecological review. Many women experience abnormal smear tests and most are not cancerous.

A cervical smear test is a straightforward test which can detect any changes of the cells in the cervix which could develop into cancer. A sample of cells is collected from the cervix by firstly opening the vagina with an instrument called a speculum, a small wooden spatula or brush can then be inserted to scrape a sample which can be collected onto a slide and sent for checking. This procedure can be a little uncomfortable but rarely painful. Results are usually sent to the clinic and then forwarded to the woman.

Recently it has been noted that African women may be less likely to attend for routine smear testing. It is important that all positive women are made aware of the importance of this procedure in reducing the risk of cervical cancer.

Smear tests are offered by most family doctor's surgeries and family planning/well woman clinics.

Menopause

The menopause (sometimes called 'change of life) is a natural process which occurs when the production of female sex hormones from a woman's ovaries starts to decline. HIV-positive women and negative women experience similar symptoms of the menopause but it is thought that since HIV can interfere with women's ability to produce some sex hormones that this may lead to an early menopause.

Many women take hormone supplements to replace those that are lost. This hormone replacement therapy (HRT) may have greater risks for positive women especially if they have lipodystrophy or high cholesterol levels. If a woman is considering HRT she should discuss this with her doctor.

References

1   Ciambrone D, Illness and other assaults on self: the relative impact of HIV/AIDS on women's lives, Sociology of Health and Illness, Vol. 23, No.4, p517-540, 2001

2   NIAID, National Institute of Allergy and Infections Diseases, May 2006, HIV Infection in Women - Fact Sheet, available at http://ww.niaid.nih.gov/factsheets/womenhiv.htm

3   Massad LS, Evans CL, Minkoff H, et al. Effects of HIV infection and its treatment on self-reported menstrual abnormalities in women, Journal of Women's Health, Vol.15, No. 5, p591-598, 2006

See also:

BHIVA, Guidelines for the management of HIV infection in pregnant women and the prevention of mother-to-child transmission of HIV, British HIV Association, 2005

HIV treatment in women

Introduction

As discussed elsewhere in this manual, the introduction of antiretroviral therapy (ART) has meant that positive people who have access to this therapy have the chance of increased good health, quality of life and life expectancy. However, adherence to ART can be difficult both in terms of the side-effects associated with some of the medications and in managing the drug regime itself.

Since most trials of drugs have to date occurred in Western countries, the majority of the participants in the trials have been men, reflecting the nature of the epidemic. It has therefore often been difficult to establish accurate information on women-specific issues related to ART. We know that most positive people worry about the long-term impacts of HIV treatment and this concern can also be amplified for women when they are considering having children and worry about the effects of ART on their unborn babies. Women tend to be smaller and weigh less than men; they also have different hormonal systems which may affect metabolic or other effects of medication. Recently more effort has gone into research which is applicable to women but there remains a gap in terms of our knowledge about how specific treatments affect positive women.

Women not taking antiretroviral therapy tend to have a lower HIV viral load than men. A meta-review of studies of viral load in women[1] found that they reported that for any given CD4 count, women's viral load was 41% lower than men's. Some studies have also found that women progress to AIDS faster than men. One study[2] comparing disease progression among male and female injecting drug users found no difference in CD4 decline or mortality between men and women, but when controlling for age and CD4 cell count, women progressed to AIDS 60% more quickly than men. Other studies however have found no difference in progression rates.

Some of the evidence and emerging data about women specific issues in relation to ART are outlined below.

Side -effects

Lipodystrophy

(for more information please see Treatments Chapter)

Lipodystrophy is the name used to describe particular changes in body shape and the metabolism caused by anti-HIV drugs. The changes in body shape which have been described are:

- Lipohypertrophy/lipoaccumulation - Fat gain on the abdomen/belly, between the shoulder blades, around the neck, or in the breasts.

- Lipoatrophy: Fat loss from under the skin most commonly in the face, in the legs and arms: can make veins look more prominent and in the buttocks can make sitting uncomfortable.

- Some people also experience a mixture of both fat loss and fat gain.

Changes which occur in the metabolism include altered cholesterol and blood lipid levels.

All of these changes have been noticed in both men and women. There remains a lack of certainty about the exact mechanisms which cause lipodystrophy and how best to approach treating these side-effects. It would appear that we are seeing two overlapping forms of toxicity: one related to the nucleoside drugs (NRTIs) or possibly solely to the thymidine analogue drugs AZT and d4T, which cause the fat loss and some of the blood lipid changes, and one possibly related to the protease inhibitors, which cause the fat accumulation and other metabolic changes, though it is unclear as yet which PIs are more likely to fat accumulation, or even if they do at all: one study found that in men, at least, visceral fat gain was no worse in HIV-positive men than HIV-negative ones; it was just made more obvious by fat loss in other areas. As with general treatment trials to date much of the early research on lipodystrophy has focused on men, however, more recently there have been some studies which attempted to investigate its effects in women and whether there are any differences between the sexes.

It appears that lipodystrophy is a problem for HIV-positive women receiving ART treatment. Some authors have suggested that it is a more common problem for HIV-positive women than for HIV-positive men however this remains uncertain[3]. It does appear, however, that lipodystrophy has a tendency to manifest itself differently in women and men, in that women appear more likely to experience fat accumulation around their waist and breasts whereas men are more likely to experience facial fat loss[4].

Non-nucleoside Reverse Transcriptase Inhibitors (NNRTIs)

Both NNRTIs have potentially serious side-effects for some particular groups of women:

Nevirapine - like most medicines nevirapine carries the risk of side-effects. However, with nevirapine there is a risk of two serious side-effects, both caused by an immune reaction to the drug. One is liver failure, which can develop within days, and the other is a severe form of rash - in reality more like severe burns - called toxic epidermal necrolysis or Stevens-Johnson syndrome (SJS). Both of these side-effects can be fatal, though liver failure has caused more deaths[5]. The group of patients most at risk of these side-effects are women with a CD4 count over 250 cells/mm[3]and women in this group should not be prescribed the drug (men have a higher threshold for risk, at a CD4 count of 400). Rash is a quite common side-effect when starting treatment with nevirapine but SJS usually involves fever too. Anyone with these symptoms should seek medical advice immediately.

Efavirenz Beckerman et al[6] reported birth abnormalities reported in women taking ART. Although causation has not been proved, there does appear to be an association between efavirenz and increased risk neural tube defects (development of the spinal cord and brain) in the foetus[7,8]. This association means that women who are intending to become pregnant should not use efavirenz and their treatment options are therefore restricted.

Ethical constraints mean that data about the effects of ART on the developing foetus are generally only available retrospectively (i.e. by examining pregnancy outcomes rather than by setting up a trial before pregnancy begins). Please see the Pregnancy section below for more information about treatment in pregnant women.

Adherence

A small study in Brazil[9] (144 women in total) looked at levels of adherence (i.e. taking at least 95% of the doses of their ART correctly) in women - half who were pregnant and half who were not. They found low levels of adherence overall with only 17.7% of the non-pregnant women adherent. However, adherence levels in the pregnant women was much higher at 41.3% but still below the levels reported in previous studies. It is not possible to generalise findings from this study, however, it does suggest that the motivation and ability to adhere to medications may be different for some groups of positive women and men.

However few studies have found a general gender difference when it comes to adherence - good and poor adherence, it appears, tends to be situational (based on events in a person's life at the time) and attempts to find 'types' of people who are more or less likely to be adherent have usually failed. See **adherence** in the NAM Treatment Directory for more on this.

References

1 Napravnik S et al. Gender difference in HIV RNA levels: a meta-analysis of published studies. Journal of Acquired Immune Deficiency Syndromes 31(1): 11-9, 2002.

2 Webber MP et al. A prospective study of HIV disease progression in female and male drug users. AIDS 13:257-62. 1999.

3 Galli M et al, Gender differences in antiretroviral drug-related adipose tissue alterations. JAIDS Vol. 34, p58 - 61, 2003

4 FRAM Study Team. The Fat Redistribution and Metabolic Change in HIV Infection (FRAM) Study Team. Fat distribution in women with HIV infection. Journal of Acquired Immune Deficiency Syndrome, Vol. 42, No. 5, p562-71, 2006

5 Sanne I et al. Severe hepatotoxicity associated with nevirapine use in HIV-infected subjects. J Infect Dis 191: 825-829, 2005.

6 Beckerman K, Watts H, Covington D et al, Assessing the risk of central nervous system birth defects associated with ART exposure during pregnancy, 13th CROI, Denver, Abstract 713

7 Fundaró C., Genovese O., Rendeli C., et al. Myelomeningocele in a child with intrauterine exposure to efavirenz, AIDS, Vol. 16, No. 2, p299-300, 2002

8 Botto L. D., Moore C. A., Khoury M. J. and Erickson J. D. Neural tube defects. New England Journal of Medicine, Vol. 341, No. 20, p1509.1519, 1999

9 Vaz MJR et al. Adherence with antiretroviral therapy during pregnancy. 43rd ICAAC, abstract H-859, Chicago September 14 - 17th, 2003.

Stigma and disclosure

Women living with HIV are often concerned about the stigma associated with their diagnosis. Although it is often assumed by workers and public that there is somehow less stigma associated with HIV than in the early days of the epidemic this does not feel true for many women (and men) living with HIV as the following quote shows: an African woman taking part in a study on stigma and discrimination[1] described a trip to her dentist:

"I have a dental problem and I go to this clinic, and I go there, two maybe three times. So eventually I told them about my condition. They explained that I would have to be the last appointment of the day. I have been to that room, and sat on that chair, and the same doctor examined me as before, but after I told them I was HIV-positive. So I went for the last appointment of the day last week, they covered the chair, the light, the doctors were wearing three pairs of gloves."

This stigma is a complex intertwining of several aspects: positive women can experience stigma and discrimination from health professionals (often through assumptions about health behaviour), additional stigmatisation of women who have been drug users or sex workers and positive women may themselves 'internalise' stigma.

The media has often represented HIV-positive women as solely as sex workers or pregnant mothers, in other words, potential infectors of others rather than people who have themselves been infected. Also, lesbian women have been perceived as not 'at risk' and therefore rarely receive mention in relation to HIV even though lesbians may be at higher risk of transmission by non-sexual means such as injecting drug use - and many also have sex with men.

This burden of stigma can be amplified when a woman is a mother as she is often reluctant to disclose her status for fear that her children experience associated stigma.

There is also evidence that positive women find it more difficult than positive men to disclose their status to sexual partners. These difficulties around disclosure can make women less willing to access services and less able to receive support they need from families and friends.

The Ousider Status study[1], which looked at stigma experienced by African people and gay men with HIV showed how African people living with HIV experienced stigma and discrimination related to their HIV infection and to racism. Often racism was associated with assumptions about people's immigration status. Positive African people are also stigmatised within the African community as HIV is often associated with sexism and homophobia. An African woman in the study describes the stigma within the African community and its effect on women needing to access services:

"*There was a lady who lived with me in the hotel. She was from Zimbabwe. She was a great friend of mine. I asked her, "Can't we go to (name of African support agency) or something together." She said, "Aye, I can't go there. I go there, and people know me, and maybe some people from home will social exclusion me and they will know that I am HIV-positive. I can't go." She never came."*

Many voluntary sector HIV projects offer women specific groups or activities which can help support women to disclose.

Disclosing to children

Many positive women are also mothers and thus must decide how and when they might decide to disclose to their child(ren). Preventative measures which help reduce the risk of vertical (mother-to-baby) transmission are well established and, coupled with the increase in life-expectancy associated with access to ART, may lead to an increased desire to have children and a consequent increase in the number of children born to positive mothers.

Parenting, a challenge at any time, brings additional pressures for positive women who will have concerns about practical issues such as what happens if a mother becomes unwell and how will she care for her children, how to adhere to medication if it is a 'secret' as well as psychological issues such as guilt or concerns her children's future. If the child is born HIV-positive there will be additional pressures associated with caring for that child.

A Dutch study[2] described how disclosure often falls to mothers as women are more likely to have care of children. Within this study there was a tendency to wait until children are older (around 16 years) to disclose and, while this may be an option as

people remain healthier for longer, for some mothers a decision must be made much earlier due to her own ill-health.

A small study of African mothers described factors which influence their decision to tell their children. These mothers were concerned that their children might be too young to understand or that the news might be too disturbing for them. They also wondered if there was a benefit in telling their children and were concerned about their own ability to disclose to them. One of the major influences was the perceived stigma relating to HIV infection and how this might impact on the children. However, despite these concerns, the mothers did want to disclose but hoped that they might be able to do this with the help of a professional. For some African parents disclosure difficulties are increased as the patterns of migration mean that some children will be living with relatives in the country of origin while their parent is living in the UK.

It is likely, however, that the decision about how or when to disclose will be an individual one within families. Mothers who are preparing to disclose their status to their children will hopefully receive support from specialist workers and other women who have experience in this area. The mother can then be supported to find cultural and age appropriate materials and ways of communicating about HIV to her child(ren).

If parents have explained the facts of HIV to their children, then the disclosure of a parent's own status to their child may leave that parent open to questioning by the child on how they became infected. Having to explain facts about their own lifestyle - for example taking drugs, being gay or bisexual may prove to be too difficult, and the parent may decide not to disclose their status in order to circumvent these questions.

For more discussion about discussing HIV with children please see the Chapter: **Children and Adolescents.**

References

1 Dodds C et al. Outsider Status, Stigma and discrimination experienced by Gay men and African people with HIV, 2004, Sigma Research. ISBN 1 872956 76 9. See www.sigmaresearch.org

2 Nostlinger. Families affected by HIV: parents' and children's characteristics and disclosure to the children, AIDS Care 16(5): 641-648

Sex and relationships

The World Health Organization defines sexual health as "A state of physical, emotional, mental and social wellbeing related to sexuality; it is not merely the absence of disease, dysfunction or infirmity.for sexual health to be attained and maintained, the sexual rights of all persons must be respected, protected and fulfilled.' In other words, positive women have the same rights to a healthy sexual life as any other woman.

At the time of diagnosis with HIV many positive women may feel that they are now less able to have an active sexual relationship. However, studies have shown that most positive women continue to have sexual relationships after their diagnosis. There is some evidence that sexual activity is related to the fact that people who have access to ART are likely to live longer, more healthy lives than in the past and therefore they may have an increased desire for an active sexual life as it is known that ill-health can impact negatively on individual's desire about sex[1].

In common with the lack of prevention work for positive women there is a lack of evidence about what positive women hope for and experience in their sexual relationships. There are a lot of

studies focussing on 'sexual behaviours' and 'reproductive health' but, in line with much of the research done for and about women with HIV these tend to focus on: how to prevent transmission to negative partners or to children; and the prevalence, treatment and prevention of sexually transmitted infections (STIs). While it important that these aspects of sexual activity are researched this focus reinforces stereotypes of positive women as being 'vectors of transmission' rather than infected people in their own right.

Current draft BHIVA guidelines[2] state that at the all HIV-positive women should, as part of their initial medical assessment, have a sexual and gynaecological history taken and given the opportunity to discuss contraception and screening for STIs. The decisions positive women will take regarding sex and relationships, however, are likely to include wider issues such as: contraception and prevention of sexually transmitted infections, whether to disclose to a sexual partner, the risk of transmission to a sexual partner.

Contraception and prevention of STIs

There are a variety of different methods of contraception available but only two will also protect women from HIV and STIs: the condom and female condom which are both associated with 'safer sex'.

Choosing to have 'safer sex' means choosing sexual activities which reduce the risk of HIV transmission. Condoms (both male and female) can markedly reduce the risk of transmission of HIV if used correctly and for this reason the draft BHIVA guidelines recommend that all HIV-positive women are advised to use condoms within sexual relationships. However, not all couples choose to have 'safer sex'. For example, in relationships where monogamous partners are untested or have tested HIV-negative other methods of contraception may be used. Some couples where both partners are HIV-positive have also made this choice although this is not recommended as they risk being infected with different strains of the virus or with other STIs.

A survey of positive people published in 2002[3] showed almost a quarter of one sample of positive people reporting that they practised safer sex less often since the arrival of new treatments as HIV was somehow seen as 'less serious' than previously and the perception that an individual with an undetectable viral load was less likely to be infectious. Another study of HIV-positive women in New York with HIV-negative partners[4] found that condom use, initially high during the first weeks of a relationship, fell during the first couple of years of a relationship. On investigation this seemed to be linked to the need to demonstrate trust and love in a relationship: allowing unprotected sex was psychologically equated with demonstrating the wish to bond. If the relationship continued longer, and the woman remained uninfected, condom use started to go up again. The risk of sexual transmission may be reduced if a person's viral load is undetectable but it is not eliminated as there is still a risk associated with unprotected penetrative vaginal and anal sex since HIV can be present at different levels in the genital fluids than in blood.

For more on all these questions, see the chapter on **HIV prevention.**

However, often it can be difficult for women to control condom use within a heterosexual relationship. It is important to remember that barriers to condom use which were mentioned earlier in this chapter such as the perceived loss of physical intimacy, and loss of spontaneity may exist for positive people too. The use of male and female condoms requires co-operation from a male partner and, in the context of 'cultural silence' about sexual relationships and women's role within them, this can add to difficulties for HIV-positive women trying to make an informed choice about their contraceptive needs. Some men (and some women) dislike condoms and some men complain of discomfort or reduced sensitivity when they are wearing them. Insisting on condom use can sometimes mean a woman risks being suspected of infidelity, distrusting her partner or may be coerced into revealing her HIV status against her wishes. Disclosing HIV status to a sexual partner can make women vulnerable to rejection or even violence.

The importance of establishing a method of protection which women can control has led researchers to investigate the potential of microbicides (see below).

Positive women are often recommended to adopt a 'belt and braces' approach to contraception, that is, to use a barrier method such as a male condom or female condom for safer sex and an additional hormonal form of contraception such as the oral contraceptive pill (OCP) to avoid pregnancy.

There is no method of contraception that will offer 100% protection against pregnancy or STIs. A brief guide to different forms of contraception follows. However, best informed advice about contraception can be obtained from Family Planning and Well Woman Clinics. Positive women will probably wish to seek advice from their HIV doctor.

References

1 Siegel K and Schrimshaw E, *Reasons for the adoption of celibacy among older men and women living with HIV/AIDS,* The Journal of Sex Research, Vol. 40, No. 2, p189-200, 2003

2 BHIVA. *Draft guidelines for the management of sexual and reproductive health of people living with HIV infection,* 2006

3 Demmer C. *Impact of improved treatments on perceptions about HIV and safer sex among inner-city HIV-infected men and women,* Journal of Community Health 27(1): 63-73, 2002.

4 Simoni J M et al. *Safer sex among HIV+ women: The role of relationships.* Sex Roles 42: 691-708, 2000.

Types of contraception available

Contraceptive methods can be grouped in to two main types:

1 Barrier

2 Hormonal

Barrier forms of contraception

As the name implies, these forms of contraception aim to put a physical barrier in place to prevent fertilisation and hence pregnancy.

Male Condom

The contraceptive effectiveness of the condom depends upon how carefully it is used. There is a 2% failure rate for properly used 'Kitemark' condoms (this means that in one year, two in 100 women will conceive who have used condoms consistently and properly for all occasions of vaginal intercourse). This failure rate rises to 15% for improperly used condoms (source: Durex).

Condoms cannot be used with oil-based lubricants. Some treatments for gynaecological conditions, like thrush, may be oil-based. It is important to check whether any cream or pessary used as a treatment can destroy latex, and to use a different method of contraception if it does (for example, the female condom which is not made of latex).

The condom requires the man to take an active responsibility for contraception. It has no health risks and it substantially reduces the risk of acquiring or transmitting HIV or other infections.

A word about nonoxynol 9 -'N9' spermicide. Nonoxynol 9 (N-9) is a spermicide which has, in the past, been added to some condoms and lubricants to reduce the risk of pregnancy and also to reduce transmission of HIV and other STIs. N-9 is now known to increase this, particularly when used rectally but also vaginally as it affects the skin lining the vagina and rectum and can cause abrasions and blisters. It is now recommended that N-9 be removed from condoms. Most condoms available via free NHS schemes are now N-9 free, however, there are still some available and individuals should always check their choice of condoms.

The female condom

The contraceptive effectiveness of the female condom depends upon how carefully it is used. There is a 2.4% failure rate when the female condom is used properly, and 12.2% when not used properly and consistently (source: Chartex). The female condom is polyurethane sheath which is inserted in to the woman's vagina and covers both her internal and external genitalia. Female condoms come with instructions for use.

The diaphragm, or cap

This method of contraception does not protect against HIV transmission for either partner and is therefore not generally recommended for use by women living with HIV.

If used properly, the cap has a pregnancy failure rate between 2-5%. It has no health risks for women who are not allergic to rubber or spermicide. This is a circle of thick rubber with a rim containing a flexible spring. The cap comes in different sizes and shapes, and has a range of names. Some caps only cover the cervix, while others also cover a large area at the top of the vagina. The cap is put in the vagina before intercourse - several hours before, if wanted - so there is no danger of forgetting it in the heat of the moment. The main contraceptive action comes from the spermicide used with the cap; however, most spermicides contain Nonoxynol 9 which is not recommended for use by HIV-positive women as it can increase the risk of transmission of HIV.

The cap can be re-used, and should be washed thoroughly after removal. It should not be shared.

The sponge

This method of contraception does not protect against HIV transmission for either partner.

Contraceptive sponges have a failure rate of up to 25%. There is no health risk, as long as you are not allergic to the spermicide. A contraceptive sponge is a soft, polyurethane foam circle which contains spermicide. It has a cord for removal. It is placed over the cervix like the cap and should be used only once.

These are often easier to use than the cap and one size fits everyone. They can be difficult to remove, and sometimes they disintegrate. This is not dangerous, but it can be tiresome to remove the bits. Sponges are expensive as they are used only once. However, most spermicides contain Nonoxynol 9 which is not recommended for use by HIV-positive women as it can increase the risk of transmission of HIV.

Spermicides

This method of contraception does not protect against HIV transmission for either partner.

Spermicides have a failure rate of up to 70%, especially for young women.

There are several different formulations and brands of spermicide. Spermicides are chemicals which are contained in cream, jelly, pessaries, foams or C-film (a papery square). These are placed in the vagina, and should be inserted as high up as possible since they aim to prevent live sperm from entering the cervix. This is easiest by using them with a cap. Some foams come with applicators to help place them high up in the vagina by the cervix.

There is no health risk, as long as you are not allergic to the spermicide. However, most spermicides contain Nonoxynol 9 which is not recommended for use by HIV-positive women as it can increase the risk of transmission of HIV.

The intrauterine device (IUD) or coil

This method of contraception does not protect against HIV transmission for either partner.

The IUD has a failure rate of about 2%. This varies depending upon the skill with which the IUD is inserted. The IUD is a small piece of plastic or copper which is placed inside the uterus (womb) which must be inserted by a Doctor. Removal is usually easy and painless, but inserting an IUD can cause discomfort. It can make periods longer, heavier and more painful. There is a slight risk that the cord from the IUD might damage a condom.

Some concerns have been raised about using the IUD in HIV-positive women since some women experience heavier menstrual bleeding with the coil and also due to positive women's increased experience of PID and menstrual problems. There is limited evidence available about these potential cautions and draft BHIVA guidelines suggest that women seeking this kind of contraception should be offered a risk assessment and screening/treatment for STIs before having it fitted.

The IUD increases the risk of Pelvic Inflammatory Disease (PID) (see *A-Z of sexually transmitted infections* above).

Hormonal forms of contraception

Hormonal forms of contraception cause changes in the woman's menstrual cycle which prevent them becoming pregnant. Since none of the available forms of hormonal contraception protect against HIV transmission they are only recommended to be used in conjunction with condoms.

Women who are not using ART may choose from any of the options below, however, there are special considerations for those women currently using treatments. Protease inhibitors and non-nucleoside inhibitors may reduce the effectiveness of hormonal contraception; however, to date there has been limited research into the effects of hormonal contraception on ART and the efficacy of the contraception. Because of this the draft BHIVA guidelines recommend that the combined oral contraceptive pill, the progesterone-only pill and hormonal implants should be avoided in HIV-positive women using ART.

The combined oral contraceptive pill

This method of contraception does not protect against HIV transmission for either partner. As described above this method of contraception is not recommended for women on treatment.

The combined pill is very effective and easy to use with only a 0.5% failure rate. It contains two hormones which mimic hormonal changes which take place in a pregnant woman and therefore prevents ovulation and conception. For 21 days the woman takes a pill containing hormones, and for the next seven days she either takes a blank pill or no pill. During these seven days she bleeds, although this is not real menstruation as she has not ovulated.

Many women like using the pill because it is a reliable contraceptive which offers confidence, control and regular light periods. However, there are some health concerns relating to the pill, and women should be advised to find out as much information as possible.

Women with conditions which can be aggravated by oestrogen should not use the pill. These conditions include breast cancer, thrombosis, sickle cell anaemia and recent liver failure. People with Hepatitis B or C or with a history of alcohol or drug use may have reduced liver function which means the combined pill is probably not suitable for them.

Some women find that taking the pill sets off vaginal thrush. This may make the pill unsuitable for an HIV-positive woman who has recurrent thrush which is hard to treat. The pill can interact with other drugs, courses of antibiotics and some other drugs can reduce the pills effectiveness as a contraceptive. HIV-positive women who use the pill should be encouraged to check with their doctor whenever they are given medication. Vomiting and diarrhoea can stop the pill from being absorbed, and reduce the contraceptive effectiveness.

The progesterone-only pill or 'mini-pill'

This method of contraception does not protect against HIV transmission for either partner. As described above this method of contraception is not recommended for women on treatment.

The mini-pill has a failure rate of 2%, which becomes less in older women. This pill works by providing extra progesterone, which creates an environment which is hostile to sperm and to a fertilised egg. However, the woman still ovulates.

The mini-pill has to be taken every day at the same time, preferably the early evening. Sticking to a rigid timetable can be difficult for some women. Some of the health problems associated with the combined pill also occur with the mini-pill, but there are fewer side-effects. It may be suitable for women who cannot take oestrogen.

Contraceptive injections

This method of contraception does not protect against HIV transmission for either partner. Progesterone only injections may be used by women currently on treatment.

Contraceptive injections have a failure rate of less than 1%.

This is a different method of introducing the hormonal changes provided by the pill. Women are given a one-off injection containing a very high dose of progesterone. The effects last on average three months and cannot be reversed during this time.

However, it is convenient, as just one injection gives long-term protection. There is no need to remember to take it.

The treatment is controversial, partly because some women have been given injections without their fully informed consent. There is disagreement about the health implications. Some women have experienced painful and persistent side-effects, including difficulty conceiving after using it. It is not possible to halt the hormone changes (whereas it is possible to stop taking the pill) and this can be a problem for women who experience side-effects. If a woman is considering a future pregnancy she should be advised that fertility can take as long as 1 year to return after she stops using injections.

Emergency contraception - the 'morning after pill'

The 'morning after' pill. This method of contraception does not protect against HIV transmission for either partner.

If a woman fears that she may have conceived, for example because no contraception was used or the condom broke, it is possible to intervene within three days of having sex. The failure rate is about three per cent.

A course of pills is given which contain a high dose of oestrogen to stop ovulation. These methods can result in some sickness. Some doctors will ask the woman to agree to an abortion if the pregnancy continues, as the foetus could have been damaged by the pill medication.

The standard treatment regime is suitable for women who are not on treatment; however, due to the considerations mentioned above, HIV-positive women on ART may be offered an emergency IUD insertion to prevent pregnancy or an increased dose of the hormonal pills.

Other methods:

'Natural' method - timed unprotected intercourse

This method of contraception carries a risk of HIV transmission both for HIV seroconcordant (i.e. both partners are positive) and HIV serodiscordant (one partner is positive and one negative). The risks associated with unprotected sex are discussed more fully in the Transmission chapter.

Women are only fertile for two days in each menstrual cycle (normally 28 days). As sperm can survive in the body for three days, there are some five to seven days in each cycle when a woman can conceive. One method of contraception is to avoid unprotected vaginal intercourse during this fertile week.

The failure rate (i.e. rate of pregnancy) is about three per cent when this method is followed carefully. However, it does require a great deal of organisation and body awareness to achieve this level of effectiveness and, given the availability of contraception methods which protect couples from transmission of HIV and other STIs using this method of contraception would require careful consideration.

Women should seek advice about contraception from a Family Planning or Well Woman Clinic or from their Doctor.

Further reading

BHIVA, Draft guidelines for the management of sexual and reproductive health of people living with HIV infection, 2006

BHIVA, 2005, Guidelines for the management of HIV infection in pregnant women and the prevention of mother-to-child transmission of HIV, British HIV Association available at http://www.bhiva.org/, 2005

NAT Campaign Briefing Paper. The need to remove Nonoxynol - 9 (N-9) from condoms and lubricants, 2003.

Disclosing your HIV status to a sexual partner

The decision about when or how to disclose your HIV status to a potential sexual partner is complex and can be stressful. Positive women will be concerned not to pass on the virus to their partner but will also have concerns about their own confidentiality and safety. Many people without experience of HIV do not have a lot of knowledge about the virus and will not know that it is possible for positive people to enjoy a good sex life with positive and negative partners.

As well as personal concerns there are also important legal considerations regarding disclosure. At the time of writing seven people within the UK have been prosecuted for infecting their sexual partner with HIV through unprotected sex. The important aspect of all of these cases is that the positive person did not disclose their status to their partner. Disclosure is covered elsewhere in this Manual.

Pregnancy and HIV - Introduction

There are many HIV-positive women who are mothers whether diagnosed before or after their children were born and the prevalence of HIV infection amongst women giving birth in the UK has risen every year since 1990. There are also many women who choose not to have a family, however, for many people living with HIV the availability of antiretroviral therapy means that they can hope for longer, healthier lives than was anticipated even fairly recently. One of the results in this difference for

positive women (who have access to treatment) can mean that the possibility of having children may seem more realistic than in previous years.

One of the difficulties for positive women who might decide to become pregnant is that there is a risk of vertical transmission (i.e. mother-to-child) of HIV. This risk is currently calculated in the UK as a one in seven chance that the baby will be infected if no preventative measures are taken. However, it is now known that highly effective preventative measures can reduce the risk of transmission to a level estimated to be below 2%.

In summary these preventative measures are:

- Treatment of mother and child with antiretroviral therapy.

- Delivery of the baby via a planned pre-labour caesarean section although vaginal delivery may be considered for women on stable therapy with viral loads below 50 copies/ml prior to delivery

- Feeding the baby exclusively with formula milk (i.e. avoiding breastfeeding).

It is also known that the risk of vertical transmission in women who have not been treated with ART is related to the health of the mother in relation to viral load, CD4 count and clinical disease stage. It is also related to obstetric factors such as length of labour and premature delivery: delivery before 34 weeks has been shown to increase the risk of vertical transmission.

However, although it is also the case that most babies born to positive women will be HIV-negative the interventions offered to reduce the risk of vertical transmission are not without side-effects and do not offer 100% protection.

The long-term effects of anti-HIV drugs on an HIV-negative child are not known, and Caesarean section is also not without danger for the mother. These risks must be balanced against the proven effectiveness of anti-HIV therapy in reducing transmission, and the well-established health consequences of being born HIV-positive.

Positive women will also want to consider any risk of transmission to a negative partner.

Negative women who are considering conceiving with a positive partner will have concerns regarding the risks of transmission of HIV to themselves and their baby. These are discussed below.

Much of the following information is based on the BHIVA 2005 Pregnancy Guidelines

Positive women planning pregnancy

Planning parenthood for positive women can feel a more viable option for many women than previously. ART means that women may expect to live longer and healthier lives than before and the risk of vertical transmission can be greatly reduced using the preventative measures listed above. However, the decision to have children remains a difficult one both on a practical and emotional level.

The attitudes of health care professional and assumptions about women's reproductive choices can make this decision even more difficult. It is important that a positive woman receives sound information and advice about the options available to her so she can choose whether or not to go ahead with planning a pregnancy.

It was previously thought that pregnancy itself could be damaging to the health of positive women as pregnancy could have a negative effect on the immune system. It now seems pregnancy is only likely to have an impact on a woman's physical health if she is already unwell or has very low CD4 counts. However, it is often not immediate health worries that are of greatest concerns to positive women. For some women even the greatly reduced risk of vertical transmission feels too high and they may decide not to start a family. Women will also have worries about longer-term issues for their child should they themselves or, in some circumstances their partner, become unwell or terminally ill.

However, for many women being diagnosed with a life-threatening condition may intensify the desire to have children, especially if she is not yet a mother. There is often, also, external societal pressure to have children and it is possible that this pressure is stronger amongst African communities.

When any woman is pregnant she will be concerned about the effect of medicines and other drugs on her unborn baby. Positive women on treatment will share these concerns and may express worries about the intra-uterine effects of ART. Due to ethical and other constraints there is little and sometimes conflicting evidence about the safety of ART in pregnancy. However, these concerns must be balanced against the health needs of the positive mother herself and the desire to reduce vertical transmission.

HIV testing in pregnancy

It is now routine for pregnant women in the UK to be offered an HIV test. This test was introduced in recognition of the fact that we have increasingly effecting methods of preventing vertical transmission and also effective treatments for positive people. Whilst the introduction of routine testing has resulted in a reduction in the number of children being born HIV-positive, this initiative also means that some woman will be given a positive diagnosis for the first time in pregnancy. For a newly diagnosed positive pregnant woman her HIV diagnosis is likely to be shocking and extremely anxiety provoking. She will have concerns about her health, the health of her baby and the HIV status of her partner. BHIVA cites two studies which compare the psychological impact of an antenatal HIV diagnosis to being bereaved. Women in this situation will be required to make complex decisions about treatment, prevention of mother to child transmission and potentially disclosure of her status to her baby's father. She should be offered care from an obstetrician experienced in this field and an HIV consultant.

Further reading

BHIVA, 2005, Guidelines for the management of HIV infection in pregnant women and the prevention of mother-to-child transmission of HIV, British HIV Association available at http://www.bhiva.org/

WHO, HIV-infected women and their families: psychosocial support and related issues. A literature review, www.who.int/reproductive-health/publications/rhr_03_07/ . 2003.

Conception

It is recommended that couples affected by HIV who are considering planning a family should have pre-conceptual care to discuss their fertility options. There are three aspects to consider: interventions that can minimise transmission risk between discordant couples during conception, the management of any fertility issues and the state of health and medication of the infected partner pre-conceptually.

In summary, BHIVA guidelines recommend:

- Self-insemination of partner's semen is recommended to protect the uninfected male partner of a positive woman and is easily performed by the couple.

- Sperm-washing is recommended to protect the uninfected female partner of a positive male.

- Fertility assessment is indicated if conception has not occurred after 6-12 months of self-insemination.

HIV serodiscordant couples where the woman is positive

In couples in which the female partner is positive and the male partner is negative, self-insemination is recommended. The woman can be supplied with quills and syringes which she can use to insert sperm ejaculated into a sterile container or, following intercourse. into a condom which does not contain spermicide. This insemination should be timed to occur within the fertile period of a woman's cycle. Help with identifying the best time for insemination can be gained from the woman's gynaecologist and may include use of a home ovulation detection kit.

Women with HIV may find it more difficult both to conceive and to carry their babies to full term. A study of French women with HIV from the early 1990s[1] found that the percentage of miscarriages and ectopic pregnancies increased significantly from 8.3% to 25.4% of those conceived before and after HIV diagnosis, respectively. Italian researchers[2] have suggested that HIV affects the placenta by interfering with the transfer of important nutrients to the foetus, or that the virus causes abnormal development of the embryo.

Some studies have also linked antiretroviral treatment to both premature delivery and low birth weight. For instance a 2004 study[3] found that in 3807 pregnancies reported between 1990 and 2003, 13% of deliveries were before 37 weeks, with a 1.5 fold increase risk if the mother took HAART during pregnancy compared with AZT monotherapy, while another study[4] found that 3% of babies had very low birth weight if the mother took protease inhibitors compared with 1% if she did not, with the likelihood increasing the earlier in the pregnancy she started to take them.

HIV serodiscordant couples where the man is positive

In couples where the man is positive and the woman is negative there are two options for assisted conception: sperm washing or donor insemination. Timed unprotected intercourse (i.e. during the fertile time of a woman's cycle) is not recommended due to the risk of transmission of HIV to the negative partner, this is discussed below.

Sperm washing: in couples in which the male partner is positive sperm-washing is recommended to reduce the risk of transmission of HIV to the female partner and child.

Sperm-washing is a relatively simple procedure which involves centrifuging semen to separate live sperm (which do not carry HIV) from seminal plasma and other cells. After the sperm is separated it is tested for HIV before being used since there is still a risk that the sample may have detectable HIV should the centrifuge procedure fail to remove all of the seminal plasma. The sample can then be used for insemination at the time of ovulation. Before sperm washing is carried out couples should be offered a sexual health screening to exclude the presence of STIs (as these can increase transmission rates and reduce fertility). The male partner will undergo semen analysis and the woman will have her endocrine levels and a pelvic scan check to ensure insemination occurs at the optimum time.

BHIVA reports that in reviewing studies which included over 3000 cycles of sperm-washing no HIV-negative women or children born as a result of the procedure seroconverted to become HIV- positive.

Unfortunately, despite it being a relatively simple and inexpensive technique, sperm-washing is not widely available within the UK. The clinic with the most experience to date is the Chelsea and Westminster Hospital, London and they will provide this procedure on the NHS although it may have a long waiting list. The availability of this technique should be discussed with the woman's doctor. Sperm-washing done privately is likely to cost several thousand pounds; this however is not due to the expense of the technique but because some men with HIV have low fertility, caused in part by mitochondrial damage in sperm caused

by NRTI anti-retroviral drugs. This means that techniques like intracytoplasmic sperm injection (ICSI) where the sperm is injected directly into the egg may have to be used. An Italian study[5] of women with HIV-positive partners whose sperm was washed and them delivered by ICSI (Vichi) was 30.7% and the delivery rate 25.5%, about half of what would be expected when the technique is used on HIV-negative men.

Clinics that perform sperm-washing also exist in Milan, Italy, where Dr Augusto Semprini invented the technique[6], Barcelona and Valencia, Spain, Belgium and France. In 1997[7], Semprini said there had been no instance of HIV infection in 350 couples he had treated in over 1,000 cycles of insemination with washed sperm. In the USA, sperm-washing is contrary to Centers for Disease Control guidelines, after an incident in 1992 where a woman became infected with HIV after artificial insemination with her partner's unwashed sperm.

Donor insemination - donor insemination involves using a sperm sample from a donor who is not the partner of the woman (often this is done through anonymous donors via fertility clinics but some people have chosen a member of the partner's family or other close friend as a donor). This would eliminate risk of transmission from an infected male partner since all sperm donors are screened for HIV and other blood-borne viruses. However, it does bring its own issues in terms of availability of samples and the acceptability of this type of conception for many couples. Recent debates over the rights of children born through anonymous donor insemination to be allowed to make contact with their biological father have reportedly reduced the availability of anonymous donated sperm within the UK.

Men taking antiretrovirals may suffer from reduced fertility and sperm viability because nucleoside (NRTI) drugs cause mitochondrial toxicity, and sperm are packed with mitochondria. This is an option that some women use if their partner is infertile or risks passing on other infectious or congenital conditions.

Timed unprotected intercourse

This method of conception (which at times has been called the 'rhythm method') involves having unprotected sex only during the fertile time of the woman's cycle in an attempt to minimise the risk of transmission of HIV. This method of conception is not recommended for couples where one or both partners are HIV-positive due to the risk of transmission of HIV. It is recognised, however, that this option is at times used by couples who are unable to access sperm washing or other support with fertility.

The exact risks of timed unprotected intercourse between partners affected with HIV are difficult to confirm due to the small number of studies done and the observed behaviour that some couples will continue with unprotected intercourse at other times of the month. In one study where couples tried to conceive in this way, and limited intercourse to the fertile period of ovulation, four per cent of women seroconverted, which is an unacceptably high risk. It is also difficult to quantify the risk of infection with other or resistant strains of the virus in couples where both partners are positive and for this reason other methods of conception are recommended.

Unpublished data by Semprini says that out of 487 couples treated with sperm-washing, 270 (55%) achieved pregnancy, but that of the remaining 45%, 58 (27%) had continued trying to have a child via unprotected intercourse. One woman seroconverted.

However a recent study from Spain[8] found no infections of the HIV-negative partner (40 women and 22 men) when 62 serodiscordant couples used timed unprotected intercourse to conceive and where the HIV-positive partner had an undetectable plasma viral load (under 50). The researchers concluded that timed unprotected intercourse with a partner with an undetectable viral load was probably safe enough to pose an acceptable risk for people wishing to conceive as long as occasions of unprotected sex were minimised.

Seroconcordant couples (both HIV-positive)

Couples where both partners have HIV may nonetheless want to continue to have safer sex to avoid the risk of HIV Superinfection (infection by second strains of HIV) or other chronic STIs such as HPV or herpes. However surveys of established heterosexual concordant couples have found condom use to be very low, even in the pre-HAART era[9].

Infertility treatment

For similar reasons as noted above, that is, increased life expectancy and reduced risk of vertical transmission, more positive women may become interested in fertility treatment. Furthermore, as explained above, they - or partners of HIV-positive men - may need it more. Historically, there has been reluctance for some treatment centres to offer fertility treatment to couples affected by HIV. For example, the results of a survey[10] published in December 2001 in the British Medical Journal highlighted a serious inequity in the availability of both infertility investigation and access to infertility treatment.

In total 57 of the 75 UK clinics (76%) responded to the questionnaire. 27 of the 57 clinics had not seen an HIV-positive person in the past year. Units that had seen an HIV-positive person in the past year were more likely than not to offer infertility investigation and treatment where the male partner was HIV-positive but this trend was not observed where the female partner was HIV-positive or both partners were HIV-positive. A total of 38 of the 57 clinics (67%) that responded to the survey said that they would not offer infertility treatment to couples where both partners are HIV-positive.

The Human Fertilisation and Embryology Act 1990 states that the welfare of the child should be considered before any course of treatment starts. BHIVA suggests that where a couple are seeking treatment ideally they should be in good health (i.e. undetectable viral load, CD4 count >400 and, for positive women, have a commitment to comply with interventions to reduce vertical transmission risks.)

BHIVA also recommends that procedures such as IVF should only be offered within research settings as it is not clear what associated risk of transmission there might be with such invasive procedures.

No category of women (including women with HIV) is excluded from consideration for infertility treatment. It should be hoped that the BHIVA guidelines and wider appreciation of the developing techniques to prevent vertical transmission will help reduce inequality of access to treatment for positive people.

References

1 De Vincenzi I et al. *Pregnancy and contraception in a French cohort of HIV-infected women.* AIDS 11(3): 333-338.1997.

2 D'Ubaldo C et al. *Association between HIV-1 infection and miscarriage : a retrospective study.* AIDS 12(9):1087-93. 1998.

3 Tookey PA et al. *Antiretroviral therapy and pregnancy outcome: UK/Ireland surveillance data 1990-2004.* 7th International Congress on Drug Therapy in HIV Infection, Glasgow. Abstract PL11.3. 2004.

4 Beckerman, K et al. *Association between Antiretroviral therapy during pregnancy and prematurity/low birth weight.* 11th Conference on Retroviruses and Opportunistic Infections, San Francisco. Abstract 2004.

5 Vichi F et al. *Intracytoplasmic sperm injection (ICSI) for HIV couples: our results with tested negative criopreserved sperm samples.* Eighth International Congress on Drug Therapy in HIV Infection, Glasgow. Abstract P387. 2006.

6 Semprini AE et al. *Insemination of HIV-negative women with processed semen of HIV-positive partners.* The Lancet 340(28): 1317-1319, 1992.

7 Semprini AE et al. *Reproductive counselling for HIV-discordant couples (letter).* The Lancet 349: 1401-1402, 1997.

8 Barreiro P et al. *Natural pregnancies in HIV-serodiscordant couples receiving successful antiretroviral therapy.* J Acquir Immune Defic Syndr. 43(3): 324-326, 2006.

9 Carballo-Diéguez A. *Persistent sexual risk behavior among heterosexual IVDU partners regardless of HIV antibody status.*Int Conf AIDS 1990 Jun 20-23; 6:225 (abstract no. S.C.547)

10 Apoola A, et al. *Access to infertility investigations and treatment in couples infected with HIV: questionnaire survey.*BMJ 323: 1285, 2001.

Considerations for pregnant women

Specialist teams

BHIVA strongly recommends that given all the considerations about methods of conception and issues around vertical transmission positive pregnant women should receive care from suitable qualified staff including their HIV specialist, obstetrician, specialist midwife and paediatrician (children's specialist). This may be more attainable for women living in areas where there are large testing and treatment centres than for women living elsewhere in the UK.

Antenatal classes

The mechanisms through which positive women aim to prevent vertical transmission of HIV (i.e. planned caesarean section and avoidance of breastfeeding) is markedly different from current ante-natal advice for other pregnant women. This can make attending antenatal classes uncomfortable as often the emphasis there can be on vaginal delivery and promotion of breastfeeding. Except in some higher prevalence urban areas it is unlikely that ante-natal sessions for positive women will be sustainable. Midwives and other staff should be sensitive to these issues and understand why some positive women may feel unable to participate in such classes and ensure they receive additional support/information as required.

Sexual health

We know that the presence of sexually transmitted infections and other genitourinary tract infections increase the risk of HIV transmission during sex. Their presence may also increase the risk of vertical transmission and complications of pregnancy. For this reason BHIVA recommends routine screening for such infections for all positive women

'Adverse pregnancy outcomes'

BHIVA reports that the risk of adverse pregnancy outcomes is slightly increased for positive women. Adverse pregnancy outcomes are events such as spontaneous abortion, stillbirth and intrauterine growth retardation. BHIVA also suggests that there may be an increased risk of premature delivery in women using combination therapy. These concerns reinforce the importance of high quality specialist support for positive women who are pregnant.

Eligibility for treatment

The legislation concerning access to Free NHS Treatment in the UK is subject to change and it is unclear how this might affect antenatal care. Staff should be aware of sources of advice in circumstances where a woman presents for care and her eligibility is uncertain.

Viral load

The risk of vertical transmission of HIV is related to the pregnant woman's viral load and, while the risk of transmission is clearly increased for those women with a high viral load, transmission can occur even when her blood tested for viral load is undetectable. At time, however, a woman with undetectable plasma viral load (i.e. viral load in the blood) can have a detectable viral load in the cervicovaginal secretions (i.e. those in the female genital tract). It is possible that this difference could account for some of the transmissions in women with very low or undetectable viral loads. It is therefore recommended that (plasma) viral load be monitored at least every three months during pregnancy and at approximately 36 weeks gestation. At the moment there is no guidance that suggests monitoring of genital tract viral load.

Antiretroviral treatment in pregnancy?

There are two aspects to consider when discussing ART in pregnancy:

- the needs of the pregnant woman's health

- prevention of vertical transmission and care of the infant

The decision regarding the most appropriate treatment in gaining successful outcomes for both the woman herself and her baby will be based on her individual clinical situation based on her previous and current treatment use, her viral load and at what time in her pregnancy she attends for care and balanced with the risk of toxicity against the risk of HIV transmission. The complexities of such a decision making process are outside the scope of this chapter and the following information should be used as a guide only.

The following information is summarised from BHIVA Pregnancy Guidelines, 2006

- If the mother is already receiving treatment when she conceives she should remain on treatment; if her viral load is not adequately suppressed her treatment regimen should be changed to attempt to achieve as low a viral load as possible. If a viral load of <50 copies/ml is not achieved she should receive zidovudine (AZT) intravenous therapy during labour (if she is not resistant to this drug).

- If a woman is not on treatment but requires commencement during pregnancy due to their stage of disease she should be started on a potent ART regime after the first trimester of her pregnancy

- If a woman does not require ART for her own health (when assessed according to BHIVA Treatment Guidelines) she may be treated with a short-term anti-retroviral therapy commencing in the second trimester with the intention to achieve undetectable viral loads of <50 copies per ml prior to delivery. A protease-inhibitor based combination is recommended. PIs have a greater barrier to resistance development than NNRTIs and can be stopped concurrently with the nucleoside backbone. In addition PI pill burden and tolerance is improving with newer formulations and there is a low incidence of severe short-term side-effects. If non-nucleosides are used, these must be discontinued 1-2 weeks prior to the nucleoside backbone to reduce the likelihood of the emergence of NNRTI resistance.

- An alternative approach, in women who do not require treatment for themselves, and who have a viral load of less than 10,000, is to use AZT monotherapy, combined with an elective caesarean section. The risk of vertical transmission is low, and this reduces antiretroviral exposure to the foetus in pregnancy. Maternal toxicity is reduced and the risk of the development of resistance in the mother, when used at this level of viral load, appears minimal.

- Women who present late in pregnancy or in labour, for whom no risk assessment has been possible should be treated with a triple combination containing nevirapine as nevirapine is rapidly absorbed via the placenta. Triple therapy is recommended as nevirapine monotherapy given in labour has been shown to cause resistance in mothers. Zidovudine should preferably be infused intravenously, and all treatments should be continued after delivery until the mother's clinical, immunological and virological status has been determined.

- If a positive mother presents after delivery post-exposure prophylaxis should be given to the infant.

Drug levels and side-effects in pregnancy

One particular protease inhibitor - nelfinavir - has been shown to have lower concentrations in pregnancy. BHIVA suggests that dose adjustment may be necessary and all pregnant women taking protease inhibitors or changing therapy should be considered for therapeutic drug monitoring (TDM) and that

there is an urgent need for extensive investigation of the pharmacokinetics of antiretroviral therapy in pregnant women to ensure efficacy, reduce toxicity and to prevent the emergence of resistance through inadvertent under dosing.

Adherence to ART

Adherence to ART is vital for the success of treatment. This is never more so than during pregnancy when a woman will be wanting to support her health as well as reduce the risks of vertical transmission. Pregnant women commonly experience nausea and vomiting in early pregnancy, this may make it more difficult for positive pregnant women to adhere to medication. Sometimes this can be managed by changing the timing of medication doses to out with those periods of nausea. In more severe cases medication to prevent sickness (anti-emetics) may be prescribed with the guidance of an obstetrician

Single-dose nevirapine

Trials of single dose nevirapine given in pregnant women to prevent vertical transmission have been shown to effectively reduce transmission rates. In resource poor settings this method was investigated since it was relatively affordable and straightforward to administer. However, research[64] has shown that even at a single dose the mother risks developing resistance across the non-nucleoside reverse transcriptase class of drugs thus seriously limiting her future treatment options.

Reference

64. Lee JE et al. Breastmilk shedding of drug-resistant HIV-1 subtype-C in women exposed to single-dose nevirapine, Clin Infect Dis: 192 (online edition), 2005

Care of infants born to positive mothers

Treatment

BHIVA states that the choice of post-exposure prophylaxis treatment for infants born to infected mothers should be guided as follows:

1. if the mother is considered to have a low transmission risk and has used Zidovudine (AZT) monotherapy during pregnancy the infant should receive Zidovudine for 4 weeks

2. if the mother is on triple therapy with a viral load of <50 copes the infant should have one single drug from the mother's regime (usually an non-nucleoside reverse transcriptase inhibitor) for four weeks

3. If the mother is only found to be HIV-positive after delivery or has had an unplanned delivery or her treatment has failed to lower her viral load satisfactorily then triple therapy should be considered for the infant. ART choice may also be guided by HIV DNA PCR results.

Testing for HIV infection

All babies share their mother's antibodies at birth and this is no different for children born to positive women. This means that all such babies will have a positive result for an HIV antibody test and may continue to have these anti-bodies in their blood up to the age of 18 months. However, this result will not mean that the baby is HIV-positive. Previously mothers faced having to wait until their children's antibodies cleared before being able to confirm their HIV status; however, an HIV DNA PCR (Polymerase Chain Reaction) test has reduced this waiting time. To establish whether a baby has seroconverted BHIVA recommends that she/he be PCR tested at one day, six weeks and twelve weeks of age. If all of these tests are negative - and the baby is not being breastfed - then the child is not HIV infected.

New and first time mothers often experience extreme emotional and physical upheaval at this time. For positive mothers this is compounded by the anxiety and distress of waiting to hear results and the subsequent decisions to be made in the event of a positive test result. The experience and support of qualified specialist staff will be important at this time and help understanding of test results.

Breastfeeding

HIV can be transmitted via breastfeeding and therefore positive mothers are advised to use formula milk feeding. This is safely achievable within the UK but does bring difficulties for positive women given the current advice to the general public to exclusively breastfeed their babies. This may lead to discomfort for a mother and, in some communities, suspicion about HIV status if a mother is choosing not to breastfeed. In areas where safe access to formula feeding is not available or affordable this is a major concern.

Further reading

BHIVA, 2005, Guidelines for the management of HIV infection in pregnant women and the prevention of mother-to-child transmission of HIV, British HIV Association available at www.bhiva.org

Resources and Contacts

ICW
(International Community of Women Living with HIV and AIDS)

ICW is a global network of HIV-positive women with representatives throughout the world. ICW publishes a regular newsletter.

UK Contact: International Community of Women Living with HIV/AIDS, Unit 6, Building 1, Canonbury Yard, 190a New North Road , London, N1 7BJ

Tel: 020 7704 0606
email: info icw.org
Website: www.icw.org

Positively Women - Positively Women is a UK national charity providing support *for* women living with HIV *by* women living with HIV. Positively Women has its headquarters in London and hosts a national resource centre with HIV information. They also publish a regular newsletter.

Contact: Free Call Back Helpline: 020 7713 0222 from Monday to Friday 10am - 1pm, and 2pm - 4pm.

www.positivelywomen.org.uk

Body & Soul - A UK charity supporting children, teenagers, women, heterosexual men and their families who are living with or closely affected by HIV and AIDS..

Contact: Body & Soul, 9 Tavistock Place, London, WC1H 9SN

Tel: 02073837678
E-mail: info@bodyandsoulcharity.org
Website: www.bodyandsoulcharity.org

Other websites

The End Violence Against Women Coalition Campaign - aims to mobilise organisations and individuals to rise up and demand that the UK Government and devolved administrations honour those obligations.

www.endviolenceagainstwomen.org.uk

Gender and AIDS - This comprehensive gender and HIV/AIDS web portal provides up-to-date resources on the gender dimensions of the HIV/AIDS epidemic:

www.genderandaids.org

International Women's Health Coalition - works in three ways to build political will and influence the policies of governments, donors, and international agencies to secure girls' and women's sexual and reproductive health and rights:

www.iwhc.org/who

UNICEF is running a global HIV campaign to build a coalition of those concerned about making sure children and families receive the support and protection they need.

www.unicef.org.uk

The Well Project - an American advocacy web-site which contains treatment and more general information about women and HIV:

www.thewellproject.org

Women and AIDS - A loose alliance of civil society groups, networks of women living with HIV, and United Nations agencies, the Coalition works at global and national levels to advocate for improved AIDS programming for women and girls.

www.womenandaids.unaids.org

Women, Children and HIV - Resources on the prevention and treatment of HIV infection in women and children targeted at health workers, program managers, and policy makers in resource-poor settings.

www.womenchildrenhiv.org

Children, adolescents and families

Routes of transmission

In the UK, the most common route of infection for children is through mother-to-child transmission, often referred to as vertical transmission. In non-breastfeeding populations, this occurs predominantly around the time of delivery. Breastfeeding increases the risk of transmission by around 4% for every six months it is continued.. However, other possible routes such as infection via blood products, organ or tissue donation, consensual and non-consensual sex and contamination with non-sterile equipment have been reported. Infection from non-sterile equipment tends to occur among children from outside the UK who have undergone surgical procedures or cultural rituals abroad.

Estimates for the risk of mother-to-child transmission (without interventions) are commonly quoted at around 15-20% in Europe and the USA. In developing countries this figure can be much higher. For example, in some African countries estimates of approximately 35% risk of transmission without interventions have been reported. The most important risk factor for transmission is maternal viral load.

The Aids Clinical Trial Group's (ACTG) 076 trial revealed that the use of AZT during pregnancy reduced the risk of mother-to-child transmission by two thirds. The use of combination antiretroviral therapy, avoidance of breastfeeding, and possibly elective caesarian section can further reduce transmission to one per cent or less in resource-rich settings.

As a result, in the UK since 1999, universal testing for HIV during pregnancy has been recommended by the Department of Health. This has resulted in a marked improvement in antenatal detection rates. It was estimated that in 2004 88% of pregnant women in London and 95% outside London had their HIV infections diagnosed prior to giving birth - a huge improvement from the year 2000, when 82% in Inner London, 65% in Outer London, and 56% in the rest of England and Wales had their infection diagnosed prior to giving birth. The Department of Health set a target of 90% uptake of HIV testing by the end of 2002.

Despite these improvements in detection rates, vertical transmission will remain as the main source of paediatric HIV infection internationally, until intervention services reach populations in endemic regions

Testing children for HIV

Methods of testing infants and children

All babies born to HIV-positive women will have maternal HIV antibodies present in their blood up to the age of 18 months. Therefore, an HIV antibody test will be unable to establish whether a child this young is infected. Waiting for antibodies to clear is a slow way of establishing the child's infection status. However, with the introduction of a test known as the PCR test (Polymerase Chain Reaction) a child's infection status can be established by age three months. Different types of PCR tests have been developed. The standard diagnostic test uses DNA extracted from the infant's white blood cells (proviral DNA PCR tests). Samples can be sent to the reference laboratory at the Health Protection Agency, Centre for Infections, 61 Colindale Ave, London NW9 5DF (020 8327 6204 or 020 8200 4400), but check for local arrangements with your hospital/regional Virology laboratory. A sample from the mother should be tested in parallel with her infant's blood, to ensure that the PCR test can detect her individual strain (subtype) of HIV.

Some centres use quantitative RNA assays (a.k.a. viral load tests) which are more easily available and may have a faster turn-around time compared to proviral DNA PCR tests. It is important to beware of false positives around the lower limit of detection with the RNA assays, none of which are licensed for diagnostic purposes in infants, and to ensure that the assay used is appropriate for the mother's HIV subtype.

Current statistics

Global figures

By the end of 2006, it was estimated that 2.3 million children worldwide were living with HIV infection. Around 1500 children under 15 years of age had acquired HIV infection each day, and 380,000 children had died of AIDS during that year. Moreover, estimates suggest that 15 million children have been orphaned as a result of the epidemic.

Global disparity is evident, with the largest numbers of HIV-positive children reported from developing countries, in particular sub-Saharan Africa and increasingly Asia. The vast majority of children acquire infection through mother-to-child transmission, although child sexual abuse, high-risk behaviours in teenagers, or transmissions due to imperfectly screened blood transfusions still occur

UK figures

Over the last ten years the epidemiology of paediatric HIV infection in the United Kingdom (UK) has changed dramatically. This is due to a number of factors (for more details see **HIV epidemiology).**

Firstly, the widespread implementation of interventions to prevent transmission from HIV-positive pregnant women to their newborn babies has resulted in a decrease in mother-to-child transmission.

Secondly, the increase in HIV in immigrants coming from high-prevalence areas has been reflected in an increase in the proportion of children born abroad. Whereas this was running at about 24% between 1994 and 1996, it was 64% in 2003-2006. Dispersal of immigrant families has resulted in increasing numbers of children living outside London.

Thirdly, the introduction and development of combination antiretroviral therapy to treat HIV infection has considerably increased the life-expectancy of those children who are

HIV-infected. This is reflected in the numbers of children surviving childhood and living into adulthood.

By March 2006, 1,846 HIV-infected children had been reported to the National Study of HIV in Pregnancy and Childhood (data available upon request from nshpc@ich.ucl.ac.uk, tel. 020 7829 8686 or 020 7905 2692). About 18% of all infected children ever reported in the UK & Ireland are known to have died, and about 10% have left the country or are otherwise lost to follow up. Around 95% of those currently living with HIV had acquired infection from their mothers perinatally.

In April 2000 the Collaborative HIV Paediatric Study (CHIPS) was established as a multi-centred cohort study of HIV-infected children in the UK and Ireland. The collaboration is between centres in the UK and Ireland that care for HIV-infected children (many of whom are enrolled in the PENTA network of clinical trials), the National Study of HIV in Pregnancy and Childhood (NSHPC), and the MRC Clinical Trials Unit, London.

This has provided more detailed information about treatment and outcomes, and includes more than 90% of children living with HIV in the UK/Ireland. Of the 1,133 children with perinatally acquired HIV in CHIPS follow-up, 11% were over ten years of age in 1996, compared with 44% in 2005.

Rates of progression to AIDS/death per 100 child years fell from 13.3 in 1996 to 2.5 in 2003-6. Similarly, death rates fell from 8.2 to 0.6 in the same reporting periods. Hospital admissions fell from 4.3 to 0.7 per 100 child years.

In addition to the number of children diagnosed with HIV infection, considerably larger numbers of children have been AFFECTED as a result of HIV infection in their parents and siblings. As Lwin and Melvin (2001) suggest this is an important but often neglected group.

This chapter addresses some of the relevant issues for children infected and affected by HIV living in the UK. It includes:

- Medical aspects of care for children infected with HIV.

- Psychological aspects of care for children infected and affected by HIV.

- Social aspects of care for children infected and affected by HIV.

Methods of testing children aged 18 months or older

For children aged 18 months plus, the standard HIV antibody test can be done. However, there are certain key points which must be considered prior to testing:

Why is the test being done?

- Parents may feel there is no point having their child tested as there is no cure for HIV infection. Many will have seen friends and family die from HIV-related diseases in their countries of origin. Health care workers need to help them understand the tremendous advances in treatments for children with HIV infection, that can now enable infected children to become independent, productive adults.

- In resource-rich countries where children have access to treatments and there is a strong suspicion that a child has been exposed to HIV, there are no tenable arguments against recommending a test. It is no longer acceptable to delay testing until HIV-related illness has developed.

- The arguments in favour of testing extend to children entering adoption and fostering systems, especially if the social situation indicates risks for blood-borne viruses, including HIV, HBV and HCV.

When is the test being done?

It is important to consider the emotional state of the parents and whether they would be able to cope with a positive result:

- What support, if any, do they have?

- Is there anyone in their immediate family or group of friends they could share the diagnosis with?

- Do they want to be referred to a voluntary organisation for advice and support?

Despite the benefits of knowing a positive diagnosis, parents may be extremely anxious about having their child tested as a positive result can often provoke difficult questions and emotions. Testing a child has important implications for the whole family, since a positive result in an infant means that the mother, and possibly the father too, is also HIV-positive. Parents may blame themselves for having passed on the infection to their child. It can also be painful accepting that their child will require regular hospital follow-up and treatment for the rest of their lives. Some parents may not wish to know about a positive diagnosis because they do not believe in HIV infection or the treatments that are available. In such circumstances, it is still valuable to have a confirmed diagnosis, so that the child can be regularly monitored and a dialogue maintained with the parents.

Where is the test being discussed?

The subject of testing a child may be raised in a number of settings, from an out-patients' department to a paediatric intensive care unit. Whatever the situation, all efforts must be made to ensure the setting is private and free from disturbance.

Parents may have concerns about confidentiality and fear the diagnosis becoming widely known. This may extend to refusing the involvement of interpreters in pre-test discussions. If the result is positive, reassurance should be given that the diagnosis will only be disclosed if consent is obtained or there are child protection concerns.

Consenting to the HIV test

Infants and young children

In the case of babies and young children, consent must be given by whoever has parental responsibility- this may be the parent(s), a carer or a local authority. Where there is disagreement on the issue of testing among those who hold parental responsibility, it may be necessary to obtain legal advice. Consent from a parent or care-giver with parental

responsibility can be verbal. Written consent is not a legal requirement, but the discussion should be fully documented.

Older children and young adults

In some instances, a young person may wish to have an HIV test without the knowledge of their parent, for example if they are sexually active or have been injecting drugs. 'Fraser competence' (previously referred to as 'Gillick' competence) is the legal framework which states that children under the age of 16 can consent to treatment without parental consent, provided the doctor believes they understand the nature of the treatment. The Fraser judgment has also been extended to HIV testing.

Fraser competence requires that:

- The child has sufficient understanding and intelligence to enable him or her to understand fully what is proposed.

- Each child must be assessed separately in relation to each different procedure. It follows that a child may be able to consent to some procedures but not to others.

- There is no specific age at which a child becomes competent to consent. This depends on the particular child and on the seriousness and complexity of whatever treatment or procedure is proposed.

- Competence is about capacity to make a decision, not about the ability of the child to make a choice that other people might consider wise.

- A person who has reached the age of 16 years should be regarded as competent to give consent unless there is evidence to the contrary, as in the case of adults. Competence should be assessed in the same way as it is in adults.

- It is good practice to involve families of 16 and 17 year-olds in the decision-making process unless the young person specifically requests that this should not happen.

- Attempts should be made to persuade them to confide in their families.

- A request from a child under the age of 16 years that the treatment should be kept confidential should be respected unless, in the opinion of the healthcare professional, there are reasonable grounds to suggest that the child is suffering, or is likely to suffer, significant harm as a result.

A young person who attends clinic with a parent and who has requested testing or might be considered to have sufficient understanding to give informed consent should be fully involved in discussions.

Many parents are not aware of these legal issues and the rights of children in consenting to testing. Some parents, for various reasons, may find it unacceptable for their child to make such decisions or be involved in discussions around HIV.

Sexual abuse and HIV testing

All professionals working in child care should have a thorough knowledge of HIV issues so they are able to discuss testing or help the child access sensitive pre-test counselling. A child or young person who has been sexually abused may already be aware of the risk of HIV and be highly anxious.

Adolescents with HIV

"Too old to be children, yet too young to be adults, adolescents needs are often underestimated or simply overlooked".
(Seery 2001)

The population of children and young people living with HIV in the UK is steadily growing older. Of the 1133 children in follow-up in the Collaborative HIV Paediatric Study (CHIPS) cohort, 44% were aged over 10 years in 2005 and 9% were 15 years or older. Improved survival as a result of advances in therapy has meant that transition services to enable successful progression from paediatric to adult clinics are increasingly needed.

Complexity of need

Young people who have acquired the infection from their mothers have different needs to young people who have become infected later in life through sexual activity or drug use.

The majority of vertically infected children will have been attending hospital for many years.

Many of the children currently in early adolescence were diagnosed to have HIV before effective treatment was available and initially were not expected to survive beyond early childhood. This has resulted in a tendency for families, and services, to shelter or overprotect these children. In turn this adds extra strain on the processes of independence, autonomy and self-esteem which are developing during adolescence.

It is well-recognised as being challenging to help adolescents come to terms with and learn to take personal responsibility for other chronic diseases such as diabetes and cystic fibrosis. However, the needs and consequences of living with HIV bring additional complexities and are not static. Voluntary and statutory agencies are now having to re-examine the services they offer to meet the specific needs of these young people.

These children are vulnerable to the effects of both HIV infection and also medicines. For example approximately 10% of children have neurological consequences from the early effects of HIV on the developing brain and CNS. Whilst these may be mild in their effects on functioning, there are some children with severe impairments of mobility which deny them independence. There are increasing numbers who are struggling with the learning and social demands of school, and accessing help can be difficult given the anxiety that still surrounds disclosing the diagnosis. There are a small but increasing number with other diagnoses as well as HIV, affecting physical and or mental health. Some will be consequences of living with HIV (e.g. lymphomas) but others have complex multi factorial causes such as depression or anorexia.

A diagnosis of HIV is still a stigmatising diagnosis, and parents may find it extremely hard to share this with their child. However a prerequisite for developing autonomy is an understanding of the diagnosis. Without this knowledge it is not be possible for the child to progress completely through the transition process.

Providing multidisciplinary approaches to care within the community as well as in health settings and which can address other disabilities and difficulties as well as direct HIV care must remain a priority for all service provision and developments for this population.

This is particularly relevant in healthcare terms in the UK. Defining adolescence is a contentious issue. In the UK, adolescence is generally considered as young people between 13-16 years of age.

All clinics should be developing transitional or adolescent clinics for young people infected with HIV. 'Transitional' care is the term used to describe the transfer of medical care from paediatric to adult HIV services. The process of transition may take place over several years starting in the pre-teen years when the young person is aware of their diagnosis.

Many young people with HIV infection are from families of sub-Saharan African origin but have grown up in the UK. This pull between two cultures can be a source of potential conflict within families and must be recognised.

A survey at the Eighth Congress on Drug Therapy in HIV Infection in 2006 looked at the information and sexual health needs of HIV-positive teenagers attending two London HIV clinics. The survey of youngsters aged 16-21 attending the Mortimer Market and Archway HIV clinics could only find 38 of them. However the majority were young people who'd lived with HIV all their lives. Sixteen of the 38 were under 18 and three-quarters of them not unexpectedly were of black African origin. Twenty-three were boys and 15 were girls.

About half were living with one or both parents but a lot of the others were living in care or in hostels. No fewer than 63% had lost one or both parents to AIDS - a reminder of the toll on African families. Four out of five were attending school or college.

Twenty-three (60%) had been born with HIV and 11 (30%) had got it through sex, with four where the source of HIV was unknown: two of the 23 young men defined themselves as gay. Three of the ones who got HIV through sex did so from being raped.

Seventeen (45%) of them were sexually active themselves and of these more than half had either had casual sex or had not disclosed their HIV to their regular partner. On the other hand three had sough post-exposure prophylaxis (PEP) for a partner. There had been seven pregnancies (five live births, two terminations) among the 15 young women.

Five (13%) said they used recreational drugs but in a reminder of the toll of living with HIV, one-third said they had sought psychiatric help for mental health problems. Twenty-one of the 38 (55%) were on HIV therapy and of these a third had a detectable viral load, two-thirds had resistance to at least one HIV drug class, and over a third said they had difficulty sticking to their drug regimen.

What the young person needs to know

Multi-disciplinary teams will have helped to support parents in providing explanations and information for their child about what is happening from a young age.

The very young child will want explanations about what happens at the hospital especially why they have blood taken or have to take medicines. Later it is possible to talk about goodies and baddies in the blood and sometimes about viruses or bugs. Providing truthful explanations, appropriate to the age and maturity of the child but which do not name the diagnosis are possible when the child is young. These can help build an understanding of health and illness. However by early adolescence it becomes increasingly important that a full and open discussion which includes the diagnosis can take place. This enables the young person to feel involved and participate in decisions and feel more in control of treatments and care. It can also help allay any confusion about what is happening to them and provides an opening for the young person to talk about any fears or concerns that they may have about themselves and the future.

Self-esteem and independence are developing during adolescence and knowledge enables these processes to continue and expand. Those young people who have been fully informed about their diagnosis mention the importance of hearing this information from their parent or at least with the parent's involvement and agreement. Planning and supporting the family and youngster during the sharing and afterwards helps the adjustment to the news and reduces long term anxiety. Situations where the young person found out or was told inappropriately have always been more upsetting.

Whilst recognising that by the ages of 12-13 most young people with HIV should have had a full and open discussion about their diagnosis there will always be circumstances which mean that exceptions will occur. The stigma which still surrounds this diagnosis and the family impact, where other family members are HIV-positive or may have died from the condition, increases anxiety about sharing the knowledge with children often for fear of who else will get to know.

Particular situations in which the sharing of the diagnosis is more difficult include those where the family live in very isolated circumstances, where the parent or carer has strong beliefs that it is wrong for the child to know and would not support them knowing and where the child has a learning or cognitive difficulty. In all these cases it may be that progress through the transitional care will be delayed or take longer. However it is likely that transition to adult services would be delayed in all of these kinds of situations anyway.

Starting the process in discussion with families

It is important to start a discussion with parents as the child progresses through primary school so that they are prepared for what to expect of this process. Giving parents ideas on how to continue telling their children more about HIV (see above) is part of this and takes time. Explaining to the parents about puberty and the changing needs and expectations of the young person, as well as how to progress with their care over the next few years, gives the family a time frame to work with. Explaining that as the young person enters early puberty it is usual to begin to give them some personal time within the clinic is advisable. This is important to give them opportunities to discuss issues such as physical and sexual development, which are not necessarily related to HIV. It also allows for opportunities for them to mention any worries or concerns of their own. This will start in quite an informal way, e.g. when they go to be weighed and measured with the specialist nurse. Parents will be reassured that young people may always have a same-sex chaperone.

Increasing knowledge and autonomy for the young person

The changes noted above also need to be explained to the young person. Greater emphasis should be given to providing opportunities for the young person to take more of a lead in consultations with the doctor as they approach adolescence. In time they should be offered the choice of part of the health consultation to be by themselves.

Once the young person knows their diagnosis of HIV then discussions around HIV issues can also begin. Some of these will be with parents in the consultation and as time goes by without

parents too. Issues of privacy and confidentiality will need to be given particular consideration during this time.

If this process is working well then both parents and the young person should feel that they can discuss freely all aspects of their care.

Medical/social review of the HIV history

The young person may wish to have an up-to-date summary of their HIV disease history as they may not remember early childhood illness, nor have understanding of their significance. This may be especially important for young people who have lost parents and cannot easily refer back to them for past events. Flow charts of the treatment history, CD4 progression and viral loads etc. may also be offered. These will also be very useful to the adult doctor during the transition process (see summary sheets below).

Communication with other professionals

Most children are unaware that with their parents' consent communication about them goes to other professionals e.g. the GP. As the young person is gaining autonomy they should be asked permission for information to be shared with other professionals.

Combined consultations / moving to consultations only with the adult team

When it appears appropriate for the individual and after discussions, and with agreement from the young person and the parents, joint consultations with the paediatrician and the adult HIV doctor will begin. In clinics where most of the young people have attended for many years the adult doctor will already be a well-known face. Parents may or may not be part of this. Over a period of time the adult doctor will take over the consultations, this may be as short/ long a time as is considered necessary. At this point many young people appreciate doctors' letters being copied to them, and specific letters with results following clinic appointments being sent directly to them. Although the young person's doctor may no longer be the paediatrician, other team members e.g. the psychologist or clinical nurse specialist may still be actively involved.

Transition of care from a paediatric to adult setting is not specific to HIV, but occurs in a number of paediatric specialities (e.g. cystic fibrosis, congenital heart disease, diabetes etc). Indeed the overall principles of helping young people to gain knowledge and independence and maintain good self esteem can be applied to all adolescents with or without chronic diseases.

However, there are important differences for young people with HIV which may make this process more difficult. Other family members are also likely to be infected and one or other parent may even have died. HIV is a sexually transmissible infection, which is a complex burden for a young person developing their sexual identity to carry. HIV remains a stigmatised condition so it is very hard to share this diagnosis with peers (unless they are also infected).

For these reasons it is especially important that young people are

- well educated about their condition and its treatment.

- confident in their ability to talk about HIV with those who they want to know about their condition.

- have a support system, so they know where to get help and advice when they need it.

- offered genuine choices as to where to continue their care (e.g. transfer to a clinic which is not treating their parents)

Legal & Ethical Issues when Working with Young People

(Extract from Supporting Change: Working Party 2005 Chair Diane Melvin)

Confidentiality v Criminalisation/transmission

There are procedures to ensure confidentiality of personal medical information within health and other systems. These exist together with systems of contact tracing for STI's. There are alo expectations that adults with sexually transmissible disease, including HIV, act responsibly in safeguarding the health of others and do not deliberately pass on these conditions to others. Recent court cases have indicated that the law is acting more punitively to adults who do not tell sexual partners about their HIV infection particularly where partners have become HIV-positive themselves. At present it is unclear at what age and in what circumstances these expectations apply to vertically infected adolescents who are in sexual relationships and what responsibilities around disclosure rest with health and other professionals who are aware of the diagnosis. Practice codes in the adult field take a cautious approach to making it a duty or requirement of workers to inform partners. They emphasise the importance of working to gain the patient's consent for partner disclosure but recognise that in some cases it is in the wider public interest to proceed with disclosing without full consent.
(More Information available from THT)

Management and treatment of children with HIV

Family-centred care

Paediatric HIV must be considered as a family condition. Appropriate services such as Family Clinics where multi-disciplinary care is provided offer good models of care for working with children and families with HIV. In essence, parents and children who are both HIV-positive should be encouraged to have their care together. There is evidence to suggest that this approach reduces distress and disturbance among the other, HIV-negative children in the family.

Many excellent resources now exist on-line, providing up-to-date information about the management of HIV infected children and families. The Children's HIV Association of the UK and Ireland has information for health professionals about many aspects of care (http://www.bhiva.org/chiva). Information about clinical trials for HIV infected children in Europe can be found through the Paediatric European Network for Treatment of AIDS (PENTA) website (http://www.ctu.mrc.ac.uk/penta/)

Internationally, WHO has played a leading role in developing policy towards rolling out antiretroviral therapy for children (http://www.who.int/hiv/pub/guidelines/WHOpaediatric.pdf)

Signs and symptoms

Common clinical features of HIV infection in children are:

- Hepatosplenomegaly (enlarged spleen or liver).

- Chronic or recurrent diarrhoea.

- Recurrent fevers

- Recurrent otitis (inflammation of the ear) or sinusitis (inflammation of the sinuses).

- Persistent swelling of the parotid glands (in the cheeks).

- Recurrent bacterial infections

- Lymphoid Interstitial Pneumonitis (LIP) (inflammation of the lung) may be found in approx 20-30% of vertically infected

children, however this is not common in adults. It often does not cause any symptoms, but it may lead to damage to the lung and chronic hypoxia (low blood oxygen). It is usually diagnosed by chest X-Ray. Causative factors may include an abnormal reaction to Epstein-Barr Virus (EBV) which is the most common cause of 'glandular fever'.

- Other respiratory diseases such as *Mycobacterium Tuberculosis* may be difficult to distinguish from LIP on X-ray.

- Other respiratory conditions associated specifically with HIV, such as *Pneumocystis* Pneumonia and disseminated CMV, usually present in children with severe immunosuppression. In particular, infants below one year of age may present with these symptoms. Septrin prophylaxis is recommended for all HIV-positive infants below one year.

- Malignancies, such as Lymphoma and Kaposi's sarcoma, are rare presentations in children.

- HIV encephalopathy can be a presentation in children with rapid disease progression. It can manifest itself with symptoms which range in severity, from loss of developmental milestones in babies, to difficulties with gait in young infants and children, to loss of concentration and faltering cognitive function in older school age children. Monitoring any deterioration is vital. Developmental assessments will capture any progression. MRI (Magnetic resonance imaging) scans and cranial (brain) imaging are useful monitoring tools.

Monitoring children with HIV infection

As with HIV-positive adults, the most common markers for disease severity and progression in children are CD4 and viral load tests. However, it should be remembered that CD4 counts and viral load results in children should be interpreted differently from adult results.

Children may present with higher viral loads than adults, and CD4 counts are generally higher in children, particularly in infants.

For this reason the **CD4 percentage** (CD4:CD8 ratio) is a more useful guide to disease progression in children less than 5 years than the absolute CD4 count. More recent data has shown that for children over the age of 5 years, absolute counts have very similar predictive value for disease progression as in adults. This is reflected in the 2006 classification system (see Table, below). This supercedes the Centers for Disease Control 1994 Classification. Monitoring children with HIV infection should take into account signs and symptoms, as well as CD4 counts and viral loads.

Treatments for children with HIV

The goals of treatment in children are to improve quality of life, restore and sustain normal growth and development, prevent complicating infections, and prolong survival into independent adulthood.

Over the past ten years, treatment options for children with HIV have changed dramatically. In resource-rich nations, access to and availability of medications is similar to those used with adults. In the UK all classes of medications are currently available for use in children. However, not all are in formulations which are "child-friendly"; by this, we mean formulations that are easy for children to take.

Clinical trials designed to evaluate the safety and effectiveness of anti-HIV drugs have been critical to incremental improvements in treatment for children.

In Europe, the Paediatric European Network for the Treatment of AIDS (PENTA) carry out such trials (http://www.ctu.mrc.ac.uk/penta/).

Additional specific research into treatments for children is urgently needed, as the results of studies in adults cannot always be applied directly to children. The main reasons for this are:

- The natural history of HIV differs between children and adults.

- Some drugs are handled differently in children's bodies, which may affect the dose that is required. Pharmacokinetic (pk) studies. This has led to increasing use of therapeutic drug monitoring in treating children with HIV.

- Young children have immature immune systems, which may be more responsive to reconstitution following treatment compared with adults.

- CD4 counts have to be interpreted differently from adults, as they can be much higher in infants than in adults - see "CD4 percentage" above.

Research studies looking at HIV treatment use in children have been relatively short-term. However, children will potentially be exposed to antiretrovirals for very long periods of time, and this exposure occurs when their bodies are growing. No-one knows the long-term effects of this.

Treatment regimens

In the UK, children starting on treatments will generally start on a triple combination. However, for young infants and those with high viral loads and very symptomatic disease, quadruple (four drug) therapies have been used. This should ideally spare at least one class of drug.

Deciding when to start treatment in children and what to start with is constantly evolving. There are no data available to suggest that PI-containing or sparing regimens have greater clinical efficacy, and this is the subject of a large international trial between PENTA sites across Europe and collaborators in the USA

Side-effects

Toxicities associated with antiretrovirals are broadly similar in children and adults. The most common side-effects in children are gastrointestinal symptoms and rashes. However, lipid abnormalities and lipodystrophy are being increasingly reported.

In the UK, for babies born to HIV-positive mothers and who have been exposed to antiretroviral therapy in utero, reporting to the British Paediatric Surveillance Unit (BPSU) is required to monitor any long-terms effects of antiretrovirals.

Dosing

Dosing of antiretroviral therapy for children differs from adults. Doses are generally calculated on weight or surface area. In some instances, paediatric doses of antiretrovirals may exceed adult doses, with children requiring larger doses. This applies particularly to protease inhibitors. Children's livers are more efficient and process drugs faster. However this varies widely from child to child. Increasingly, therapeutic drug monitoring is being used to individualise treatment.

Adherence to treatments

A major consideration for starting treatment in children is the child and family's readiness and motivation to embark on often complex medication regimens. In other words, their ability to start and maintain therapy. The importance of supporting adherence cannot be overemphasised.

Essentially, children rely on adult caregivers for their medications and thus the support needs required to aid children in adhering to combination therapies can only be managed by considering the family unit as a whole. Each is dependent on the other and each has an important role to play in maintaining high adherence rates. Children as a group cannot be categorised under a broad umbrella of "paediatrics". Age-specific differences exist, which require careful consideration when planning and starting antiretroviral therapy.

Children as a group are known to be a difficult population to administer medications to. The issues surrounding taking antiretroviral therapy for an infant will differ greatly from that of an adolescent. As such strategies to aid adherence need to be age specific and individually focussed. Further information can be obtained from the Children's HIV Association website - www.bhiva.org/chiva

Other medical management issues

Immunisation schedule for HIV-positive children

Routine immunisations (with certain alterations) are recommended for all children with HIV. Live vaccines should be avoided with the exception of the MMR vaccine. BCG is not recommended because of the risk of dissemination of BCG in the immuno-compromised individual. Inactivated polio vaccine has now replaced live (oral) vaccine in the UK. Influenza vaccines are recommended annually, with two doses in the first season and one thereafter. Children with damaged immune systems may not always respond adequately to vaccination. If a child with HIV infection has come into contact with measles or chickenpox then medical advice should be sought.

The current approach is to restore immunity with ART then to immunise the child. Passive immunotherapy may be offered if the child has a very low CD4%.

Please refer to the Children's HIV Association website for additional details (www.bhiva.org/chiva)

Sharing information

"The right time"

Sharing information is a process, not a one-off occasion. Parents vary greatly in their views regarding the age that their child is mature enough to cope with being told.

Openness in family communication

Parents usually want to be open and honest with their children and do not like having to hide literature on HIV, or stop telephone conversations when their child comes in to the room.

In order to promote open family communication to resolve problems, some parents may decide to tell their children to actively encourage the expression of their feelings and develop their views and plans for the future.

Another reason parents may wish to be 'open' about their status is to explain changes in the household. The parent may feel it is unfair for their children to be the recipient of all these changes without knowing why it is happening. The children may also react to these changes by questions to the parent, or by exhibiting significant behavioural changes.

Inadvertent disclosure of a person's status

Occasionally, if a parent is recently diagnosed and believes they are going to die, they may share information about their illness.

Parents who have been through the process of disclosing their status to other significant people may find it easier to disclose it to their child. Parents may be pressured by these people into telling the child; they may be worried that the child will be told inadvertently by someone else, or that he or she will ask other people. The parents' decision may also be influenced by the presence of other adults who are available to provide support to the children.

Parents may not have ultimate control in the decision to disclose their illness to their children due to pressure from professionals. This pressure may be due to professional's view that withholding information is not healthy or because they may have serious concerns about the child's emotional welfare.

Unfortunately in some situations professionals have highlighted their concerns because of changes in the child's behaviour, signifying that the child is aware of something happening in the family. In this case it may only be necessary for the parent to tell the child they have an illness (not specifically HIV) for the child's behaviour to improve.

Research into families affected by life-threatening illnesses often found that children had suspected something and that their fantasies about what was happening were worse than the reality of the situation.

Another area that some child care professionals stress is the rights of the child. This school of thought believes that the child should be told about HIV status, whether it is their own or their parents, as a matter of right.

A balanced approach is desirable: it is crucial that parents are encouraged to think about these issues so that they are prepared to give truthful answers to direct questions from their children.

Concerns about sharing information

Many HIV-positive parents worry about telling their child about their status because of stigma and discrimination. The parent may fear rejection from their child because of negative messages the child may have received about HIV. If the child doesn't reject them, parents may feel the child will view them as having done something bad or wrong.

Because of the widely held view that 'HIV equals AIDS equals death', parents may worry that in telling their child, the child may assume their parent will die soon or is dying. Parents often feel unable to cope with talking about the possibility of their own death, and death itself may be a taboo subject.

Confidentiality is often a major concern of parents who feel their child or children may not be able to keep their illness private. Parents often say that they are most concerned about the impact on their children of others learning of their HIV status, as the child may experience discrimination at school or become isolated from their friends. Parents also worry that the child will tell their siblings or relatives, who in turn may not yet have been told by the parent.

While some parents feel that their child would be able to keep their status confidential, they believe that such a burden on their children is unacceptable. It is difficult to know what impact keeping a secret such as this may have on a child or young person.

Children can be trusted with information about important things in their family life, such as drug use, child abuse, domestic violence, etc. In these situations, children and young people report various negative impacts, such as withdrawal from their friends, not inviting other children home, a feeling of difference from other children or generally having to cover up. Because of the stigma attached to HIV, the impact of telling an outsider about HIV in the family may be more detrimental than telling someone about other family matters.

Some parents decide not to tell their children until they are seriously ill, or may decide they never want to tell their children. Parents feel that telling a child will change that child's life forever, and they want the child to have 'as normal a life as possible' without having to worry constantly about their parent, or who will look after them. The child or young person could become burdened by the knowledge and may, for instance, start taking on more responsibility in the house or checking on the parent's movements and health.

Discussing their status with the child or a young person may be too difficult for some parents because they don't know how to explain something as unclear as HIV. No-one can say exactly if they will get ill, or if they do, if and when they might die. Parents may not want this emotional uncertainty about the future to hover over their children.

Some parents feel that there may be a possibility of a cure, so they don't want to subject their children to the emotional trauma of being told about their parent having a life-threatening illness today, when a cure could be found tomorrow.

If parents have explained the facts of HIV to their children, then the disclosure of a parent's own status to their child may leave that parent open to questioning by the child on how they became infected. Having to explain facts about their own lifestyle - for example taking drugs, being gay or bisexual may prove to be too difficult, and the parent may decide not to disclose their status in order to circumvent these questions.

How much harm can withholding information cause?

Research into children's reactions after they are told their parent has a life-threatening illness, such as cancer, has shown that it is usually better for the child to be told. However, some parents and professionals feel this to be of limited value in the context of HIV, as most other life-threatening illnesses do not carry the same stigma and discrimination.

The decision whether or not to disclose a parent's status is also influenced by the child's age and its family background. For example, very few parents would decide to tell a three-year old about HIV, but may consider telling an older child. If family or cultural norms mean that the child or young person is not involved in family matters, trying to bring a degree of openness about a complex issue such as HIV may prove to be difficult for parents.

Another reason why a parent may choose not to disclose their status may be their emotional state or that of their child or children. The parent may want to be emotionally calmer before disclosing their status in order to help the child or young person through their emotional response and reduce the possibilities of over-dramatising the situation.

In other circumstances, the child or young person may just be achieving a sense of stability which the parent may not want to disrupt; for example, if a child is coming to terms with the death of the father, the mother may not want to tell the child she also has a life-threatening illness. The child or young person may recently have been told about a parental separation or of a family secret such as parental drug use, leaving the child or young person emotionally unsettled. Being told about the parent's HIV status at this point would probably be detrimental.

Children and young people - what to tell them

Many HIV-positive parents worry about telling their child about their status because of stigma and discrimination. The parent may fear rejection from their child because of negative messages the child may have received about HIV. If the child doesn't reject them, parents may feel the child will view them as having done something bad or wrong.

Because of the widely held view that 'HIV equals AIDS equals death', parents may worry that in telling their child, the child may assume their parent will die soon or is dying. Parents often feel unable to cope with talking about the possibility of their own death, and death itself may be a taboo subject.

Confidentiality is often a major concern of parents who feel their child or children may not be able to keep their illness private. Parents often say that they are most concerned about the impact on their children of others learning of their HIV status, as the child may experience discrimination at school or become isolated from their friends. Parents also worry that the child will tell their siblings or relatives, who in turn may not yet have been told by the parent.

While some parents feel that their child would be able to keep their status confidential, they believe that such a burden on their children is unacceptable. It is difficult to know what impact keeping a secret such as this may have on a child or young person.

Children can be trusted with information about important things in their family life, such as drug use, child abuse, domestic violence, etc. In these situations, children and young people report various negative impacts, such as withdrawal from their friends, not inviting other children home, a feeling of difference from other children or generally having to cover up. Because of the stigma attached to HIV, the impact of telling an outsider about HIV in the family may be more detrimental than telling someone about other family matters.

Some parents decide not to tell their children until they are seriously ill, or may decide they never want to tell their children. Parents feel that telling a child will change that child's life forever, and they want the child to have 'as normal a life as possible' without having to worry constantly about their parent, or who will look after them. The child or young person could become burdened by the knowledge and may, for instance, start taking on more responsibility in the house or checking on the parent's movements and health.

Discussing their status with the child or a young person may be too difficult for some parents because they don't know how to explain something as unclear as HIV. No-one can say exactly if they will get ill, or if they do, if and when they might die. Parents may not want this emotional uncertainty about the future to hover over their children.

Some parents feel that there may be a possibility of a cure, so they don't want to subject their children to the emotional trauma of being told about their parent having a life threatening illness today, when a cure could be found tomorrow.

If parents have explained the facts of HIV to their children, then the disclosure of a parent's own status to their child may leave that parent open to questioning by the child on how they became infected. Having to explain facts about their own lifestyle - for example taking drugs, being gay or bisexual may prove to be too difficult, and the parent may decide not to disclose their status in order to circumvent these questions.

Children & young people's reactions to HIV in the family

Children will have different reactions when they are told that a family member is HIV-positive. Because children's reactions differ to those of adults, it is often useful for a parent to have advice or support from someone who is experienced in working with children and young people. Children's reactions to being told this type of information will also be influenced by their age, their ability to express themselves and family permission to do this, as well as their own thought processes.

Some parents will need assistance in recognising that the child or young person may react negatively to this type of information. These parents may need help in relating their own grief reactions to being told about their HIV diagnosis with the reactions of the child.

Children's responses, like adult responses, will often occur over a period of time. They will experience reactions which are known as the grief cycle because they are experiencing a loss, even though this may not be the physical loss of a person. They may be losing what they see as their normal family life. They may think about the person dying, and they may lose the stability and security of being in the family home, or lose certain types of interactions with the person with HIV. If it is the child or young person who has HIV, they may lose their hopes for the future, hopes of having a family, employment or education. These fears need to be addressed with honesty and optimism.

For some children or young people who have guessed a family member is ill or has HIV, their reaction may be of relief that it is confirmed and relief at not having to pretend that they didn't know.

A child or young person may appear to have no reaction at all to being told. This is not because they don't understand the implications of the information, or that they have no strong reactions to the information. They may need to time to think about everything by themselves, or they may worry about how their parents will cope with their reaction.

Children and young people may even feel unable to react in front of their parents in case of upsetting them because showing any emotions is not normally acceptable. The child/young person may be in such a state of shock that no emotions surface.

If the parent or another adult can be supportive to the child or young person, the child can then discuss their feelings, fears and questions, and express some of the emotions they are experiencing.

Supporting them

Currently there are different levels of responses to support and services for children and young people affected by HIV. Parents may seek support from within their own networks, such as friends, church or community groups. Because of fears of breaches of confidentiality and experiencing stigma, parents often look for alternative avenues of support for their children from voluntary and statutory agencies. Sometimes the child or young person may seek sources of support, with or without their parents' knowledge.

Some parents decide to tell someone at their child's school about HIV in the family. This can be a source of support for them in case they are unable to participate as actively in school activities as previously.

Schools are often able to provide support for the child or young person. The parent may not yet have told the child, but may feel

they should inform the school in case their child exhibits inappropriate or unusual behaviour, such as lack of attention or attention seeking. If the parent has already told the child or young person, they may feel that this will help their child who can talk then to someone else about their feelings.

There is often concern about the impact of knowing about the status of a family member on the child or young person. The school can often provide a link between the family and child-focused support services, such as educational social workers, child guidance clinics, or the school psychological service.

Families often have a strong link with community or hospital based medical staff, who become key sources of support. Hospital social workers, psychologists, play therapists and counsellors can also be accessed via this route.

Other avenues of support often include statutory or voluntary childcare agencies. These offer a wide range of experience and services for helping children with different problems.

One of the difficulties facing many families affected by HIV is the lack of knowledge about the needs of children in adult-focused HIV agencies. The response of some HIV agencies are encouraging with some work and creative partnerships developing between HIV agencies and child care agencies.

As the response of both HIV agencies and child care agencies to HIV and children develop, services are likely to become both HIV-aware and focused on the needs of children.

The care of children and young people affected by HIV & AIDS

Planning for care

There are considerable practical issues that parents need to address when making a plan for the care of their children. Professional help, such as children's social workers or lawyers should be sought to ensure that the plan is feasible and families are helped to access all the services they require.

The aim of planning is to enable parents who have a life-threatening illness to consider who might care for their children if they became unable to or if they should die. This may involve arrangements for emergency, respite, short term or long term care of the child or young person. Planning is important situations where one parent has died, if both parents have HIV, or if the children are not living with their parent,, for instance in another country, or in foster care.

Introducing the idea of planning to a parent will be dependent on various factors such as how long they have been diagnosed, their state of health, contact with other parents affected by HIV, relationships with professionals and timing.

The empirical experience of parents and workers in making plans for the care of children has shown it to be better to start the process as early as possible. This acknowledges the complexity of the emotions that can arise for parents and the time they may need to process them. It also allows time to arrange practical tasks, such as making wills, looking at accommodation or finding an alternative carer.

Some parents may have made practical arrangements for their children without input from a worker who has a child focus. It may still be beneficial for parents to review these arrangements

with a child-focused worker who can then act as a sounding board, or who can provide useful information about the emotional and practical implications for parents, their children or carers. Topics may include what the parents expect of carers, or how the child or young person may react to the changes in living arrangements.

At an appropriate time, the child or young person should be involved in the process. This will depend on the age and maturity of the child, and the normal family decision-making process and cultural background of the family.

The child or young person may have very definite views or feelings about plans for themselves. Even if their views are unrealistic or unsuitable, this needs to be discussed with them. If the child or young person is involved in making decisions about their life, they will be more emotionally prepared for any change in living arrangements.

Impact on the parent

After being diagnosed, parents often ask themselves 'What will happen to the children if I die?' Subsequently, some parents will start to making plans for the care of their children. Many parents assume that a relative or friend will care for their children, although they may make no definite arrangements.

Sometimes the thought of not being around to care for the children causes so much emotional pain that the parent will not be able to start making any plan. In other situations, parents defer making a plan because they believe there will be time in which to do it.

Emotionally, very few parents ever believe that someone can care or love their child or their children as well as they would, while providing a similar lifestyle for their children. This often results in parents being ambivalent about the carer's abilities and lifestyle. It is also extremely difficult for a parent to acknowledge that someone else could 'take their place'.

Many parents find it difficult to involve their children in planning because they feel unable to cope with possible emotional reactions of their children. Instead the parent may try to find out indirectly what the child may want. It is better in this situation for the parent to have an idea about who the carer will be, rather than asking the child a very open question.

Any response from the child will evoke both positive and negative emotions in the parent.

Impact on children

Parents often worry about how their children may cope emotionally with a change in living arrangements. Most parents want a relationship to develop between the carer and their children, so that in an emergency there is less emotional trauma to the children who can be cared for by someone who is familiar and trusted.

The child or young person will be more emotionally able to cope if they are involved in the decision about the carer or told about the intended plan by the parent. They can prepare themselves emotionally for a change as well as making feeling a part of the process.

Parents may decide to tell their child that the reason for making a plan is because they have a life-threatening illness. Allowing discussions about the impact of this news often decrease negative impact on the child because they are able to express their feelings and the changes. Someone other than the parent may act as a confidant for the child or young person. The planning process needs to address the emotional needs for the child or young person so they can keep in contact with their parent. The child or young person may need regular information about their parent to help decrease their anxiety and to promote this emotional bonding.

A plan should incorporate possible changes, such as the parent being ill or having to go to hospital. This may result in the carer being responsible for preparing the child for visits to see their parent. The emotional response of children may vary; sometimes the child or young person appears to lose interest in their parent or be unable to communicate with them while in hospital, or the child may be overwhelmed or frightened.

Practicalities of planning

Planning for the care of children is a process where parents (and if appropriate their children) decide who will care for the children when they need a break, if they should become ill or if they die.

The plan may involve looking at various options for the care needed - either respite, or a continuum of short, medium or long term/permanent care.

Respite care gives parents planned breaks away from their children. Short-term care may be necessary if the parent has to have a longer break, go into hospital or is ill intermittently.

Permanent care enables another person to provide care for a child or young person whose parent is permanently incapacitated or has died.

This section focuses on the directions that parents may consider before making a decision about a plan for the care of their children, discussing the current legislative framework of the Children Act 1989. Some families will need no input from local authority or voluntary agency children's workers, while other families may be dependent on support or services from agencies to arrange the best plan for their children.

Planning usually takes one of four directions:

- The parent has a family network or friends who are able to provide some form of support.

- The parent(s) decide the child or young person will best be cared for in their own family home. This could mean a carer coming into the home or alternatively a carer living nearby providing close support to the family.

- Childcare will need to be accessed from the local authority if there is no one available within the parents' network to provide any form of support.

Planning when family or friends are available

If there are family members or friends available to provide support, the parent will normally consider them as the first option. Normally this is also given first priority by children's social workers. This philosophy is embodied in the Children Act 1989 which states that 'children are normally best looked after within their own family' and 'placements with relatives will often provide the best opportunities for promoting and maintaining family links in a familiar setting.' (Children Act 1989 and Volume 3 of the Children Act Guidance and Regulations - HMSO 1991) There would have to be significant concern for Social Services to look outside family members for care of children, if they were available.

When the carer is not a relative and the child stays with the person more than 28 days, they should inform Social Services Children and Family section. Social Services may inquire into the situation to ensure the child is cared for and safe. This is known as a private fostering.

If a relative or friend continues to provide care for the child or young person, Social Services could assess approving' this person as a foster carer and provide financial assistance. This involves a comprehensive assessment of the carer (including a police check to ensure the carer does not have a record of offences against children) and how the carer could meet the needs of the family.

These more formal arrangements may result in the family providing regular short term help, foster care or permanent long-term care. Practical issues such as making wills and guardians or housing may need to be taken into account.

From the parents and the child's point of view asking a relative to provide some form of care is often the best way of maintaining family links. The continuity for a child being in a familiar setting, the relationship between the child and relative and the advantage of the carer sharing the same race, culture and language should not be underestimated.

If families or friends are available to provide care for the children, there may not be any need to be in contact with agencies such as Social Services.

Planning when local authority carers are needed

Many parents are hesitant about approaching Social Services for help, because they think their child will be taken away, that there will be too much state intervention, or that Social Services is connected to other agencies such as the DWP or the Home Office. Parents should be reassured that local authorities have a legal 'duty to promote the upbringing of children within their own family, by providing a range and level of services appropriate to those children's needs'. (Section 17(1) of the Children Act 1989).

Parents should be given information about their rights and the roles of Social Services, so that they feel confident about contacting statutory or voluntary agencies to access the services to which they are entitled and can make informed decisions.

Social Service carers may be the only option where there are no family or friends able to provide any form of support. If family or friends are able to provide a limited response, Social Service carers may provide complementary services such as foster carers providing short-term or respite care, while the family provides long-term care. Foster carers from voluntary childcare agencies or Social Services are assessed and provided with training and support in order to be 'approved' as foster carers. In making such arrangements, Social Services need to consider keeping children together, if this is in their best interests, while trying to place the child in a familiar neighbourhood and taking into account the child's race, religion, culture and language.

Childminders

Many families already have childminders who care for their children during the day. Under the Children Act 1989 childminders are now legally able to care for a child for overnight stays. This may be an option for emergency or specific situations. Parents will need to consider what information will be given to the childminder about their need for this type of care.

Residential care

Occasionally, a plan might involve the child or young person being accommodated in residential care.

Planning when children are cared for in their own home

Many families want their children to be cared for in their own home. This may involve a relative or friend moving into the family home to act as the carer, or the children caring for themselves. This plan provides maximum continuity for the family, by enabling the children to be cared for by a familiar person, within familiar surroundings while continuing their normal routine. Financial assistance may be needed from Social Services for this plan and this must be included as part of the planning process.

Sometimes the long-term plan involves the child or young person caring for themselves in the family home. Parents may regard their children as capable, independent and mature enough to establish their own home. Landlords may offer an interim tenancy in the child's name at 16 years and a proper tenancy at 17 years. Benefits may be claimed if the eldest child is old enough, perhaps with additional financial support from Social Services to help cover any shortfall such as upkeep on the family home.

This option needs detailed planning and careful consideration in looking at the practicalities of a young person being carer for themselves and any siblings. For example, who will sign contractual agreements with telephone, gas, or electricity companies?

The emotional impact on a young person being a carer will also need to be fully discussed. The young person should receive support to minimise the pressure of being responsible for managing the household while acting as a parent to other siblings. These responsibilities may also impact on the young person's social and educational development.

An adult may be the identified carer whilst staying in their own home. This adult becomes the support person for the child/young person, whilst ensuring that the children have adequate care. They may act as a guarantor for contractual agreements or take on the role of a carer as necessary, for example going to parent/teacher meetings. Alternatively, Social Services may seek a carer to move into the family home. This is not a very common arrangement, but more agencies are viewing this as a way of meeting the families' plan.

Planning for adoption

Adoption involves a child becoming a permanent part of another family. Legally the links between birth family and the child are broken. Currently more birth families are continuing contact with their child in a change towards greater 'openness' in adoptive situations. This openness may mean contact by arranged visits, telephone, letters or photos between both families.

Adoption may be by a close relative, distant relative, friend or non-relative. The local authority has different roles and processes in each of these situations. The application for adoption needs to be heard formally in court, with an advocate for the child (known as a guardian ad litem) looking at the child's need. The court must be satisfied that making an adoption order is in the best interests of the child.

When there are no plans

If there are no plans made and the parent is unable to care for the child or dies, Social Services will assume legal responsibility for the children. Social Services will prioritise seeking family, relatives or close friends to care for the children.

Seeking family members to provide care may be contrary to the unwritten wish of the deceased parent. The carer may not be who the deceased parent would have chosen, however, these may be options that the Social Services feel most appropriate.

In the event of no-one being suitable or available from within the family network, Social Service will locate a long term/permanent carer for the child or children. Social Services should try to keep siblings together and find a carer who reflects the cultural, linguistic, religious and racial background of the children. Often the process of finding a suitable long term/permanent carer is lengthy, and in the interim the children could live with several short-term carers.

The child's cultural identity

A significant number of black and minority ethnic parents prefer carers to be from a different cultural background to their own. This may be due to fears of family in their home country wanting to take the children back to the country of origin or finding out about their HIV status when they have not disclosed it to their family. Parents may perceive that bringing a child up in a white family will bring more benefits to the child and also think the child will assimilate more quickly into white culture.

The current practice in fostering is to place children with a carer that reflects the child's background. There should be discussion with these parents about the reasons for their preference for culturally different carers - and about the negative impact on children who lose their own cultural heritage, language, contact with their community and perhaps even family links.

Arranging for children to be fostered

What is foster care?

Fostering (or foster care) is the term used to describe an arrangement where a carer looks after somebody else's child. Usually, this is in the home of a foster carer.

Arrangements may be made privately between the child's parent and the foster carer or, more commonly in the UK, the arrangements may be made at the request of the parent, via the local authority social services department. Foster care can provide support to families with children in a range of circumstances.

Emergency or short-term fostering

There are situations in which arrangements need to be made, sometimes at short notice, for a child to live with a foster family because the parent is temporarily unable to care for the child.

Respite care (Short-term breaks)

This is an arrangement whereby the parent can have a break from the pressures of caring for children. Usually, particularly for young children, arrangements are made for foster carers to provide family based respite care (rather than, for example, placing the children in a children's home). A typical arrangement could be that the child goes to stay with the foster carer one weekend a month. Ideally, a flexible arrangement would mean that if the parents were ill, or there was an emergency, then the children would be able to stay with the same foster carers, whom they already knew and whom the parents trusted.

Long-term foster care

This is an arrangement to provide care for a child for the foreseeable future. It could be for a teenager, until he or she becomes independent, or for younger children whose own parents are unable to care for them.

An arrangement for children to be cared for on a long-term basis through the social services department involves careful selection by the department's social workers of a foster family who would be likely to provide a secure environment until they were adults. Parents would be closely involved in this process. Important considerations would include where the foster family lived; their ethnic, religious and cultural backgrounds, including languages spoken; their willingness to maintain contact in the future with significant people in the children's lives; and, in the case of a parent who was HIV-positive, their commitment to share care with the parents until he or she was no longer able to provide day-to-day care.

In a long-term foster care arrangement set up by the social services department, a social worker would have responsibility for visiting the children at regular intervals and the foster family would receive financial and social work support. The children would continue to use their family name and identity and maintain their legal relationship with members of their birth family. Adoption is sometimes suggested rather than foster care for young children who will be unlikely to have any family contact after the death of their parents. A discussion regarding adoption should take into account whether this would better promote the children's welfare, particularly in the light of the child's ethnic and cultural background. Legal adoption as

developed in the UK is not well understood in some communities, where informal adoption is more usual.

Parents' involvement in foster care

Unless there are exceptional circumstances (such as issues of child protection), then parents who have requested that their children be accommodated by the local authority with foster carers will retain full parental responsibility. The local authority cannot make any decisions about the children without the parents' agreement.

Contact between parents and children while they are accommodated with foster carers is very important and a local authority will help with the transport or the cost of transport to ensure that contact is maintained.

Except in an extreme emergency, parents would have the opportunity of meeting foster carers before their child was placed so that they could be satisfied with the choice of placement and pass on important information to the carers.

Can friends or relatives foster?

Friends or relatives can foster children. In fact, before arranging for children to be placed with foster carers registered with the local authority, a social worker would always check out with parents whether there are friends or relatives who might be able to care for the child. Clearly such an arrangement is usually easier for children and young people, who would not have to adjust to living with strangers at a time when they might already be worried about their parents' health.

There are a number of different ways of making arrangements for children to be fostered by friends or relatives.

Arrangements may be private and informal, with children moving to stay with relatives or friends for short or longer periods. In certain circumstances (but not always), the social services department should be notified of the arrangement.

The arrangement may be made privately but with financial or practical assistance from the social services department.

The arrangement may be made through the social services department. This means that the local authority would take responsibility for accommodating the children, but instead of placing them with registered foster carers not known to the children, would place the children instead with friends or relatives. The regulations permit children to be placed with friends or relatives in an emergency for a period of up to six weeks, even though the foster carers have not been registered. However, if the arrangement is likely to be a continuing one (on a respite care or long-term basis), then the relatives or friends would apply to the local authority to be 'approved' as foster carers.

The advantages of children being fostered through the social services department are that carers receive continuing financial help (until the children are independent) as well as social work support. The main disadvantages are that there is inevitably quite a lot of bureaucracy involved; prospective foster carers may find the procedures quite personal and possibly intrusive; and there will need to be a social worker involved in visiting from time to time throughout the period the children remain with their foster carers.

Local authority information on foster care services

If there is already a local authority social worker involved with the family, then he or she can make enquiries about the availability of foster carers on behalf of the parents and children.

If the family is not already in touch with the local authority, then an enquiry can be made to the local area or neighbourhood office of the social services department. The enquiry may be handled by the duty officer in an Assessment Team or by a duty officer in a Children and Families Team.

An enquiry can be made about the availability of foster care and how to access the service without giving identifying information in the first instance.

It would be important to check what the local authority policy is with regard to providing information to foster carers about a parent's or child's HIV status. The local authority must ensure that the foster carer has information which is relevant to promoting the child's health. Most foster care agencies would not expect a parent to divulge his or her own HIV status, but would ask a parent's permission to divulge a child's HIV status to the foster carer (who would have to respect the confidential nature of the information).

The initial response from the local authority may be that there is no suitable foster carer available, taking into account the child's or parent's HIV status, the cultural and ethnic background, the number of children in the family, etc. However, the local authority has a duty to provide accommodation for children 'in need' and therefore should contact other foster care agencies, voluntary and statutory, to try to obtain the appropriate provision.

The local authority has a duty to ensure that wherever possible children stay within their family and community network: therefore the possibility of friends or relatives being able to care for the child, perhaps with help regarding finance and housing, should always be explored in the first instance.

Guardianship and parental responsibility

Choosing who is to be legally responsible

Parents will be influenced in their choice of future carer for their children by the adult's ability to provide financial, emotional and practical support. The parent may have some idea of the type of person they would like to have legal responsibility. Often parents will choose a relative or close family friends.

The following are some of the common questions which parents should think about before appointing someone to be legally responsible for their children.

- How do my children feel about this person and how does the potential guardian feel about being appointed?

- How has the person brought their own children up? Is this similar to the way I would want my children raised in relation to culture, religion, expectations of education, manners, relationships, roles, behaviour and boundaries?

- Do I need more than one guardian? For example, if I choose my parents should I also choose another guardian who is younger in case my parents die? Would having two guardians help ensure that there are some safeguards about what is happening to my child - two carers can share responsibility? Or will it confuse the issue more because two people may have different expectations?

- Is this person able to take responsibility for my child or are they not used to children? If they have they their own family or other responsibilities to think of how will they cope with the added responsibilities of my children?

- Are there financial implications for the potential guardian, which may need to be discussed with Social Services?

- Is the guardian willing or able to have the children living with them? Where might the children live if not with the guardian? Does the guardian have space for all the children?

Are there reasons for not wanting someone in my family/relatives to have legal responsibility for my children? If there are, who

else could take on this role and perhaps ensure there is contact with the family?

Sometimes parents may not wish to consider a potential carer who they feel is not in the situation to care for their children, for example, a younger sibling. However, the worker should highlight the fact that this might not be needed for many years and in the meantime the sister's situation may have changed positively. Also the parent needs to be reminded that wills can be changed if they change their mind or decide to include someone else as guardian.

If parents do not appoint a guardian before they die, the wishes of the deceased parent may not be considered by the Social Services in arrangements for the care of the children.

Planning for sustained care

One of the most important tasks of making a plan for the care of children affected by HIV involves granting another person parental responsibility or appointing a guardian. These are two ways in which parents can ensure another person has legal responsibility for their child's welfare, upbringing and safety. The decision to make someone legally responsible for their child needs to be very carefully thought out by the parent.

If parents do not appoint someone to have legal responsibility for their child, another person may assume responsibility and could apply for legal recognition of their role. If no one comes forward, Social Services will act to make arrangements for the children. Any current arrangement that the deceased parent may have made will be assessed and may be changed.

The role of a guardian

A guardian appointed under Section 5 of the Children Act 1989 has parental responsibility for the child or young person. The guardian has the right to consent or withhold consent to free the child for adoption, to agree or withhold agreement to the child's adoption and to appoint a guardian for the child or young person in case of their death. Their duties end when the child reaches 18 years old, or when the child dies.

Who can be a guardian?

A guardian can either be appointed by a court, or by the parent (known as a testamentary guardian). This is possible for any child until they are 18 years old.

The court can appoint a guardian if;

- the child has no parent with parental responsibility for him, or

- a residence order has been made with respect to the child in favour of a parent or guardian of his who has died while the order was in force under section 5 (1).

There may be more than one person appointed as guardian but the court cannot appoint the local authority as guardian. Anyone with an interest in the child can make an application to the court for guardianship. The court must consider the child's welfare and other factors. To do this, the court may ask for a welfare report from a guardian ad litem.

Parents can also appoint a guardian through either a will or a written statement. Because the written statement needs to satisfy the requirements of the law, it is important to seek legal advice on preparing it. One or more guardians may be appointed by the parent.

Parental responsibility

The Children Act 1989 has defined parental responsibility as 'all the rights, duties, powers, responsibilities and authority which by law a parent of a child has in relation to the child and his/her property' (S3(1)).

The following people automatically hold parental responsibility:

- Any mother.

- A mother and father who were married to each other at the time of the birth, even if they separate or divorce.

- The unmarried father does not have parental responsibility unless he acquires it by the following means:

By a formal agreement with the mother. This must be made on a specific form and recorded in a certain manner. Forms are available from legal stationers, Citizen Advice Bureaux, law centres or specialist services such as THT.

By being appointed guardian either by the court or through the mother's will.

Through a parental responsibility order made by the court. The court must be satisfied that making an order would be better than not making an order.

By being granted a residence order by the court - the court is obliged to grant a parental responsibility order (Children Act 1989).

More than one person may have parental responsibility at one time, which does not cease just because another person gains parental responsibility. They may act independently from one another unless the action requires the consent of other parties with parental responsibility. If there is disagreement about an action, for example schooling, then the person not in agreement may as a last resort go to court to try and stop the action.

Sometimes parental responsibility is granted to people or statutory bodies for specific periods of times and in specific instances. For example, if a relative has cared for the children and is granted a residence order, then this person gains parental responsibility for the length of time the children are with them. Other specific instances are when there are emergency orders, and care orders where the local authority are granted parental responsibility.

These people or statutory bodies do not have the full parental responsibility. A local authority is also not able to bring the child up in any religious persuasion other than what the child is used to. Parents still have parental responsibility if there is an emergency protection or care order.

African families in the UK

Language problems

Service users may have a working knowledge of English, but they may require translation and interpretation services to deal with complex issues or difficult language. Some voluntary agencies are able to provide interpreting services.

In situations where there are few people who speak the required language, care needs to be taken to maintain confidentiality for the service user. Some African families may be wary of interpretation services because of a fear of identification.

Recognising specific problems

On top of the range of difficulties which arise for all families living with HIV, African families are likely to experience additional problems which may include poverty, racism, language and cultural barriers and uncertainty over immigration status. Many of the families have come to the UK, mainly from sub-Saharan Africa, and can be cut off from relatives and isolated from the usual community support systems.

For most families who have come to the UK seeking asylum, the National Asylum Support Service will be involved. It is important to encourage families to fully disclose health issues including HIV in order to ensure the families are not dispersed inappropriately.

Medical issues

Because of the language barrier, past experiences and the insecurity of their present situation, many African people find it difficult to press for information or to assert their wishes in regard to treatment for themselves or their children.

Social factors

Information about how voluntary and statutory agencies operate in the UK and an accurate and sensitive needs assessment should be carried out.

Service provision needs to adjust to the needs of African families with children, for example through provision of acceptable diet, crèche facilities, appropriate decor, reading materials, videos etc. to reflect and enhance the positive identity of service users, especially children.

Empowerment and advocacy for African families will be promoted by recruiting workers and volunteers of relevant backgrounds and by encouraging user participation in developing and running services.

Specific groups who may be particularly isolated and vulnerable, including those newly arrived in the UK, prisoners and detainees.

Specialist HIV pædiatric/Family HIV Clinics

St Mary's Family HIV Service
6th Floor, QEQM Wing, South Wharf Road, London W2 1NY
020 7886 6349

Great Ormond Street Hospital for Sick Children
Great Ormond Street, London WC1N 3JH
020 7242 9789

Penta Clinic
St Georges NHS Trust,
Tooting, London
020 8725 3353/4

Guys & St Thomas's Hospital - Harrison Wing
Lambeth Palace Raod, London SE1 7EH
020 7188 6666

Royal Free Hospital
Pond Street, London NW3 2QG
020 7794 0500

Chelsea and Westminster Hospital
Fulham Palace Road, London
020 8846 6161

Newham General Hospital
Department of Sexual Health
The Greenway Clinic
Glen Road
London E13 8RU
020 7363 8146

References

http://www.unaids.org/en/HIV_data/Epidemiology/epi_slides.asp [accessed Feb 2007].

Gibb D, et al. Decline in mortality, AIDS and hospital admissions in perinatally HIV-1 infected children in the UK and Ireland. BMJ; 327: 1019-1025

Lwin R and Melvin D (2001). Paediatric HIV Infection. J.Child Psychology. Psychiatry 42(4): 427-438

Haemophilia

What is haemophilia?

Haemophilia is a general term for a family of inherited blood-clotting disorders. In haemophilia, there is a life-long defect in the clotting mechanism of the blood caused by a deficiency in one of the thirteen proteins in the blood called *clotting factors*. These work in a chain reaction whenever there is tissue damage to form a blood clot. If one of the factors is missing or defective, the process of forming a clot is slowed down or affected in other ways.

The best known bleeding disorder is so-called *classic* haemophilia, or haemophilia A, which is caused by a deficiency in factor VIII (NB most clotting factors are referred to using Roman numerals). A smaller number of people are missing factor IX. This is called haemophilia B or Christmas Disease, after Stephen Christmas the first person diagnosed with the condition (CHS 2001). In the UK approximately 6,000 people have a diagnosis of haemophilia A with around 1,100 with haemophilia B.

A more common bleeding disorder is von Willebrand's Disease (vWD) named after the Finnish doctor Erik von Willebrand (1870-1949). This is caused by a deficiency of or a defect in von Willebrand's Factor, which works closely with Factor VIII and the proper functioning of platelets in blood clotting. There are around 3,500 people diagnosed with vWD in the UK, although it is thought to affect as many as 1-3% of the population. It often goes undiagnosed, as it is usually less severe and less well known than haemophilia.

There are differing degrees of severity in both forms of haemophilia and vWD. This severity is measured by the amount of the clotting factor people have and is described in a rather complicated way because a figure was set as the normal amount in a person and described as a level of 100%. In reality most people have a clotting factor level of between twice this level and half of it described as between 200% - 50% of this specified normal amount.

In people with haemophilia this level can vary from 25% (mild haemophilia) to less than 1% (severe haemophilia). With moderate to mild haemophilia of both types, bleeding usually only happens after an injury, and treatment need only be administered if there is a bleed. With severe haemophilia, bleeding happens spontaneously, and must be treated very promptly. vWD is rarely as severe as haemophilia, usually causing only bruising or prolonged bleeding with cuts, tooth extractions, or nose bleeds etc. However, there is a rare and severe form of the condition that can be just as serious as severe haemophilia. There is also not a perfect correlation between clotting factor levels and the number of bleeds people experience, some people with mild to moderate levels of a clotting factor can experience as many bleeds as a person with severe haemophilia and a few fortunate people with very low levels of a clotting factor have very few bleeds (CHS 2001).

There is also an extremely rare condition called 'acquired haemophilia' in which a person develops antibodies to one of the clotting factors in their own blood.

Haemophilia and HIV

Patterns of inheritance

Haemophilia is an inherited genetic condition. However, approximately 30% of people with it are unable to trace back any family history, suggesting a spontaneous gene mutation. The cells of human beings contain chromosomes which have genes on them. These genes are the things that carry the information needed to generate the features of a person such as an ability to make clotting factors. Most people have 23 pairs of chromosomes and the one that defines gender is described as either **XX** for women or **XY** for men. The Y chromosome is described as a **Y** because it is literally missing a leg that would turn it into an **X** and the blood-clotting gene is on this missing leg.

Some genes are 'dominant' over others. This means that we only need one copy of the gene - inherited from either the father or the mother - for it to work and decide how the body functions.

The haemophilia gene is not dominant but 'recessive'. Generally recessive genes only work if we inherit a copy of the gene from *both* parents.

However because the blood-clotting gene is on the 'missing leg' of the **X**, men inherit it exclusively from their mothers. Women have two **X**'s so have one copy of the gene if the other chromosome is defective.

However men possess only one **X** chromosome. If it is the recessive haemophilia gene rather than the dominant normal gene then the single copy on that chromosome will decide those features in that man, because there is no dominant gene on the **Y** chromosome to correct it.

This means that women can carry the gene for haemophilia without suffering the symptoms. Any son of such a carrier would have a one in two chance of inheriting the condition from them. Their daughters would have a one in two chance of being also becoming a carrier of the disorder. A man with haemophilia cannot pass it on to his sons but will inevitably pass it to his daughters who will become carriers. Thus haemophilia is usually only expressed in men however carriers may have a lower than normal level of factor VIII or IX but it is only usually a cause for concern at times of major operations or childbirth and even then treatment may not be required. This description of bodily genetics is highly simplified and as human beings are extremely complex organisms do not expect the case of every person with haemophilia to follow this pattern exactly.

Von Willibrand's Disease (vWD) is inherited in a more complex manner, and can affect men and women equally. Over 67% of cases of diagnosed vWD occur in women, mainly because heavy and prolonged periods are amongst the most recognisable and frequent symptoms of the condition (Lee). Paradoxically this may also be a reason why vWD is rarely diagnosed, as few doctors are aware that clotting disorders can affect women. Menorrhagia, slow healing cuts and easy bruising experienced by women with vWD are often dismissed as *just a part of life*, and not recognised as symptoms of a potentially serious clotting disorder.

The most well-known example of haemophilia passed through a family is to be seen in the extended family of Queen Victoria. The British Royal Family was, by the end of the nineteenth century, related to the majority of the royal families of Europe. Victoria had nine children and, unbeknown to her, she was a carrier of the haemophilia A gene. Although only one of her sons, Leopold, actually developed haemophilia, she passed the gene on to her daughters as eventually the condition emerged in the Spanish, Greek and Russian royal families and many smaller princely families (Zeepyat). The condition was a factor in both the communist revolution in Russia in 1917 and the civil war in Spain by adding to an environment of uncertainty about the strength and future of the monarchy in both countries (Potts).

The effects of haemophilia

The common misconception about haemophilia is that when someone has a cut (e.g. whilst shaving) they are in danger of bleeding to death. Whilst such cuts need to be treated, they are seldom a major problem. The real danger lies in internal bleeding into muscles, joints and body cavities. Internal bleeding can occur spontaneously or as a result of an injury. Once an internal bleed starts, without treatment it can cause irreparable damage to the joints or muscles. Blood is toxic to bone; therefore untreated bleeds into joints can cause chronic arthritis.

Bleeding episodes cause the joint or muscle to swell, causing acute and often permanent damage and can be excruciatingly painful as blood pumps uncontrollably into the area. Bleeds into the vital organs can be fatal. The pain, arthritis and the limited movement after frequent bleeding lead to a need for surgery to the joints. Ankle and knee replacements are common in adults with haemophilia although the hope is that the next generation will have far less surgery after a lifetime of prophylactic treatment to prevent bleeding. This is why so many adults with haemophilia have difficulty walking or an unusual gait.

Treatment for haemophilia

Prior to the Second World War the only treatment available was bed rest, and waiting for the bleed to stop and the blood to drain away. This could take weeks, or even months. Some, more alternative remedies, such as snake venom and peanut oil were available, but with questionable effectiveness. During the war, large quantities of blood plasma were collected to treat heavy casualties on the battlefield. During the process of storing this plasma at low temperatures, thick, brown sediment was seen to form. This *cryoprecipitate* turned out to be very rich in clotting factors, and so formed the basis of the first effective haemophilia therapy. During the seventies it became technologically possible to isolate individual factors and pool them to create batches of factor concentrate. These concentrates could then be self-administered intravenously at home, either at the onset of a bleed to stop it, or alternatively prophylactically, in an attempt to prevent bleeds altogether.

The development of factor concentrates and home treatment was heralded as one of the major breakthroughs and success stories of post war medical technology. The effect of concentrates was to transform the lives of people with haemophilia. Home treatment with factor concentrates meant not having to automatically face all the most serious problems of haemophilia, such as acute and chronic pain, crippling disability and the prospect of spending over one quarter of one's life confined to bed. People with haemophilia could now become active, independent members of the community, able to engage in all aspects of society.

The treatment of von Willibrand's Disease is dependant on the type of von Willebrand's and severity of the bleeding. For some women with mild type 1 disease oral contraceptives may be the only treatment they require. Desmopressin is used mainly for people with mild type 1 von Willebrand's, to boost the levels of clotting factors in the blood. Tranexamic acid is used for minor bleeding problems such as nose bleeds and may be used in conjunction with Desmopressin or factor concentrates to help stabilise a clot. Usually only people with severe vWD are treated with cryoprecipitate or Factor concentrates.

Factor concentrates, like many blood products, are made from pooled plasma. They are produced by a number of commercial pharmaceutical companies, the Red Cross and, in England, by the Bio-Products Laboratory (BPL). It can take up to 30,000 donations of blood to make one batch of factor concentrate. As a result of relying upon such a huge donor pool, blood products have always been susceptible to contamination by viruses. Injecting factor concentrates has been likened, in terms of the risks of exposure to HIV, to having unprotected sex, or sharing needles with tens of thousands of people every time you take treatment. All people with haemophilia treated with factor concentrates during the 1970s and early 1980s were exposed to infection with the hepatitis viruses B and C.

This was already a problem in the UK, where donations were always voluntary, but in the USA, and some other countries where blood donors have usually been paid, the rates of infection were far higher. It was as a result of the use of hepatitis infected, imported commercial factor concentrates that, in 1977, the then Labour Government made a commitment to UK self sufficiency in factor concentrates and other pooled plasma blood products.

Scotland did become self-sufficient, but England and Wales did not. During this period pharmaceutical companies pioneered various systems of treating concentrates in an attempt to eliminate viral contamination such as the hepatitis viruses. The most successful was heat treatment, a form of pasteurisation developed in 1978 by Behringewerke Atkionsgesellschaft in Germany. However, despite the high incidence of hepatitis in the haemophilia population, heat treatment was not prioritised, mainly because of cost. As a result of a drug company and public health policy failure to recognise the need to virally inactivate factor concentrates, HIV was spread unknowingly to tens of thousands of people with haemophilia worldwide through what was then being hailed as a life saving treatment.

Haemophilia and AIDS

Despite the fact that it was known that a person with haemophilia died in the United States in 1981 from what is now termed an AIDS-related illness, the association between factor concentrates, AIDS and viral contamination was not made until 1983. In early 1984 in Britain there were at least two reported cases of AIDS in people with haemophilia and later that year, after months of prevarication by the pharmaceutical companies and authorities over whether to heat treat factor concentrates or not, the Haemophilia Foundation in the USA instructed the 20,000 people with haemophilia in the United States to refuse to use all non heat-treated product. The UK Haemophilia Society threatened to follow suit. By the end of 1984 all imported, commercial concentrate in the UK was heat-treated. By mid-1985 domestic product was also treated to destroy the virus. Earlier there had been an attempt to encourage donors who may have been at risk of exposure to AIDS, such as people who had lived in sub-Saharan Africa, gay men and intravenous drug users, not to give blood.

When the test for HIV was pioneered, people with haemophilia were routinely tested. The enormity of the disaster became clear. In the United States, around 10,000 of the 20,000 people with haemophilia were diagnosed as seropositive. In the United Kingdom of the 7,000 people with haemophilia 1,246 were infected, representing 42% of those with severe haemophilia and 6% of those with moderate or mild haemophilia (UKHCDO). As a general rule, people were infected in proportion to the amount of commercial concentrate used, the more severe the haemophilia, the more concentrate used, the more the risk of infection. HIV infection through blood products is discussed in more detail in *HIV transmission*.

The UK Haemophilia Society eventually assumed the responsibility of advising and assisting people with haemophilia affected by HIV in the UK. In 1984 the Society was a small organisation with one full-time employee. The HIV recompense campaign in effect forced the Society to come of age.

Living with HIV and haemophilia

Most adults with haemophilia in the UK have had to incorporate HIV and viral hepatitis into living with their haemophilia. In the early years of the HIV/AIDS crisis, this, along with the compensation campaign, led to charges from certain quarters of separatism and allegations that the haemophilia community was claiming to be more deserving than other people affected by HIV. However, within the haemophilia community in the UK, with the possible exception of a few healthcare professionals, there were

no public assertions that they were the *innocent victims* of HIV/AIDS. The Haemophilia Society's policy has always been that all the communities affected by HIV should be treated equally, but at the same time have their specific and differing needs met. Since haemophilia affects a range of people with different backgrounds it should not, though, be assumed that they are not affected by the prevalent views and circumstances within society. Homophobia and indeed homosexuality are as common amongst people with haemophilia as everybody else.

The haemophilia community has responded differently to the AIDS crisis from other affected communities. People with haemophilia are already living with a pre-existing, potentially disabling and fatal condition. Many people, and particularly those with severe joint damage, have a major disability, which, in its own right, affects mobility, and care needs. Even before HIV, 30% of people with haemophilia were already dependent upon state benefits and because of the genetic nature of the condition, the associated poverty, like the disease itself, tends to run through families.

Once blood products were heat-treated, the haemophilia community effectively ceased to be at risk of HIV infection from their treatment. Those with haemophilia and HIV are therefore a finite group of people. After mid-1985, at the very latest, no person should have been infected with HIV in the UK through the use of factor concentrates. Naturally people with haemophilia remain as much at risk of contracting HIV sexually or through sharing needles as everyone else.

A primary concern for the haemophilia community has also always been the safety of the blood product supply. The extent to which people with haemophilia rely upon uncontaminated factor concentrates cannot be underestimated. This concern has been long-standing and about much more than just HIV. After contaminations with hepatitis viruses, HIV and recent concerns about transmission of variant Creutzfeldt-Jakob Disease (vCJD). In September 2003 the Department of Health conducted a patient notification exercise asking haematologists to inform all their patients who had received blood products made from British blood donors that they was a risk of contracting vCJD. No person with haemophilia had contracted the disease but one person had died of vCJD after receiving a blood transfusion from a donor who went on to develop and die from the disease.

These concerns have led to ongoing campaigns for the widespread use of recombinant factor concentrates, manufactured from transgenic animal cell cultures. Not being produced from human blood, these factor concentrates should be free of human viruses. From April 2003 in Britain a three-year programme of funding began to make recombinant factor concentrates available to everyone with haemophilia A and B who wanted it. Recombinant factor products are not effective in people with von Willebrands and so products made from plasma continue to be used.

People with haemophilia usually attend specialist centres seeing a consultant haematologist for their haemophilia so when they were diagnosed with HIV they often had a pre-existing life-long relationship with a hospital. Many Haemophilia Centres have incorporated control of HIV-related health issues into their general management of haemophilia while others have referred their patients to HIV clinics. Some are still treated for their HIV by haemophilia consultants while other centres have joint clinics with HIV clinicians. It is also worth noting that over 95% of those with haemophilia and HIV are co-infected with Hepatitis C - with all the attendant health and treatment complications that can ensue (see below).

People with haemophilia and HIV are scattered across the country and even though it is possible to speak of the haemophilia community as a generic term, the community exists around a medical and not a social condition. Haemophilia is neither confined to, nor generally more prevalent in any one social or ethnic grouping. HIV has also affected people with haemophilia of all ages. From a health education perspective the response has had to reflect this diversity. Elderly as well as paediatric HIV has had to be tackled, as has HIV in schools. They are also predominantly heterosexual men, which historically is not the case for HIV epidemic in England and Wales and so often had different specific needs for information and support. The ability for men with HIV to have children as safely as possible with their partner is an obvious example of something which has been an issue for many years but only recently started to become part of the services of some HIV clinics.

All these differences, and the small number of people still alive probably accounts for the lack of integration between people with haemophilia and HIV into the more general community of people with HIV. However, the rest of this manual remains relevant for them as they will not only have similar concerns regarding adherence, side-effects and safer sex but will also have to bear the same discrimination and ignorance as everyone else with HIV.

Treatment issues

As a group, people with haemophilia and HIV seem to be responding well to combination therapy. Everyone has now been living with a positive diagnosis for over twenty years. However, antiretroviral therapies have a few particular problems for people with bleeding disorders. In addition to the normal side-effects of HIV medicines there is the complication of bleeding related to the use of protease inhibitors. There are also some haemophilia-specific issues for people with HCV coinfection.

Protease inhibitor-related bleeding episodes

Since 1996 there have been reports that protease inhibitors cause an increase in spontaneous bleeding for people with haemophilia and other clotting disorders (FDA). The reasons for this remain unclear, as all other factors such as platelet counts and prothrombin times remain normal. Studies have also shown that people with haemophilia and HIV on PIs tend to increase their use of clotting factor concentrates by up to or in excess of 50%. Figures suggest that between 16 - 52% of people with haemophilia and HIV on PIs develop these side-effects to a greater or lesser degree (Martinez; Stanworth).

The cause of this side-effect has not been identified and the sites of these bleeds are often abnormal or in places in which the person with haemophilia has rarely if ever experienced bleeds in the past. Most people with severe haemophilia are prone to spontaneous bleeds into weight- bearing joints, especially knees and ankles, as well as elbows and some larger muscles. However, PI related bleeding seems to occur in additional areas such as toe and finger joints, and smaller muscle groups in the face, hands, and feet. The incidence of these atypical bleeds seems to drop off after people discontinue treatment with PIs (Yee; Stanworth) but should be expected to return if someone recommences therapy including PIs.

The management of these complications seems to involve a significant increase in clotting factor prophylaxis. Most people with haemophilia and HIV seem to manage fairly well with this, although it may not fully control all the atypical bleeding. For many the trade-off between improved health and an increased incidence of bleeding is worthwhile. For others it has been a major deterrent to starting treatment. The bleeding seems to occur equally in people with haemophilia A, B or von Willebrands disease and for all PIs. The bleeding seems to diminish or disappear after a few months of treatment in the majority of people with haemophilia (Wilde) but for a small minority, the bleeding is so extreme that the only course is to stop PI therapy altogether, and to look at alternative regimes (Stanworth). Many people with haemophilia take PIs and have no problems of excess bleeding, though and the fear of it should not be seen as a reason to deny access to these important medications.

Tipranavir and bleeding

However in 2006 the issue arose again in connection with a specific protease inhibitor, namely the then fairly recently-licensed salvage PI tipranavir (*Aptivus*).

It was found that tipranavir might be associated with an increased risk of bleeding within the skull when boosted with low-dose ritonavir (*Norvir*), according to a warning issued by tipranavir's manufacturer Boehringer Ingelheim.

The company issued a 'Dear Healthcare Provider' letter in the United States, explaining that 14 cases of intracranial haemorrhage have been identified in 6840 patients receiving ritonavir-boosted tipranavir as part of an anti-HIV combination in clinical trials. Eight of the patients had died.

The manufacturer claims that most of the patients had other risk factors for intracranial haemorrhage - including blood clotting disorders.

Other risk factors included lesions in the brain, head injury, recent brain surgery, , high blood pressure and alcohol abuse, as well as use of medications that can increase bleeding. It took a median of 525 days from the start of treatment with ritonavir-boosted tipranavir for the haemorrhage to occur.

The company has advised that patients who may be at risk of bleeding due to haemophilia or other clotting disorders, surgery, injury, other conditions or other medications should use ritonavir-boosted tipranavir with caution.

Intracranial haemorrhage is a serious emergency medical condition, which causes dangerous increases in the pressure within the skull. Bleeding can occur within the brain, or between the skull and the membranes that surround the brain tissue.

Patients given tipranavir in clinical trials did not show any blood clotting abnormalities. However, some test-tube studies and animal experiments did find some reductions in the ability of blood clots to form. Boehringer Ingelheim is carrying out more investigations into the link between tipranavir and bleeding.

Hepatitis C complications

Another major issue is the tolerance of drug regimes by people with active HCV related hepatitis. Over 5,000 people with haemophilia have HCV infection acquired from blood products in the UK - this includes the vast majority of those who are HIV-positive. A number were also infected with hepatitis B which may have become a chronic infection. The section below looks only at the haemophilia specific issues regarding hepatitis coinfection and not at all the general issues for people with HIV and viral hepatitis which are covered elsewhere.

The initial problem for people with haemophilia and HCV, with or without HIV, has been the efficacy of having a liver biopsy. This is where a needle is inserted through the skin and a section of the liver taken away for analysis in order to understand how well the liver is coping with the hepatitis virus. A biopsy result can be very important in deciding whether to take treatment for viral hepatitis. In people with haemophilia a biopsy should always be done under the cover of treatment and can be done with the guidance of an ultrasound to follow the path of the needle inside the body. Despite this, a number of haemophilia clinicians are understandably reluctant to perform biopsies on people with haemophilia.

The treatment of choice for people with haemophilia and HIV is pegylated interferon, as it is for everyone with hepatitis C. The only haemophilia-specific issue with treatment concerns potential bleeding issues with interferon. Whether the use of interferon has no effect, increases the number of bleeds someone has, possibly from the subcutaneous injection, or reduces the number of bleeds as the person is less active if they are experiencing major side-effects is unsubstantiated but has been discussed at meetings of people with haemophilia.

For those whose liver disease is more advanced, liver transplants can be an option. There are a few centres in the UK that will offer transplants to co-infected people with haemophilia, and there are people with haemophilia, HIV and HCV living comfortably over three years after a successful liver transplant but so few operations have been done since the advent of HIV combination therapy, it is difficult to estimate survival rates.

In addition, the liver transplant also *cures* the haemophilia (Factor VIII & IX are synthesised in the liver). However, the new liver will once again be infected by HCV, although with treatment advances, and the slow progression of HCV, the limited evidence so far suggests that those who have successfully received transplants can have several years of reasonably good quality life ahead.

Effectively, the clinical management of HIV in those with haemophilia actually involves the management of three chronic and life-threatening illnesses. Psychologically, the stress of this cannot be underestimated. For the person with haemophilia and HIV/HCV co-infection, their families and their carers, the problem of overcoming one illness, only to be faced with another, and then when that is apparently under control, to be faced with yet another, can be devastating. However their continued survival and ability to cope with these conditions on top of the usual work, and life stresses can also be seen as a sign of resilience.

Psychosocial issues

Haemophilia, HIV and women

HIV has had a significant, but still largely unrecorded impact on women in the haemophilia community. Women with bleeding disorders often find it difficult to have their conditions taken seriously because of the pervasive belief that haemophilia can only affect men. As explained above there are women with bleeding disorders and for those seriously affected they may have received blood products as part of their treatment and six were infected with HIV, many more with hepatitis C.

Over 60 women partners of people with haemophilia were also infected through sexual intercourse, some prior to the availability of the test for HIV over twenty years ago.

Historically in society the burden of caring has been taken up by women and this will have been the case in haemophilia. There may also have been feelings of guilt for mothers of children with haemophilia A or B from the genetic inheritance of haemophilia, the ineffective blood clotting gene coming from the mothers chromosomes and not the fathers, compounded if they were also the primary injector of treatment in children with haemophilia.

Mothers, wives and partners and siblings have often provided the care of men with haemophilia and took up the burdens of HIV as well. With HIV, this burden was exacerbated - not only by the illnesses associated with HIV infection, but also the culture of secrecy that grew up around it. It was no longer possible to discuss with friends and family - the normal sources of informal support - the reasons for and nature of the illness affecting their family member. It often had to remain a secret, even after the death of the infected individual. (Latimer).

Support for families and individuals living with haemophilia and HIV

For many, the main source of support in all areas remains the Haemophilia Centre. Many have helped establish and run support groups, provided counselling, etc. However, the nature of the transmission of HIV to the haemophilia community has also made it difficult for some to trust their centre, or feel comfortable receiving anything but the most basic medical support from them.

The Haemophilia Society continues to offer advice, support, information and services to people with haemophilia and affected by HIV, and continues to advocate for access to the best possible treatments, both for haemophilia and for HIV and Hepatitis C. The Society is involved in networking with other disabilities organisations, including HIV organisations, to campaign and advocate for the rights and needs of all those living with disabilities. However, the organisation is not HIV specific, and is necessarily geared towards the wider needs of the haemophilia community.

Birchgrove, initially a self-help group of people with haemophilia and HIV in South Wales has provided advocacy, advice and a regular national newsletter since 1990. In 2005 it changed its services, discontinuing the newsletter, but it still provides a website with back issues and news items. The group also sponsored the planting of 1200 trees and an inscribed rock at Stratton Wood near Swindon to celebrate the lives of the people infected with HIV through blood products. Details of how to visit the wood can be found on the Birchgrove website.

The Macfarlane Trust is the body set up to administer the *recompense* payments and the hardship fund set up by the Government for all those infected and affected by HIV within the haemophilia community. The Government was very specific in stating that it was not compensation, because that would imply fault and there was no admission of negligence when the case was settled out of court. It was initially set up to administer a hardship fund and was then used as the vehicle to make the out-of-court settlement payments. The Trust provides regular payments to those with haemophilia and HIV and partners who were infected. The dependants and those who have been bereaved are entitled to some specific grants from the Trust and may apply to the hardship fund for help. In addition, the Trust makes one-off grants to those with particular needs and organises events for people with haemophilia and HIV to meet up, share experiences and look toward the future. Its website also provides a bulletin board restricted to recipients of the Trust's regular payments allowing people to communicate and share feelings with one another.

Conclusion

Haemophilia is a genetic condition and so it was not unusual for more than one person in a family to have been infected with HIV. This had a devastating effect on families and many of those who have survived saw and helped care for other family members who died. Anyone who had friends amongst other people with haemophilia, attended the boarding school that specifically catered for people with bleeding disorders or got involved in Birchgrove may well have dealt with multiple bereavements similar to those experienced by gay men infected in the 1980s and 90s. As of January 1st 2000 over 800 of the 1246 originally infected had died (UKHCDO).

The infection of the haemophilia community with HIV through contaminated factor concentrate is one of the most devastating post-war health care disasters. The lurking fear is that it may have been a catastrophe that could have been avoided or minimised at the very least. The failure of governments worldwide to address the AIDS epidemic contributed to the high death toll amongst people with bleeding disorders. Had AIDS been taken seriously in 1981, it is probable that significantly fewer people with haemophilia would have been infected. If governments and drug companies had considered seriously the risks posed by viral hepatitis in the late 70's, even fewer would have contracted HIV infection.

Politicians have paid their price. What was perceived as a heartless approach to the issue of compensation certainly did not help Mrs Thatcher prior to her resignation as prime minister; the Irish Government collapsed over their inability to deal effectively with the problem of infections in blood products; criminal prosecutions were brought against bureaucrats in the French health service, whilst the former French Prime Minister, Laurent Fabius, and two of his ministers were unsuccessfully tried in 1999, accused of delaying the introduction of screening measures for HIV in blood and plasma during 1985. In Canada, scandals have rocked both former government ministers and the Canadian Red Cross as a result of the Krever Report into the use of contaminated blood and blood products.

Throughout the world governments have been forced to make payouts to HIV-positive people with haemophilia, some larger and some smaller. As ever, the haemophilia community has had to fight tooth and nail with drug companies and governments to have their case recognised and litigation continues even today with over 2000 people with haemophilia, HIV and/or HCV from the UK and other countries, taking legal action in America against the companies that produced blood products during the

1970s and 1980s. Where there has been financial recognition, such remuneration is a scant recompense for the ruin of lives and the thousands of deaths.

Sustained pressure from haemophiliacs and their advocates in the UK has borne fruit. On 19 February 2007 - in the case of HIV, some 23 years after the event - Lord Morris of Manchester announced the Archer Independent Public Enquiry into how a generation of people with haemophilia were infected with HIV and/or hepatitis C and its consequences.

The Haemophilia Society Chairman, Roddy Morrison, said: "The Archer Enquiry's importance to the haemophilia community cannot be overstated. All across the United Kingdom those infected and their families will rejoice that all the facts are finally to be brought out into the open.

"It is particularly important that the inquiry will be examining the consequences of the disaster for the haemophilia community for those living with infection/s. Many have suffered unduly with financial hardship; some have even had to give up their homes. Many more have found themselves to be uninsurable, unemployable and unable to make adequate provision for their dependants.

"It is an historic day for us: The first time that we have had the opportunity to make our voices heard. An entire generation of people with haemophilia have gone unheard."

Contacts

The Haemophilia Society

First Floor
Petersham House
57a Hatton Gardens
London EC1N 8JG

tel: 020 7831 1020
website: www.haemophilia.org.uk

Birchgrove

www.birchgrovegroup.org

The Macfarlane Trust

Alliance House
12 Caxton Street
London SW1H 0QS

tel: 020 7233 0057
website: www.macfarlane.org.uk

References

CHS (2001) All About Hemophilia available at:

http://www.hemophilia.ca/en/13.1.php

(accessed on 5-8-2005)

DoH (2004) available at
http://www.dh.gov.uk/PublicationsAndStatistics/PressReleases/PressReleasesNotices/fs/en?CONTENT_ID=4088953&chk=4BSn4F

(accessed on 5-8-2005)

FDA Food and Drug Administration Advisory Reports. Reports of Increased Bleeding amongst HIV-positive Hemophiliacs Treated on Protease Inhibitors. 1996.

Haemophilia Society see http://www.haemophilia.org.uk/

Latimer P. What are the Ethical Dilemmas Experienced by Women Carers Who Have Suffered Haemophilia & HIV Bereavement? MA Thesis, 1997.

Lee CA. & Brettler DB. Guidelines for the Diagnosis and Management of Von Willibrand's Disease. Haemophilia, 3: Supplement 2, 1997.

Martinez, PR et al. Incidence of Increased Number of Bleeding Episodes in HIV-positive Haemophiliacs Treated with Protease Inhibitors. Conference Abstract, XXIII Congress of the World Federation of Hemophilia, 1998.

Potts & Potts. (1998) Queen Victoria's Gene. Sutton Publishing Ltd.

PHLS (1998) Communicable Diseases Report, December.

Stanworth MJ et al. Increased Bleeding in HIV-Positive Haemophiliacs Treated with Antiretroviral Protease Inhibitors. Haemophilia; 4: 109-114, 1998.

UKHCDO (2004) The impact of HIV on mortality rates in the complete UK haemophilia population. AIDS, 18: 525-533.

Yee TT, et al. Protease Inhibitors and Unusual Bleeding in Haemophiliacs. Haemophilia, 3; 219 - 221, 1997.

Wilde JT, Lee CA, Collins P, et al. Increased bleeding associated with PI therapy in HIV-positive patients with bleeding disorders. British Jol of Haematology 107: 556-559, 1999.

Zeepvat C. (1998) Prince Leopold: The Untold Story of Queen Victoria's Youngest Son. Sutton Publishing Ltd.

HIV and prisoners

People living with HIV within a prison system face a unique set of circumstances: those of providing for healthcare needs in a difficult environment to a crowded population, many with mental health, drink and drug abuse histories. Stigma and discrimination within the UK prison system causes many HIV-positive prisoners not to disclose their status. Although the UK has relatively low numbers of HIV-positive prisoners, the numbers passing through UK prisons and the persisting refusal to contemplate needle exchange in England and Wales mean that bloodborne infections continue to pose a serious risk to prison inmates.

Prisoners are up to five times more likely to contract HIV than the general population, and more likely still to be infected with hepatitis C and other blood-borne viruses and infections. The Department of Health's anonymous 1997 sero-survey points to an HIV rate among male prisoners four times that of the general population. Women prisoners were 13 times more likely to test positive for HIV than the wider population.

The number of prisoners in England and Wales has increased by more than 25,000 in the last ten years, reaching 76,524 in July 2005 (Home Office), 4,570 of whom were women. In October 2005 the prison population in Scotland was 6,929 (Scottish Prison Service) and 1,394 in Northern Ireland (Northern Ireland Prison Service).

At the start of 2005 there was a total UK prison population of nearly 85,000 or one in 700 of the entire population, the highest rate in Western Europe.

All but 30% of these prisoners will be released back into the community at some stage. Almost 200,000 people will pass through prison annually, impacting on an estimated 1.5 families and friends. Health problems created in prison then become problems for the community as a whole.

The nature of the prison population is also changing. Research published in *The Lancet* (Fazel) for the first time looked at the long-term trends in suicide rates in English and Welsh prisons. The overall suicide rate among prisoners was five times greater than the general population, and in the 15-17 year-old age group, 18 times higher. The study points to the shift of care from psychiatric hospitals to community-based services, including eventually prison.

Together with mental health problems (around 70% of prisoners have a diagnosable mental illness), many prisoners have faced social exclusion and exclusion from education. More than half of the prisoners have a reading ability at or below that of an average 11 year-old, according to the Prison Reform Trust (Factfile May 2005). The UK prison population is a marginal and vulnerable group, disproportionately vulnerable to blood-borne infections.

HIV and AIDS in prisons is becoming an important topic worldwide. In countries with low HIV prevalence prisons can be places where HIV infections gain critical mass and move into the wider community. In countries of high HIV prevalence, prisons can act as an incubator, with a reservoir of infected prisoners often many times higher than the rate of the outside world.

When talking of prison health care equivalency is the watchword. Access to antiretroviral drugs and harm reduction efforts like needle exchange programmes (NEPs) and condoms, successfully applied in the wider community should be available to prisoners. This concept is well enshrined in human rights guidelines through United Nation resolutions, World Health Organisation directives and the 2004 Dublin Declaration.

The equivalence approach to prisoners' rights to health falters where countries' attitudes to sex are homophobic and repressive. The distribution of condoms in a prison setting is one issue. Many prison authorities do not acknowledge homosexual activity and as is the case in many countries such as Cameroon, Nigeria, Malawi, Jamaica - all with high rates of HIV - homosexuality is prohibited and punishable by national law.

Mandatory testing in prisons appears to be gaining ground in some quarters. In the US a number of states already have mandatory testing and a number are increasingly considering its implementation, particularly since the advent of 'fast test' oral swabs. 'Exit testing' and 'spouse notification,' are attempts to protect the outside community with programmes that would be unacceptable outside of prison walls.

When HIV outbreaks have been identified in prisons like Glenochil in Scotland or Alytus in Lithuania, the sharing of needles for drug injection has been a clear source of transmission. A recent report by the US, Centers for Disease Control and Prevention on the Georgia state prison system (CDC) showed that nerarly one in ten HIV-positive inmates acquired their infection in prison. When people enter prison negative and leave HIV-positive, one of the routes of transmission is sex between men, along with shared needle use and tattooing.

HIV in prisons: the UK perspective

HIV prevalence

England and Wales have the highest per capita prison population in western Europe -143 people in prison per 100,000 in January 2007. The prison population in England and Wales has increased by 90% since 1993 when the prison system held 41,000. Now 80,000 plus are held in 139 jails across England and Wales. Almost 200,000 people will pass through the system annually. Scotland held 6,447 prisoners in January 2007.

There is a great deal of uncertainty about the prevalence of HIV in the UK prisons. The Department of Health's 1997/8 anonymous serosurvey is widely regarded by the Home Office as a benchmark study of HIV prevalence in prisons (Department of Health). Prisoners in eight of the 135 prisons in England and Wales were surveyed to determine the prevalence of and risk factors for transmission of blood-borne viruses in prison. Among the 3,930 tested, nine men and five women prisoners tested HIV-positive, giving an overall infection rate of 0.32% and 1.2% respectively.

In Scotland there are 4,303 people living with HIV according to Health Protection Scotland April 2005. The official HIV rates mirror those in England with a male inmate prevalence of 0.3%. The female HIV-positive rate was put at 0.6%.

England and Wales

The control and treatment of blood-borne infections, namely HIV and hepatitis C, in English prisons is at a crossroads. In 2006 the Prison Reform Trust and the National AIDS Trust produced a comprehensive report called for prison health to line up with public health and described prison healthcare as "sub-standard and inconsistent." (Prison Reform Trust, 2006).

During 2007 English and Welsh HM Prisons are introducing disinfectant for cleaning injecting equipment throughout its prison estate, which follows the devolution of prison healthcare to local Primary Care Trusts in 2006. In the meantime the Home office is facing a challenge to its lack of harm reduction programmes for prison needle users in the European Court of Human Rights.

Although the official prevalence for HIV rate is lower than in some other European countries, such as Spain and France, the UK has the highest levels of imprisonment in Western Europe the data that public health and prison officials are working with is long past its sell by date.

In the Department of Health's 1997/8 anonymous sero-survey, prisoners in eight of the 135 prisons in England and Wales were surveyed to determine the prevalence of and risk factors for transmission of blood borne viruses in prison. Among the 3,930 tested, nine men and five women prisoners tested HIV-positive, giving an overall infection rate of 0.32% and 1.2% respectively. HIV prevalence for men is 15 times higher than in the wider community. However this figure may overestimate or underestimate the current prevalence given the growth in the prison population since 1997.

Hepatitis C rates in the English and Welsh prison system are also disproportionately higher than the wider population. *The Hepatitis C Action Plan for England*, published by Department of Health in July 2004, estimated that 0.5% of the general population in England (approx 250,000 people) has been infected with Hepatitis C but that eight per cent of the prison population is believed to be HCV-infected - more than ten times the rate of the general population.

The *Action Plan* says that there is variation in the current delivery of care across the country for people with Hep C:

> "*Some groups of the population suffer from these inequalities more than others. There is a higher prevalence of chronic Hep C among prisoners because the majority (60%) of injecting drug users pass through the prison system at some point. A window of opportunity exists while they are in prison to take preventative action and improve their access to healthcare services.*"

In Scotland the sheer weight of numbers of blood-borne transmissions has forced the prison authorities to react with pragmatic programmes of prevention. In England and Wales determining accurate levels of infection is a vital platform for prisoner health care.

Harm reduction

The policy and campaign group the National AIDS Trust and Prison Reform Trust published its report in 2006: *HIV and hepatitis in UK prisons: addressing prisoners' healthcare needs*. Researchers sent questionnaires to 139 prisons and detention centres in England and Wales 63 were returned. None had needle exchange programmes and disinfectant to clean 'injecting gear' was available in eight of these prisons. Understanding of harm reduction was found to be limited.

Condoms

The prevalence of sexual activity in prisons varies, although consensual sex is accepted as a fact of prison life. Strang et al report that two per cent of men said they had sex with other men in prison. In the late 1990s the Public Health Laboratory Service found that three per cent of male prisoners reported having sex with another man in prison. More recently the Howard Journal of Criminal Justice Study (Banbury) reported that one per cent of men had experienced forced penetrative sex attacks out of 200,000 men who pass through the prison system annually.

Under the Sexual Offences Act, according to HM Prison Service, homosexual activity in prison is prohibited by law, prisons being classed as a public place; *ipso facto* providing condoms or other safe sex materials would be condoning illegal activity. Despite this stance there have been developments regarding recommendations made to the Home Secretary by the AIDS Advisory Committee of the House of Commons.

Following the Home Secretary's rejection of the committee's recommendations on condom provision, the prison service directorate of health sent out a 'dear doctor' letter to each prison establishment, which states that each doctor had the clinical freedom to prescribe condoms to prevent infections.

Because of the prescription process condom distribution is generally regarded as patchy and slow with prisoners resorting to use home-made devices such as latex gloves, (Positive Nation, 2005). Confidentiality is often compromised.

Needles

Injecting drug use in English and Welsh prisons is widespread and well documented. In 2003 the Home Office Research Directorate reported two per cent of prisoners injecting. The Howard Journal of Criminal Justice put the figure at 6.7%. In 2004 a random drug test of 6,500 prisoners in Scotland showed 32% of inmates had tested positive for heroin, either 'chased' (smoked) or injected.

Such levels of injecting and the concomitant risk of blood-borne infection have led Scotland to rethink its approach to mandatory drug testing (MDT) in its prison system. In England and Wales the Prison Service is still committed to mandatory testing as part of its *Tackling Drugs Together* initiative.

One issue with MDT is that urine samples are taken for the test that can detect cannabis for up to 30 days after smoking, while heroin and cocaine both of which can be injected leave the system in a few days. Some prison staff feel this has led to an increase in class A drug usage and the consequent rise in injecting use.

The England and Wales Home Office refuses to consider a trial of an in-prison needle exchange programme. The prisons drug strategy, revised in 2002, is largely aimed at reducing the supply of classified drugs into prisons. The strategy also aims to reduce the demand for drugs among prisoners through treatment interventions such as managed withdrawal through detoxification, drug rehabilitation programmes and support, and mandatory and voluntary drug testing programmes to encourage prisoners to remain drug free.

The Home Office stance on needle exchange has been challenged by prisoner John Shelley serving a sentence in HMP Long Lartin. He claims that the refusal of the Prison Service to consider NEPs represents a real and immediate risk to his health.

At a judicial review of his case in the High Court it was argued that treatment in prison was not "equivalent to that available in the community". His solicitors also argued that the harm reduction measure of disinfectant tablets was not proven to be safe and offered a false sense of security for prisoners, having not been scientifically proven.

Regarding the issue of needle exchanges in prison Shelley's solicitor has commented, "NEPs were a discussion society had a decade ago. Society generally agreed that NEPs should be implemented. We don't think that it's right for the Home Office to reargue the issue and come to a different conclusion." (O'Connor, Positive Nation, 2005). The High Court refused the case permission to continue

The solicitors for Shelley have now taken the case to the European Court of Human Rights. A supporting document by the National AIDS Trust was submitted in February 2007. In it the NAT refers to the UK Health Protection Agency's (HPA) document *Shooting Up*, published in October 2006. The document looks at infectious diseases in Intravenous drug users in the UK.

The report says the UK's relatively low prevalence rate of HIV among IDUs is "a result of proven community and public health responses including needle exchanges." According to the AIDS rights organisation 99% of local authorities provide needle exchanges. The NAT and Shelley's lawyers argue that equivalency in healthcare for prisoners is enshrined in the Human Rights Act as are the rights to health and life, in articles1-4. One other submission was made by 'interested parties': a joint effort by the Irish Prison Reform Trust together with the Canadian HIV and AIDS Legal Network.

Vaccination

One initiative proves that prison can be a window of opportunity in improving public health. There is an ongoing national programme to immunise prisoners against hepatitis B infection run by the Health Protection Agency (HPA) and HM Prison Service. According to the HPA the vaccination scheme has had "a major impact on public health, both in prisons and the community," (*Infection inside: the Prison Infectious Disease Quarterly*, Feb 2006).

According to the HPA, prison was the most common source of hepatitis B vaccination among IDUs in the UK (37%) compared to 14% from needle exchange services. The HPA has projected that if 50% of prison receptions were vaccinated from 2006 onwards, the number of acute hepatitis B infections among the IDU population may be reduced by 80% over 12 years. The HPA says that their projections on prison healthcare will estimate the cost of identifying a new case of hepatitis C if a screening programme was introduced in England and Wales. A study in 2002 looked at the cost of Hepatitis B vaccines in a prison setting (Pisu, M et al, *Vaccine*, 2002).

Prison Health Care transfers to local PCTs

The vaccination programme for hepatitis B (HPA, *Infection Inside*, Feb 2006) shows that in many cases vaccination is either not being carried out or not reported. One obstacle to vaccination is a lack of clear guidance at local level. Despite the HPA issuing national guidance on vaccination in the 'green book', each primary care trust can interpret the guidance differently. This, says the HPA. is adding unnecessary complexity and putting a barrier to achieving higher vaccination coverage.

Despite this barrier to national treatment, most public health observers have welcomed the recent moves on prison health which have led to the biggest upheaval since the formation of the NHS.

At the start of April 2006, health responsibility was fully handed over from prisons to Primary Care Trusts (PCTs).

All UK prisons have some form of medical centre, with access to regional hospitals for patients who require more intensive care.

Scotland

Despite political opposition, the Scottish Prison Service has for a long time been aware of and studied the implications of needle exchange programmes (NEPs). To a certain extent its hand has been forced: 80% of Scottish inmates are drug users compared to 40% in England and Wales.

In 2007, Aberdeen's Craiginches prison should pilot the UK's first needle exchange programme. Craiginches houses 230-250 inmates.

The move is primarily to prevent the spread of hepatitis B and C and HIV viruses. As well as exchanges, needle injecting kits could include swabs, filters, and a sharps disposal box.

Audrey Mooney, Craiginches' governor, told the *Scotsman* Newspaper in 2003: "Ninety-eight per cent, sometimes 100% of our population coming into prison indicate to us that they have taken illegal drugs".

The Scottish Prison Service made a philosophical leap in introducing NEPs in its paper, *The Direction of Harm Reduction in the SPS; from Chaotic Drug Use to Abstinence.* The report recommended the introduction of sterile injecting equipment as part of overall healthcare. The report said: "It could be argued that the refusal to make sterile equipment available to prisoners is actually condoning the spread of HIV and HCV to prisoners and, indirectly, to the community at large." 50% of Scottish inmates had used drugs while in prison (Daily Mirror, Jan 2007).

In 2006 the Scottish Executive produced its Hepatitis C Action Plan. It stated that HCV prevalence among IDUs in Glasgow was between 45% and 62%, according to recent studies. The SPS has developed a harm reduction awareness session which all prisoners attend on admission. This is repeated pre-release for prisoners who are serving longer sentences. The awareness session provides prisoners with information on overdose risk due to loss of tolerance, blood-borne viruses, and ways of getting treatment in prison.

The incidence of Hepatitis C in Scottish prisons was put at eight per cent among male prisoners and 14.8% among female prisoners (Gore, Bird et al, *Nursing Service Review,* 2003). However according to the *Hepatitis C Action Plan for Scotland 2006,* it is suggested that as many as one in five prisoners in Scotland are Hepatitis C positive.

The SPS has also been piloting a needle replacement scheme at reception in several prisons over the past year, to support the schemes now existing in many police custody suites in Scotland. This involves offering sterile needles to known injectors when they leave prison. It is expected that the Craiginches prison scheme will be expanded further in 2007-08 to incorporate further pilot in-prison needle exchange schemes. These activities will be 'robustly' evaluated over a significant period of time

The effectiveness of needle exchanges within the wider community in Scotland has been well documented.

HIV outbreak in UK prison - the Glenochil outbreak

Between April and June 1993 needle sharing at Glenochil Prison, Scotland resulted in 14 HIV infections and a wave of apprehension which is still felt in UK prison system to this day. In 2001 Stephen Kelly, one of the men infected in the outbreak, became the first person to be tried and convicted in Scotland of having 'recklessly injured' his former partner by infecting her with HIV.

To understand the behaviour at Glenochil is to understand the potential risks that prisoners and society are facing. There were eight definite HIV seroconversions among inmates at Glenochil prison and a further six seroconversions possibly took place. Drug injecting and needle and syringe sharing were identified as risk factors. At the end of June 1993 intensive HIV testing and counselling was implemented

There were 636 inmates at Glenochil between 1 January and 30 June 1993. By the time of the intensive HIV testing and counselling 66 had been released and 192 had been transferred to other prisons.

In total 227 men were counselled and 162 (71%) decided to be tested for HIV infection. In total, one third (76) of those counselled had ever injected drugs, and 33 (43%) reported injecting in prison. All twelve men who were found to be HIV-positive were among the 27 in this latter group who were tested for HIV.

The primary objective for the counselling was to prevent the further spread of infection, not to determine HIV prevalence among the prison population.

The prevalence of HIV among the 27 who had injected while in prison and had opted for testing was 44% (12/27). In addition, two other inmates, who did not opt for counselling also reported having injected while in Glenochil. In total 34 men who had injected outside prison but who had not injected while in Glenochil came forward for HIV testing. None of these men were found to be HIV-positive. Being HIV-positive was significantly associated with injecting while in Glenochil prison in the early months of 1993.

Thirteen of the 14 men who were found to be HIV-positive were from Glasgow. HIV prevalence in Glasgow among injecting drug users was 1.8% according to a community survey conducted in 1990. The introduction of needle exchanges in Glasgow in 1988 appears to have prevented the rapid spread of HIV among injecting drug users outside of the prison setting.

Shared needles and syringes

Of the 76 men who claimed to have injected at some time, seven had begun injecting while serving their current sentence. All of the seven injected with used equipment.

Injecting in prison appeared to occur at a much reduced frequency; weekly or monthly, as opposed to daily when on the outside. When on the outside, two men admitted to always sharing needles and syringes. In prison, 20 men admitted to always sharing injecting equipment.

Of the twelve men who were found to be HIV-positive, ten said that they always injected with used equipment in prison, and eight claimed they never did so outside prison. Some prisoners estimated that up to 30 inmates would use the same needle and syringe.

The cleaning methods adopted by many of the inmates were mostly ineffective. Seventeen would rinse the needle and syringe with hot or cold water, three used bleach, three used hairdressing liquid, one used boiling water and seven used a combination of techniques.

Between one quarter and one third of men who injected drugs between January and June 1993 became HIV-positive while in prison.

Only one of the 227 inmates counselled for HIV admitted to having sex with another man while in prison. Of the 33 inmates who had injected drugs while in prison, the median number of female sexual partners in the 12 months before incarceration was three. All except one said they never used condoms.

Northern Ireland

The first study of blood borne viruses in Northern Ireland prisons was reported in *Eurosurveillance* in January 2007 (Danis). The absence of this information was considered a barrier to the development of appropriate public health interventions, including immunisation policy, and health protection measures said researchers.

Data from other studies are difficult to extrapolate to the Northern Ireland (NI) prison population, as this specific population is likely to differ from that in other European countries, given the unique Northern Irish sociopolitical and security situation. Prior to the Good Friday Agreement in 1998, which resulted in cessation of paramilitary activity, the majority of prisoners in NI had been imprisoned for paramilitary activity (criminal activity by members of an illegal armed organisation). Prior to 1998 prevalence of blood-borne virus infections was low in NI outside prisons, and this was thought to be due, in part, to the prevailing security situation: injecting drug use and drug dealing were not tolerated by the paramilitary organisations.

In three Northern Ireland prisons 633 prisoners completed questionnaires and 658 agreed to have anonymous oral samples taken. The median age was 26 and 11 sampled were women. Seven inmates tested positive for HCV 9 (1.06%) five (0.76%) for HBV and none for HIV. Of the sample 11% reported using drugs, (20% of those started in prison) and nine men (1.4%) reported sex with men, three of those in prison.

As reported in the background Northern Ireland's low prevalence rates compared to the UK and other European countries reflect the unique political situation there. However, the numbers of blood borne diagnoses have been increasing in the wider community in recent years, particularly since the Good Friday agreement

The prevalence of drug use among NI prisoners was 11%, compared with 43% and 24% recorded during similar studies in ROI and Great Britain respectively. This may well start to change now as evidence points to increasing levels of injecting drug use in the community.

References

Allison E, Health Officials and Prison Service Clash over HIV Prevention, The Guardian, April 13, 2005

Banbury S, Coercive Sexual Behaviour in British Prisons as reported by Adult ex-prisoners. Howard Journal of Criminal Justice Study, 43 (2):113-130, 2004

BBC News - Prison care moves to Primary Care Trusts, 2006

Daily Mirror - State of British prisons in numbers, January 2007

Dublin Declaration on HIV/AIDS in Prisons in Europe and Central Asia, February, 2004

Gore, Bird et al. Hepatitis C in Scottish Prisons, Nursing Service review, 2003

Health Protection Agency, 'Shooting Up,' October 2006

Health Protection Scotland, April 2005, national HIV/Aids prevalence

Home Office Research Directorate, 2003

Irish Prison Reform trust/Canadian HIV/Aids Legal Network, submission to Court of Human Rights, J Shelley case.

K Danis, Blood borne infections in Northern Ireland prisons Eurosurveillance, January 2007

Northern Ireland Prison Service, prison population facts, see http://www.niprisonsservice.gov.uk/

O'Connor, C, Positive Nation, 2005

Pisu, Me et al, Vaccine, Cost Effectiveness of Hepatitis C in Prisons, 2002

Prison Infectious Diseases Quarterly (Health Protection Agency/Prison Reform Trust), Feb 2006

Prison Reform Trust, Fact File, May 2005

Prison Reform Trust, press release, 2006

Scotsman Newspaper, HMP Craiginchie Prison (Aberdeen), 2003

Scottish Health, Hepatitis C Action Plan, 2006

Scottish Prison Service, prison population, see http://www.sps.gov.uk/

Scottish Prison Service, the Direction of harm reduction in SPS: from chaotic drug use to abstinence

Seena Fazel, Benning R, Danesh J. Suicides in male prisoners in England and Wales, 1978-2003. Lancet 2005; 366:1301-2

TB/AIDS in Moldovan Prisons, International Aids Conference, Toronto 2006

The Hepatitis C Plan for England, UK Department of Health, July 2004

UK Department of Health, Anonymous HIV prevalence monitoring programme England and Wales to1997

US Centers for Disease Control and Prevention (CDC) Georgia State Prisonshttp://www.cdc.gov/nchstp/od/nchstp.html

Valette D et al. National Aids Trust/Prison Reform Trust; HIV and Hepatitis in UK Prisons: addressing prisoners' healthcare needs, October 2005

HIV in prisons: the global perspective

At any given time, there are approximately ten million people imprisoned worldwide - two million of them in the USA alone. Prison populations come largely from the most marginalised groups in society, people in poor health and with chronic untreated conditions, the vulnerable and those who have engaged in activities with high risk of HIV exposure, such as injecting drugs and sex work. At some point, the vast majority are released into the wider community.

The situation is exacerbated by high rates of tuberculosis (often multi-drug resistant), sexually transmitted infections and hepatitis B and C. According to the World Health Organisation's European Office in 2002 TB prevalence in prisons in the Russian Federation was 9.8%, syphilis incidence 1.2%, and 20-40% of all prisoners were living with hepatitis C.

Evidence of high HIV prevalence in prison is widely available. Globally, most prisoners are men, but women prisoners are also at risk of HIV. In Brazil, Canada, UK and the United States, women prisoners are more likely to be HIV-positive, largely because a high proportion is incarcerated for drug use and sex work.

A large proportion of prisoners are drug users. In Europe this can range from 30% (Italy) to 70% (Portugal). According to the UN Office on Drugs and Crime, (UNODC), up to half of all inmates of some prisons in the Russian Federation are injecting drug users, while in Kazakhstan the proportion is close to two-thirds.

In many countries detention centres are breeding grounds for HIV infection. Overcrowding, homosexual relations, gang violence, lack of protection for the weakest inmates, and corrupt prison management create an environment that increases vulnerability to HIV transmission through unsafe sexual practices, sharing of injecting equipment or crude substitutes, tattooing, violence and rape.

According to data from the Canadian HIV and AIDS Legal Network, prisons are overcrowded in over 100 countries, with prisons housing four to five times the numbers of inmates originally planned. As a consequence, around the world the percentage of people with HIV and AIDS in prisons is significantly higher than in the community.

When it comes to data on the prevalence of HIV among prisoners and prevention and treatment programmes within prisons, information is highly variable. Within Europe, surveillance of HIV-positive prisoners and approaches to harm reduction varies widely, and in the USA approaches differ from state to state.

For the rest of the world, in particular the developing world, any data is at a premium. The Canadian HIV and AIDS Legal Network, at the 2004 International AIDS Conference, reported that a survey of international information on HIV in prisons and HIV among indigenous intravenous drug user (IDU) populations produced only 29 countries with any information.

The Conference Summary commented: "The risk of HIV in prison has similarly not been the subject of intensive investigation by prevention researchers in developing countries. The triple stigmatisation of incarceration, drug injecting and HIV or hepatitis C infection has all but guaranteed a low priority to programming in this area."

Internationally the terminology in surveying prisons is problematic; prisons, juvenile prisons, prisons for mentally ill offenders, pre-trial and remand centres, police detention centres - all may be included or discounted by national authorities. Prison populations are dynamic, with occupation rates varying in terms of overall incarceration rates and length of imprisonment.

However, the accumulation of data must be a priority, according to UNAIDS.

Forcing the issue is the growing realisation that prisons are not just repositories of blood-borne viruses but have been the springboard for fuelling the epidemic of HIV and AIDS TB and Hepatitis. "Prisons are HIV factories," said Elizabeth Pisani of Family Health International. "We are introducing a population that we know to be infected with the virus into an environment where people shoot up drugs and have anal sex." (Associated Press, 1 December 2004)

Turning point?

At international AIDS conferences the issue of HIV and AIDS in prisons has historically received little attention. A turning point may have come with the XV International AIDS Conference 2004 held in Bangkok, Thailand. Before the official conference started, a one-day satellite meeting debated issues related to HIV and AIDS in prisons. At the conference itself, two oral sessions and a large number of poster presentations were dedicated to HIV and AIDS in prisons.

In addition, three United Nations agencies released an important policy briefing on reduction of HIV transmission in prisons. Although most activities focused on HIV prevention, delegates also debated the question of how HIV treatment, including antiretrovirals (ARVs), can best be made available to inmates.

At the Bangkok conference and afterwards, delegates heard that the latest epidemiological data in countries such as Vietnam and Cambodia increasingly pointed to prisons and detentions centres as being engines of the epidemic, driving HIV into the wider community (Rich 1999). Two previous and well documented examples have been Thailand and Lithuania.

In Thailand the first wave of HIV infections was observed in 1988 among IDUs. The infection rate rose from a negligible percentage at the beginning of 1988 to over 40% by September of that year. This was fuelled in part by transmission of the virus, as many IDUs moved in and out of prisons (Jurgens). A more recent study concluded that IDUs in Bangkok continue to be "at significantly increased risk of HIV infection through sharing needles with multiple partners while in holding cells before incarceration" (Buavirat).

In Lithuania, random checks undertaken in 2002 by the state-run AIDS Centre found that in Alytus Prison, 263 prisoners tested positive for HIV antibodies. Tests at Lithuania's other 14 prisons, which house 11,700 convicts, found only 18 cases of HIV infection. Before the tests at Alytus prison, Lithuanian officials had listed only 300 cases of HIV infection in the whole country, or less than 0.01% of the population, the lowest prevalence in Europe. It is believed that the outbreak at Alytus

prison was also due to sharing of drug injection equipment (Dapkus). In 2002 7,000 prisoners, 60% of the country's total prison population, went on hunger strike demanding better treatment for HIV prisoners.

Setting benchmarks standards of care

The situation has called for a drastic response, with the UN and the WHO in particular trying to set bench marks for prevention and care in prisons. In February 2004, the Dublin Declaration on HIV and AIDS in Prisons in Europe and Asia stated: "Under national and international law, governments have a moral and ethical obligation to prevent the spread of HIV and AIDS in prison." This includes the rights of inmates to protect themselves by using preventative measures against HIV transmission.

A wide-ranging study carried out by the Canadian HIV and AIDS Legal Network has shown that needle exchange programmes (NEPs) have been effective in reducing transmission in six countries who have either implemented NEPs fully into their prison system or on a trial basis. Germany, Spain, Moldova, Kyrgyzstan, and Belarus were looked at.

Italy, Portugal and Greece are considering NEP trials. Canada and Australia have also conducted NEP trials.

WHO: effectiveness of harm reduction

Despite the reluctance within some administrations to tackle the issue, the chain of evidence linking IDUs, unprotected sex and HIV infections continues to grow. In May 2005 the World Health Organisation's status paper on prisons, drugs and harm reduction was published.

It states: "Two of the greatest public health problems facing all societies overlap: the epidemic of HIV and AIDS and the pandemic of harmful use of psychotropic substances such as alcohol and illegal drugs." An estimated 10% of all cases of HIV infection worldwide result from unsafe injecting behaviour, according to WHO. In countries in Eastern Europe and Central Asia up to 90% of the people reported to be infected with HIV are injecting drug users. According to the European Monitoring Centre for Drugs and Drug Addiction (EMCDDA) Annual Report for 2003, levels of Hepatitis C among injecting drug users in the 15 countries that were members of the EU before May 1 2004 plus Norway varies between 30% and 79%. At the relatively low end is the UK at 32%; Italy is highest at 79%.

The WHO report proposes a continuum of approaches including information, education and communication, together with detoxification and drug substitution therapy, and goes on to define 'harm reduction' measures. On the issue of needle and syringe exchange in prisons it states: "While acknowledging that in prisons needle and syringe exchange schemes are still controversial, programmes have been introduced in six European countries: Belarus, Germany, Kyrgyzstan, Moldova, Spain and Switzerland. In Spain needle exchange has been introduced in all prisons."

An evaluation of eleven programmes (Stover & Nelles) showed that syringe distribution did not support fears that were expressed before the scheme was introduced.

References

Associated Press, Prison Drug use, Unsafe Sex fuelling Asia AIDS Epidemic, December 1, 2004

Buavirat et al, risk of prevalent HIV infection associated with incarceration amo9ng injecting drug users in Bangkok, Thailand. British medical Journal, 326,2003

Canadian HIV/AIDS legal network, Human Rights at the Margins, satellite seminar, 15th International Conference on AIDS, Bangkok, see www.AIDSlaw.ca/bangkok/2004

Dapkus L, prisons rate of HIV infection frightens a nation, Associated Press, August

European Monitoring Centre for Drugs and Drug Addiction (EMCDDA) Annual report, 2003

Jurgens, R. HIV/AIDS in Prisons :Final Report, Canadian HIV/AIDS Legal Network, 1996

Stover H, Nelles J. Ten years of Experience with needle and syringe exchange programmes in European Prisons. International Drug Policy 1'4: 437-444,2003

United Nations Office on Drugs and Crime, drug use in Russian proisons

World Health Organisation, TB Prevalence in Prisons, European Office

World health Organisation, Status paper on prisons, drugs and harm reduction, may 2005 see:www.euro.who.injt/document/e85877.pdf

Europe

High HIV prevalence rates in prisoners have been reported in some European countries, such as Portugal (11%). In contrast in other western European countries (such as England & Wales and Scandinavia), where successful prevention interventions were targeted at injecting drug users (IDUs) early in the epidemic, HIV prevalence is around or below one per cent.

The degree of HIV transmission within prison walls has never been determined in Europe, according to a report *HIV transmission in part of the US prison system: Implications for Europe* (Weiland et al, HPA London, ENDIPP, 2006). It concludes that current HIV prevention and harm reduction provision in Europe remains scarce and frequently inferior to provision in the community.'

Despite the gap in knowledg, within prison walls the link between IDUs in the community and prisons is well proven. The European Monitoring Centre for Drugs and Drug Addiction (EMCDDA) annual report 2005 states that HIV prevalence among IDUs, mostly those in drug treatment, showed wide variation within and between countries, ranging from 0 % in Bulgaria, Hungary, Slovenia and Slovakia to 37.5 % in one city in Italy (2003, Bolzano - '*Users in Treatment and Prisons*'). Similarly in Germany, Switzerland, Austria and the UK, HIV among IV drug users was less than 5% (World Drug Report 2005). The highest prevalence rates in national samples (over 10 % in 2002-03) were found in Italy (65%), France (19%) Latvia, Portugal and Spain (66%). HIV prevalence was less than 1 % in the Czech Republic, Greece, Hungary, Slovenia, Slovakia, Finland, Romania, Bulgaria and Norway. (EMCDDA 2005)

As a rule HIV prevalence among injecting drug users in general society is reflected in the HIV rates in a society's prisons and are a vital tool in understanding HIV in a correctional setting. However there is a lack of systematic documentation and research specifically on health issues in European prisons and an even greater lack of knowledge on HIV prevalence and transmission. However, there are some valuable starting points in gathering information which could support health planning and policy making.

The Health in Prison Project (HIPP) of the World Health Organisation Regional Office for Europe recently launched a Prison Health Database, which has been developed in collaboration with the European Monitoring Centre for Drugs and Drug Addiction (EMCDDA) and the European Network on Drugs and Infectious Prevention in Prison (ENDIPP). The database includes a large number of relevant indicators on prison health.

Currently, several studies on the prevalence of blood-borne infections and related risk behaviours in prisons are being finalised in different European countries, according to *Eurosurveillance*. They are based on the WASH (Willing Anonymous Salivary HIV/hepatitis C surveillance) method, and

have been carried out under guidance of the EC funded ENDIPP Network. These studies are so-called second generation surveillance, merging information on prevalence with information on knowledge, attitudes, behaviour and practices of prisoners and prison staff (Zaba et al. AIDS, 2005).

Surveys have been carried out in Armenia and Belgium using saliva for blood-borne virus detection and in Poland and Estonia using full blood samples, while another survey is ongoing in Germany using dried blood spots (Weilandt C et al. *Int' Journal Prison Health*, 2007).

The UN Office on Drugs and Crime (UNODC) has recently published another, more general, framework for effective national responses regarding HIV and AIDS prevention, care, treatment and support in prison settings. This framework sets out principles and actions for management of prisons but also for treatment of prisoners. Its objectives include aspects of prevention, treatment, and support regarding HIV and AIDS among prisoners that equal the very same standards available to people in the community outside of prison.

HIPP is about to publish an international guide, "Promoting Health in Prisons: The Essentials", which will outline key points regarding health promotion in prisons in general, and will also touch issues related to other infectious diseases

Harm reduction measures are inconsistent

It is not only prevalence rates that vary. National approaches to harm reduction within prison systems, such as condom distribution, bleach for cleaning injecting equipment and needle exchanges might be acceptable in one country but not in another. Spain has needle exchanges throughout 39 prisons; in France such a move has been considered and so far, rejected.

The Needle Exchange Programmes (NEPs) tried in prisons in Germany, Spain, Luxembourg and Switzerland have not led to any increases in drug addiction, nor have they caused any security incidents linked to the possession of syringes according to the studies (HIV and AIDS Legal Network, 2004, Stover et al, Dolan et al). There are plans to introduce NEPs in prisons in Scotland and Portugal.

Although western Europe is seen as being at the forefront of harm reduction programmes in prisons the approach remains a loosely stitched patchwork of approaches. The use of bleach in prisons to clean injecting gear is now a relatively common practice across the region. The UK is rolling out bleach in its prisons during 2007. However, as with condom distribution, the means of distribution, confidentiality and accessibility can all affect the uptake and effectiveness of these measures. Again, a wide variety of approaches and understanding are seen in Europe. The HIV outbreaks at Glenochil and Alytus, Lithuania are a constant reminder of the tinderbox nature of prison, blood-borne infections and ignorance.

Portugal will roll out a needle exchange programme by 2008, as part of a package of measures "to reduce the consumption of drugs and diminish their harmful social and health effects", according to Portuguese government (*Agence France Presse, 2006*). The Portuguese government legalised the possession of drugs in 2001.

The latest available data on HIV prevalence in Portugal is included in the US State Department report on Human Rights 2006, which quotes the Portuguese Director General of Prisons saying that 20% of prison population have Hepatitis C and that "at least" 10% are living with HIV. Twenty-five prisoners died from AIDS-related illness in 2005; in 2002 there were over 60 deaths. One study in 2002 put the HIV rate at a prison in Porto at 11.1% of inmates (Moragado 2002).

Central Europe

Data regarding the prevalence of HIV infection in **Poland** are collected by the National Institute of Hygiene. In 2005 the incidence of newly-reported cases of HIV infections among drug users was decreasing (in 2004: 187 cases, in 2005: 129 cases), whereas new infections in the general population remained stable. No national data are available for HCV and HBV infection rates among IDUs.

In 2005 a seroprevalence cross-sectional study among IDUs was carried out in three places in Poland (the City of Wroclaw, Lubuskie region and Warminsko-Mazurskie region). Biological tests indicated HIV prevalence of 24.1% and HCV prevalence of 57.9%. In 2001there were 981 prisoners who were HIV-positive out of a prison population of around 80,000. (*Prison Healthcare in Czech Republic,Hungary and Poland* Morag McDonald, 2001).

Testing in Poland is voluntary with pre- and post-test counselling. The situation is the same in the **Czech Republic** with voluntary testing (only seven people, of those tested, were known to be HIV-positive out of the 68,000 prison population). HIV testing is mandatory in **Hungary**; the testing is anonymous and forms part of the prison admission procedure. HIV-positive inmates in Hungary are placed in a unit in Budapest, which is at the only hospital offering specialised HIV treatment in Hungary. According to prison authorities there were only eight prisoners in Hungary who had tested HIV-positive (McDonald, Helsinki 2001)

Ireland

Despite a 1999 study showing 90% of all IDU inmates were living with HCV and the HIV rate was far higher than in the wider community, the Irish Justice Department created a zero-drug-tolerance regime and introduced mandatory testing for drug use. No needle exchanges or bleach distribution programmes exist despite continued calls from the Irish Prison Reform Trust. A Irish prevalence study (Allwright et al, *BMJ*, 2001), randomised across 15 prisons, showed an HIV prevalence of 2%, hepatitis C prevalence of 37% and hepatitis B prevalence of 8.7%. At the time Ireland held 2,680 prisoners.

The Baltic states - Estonia, Latvia and Lithuania

Estonia has a small population of 1.3m, but possibly the highest HIV rate in European prisons at 17% (UNAIDS). IN May 2000 the first case was detected in Estonian prisons, in 18 months 800 prisoners had tested HIV-positive (Integration-Project Estonia). The total prison population in Estonia is 4,433 in October 2005, at 333 prisoners per 100,000 of population the highest in Western Europe (World Population list 2006).

Latvia has 6.2% prevalence in prison, and in Lithuania, the largest country, with a population of 3.4m, 15% of prisoners has HIV. According to the UNAIDS country report in 2006, 28% of all newly diagnosed HIV cases in Latvia were from prisons. The report said that HIV prevention strategies were 'fragmentary and ad hoc but harm reduction facilities are not available at all.'

On 13-14 March 2007, the United Nations Office on Drugs and Crime (UNODC), together with governments of the Baltic States, organised a meeting to share current approaches in HIV prevention and drug services. It brought health care and prison authorities, substitution therapy providers, drug user organisations and other NGOs from three countries to Vilnius, Lithuania. Blood-borne infections in prisons in the Baltic States have been of epidemic proportions. $5m dollars was pledged by the Dutch government for Harm reduction among IDUs and prisons in the region.

Approaches in prisons in the region do not include substitution therapy or needle exchange (Estonia had been implementing pilot substitution therapy programmes in the past). Increasingly acknowledged drug use in prisons is addressed mainly through increased security measures and partly through information dissemination. However Estonian, and to a lesser extent, Latvian and Lithuanian prison authorities are becoming more open to considering the introduction of evidence informed experiences like substitution therapy and even needle exchange, according to the UNODC.

A European Quaker Council mission to Tartu Prison, the most modern in the country, inspected the facilities for the small number of women incarcerated there. Tartu houses 17 female inmates, five of whom were HIV-positive. The prison holds 550 men. A similar inspection of Tallinn prison revealed 160 positive prisoners, around 10% of total inmates. Although the numbers are dropping for IDUs who are testing positive for HIV, in 2001 80% of new HIV cases were in people aged 15-24

Lithuania health authorities report that 64.6% pf people with HIV status have spent tie in prison. In 2002 Lithuania, Alytus Prison was the site where public health authorities around the world realised the consequences of incarceration without harm reduction. HIV tests revealed 263 prisoners had tested HIV-positive through intravenous transmission. Before that there were only 300 reported cases of HIV in the whole of the country. Tests at Lithuania's other 14 prisons found only 10 other cases of HIV.

Germany

Health experts from all the German states met for the first time in Bonn in 2006 to discuss a common approach to dealing with drugs and infectious disease in prisons. Their report has not yet been published. Only sporadic data are available on the prevalence of AIDS in German prisons.

Estimates published in the *British Medical Journal* suggested that 1-3% of prisoners in Germany may be HIV-positive and that many of those probably became infected while in jail. Prisons in Germany are not supervised by the federal government but are managed by the 16 German states. Medical policy and practice therefore vary considerably.

In 2006 115 out of 4000 inmates in Berlin's prisons were registered as HIV-positive, while in Munchen-Stadelheim prison 11 out of 1700 were. Out of about 60,000 prisoners in Germany, between 600 and 2,000 may be HIV-positive according to UNAIDS, and most of these are thought to have contracted HIV or hepatitis B virus, or both, in prison. A high prevalence of hepatitis C (HCV) virus infection of up to 80% has been reported for injecting drug users (IDUs) in prison communities.

A study by F Myer et al, *Epidemiology and Infections*, 2006) looked at hepatitis C in Germany's largest institute for young offenders, about which little was known. In 2002, all 1176 inmates age 16-24 were asked to participate in the study of which 95% agreed: 8·6% tested positive for HCV. Hepatitis C was significantly more common among immigrants from the former Soviet Union than among German inmates (31% vs. 6% respectively). HIV co-infection was found in five individuals, all of whom were German. In conclusion, the prevalence of hepatitis C was relatively low among inmates of German young offender Institutions although there were significant differences in relation to the country of birth. The data highlight the need for educational programmes for young offenders in order to prevent the further spread of blood borne infections.

The Prevention of blood-borne virus infections among drug users in an open prison by vending machines, (Heinemann et al, 2001), looked at the uptake for clean syringes in a German study. The study looked at the feasibility and acceptance of a needle exchange pilot project in an open prison for males in Hamburg. Many prisoners reported insufficient supply of syringes after the start of the programme, mainly due to frequent breakdowns of the vending machine, and because of this the frequency of needle-sharing decreased significantly. Among the interviewed staff members, unfavourable attitudes towards the project did not improve during the first year. The authors suggested that, should the programme be extended to other prisons, the supply of syringes by medical staff or drug services be considered, in order to increase staff acceptance of the programme.

This study was followed up by another by K Stark et al, (*Epidemiology and Infection*, 2005) in two prisons in Berlin. Here provision of sterile injection equipment for injecting drug users (IDUs) started in 1998. To assess the programme's impact, the frequency of injecting drug use and syringe sharing, and the incidence of HIV, HBV, and HCV infection were determined in a follow-up study. Of all 174 IDUs, 75% continued to inject. After the project started the level of syringe sharing declined from 71%

during a 4-month period of previous imprisonment to 11% during the first 4 months of follow-up, and to virtually zero thereafter.

Baseline seroprevalences were 18% for HIV, 82% for hepatitis C, and 53% for hepatitis B. HIV and HCV seroprevalence at baseline was significantly associated with drug injection in prison prior to the project start. There were no HIV and HBV seroconversions, but four HCV seroconversions occurred. The provision of syringes for IDUs in appropriate prison settings may contribute to a substantial reduction of syringe sharing. However, the prevention of HCV infection requires additional strategies said the researchers.

Italy

The Italian Ministry of Health reports that 13.8% of IDUs in Italy are living with HIV in 2004. However statistics on HIV infections in Italy are difficult to assess as only seven of the 20 regional departments of Italy perform HIV reporting.

However data do exist. A study in the *Journal of Medical Virology* (Babudieri S et al, 2005) looked at that correlates of HIV, HBV, and HCV infections in a prison inmate population. A total of 973 prisoners were enrolled; 87% males with a median age of 36 years, 30.4% were intravenous drug users (IDUs), and only 6 (0.6%) men who (openly) had sex with men. In this sample, high seroprevalence rates were found. The HIV rate was 7.5%; HCV 38.0%; anti-HBc antibody (an indicator of present or previous HCV infection) 52.7%, and Hepatitis B surface antigen (a marker of chronic infection) 6.7%. HIV and HCV seropositivity were associated strongly with intravenous drug use. After excluding IDUs and male homosexuals, HIV prevalence remained nonetheless relatively high (2.6%).

Tattoos were associated with HCV seropositivity. The number of imprisonments was associated with HIV infection, whereas the duration of imprisonment was only associated with hepatitis B. In conclusion, a high prevalence of HIV, HCV, and HBV infections among inmates was observed.

Frequency of imprisonment and tattoos were associated, respectively, with HIV and HCV positivity. Although it is possible that the study population is not representative of Italy's prison inmate population, the results stress the need to improve infection control measures.

Another study in Bologna Prison showed 12.5% HIV prevalence (Sabbatani, et al 2003).

Spain

HIV among inmates in Spanish prisons has been of epidemic proportions; a prevalence of 47% among 639 needle-using prisoners in Leon was reported in 1998. *(European Journal of Epidemiology*, 1998). In 1996 the Spanish Ministry of health estimated that 23.9% of Spanish prisoners (excluding Catalonia) were HIV-positive.

Since then, however, prevalence has dropped. In 2003 the estimate had decreased to 12%. In the wider community 29.3% of IDUs had HIV in 2004. Hepatitis C infections in the same period fell from 48% to 37%.

The drop in the number of prisoners with HIV is partly attributable to the decision made by the Spanish Prison Authorities who made a bold move in 2001 and ordered NEPs to be implemented in all Spanish prisons. This followed a successful pilot scheme in Bilbao begun in 1997.

Sterile injecting equipment is distributed 'hand to hand' (unlike vending machines in other schemes) and all prisoners are eligible to receive them, not just those designated as IDUs. Additional preventative information is provided by the NEP team who are either medical staff or external health professionals. According to a report by Menoyo, Suarez and Bianco, needles have not been used as weapons, with staff and inmates adapting well to the system.

In 2003 Spain had needle exchange points in 38 prisons, had 18% of its prisoners on methadone maintenance programmes, and had distributed 2.3 million condoms.

For a detailed plan and guidelines used for the implementation of needle exchange programmes in Spanish prisons see the *Needle Exchange in Prison Framework Programme* by the Ministerio Del Interior/Ministerio De Sanidad y Consumo (2003). The HIV and AIDS Legal Network described this study as "essential to see how a successful needle exchange programme can be established in a prison." Another document on the same issues is entitled *"Elements key for the installation of programmes of exchange of syringes in prison"* (Elementos clave para la implantacion de Programmeas de Intercambio de Jeringuillas en Prision)

Although the needle exchange programme has stemmed the tide of prison infection, EMCDDA reports that among voluntarily-tested recent IDUs (those who have injected in the last 12 months prior to admission to treatment) in the wider community, the HIV infection rate was 29.3% in 2004 (23.5% among male and 30.9% among females). However HIV prevalence among young tested IDUs (under 25) decreased from 20.3% in 1996 to 13.1% in 2000 and 7.1% in 2004.

A study in Spanish prisons in 2006 looked at the rate of drug resistance of inmates receiving ARVs (Garia-Guerrero 2006). Fifteen prisons were randomly selected and 38 HIV-positive prisoners from each prison were also randomly enrolled. Genotype testing was used on 184 prisoners. Each prisoner had a viral load below 2000 copies before the trial. Valid sequences were obtained from 133 inmates.

One or more key resistance mutations were detected in five (11.6%) of treatment-naive and in 35 (38.6%) of treatment-experienced prisoners. Among treatment-naïve and experienced inmates, resistance to nucleoside reverse transcriptase inhibitors was found in three (6.9%) and in 20 (22.2%) patients, respectively, resistance to non-nucleoside reverse transcriptase inhibitors in three (6.9%) and in 21 (23.3%) patients, and resistance to protease inhibitors in three (6.9%) and in 14 (15.5%) patients. Multi-drug resistance was detected in one of the 43 (2.3%) treatment-naive patients.

The researchers concluded; 'these findings support the use of resistance testing in HIV-infected inmates who must begin antiretroviral therapy, given the high rate of primary resistance to drugs frequently included in the initial treatment regimens.'

Another study in 2005 looked at the levels of adherence to ARV therapy. One hundred and seventy-seven HIV-infected inmates at two Spanish prisons were selected for the trial (Blanco 2005). A total of 23.4% of prisoners were non-adherent to their regimens. The researchers found that predictors of poor adherence included no visits in a month, depression, cannabis consumption and robbery. Although adherence was higher than in the wider community, variables such as adaptability to prison had no effect on adherence.

France

There are no national estimates on prevalence rates for drug-related infectious diseases among injecting drug users in France. However a few local studies have been carried out in the last few years. Data on HIV, HBV and HCV prevalence rates based on self-reports of drug users are available on a yearly basis from low-threshold services, needle exchange programmes and drug users outside of treatment (street surveys) from 12 cities in France. A study in 2001 estimated HIV prevalence among prisoners at 8%.

Outside of prisons in 2003, the HIV-positive rate from the latest known serological test of drug users who were currently injecting was 14% for HIV, 9% for HBV and 55% for HCV.

French prisons and HIV have a poor track record. In spite of repeated warningsissued in 1984 and 1985 about the high incidence of HIV infectionin prisons, blood donation continued in several large prisonsuntil December 1986 which led to the HIV infection of 4,000 blood transfusion recipients. In Bastia (Corsica) and Fort-de-France(Martinique) blood donation in prisons was discontinued onlyin 1990.

A 1992 report by the General Inspectorate of Judiciary servicesand the General Inspectorate of Social Affairs said that in1985 blood donated in prisons represented only 0.37% of thetotal donated in France, but was the source of about a quarterof contaminated donations.

According to the French HIV and AIDS organisation AIDES, drug users account for 30 % of the French prison population and the prevalence of HIV and AIDS is four to six times higher in prison than in the outside world, and that of hepatitis C ten times higher. However, access to harm reduction equipment is still prohibited in prison. No syringe exchange programme has been put in place in French prisons, says AIDES.

In France, though access to substitution treatments in prisons has improved overall, the situation is still very uneven between prisons. Drug users in prison are still not offered the full range of substitution treatments available in the outside world. AIDES claims that by refusing to tackle drug use as a public health issue, France has fallen well behind its European neighbours and demands the implementation of syringe exchange programmes in prisons and greater consistency in the prescription of substitution treatments in prison.

In 2002 the French government introduced a law, the *Suspension de Peine*, whereby terminally ill prisoners could be released from prison if they presented no risk to society. ActUp Paris say that three years after the law was passed there has been little impact. In January 2005 the French government introduced a proviso that prisoners given release under the system could have the order revoked without recourse to medical opinion, for example if they failed to pay outstanding fines.

A 2000 study aimed to estimate the frequency of risk behaviour for HIV transmission in prison and to identify the factors associated with reincarceration (Rotily 2000). Multivariate analysis showed that re-imprisonment was significantly more frequent among prisoners not receiving opiate substitutes at the time of their imprisonment.

References

BMJ, Germany HIV prevalence, Feb 1995, 310-282

Agence France Press, Portuguese Government acts to reduce impact of drugs, 2006

AIDES, website

Allwright et al, Irish prevalence study, BMJ 2001

Babudieri S et al, HIV in Italian prisons, Journal of Medical Virology, 2005

Blanco et al, ARV Adherence in Spanish Prisons, Int' Journal of STD/AIDS, Feb 2006

Bolzano, Users in treatment and Prisons, 2003

Dolan K et al, ???

Elements Key for the installation of programmes of Exchange syringes in Spanish prisons ???

EMCDDA Annual report, 2005

European Journal of Epidemiology, HIV rate in Leon Prison, Spain,1998

Garcia-Guerrero et al, HIV drug resistance in Spanish Prisons, European Journal of Microbiology and Infectious Diseases, Oct, 2006

Health In Prison Project, HIPP (WHO)

Heinemann et al, The prevention of bloodborne virus infections among drug users in an open prison by vending machines, 2001

Integration project Estonia

McDonald M, Prison healthcare in Czech Republic, Hungary and Poland, 2001

Menoyo, Suareez and Bianco, Needle exchanges in Spanish Prisons.

Ministerio Del Interior/Ministerio De Sanidad y Consumo, Needle exchange in Prison, framework programme, 2003

Moragado, HIV rate in Port Prison, Int Cong AIDS, 2002

Myer, F et al, Hepatitis C in Germanys largest Institute for Young Offenders, Epidemiology and Infections, 2006

Rotily et al, French prison HIV prevalence, 2001

Rotily et al, HIV risk behaviour in French Prisons, la Presse Medicale 2000

Sabbatani et al, HIV prevalence in Bologna Priosn, Italy, 2003

Stark K et al, provision of sterile injecting equipment in two German prisons, Epidemiology and Infections 2005

UNAIDS, Country Report, Latvia, 2006

US State Department on Human Rights, conditions in Portuguese Prisons, 2006

Wartelle-Bladeau C, preventative measures for Prisoners (France), VHPB, Nov 2004

Weiland et al, HIV transmission in part of the US prison system: implications for Europe, HPA/ENDIPP, 2006

World Drug Report, 2005

Zaba et al, International Journal of prison health, surveys for bloodborne viruses in European prisons, 2007

Eastern Europe and Central Asia

At the International Conference on AIDS, Toronto, 2006 one speaker described prisons as 'incubators' for HIV and AIDS. Nowhere is this more true than in the Eastern Europe/Central Asian region. In the Russian Federation and the Ukraine, the proportion of people behind bars who are living with HIV is far higher than the rest of Europe and in much of the world.

One study presented at Toronto found HIV rates in Ukraine prisons varied from 16% to 91% of prison populations. Even in countries where overall HIV infections rates are comparatively low, prisoners are bearing the brunt of HIV and AIDS. Against this background tuberculosis infections are notoriously high in the region's prisons with multi-drug-resistant TB strains an increasing problem.

Moldova and Belarus

In **Moldova** harm reduction programmes started early in the country's HIV epidemic and appear to have had an impact. At Toronto, D Laticevschi of the TB/AIDS Programme Moldova reported that HIV prevalence in Moldova nationally was 0.1%. Needle exchanges were in place for 30% of prisoners along with substitution therapy for drug users and peer-based education surrounding HIV.

Moldova had been projected to have 25,000 HIV infections in 2005, but with interventions this was down to 2,500, he claimed. Prevalence in prisons decreased from 3.2% in 2001 to 2% in 2003. Crucially, antiretrovirals are widely available in Moldova, unlike in many countries in the region.

In **Belarus** again the prevalence rate in prisons is out of proportion to the rest of the country. In November 2006 *All Russian News* reported that 1,098 prisoners were HIV-positive, 15% of the overall population living with HIV. Needle exchanges schemes are now operating. In Svetlogorsk the needle exchange programme claims to have reduced transmission from 92% to 35%

Central Asia

Central Asia comprises the countries known as the 'stans', Kyrgyzstan, Kazakhstan, Uzbekistan, Turkmenistan and Tajikistan. In the *International Journal of Prison Health*, March 2006 Gesa Walcher described the situation in Central Asian prisons as an 'epidemiological pump' for HIV and TB in the region. It estimated that up to a third of Central Asian people living with HIV are with the regions penitentiary system

The biggest HIV epidemic in central Asia is in **Kazakhstan**. It is thought that at least 1227 prisoners in local penitentiaries are HIV-positive (WHO 2005), about 10% of the overall number of Kazakhs living with HIV, which was estimated to be 12,000 in 2006. In 2002 mandatory testing and isolation for HIV-positive testing prisoners was said to have ceased, although according to Human Rights Watch prisoners are still kept in isolation.

In March 2007 the Kazakhstan government fired the health minister after an outbreak of HIV among 100 children infected through using contaminated blood products. In 2007 Reuters reported that Kazakhstan, despite huge oil revenues, was doing little to restructure a crumbling and corrupt health system.

In **Uzbekistan**, the HIV epidemic is one of the youngest in the world. According to UNAIDS over 90% of the country's HIV infections have been diagnosed since 2001. Although the prevalence rate is low compared to the total population of 26 million, the growth of HIV infections has been described by UNAIDS as one of the most 'dynamic' internationally. Estimates of those living with HIV vary from 5,000 to 30,000 although the WHO estimates 30% of those with HIV are in Uzbekistan prisons. USAID estimates 20% of women prisoners are HIV-positive. According to Amnesty International in 2006 of the 25 prisoners on death row in Tashkent prison, 20 have active TB.

In **Kyrgyzstan** official statistics released in June 2006 said the country has 865 people living with HIV, although unofficial estimates put the true figure at ten to 15 times that. According to IRIN news prisons have seen the largest rise in prevalence rates. The government says it has had success with needle exchange programmes and is now extending these into prisons.

In **Tajikistan** the British NGO Christian Aid/Act Central Asia, urged faster reform of the prison system. Tajik prisons, home to 13,000 inmates according to official figures, saw almost 90 deaths due to infectious diseases in 2005. The deputy of the correction department in the Ministry of Justice, Bakhrom Abdoulkhakov, said in 2006. "87 people have died in institutions of confinement due to infectious diseases, in particular tuberculosis," he added. More than 3,700 tuberculosis cases were diagnosed in Tajikistan between January and November 2005 - a leap of 33% over the same period the previous year, the health ministry said. A Global Fund grant enables condom distribution, HIV education materials and a pilot programme for a needle exchange at one of Tajikistan's prisons

The Russian Federation

Although the epidemiology suggests the potential for a surge in new HIV infections in other parts of eastern Europe and central Asia, nearly 90% of HIV cases were reported from the Russian Federation. In Russia there were 35,000 new HIV cases in 2005 (epidemic update 2006). The official total of people living with HIV is 350,000, which only counts people who have come into contact with the HIV diagnosis reporting system. UNAIDS has estimated that 940,000 people were living with HIV in the Russian Federation at the end of 2005.

A United Nations inspector in the early 1990s commented he would need "the literary skills of Dante and the artistic skills of Hieronymus Bosch" to describe the situation in the prisons he visited. The emergence and rapid spread of multi-drug resistant TB was identified in the mid 1990s in Russia . Rates of MDR-TB as a proportion of all TB cases have been recorded ranging from 34% to 80% in Russian jails. In the summer of 2005 280 prisoners at Lgov prison, south of Moscow, slashed their bodies, faces and hands with razor blades in protest at conditions.

One difficulty in writing about HIV in prisons in this region is illustrated by the decline in new HIV diagnoses in Russia. After peaking in 2001 at 87,000 they have levelled off at 33,000 - 36,000 in 2003/4. The UNAIDS 2006 Epidemic Report comments, "a partial explanation for the decline in HIV diagnosis after 2001 is that fewer tests have been carried out in some population groups at high risk of HIV infection; prisoners and injecting drug users."

In 2004/05 51% fewer tests were carried out in Russia among injecting drug users and 30% fewer among prisoners. One factor may be that many in these population groups have already tested HIV-positive. Factors specific to prisons are; a decline in prison population and government orders to release those with HIV and AIDS early. Also saturation point in these groups may have been reached especially among IDUs using non-sterile equipment.

However transmission rates among sex workers and IDUs vary from region to region suggesting that saturation levels have not been reached altogether. In Volgograd IDUs have an HIV prevalence of 3% which rises to 12-14% in Moscow (Rhodes et al, 2006). There is 30% infection rate in St Petersburg (Shaboltayl, 2006) and 70% in Biysk (Pasteur Institute, 2006). Among sex workers in St Petersburg 48% in one study tested positive for HIV (Kozlov et al, 2006).

Given that IDUs and sex workers face high odds of arrest and imprisonment HIV prevalence in Russian prisons has unsurprisingly risen from 7,500 in 1999 to 32,000 in 2006 according to the Ministry of Health and Social Development in 2006. A study by Rhodes and colleagues in 2006 found that among IDUs those that had been in prison had a greater risk of HIV. The UNAIDS Epidemic Report of 2006 said that no clean needle exchanges exist in Russian prisons. It commented: "Unfortunately in this region such public health approaches to harm reduction are overshadowed by more traditional law enforcement approaches to drug use."

In 2004 a Human Rights Watch (HRW) report, *"Lessons Not Learned: Human Rights Abuses and HIV and AIDS in the Russian Federation"*, April 2004, recommended that Russia stopped the practice of segregating HIV prisoners from other inmates in correctional facilities. HRW argued that the system for mandatory HIV testing be replaced with a voluntary scheme. It asked Russia to commit to the principle that healthcare should be the same as for the wider public.

In 2004 the St Petersburg prison system held 18,000 prisoners, a decline from 28,000 in part due to procedural changes to arbitrary imprisonment of drug users, and partly due to a move from heroin to other non-injectable drugs. The number of pre-trial prisoners was reduced from 190,000 in 2003 to 120,000 in 2006 (BBC World News). New legislation limits the amount of time an inmate may be held in a SIZO (pre-trial) prison without a hearing to six months.

All inmates are tested for HIV although obligatory testing was changed in 2001. A 2000 survey found that 47% of 9,727 inmates in a St Petersburg prison system were HIV-positive (Rhodes et al, 2004).

Human Rights Watch reported that a 2001 order eliminating mandatory segregation had been interpreted in St Petersburg to allow individual facilities to house HIV prisoners as they wanted. In all but one prison and the Kresty detention centre, prisons still had separate wards for HIV prisoners, but they were voluntary. One of the main objections to segregated facilities is the false sense of security it gives other prisoners, who wrongly assume all HIV-positive inmates are being segregated, according to the Canadian HIV and AIDS Legal Network.

One prisoner, Fyodor N told Human Rights Watch that care on a HIV segregated ward was no different than other parts of the prison, although they were given vitamin tablets that had passed an expiry date. "I was kept in an HIV isolation ward after I got my result. The people who were kept there went crazy. Many were serving long sentences and thought they would die there; so some of them did everything possible to die sooner."

One study concluded that prisons were "the major drivers of the tuberculosis and HIV epidemic in Russian prisons" and that novel strategies were needed to reduce the spread of blood-borne diseases.

Prisoners with TB were studied in order to identify the prevalence of HIV, and risk factors for HIV and other blood-borne virus infections; and clinical and social factors that might compromise TB treatment effectiveness and/or patient adherence and, hence, encourage treatment failure. A 1-year cross-sectional prevalence study of 1,345 prisoners with TB was conducted at an in-patient TB facility in Samara, Russian Federation.

HIV/HBV and HIV/HCV co-infection occurred in 12.2% and 24.1% of prisoners, respectively, and rates were significantly higher than in the wider population. Overall, 48.6% of prisoners used drugs, of which 88.3% were intravenous users. Two-thirds of prisoners (68.6%) had received previous TB drug therapy (frequently multiple, interrupted courses) and were significantly more likely than the general population to have had previous therapy consistent with the high drug-resistance rates seen.

A study of 63 harm reduction schemes underway in Russia by the World Bank in August 2006 added to a growing body of evidence that education, needle exchange programmes and medical and social services are a cost effective tool in a prison setting.

Despite these programmes the political climate in Russia regarding harm reduction, specifically substitution therapy, is difficult. Russia's leading clinicians of psychiatry and narcology published an attack on substitution therapy in the Medical Newspaper in 2005, rejecting methadone substitution, and needle exchange in Russian remains funded almost entirely by foreign donors.

Ukraine

HIV-ppositive people are regularly abused among the police and health care systems according to the Human Rights Watch report *Rhetoric and Risk; Human Rights Abuses impeding Ukraine's fight against HIV and AIDS"* in March 2006.

Ukraine has, on paper, comprehensive HIV legislation, the model for the region. After a visit to the Ukraine in 2005 HRW observers reported that *people living with HIV were being refused treatment and transport in ambulances.* There have been reports of IDUs arrested and beaten at needle exchanges as well as outreach workers being arrested. A study in 2005 found that 2,540 TB patients, 420 of them co-infected with HIV, had had treatment terminated by hospitals because of drug use (A. Ovsepyass, *All Ukrainian Network of people living with HIV*).

The Ministry of health has ordered the distribution of antiretroviral drugs to 30 patients in Kherson Prison. According to Human Rights Watch, in theory, access to antiretroviral is based on clinical decisions; in effect, health staff cite 'lack of motivation and commitment to adherence' as a bar to treating IDUs and inmates.

Prison health care is provided by a parallel health system under the State Department for the Penitentiary System. Inadequate coordination among parallel systems means that people in need of comprehensive health care services often fall between the gaps.

Ukraine has an estimated 370,000 people living with HIV in 2005, the worst affected country in Europe. Ukraine has adopted a very repressive approach to drug addiction, according to the Canadian HIV and AIDS Policy & Law Review. Consequently any harm reduction measures for prisoners are few.

HIV prevalence among injecting drug users is very high, up to 66% in the city of Mykolayiv (Ministry of Health Ukraine 2006). In the capital, Kiev, in one study of IDUs 49% were HIV-positive (Min of health 2006). The latest figures show an alarming rise in the general population in the first half of 2006 almost half (41%) were women and the Ukraine now has one of the highest rates in Europe among pregnant women; 0.31% in the first half of 2006.

In April 2006 The World Bank announced that it was suspending a $60 million project that aimed to curb the spread of tuberculosis and HIV and AIDS in Ukraine because of the government's failure to launch the programme and distribute funds.. Up to April 2006 the government had spent 2% of the $60 million allocated in January 2004 to be dispersed over a four-year period. The programme was aimed at providing funds for medicines, training health care workers and other prevention measures targeted at high-risk groups such as injection drug users, commercial sex workers and prisoners.

The situation in the Ukraine's prisons appears to be one of spiralling infections. Up to mid-2006 Ukrainian jails held 4,300 HIV registered inmates - 1530 had been diagnosed in the first six months of 2006. The Ukrainian AIDS Centre estimates that the HIV prevalence rate has risen to 9% in 2003 to 14% in mid-2006.

The WHO put the number of inmates who had active TB at 14,000, 7% of the Ukrainian prison population. TB rates in the Ukraine have tripled since independence from 32 per 100,000 in 1991 to 91 per 100,000 in 2002 (V. Lekahn et al, 2004). Forty per cent of deaths in Ukrainian jails are attributable to TB.

Drug injecting is common in the Ukrainian prison system. In 2005 the Ukraine - Helsinki Human Rights Union reported that the Ukraine State Department recognised that unsafe injection use was taking place in prison and had taken steps to launch two pilot needle exchange programmes in two prison colonies in Kiev and Mykolaiv in 2006.

Another element in Ukraine has to be factored in: sex between men. Gay sex in Ukraine has not been studied and although the law prohibiting homosexual sex was repealed in 1991, stigma in Ukrainian society still surrounds homosexual sex. In Odessa and Mykolayiv limited sentinel surveillance of this group showed an HIV prevalence of 28% and 9% respectively.

References

Abdoulkhakov, Tajikistan, 2006, Ministry of Justice

All Russian News, Belarus prisoners HIV-positive, November 2006

Amnesty International, Uzbekistan HIV prisons, 2006

Associated Press/Kiev Post, Ukraine loses World bank HIV funds, 2006

BBC World News (Parsons, R). Ray of Hope Enters Russian Prisons, April 2003

Dolan J et al, peer based education programme in Siberia, 2004

EuroHIV, HIV rate Russian federation, 2006

HIV/AIDS Policy & Law Review, Ukraine repression of drug use, 2005

HIV/AIDS Law Policy & Law Review, substitution therapy problematic in Russia, December 2006

Human Rights Watch, Lessons Not Learned, Human Rights Abuses and HIV/AIDS in the Russian Federation, April 2004

Human Rights Watch, Rhetoric and Risk, Human Rights abuses impeding Ukraine's fight against HIV/AIDS, March 2006

Int Conf on AIDS, Toronto, Incubators quote?

IRIN News, Kyrgyzstan prison prevalence, June 2006

Journal Of Public health, Drug Resistant TB, Russian federation, 2005

Kozlov et al, HIV among sex workers in St Petersburg, 2006

Laticevschi D, HIV prevalence Moldova, TB/AIDS Programme Moldova, Int Conf AIDS, Toronto

Lekahn v et al, TB in Ukraine jails, 2005

Ministry of health Ukraine, HIV among injecting drug users, 2006

New York Times/Reuters, contaminated blood products in Kazakhstan, 2006/7

Ovsepyass, HIV/AIDS treatment failures, All Ukrainian Network Of People Living with HIV

Pasteur Institute, HIV prevalence in IDUs in Biysk, Russian federation, 2006

Rhodes et al, HIV in St Petersburg Prison System, 2000

Rhodes et al, IDUs in Russian prisons, 2006

Ruskin, St Petersburg Health Department, 2004

Russian federation, Ministry of health and Social Development, HIV in Russian Prisons, 2006

Shaboltayl, HIV among St Petersburg IDUs, 2006

Ukraine - Helsinki Human Rights Union, two NEP pilot schemes in Ukraine prisons, 2005

Ukrainian AIDS Centre, HIV prevalence rate, 2003-2006

UNAIDS 2006 Epidemic Report, HIV prevalence in Russian Federation Prison System

Walcher Gesa, HIV in Central Asia, Int Journal pf Prison Health, Mar 2006

Walker, Needle exchange in Belarus, abstract, Int Conf AIDS, 2000

WHO 2005 Kazakhstan HIV prison rate

World Bank, Needle exchanges cost effective in Russian August 2006

World Bank, TB/AIDS project Ukraine, April 2006

The United States

The United States has more people behind bars both in absolute terms and per head of population than any other nation; 922 per 100,000 or nearly one in a hundred US citizens, according to the US Bureau of Justice's statistics. This country, with five per cent of the world's population, has 25% of the world's incarcerated population. At the end of 2005 over 2.2 million were in prisons and altogether seven million people, or one in 32 US adults, were under US legal jurisdiction, whether on probation, parole, in state or federal prisons or in county jails.

Prisoners' health and its impact on the wider community is an increasing public health concern. The first thorough study on HIV transmission in US State prisons was completed in 2006 and showed that almost one in ten HIV-positive prisoners in the state of Georgia had contracted the virus while in prison.

The rate of growth of the US prison population has been rapid and rising. Inmate numbers have quadrupled since 1980, largely as a result of mandatory sentencing driven by the US government's war on drugs. US prisoners living with HIV are now officially counted at 23,046 at the end of 2005 (US Justice Dept): around the same figure as Germany's total population of people with HIV.

The US Department of Justice reported in late 2006 that the number of HIV-positive state and federal prisoners had decreased for the fifth consecutive year, as have deaths from AIDS. At the end of 2004 HIV-positive inmates stood at 23,046 compared to 25,807 in 1999. The average sero-prevalence of 1.9% in US state prisons is relatively low compared to four per cent and 16% respectively for France and Spain. (WHO Global report). The prevalence rate however for African-American women prisoners is 3.4%.

While the number of AIDS related deaths dropped from 282 in 2003 to 203 in 2004, the number of AIDS cases increased from 5,944 to 6,027, a rate three times than that of the general US population, (0.51% v 0.15%). African-Americans account for two thirds of these AIDS-related deaths in prisons (Marushak et al. 2006).

These figures may under-report the US prison HIV rate. A lack of universal screening (due to be introduced during 2007), limited access to healthcare and brief periods of incarceration in local jails could point to higher numbers.

In areas of low prevalence, such as North Dakota and Montana, just 0.2% of the total prison population are HIV-positive.   This contrasts to 7.6% in New York.

As well as African Americans, women are over represented among HIV-positive prisoners. Although only accounting for 5-10% of the prison population, women have a higher HIV prevalence rate than male prisoners: 2.8% compared with 1.9% in 2003. More than 10% of all female inmates were known to be HIV-positive in two states, New York and Maryland (14.6% and 11.1%, respectively, Manuschak, Sep 2005). In all states, less than 10% of male inmates were reported to be HIV-positive. Only New York reported higher than 5% seroprevalence among male prisoners.

The Georgia state report

In 2006 the US Centers for Disease Control and Prevention (CDC) concluded a study which has caused a major impact in the US public health community. The report, "HIV Transmission Among Male Inmates in a State Prison System - Georgia, 1992-2005," (CDC, *Morbidity & Mortality Weekly Report April 2006*) was hailed by some as a landmark report.

The study shows HIV transmission rates in Georgia state prisons from 1992 to 2005. Eighty eight prisoners who tested HIV-negative on entry to the Georgia penal system have since tested positive indicating seroconversion during incarceration. Mandatory testing has been in Georgia prisons since 1988. Risk behaviours in prison, specifically sex between men and tattooing, were associated with HIV seroconversion.

Data were gathered in the Georgia prisons from mandatory testing of all inmates at intake followed by inmate requested tests, or annual voluntary HIV testing, which was offered between 2003-2005. Investigators analysed data collected from cases and control subjects through computer-assisted self interviews.

This CDC report includes a wealth of information about the prisoners, reported risk activities, precautions practised, and knowledge about and suggestions for prevention of transmission of HIV in prison.

In October 2005, the Georgia Department of Correction housed 44,990 male inmates of whom 856 - nearly two per cent - were reported to be HIV-positive. Of that 856, 780 (or 91%) were infected before incarceration, and 732 (or 86 %) were black, the report states.

From July 1988 to February 2005, a total of 88 male inmates who were HIV-negative when sentenced contracted HIV while in

prison. Not surprisingly, the CDC identified sex between male inmates and sharing needles for tattoos and drug use as the most common risk behaviours for HIV inside prison walls. Characteristics associated with prisoners' HIV seroconversion were male-male sex in prison, tattooing in prison, age over 26 at interview, more than five years served of current prison sentence, black race, and a body mass index less than 25.4kg/m^2 on entry into prison.

One third of HIV prisoners said they had sex with male staff and one fifth with female staff . One-third of inmates also said they used some kind of barrier - like rubber gloves or plastic wrap.

In March 2007 the public affairs director for the state Department of Corrections, said Georgia has no immediate plans to implement any new HIV initiatives .

'Contraband' condoms

The Georgia Department of Corrections take the view that condoms are considered "contraband" in Georgia prisons and sex between inmates is forbidden by both state law and prison policy.

Condom access programmes have been successfully introduced in the prison system in the state of Vermont and a portion of the prison system in Mississippi. Additionally, such programmes have been employed in large and complex jail systems in New York City, Philadelphia, Washington, DC, San Francisco and parts of Los Angeles County, among others. Fears by correctional officers and system officials that such programmes might create safety or management problems or might encourage more sexual activity have proven to be unfounded.

The largest such evaluation published in the scientific literature, based on interviews with more than 307 inmates and 100 correctional officers, reported that after implementation in the Washington, D.C. Central Detention Facility, "condom access was unobtrusive to the jail routine, no threat to security or operations, no increase in sexual activity and accepted by most prisoners and correctional officers."

African Americans disproportionately represented

African Americans account for 13% of the US population but more than half of new cases of HIV.

The Georgia report and the numbers of African American men and women who are behind bars has provoked community leaders and elected officials to push harm reduction in US prisoners on to the political agenda.

According to the Department of Justice in 2004 female prisoners in state prisons were more likely to be HIV-positive than males. Black (non-Hispanic) women inmates had an HIV seroprevalence of 3.4%. African American men with a prevalence rate of 1.8% are also over represented in terms of HIV infection: African Americans comprised two-thirds of all prisons deaths from AIDS related illness, compared to 39% of total AIDS deaths in the US. (Maruschak L). A report from Maryland showed that of 888 AIDS cases in the state's prisons, 91% were African Americans. (*Journal Urban Health,* 2001).

In November 2006 the influential National Minority AIDS Council (NMAC) released a report calling for US policy-makers to implement a strategy for combating HIV and AIDS among the country's black community. The report called on US prisons and jails to make condoms available and to implement HIV prevention and education campaigns. Democratic representative Barbara Lee told the *San Francisco Chronicle* that 'the NMAC plan offers a clear blueprint.'

Lee had unveiled legislation in September 2006 aimed at putting condoms into federal prisons. The bill also calls for prisons to allow community organisations to come into prisons to conduct HIV and sexual health counselling, testing and treatment as well as condom distribution.

In California, with an estimated prison population of 162,000, the local authorities in Los Angeles and San Francisco permit the distribution of condoms. However a similar bill to Lee's in California was vetoed by Californian Governor Arnold Schwarzenegger. The Bill had been approved by the Californian State Senate in August 2006, but was vetoed by the governor in October 2006.

Mandatory testing in prisons

There is no specific CDC recommendation on how prison inmates should be tested, but the agency does identify them as a high-risk group that should be targeted under the Advancing Health Prevention (AHP) scheme Introduced by CDC in 2003. Over 200,000 HIV 'fast tests' have been used in prisons.

The *New England Journalof Medicine* (NEJM - Jan 2007) reports that 20 states conduct HIV tests among all inmates and the remaining states test for high-risk groups, at inmates' request, or under specific circumstances.

Mandatory testing for HIV in prisons raises a number of issues. The earliest public policy debates on HIV in prisons in the US focused not on care and prevention but on whether to mandate universal testing. In 2003, 19 state prison systems and the Federal Bureau of Prisons had mandatory HIV screening policies for their incoming inmates. (Maruschak Bureau of Justice March 2006).

The question of prisoners' ability to make a free informed consent to a HIV test is problematic, according to the *NEJM*. Inmates negotiate for privileges, better conditions, and, ultimately, release. Where HIV testing is not mandatory, prisoners require more information than others to make informed decisions about taking the test. Prisoners must understand the institutional consequences of a positive HIV antibody test result, such as segregation and loss of access to activity programmes, visitation, and jobs.

In 2004 a court decision in Alabama, where HIV-positive patients had been segregated, allowed these inmates to integrate into the wider prison population for work and education programmes. In 2006 only two or three inmates continued to participate in these activities. Many US prisons have policies of segregating prisoners who refuse testing with the policy that they can join the general population only after they have been "medically cleared."

Despite the downsides there is evidence that HIV testing has benefited inmates in institutions that offer antiretroviral therapy and prophylaxis against opportunistic infections. Voluntary testing increasingly has become available to prisoners.

A review of HIV infections identified through voluntary counselling and testing programmes for prisoners in 48 project areas in the United States between 1992 and 1998 found a steady increase in the use of testing services. (Sabin et al, *Journal of Urban Health*, 2001). There were 16,797 reactive tests (3.4%), 56% of which involved individuals who had been unaware of their serostatus at the time of testing. Acceptance rates for seroprevalence testing by new inmates in Maryland and Wisconsin have been reported at 47-83%. (Shuter J, *National Commission on Correctional Health Care* March 2002) In 2003, 45 of 49 responding state prison systems and the federal prison system reported testing for HIV at inmates' request. (Maruschak, *Bureau of Justice*, 2003).

In April 2006 New York City health officials introduced a new computerised medical screening process for inmates arriving at city jails. Inmates are assigned an identification number that remains the same from incarceration to incarceration, said Louise Cohen, the deputy commissioner with the Department of Health and Mental Hygiene in charge of supervising jail health care. She said that this allowed workers to quickly access the medical histories of repeat offenders and that the $200,000 system also lets workers generate requests for specialised care faster and more accurately.

New York City Health Commissioner Dr. Thomas Frieden said the New York Health Department is looking to expand inmate testing for HIV and STDs. Ten per cent to 20% of the approximately 14,000 city inmates at any given time are HIV-positive, according to health officials.

In addition to using the rapid-result HIV test, Cohen said her department has launched a pilot programme that assigns patient care coordinators to all HIV-positive inmates in one jail - Rikers Island. If successful, the programme will expand to other jails. This network of caseworkers will track all HIV-positive inmates and link them to community care after their release.

Apart from New York, 39 states test inmates if they are involved in an incident that caused bleeding, and three states (and all prisons run by the Federal Bureau of Prisons) impose mandatory testing of inmates upon release. Local and city prisons generally do not enforce mandatory testing however.

Both the World Health Organisation and the US Department of Justice oppose mandatory testing in prisons, and AIDS organisations have long campaigned for it to be banned. They argue that mandatory testing removes the basic human right of choice, and can lead to discrimination and segregation within the prison. It also results in lower levels of counselling being given to the prisoner at the time of the test. If an inmate can make a personal decision about whether to get tested, they will require far more knowledge about the causes and dangers of HIV before they can make an informed choice. With a compulsory test, there often seems little point in counselling a prisoner, as they will receive a test whether the individual concerned deems it necessary or not.

There is currently very little evidence showing that mandatory testing in prisons is effective as a public health measure, so most AIDS organisations advocate a voluntary opt-out policy similar to that offered to pregnant women.

Exit testing and spouse notification

A proposal before the state legislature in Indiana will make HIV antibody tests mandatory for inmates entering and leaving the state's prisons for HIV and Hep C. The new law was voted for in February 2007. Inmates have been tested on entering prison since 2002, and the new move would 'close the loop', according to advocates for the bill.

The $525,000 costs are a bone of contention and the bill has been temporarily stymied due to the expense. Only Missouri and Alabama do both entry and exit tests. Alabama continues to segregate HIV-positive prisoners from the rest of the prison population (se below).

Dr Elton Amos, the Indiana State Department of Corrections medical officer, has stated that he saw no evidence that Indiana inmates had contracted 'HIV or other viruses while incarcerated' (*The Indianapolis Star*, March 2007). Exit testing said Amos would not help his department as they were only concerned with the care of inmates while incarcerated.

At the time of writing (March 2007) the Kentucky state legislature is considering a law that would require testing of inmates as they left prison, with the results given to offenders' spouses or partners. The proposal has the backing of a number of Kentucky state church groups alarmed at the rise of infections, particularly among black prisoners and their families, according to the *Louisville Courier & Journal*. Some health-care professionals have argued, however, that the bill does not go far enough. They want to see inmates tested when they first get to prison, which would lead to earlier treatment. Barry Zack, executive director of a California-based agency called Centerforce that works with prisoners and their families told the *Courier & Journal*; It's "immoral and unethical" to test only when inmates get out, Zack said, because many with HIV won't have access to the medical care they need.

The proposed law's sponsor, Senator Dan Seum, acknowledged that Louisville religious leaders originally approached him about testing inmates when they entered prison, as 18 other states do.

But Seum said that would potentially triple HIV treatment costs for state inmates to $3.6 million a year. If they are diagnosed with HIV as they go in, "you've got to give them medical attention," Seum was reported as saying. "Now you're talking about millions."

Hepatitis C and TB

During 1997, 20% to 26% of all people living with HIV in the United States, 29% to 43% of all those infected with the hepatitis C virus, and 40% of all those who had tuberculosis disease in that year passed through a correctional facility, according to a study published in 2002 (Am J Pub H).

These results have implications for the optimal planning of preventive and therapeutic measures. Effective HIV treatment must also focus on HCV and TB.

In 2004 testimony presented to the New York State Assembly in April 2004 put the HCV rates at 23% for women and 13.6% for male inmates, while several studies in Texas have found HCV prevalence of between 20 and 50% among prisoners in the state.

References

Austin Chronicle, Texas prisons and HIV transmission prevention, October 2006

Colton C, HIV and hepatitis C co-infection: Where Do We Stand, October 2006

Correctional Association of new York, HIV/Hep C in Female prisoners??

Corrections Service Alabama, inmate AIDS Deaths 1999-2002

Human Rights Watch, Limestone correctional Facility, Alabama, February 2005

Hylton W, Hepatitis C in US Prisons, Harpers, August ???

Indianapolis Star, HIV Exit testing, March 2007

Journal of Urban Health, AIDS deaths in Maryland 2001

Louisville Courier & Journal, Kentucky considers exit testing, march 2007

Maruschak L et al, (US Bureau of Justice Statistics) US deaths from AIDS, 2006. HIV among female inmates, Sep 2005, testing for HIV and inmates request, 2003 HIV among female prisoners in New York State, Spe, 2005

New England Journal of Medicine, Mandatory HIV testing in US prisons, Jan 2007

New England Journal of Medicine, Sex, Dugs, Prisons and HIV, January 2007

New York State Department of Correctional Services, HCV/HIV Co-infection, Dec, 2003

New York Times, Alabama limestone Correctional facility, August 2005

Sabin et al, HIV testing of prisoners, Journal of Urban health, 2001

Shutter J, National Commission on Correctional Health Care, March 2002

Southern Voice Newspaper, Georgia, HIV in Prisons, 2006

The Body, HIV Testing in New York Correctional facilities, April 2006

US Bureau of Justice Statistics, US prison population, 2005

US Centers for Disease Control and Prevention (CDC), HIV Transmission Among male Inmates in A State Prison System - Georgia 1992 - 2005, CDC, Morbidity & Mortality Weekly Report, April 2006

WHO Global Report, US prison HIV sero-prevalence.

Canada

Canada had a prison population of 34,000 in 2004 according to Statistics Canada, a rate per 100,000 of 107, compared to its neighbour, the US, with a rate of 738 per 100,000. A study in 1999 (Ford et al) showed an increase of HIV prevalence of from one to two per cent over four years. In 2001 the correctional service of Canada put the HIV infection rate at 1.7% for men and 4.7% for women. Hepatitis C rates were 23.4% for the same period, (*CSC Infectious diseases, prevention and control.*). HIV rates in provincial prisons can be as high as 8% according to Ralf Jurgens of the Canadian HIV and AIDS Legal Network in 2004.

Corrections Canada told local news services in January 2007 that more than 3,300 male and female inmates in Canada's 54 prisons had hepatitis C in 2004, and almost 2,500 were released into the community that year. Almost 200 prisoners were infected with HIV. The annual cost of treatment is C$29,000 per inmate for HIV and C$26,000 each for hepatitis C. In Canada prisoners are likely to be 30 times more likely to be infected with Hepatitis C and 10 times more likely to have HIV than people on the outside.

In September 2005 the Correctional Service Canada (CSC) started a one-year pilot programme for safer prison tattoo parlours using safe and clean equipment. The move was applauded by many public health experts. Tattoo shops were set up in six federal prisons, run by prisoners and supervised by staff. Tattoos were not allowed below the wrists or above the collarbone, and gang tattoos were forbidden. Prisoners were given training on infection prevention and taught to be peer health educators.

In December 2006 the Canadian government decided to close prison tattoo parlours citing them as "a waste of taxpayers' money". The decision to close the Tattoo parlours was premature according to David Butler Jones the head of the Public Health Agency of Canada, who said the year long programme was not enough time to see if rates of HIV and Hepatitis C had been reduced. Each site costs $C100,000 to run, which the Canadian HIV and AIDS Legal Network said was equivalent to preventing just five HIV or Hepatitis C infections at each site. A spokesperson for the Legal Network commented: "Prisoners are sentenced to serve time, not to be infected with potentially fatal diseases." They added that safe tattooing facilities were a public health issue, as well as a fiscal issue.

The CSC came under criticism in July 2006 for the way it dealt with a prisoner who died in custody of AIDS related complications. An inquest into the death of Eric Boyer, 36, who died at Archamault Prison, found that steps had not been taken to prepare his case for medical parole, until four days before his death.

The Coroner at the inquest made two recommendations: That Archambault Institution revise its guidelines on medical parole and that CSC put in place an expedited process for presenting terminally ill prisoners to the parole board. According to the Canadian HIV and AIDS Law Review at least another two prisoners have died in similar circumstances and earlier recommendations have not been put into practice.

References

Correctional Service Canada, infectious diseases prevention and control, Hepatitis C rates, 2001

Jurgens R, Canadian Legal HIV/AIDS Network HIV rates in Canada prisons, Statistics Canada, prison population, 2004

Latin America

Addressing the issues of HIV transmission, prevention and treatment in the prisons of Latin American presents huge challenges. Societies in the region are dealing with crime, often violent, that is perceived to be out of control. Gang culture and its influence within Latin American prisons have sapped political and public support for dollars spent on prison health. This is in a region where the highest ever HIV prevalence in a single prison was recorded in Caseras jail, Buenos Aires in 1996 (see Argentina): half of the prison population were thought to be HIV-positive.

The Sao Paulo prison system, in Brazil is notorious for under-staffing, extreme overcrowding, deaths in custody, and lack of medical and sanitation facilities. The United Nations special rapporteur against torture reported in April 2006 that torture and ill-treatment were widespread in Brazil's prisons and detention centres

A Latin American 'machismo' culture creates stigma and prejudice around homosexuality and difficulty identifying HIV prevalence rates among men having sex with men. The 2006 *AIDS Epidemic Update* states: "The role of unprotected sex between men in many of Latin America's epidemic tends to be publicly denied and ignored in HIV strategies."

Information and surveillance are inconsistent. Brazil has had a number of controlled studies of infection rates and routes within its prisons. Yet other countries are a blank. The HIV risk behaviours of vulnerable and ethnic minorities outside urban areas are little understood such as the Mayan population of Guatemala and the Garifuna Indians of Honduras.

Brazil, Mexico, Argentina and Colombia have the highest number of people living with HIV, but small Central American countries such as Belize, Guatemala and Honduras have higher HIV prevalence.

These rates of HIV infection are hugely amplified within the prison systems of the region. In Argentina, for example, the overall adult prevalence rate is 0.6% of the population. Yet in 2004 between 17% and 24% of prisoners in Buenos Aires province were found to be HIV-positive (UNAIDS fact sheet 06).

The link between HIV infections and intravenous drug use (and consequently prison time) is particularly prevalent in the region. The rate of HIV among IDUs has been found to be 24% in Uruguay, 15% in Asunscion, Paraguay and 16% in Bogota, Columbia (Aceijas et al 2004).

Mexico

Mexico has the second largest prison population in Latin America after Brazil. The latest figures for 2006 show that Mexico has a prison population of 214,000, (196 inmates per 100,000) with prisons operating at 125% of capacity.

Although Mexico's overall national prevalence rate is low compared with some other Latin American countries, at 0.3%, because of its large population (104 million) there are 180,000 people living with HIV in Mexico (2006 AIDS Epidemic Update). One study (see below) has put the HIV prevalence rate at Durango Penitentiary at 6%, a massive concentration of infection compared to the wider community.

Mexico is putting effort into mass media campaigns to educate people about HIV and to challenge homophobia. The head of Mexican HIV agency CENSIDA, Dr Jorge Saavedra, is a gay man living with HIV whose appointment created huge media commentary at the time. Evidence of outreach work in prisons, though, is hard to find.

Sex between men is believed to account for more than half (57%) of these HIV levels (Bravo-Garcia et al, 2006), which makes the prison environment in Mexico a potential source of new infections. The HIV rate was 4% among injecting drug users in Tijuana (Magis Rodriguez et al, 2005). Another study (Patterson et al 2006) found HIV rates of up to 16% among injecting female sex workers in the same region.

Under-reporting, unprotected sex between men, and high rates of HIV infection equal a much more problematic situation in Mexico's prisons. Although CESIDA asserts that there is 100% access to antiretrovirals, AIDS activists in Mexico contend this is far from the case. Nuar Luna, a prominent AIDS activist, told *Science* in 2006 that the biggest challenge Mexico faces is unequal access to quality care. "If you have influence and you have money, you have access."

One important study in Mexican prisons investigated hepatitis and HIV infections in inmates of a state correctional facility in Mexico. Researchers at Durango University sought to determine the prevalence and associated characteristics of hepatitis A, B, C and D viruses and HIV infections in a prison in Durango, Mexico. *(Epidemiology and Infection, 133, 2005).* They found prevalence rates of 10% for HCV and 6% for HIV among the inmates.

An association between HBV infection and age over 30 was found. HCV infection was associated with being born in Durango City, a history of other hepatitis infections, ear piercing, tattooing, drug abuse history, intravenous drug use and lack of condom use. The study concluded that the prevalence of HAV, HBV, HDV and HIV infections in inmates in Durango, Mexico were comparable to those of the Mexican general population and blood donors, but lower than those reported in other prisons around the world. However, HCV infection in inmates, at 10%, was higher than that reported in Mexican blood donors but lower than those reported in other prisons of the world according to the study.

Belize

Belize has the highest per capita HIV infection rate in Central America. A survey conducted in Belize Central Prison in 2004 revealed an HIV infection rate of 4.9% or one in 20 of inmates surveyed, compared to HIV prevalence in the general population of 2.5% at the end of 2005. (Ministry of Health: *HIV seroprevalence in inmates at the Kolbe Foundation, Central Prison;* June 2005).

According to the World Health Organisation in 2005, an estimated 3,600 Belizeans are living with HIV. In a small country like Belize, that represents 2.5% of the adult population of 240,000, nearly double the per capita HIV infection rate of neighbouring Guatemala, and eight times the rate in Mexico. Because of stigma and discrimination in Belize the WHO say the numbers are likely to be unreported, in such a small country the population find it hard to believe the HIV test results are confidential.

The National AIDS Programme (NAP) has completed fieldwork in 2006 determining HIV seroprevalence and risk factors at the Kolbe Foundation, Belize Central Prison. The Belize government introduced universal antiretroviral treatment in the wider community in 2003 on a first come first served basis. The NAP organises all drug allocations and is now working closely with a community group at the Belize Prison, where 12 prisoners in 2006 were on antiretrovirals.

An interesting project in Belize is the 'Youth for the Future' scheme which looks for cooperation from gang members. There are strong links between the gang lifestyle and Belize's high prevalence of HIV. Most gang members have been in prison at some time.

Although many Latin American countries have problems with gangs, a 2005 report by the non-partisan US Congressional Research Service quoted in *Science* magazine, reported "the largest and most violent" ones are in Central America and Mexico. According to the report, several factors have led to an increase in gangs: weapons left over from the many civil wars in the region, a stepping-up of US deportation of illegal immigrants, and huge income inequalities in Belize and its neighbours. Youth for the Future is one of the few efforts that explicitly targets gang members as "at-risk youths" for HIV infection.

Gang members often share one woman, the project says in the *Science* magazine, and transactional sex or "Give some, get some," in local parlance for a meal or protection is also the norm. Condom use is also low. Supported by the United Nations Population Fund and a grant from the OPEC Fund, Youth for the Future maintains a resource centre, education work and distribution of free male and female condoms. "They have done tremendous work," says epidemiologist Paul Edwards, head of the Ministry of Health's National AIDS Programme. "These kids have a lack of education and don't make the best decisions possible."

No study has ever assessed HIV prevalence in gang members in Belize. Most long term gang members have been incarcerated in the country's Central prison at some point. Youth for the Future plans to start offering HIV counselling and testing, and hopes to recruit gang members to participate in a prevalence study

Brazil

Brazil dominates the South America HIV epidemic by its size of population (184 million, by far the largest in South America), and the number of HIV-infected people who live there, 620,000 at the end of 2005 (UNAIDS). The country has pioneered universal access to antiretroviral treatment, and this and prevention work have helped keep the HIV epidemic stable in recent years, but the escalating cost of the drugs poses a tremendous challenge and the health of Brazil's prison population, treated with apathy in most quarters, could continue to be bottom of list of priorities.

According to the Ministry of Justice, Brazil's prison population grew by 84% between 1995 and 2003, as governments eager to stem the crime wave tearing through Brazilian cities encouraged the justice system to get suspects behind bars. According to

United Nations figures the Brazil prison population had reached 385,000 or 203 prisoners per 100,000 of overall population. Amnesty International estimates the prison system has a capacity for 180,000 prisoners. The Panos Institute estimates that 70% of men in Brazilian jails are sexually active, via prostitution, conjugal visits or sex with men.

There is evidence that the high prevalence of HIV among the nations IV drug users is falling in some regions. In the recent past HIV prevalence ranged from 25% of IV drug users in Sao Paulo to 75% in a particular Sao Paulo network (MAP 2000). Now rates appear to be falling in some areas as crack cocaine is being smoked, rather than injected (Fonseca et al 2006).

However one cross-sectional study across a number of states found a 37% level of HIV prevalence among injecting drug users and those levels were significantly associated with incarceration and having unprotected sex with other men (Caiaffa et al, 2006)

The high levels of HIV and AIDS found in Brazil's prisons bear out these contributory factors. In a study in 1995 researchers found that 80% of male prisoners had been exposed to TB, as had 90% of female prisoners (*Comissão Parlamentar Inquérito* CPI). Another report (Biancarelli) found 2-4% of inmates in a prison in Sao Paulo had developed active TB. Multi-drug-resistant strains of TB were found in 3.4% of prisoners in Rio de Janeiro's penitentiary sanatorium, compared to 1.3% in the wider community (J. Braz, *Brazil Journal of Microbiology*).

In 1997, researchers at the University of São Paulo estimated that some 20% of Brazil's prison inmate population was living with HIV, after having collected data from around the country. According to their research, the highest levels of HIV infection are found in the prisons in the southeast of Brazil, an area that includes São Paulo, in some instances affecting some 30% of the inmate population (*Correio de Paraiba*, Pessoa, Dec 1997). The lowest levels of infection are found in the northeast, where only 2 to 3% of inmates are infected.

One of the studies done to ascertain transmission rates and routes of infection was in 2001 the '*Correlation between HIV and HCV in Brazilian Prisoners: evidence for parenteral transmission inside prison.*' MN Burrattini et al Sao Paulo university).

A total of 631 prisoners from a Brazilian prison with 4,900 inmates at that time were interviewed and their blood drawn. Risky behavior for HIV infection was analysed, and serological tests for HIV, hepatitis C and syphilis were performed. Prevalence rates were: 16% for HIV, 34% for HCV and 18% for syphilis 18%. The study showed that the risk of acquiring HIV infection increased with the time of imprisonment, peaking around three years after incarceration.

A study of 229 women in Sao Paolo state penitentiary found prevalence of 13.9% for HIV, 16.2% for HCV and 22.8% for syphilis.

A presentation at the 2002 International Conference on AIDS in Barcelona by Tourinho et al showed that although sexual activity was high and prison authorities claimed condom distribution, a quarter of prisoners had no access to condoms. Although Brazil has a national condom distribution strategy (in February 2007 condom dispensers were installed in some Brazilian schools), distribution in prisons is uneven according to press reports.

Back in 1998 Human Rights Watch described HIV and TB as reaching 'epidemic' levels in the Brazilian inmate population. It said at the time: 'By denying inmates proper treatment, the prison system not only endangers inmates' lives, it facilitates the transmission of such illnesses to the general population through conjugal visits and upon prisoners' release. Since prisoners are not entirely cut off from the world outside, the unchecked spread of disease among inmates represents a serious public health risk.

Argentina

There are 130,000 people living with HIV in Argentina according to UNAIDS, or 0.3% of the population, a figure lower than the US and not vastly higher than the UK's 0.2%. And yet

Argentina has the distinction of having the highest rate of HIV infection at a single prison ever recorded. Fifty per cent of prisoners at Caseras Penitentiary in Buenos Aires were infected with HIV in 1997. More recently as much as one-quarter of inmates in Argentinean prisons have been found to be HIV infected (Argentine Ministry of Health, 2004).

With a prison population of 54,000 (min of Justice 2004 and extremely high transmission rates of HIV among prisoners and drug users, the epidemic in Argentina means that the marginalised sections of the population continue to be highly vulnerable.

There has been an enormous rise in the use of 'pasta bas?.' crack cocaine in Argentina. Also known as 'paco', it is a chemical by-product of coca leaves left over from the production of cocaine, which has become popular in Argentina since the financial crash of 2001. Pasta bas? or paco sells for as little as 30 US cents a hit. Consequently the profile of HIV transmission has altered since 2001, as more addicts turn to smoking paco. In Buenos Aires for example injecting drug users accounted for only five per cent of new infections between 2003 and 2005 (Cohen 2006).

This drop in new infections has not been reflected in the mortality rate for HIV-positive drug users, which continues to be high. Researchers suggest injecting drug users have gone further underground and into the country's and become further marginalised, or into the prison population. (Rossi et al, 2006).

In 2002 at the *International Conference on AIDS* a study on risk reduction in Rosario Penitentiary (abstract no. F11880) reported that drug use in Argentinean prisons is a hidden problem. In 2001 an innovative programme run by the Argentinean Harm Reduction Association (ARDA) and the Drug Abuse and AIDS Advanced Study Center (CEADS) began in the city's prisons.

The programme involved, for the first time in Argentina, harm reduction interventions related to drugs. The campaign used prisoners' language: "Si you are inside, no, you don't have a reason not to care", to convey information about drugs, injection use, tattoos, using of condoms, distribution of condoms, and workshops where disinfection techniques and delivering of bleach is involved.

ARDA/CEADS say that one outcome of the project was that they obtained a resolution from the Regional Penitentiary System recommending free access to condoms in prisons. Although the programme says that needle exchanges are a non-starter in Argentina, they say this could be solved by education on disinfection techniques, something 'without antecedents' in the Argentinean jail system. However condom dispensers have now been allowed.

Honduras

A Honduran Health Ministry study published at the end of 2000, in which more than 2,000 inmates from the country's three biggest prisons submitted to blood testing showed that 6.8% of the sample was HIV-positive - suggesting almost 800 HIV-positive prisoners in a small country. This is five times the national prevalence rate. The prison population stood at 11,589 at December 2005 according to National Prison Authorities.

The HIV rate in the wider community is difficult to assess but appears to be growing; HIV prevalence in antenatal clinics were 1.4% in 2004; this was up to 3-4% in Valle de Sula region in 2006 (Ministry of Health). The epidemic seems especially severe among ethnic minorities in Honduras such as the garafuna people, descendants of west African slaves where prevalence rates of 8-14% have been found (Secretariat of Honduran health 1998).

Recently the Canadian Red Cross organisation has launched a pilot programme to educate the inmates of Comayagua Prison about HIV, how it is and is not transmitted and how to avoid it. The Honduras Prison system is woefully underfunded, housing the country's most neglected high risk group for HIV and AIDS, says the Red Cross.

'The general attitude is that these people have committed crimes against society, that they have to pay, and that they should pay in the worst way possible,' a warden told the Red Cross.

A Honduran Health Ministry 2004 study characterised conditions in Honduran prisons as 'deplorable.' 'The frequent outbreaks of violence and death that occur in these installations are a reflection of the subhuman conditions in which the Honduran population lives', said the study. The prison, built for 250, currently had 598 inmates. The Red Cross say that HIV and AIDS prevention was almost nonexistent in Honduran prison system before they went in, and with the support of the Canadian International Development Agency, launched its programme.

In July 2006 *Science* magazine reported a story of Father Alberto Gauci, a Catholic priest who is trying to help slow HIV infections at a men's prison in Juticalpa, Honduras. Gauci is on a mission   to build a new prison in Juticalpa, where he runs an HIV and AIDS orphanage and hospice.

The existing prison, built more than 100 years ago for 90 inmates, currently holds more than 400 men who sleep at least two to a bunk. More than five per cent are 'known to have AIDS', says *Science*. In December 2005, no HIV tests or anti-HIV drugs were available. "The church has to play a role because people have lost all hope with politicians here," says Gauci, "Illness is spreading in the prison in a very accelerated way."

References

Aceijasd et al, HIV and IDUs in South America, 2004

AIDS Epidemic Update, unprotected sex between men, 2006

Argentine Ministry of Health Inmates in prison with HIV, 2004

Argentine Ministry of justice, prison population 2004

Belize Ministry of health, HIV seroprevalence in Inmates at the Kolbe Foundation Central Prison, June 2005

Biancarelli, TB in prisons, Brazil Journal of Microbiology

Bravo-Garcia et al, sex between men, Mexico, 2006

Burrattini M N, et al, Correlation between HIV and HCV in Brazilian Prisoners: evidence for parental transmission inside prisons, 2001

Caiaffa et al, incarceration and unprotected sex in Brazilian prisons, 2006

Cohen, new infections among drug users in Buenos Aires, 2006

Comissao Parlamentar Inquerito, TB in Brazilian Prisons,

Craviato P, patterns of heroin Consumption in a jail on the Northern Mexican border, barriers to treatment, 2003

Epidemiology and Infection133, 2005, Hepatitis and HIV in Durango prison Mexico,

Fonseca et al, crack cocaine brazil, 2006

Hiv rates in pregnant women screened at Tijuana Hospital, Mexico, JAIDS, jan, 2006

Honduran Ministry of health, HIV sample among Honduran prisoners, 2000

Magis Rodriguez et al, HIV rate among injecting drug users in Tijuana, 2005

MAP 2000, HIV in IDUs Sao Paulo region, Brazil

Ministry of Justice Brazil, prison population, 1995-2003

Panos Institute, sexual activity in Brazilian jails

Patterson et al, HIV rate among female sex workers, Mexico, 2006

Risk reduction at Roasario Prison Argentina, Int'l Conf on AIDS, 2002 (abstract F11880)

Science Magazine - Gangs/HIV in Central America and Mexico ??

Science magazine, new prison in Juticalpa, Honduras, July 2006

Strazzz I et al, The Vulnerability of Brazilian female Prisoners to HIV Infection, Sao Paulo University

Tourinho et al, Condom distribution in Brazilian Prisons, Int'l Conf AIDS, 2002

UNAIDS 2006 national HIV prevalence

UNAIDS Fact Sheet Argentina HIV prevalence in Buenos Aires Province

WHO, Belize national HIV prevalence, 2005

The Caribbean

The Caribbean has the highest percentage of population living with HIV outside of Sub-Saharan Africa, according to UNAIDS figures. At the beginning of 2006, 333,000 people were living with HIV in the Caribbean. Haiti and the Dominican Republic, the two countries sharing the Island of Hispaniola, accounted for 85% of this figure.

The total prison population for the region is around 105,000, (including Cuba where estimates vary wildly and with no official figures; the World Prison List 2006 estimates 55,000 prisoners in Cuba). Incarceration rates are much higher than western Europe.

HIV surveys of prisons in six small Eastern Caribbean countries in 2004/05, Antigua and Barbuda, Dominica, Grenada, St Kitts and Nevis, St Lucia, and St Vincent and the Grenadines, showed rates ranging from a low of 2.0% to a high of 4.1%. The countries were surveyed by the Caribbean Epidemiology Centre (CAREC), January 2007 report. HIV infections in prisons of these islands are around three times higher than in the wider populations.   In the Dominican Republic HIV in prisons, according to COPRESIDA, the Dominican HIV agency, was 19%.

Behind the figures though, prisoners and health and prison authorities face desperate conditions on most islands. Many of the regions jails are breeding grounds for a range of conditions, including HIV, Hepatitis C and TB.

Complex and little understood

The frequency of sex between men and injecting drug use in the wider Caribbean community are reported to be comparatively low, but homophobia and social taboos means that the problem may be larger than identified. UNAIDS reports that, of the Caribbean countries that submitted data for its 2006 global report, over three-quarters had laws that "may hinder the provision of prevention and treatment services to vulnerable and high-risk populations such as those in the prison system."

In Jamaica such an environment contributed to the 'Condom riots' in two Jamaican prisons in 1997 which still leaves a shadow over HIV prevention work on the Island.

Many Caribbean countries share common traits in terms of routes to HIV transmission. Unprotected heterosexual sex is the major driver and intravenous drug use is not as important a factor as in neighbouring regions. However in Puerto Rico and Bermuda IV drug use is highly significant factor in transmission. In Puerto Rico, in the wider population, HIV prevalence among injecting drug users has been found to be 30-45% *(Monitoring the AIDS Pandemic 2000)*.

Internal migration within the Caribbean is a factor, and many of the region's prisons house large numbers of non-nationals. In the Bahamas and Turks and Caicos Islands 25% of HIV cases are from Haitian migrant workers (Bahamas Ministry of Health, TCI Surveillance Evaluation).

Tourism-dependant economies are also among the most affected. Sex workers, and its occupational risk of prison, are among the most vulnerable. The 'Hanki Panki' sex workers in the Dominican Republic and Barbados and the 'Beach Boys' in Jamaica are a well-documented, potentially at risk population. (COPRESEDA, CAREC)

These factors contribute to a complex and little understood picture. Inadequate surveillance is a barrier to greater understanding of the epidemic in the region and this is particularly true for high risk groups including the inmates of prisons in the Caribbean.

The CAREC conclusion to its 2007 report reads; "it is imperative that prevention programmes must be tailored to high risk groups. This is going to require us as a region to divorce personal/moral issues from decision making and employ ethical and public health principles to our practices."

Haiti

Haiti has the highest number of people living with HIV - 190,000, a national HIV prevalence of 3.8%, according to UNAIDS in 2006. However new infection rates overall have decreased in recent times: the Haitian Health Ministry recently claimed they had halved in the last ten years.

Rated as the poorest country in the western hemisphere, Haiti has improved condom supply (15m in 2003 compared to 1m in 1992; *Science* magazine 2006). Organisations such as Zanmi Lasante have provided antiretroviral care through decentralised primary care services, bypassing the crisis-plagued government. It is doubtful to most observers that health care in Haiti's prisons have followed suit.

In November 2005 the Haitian prison population stood at 3,670, a rate of 43 per 100,000 (US State Dept Human Rights Report). Conditions in Haiti's prisons are severe, infectious diseases, particularly tuberculosis, are frequent - the Amnesty International report 2004; "Conditions in prisons and other places of detention were harsh and in many cases amounted to inhuman and degrading treatment. Overcrowding was commonplace. Several prisons across the country had not been repaired after they were attacked and partially or totally destroyed during the rebellion earlier in the year.'

Haitian HIV and AIDS activists point to the absence of any legislation to regulate the status of people with HIV and AIDS. Although a bill on the rights of people living with HIV has been pending before the health committee of the Haitian parliament, this is yet to be ratified because of political instability.

According to the Panos Institute, the absence of a legislature to help enforce the national strategy means that on the ground, much work, such as in preventing HIV and AIDS in prisons, remains stalled. "We set up a programme to combat HIV and AIDS among prison inmates that should have started in January 2004. But it has been postponed to due to the political instability," Pierre Esperance, who leads the National Coalition for the Defence of Haitians' Rights, told Panos.

According to the Health through Walls charity their primary focus has been the National Penitentiary, Haiti's largest prison facility, located in the capital Port-au-Prince. The prison holds approximately 2,000 prisoners. Since 2001 Health through Walls has visited the prison every two months bringing donations of medications and other equipment. Responding to a request from the medical director of prisons, one of the first projects was the establishment of a laboratory in the prison for the diagnosis of tuberculosis. Training on specimen collection, analysis, and diagnosis was provided to the prison health care staff. Antiretroviral provision is unknown - in the wider community ARVs are only reaching 12% of the population. (WHO)

General health and nutrition standards are still poor according to a report in the *New York Times* in January 2007. A newly released investigation into a deadly outbreak of Beriberi in Haiti's National Penitentiary uncovered evidence that the combination of the manufacturing process used in US processed rice and the traditional Haitian rice cooking method has been killing poor young men behind bars and leaving others morbidly ill through lack of vitamins B1 and B2. According to prison authorities they had tried to distribute Vitamin B supplements, they were aware of the Beriberi outbreak, but the prison never had enough to go around the inmates nor regular supplies.

Jamaica

In Jamaica an HIV diagnosis in the prison system is a dire prospect. Unprotected sex between men and homosexuality within the wider Jamaican community are the source of stigma, neglect, violence and homophobia. This discrimination is magnified within the Jamaican prisons system. Such attitudes combine to make HIV education and prevention in prisons a volatile issue. The country still reverberates from the 'condom riots' of the summer of 1997 which saw 16 inmates murdered after four days of rioting.

Jamaica has a population of 2.6 million and 1.5% of the adult population, 22,000 people, is living with HIV. The two main prisons on the island, St Catherine's District Prison and Kingston General Penitentiary, remain severely overcrowded, having been built for 650 and 850 inmates respectively but currently housing approximately 1225 and 1378. The total prison population in mid 2006 was 5,000 (World Prison Population List 2006).

conditions in Jamaican prisons are generally desperate, cruel or degrading according to Amnesty International

HIV prevalence in prisons is estimated at 12% (World Bank/Pan American Journal of Public Health 2004), a very high level for the Caribbean. Despite this, in June 2006 Jamaica decided not to distribute condoms in prisons, according to the Caribbean Net News. The decision came after Health Minister, Horace Dalley, called for condoms to be distributed to all correctional institutions to stem the spread of AIDS.

The Jamaican government had been divided over this issue. The Health Ministry believed condoms would help prevent HIV and AIDS in penal institutions, but the National Security Ministry, which has responsibility for prisons; disagreed, arguing it would encourage sexual activity. Both ministries met to settle the matter and an agreement was reached not to distribute condoms. Violence has broken out in the past over mere suggestions that men have sex with men in the facilities,

The Dominican Republic

Sharing the Island of Hispaniola with Haiti, the Dominican Republic has HIV rates estimated at 1.1% (66,000 according to CAREC). Compared to Haiti whose infection rate is over 3%. However access to antiretrovirals is even more difficult to obtain in the Dominican Republic than in neighbouring Haiti (Science July 2006, vol 313). The hotels and casinos of the capital city, Santo Domingo, are a destination for many tourists and the sex trade is booming, as are HIV prevalence rates among sex workers; the Dominican Ministry of Health estimates that this group has an HIV rate of 3.6%, but some researchers put the levels nearer 11% (Cohen 2006).

The prison population has an HIV incidence of 19% says CAREC, the highest recorded in the Caribbean and a huge inflation of the problem in the wider community. Beyond this estimate surveillance in the public health sector in Dominica is very weak.

An insight into the difficulties faced by health work in the prison systems of the Caribbean was provided by Dr John May of the Health through Walls charity which supplies expertise and antiretrovirals to prisons in the region. La Victoria, a prison in Santa Domingo, has a population exceeding 4,000 prisoners. The rate of drug-resistant tuberculosis is known to be one of the highest in the world here, where prisoners jam together against the bars of narrow cell doorways for air, but doctors at La Victoria prison don't have any idea how many prisoners have the virus according to Dr May.

Cuba

Prison conditions in Cuba are notoriously difficult to gauge. Propaganda and counter-propaganda present images ranging from a holiday home to a dumping ground. Prisoner numbers range from the 30,000 claimed by the government to the hundreds of thousands claimed by one US-based Cuban exile group. The World Prison Population list estimates 55,000 people in the Cuban prison system.

In Cuba, some people living with HIV in prisons have had a unique experience. During the 1970s 300,000 Cuban soldiers fought in Angola and other parts of Africa. Some who returned were HIV-positive and were shut away in sanatoriums, drawing worldwide criticism. Cuba stopped quarantining people in 1993 but still requires mandatory testing for groups such as pregnant women, army recruits and prison inmates. Cuba says its approach has been vindicated by the lowest rates of HIV infection in the Americas. UNAIDS says that at the end of 2005 Cuba had an HIV rate of 0.1% - half that of the UK

Cuba is the only country in the region with 100% access to ARVs, an achievement made easier by a low national HIV prevelance and local manufacture of generic versions of antiretrovirals.

Trinidad & Tobago

Trinidad and Tobago (T&T) is home to an estimated at 30,000 people living with HIV according to the UNGASS report for 2006, a prevalence of 3.2%, one of the highest in the region. Back in 1993 the prison rate was 4.9% (Doland et al). According to the National Prison Authority, T&T held 4,090 prisoners in mid 2006, a rate per 100,000 of 296.

Prison conditions at two of the three largest men's prisons generally met international standards concluded a report from the US Department of State released in 2003. However, conditions were poor at the Frederick Street Prison in Port of Spain, which dates from the 1830s. It was designed for 250 inmates but housed approximately 800 prisoners in December 2002. Diseases such as chickenpox, tuberculosis, HIV and AIDS, and viruses spread easily, and prisoners had to purchase their own medication.

Overcrowding was a problem in four out of eight facilities, where 2,290 inmates were housed in prisons built for 980. A new maximum security prison opened in late 1998 has a capacity of 2,450. However, at year's end, it was not fully operational, held approximately 800 inmates, and had done little to relieve the overcrowding in the detention system.

Guyana

Although situated on the South American mainland Guyana is part of the CARICOM, group of countries, and is ethnically and culturally closer to the Caribbean than Latin America.

The US Census Bureau of Population Department predicted Guyana's rate of population growth would be the lowest in the region because of deaths from AIDS. However there has been some stabilisation in the epidemic. The PEPFAR report on Guyana for December 2006 reported that a survey of 4,400 pregnant women showed a prevalence of 1.5%. The last time the survey was carried out in 2004 it had been 2.3%. In the late 1990s the rate was around 7%.

Reflecting the lack of data in the wider community, the Guyanese prison population's rate of transmission and subsequent treatment is unknown. However some initiatives have been developed to help the country's 1,500 prisoners.

Through aid from PEPFAR an HIV counselling and testing service had been set up at Mazarani Prison starting in January 2007. In 2006 the GUM clinic in Guyana had started a testing and treatment prison programme working with the national TB programme. Monthly prison visits were undertaken by a doctor and pharmacist and twice monthly visits by counsellors for testing prisoners. The programme includes testing prison officers. The testing uses 'fast result' tests, followed by TB screening, if positive, before antiretrovirals are prescribed.

The University of Guyana started a workshop programme in March 2006 called "Slashing Stigma" at the Camp Street Prison. The four-week project aims to eliminate stigma and discrimination against people living with HIV and AIDS. On completion of the course each participant will be given a certificate of completion and will be asked to sign the petition to end the stigma against people living with HIV and AIDS.

References

AIDS Presidential Council of the Dominican Republic (COPRESIDA), HIV prevalence in prisons report, Jan, 2007

Amnesty International Report, conditions in Haiti's prisons, 2004

Bahamas Ministry of health, TCI Surveillance Evaluation, Haitian migrants in prison

Boadle A, Cuba fights HIV with ARVs not quarantine, Reuters News Service, Nov 2005

Caribbean Epidemiology Centre (CAREC) regional HIV prison, prevalence, Jan 2007

Caribbean Net News, Jamaica refuses condoms in prisons, June 2006

Cohen J, condom supply in Haiti, Science magazine, 2006

Cohen, HIV prevalence among Dominican sex workers, 2006

COPRESIDA, CAREC, male sex workers and risk of HIV transmission

Cuban Prison Population, World Prison List, 2006

Djumalieva D, et al, crack cocaine use Trinidad & Tobago, International Journal STD/AIDS, 2002

Doland K et al, Trinidad & Tobago, HIV in prisons, 2004

Dominican Ministry of health, HIV prevalence among sex workers, 2006

Guyana Chronicle HIV/AIDS in prisons, Guyana, October 27, 2005

Haitian Health Ministry, national HIV prevalence, 2006

Health Through Walls NGO, HIV/TB treatment in Haiti prisons, 2006

Human Rights Watch, Jamaican condom riots, 2004

Jamaica, Dominican Republic

Monitoring the AIDS Pandemic, HIV among injecting drug users, Puerto Rico, 2000

National Prison Authority, Trinidad & Tobago, prison population, mid, 2006

New York Times, beriberi outbreak in Haitian prison, Jan, 2007

Palm Beach Post, conditions and HIV treatment in La Victoria Prison, Dominican Republic, October 2006

Pan Caribbean Partnership Against AIDS (PANCAP) Institute, Cuba manufactures generic ARVs

Panos Institute, prevention of HIV in prisons, Haiti, 2005

PEPFAR report, HIV survey of pregnant women in Guyana December 2006

Reuters News Agency, Jamaican condom riots, 2004

Stabroek News, HIV prevalence in Guyana prisons, August 6, 2006

UNAIDS Country File, Haiti, national HIV, 2006

UNGASS Report, Trinidad & Tobago, national HIV prevalence, 2006

US State Department Human Rights Report, Haitian prison population, 2005

US State Department Report, conditions in Trinidad & Tobago prisons, 2003

World Prison Population List, Cuba prisoners, 2006

Sub-Saharan Africa

For the purposes of clarity this section will divide reports on Sub Saharan African prisons by region: South, South-East, East, West and Central Africa, and by country - where information exists.

TB/HIV in Africa a 'noxious synergy'

See **HIV and Tuberculosis** for more information

The lethal combination of HIV and TB in Sub-Saharan Africa meets an ideal breeding ground in the region's prisons. In South Africa 70% of people living with HIV also carry tuberculosis.

"Together TB and HIV display a noxious synergy that has led to explosive outbreaks of TB in areas of high HIV prevalence" reported Paul Farmer in a WHO report on multi-drug resistant TB. Farmer identifies prisons as one of the sites for the 'strikingly non-random occurrences' of MDR-TB.

Southern Africa

South Africa

With the highest number of HIV infections in any country and one of the largest prison populations in the world, South Africa's 240 prisons continue to be 'factories' for HIV transmission.

Accurate surveillance of HIV in South African prisons is notoriously unreliable, though there have been some studies. One such found that approximately 41% of the inmates in South Africa's "overburdened" prison system are HIV-positive, according to a 2003 study conducted by the nongovernmental Institute for Security Studies (http://www.iss.co.za/).

It showed that since 1995, reported cases of HIV and AIDS in South African prisons have risen by 750%, and the number of natural deaths in prison has risen by about 600% over the same period. According to the South African Press Association, about 90% to 95% of the natural deaths were believed to have been AIDS.

Maria Mabena, acting director of health at the Department of Correctional Services (DCS) said that there were 5,285 HIV cases in the prison system in 2002, compared with 623 in 1995.

Between 1996 and 2000, departmental statistics show that the system has experienced a 40% increase in the number of HIV and AIDS cases, Mabena said. She added that the DCS is realising the importance of giving prisoners access to condoms, counselling, HIV testing and treatment. However, the South African government's policy of "discouraging use of antiretroviral drugs in the public sector" has not helped the effort to treat the country's large HIV-positive prison population.

Despite this situation advocates of access to antiretrovirals have seen a number of breakthroughs over the last 18 months - although they say these moves by the South African Correctional Services will come too late to stem the terribly high mortality rate among South Africa's 157,000 prisoners (World Prison List 2006).

Prisoners go to High Court for ARVs

The case began in March 2006 when a group of South African prisoners at the Durban-Westville prison staged a hunger strike to protest at the lack of availability of antiretroviral drugs. Fifteen of the protesting prisoners then launched a court action claiming that their CD4 counts were at a level when ARV treatment would normally begin.

The South African government called the protest 'opportunistic' and said it had plans to introduce ARVs into prisons. Since the effective replacement of health minister Manto Tshabalala-Msimang by Deputy President Phumzile Mlambo-Ngcuka as head of the country's AIDS strategy at the beginning of 2007, ARV provision has accelerated outside prisons in South Africa and WHO now estimates that 330,000 of six million south Africans who are HIV-positive are receiving ARVs or about a quarter of those who need them.

With the help of the AIDS Law Project at Witwatersrand University and the Treatment Action Campaign (TAC), the case brought to court claimed that the correctional service Department had failed to provide the 15 inmates with the necessary drug treatment. Prison hospitals are not on the list of authorised institutions to distribute antiretrovirals.

In June the Durban High Court ruled that the prisons department must remove restrictions on access to HIV and AIDS drug treatment in the Westville prison and to take steps in ensuring that all prisoners who need ARVs are immediately assessed for treatment. The government appealed against the ruling and the order was suspended.

In July the AIDS Law Project, acting on behalf of the prisoners and TAC, argued that it would be 'outrageous' to allow the order to remain suspended until the appeal is heard as this could take up to a year. Given the health of the prisoners the case, the issue was one of life and death, said the Project. On the 25th July Judge Thimba Pillay, who made the original decision, ordered that the judgement be implemented forthwith. Pillay added that on the government's own estimates of HIV mortality in prisons, nine prisoners per month would have died since 2005 of AIDS related illness.

On the 6th August 2006 one of the group identified as 'MM' had died of AIDS related infections after drugs were provided too late, according to TAC.

In September 2006 an appeal was refused by the High Court in Durban ruling against the Department of Correctional Services Department of the South African government. The Correctional Service had been ordered by the courts to supply HIV antiretrovirals to inmates in Westville Prison Durban. Only four facilities are accredited prison based ARV sites out of 240 prisons; all the other 240 South African prisons transport prisoners to local hospitals for ARV treatment.

In October 2006 the Correctional Services said it aimed to test 12,500 prisoners and prison warders over two months so they could plan treatment interventions for inmates with HIV. The plan was met with a mixed response by AIDS activists; the AIDS Law Project welcomed further information on HIV prevalence in prisons, but said that the survey did not address the fact that

drug therapy was needed immediately to save lives. The initiative has funding from PEPFAR.

Jali Commission

A much anticipated insight into South Africa's healthcare in its prisons came In October 2006 from the Jali Commission, which investigated corruption and maladministration in the South African prison system, It reported after hearing from 516 witnesses over two years. The reported reminded the world that 'The rights of prisoners are also enshrined in the Bill of Rights of the South African Constitution.'

After sacking or sending to trial dozens of guards and executives from the South African Prison system, the report was published and it made harrowing reading. The report looked at sexual violence in prisons, where it admitted sex was a tradable commodity, with young prisoners sometimes sold to the highest bidder and with warders themselves implicated in many of the sexual assaults. Abuse, said the report, was 'rife.'

"If the department keeps on ignoring the fact that sexual abuse is rife in our prisons and that there is an extreme likelihood that prisoners that are exposed to violent, unprotected sex would in all likelihood contract HIV, then it is effectively, by omission, imposing a death sentence on vulnerable prisoners."

Evidence also revealed that homophobia is a very real issue among prison warders whose prejudice impacted negatively on how they protected prisoners who are sexually abused by their co-prisoners.

The report revealed that 40% of prisoners are incarcerated for less than one year and that on average 25,000 prisoners are released every month. The enquiry also briefly looked at medical parole, for prisoners on their 'deathbed' with chronic disease. The report recommends diversity training on cultural differences and homophobia as well as screening for vulnerable targets.

Namibia

A 30-year-old law in Namibia prohibiting homosexuality is preventing condom distribution in the country's prisons and hindering HIV prevention efforts, according to HIV and AIDS advocates in Namibia (South Africa's Mail & Guardian (http://www.mg.co.za/articlePage.aspx?articleid=260457&area=/insight/insight__africa/), 2006). Namibia housed around 5,000 prisoners in 2001, the last time figures were available. National prevalence for HIV was put at 19.6% in 2005.

According to Namibian officials, condom distribution in prisons would promote sex between men, and is outlawed under the 1977 Criminal Procedures Act. Ignatius Mainga, a spokesperson for the country's Ministry of Safety and Security's prison services, said, "By giving (prisoners) a condom, you are telling them to go ahead and do it." Mainga added that the "majority" of cases involving men who have sex with men in prison are consensual and that inmates do not want condoms because they do not "want to be seen as having sex with other men."

However, Michaela Hubscle, former deputy minister at the now-closed Ministry of Prisons and Correctional Services, said that instances of rape still occur between men in prison and condoms are needed to protect inmates. "We are sitting on a time bomb," he said. "The prevalence rate will increase if we do not protect those who enter prison HIV-negative, and those who are positive from re-infection."

Lesotho

Lesotho, a country of 1.85 million people, had around 3,000 prison inmates in 2005, according to the Lesotho Prison Authority, 1,000 of which are in Maseru Central Prison, a prison designed to hold 700, in the country's capital. Adult HIV prevalence in Lesotho has remained stable but high according to UNAIDS with almost one in four living with HIV (UNAIDS 2006).

Matete Mahao, Lesotho's divisional commander of correctional services, reported on the Africa News 24 website in April 2005 that at least one prisoner dies weekly from AIDS related diseases at this, Lesotho's largest prison. He said that the main contributing factor to the deaths and the spread of HIV and AIDS was sex between men, which, he said, was not a new phenomenon in Lesotho's male prisons.

Botswana

A project to screen prisoners and guards for tuberculosis in Botswana has implications for those with HIV. Eighty-six per cent of TB patients in the country are also infected with HIV (Samarandi et al).

The Study (Notha)was the first to determine the prevalence of TB among Botswana prisoners and prison guards, and to investigate the risk factors for TB in prisoners. Studies in African prisons have found TB rates five to ten times higher than local/national rates. Screening was offered at four prisons in the prison system in the capital Gaborone during 2002. Those who agreed to participate were administered a questionnaire in English or Setswana for demographic, treatment history and symptom information.

Three sputum samples were requested from any prisoners or guards reporting cough for smear microscopy and culturing. Chest x-rays obtained for anyone with a cough who was unable to produce sputum samples.

1027 prisoners (or 88% of the prison population) were screened, including 20 who were on treatment at the time the screening began. Ninety-six per cent of the prisoners were male. The median age was 26 years. Eighty-three per cent of prisoners were incarcerated for the first time. The median duration of incarceration was 15 months with a wide range from 1 day to 22 years.

Out of 1027 prisoners, 509, or nearly half, reported a cough. Sputum was obtained on 371 (73%). Thirty-three chest radiographs were obtained on those with a cough who were unable to produce sputum. None was counted as a clinical case.

A total of 41 cases, or four per cent of prisoners, were identified with active TB: 19 prisoners were identified during screening, including eight who were smear-positive and eleven who were smear-negative but culture-positive. Twenty were already on TB treatment at the time the screening began. The prevalence of active TB in prisoners was found to be nearly 3.8% (3797 cases/100,000 population).

Three factors remained significant in the same model. Incarceration for more than six months was associated with a more than five-fold increased risk of TB when compared with those incarcerated for six months or less. Being a first time offender in residence in one particular prison was associated with nearly four times the increased risk of TB compared with residence in one of the other large facilities.

Results for prison guards were similar to those of prisoners. 263 out of 288, (91%) of prison guards were screened. Only 45, or 17% reported any cough, and sputum was obtained on 25 (56%) of those with cough. A total of seven cases of TB were identified of which five were on treatment at the time of screening. Two new cases, both smear-negative but culture-positive, were identified through screening. No new cases were identified through chest radiography.

Dr Notha comments: "This project found critically high rates of TB among prisoners and guards in Botswana. The two-month incidence of 1850 among prisoners was nearly 18 times the two-month incidence in the general population. The two-month incidence among guards was more than seven times the two-month incidence in the general population.

"Longer incarceration has been associated with a risk of TB in other prison studies and suggests that transmission within prison settings is causing high rates of TB.

"Several recommendations follow from these findings," concluded Dr. Notha. "First, a programme to screen for TB should be initiated. This should include prisoners at prison entry or transfer. However, since TB was associated with the duration of incarceration, screening at entry alone may be insufficient and screening on a periodic or ongoing basis should also be considered. Prison guards should also be screened on a periodic basis. Contacts such as cellmates of newly identified smear-positive cases should be evaluated for active disease.

South-eastern Africa

Zambia

Zambia had a prison population of 14,000 at the end of 2005, according to national prison authorities. Two pieces of research have stood out in a country with a very high HIV prevalence: "Behind walls", a study of HIV risk behaviours and seroprevalence in prisons in Zambia, and a study in the British Medical Journal (Simooya).

These papers reported on a survey of HIV seroprevalence and risk behaviours in Zambian prisons. The prevalence rate of HIV was 27%, compared to a national average of 19%. The authors said: "Some inmates may be getting infected inside prison. Only four per cent of inmates agreed in one-to-one interviews that they had sexual relations with other men, but indirect questioning suggested that the true figures were much larger. No condoms were available in any prison."

Seventeen per cent of prisoners had been tattooed in prison, and 63% reported sharing razor blades. The report said that in 2004 alone some 449 inmates had died of AIDS related illness.

A 2003 study at Kamfinsa prison, which houses 10,000 male and female inmates, put the HIV incidence level at 24% after 200 inmates were tested (Pupwe).

Reiterating the human cost of HIV in prison, a controversy took place in 2004 in Zambia concerning the release of prisoners in the advanced stages of AIDS. Zarina Geloo from Lusaka reported to *The Real Cost Of Prisons*: weblog that since late 2001, more than 300 sick inmates have been freed by President Levy Mwanawasa on compassionate grounds. The Commissioner of Prisons, Jethro Mumbuwa, says that Zambia's jails simply lack the resources to look after convicts who are seriously ill.

Many of the former inmates had been given life sentences for serious offences, and protests from the victims of their crimes might have been expected. But surprisingly, some of the strongest opposition to the releases has come from the prisoners' families. "Why, why give me this shell?" asked the wife of HIV-positive ex-prisoner Samson Nkumba (not his real name). "They (the government) must keep him, because I cannot do what they have failed to do. I cannot afford ARVs," she added.

At present, Zambian courts do not take HIV status into consideration when sentencing. There are no voluntary counselling and testing facilities in prisons, and HIV tests are only conducted when a prisoner falls ill repeatedly.

Zambia's Permanent Human Rights Commission insists that no prisoner should be forced to test for HIV. Instead, it recommends that prisons be reformed to ensure that HIV-positive inmates receive the treatment needed to keep them alive.

Mozambique

Mozambique housed approximately 10,000 prisoners out of a population of 19 million at the end of 2004, according to the US State Department of Human Rights. The country's HIV prevalence was 12%.

In September 2006 a challenge came to prevailing attitudes to HIV in the Mozambique prison system. The chief medical officer of the Machava General Hospital, Dr Noorjehan Abdul Magid, told theUnited Nations Integrated Region Information Network (IRIN/PlusNews); "Of the tests I've conducted, I've established that although certain inmates were infected before they were detained, the majority had been infected in prison."

Dr Magid, who treats most of the HIV-positive inmates in Mozambique's Machava Central Prison, added: "Homosexual relations are a common practice existing inside prisons."

Homosexuality is taboo in Mozambican society and officials at Machava prison in the capital, Maputo, have refused to distribute condoms, saying there was no homosexual activity in the jail. However according to staff and inmates who talked to *IRIN/PlusNews*, sex between prisoners is a reality, and little is being done to prevent it.

"Some of the younger inmates are forced to sleep with the older ones in exchange for food and protection," said Júlio Vicente Mundai, 41, a mechanic serving an eight-year sentence for stealing a car. Mundai discovered his positive status after taking a voluntary test in jail. Because prison regulations prohibit conjugal visits, many HIV-positive inmates said they were infected before they were arrested to avoid admitting to homosexual activity in prison.

Malawi

According to UNAIDS, HIV prevalence in Malawi is at 15%. Malawi, with its Banja la Mtsogolo (Family of the Future) programme, aims to educate over 5,000 prisoners in 21 jails about HIV. The initiative also incorporates treatment for prisoners who have sexually-transmitted infections.   In 2003 a proposal in the Malawian parliament proposing the introduction of condoms in the country's 23 prisons was met with hostility from Malawi's evangelical church leaders. Zomba central prison has been highlighted by Amnesty International for abuses involving young offenders, some of them children, incarcerated with adults. Amnesty said in the past the 49% of people treated at Zomba tested positive for HIV.

East Africa

Uganda

A study in 2004 by the Ugandan Prison Service and the Mulago Medical School revealed that 40% of deaths in Ugandan prisons were due to tuberculosis. A further 20% of deaths were attributed to AIDS. The survey was commissioned by the European Community. Overcrowding and unsanitary conditions were cited as major factors.

In 2006 the *Behind the Mask* website for gay and lesbian issues in Africa reported on the case of Benjamin Buloba who died in Luzira prison in 2004. Although it was widely suspected he died of internal bleeding because of rape, the official cause of death was respiratory failure.

Mary Kaddu, the Ugandan assistant commissioner for prisons, told the *Ugandan Monitor* newspaper: "We are carrying out a study to ascertain whether homosexuality is a myth or reality in Ugandan prisons." Although the Ugandan national AIDS policy prescribes accessibility of condoms to sexually active people, Kaddu conceded that condoms were not available for prisoners, saying that male and female prisoners were kept in separate facilities.

A community based organisation has taken it upon themselves to help vulnerable women and prevent the spread of HIV in Ugandan prisons.

Kenya

Kenya's HIV prevalence is 6.7% to 9%, according to UNAIDS, but it is estimated that the HIV rate in the drug injecting population is 68-88%. In Mombasa a seroprevalence study among injecting drug users found that 49.5% were HIV-positive and 70% had hepatitis C. (Ndetei).

At Lodawar Prison in the remote Turaka region of Kenya inmates are being educated about HIV through films, which avoid the problem of illiteracy rates in the region. Ruth Eripete, a counsellor with a mobile voluntary counselling and testing (VCT) unit run by Merlin, a UK-based healthcare NGO, said one of the benefits of educating prisoners was that after their release they would carry the message to people in remote areas of northern Kenya, which government and relief agencies often could not reach because of poor roads and sporadic ethnic clashes.

The prison, built to hold 112 inmates, now regularly accommodates more than 300 prisoners accused of crimes ranging from murder to cattle rustling and petty theft. Merlin has visited the prison twice to conduct HIV and AIDS education and provide VCT.

West Africa

Ghana

New research into HIV prevalence has come from three prisons in Ghana that has uncovered HIV rates of 19% among inmates and 8.5% among prison officers out of those who participated in the study (Adeji). This is in a country with a relatively low rate of national HIV and AIDS prevalence, put at 2.3% in 2005 by UNAIDS.

Overall, almost one in three of the inmates in the study reported having sex with other men, inside or outside the prison, while a small percentage said they injected drugs. Tattooing might also be a cause of HIV transmission. It appeared, say the researchers, that many of the inmates had acquired the virus in prison and although a majority of them had been imprisoned for 10 years, none had reached the symptomatic stage of AIDS. This, researchers said, indicated relatively recent infection.

Nigeria

In November 2006 the HIV prevalence rate in Nigeria (http://english.peopledaily.com.cn/data/nigeria.html)'s prisons had reached 8.2%, far higher than the nation's average of 5.6%, according to Deputy Controller of Prisons of Nigeria Stella Orisakwe (Xinhua News Agency). By the end of 2005 Nigeria had a total prison population of 40,000 out of a population of 137 million (World Prison Population List).

Although, as in other parts of Sub-Saharan Africa, the HIV epidemic has been fuelled primarily by sexual transmission, injecting drug use is becoming more common. In Kana state and River State, Nigeria, prevalence in the wider community was 3.8% to 7.7% among drug users in the same states the rate was 14.3% (Lawal).

Ivory Coast

In March 2007 Agence France Presse reported that the AIDS epidemic was fuelling the spread of tuberculosis in Côte d'Ivoire. In 2006, there were 21,204 TB cases detected in Cote d'Ivoire, compared with 16,031 in 2002, and the cases were connected to the country's high HIV and AIDS prevalence, according to the latest statistics. In addition, TB incidence in the country is 393 cases per 100,000 people, compared with the average of 290 cases per 100,000. However, the prevalence of HIV in the country's prisons remains unclear.

Central Africa

Burundi

In Burundi, Prisoners at Mpimba Prison have formed an association for inmates living with the HIV virus. The

'Turemshanye' (Support One Another) association got together in January 2007 to give help to access food, ARVs and psychological support. Turemshanye has 60 members. The Turemshanye organisation was also needed because many HIV-positive prisoners' families gave up on them, particularly when they were not expected to survive a long sentence.

The Mpimba jail was built to accommodate 800 prisoners but currently holds more than 3,000. Burundi holds 8,000 prisoners in 2005 out of a population of 6.2 million, according to the Burundi Ministry if Justice.

The Burundi chapter of the Society for Women against AIDS in Africa (SWAA) helps the prisoners with food. The women's organisation also provides ARVs, and twice a week brings a doctor to Mpimba to treat opportunistic infections. The government's treatment programme bypasses prisoners, and the group is now lobbying for inclusion in the national rollout.

Despite the existence of the 60-member Turemeshanye, Ndabihawe noted that stigma remained high in the jail and many inmates were reluctant to join the group, as this would confirm their HIV status to the rest of the prisoners. "Those who accept to come in the open have no choice," he said. "Rather than dying unattended, they accept their status."

"Some inmates may develop high-risk behaviour such as homosexuality," said a spokeswoman for SWAA, adding that poor living conditions forced some female inmates to sell sex for money. Condoms are not distributed by prison officials, but SWAA offers them to prisoners who request them, who are mostly female inmates.

Cameroon

A report in IRIN looked at the spread of HIV and TB in Cameroon prisons. According to a study by the German based group GTZ (2004) and the University of Yaoundé, an average of two people per cell was found to be living with TB at New Bell prison. New Bell is in the city of Douala which houses 3,000 inmates in a prison built to hold 700. The prison budget for medicines in 2004 was US$550 for the 3,000 inmates.

According to the researchers, HIV prevalence at New Bell increased to 12.1% in 2005 from 11.5% in 2004, although they warned because of stigma those figures might be higher. Although workers from the SunAIDS organisation enter the prison regularly for counselling and testing, and samples are tested at Douala hospital, the study called for quarantine facilities and diagnostic and treatment centres in the prisons of Cameroon.

An insight into the plight of homosexual menin the Cameroon prison system was related to *INRI/PlusNews* in October 2006. 'Alim' was one of 30 men arrested at a bar in Yaoundé in May 2005; Alim was one of nine men transferred to Yaoundé Central Prison with a one year prison sentence. Homosexuality is a crime under Cameroonian law. Alim died in the prison in October of 2005. He was HIV-positive before he entered the prison. The group of men claimed they had been raped and assaulted. Their advocate is bringing the matter to the Supreme Court.

International human rights groups provide aid in the form of medication and food for Cameroonian prisoners criminalised for their homosexuality but physical abuse continues, said the Association for the Defence of Homosexuals (ADEPHO).

Rwanda

Kigali Central Prison (KCP), in the capital of Rwanda, has the nation's highest number of HIV-positive prisoners, says a report by UNRI. "The prison holds more than five times the recommended capacity, with most inmates awaiting trial for crimes related to the 1994 genocide, in which the government estimates some 937,000 Tutsis and moderate Hutus were murdered. A national demographic health survey in 2005 found that three per cent of the Rwanda's eight million people were living with HIV. But 16.5% of women and 15% of men among KCP's 60,000 inmates

are HIV-positive, according to the National Commission for the Fight against HIV and AIDS (CNLS).

HIV-positive inmates say they were infected before they were jailed because Rwanda's prison regulations do not allow conjugal visits. Said one prisoner, "basically, men sleep with men."

There have also been reports of inmates engaging in sexual activity while working outside of the jail, and of prisoners bribing their guards to allow visits from family and friends. "I have come across men who have three-year-old biological kids, yet they have been in jail for 10 years," said journalist Sula Nuwamanya.

Rwanda does not provide prisoners with condoms, but Nathan Gasatura of CNLS acknowledged that "if you suspect there are sexual practices going on, then it would only be wise to provide them [inmates] with condoms".

Although prisoners do not receive ARVs, the authorities started paying more attention to HIV prevention and counselling about three years ago. The International Committee of the Red Cross (ICRC) informs prisoners about HIV and the dangers of high-risk behaviour, while the NGO Population Services International (PSI), a health NGO in low-income countries, offers voluntary counselling and testing (VCT), and trains peer educators to influence behaviour change and provide post-VCT counselling.

"With all the justice and reconciliation initiatives going on, thousands of genocide suspects are being released and returning to their towns and villages," Gasatura said. "What these people bring back to their communities is of much concern to us. We also look at it from the perspective that these are fellow Rwandans who need as much care as any one else."

References

GTZ/University of Yaoundé. HIV prevalence in New Bell Prison, Douala, Cameroon, 2004

Institute for Security Studies, HIV among South African prisoners, Feb 2003

IRIN Report - Kigali Central Prison, Rwanda, 2005

IRIN/PlusNews - HIV in Mozambique prison system, September 2006

IRIN/PlusNews - Homosexual criminalisation, Cameroon, October 2006

IRIN/PlusNews - United Nations World Food Programme, Burundi, November 2006

Jali Commission, conditions and treatment in South African prisons, Oct 2006

Lawal, R. UNDOC study on drugs and HIV/AIDS in Nigeria, 2003

Lesotho Prison Authority, prison population, 2005

Ministry of Safety and Security, condom distribution in Namibia prisons.

Ndetei, D. Study on the linkage between drug use and HIV/AIDS in Kenya, UNDOC, 2004

New Vision News, Sisters United - work in Luzira Prison, August 2006

Notha M, Rapid TB assessment in a prison system - Gaborone, Botswana, 2003

Pupweo O, HIV Incidence Kamfinsa Prison, Zambia. Int'l Conf on AIDS (Abstract c10950), 2004

Rwanda National Commission for the Fight Against HIV/AIDS (CNLS), demographic health survey, 2005

Samarandi et al, TB screening in Botswana, 2006

Simooya O et al. "Behind walls": a study of HIV risk behaviours and seroprevalence in prisons in Zambia. JAIDS, 15: 1741-1744, 2001

Simooya O, Sanjobo N. Study in Zambia showed that robust response is needed in prisons. British Medical Journal, 324(6 April): 850, 2002

South African Department of Correctional Services (DCS) HIV prevalence in prisons, 1996-2002

South African Press Association, AIDS deaths in S African prisons, Feb 2003

The Real Cost of Prisons weblog, Zambia - early release, 2004

Ugandan Monitor, Sex in Prisons, 2006

Ugandan Prison Service, TB/AIDS deaths in prison, 2004

UN Intelligence report/Plus news, S African Correctional Service ARV legal challenge, September 2006

UNAIDS - Ghana national HIV prevalence, 2005

UNAIDS - HIV Prevalence in Malawi, 2006

UNAIDS 2006, HIV prevalence, Namibia, 2006

World Prison List - Nigerian prison population, 2006

World Prison List, South Africa prison population, 2006

Xinhua News Agency - HIV/AIDS prevalence rate in Nigeria, November 2006

Asia

(including Iran)

In March 2007 Asian health officials at the United Nations called on the international community to increase its involvement in fighting the HIV and AIDS epidemic. More than 8.5 million people are living with HIV in the region, and about 630,000 people in the region died of AIDS-related illnesses last year. The UN ambassador from Mongolia briefed reporters: "HIV and AIDS is often overlooked compared to Africa.how many more infections do we need before we take action."

Adeeba Kamarulzaman of the Malaysian AIDS Council said that most people in the region with HIV, and most prisoners, are part of marginalised groups that do not receive adequate support such as commercial sex workers, men who have sex with men and injection drug users.

One worrying example is **Afghanistan**, where says the UNAUDS 2006 epidemic report, conditions are favourable for HIV's rapid spread. Evidence from a new study (Todd et al 2006) show that men in prison are at the nexus of this potential epidemic. Four per cent of IDUs have tested positive for HIV in Kabul, 54% had spent time behind bars and 32% had injected drugs in prison.

The 2006 Epidemic report from UNAIDS reports 'risk behaviour is commonplace in **Indonesia**'s prisons.' New studies have found HIV prevalence among inmates of 13% in West Java, 18% in Jakarta and 36% in Banten (Ministry of Health Indonesia). The growth rate of HIV infections has been highly disturbing; in 1998 there no recorded cases of HIV, then in 2002 40% of IDUs in rehabilitation centres in Jakarta were infected. Without doubt prisons in Indonesia are one of the major drivers of the epidemic in Indonesia. Not all of the regional developments in preventing HIV have been negative. There have been a number of initiatives, to prevent the spread of HIV into the general population, and to control and reduce HIV infections in vulnerable groups.

In **Taiwan** the Department of Health (DOH) began to provide methadone therapy for drug-addicted prison inmates in northern Taiwan in 2007. DOH data indicate 40,000 out of 60,000 inmates are incarcerated for drug-related crimes, and 6,000 are HIV-positive. Overall the harm-reduction efforts in Taiwan seem to be having major impact: The DOH started providing methadone therapy for HIV-infected drug addicts and launched a clean needle programme in other areas.

In **Cambodia,** with the highest HIV prevalence in the region, 1.6% of the population, there has a lot of important work with prevention in armed forces and sex workers. Prisons have been ignored and AIDS is the leading cause of death in Cambodian prisons according to a 2004 report. Official figures stated 15 and 20 deaths from AIDS in 2002 and 2003 respectively among prison inmates. LICADHO, the Cambodian League for the Promotion and Defence of Human Rights, said the numbers were definitely underestimated. Prison authorities do not make diagnoses of AIDS but list illness as symptoms, colds, sore throats, bronchitis. Even LICADOH's own medical officers who have access to prisons do not have the facility to carry out blood tests. Given these factors and the doubling of the prison population from 2,933 in December 1998 to 5,701 in December 2003, HIV in Cambodian prisons will continue to be a major health concern.

One feature of Asia has been the related epidemics of injection drug use and HIV and AIDS in cross border areas - The Golden Triangle being the prime starting point. Beyer and colleagues described a heroin trans-shipment route from the Golden Triangle of **Thailand**, **Myanmar** and **Laos** into **Vietnam**, **China**and finally **Hong Kong**. In the wake of the route lay injecting drug users increasingly infected with HIV. Inevitably many IDUs will spend time in a correctional facility.

Cross border patterns of HIV epidemiology are also seen between Northern Vietnam and Southern China. The HIV epidemic, here and in other Asian border regions is fuelled by complex patterns of small scale cross-border movement of drug dealers and drug users. Hammet and colleagues (JAIDS vol 38, Feb 2005) reported the first cross border HIV prevention project targeting IDUs where the same interventions are being implemented in both countries (see Vietnam below).

China

China has an estimated 1.5 million people in its 670 jails, according to the World Prison Population List. The country has approximately 840,000 HIV-positive people, of whom 80,000 have developed symptomatic AIDS. Yunnan Province in Southwest China is the worst hit region, followed by Henan Province, Xinjiang-Uighur region, Guangxi province and Guangdong province.

In December 2004 the Chinese Ministry of Health announced that it would start HIV testing among the country's prison population. The China News Agency reported that the Health Ministry worked with the Ministry of Justice to carry out the testing until March 2005.

If an inmate is found to be HIV-positive, the health authority test his family members, the Ministry said. HIV-positive inmates and AIDS patients will receive proper treatment, it added.

One of the few methodologically sound studies of HIV in China's prison system was reported at the International AIDS Conference in 2002 (Bao). The study reported that between 1991 and 1999, 12,998 serum samples were taken among the offenders serving in the Shanghai prison system. Thirty HIV-positive samples were identified, with a resulting prevalence rate of 0.23%. The majority of the positives were from among inmates of Xinjiang origin and Uighur nationality.

The progression of the disease within the Shanghai Prison System can be divided into two stages, the study concluded. The first stage (1991-1997) included a few individuals with foreign associations who were infected outside of the prisons and then imported the virus into the prison environment. During the second stage intravenous drug users began to appear HIV-positive in the surveillance records.

China: Guangdong

In November 2005 *China.org,cn,* part of the Chinese state controlled media, announced that two separate prisons were to be built in Guangdong province in southern China, by the Guangdong Bureau of Justice specifically to house inmates with HIV. Officials were quoted as saying 514 HIV 'carriers' and 20 patients with AIDS were serving in Guangdong prisons.

Such a strategy was ruled out by the Chinese Ministry of Foreign Affairs, according to Agence France Presse. In 2005 the government said it would improve existing facilities, provide free examinations and better medical care. It was claimed in late 2005 that there were around 1,000 AIDS cases among prisoners in the state.

Statistics from Guangdong Provincial Bureau of Public Health indicated that the number of AIDS patients in Guangdong reached 5,051 by the end of 2004. However, observers said that the figure was, in fact, nearer to 40,000. This number could grow in the future. According to the *China Daily News Service* November 2005, some epidemiologists forecast that the prosperous province could have around 500,000 people living with HIV by the end of 2010.

In March 2007 Hong Kong and China's Guangdong province will increase joint HIV surveillance and prevention efforts, which they began in 2003. Both state governments reported record numbers of HIV cases in 2006, *China Daily News* reports. Officially the Hong Kong Department of Health reported 373 new HIV cases last year, an increase of 19% from 313 cases reported in 2005. Guangdong reported 4,823 new HIV cases from January 2006 to October 2006, an increase of 8.4% from the same period in 2005

Currently, Guangdong has the fifth largest population of AIDS patients and HIV-positive people in China.

China: Henan

Henan is the Chinese province worst affected by HIV. Unhygienic blood donation centres led to large-scale infection among the local population because blood was purchased from poor rural inhabitants, many of whom earned a living by frequent donations. Henan officially had 25,000 people living with HIV at the end of 2004 with 11,815 AIDS cases according to the *Xinhua News Agency*, many infected in the 'sale of blood' scandal. However other estimates put the figure much higher, up to 500,000 people living with HIV in Henan. (Guardian 2001).

It is alleged that separate detention facilities for HIV-positive prisoners have been built in the province.

Beijing

The Chinese authorities announced in mid 2005 that prisoners in Beijing correctional facilities would receive compulsory HIV and AIDS tests, with inmates receiving a positive test receiving free medical treatment. The treatment will continue after the prisoners finish their jail terms, according to an official with the Beijing Prison Management Bureau as reported in *China News*.

According to the official at the prison management bureau, all HIV and AIDS prisoners in Beijing will be put in the city's Jinzhong Prison, where an attached hospital can provide medical treatment. A high proportion of HIV-positive inmates are drug addicts and Chinese law requires that they should be cured of their addiction as soon as it is discovered. Those found to be taking drugs after this will be sentenced to three years re-education through labour.

The China Daily News also in August 2005 added to the story by saying that testing prison populations was identified as a national priority by health authorities at the end of last year, and tests conducted in east China's Shangdong Province amongst inmates of correctional facilities found 21 people to be HIV-positive, provincial authorities said on July 26.

Malaysia

Malaysia recorded 70,559 cases of HIV from 1986 to 2006 , according to the Malay Ministry of Health statistics released in July 2006. According to the Ministry, 6,000 new HIV and AIDS cases are reported annually, 70% of which involve injection drug users.

HIV-positive prisoners now makes up about 4.35% of the prison population, which stood at almost 36,000 in 2004 (World Population List 2006). Almost half of Malay prisoners are convicted on drug charges. Malay prison authorities have set up guidelines on how to deal with HIV-positive prisoners. Staff are also sent for courses to educate them on HIV.

In 2006 the Malaysian government announced it would be setting up the first 'medical prison' in the country to hold prisoners mostly infected with HIV and TB. The move came after the National Prison Advocacy on Drug Use and HIV seminar organised by the Prisons Department and the Malaysian AIDS Council and attended by, among others, eight prison directors from all over Malaysia. These directors also presented their reports on the HIV and AIDS situation in their respective prisons.

Findings from a survey of Salrangor state showed that most cases reported in the region were from prisons and drug rehabilitation centres (DRCs). The study found that the overall rate for TB/HIV was from 12% to 15% in HIV-positive prisoners. Sputum screening covered 30-97% of the HIV prisoners in each facility and chest x-rays 46- 50% of these inmates.

Vietnam

According to the UNAIDS Epidemic Update, 2006, 260,000 people were living with HIV in Vietnam in 2005. Although a relatively low national rate of HIV, infection has been concentrated in a few at-risk communities such as injecting drug users and sex workers. HIV prevalence among IDUs was at 30% in Han Phong in 2006 (Phan et al).

Human Rights Watch says that officials adopted an increasingly harsh stance towards high-risk groups for AIDS, such as drug users and prostitutes, who were deemed "social evils." In late 2001, the government announced plans to send all of Vietnam's one hundred thousand registered drug addicts to compulsory drug detoxification centres for up to two years. As many as seventy-five thousand drug users remained in detention during the year in seventy-one crowded drug detoxification camps.

Vietnam has the thirteenth highest global TB burden, with roughly 221,000 people living with the disease, according to the NTCP. About 145,000 new TB cases are detected annually, and 70% of people with the disease are between ages 15 and 55.

Perhaps unsurprisingly, in January 2007 it was reported that tuberculosis is becoming more difficult to treat in Vietnam because 10% of people living with the disease also are HIV-positive, according to statistics from the National TB Control Programme (NTBCP), the *Vietnam News* reports. An increasing number of people with TB also are developing drug resistance.

HIV Status Among IDUs in a Border region of Southern China and Northern Vietnam (*JAIDS* VOL 38, 2005) claimed to be the first prevention project to straddle two countries. The intervention, at four sites in china and six in Vietnam, used paid peer educators, distribution of risk reduction information, and used/new needle exchanges. HIV prevalence among IDUs in the China border area was 17% and 46% in the Vietnam border region.

Thailand

The Corrections Department of Thailand estimated that in 2006 that it housed 740 known HIV and AIDS cases, reported the Bangkok Post. The figure was immediately questioned by the UNAIDS country coordinator for Thailand, Patrick Brenny, who put the number at about 4,800 cases in prison.

A United Nations Development Report ahead of the Bangkok International Conference on AIDS said that the Thai government's 'War on Drugs' was counter productive in terms of restricting the spread of HIV. Two thirds of Thailand's 220,000 prisoners are drug users, the report said. The draconian action against drug users has driven users underground away from accessing HIV programmes and put them together in prisons.

Although Thailand has had success with widespread condom and antiretroviral distribution programmes, the government's stance on drug users has attracted criticism from HIV workers. Human Rights Watch reports: "The Thai government has rejected similarly effective HIV prevention programmes in favour of policies of arbitrary arrest, mass incarceration, and forced drug treatment.

Methadone is severely limited in Thai drug treatment centres. An estimated one per cent of Thai drug users were receiving HIV prevention services as of February 2004, including those who obtained condoms through the 100 per cent condom programme.

Myanmar

In the words of the UNAIDS Epidemic Update 2006 Myanmar is facing a 'serious' epidemic with 360,000 people living with HIV, an adult prevalence rate of 1.3%. This rate climbs to 43% among injecting drug users. The UNAIDS regional office estimate, though no official figures are available that Myanmar spent $147,000 on HIV in 2005, equivalent to $0.01 per person. In contrast neighbouring Thailand spent $1.47 per person on HIV intervention in the same period. The prison population in Myanmar is estimated at 60,000 in 2004 by the World Prison Population list.

In the face of pressure from the Myanmarese military junta, many international medical charities are winding up operations in Myanmar. In 2005, the Global Fund for HIV and AIDS, Tuberculosis and Malaria cancelled its US$37.5 million programme in the country, blaming government restrictions on its movements that made functioning nearly impossible. Médecins

Sans Frontières was forced to pull out of Karen and Mon states in 2006 for similar reasons.

In October 2006 the International Committee of the Red Cross (ICRC) was ordered to close all of its offices outside of Yangon, after the organisation reported rampant infection of HIV and other infectious diseases among inmates in the country's prisons.

According to UNAIDS, the western part of the country is most neglected where HIV and AIDS treatment is concerned. The agency reported recently that not a single AIDS patient received free antiretroviral drugs from the government. UNAIDS have reported 60-70% of IDUs had HIV with very high rates along the Myanmar - China border; in the Kachin and Yunnan provinces respectively. Yunnan province contains 80% of China's HIV population mostly ethnic Kachin people. The Golden Triangle of opium manufacture and transhipment has seen an epidemic of injection of heroin and a resultant rise in HIV rates along the cross-border shipment routes.

While little is known about medical practices in Burma's extensive prison system, testimony from ex-prisoners has begun to shed light on the issue according to the *Burmanet* website. It reports: "It is known, however, that prisoners have been used for blood donation, and that donation drawing equipment is re-used repeatedly. Condoms are not provided, as sex in prisons is a further crime under the still active-British penal code, ensuring that any sex which does occur in prisons is unsafe."

National League for Democracy leader, U Hla Than, an elected member of the Burmese Parliament, the body which won the 1990 election, died in Insein prison hospital ward in 1996. The present Myanamese government claimed that U Hla Than died of tuberculosis. Aung San Suu Kyi, who has spent many years under house arrest has stated, however that his death was due to complications of AIDS, which he contracted from unsterilised blood collection equipment in Insein Prison

The government has drawn up a HIV strategy for implementation in 2007. However the National Health and Education Committee (NHEC), an organisation set up by Myanmarese pro-democracy activists in exile, is active in border regions.

Burmanet published a report on the work of the NHEC in January 2007: Lamlhing Touthang, a Namphalong-based health worker, recently returned home after participating in an NHEC-organised, month-long HIV care training camp in Manipur, India. On her return she was interrogated for more than five hours by Myanmarese military intelligence officials

India

India houses 332,112 prisoners out of a population of over one billion, according to the UN Human Rights Commission, making its incarceration rate of 31 per 100,000 one of the lowest in the world.

India has the second-largest number of people living with HIV of any country in the world and a complex HIV epidemic focused on different populations in different areas. HIV and AIDS prevalence among injecting drug users varies across Indian states, as it does amongst other risk groups and the general public. According to the country's National AIDS Control Council Manipur and Chennai have rates of 58% and 64% respectively, while rates in Delhi and Mumbai are 14% and 25%. In Karnataka and West Bengal states it is only 3%.

Unlike many other Asian countries, advocates have been able to use the legal system to challenge ill treatment of HIV-positive prisoners and establish common law precedent.

In two cases, highlighted at the 2006 International AIDS Conference, the right to antiretroviral treatment in some circumstances was established.

In the first, The first PNM v. State of Maharashtra, an HIV-positive man on ARVs was sentenced to 10 years. ARVs were not provided by the Jail authorities. He appealed to the Indian High

court and treatment was restarted - after a two month gap off drug therapy.

In the case of LX v. Union of India, LX, a remand inmate in Tihar Jail, Delhi, was diagnosed HIV-positive and put on ARVs. Bailed in May 2000, he was told his ARVs would then stop. LX brought his case to the High Court and In January 2001 the Court ordered his ARVs to be supplied pending final judgement; in 2004 a final trial directed continuing ARV therapy.

However, another less positive consequence of the British legal system inherited by India is the persistence of 19th century British legislation criminalising homosexual acts.

The law, enacted in 1861 and known as Section 377, makes "carnal intercourse against the order of nature with man, woman or animal" punishable by up to 10 years in prison and, when strictly interpreted, makes it illegal to distribute condoms to gay men and men in prison.

Pakistan

Until recently Pakistan had avoided the HIV rates of its neighbour India. Now, however, the country has seen its first fully fledged outbreak, in Larkana in 2004 among injecting drug users, where prevalence stood at 27%, according to researchers (Shah). According to the latest figures from the National AIDS Control Programme HIV prevalence amongst IDUs had gone from 0.4% in December 2003 to 7.6% in 2004. Pakistan had 89,370 prisoners in 2005 out of a population of 153 million, according to the Pakistan Human Rights Commission.

'Anecdotal' evidence that unprotected sex between men in prisons and hostels was spreading HIV was reported in the *Pakistan Tribune* in November 2006. However little other evidence on HIV prevalence in Pakistan jails exists in a country were stigma is stifling even discussion of the issue.

In March 2007 the Pakistani government acted and launched a project to combat HIV and AIDS in four of the country's prisons. The Ministry of Narcotics Control, in collaboration with the United Nations Office on Drugs and Crime (UNODC), has launched a three-year, $500,000 initiative. According to Pakistan's Business Reporter, 75% of the country's inmates are imprisoned for drug related crimes. The ministry also said it was planning to increase access to treatment for IDUs as part of the programme. Officials estimate there are 500,000 heroin users in Pakistan, as supply has increased following the turmoil in neighbouring Afghanistan. UNODC is expected to produce a report on HIV transmissions later in 2007.

Iran: unexpected liberalisation

Two-thirds of Iranians living with HIV have used drugs intravenously, according to the Iranian Ministry of Health's AIDS department head Dr Mitra Motamedi. The injecting of heroin has grown recently, as smoking opium has fallen away. In a country of 68 million there are 3.7 million drug users, rated the highest level in the world, (*IAACAP Conference* Kobe, 2005).

Iran has a large prison population of 148,000, or 218 per 100,000, according to the World Prison Population List. Prisons are the main source of HIV according to Dr Minoo Mohraz head of infectious diseases of the Ayatollah Khomeini Hospital, Tehran. Iran has possibly the highest HIV rate in any prison system outside of sub-Saharan Africa. She told IRIN News service that as many as 10,000 inmates might be detained in a facility built for 2,000.

"Sometimes as many as 500 inmates share the one syringe, No-one knows or cares of the consequences," one ex-prisoner told the BBC News in 2003. The report said that a pilot project in Kermanshah, in Western Iran, was offering clean needles, condoms and counselling.

A report by *IRIN* quoted a former government official, who said that of 400 inmates tested   in a prison in Kermanshah Province, 146 (36.5%) tested positive.

In 2006 a report in the *Pittsburgh Post Gazette* talked of a turnaround by the Iranian authorities, with condoms and clean needles being provided in clinics and prisons. A state backed magazine profiled HIV-positive Iranians in a monthly column, and methadone had been used as heroin detoxification.

Dr Hamid Setayesh, UNAIDS' Iran coordinator, commented: "They're passing out syringes and condoms in prisons. This is unbelievable." Setayesh sent questionnaires to influential Shiite Muslim clerics to garner their views on the government's role in HIV and AIDS prevention, and found that nearly all were in favour of the government's HIV efforts.

One of the biggest successes has been recent amendments to relevant legislation. Dr Parviz Afshar, head of Iran's prison service, told the International Conference on AIDS in Asia and the Pacific in 2005 that while the anti-narcotics law of 1988 saw drug users as 'criminals', the draft of a new law (2005) would now frame users as 'patients'.

This shift towards decriminalisation of drug use is thought to have already contributed to a reduction in the prison population from 170,000 to 130,000. The inclusion of harm reduction options for public services in new legislation is also a significant step.

The first methadone maintenance treatment (MMT) clinic in Iran was set up in 2002. Three years later there are 15 clinics in medical universities, two in drop-in-centres and five in prisons across Iran. The government hopes to have 35,000 patients on MMT by the end of this year, in 700 private clinics, said Dr Afshar.

References

Agence France Presse - New HIV prisons in China, November 2005

AIDS Epidemic Update - National HIV prevalence, Vietnam, 2006

Amnesty International - China country report, AIDS activists arrested, 2005

Bangkok Post - HIV prevalence in prisons, Corrections Department of Thailand, 2006

Bao, J. Analysis of 30 cases of HIV in Shanghai prison system, Int'l Conference on AIDS, 2002 (Abstract TuPeD3698)

Bayer et al. Increasing incarceration rates for IDUs and HIV care in Thai prisons, AIDS & Behaviour, 2003

BBC News - HIV prevention pilot project in Kermanshar, Iran, 2003

Bernama Daily Malaysian News - HIV prevalence amongst prisoners, July 2006

BurmaNet website (www.burmanet.org) - Conditions in Burma/Myanmar prisons, January 2007

Business Reporter, Pakistan - Imprisonment for drug-related crimes, 2006

China Daily News Service - HIV prevalence forecast, November 2005

China News Agency - mandatory HIV testing in China prisons, December 2004

Guangdong Provincial Bureau of Public Health - HIV prevalence, 2004

Guardian - Henan blood scandal, September 2004

Hammet et al. HIV status among IDUs in border region of Southern China and Northern Vietnam, JAIDS Vol 38, February 2005

Human Rights Watch - Vietnam prisons and marginalised populations, 2002

IAACAP Conference, Kobe, Japan - Drug use in Iran, 2005

IRIN News Service - Iran prison overcrowding, 2006

LICADHO - AIDS in Cambodian prisons report, 2004

Malay Ministry of Health - National HIV statistics, July 2006

Mansuri, S. Lawyers Collective HIV/AIDS Unite - report on conditions and lack of access to legal protection ensuring ARV treatment, Int'l Conf AIDS, Toronto, 2006

MAP - HIV rates in West Java Prison, 2004

Ministry of Health Indonesia - HIV prevalence among inmates, 2006

Ministry of Health, Iran (AIDS Department) - Drug use among people living with HIV, 2006

NACO - HIV prevalence levels by state, India, 2003

Pakistan Human Rights Commission - Prison Population 2004

Pakistan Tribune - Unprotected sex between men in prisons, November 2006

Phan et al. HIV among sex workers and IDUs in Han Phong, Vietnam, 2006

Pittsburgh Post Gazette - Provision of condoms/ clean needles in Iran prisons, 2006

Radio Free Asia - Hunan Province AIDS prison facility, 2006

Rai et al. HIV AIDS in Pakistan: The Battle Begins, Retrovirology, 2007

Shah et al. HIV prevalence among IDUs in Lakarna Pakistan, Int'l Journal STD/AIDS, 2004

Singh. HIV inmates in Delhi Prison, Int'l Journal STD/AIDS, 1998

Sunday Star - Prison/HIV conference, Malaysia, September 2005

Thaisri et al. HIV among IDU inmates in Bangkok Central Prison, BMC Infectious Diseases, 2003

Todd et al. IDUs in Afghanistan prisons risk of HIV transmission, 2006

UNAIDS - Epidemic update, Afghanistan, 2006

UNAIDS Epidemic Update - Myanmar, 2006

UNAIDS Regional Office - Myanmar HIV spend, 2005

Venugopalan B. HIV/ TB Co- infection In Prisons And Drug Rehabilitation Centres In Selangor State, Malaysia (2000-2002). Int Conf AIDS. 2004 Jul 11-16; 15: abstract no. WePeC6030.

Vietnam News - National TB control programme, January 2007

WHO Mission to Vietnam - At risk populations, Vietnam, October 2006

World Prison List - China prison population, 2006

World Prison List - Iran prison population, 2006

http://www.china.org.cn/ - Separate HIV prison proposal by Guangdong Bureau of Justice, November 2005

Xinhia News Agency - Henan sale of blood scandal, 2004

Zaheer, K - Reuters. Homosexuality and human rights in India, November 2006

The law and HIV

Confidentiality

The law of confidentiality

If a person believes that information relating to him or her is being unlawfully disclosed, it may be possible for them to rely upon the civil law of confidentiality.

If someone reveals, or attempts to disclose, information relating to an individual's HIV status without that person's consent, and the discloser of the information received it on trust or as part of a contract or agreement with the sero-positive person, then it is likely that a breach of confidence has occurred. In such circumstances the person concerned may be able to get an injunction preventing disclosure and/or awarding damages. They may also be able to get a declaration from the court stating that the information is confidential (see *Remedies* below).

In law, a duty of confidence arises "whenever the party subject to the duty is in a situation where he knows or ought to know that the other person can reasonably expect his privacy to be respected." (*Campbell v MGN Ltd* [2004] 2 AC 457, *per* Lord Hope of Craighead at para 85).

The law of confidence does not only apply to professional and business relationships: the courts have been willing to protect highly personal information disclosed without authority by spouses and friends. (*Argyll v Argyll* [1965] 1 All ER 611, *Stephens v Avery* [1988] 2 All ER 477).

The law of confidentiality does not provide absolute protection, however, and is subject to three important "limiting principles" (see *Attorney-General v Guardian Newspapers Ltd (No. 2)* [1990] 1 AC 108, *per* Lord Goff of Chieveley at 282):

1 It only applies to information which is actually confidential. Once information enters the public domain, it is no longer protected by confidentiality.

2 It does not apply to useless or trivial information.

3 Although it is in the public interest that confidential information should be protected, that public interest may sometimes be outweighed by another public interest favouring disclosure. In such cases, the public interest in confidentiality must be balanced against the public interest in disclosure.

An example of the third "limiting principle" arose in *W v Egdell* [1990] Ch 359, where the Court of Appeal accepted that, in that particular case, it was in the public interest for a medical practitioner to disclose details of an individual's health status to a third party. In that instance a consultant had disclosed to the Home Secretary his medical report on a patient who was seeking release from a mental hospital. That medical report suggested that the patient may still have been dangerous and was therefore questioning whether he should be released.

The general principle is however that it is in the public interest to maintain confidentiality. Sometimes there are said to be competing public interests, i.e. the public right to know, as opposed to the public's interest in the maintenance of confidential information. This is best illustrated by the case of *X v Y* [1988] 2 All ER 648. In that case, a national newspaper sought to disclose the names of two HIV-positive doctors. The Health Authority sought a permanent injunction preventing the paper from publishing the names. The judge, in allowing the injunction, stated:

"I keep in the forefront of my mind the very important public interest in freedom of the press. And I accept that there is some public interest in knowing that which the defendants seek to publish. But in my judgement those public interests are substantially outweighed when measured against the public interest in relation to loyalty and confidentiality both generally and with particular reference to AIDS patients' hospital records."

A similar approach was taken in the more recent case of *H (A Healthcare Worker) v Associated Newspapers Ltd* [2002] EWCA Civ 195, where a dentist who had been diagnosed as HIV-positive was granted an injunction preventing a newspaper from publicly identifying either him or the health authority for which he worked.

It would appear from such cases that there are three principles which justify, in the public interest, the disclosure of confidential information (see Kennedy and Grubb, Medical Law (3rd edn), Chapter 8, 2000). These are:

- The disclosure is to be made only to those whom it is necessary to tell so as to protect the public interest.

- To justify the disclosure any risk must be real and not fanciful.

- It may be that only a risk involving physical safety of the public justifies disclosure.

Confidentiality and medical professional standards

Unsurprisingly, professional standards and guidance adopted by medical bodies pay considerable attention to confidentiality. The General Medical Council has published both general guidance on confidentiality, along with general guidelines on serious communicable diseases which themselves address the issue of confidentiality. These are not the only such guidelines - for example, the Nursing and Midwifery Council also publish a *Code of Professional Conduct* which covers confidentiality, as does the Society of Sexual Health Advisers' *Manual for Sexual Health Advisers*. The approach taken in all these publications is essentially identical, and the GMC guidance - which is the most detailed - is often referred to as a general source of guidance even though it, strictly speaking, is addressed only to doctors.

More recently, the British HIV Association has recently been working on HIV-specific guidance. A draft paper, "HIV transmission, the law and the work of the criminal team" was posted on the BHIVA website (www.bhiva.org) in early 2006 for consultation. The paper attempts to set out the relevant legal rules, ethical standards and best practice. It is hoped that a final version will be published in due course.

What do the professional standards say?

The GMC's guidance on confidentiality stresses the importance of protecting confidentiality and of obtaining consent to disclosure. Of particular interest are the circumstances in which, according to the GMC guidance, it is permissible to breach confidentiality "in the public interest". The guidance sets out, first, a general rule on disclosure in the public interest (at para 22):

"Personal information may be disclosed in the public interest, without the patient's consent, and in exceptional cases where patients have withheld consent, where the benefits to an individual or to society of the disclosure outweigh the public and the patient's interest in keeping the information confidential. In all cases where you consider disclosing information without

consent from the patient, you must weigh the possible harm (both to the patient, and the overall trust between doctors and patients) against the benefits which are likely to arise from the release of information."

It then goes on to set out a specific rule on "disclosures to protect the patient or others" (at para 27):

"Disclosure of personal information without consent may be justified in the public interest where failure to do so may expose the patient or others to risk of death or serious harm. Where the patient or others are exposed to a risk so serious that it outweighs the patient's privacy interest, you should seek consent to disclosure where practicable. If it is not practicable to seek consent, you should disclose information promptly to an appropriate person or authority. You should generally inform the patient before disclosing the information. If you seek consent and the patient withholds it you should consider the reasons for this, if any are provided by the patient. If you remain of the view that disclosure is necessary to protect a third party from death or serious harm, you should disclose information promptly to an appropriate person or authority. Such situations arise, for example, where a disclosure may assist in the prevention, detection or prosecution of a serious crime, especially crimes against the person, such as abuse of children."

The guidance stresses that the obligation of confidentiality continues after the death of a patient, although it is unlikely that a court would uphold a claim for breach of confidence in such circumstances: "as the confidence is prima facie a personal matter, the legal duty ends with the death of the patient" (Mason, McCall Smith and Laurie, Law and Medical Ethics (7th edn 2006), para 8.79).

What do these rules mean in practice?

The rule about "disclosures to protect the patient or others" is of key importance here. It suggests that medical professionals may, as a last resort, disclose a person's HIV status where it is felt that they are putting a third party at risk. For that reason, the GMC guidance on serious communicable diseases reiterates the principle with specific reference to HIV (at para 22):

"You may disclose information about a patient, whether living or dead, in order to protect a person from risk of death or serious harm. For example, you may disclose information to a known sexual contact of a patient with HIV where you have reason to think that the patient has not informed that person, and cannot be persuaded to do so. In such circumstances you should tell the patient before you make the disclosure, and you must be prepared to justify a decision to disclose information."

It is important to note that this guidance refers only to *known* sexual contacts. There may be cases where a health professional believes that an HIV-positive person is generally taking risks and engaging in unprotected intercourse with a person or persons unknown. In such a case, disclosure would not be justified, largely for the reason that there is no-one to disclose to.

Because the rule about "disclosures to protect the patient or others" refers to the "prevention, detection or prosecution of a serious crime", it is sometimes thought that the criminalisation of reckless HIV transmission (on which, see below) gives a green light to disclosure under this heading. However, it must be remembered that this type of disclosure must be to protect a third party from death or serious bodily harm. If it is thought that reckless transmission *has already taken place*, then the harm is complete and disclosure cannot be justified in this way. This means (in the present author's view) that it is not permissible to rely on this principle to report a case of alleged reckless transmission to the police without the consent of the individual who is believed to be the "victim" of that crime. That person, is, of course, entitled to make a complaint themselves.

It is possible, of course, that reporting an alleged crime might be justified under the general principle of disclosure in the public interest - "where the benefits to an individual or to society of the disclosure outweigh the public and the patient's interest in keeping the information confidential". That principle, however, requires a careful balancing act, and medical professionals will bear in mind that such disclosures might seriously compromise patient trust, care and treatment, while a prosecution is highly unlikely to proceed without a willing complainant.

Could medical professionals ever be required to breach confidentiality?

In certain circumstances, it is possible that a medical professional who did *not* breach confidentiality in order to protect a third party from the onward transmission of HIV could face civil liability (that is, liability to pay damages, rather than the risk of a criminal prosecution).

It has to be stressed that such a case is highly unlikely. For one thing, it might be impossibly difficult to prove that the failure to breach confidentiality *caused* the onward transmission of HIV, because it would be difficult to establish whether transmission had taken place before or after the point at which confidentiality should have been breached. There are, however, five reported cases in English-speaking countries where doctors have been found liable to pay damages to the sexual partner of one of their own patients after that patient had transmitted an STI (HIV in four cases, hepatitis B in another) to their sexual partner (two in the US, two in Australia and one in Canada). But four of these claims were based on negligent advice given to the doctor's own patient - meaning that they were not aware of the risks they posed to their sexual partner - rather than any suggestion that confidentiality should have been breached.

The fifth and most recent case (*Harvey v PD* [2004] NSWCA 97, an Australian decision) is more complex, because it involved two patients (one HIV-positive, one not) who were patients of the same doctor. They requested HIV tests in a joint consultation, but their doctor did not discuss how those results would be communicated. They were communicated separately, which led to one partner being able to deceive the other into believing he had tested negative. In that case, the doctor was held liable to pay damages to the patient who subsequently contracted HIV from her partner, although based on the negligent manner in which the original consultation had been carried out rather than any failure to breach confidentiality (which would probably not have been possible given a specific New South Wales law on confidentiality in HIV cases). Liability here was based on the fact that the doctor owed her a duty of care *as his own patient*.

On the basis of such case law as exists, and applying the general principles which govern this area of law, it has been suggested that the UK courts would be likely to approach the problem as follows:

Onward transmission may result from a failure to properly advise a HIV-positive patient. **Almost certain that UK courts would impose liability.**

- The patient is properly advised but a doctor is aware that an identifiable third party who is also a patient of theirs is nevertheless at risk of infection. **Probable that UK courts would impose liability.**

- The patient is properly advised but a doctor is aware that an identifiable third party who is **not** a patient of theirs is nevertheless at risk of infection. **Possible that UK courts would impose liability, but unlikely.**

- The patient is properly advised but a doctor is aware that unidentifiable third parties may nevertheless be put at risk. **Almost certain that UK courts would not impose liability.**

It must be stressed that this is very much speculative (the legal principles involved are discussed further in J Chalmers, "Criminalisation of HIV transmission: can doctors be liable for the onward transmission of HIV?" (2004) 15 International Journal of STD & AIDS 782-787). However, the possibility of legal liability has, understandably, exercised minds in the wake of criminal prosecutions for the reckless transmission of HIV, and has been a key factor in BHIVA's draft guidance.

Confidentiality and the Venereal Diseases Regulations

Although, as noted earlier, the protection of confidentiality is not an absolute one, that does not settle the matter. This is because there is specific legislation concerning confidentiality in respect of STIs, in the shape of the National Health Service (Venereal Diseases) Regulations 1974, which apply to England and Wales only.

The Regulations - applicable to Strategic Health Authorities, NHS Trusts, NHS Foundation Trusts and Primary Care Trusts - provide that information about persons diagnosed with sexually transmitted infections shall not be disclosed except:

"(a) for the purpose of communicating that information to a medical practitioner, or to a person employed under the direction of a medical practitioner in connection with the treatment of persons suffering from such disease or the prevention of the spread thereof, and

(b) for the purpose of such treatment and prevention."

The provisions of the Regulations are replicated in the NHS Trusts and PCTs (Sexually Transmitted Diseases) Directions 2000, which apply to members and employees of all NHS Trusts and Primary Care Trusts.

The history and purpose of the Regulations

The Regulations are often regarded as providing a special, heightened level of confidentiality in respect of STIs. They may - arguably - have this effect, but that appears to be an accidental consequence of bad drafting rather than a deliberate outcome. Their history is not well documented, but can be traced through files in the National Archives (primarily MH55/1367 on the 1948 regulations, and MH154/203 on the 1968 regulations).

VD clinics were established under the control of local authorities in 1916 by the Public Health (Venereal Diseases) Regulations 1916. Those regulations included a provision that any information obtained by local authorities through such clinics should be treated as confidential. When the NHS - which took over responsibility for VD clinics - was established, the 1916 regulations were repealed as unnecessary. That led to public concern that information about VD diagnoses was no longer confidential. The Ministry of Health was adamant that this concern was unjustified - the normal rules of medical confidentiality being applicable - but eventually gave in and made a regulation in 1948 to the effect that such information should be treated as confidential. It is clear that the Ministry thought this was a redundant and unnecessary regulation, which no doubt explains why no equivalent regulations were made in Scotland then or since.

In the 1960s, concern developed that confidentiality might inhibit effective contact tracing (partner notification, as it is now better known), for which the Ministry was attempting to develop national standards. This is because it was felt that for contact tracing to be fully successful, it was necessary for the index patient's clinic to know whether contacts had been traced and what diagnoses, if any, had been made.

Accordingly, the National Health Service (Venereal Diseases) Regulations 1968 were made. The purpose of these regulations was to allow staff at one clinic, once a contact had been traced and tested for STIs, to pass back their results to the clinic at which the index patient had been diagnosed without any need to obtain consent for this. (It is notable that the Ministry seemed to think there was no problem of confidentiality where both patients were tested at the same clinic.) There was some difficulty in finding appropriate wording for the regulations, but eventually it was decided to say that information obtained by clinics "shall be treated as confidential except" where the criteria set out in paragraphs (a) and (b) (quoted above) applied.

In 1974, the Regulations were re-enacted as a result of NHS re-organisation, amended in order that they would apply to all STIs and not just the narrow category of venereal diseases (defined in the earlier regulations as gonorrhoea, syphilis and soft chancre). Additionally, the phrase "shall be treated as confidential except" was replaced with "shall not be disclosed except". It is not clear why the wording was changed in this way, and the explanatory note to the regulations gives no indication of any intention to strengthen the protection against disclosure which they provided.

The history of the regulations is important because it demonstrates that their purpose is often badly misunderstood. They were intended to *weaken* confidentiality (to assist in contact tracing) and not to strengthen it. The 1968 wording made this clear, because criteria (a) and (b) were simply presented as an exception to confidentiality, which would have meant that the other, general, exceptions to confidentiality remained available. The 1974 rewording, however, suggests that there is an absolute prohibition on disclosure except where criteria (a) and (b) are satisfied. This has caused confusion as to both the purpose and effect of the regulations.

The future of the Regulations

In August 2006, the Department of Health published a consultation on the Regulations (Department of Health, *Policy Consultation on Confidentiality and Disclosure of Patient Information: HIV and Sexually Transmitted Infections (STIs)* (2006)). The consultation paper noted that the proper interpretation of the regulations had recently been a contentious subject in a High Court decision involving the Health Protection Agency (HPA), where the HPA had sought advice from the court on the action it should take involving an identified HIV-positive patient whom the HPA was concerned might be putting multiple partners at risk through unprotected intercourse. The judge did not make a decision in that case - stressing that, although the court would be prepared to rule on the legality of specific action which the HPA intended to take, the HPA had not put forward any such proposals, and it was not the court's function to act as an advisory body on hypothetical questions. This meant that the proper scope of the Regulations remained unresolved.

The consultation paper noted that the common law duty of confidentiality can be breached in the public interest in limited circumstances, the importance of confidential information to public health monitoring, and the importance of confidentiality (and patient confidence that confidentiality will be maintained) in the effective provision of sexual health services.

Against that background, it posed questions about whether a breach of confidentiality to protect a third party could ever be justified, and who should take any decisions about such disclosure. The consultation closed at the end of October 2006: at the time of writing, no announcement had been made about any changes to the Regulations as a result of the consultation process.

Remedies against breaches of confidence

The GMC guidelines do not have legal force, although earlier versions have been referred to by the courts in deciding cases, and they can be considered as indicative of public policy. As such, any breaches could be seen as a breach of duty and/or evidence of negligence. In practice, allegations of breach of confidence are more likely to be dealt with as complaints or disciplinary matters than by resort to the courts, although the option of legal action is always open.

Injunction

The main weapon available to a person seeking to prevent an unlawful breach of confidence is an injunction (in Scotland,

"interdict"). It is possible to get an interlocutory injunction (in Scotland, "interim interdict") which is a provisional order before a permanent injunction is granted at a court hearing. These interlocutory injunctions can be applied for *ex parte*, that is without the person seeking to disclose the information being present.

Damages

Damages or compensation can be claimed where the breach of confidence has already occurred. If someone suffers foreseeable economic loss as a result of the breach of confidence, such as the loss of their job, that person could claim damages (*Seager v Copydex* [1967] 1 WLR 923). Despite earlier doubt, damages for mental distress now appear to be available in such cases (see, e.g., *Archer v Williams* [2003] EWHC 1670).

It is unclear whether it would be possible to get damages for distress for a breach of confidence. The Law Commission has recommended that damages should be available for the mental stress caused by a breach of confidence (Report No. 110, Breach of Confidence (Cmnd 838, 1981), but its proposals have not been made law.

Declaration

A declaration (in Scotland, "declarator") is the method used by the court to declare the legal relationship between the parties. The court can therefore assert that certain information is confidential. Declarations are to an extent toothless; they cannot be enforced and nor do they carry any sanction. However, they are however useful in breach of confidence cases as a means of identifying that the information threatened with disclosure is confidential.

Access to medical records

Historically an individual did not have a right to see his or her medical records. The position has gradually altered due to a number of pieces of legislation, the most important of which is now the Data Protection Act 1998. This covers both computerised and (some) manual records, and as such is a significant advance on its predecessor (the Data Protection Act 1984), which only regulated records held on computer.

There is specific legislation on access to manually held health records in the form of the Access to Health Records Act 1990. However, "since the passing of the Data Protection Act 1998, the terms of this Act are now redundant except in so far as they relate to a deceased person" (Mason, McCall Smith and Laurie, *Law and Medical Ethics* (6th edn 2006), para 8.67), and so this legislation is not discussed further here.

Data Protection Act 1998

The Data Protection Act 1998 enables an individual (the data subject) who believes that personal information relating to him/her is being electronically stored, to apply to discover if the information is being stored and if so, to have access to it (the "right of access to personal data"). It also confers a right to have inaccurate personal data rectified, blocked, erased or destroyed, and a right to prevent data processing which is likely to cause unwarranted damage or distress.

There are a number of exceptions to the right of access. Most importantly, medical information may be exempt if applying the right "would be likely to cause serious harm to the physical or mental health or condition of the data subject or any other person" (Data Protection (Subject Access Modification) Health Order 2000, reg 5(1).

Further information about data protection is available from the website of the Information Commissioner's Office (www.informationcommisioner.gov.uk).

Access to Medical Reports Act 1988

Under this Act, a person has the right to see a medical report prepared by a doctor, "who is or has been responsible for the clinical care of the individual" (i.e. their own doctor), for employment or insurance purposes. Any employer. potential employer or insurance company who wants a medical report from a person's doctor, must first obtain the individual's consent and inform them of their right of access under the Act. The person concerned has a right to see the report before it is sent to the employer or insurance company if they have asked to do so, in writing, when giving their consent to the report. Once the report has been sent, the individual may still seek a copy of it for up to six months. There is no right to amend or correct the report unless the doctor agrees to do this, but there is a right to prevent the report being sent at all.

The Act allows circumstances where non-disclosure by the doctor is possible. If a person feels that they have been wrongly refused access to a medical report, they may apply to the county court, which can order disclosure (section 8).

Although an employer or insurance company can circumvent the Act by appointing their own doctor to prepare reports, such a report might still be accessible under the provisions of the Data Protection Act 1998.

Disclosure of HIV status at a police station

For solicitors who advise on the telephone or who attend detainees at a police station a question may arise as to whether an HIV-positive detainee should disclose their status to the police.

In some circumstances the decision may be taken away from the detainee - for example, if another person at the scene of the arrest discloses the fact to the arresting officers, or if the arrested person has medication on them from which an HIV-positive status can be inferred.

Detainees may be eager to disclose their status if they need access to medication. On arrival at a police station all medication and indeed most other property will be removed from the detainee. Access to medication will not be permitted without the sanction of a Divisional Surgeon.

It is generally inadvisable for an HIV-positive detainee to disclose their status to the police. In the first place, general experience has shown that HIV-positive detainees are treated less considerately during the course of their detention. Secondly, adverse inferences relating to the alleged offence for which the person has been arrested may be drawn - for example, if a man has been arrested for an alleged offence of sexual misbehaviour and discloses that he is HIV-positive he may suffer an attitude of 'Oh well, he must be gay and must therefore have committed the offence'. Thirdly, it has been routine police practice for an individual's HIV status to be recorded on the police national computer (PNC).

This practice has been a source of considerable disquiet, since it means that HIV-positive people who have come into contact with the police and whose status has been ascertained - not necessarily with their consent - can be readily identified. When there are regular calls for controls on 'irresponsible people with AIDS', it is clear why the central recording of 'criminals or semi-criminals' who are HIV-positive causes so much concern. In mid-1991 there were press reports that the police in Cleveland took the recording of detainees' HIV status one step further by displaying photographs of people suspected of being HIV-positive on a police station noticeboard.

The practice of recording HIV status on the PNC was the subject of a complaint in 1992 by, amongst others, The Terrence Higgins Trust, to the Data Protection Registrar (DPR) - the public official who is responsible for the regulation of the storage and use of personal data (information about living individuals) on computer. The basis of the complaint was that the information was excessive and irrelevant and therefore held in breach of the Fourth Data Protection Principle, which provides that 'personal data held for any purpose or purposes shall be adequate, relevant and not excessive in relation to that purpose or those purposes'.

The Registrar, in his eighth annual report, concluded:

It appears to me that there is a small, but foreseeable, risk of infection with HIV/AIDS which could arise in connection with policing activities. Accordingly, I am satisfied that, in general the holding of a factual warning signal, including an indication of HIV/AIDS status in the PNC conviction records, is neither excessive nor irrelevant to policing purposes.

In practice an individual's HIV status should have no relevance at all to their arrest or detention. The police should already have in place procedures to reduce the risk of contracting infections during arrest and detention without such procedures being dependent upon ascertaining the detainee's health status. Furthermore, even if such procedures are not implemented the information that an individual is HIV-positive invariably becomes available after a 'risk' situation has passed. For example, if the police are dealing with someone injured and bleeding after a fight or car accident it is very unlikely that personal details sufficient to carry out a PNC check and ascertain health details will be obtained until after the immediate emergency has passed.

For these reasons The Terrence Higgins Trust, amongst others, made further representations to the DPR after the publication of his eighth annual report arguing against permitting the police to record an individual's HIV status on the PNC. These representations were instrumental in achieving a change of view on the part of the Registrar, who in his ninth annual report, stated:

I have reviewed the position which I took last year. The new factor is that there is now a firm policy on procedures, which should be adopted by police forces, to avoid the risk of HIV infection. Once these procedures are in place, whilst I would look at the facts of each particular case, the holding of HIV markers would seem to be irrelevant. Such markers would also possibly be excessive in view of the danger that they may encourage a false sense of security. This might undermine the hygiene procedures and put police officers at risk.

I have concluded that I should hold to my original view until there has been sufficient time for the necessary training and education activities for police officers to be put in place... I would expect an early development of the required courses and materials.

In his tenth annual report published in July 1994 the Registrar indicated that such training should have been completed by December 1993 and expressed some impatience with those police forces that were still retaining HIV markers on the PNC. The Registrar indicated that he might be obliged to take action if the retention of such information persisted as he regarded it as a breach of the Fourth Data Protection Principle.

In 1995 it was confirmed by the Office of the Data Protection Registrar that all police services had agreed to comply with the Registrar's requirement and to remove HIV markers from the Police National Computer.

In the situation where a detainee wishes to disclose their HIV status with a view to obtaining access to medication it is recommended that the detainee be advised to request the attendance of the Divisional Surgeon, explain the circumstances to them, insist that they treat the disclosure of HIV status as confidential, and ask them to authorise access to medication. As a matter of practice Divisional Surgeons routinely disclose information about a detainee's health to the police and indeed an officer may be present or nearby when the examination is carried out. However, Divisional Surgeons are not, despite their common title of 'police doctors', employed by the police, but are independent General Practitioners, and as such, it is submitted, subject to the same rules of confidentiality as if they were the detainee's own doctor. If a detainee specifically forbids disclosure, therefore, this will serve to remind the doctor of the duty of confidentiality and to emphasise the possible disciplinary consequences if disclosure occurs.

One final note of caution needs to be sounded with respect to advising an HIV-positive detainee at a police station and trying to ensure that their status is not needlessly disclosed. Very few telephone conversations between a detainee and their advising solicitor are confidential and, indeed, many outgoing telephone lines from a police station are routinely taped. Consequently, such matters should not be discussed over the telephone but only during a personal attendance at the police station.

HIV testing in police custody is discussed in HIV testing: HIV testing and consent.

Disclosure of HIV status during criminal proceedings

A defendant's HIV status is a factor that is potentially relevant in all prosecutions. It may be directly relevant to the commission of the alleged crime - for example, inadequate state benefits or financial support have, on more than one occasion, been the impulse for the commission of an offence of dishonesty.

Furthermore, the HIV status of a defendant may provide grounds, particularly in less serious cases, for an approach to the Crown Prosecution Service (CPS) to see if they will deal with the defendant either by withdrawing the charge altogether or by coupling such a withdrawal with a non-conviction option such as a bind-over or a caution. Binding over is a general power the criminal courts have. To bind over a defendant means, effectively, to require them to give an undertaking to the court to be of good behaviour for a stated period (normally a year). A sum of money is also specified and if the defendant breaches the bind-over they become liable to forfeit the sum or part of it.

It is of course fundamental that the defendant consents to and co-operates with such an approach, or indeed any disclosure of their health status (for example for the purposes of mitigation) which may take place during criminal proceedings. It is advisable for information relating to HIV status to be volunteered by the defendant rather than asked for. If sought, the questions should be qualified with an explanation as to how the disclosure of the information may assist the client and an assurance that the questions need not be answered if that is the client's wish.

As mentioned in the preceding section HIV status may, unfortunately be established during criminal proceedings without a defendant's co-operation and consent, for example when a search is conducted at a police station and medication or a medical appointment card is discovered, which indicates that the detainee is HIV-positive.

This information is then likely to be recorded on the detainee's Custody Record (the record of a detainee's detention at a police station). In such a case the proper course is to establish with the client whether any further, beneficial, use can be made of the information.

Having established HIV status and the client's informed consent to disclosure, the next consideration is whether disclosure is likely to be of benefit to the client - that is, whether it is likely to lead to the discontinuance of the prosecution and the avoidance of a criminal conviction. Such a resolution is less likely where the offence is serious or indeed where the defendant is, relatively, healthy.

It is also important to take into account the nature of the alleged offence and the possible ignorance of the prosecutor with whom you are dealing. The latter factor is, of course, quite unpredictable. For example, where the allegation is one of sexual misbehaviour, disclosure may have the wholly undesirable result of encouraging rather than discouraging a prosecution on the basis that the defendant's behaviour may have transmitted the

virus and put others at serious risk. This is an attitude that has been displayed in cases of alleged sexual misbehaviour even where the activity complained of is not capable of resulting in HIV transmission. An attempt can, of course, be made to counter such attitudes by providing the prosecutor with more realistic information, but this type of prejudice and misinformation can be difficult to tackle.

The CPS has certain criteria to consider in establishing whether to charge a potential defendant or to proceed with a prosecution. These are set out in The Code for Crown Prosecutors which is published on behalf of the Director of Public Prosecutions. These criteria place an obligation on the prosecuting authorities to consider, amongst other points, the defendant's health and also whether the pursuit of a prosecution "is likely to have a bad effect on the victim's physical or mental health, always bearing in mind the seriousness of the offence" (s5(10)(f) of the Code). The latter consideration is important given that it is well established that stress can result in a deterioration in the health of a person who is HIV-positive.

An approach to the prosecuting authorities suggesting that, through reasons of health, a prosecution ought not to be continued should be in the form of a letter referring the prosecutor to the criteria relied on and any additional points of assistance relating to the particular defendant (age, previous good character, etc.) and should be accompanied by a medical report confirming an HIV-positive diagnosis, describing the defendant's current state of health and treatment and, if the supervising doctor is willing, expressing the likely adverse effect of continuing the prosecution. On the issue of confidentiality, it is important to state in the letter that the information disclosed about the defendant is not to be passed to any other party under any circumstances.

The approach will either be met with a refusal to halt a prosecution, an agreement to do so (possibly coupled with a caution or bind-over) or a request for further information (clarification of the defendant's state of health or, in exceptional cases, a request for an independent medical examination).

If the initial approach is met with a refusal, it is always worth considering a further appeal later in the proceedings, especially if there have been developments in the defendant's state of health which can be attested to in a further medical report. Further approaches will, of course, only be possible if the case is continuing for some time and not, for example, being dealt with by way of a guilty plea at the first hearing.

A defendant's HIV status as a point of mitigation

If there seems to be no possibility of the prosecution discontinuing the case, then the material gathered for the purposes of making the relevant representations to the CPS can be used, in the event of a guilty plea or conviction, for the purposes of mitigation. There are a number of Court of Appeal authorities (three of them, confusingly, involving appellants named Moore) which specifically consider the relevance of an HIV diagnosis as a point of mitigation.

R v Moore (Archibald) ((1990) 12 Cr. App R. (S) 384), where the appellant had been convicted of two substantial burglaries and asked for three other offences to be taken into consideration. The appellant had been diagnosed in 1986 as HIV-positive and the lower court apparently found that there was a likelihood that he would develop AIDS within about two years. The Court of Appeal accepted that his treatment would be more difficult in prison, but Lord Lane C. J. ruled as follows:

We ... are asked in this case to mitigate the penalty of five years imprisonment imposed upon the appellant because this man is HIV-positive and it is suggested, but not based upon any medical evidence apart from second hand evidence via the defendant himself, that his life expectancy may thereby be diminished. As I say, we have no medical evidence as to the length of life expectancy.

Nevertheless, assuming that such evidence does exist, we do not consider that it is the function of this court to base its decision upon possible medical considerations of this sort. ... We do not know what the future may hold with regard to medical science and medical expertise. We do not know what the future may hold with regard to this particular appellant. If the time should come when it is no longer possible, for practical reasons, or for reasons of humanity, to hold this appellant in prison because of his physical condition, then that is the job of the Home Office... [it] is not for this court.

A very similar line was taken by the Court of Appeal in *R v Stark* ([1992] Crim L R at 384). In this case the defendant pleaded guilty to possessing heroin with intent to supply. The defendant had been in possession of 27 grams of heroin with an estimated street value of £2,500. He was sentenced to four years imprisonment. Before the Court of Appeal it was emphasised that the appellant had been diagnosed as being HIV-positive some time previously and more recently AIDS had developed. His life expectancy was estimated at between twelve months and two years. It was accepted that his condition made life in prison 'particularly hard'.

The court was asked to reduce the sentence to allow the appellant to be released and to die with dignity, but declined to do so, holding that the appellant's record clearly indicated that there was a grave risk that the appellant would continue to traffic in drugs as long as he would be able to do so. As in Archibald Moore, the court held that it was not their function to manipulate a sentence in such circumstances - it was a matter for the exercise of the Royal Prerogative of Mercy.

The third authority, *R v Moore (Richard)* ((1993) 15 Cr App R (S) 97) confirmed the approach taken by the Court of Appeal in Stark and held that it was not for the Court 'to alter an otherwise proper sentence to achieve a desirable social end'. The latter part of that phrase possibly reflects a more compassionate view of the appellant's circumstances and certainly the Court directed that all the medical reports before them should be forwarded to the prison authorities to effect a consideration as to whether the Royal Prerogative should be exercised in the appellant's favour.

In the later case of *James Moore* (Court of Appeal, 27th June 1994), the Court of Appeal did, however, take account of the fact that Moore had "advanced HIV disease" and might need hospice-type care before very long. Accordingly, the court reduced the sentence imposed to below four years, in order to ensure that he would not be categorised as a "long-term prisoner", meaning that the Home Secretary would have the power to release him on license on compassionate grounds if appropriate, without the need to first consult with the Parole Board.

These decisions, and others concerning the ill-health of the defendant, were subsequently reviewed by the Court of Appeal in the case of *R v Bernard* [1997] 1 Cr App R (S) 135, where the court made the following statement of principles (pp.138-139). (The case of *Wynne*, referred to by the court in the extract below, involved a defendant suffering from cystic fibrosis.)

(i) a medical condition which may at some unidentified future date affect either life expectancy or the prison authorities' ability to treat a prisoner satisfactorily may call into operation the Home Secretary's powers of release by reference to the Royal Prerogative of mercy or otherwise but is not a reason for this Court to interfere with an otherwise appropriate sentence (*Archibald Moore*);

(ii) the fact that an offender is HIV-positive, or has a reduced life expectancy, is not generally a reason which should affect sentence (*Archibald Moore* and *Richard Moore*) [That is also implicit in the later case of *Attorney-General's Reference (No 58 of 2005)* [2005] EWCA Crim 2721, where the defendant's HIV-positive status is referred to merely in passing.];

(iii) a serious medical condition, even when it is difficult to treat in prison, will not automatically entitle an offender to a lesser sentence than would otherwise be appropriate (*Wynne*);

(iv) an offender's serious medical condition may enable a court, as an act of mercy in the exceptional circumstances of a particular case, rather than by virtue of any general principle, to impose a lesser sentence than would otherwise be appropriate.

(These principles were reaffirmed and applied in the subsequent case of *R v Veiga* [2003] EWCA Crim 2420.)

The fourth point is particularly important: in practice it may not matter very much whether a reduced sentence is imposed as an "act of mercy" rather than "by virtue of any general principle": the result is the same.

The Home Secretary has a statutory power to release a prisoner early on license "if he is satisfied that exceptional circumstances exist which justify the prisoner's release on compassionate grounds" (Criminal Justice Act 1991, s36). Where the prisoner is a long-term prisoner (sentenced to more than four years), this should normally only be done after consultation with the Parole Board, except in exceptional circumstances.

Some more general sentencing principles which may be relevant should be noted.

There are authorities, for example, that urge leniency where it can be established that an offence was committed in circumstances of severe emotional stress (*R v Law*, Court of Appeal, 24 April 1975), or where an offence of dishonesty is committed as a result of severe financial difficulties (*R v Oakes*, Court of Appeal, 4 November 1974); note this was a case where overspending by the defendants' partners caused the financial difficulties.

The courts may also take into account any physical disability or illness which would subject the defendant to an exceptional degree of hardship if sent to prison (*R v Herasymenko*, Court of Appeal, 12 December 1975). The court may also take into account the possibility that a defendant may be placed in a segregation unit under Rule 43 of the Prison Rules if imprisoned (*R v Holmes* (1979) 1 Cr App R (S) 233. This latter point may be of significance to an HIV-positive person at risk of imprisonment as such a person is likely to be segregated if their health status is known to the prison authorities, but its importance is limited by the fact that the Court of Appeal has suggested that the likelihood of segregation is only a relevant factor where the defendant is exceptionally vulnerable (*R v Parker* [1996] 2 Cr App R (S) 275).

In very general terms the courts will not take into account the possible adverse effects on immediate family if a defendant receives a custodial sentence (*R v Ingham*, Court of Appeal, 3 October 1974). This would appear to cause difficulties with mitigation for a defendant who is the partner or carer of a PWA or HIV-positive person. However leniency may be shown as an "act of mercy" where a custodial sentence would clearly cause an unusual measure of hardship. For example, *R v Renker* (Court of Appeal, 29 June 1976), where the defendant was the carer of a child with leukaemia or *R v Haleth* ((1982) 4 Cr App R (S) 178) where the defendant was the sole surviving parent of a child with kidney disease.

The transmission of HIV as a criminal offence

Introduction

For many years, there were in the UK - in contrast to many other countries - no criminal prosecutions for the transmission of HIV. The position has now changed, with the first conviction taking place in 2001.

Neither English nor Scots Law carry legislation specific to accommodate criminal prosecutions for HIV transmission, and more general criminal offences have been used to cover such cases.

Timeline of developments in the criminalisation of HIV transmission in the UK

- 1888: In the leading case of *R v Clarence*, it is held that the transmission of an STI cannot amount to the offence of "inflicting grievous bodily harm" under the Offences Against the Person Act 1861 (England and Wales), because the term "infliction" implies some sort of attack, rather than simply causing harm.

- 1992: Media outcry after a HIV-positive man is accused of deliberately infecting four women with HIV. It is thought that no criminal law applies, and so no prosecution is brought. The Home Secretary states in Parliament that he has no plans to legislate to make the deliberate transmission of HIV a criminal offence.

- 1993: The Law Commission publishes a review of the law on offences against the person, proposing that there should be offences covering the reckless and intentional transmission of diseases, including HIV.

- 1997: The House of Lords decides, in *R v Ireland*, that a man who causes psychiatric injury to a woman by means of silent telephone calls can be guilty of "inflicting grievous bodily harm". Commentators subsequently note that this seems to have the effect of overruling the decision in *R v Clarence*, and opens the door to prosecutions for the reckless transmission of HIV under English law.

- 1998: A prosecution is brought in York for the transmission of hepatitis B, but the trial judge rules (seemingly on the basis of *R v Clarence*) that this cannot be a criminal offence.

- 1999: the Home Office publishes a consultation paper following on from the 1993 Law Commission proposals, suggesting that there should be legislation to make it an offence to deliberately - but not recklessly - transmit HIV or other diseases.

- 2001: First conviction in the UK for the transmission of HIV: Stephen Kelly is convicted in Scotland (where a different system of criminal law applies) of having recklessly injured his girlfriend by infecting her with HIV. (The relevant Scottish offence does not have a precise name and is sometimes described as "culpable and reckless conduct".)

- 2002: A prosecution is brought in London for the transmission of viral herpes (Sullivan) but is dropped after the judge hears that the complainant had sought hospital treatment for the symptoms of herpes ten months before having sex with the defendant.

- February 2003: the first English prosecution for the transmission of HIV (Mvula) is abandoned after evidence that the defendant did not know she was HIV-positive at the time of the alleged offence.

- October 2003: the first English conviction for the transmission of HIV - Mohammed Dica is convicted of two counts of "unlawfully and maliciously inflicting grievous bodily harm".

- January 2004: Kouassi Adaye pleads guilty to one charge of inflicting grievous bodily harm by transmitting HIV.

- May 2004: Court of Appeal hears an appeal against Dica's convictions and confirms that the reckless transmission of HIV is an offence under English law - *R v Clarence* no longer representing the law - but quashes Dica's convictions and orders a retrial on the basis of a misdirection by the trial judge on the effect of consent. The court confirms that consent by the complainant to the risk of infection is a valid defence to a charge of recklessly transmitting HIV.

- May 2004: Very shortly after the Court of Appeal's decision in the Dica case, Feston Konzani is convicted of three counts of inflicting grievous bodily harm by transmitting HIV. His appeal against conviction is dismissed in March 2005.

- March 2005: After a fourth trial (the second having been abandoned for unspecified legal reasons, and the third abandoned after the jury failed to reach a verdict), Mohammed Dica is convicted of one count of inflicting grievous bodily harm by transmitting HIV (one of the complainants in the first trial having felt no longer able to give evidence).

- April 2005: Paulo Matias pleas guilty to one charge of inflicting grievous bodily harm by transmitting HIV, and is sentenced to three years imprisonment. It is understood that he died nine months later from complications caused by HIV and hepatitis C, including cirrhosis of the liver.

- May 2005: Two further Scottish prosecutions for the reckless transmission of HIV are halted, at least temporarily: one (Giovanni Mola) because the accused is no longer in Scotland and cannot immediately be brought back from Italy to stand trial; a second (Christopher Walker) because the accused is found unfit to stand trial and is ordered to be detained in a psychiatric hospital.

- July 2005: A 20 year old woman - the first to be convicted of the offence - is sentenced to two years youth detention after pleading guilty to inflicting grievous bodily harm by transmitting HIV. Her name cannot be published due to a court order obtained by social services to protect the identity of her child.

- December 2005: Derek Hornett pleads guilty to one charge of inflicting grievous bodily harm by transmitting HIV and is sentenced to three years and three months imprisonment.

- April 2006: An unnamed man pleads guilty to a charge of inflicting grievous bodily harm by transmitting HIV to another man. This is the first (and, so far, only) UK conviction for the homosexual transmission of HIV.

- June 2006: Sarah Porter pleads guilty to a charge of inflicting grievous bodily harm by transmitting HIV and is sentenced to 32 months' imprisonment. The case attracts lurid media coverage, where it is noted that a complaint had been made to the police by a sexual partner of Porter's who was *not* HIV-positive, but that the police had obtained personal information (such as diaries) belonging to Ms Porter and had tracked down her previous sexual partners to construct a case against her.

- January 2007: An unnamed Zimbabwean man pleads guilty in Bournemouth to a charge of inflicting grievous bodily harm by transmitting HIV. He is sentenced to three and a half years imprisonment, with a recommendation that he be deported at the end of his sentence.

- February 2007: Giovanni Mola is convicted after a trial under Scots law where he pled not guilty to having recklessly transmitted HIV and hepatitis C by sexual intercourse. A sentencing hearing was pending at the time of writing.

The current legal position

It is now clear that, in both England and Wales and in Scotland, the reckless transmission of HIV is a criminal offence. "Recklessness" means that the defendant was aware that he was running an unjustified or unreasonable risk. The offence is not limited to HIV, but applies to other serious sexually transmitted infections.

It is probably not essential that the defendant has received a positive result from an HIV test, if he knew that for some reason he was at a particularly high risk of being HIV-positive. In the Kouassi Adaye case, it appears that Adaye had been diagnosed with a number of STIs and advised that he was at a high risk of being HIV-positive but did not attend a testing appointment. However, Adaye pled guilty and no court has yet confirmed that a person can be criminally reckless in the absence of a positive test result. It should, however, be clear that declining to take an HIV test cannot be regarded as providing any sort of immunity from criminal prosecution.

If HIV is not transmitted, there will be no offence under English law unless the defendant had intended to transmit HIV - which would be extremely difficult to prove. In Scotland, it might be at least theoretically possible to bring a prosecution in such circumstances - the trial judge in the Mola case expressly told the jury that although there had been actual transmission in that case, it was not an essential part of the crime.

Following the Court of Appeal decisions in the Dica and Konzani cases, if the HIV-positive person discloses the fact that they are HIV-positive to their sexual partner, and their partner consents to the risk of transmission, this will be a defence to a criminal charge. It is not yet clear whether the use of condoms, without disclosure, will operate as a defence, although the Court of Appeal did suggest in the Dica case that a person who used condoms might not be said to be legally "reckless", while the trial judge in the Mola case told the jury that - given that Mola had been given medical advice that he did not need to disclose provided that he used condoms - he could not be considered "culpable and reckless" unless the jury accepted the complainer's claim that he had persistently refused to do so. Given that only a very small fraction of cases of HIV transmission will result in prosecutions being brought, it is thought that a prosecution for HIV transmission by protected intercourse is unlikely - and if no transmission occurs then there can normally be no prosecution anyway, at least in England and Wales.

Prosecutions for HIV transmission by way of unprotected oral sex are also thought to be unlikely. One Canadian court has taken the view that unprotected oral sex is insufficiently risky to be caught by the criminal law (*R v Edwards* 2001 NSSC 80): the point has not arisen in the UK. (In Canada, it only arose because (a) prosecutions are possible in Canada for exposure as well as transmission, and (b) the prosecution in Edwards had alleged both unprotected anal sex - denied by the defendant, and unprotected oral sex - admitted by the defendant. The court therefore had to decide whether the defendant's admission was enough in itself to justify a conviction, and held it was not.)

Confidentiality and criminalisation

Prosecutions may involve leading evidence of confidential information: although doctor-patient (and similar) communications are legally confidential, they are not "privileged" and thus protected from disclosure to a court. In the Stephen Kelly case, concern was raised over the fact that the police were able to use Mr Kelly's blood samples, given under strict rules of confidentiality as part of a confidential clinical trial, to convict him. A Guardian editorial at the time expressed concern that such an apparent breach of confidentiality risks "[u]ndermining confidentiality (and) strikes at the heart of serious research". In reality, without the unique gene sequencing carried out by the University of Edinburgh's laboratories as well as the insistence that medical and scientific records be released, the case could not have been brought. When use of the records as evidence was challenged in court, the trial judge, Lord Mackay of Drumadoon said:

"'The interests of the accused required to be balanced against the public interest. In my opinion, when that exercise is undertaken, the balance is in favour of the evidence being admitted.In the absence of any irregularity in the obtaining of the evidence and, having regard, in particular, to the facts that the accused voluntarily undertook all the tests and that he authorised the Ruchill team to release the first test to the prison medical authorities, I have reached the view that the circumstances of this case warrant the objection being repelled."

The position elsewhere

Recently, the Global Network of People Living with HIV/AIDS Europe and the Terrence Higgins Trust conducted a "rapid scan of the laws and rates of prosecution for HIV transmission within signatory States of the European Convention on Human Rights" (*Criminalisation of HIV Transmission in Europe* (2005), available online at http://www.gnp-plus.net/criminalisation/rapidscan.pdf)

Of 41 countries where it was possible to establish the position, 36 criminalised the actual or potential transmission of HIV, 14 of which had legislation which was specific to HIV itself. 14 countries, had, however, seen no prosecutions; 15 had seen five or less. Denmark, Finland and the Netherlands had seen between 10 and 19; Austria, Sweden and Switzerland had seen 30 or more cases.

Where prosecutions had taken place, they were predominantly of men (92% of cases where data was available). A majority of cases (54%) involved HIV transmission through heterosexual sex; 45% concerned homosexual sex and 1% injecting drug use.

Criminalisation: the policy arguments

Prosecutions: why, and why now?

The (relative) flurry of prosecutions since 2001 has led to an obvious question: why now? Many other countries saw - and continue to see - prosecutions for HIV transmission or exposure from a much earlier stage. The criminalisation of HIV transmission does not, however, represent any shift in policy in the UK. As the timeline demonstrates, the authorities - at least in England and Wales - were simply not able to bring prosecutions until relatively recently. Now that the effect of more general changes in the law has been properly recognised, it is clear that such prosecutions are possible. It is this rather than any change in policy which explains the timing of prosecutions

Because the legal change has come about in this way, it means that there has been none of the public debate which might have been expected to accompany proposals for legislation. It is not, therefore, clear what purpose prosecutions are intended to serve. However, these prosecutions simply apply the general principle of law that it is a criminal offence to recklessly cause serious harm to another person - and it is fair to say that the underlying rationale of that general principle is not always that clear either, perhaps because the principle itself is felt to be relatively uncontroversial. The question, therefore, is perhaps not whether the reckless transmission of HIV *should* be criminalised, but whether it *should not* be: in other words, why should it be made an exception, and treated differently from other forms of harm?

Arguments have sometimes been made describing HIV transmission as a private matter between two individuals, or suggesting that it must be inappropriate to prosecute cases based on one person's word against another. Such arguments are unattractive, because they seem to apply equally to (for example) domestic violence or rape. Two arguments against criminalisation carry more weight, however: first, that it might deter people from taking HIV tests - itself resulting in those people not receiving proper treatment and being more likely to pass on HIV themselves; and secondly, that prosecution is likely to operate is a discriminatory fashion.

Deterring testing

Shortly after Stephen Kelly's trial, an article was published arguing that his conviction "risks a one-third increase in new HIV infections in Scotland" (SM Bird and AJ Leigh Brown, "Criminalisation of HIV transmission: implications for public health in Scotland" (2001) 323 *British Medical Journal* 1174-1177). The authors argued that if Kelly's case could result in a significant decline in the uptake of HIV testing - they suggested 25% - which would in turn lead to a significant increase in new HIV infections.

The argument made in that article was open to the objection that it was based entirely on a series of assumptions made without any supporting evidence, not just about any possible decline in testing, but also about levels of disclosure and condom use (see J Chalmers, "The criminalisation of HIV transmission" (2002) 28 *Journal of Medical Ethics* 160-163). In the event, the number of HIV tests carried out in Scotland in the four months immediately after Kelly's conviction was around 16% higher than in the same period of the previous year (R Fieldhouse, "No decline in HIV testing in Scotland following Stephen Kelly case", *AIDSMap,* 10 July 2002).

Nevertheless, it is difficult to isolate any specific effect which criminalisation might have on testing rates, and it remains possible that criminalisation is having a deterrent effect, perhaps specifically among individuals who are aware that they are at a particularly high risk of being HIV-positive.

Selective prosecution

One significant concern about prosecutions for HIV transmission has been that patterns of prosecution may be discriminatory and/or disproportionately affect certain groups.   For example, one critic of criminalisation has noted the "potential for discrimination against certain categories of people", observing that "it is a matter of record that the only people so far prosecuted and convicted in England and Wales have been men of black African origin who have transmitted HIV to their partners" (M Weait, "Criminal law and the sexual transmission of HIV", (2005) 68(1) *Modern Law Review* 121-134, at 134). The record is stark, although it may be objected that the first Scottish case was a prosecution of a white man, while in England the CPS had unsuccessfully attemptedto prosecute white men for the transmission of hepatitis B and viral herpes prior to the *Dica* case (assuming, in respect of the hepatitis B case, that the lack of any media reports of the defendant's ethnicity means that he was white). The picture has now changed slightly, and the ethnicity of those convicted in England and Wales is no longer uniform.

The picture can, however, be interpreted differently. One of the striking features of the UK prosecutions to date is that there has only been one conviction for male-male transmission of HIV. In other words, it appears that homosexual transmission has, by and large, not attracted the attention of the police and CPS. The question may not be why black defendants are over-represented in prosecutions, but instead why the authorities have not taken an interest in prosecuting cases of homosexual transmission (or why such cases have not come to the attention of the police). The profile of those defendants prosecuted for *heterosexual* transmission of HIV is roughly consistent with the available data on HIV prevalence: according to the Health Protection Agency, 70% of heterosexuals living with diagnosed HIV are of black African ethnicity, 18% of white ethnicity, 3.7% of black Caribbean ethnicity and 1.4% of Indian, Pakistani or Bangladeshi ethnicity. (See Health Protection Agency, *A Complex Picture. HIV & Other Sexually Transmitted Infections in the United Kingdom: 2006* (2006), 22.) There has been little, if any, discussion of the fact that those prosecuted in the UK have predominantly been men rather than women.

A related question is why prosecutions have focused on HIV in particular. The law certainly is not limited to HIV, and it is significant that in giving judgment for the Court of Appeal in the *Dica* case, Lord Justice Judge remarked at the outset of his judgment that "we understand that there have been significant recent increases in the recorded rates of syphilis and gonorrhoea, and that a significant proportion of sexually active young women, and many young men, are infected with chlamydia. although we agreed to accept submissions from the Terence Higgins Trust, the George House Trust and the National AIDS Trust in relation to HIV, and some of the problems faced by those with this condition, for which we are grateful, the issues which arise in this appeal are not confined to that devastating disease."

However, since the *Dica* case, there have been no attempts in England and Wales - or at least none that have come to public attention - to bring prosecutions in respect of STIs other than HIV. Such prosecutions would be possible provided the particular infection amounted to "grievous bodily harm" - given the lack of prosecutions, there has been no discussion in the courts of which STIs would and would not fall within that category. The CPS consultation (discussed below) indicated that the CPS's policy on such cases was intended to cover, in addition to HIV, chlamydia; genital herpes; gonnorhoea; hepatitis A; hepatitis B; hepatitis C; LGV; NSU and syphilis.

That does not indicate that prosecutions in respect of STIs other than HIV are likely to be frequent: given the seriousness of HIV infection it seems fair to assume that prosecutors will continue to view the reckless transmission of HIV as generally more serious than the reckless transmission of other STIs. By way of comparison, in Canada, where prosecutors have been active in bringing prosecutions for the transmission of HIV, there used to be a specific criminal offence of knowingly transmitting a venereal disease. That offence was repealed in 1985, in part because there had not been a prosecution since 1922 (see *R v Cuerrier*, (1996) 141 D.L.R. (4th) 503, at 526) - and so Canadian prosecutions in respect of HIV have, like English prosecutions, been based on the general law of offences against the person.

The Crown Prosecution Service consultation

In September 2006, the Crown Prosecution Service issued a consultation on a draft policy regarding "cases involving the intentional or reckless sexual transmission of infections which cause grievous bodily harm".

This was not a consultation on whether such cases should be within the criminal law. Now that it is clear that the transmission of STIs *can* be prosecuted, the CPS has no power to change the criminal law - and if the CPS were to decide that such cases would *never* be prosecuted, that policy could be challenged in the courts (see *R v Commissioner of Police for the Metropolis, ex p Blackburn* [1968] 2 QB 118). Instead, it was a consultation on the circumstances in which it would be appropriate for the CPS to bring a prosecution.

The draft policy set out the general principle known as the "Full Code Test" (the Code being the "Code for Crown Prosecutors") which applies to all CPS decisions to prosecute. That test has two stages: the CPS must decide first whether there is a "realistic prospect of conviction" and secondly, whether a prosecution is "needed in the public interest".

The draft policy acknowledges that not all transmissions of HIV or other STIs are reckless - factors such as condom use, the defendant's awareness of his or her infection and the medical or professional advice which they received may all affect this. Although the draft policy does not go so far as saying that a prosecution would *never* be brought where there had been "correct and consistent" (the CPS's phrase) condom use, it acknowledges that this would be a "significant factor" in determining whether or not there was evidence of recklessness. It acknowledges that "sexual transmission of infection usually takes place in a private setting where the victim is the only witness", which creates difficulties of proof, and suggests that the CPS will not prosecute without scientific or medical evidence that the defendant infected the complainant.

It is clear that the draft policy has been heavily influenced by the CPS's policy on prosecutions in cases of domestic violence. While some of this is clearly relevant (for example, the CPS has had to give careful consideration to when it should bring prosecutions for domestic violence against the victim's wishes, and similar issues might arise in respect of HIV transmission), it is less obviously relevant in respect of other issues, which means that the discussion of the public interest test is flawed at some points (see the references to previous and planned violence / threats at para 6.2). The draft policy does, however, single out four particular public interest factors: (i) medical/clinical advice received by the defendant; (ii) the use of condoms (noting that some defendants may have "limited ability" to ensure that these are used); (iii) the "context" of sexual behaviour and (iv) the "age, vulnerability and understanding. of the defendant".

At the time of writing, it was understood that a final policy would be published in "early 2007". Similar CPS policy statements - for example, in respect of homophobia and domestic violence - have been issued against a background of pressure on the CPS to demonstrate that they take such offences seriously and will actively bring prosecutions. The STI consultation is significantly different, because the pressure on the CPS is largely pressure *not* to prosecute, or at least to prosecute less. How that is reflected in the published policy remains to be seen. Beyond the statement that medical or scientific evidence will be regarded as essential, the draft policy would not commit the CPS to declining to prosecute any particular category of cases.

The risk of HIV transmission in the context of other criminal offences

In cases of assault by - for example - stabbing with a syringe, or biting, the transmission (or risk of transmission) of HIV or another blood-borne virus is likely to be considered an aggravating factor in determining the sentence to be passed. This will be so even where transmission is threatened by an assailant but does not occur because of the certain distress

caused to the victim having to wait for an antibody test. For example, in *R v Schwartzkopf* [2003] EWCA Crim 2997, where the accused had headbutted a custody officer and said "Have some hep C you bastards" before biting the officer on his leg, the Court of Appeal commented:

We, of course, must also look at the aggravating factors of this particular offence. The appellant threatened to inflict a life threatening disease upon his victim. He inflicted a 6 month period of waiting upon his victim, during which the victim did not know whether or not he may have contracted hepatitis C. That must have been a dreadful period of anxiety, not only for the victim but for his family and friends. The victim was a public servant, in a particularly vulnerable position, vulnerable to just this form of attack. Biting is a very nasty, painful and dangerous form of wounding, particularly when perpetrated by an intravenous drugs user.

With respect to sexual offences the Court of Appeal suggested in the case of *R v Malcolm* (1987) 9 Cr App R (S) 487 that HIV would only be an aggravating factor if the victim of the sexual offence had a valid reason for believing that he or she had contracted it from the offender or where that actually happened. However, the court has more recently regarded it as an aggravating factor without any reference to any such restriction: *R v Steward* [2005] 1 Cr App R (S) 5

In the context of consensual sexual offences (for example, those involving a person who is under the age of consent), the failure to use a condom or otherwise engage in acknowledged safer sex practices may be regarded as an aggravating factor, even when the virus is not actually transmitted.

Mandatory testing for HIV

In February 2005, the Scottish Executive published proposals for "blood testing following criminal incidents where there is a risk of infection". The background to these proposals was that the Scottish Police Federation had petitioned the Scottish Parliament, arguing that its members were at a "special and increasing" risk of being infected with blood-borne viruses such as HIV, hepatitis B and hepatitis C. The petition called for legislation "which will make it compulsory for assailants and others who have caused police officers to be exposed or potentially exposed to such risk to submit to a blood test or test(s)" - the results of which would then be made available to the police officer concerned. The Executive produced proposals which would largely have satisfied this request, and made similar rights available to other victims of crime. Similar proposals had previously resulted in legislation of parts of Australia and Canada.

There are obvious difficulties with such proposals, not least that for such results to be of any practical use they would have to be obtained very quickly, almost certainly before the "assailant" had been convicted of any crime. The Executive's argument in favour of the proposals was unclear - on the one hand reference was made to "reducing anxiety", while elsewhere it was claimed that the results of such tests could be of medical assistance, at least in informing decisions to commence (or discontinue) PEP. There was strong opposition to the proposals, which it was argued would have little, if any, real benefit and might violate the European Convention on Human Rights and thus be outside the competence of the Scottish Parliament (see J Chalmers, "Mandatory HIV and hepatitis testing" (2005) 332 SCOLAG 116-119).

In March 2006 the proposals were shelved, with a review promised for two years' time. It is likely, therefore, that the issue will arise again (and possibly outside of Scotland) in the near future.

Promoting safer sex lawfully

What British law allows

A number of agencies have been concerned to promote information about safer sex practices by using sexually explicit text and images. The rationale behind such a strategy is to ensure that the information is clear and does not rely upon ambiguous metaphors, and also to make the information as attractive as possible to a target audience.

British law, however, places controls on the use and distribution of sexually explicit material. The principal piece of legislation is the Obscene Publications Act 1959 (amended 1964).

The Obscene Publications Act 1959

Section 2 of the Act makes it an offence to publish an obscene article or to have an obscene article for publication for gain. The latter prohibition may have only limited relevance to the distributors of safer sex information as the vast majority of such information is distributed free rather than as a commercial exercise.

- An 'article' is defined (s. 1(2)) as anything containing material to be read, looked at or listened to. 'Publishing' includes distributing, circulating, selling, hiring, showing, playing, giving, lending and offering for sale or hire (s. 1(3)).

- The test of obscenity is contained in s.1 of the Act. The effect of the article taken as a whole must be to 'tend to deprave and corrupt [a significant proportion of] persons who are likely ... to read, see or hear the matter contained' in the article.

There have been attempts to define the term 'deprave and corrupt', but such definitions have been largely tautological. In the 'Lady Chatterley' case, 'deprave' was defined as ' to make morally bad, to pervert, to debase or corrupt morally'. 'Corrupt' was defined as 'to render morally unsound or rotten, to destroy the moral purity or chastity of, to pervert or ruin a good quality, to debase, to defile'.

These appear to be strong words - the suggestion is that what is being prohibited is something which might destroy the fabric of society. However, prosecution policy has rendered the phrase 'deprave and corrupt' largely devoid of any real meaning. In practice the legislation is applied by having an effective blacklist of forbidden images.

Text is largely left untouched since a number of unsuccessful prosecutions. The blacklist is not static, however, but constantly changing as publishers seek to push the boundaries of permitted images forward and the prosecuting authorities seek to re-impose what they feel to be the appropriate limits.

For example, it was considered, until relatively recently, that an image of an erect penis was not permissible. The early 1990s, however, have seen an explosion of sexual guidance videos, which contain such images and yet have been certified by the British Board of Film Classification, and have to date not been the subject of any prosecutions.

These constant shifts in what is and is not permissible make it difficult to give certain advice to agencies which are preparing explicit safer sex material. Text is certainly less at risk from prosecution than images. There are also certain concepts within the Act which may be of assistance.

Arguments supporting sexually explicit materials

First, it is arguable that careful targeting of a specified audience (for example, only distributing safer sex material for gay men at gay venues) will lessen the risk of prosecution since the Act requires the corruption of persons who are 'likely to', as opposed

to 'conceivably might', see the article. Consequently, it might be argued that if the target audience has regularly experienced such imagery then there is no risk of corruption. However, in DPP v Whyte [1972] AC 849, the House of Lords held that the Act was not merely concerned with the once and for all corruption of the wholly innocent, it equally protected the less innocent from further corruption and the addict from feeding or increasing their addiction.

Secondly, in the case of R v Calder and Boyars Ltd [1969] 1 QB 151 (the prosecution of *Last Exit to Brooklyn)*, the Court of Appeal added the requirement that a 'significant proportion' of the likely readership would tend to be corrupted. This requirement was imposed to protect the publisher from speculation by a jury as to the possible adverse effect of an article on a young person who might just happen to see it. Targeting safer sex information is, again, therefore advisable. The 'significant proportion' test does not, however, require the prosecution to prove that a majority, or substantial number of readers or viewers would be adversely affected.

Thirdly, the article in question must be viewed as a whole. Any isolated items of an apparently offensive nature must be viewed in their context. This may be of significance if safer sex material uses an explicit sexual image to attract the interest of its intended recipient, but otherwise contains text.

Finally, even if a prosecution is brought under s.1 of the Act there would, with safer sex material, be a chance of a 'public good' defence succeeding under s.4 of the Act. This states that the publication may be justified as being for the public good on the grounds that it is in the 'interest of science, literature, art or learning, or other objects of general concern'. It is possible to call expert evidence on the merits of a publication.

Some of the case law on this section appears to be unhelpful to the application of the 'public good' defence to sexually explicit material. In the case of Attorney-General's Reference (No. 3 of 1977) [1978] 1 WLR 1123 (following DPP v Jordan [1977] AC 699) the Court of Appeal considered the relevance of calling expert evidence to establish that certain magazines contained material which had merit in the field of sex education or had value in teaching about sexual matters, with a view to founding the 'public good' defence. The Court ruled that expert evidence was not appropriate in such a case and that the provision of information about sexual matters did not fall within the scope of the 'public good' defence.

However, it is arguable that the ruling was largely expedient and sought principally to control pornography dressed up as sex education material. Safer sex information may still be regarded as possessing scientific interest if it extends an existing body of knowledge or presents known facts in a systematic way. It would certainly be arguable that safer sex information should be within the scope of the 'public good' defence.

The Act contains not only provisions to prosecute obscene material but also to seize it without prosecution (s.3). This power is frequently used because its use effectively places the onus upon the loser of the material to take action for its recovery. However the power of seizure only applies to material which is kept for publication for gain and freely distributed safer sex information will, consequently, be exempt.

Other relevant legislation

There are a number of other statutory provisions which may cause difficulties with the distribution and display of safer sex information. It should be noted that with respect to some of these provisions the test adopted is whether the material is 'indecent' rather than 'obscene'. Indecency is accepted to be a lower standard than obscenity and therefore more articles will be prohibited under legislation containing this test. Furthermore, such legislation does not contain provisions parallel to the 'public good' defence and the material would be, consequently, viewed in isolation rather than in the context of its overall purpose.

The Video Recordings Act 1984

This legislation makes it an offence to distribute a video which has not been certificated by the British Board of Film Classification. Any new video has, therefore, to be submitted to the Board before its release. From the early 1990s (under the leadership of James Ferman), the Board has taken a liberal attitude to the certification of sex education videos containing explicit sexual imagery. This has extended to *The Gay Man's Guide to Safer Sex*, which was published in association with The Terrence Higgins Trust in 1992, and which received an 18 certificate from the Board.

The BBFC may also grant an R18 certificate, meaning that a video may only be supplied to adults in licensed sex shops. Prior to 1999, that classification was rarely used and the BBFC regularly refused to grant any certificate to material considered pornographic. However, in 1999 the Video Appeals Committee allowed a number of appeals against the BBFC's decision to refuse certificates to certain videos, and an attempt by the BBFC to overturn that decision in court failed (R v Video Appeals Committee of the British Board of Film Classification, ex parte the British Board of Film Classification [2000] EMLR 850).

The guidelines for R18 classification have since been revised (current information is available on the BBFC's website at http://www.bbfc.co.uk/) and the number of videos granted an R18 certificate has since grown dramatically - 1387 in 2004 compared to 29 in 1999. R18 videos may not be sold by mail order within the UK, a restriction which has recently survived a challenge in the courts (Interfact v Liverpool City Council [2005] EWHC 995), although it was noted in that case that such material may in practice be ordered from sellers based outside the UK.

Certification by the Board does not, however, preclude a prosecution under the Obscene Publications Act since the two pieces of legislation are not directly linked.

Importation of safer sex material

Section 170(2)(b) of the Customs and Excise Management Act 1979 (when read together with section 42 of the Customs Consolidation Act 1876) prohibits the importation of any obscene or indecent articles. However, the European Court of Justice ruled in 1986 that the principle of free movement of goods under European law meant that the UK could not restrict the import of goods on the basis that they were indecent or obscene when such goods could lawfully be manufactured and sold within the UK.

The consequence of the ruling was accepted to be (according to a later statement in Parliament by the then Chancellor) that "Customs could continue to seize obscene material but [could] not, with the exception of material involving children, seize indecent material". Furthermore, although the decision "related solely to material imported from the [European] Community, Customs and Excise consider that it would be inequitable and impracticable not to apply the same standards to all imports" (HC Debs 3 May 1989, col 105).

Post Office Act 1953

This makes it an offence to send any indecent or obscene article through the post. S.11 of the Act defines obscene as 'offending, shocking, lewd or indecent', which is a clearly different test from

that contained in the Obscene Publications Act. The legislation does not apply to alternative distribution systems such as 'Red Star', FedEx, DHL etc.

Unsolicited Goods and Services Act 1971

It is an offence under s.4 of the Act for a person to send any book, magazine or leaflet which they know or ought reasonably to have known was unsolicited and which describes or illustrates human sexual technique. Safer sex material should only, therefore, be sent when requested and not unsolicited.

Indecent Displays (Control) Act 1981

It is an offence under this legislation to display, in public, any indecent article. This may cause problems with, for example, a safer sex roadshow, which is displaying posters containing sexual imagery.

At the time of writing there have not been any prosecutions of safer sex material under any of the afore-mentioned statutory provisions, although the police and prosecution authorities have shown interest in a number of items including the video, *The Gay Man's Guide to Safer Sex*, and a German safer sex poster showing two men engaged in an act of oral sex.

Safer sex information in counselling and outreach

As with safer sex material there is a similar desire to explain safer sex practices in clear language, which avoids medical jargon. There is also a perceived need to target certain groups, for example gay men who make use of public lavatories for the purpose of sexual contacts, who may be most in need of the information.

It is an offence under s.43 of the Telecommunications Act 1984 to send by means of a public telecommunications service a message that is 'grossly offensive or of an indecent, obscene or menacing character'. 'Obscene' is not defined in the Act, but arguably, the definition will be the one contained in the Post Office Act 1953.

Presumably a prosecution under this provision might be possible if it was felt that advice, or counselling, relating to safer sex as given by counsellors to members of the public over the telephone was 'obscene', but it is very difficult, given the one to one nature of counselling, to envisage a complaint ever arising to provide grounds for a prosecution.

In the past, there was frequent concern that providing advice to a person who might engage in a sexual act which was criminal because one of the parties was underage might result in criminal liability, in that the advisor might be viewed as an accessory to the offence.

Matters are now somewhat clearer as a result of section 73 of the Sexual Offences Act 2003, which applies to a specified list of child sexual offences and provides as follows:

Exceptions to aiding, abetting and counselling

(1)   A person is not guilty of aiding, abetting or counselling the commission against a child of an offence to which this section applies if he acts for the purpose of-

(a)   protecting the child from sexually transmitted infection,

(b)   protecting the physical safety of the child,

(c)   preventing the child from becoming pregnant, or

(d)   promoting the child's emotional well-being by the giving of advice, and not for the purpose of obtaining sexual gratification or for the purpose of causing or encouraging the activity constituting the offence or the child's participation in it.

Sex education: the legal and political context

The 1996 Education Act

Sex education became compulsory in maintained secondary schools in England and Wales, as a result of Section 241 of the 1993 Education Act. In response to this legislation, the Department for Education issued guidance to schools on sex education (DfE 5/94). This explained how changes to the provision of sex education in the 1993 Education Act affected schools. In November 1996 various Education Acts including the Education Act 1993 were consolidated into a new act, the Education Act 1996.

Section 352-(1) of the Education Act 1996 requires governors of maintained secondary schools and special schools providing pupils with secondary education to provide sex education (including education about HIV/AIDS and other STIs) to all registered pupils

- Section 371-(3) requires governors of maintained primary schools to consider whether and what sex education the school will provide beyond the provisions in the National Curriculum and to make and keep up-to-date a written statement of their decision

- Section 405 grants parents the right to withdraw pupils in all maintained primary and secondary schools from all or part of sex education provided outside the National Curriculum

- Section 404 requires all maintained schools to make and keep up to date a written statement of their policy on sex education, and for this policy to be made available to parents free of charge. The existence and implementation of school sex education policies are monitored by OFSTED and OHMCI Wales as part of school inspection.

In addition Section 403 (1) requires that the LEA, governing body and head teacher 'shall take such steps as are reasonably practicable to secure that where sex education is given to any registered pupil at the school it is given in such a manner as to encourage those pupils to have due regard to moral considerations and the value of family life'.

Section 351-(1) requires all maintained schools to offer a curriculum which:

- (a) promotes the spiritual, moral, cultural, mental and physical development of pupils at the school and of society;

- (b) prepares such pupils for the opportunities, responsibilities and experiences of adult life.

Circular 5/94 and WO 45/94

Circular 5/94, also contains advice from the Secretary of State for Education, on how certain aspects of the teaching of sex education should be handled. The guidance is advisory only. It does not constitute an authoritative legal interpretation. Teachers are not obliged to follow its advice unless instructed to do so by their head teacher. The Welsh Office issued an equivalent circular on sex education, WO 45/94.

Responsibilities of school governors

Primary schools

Since 1993 it has been the responsibility of the governors of primary and middle-deemed primary schools to decide whether the school should provide sex education in addition to that in the National Curriculum (Science); to keep a written statement of this decision; and to develop a policy outlining where and how sex education will be provided. This policy should be made available to all parents. Voluntary aided primary schools are encouraged to develop a sex education policy if they decide to provide sex education in addition to that within National Curriculum (Science).

Middle schools

Where these are deemed primary, sex education is discretionary as outlined above. Where they are deemed secondary, sex education is compulsory as described below for secondary schools.

Secondary schools

Secondary schools including middle-deemed secondary schools are required to provide sex education. This must include education about HIV/AIDS and other sexually transmitted infections to all registered pupils. Parents have the right to withdraw pupils from all or part of that sex education as long as it is outside the National Curriculum. Since 1993 school governors of secondary schools have been required to develop a policy explaining how and where sex education will be taught, and to make that policy available to parents. Governors of voluntary aided secondary schools are encouraged to develop a sex education policy outlining the content and organisation of sex education provided in addition to that in National Curriculum (Science).

Special schools

In those special schools which cater exclusively for primary or for secondary age children, the responsibilities of governing bodies correspond to those of primary or secondary schools as outlined above. In all-age special schools, the governing bodies are required to adopt separate arrangements for children under and over the age of 11 corresponding to those applying to primary schools and secondary schools. In addition, the governors should ensure that their written policies explain any distinction they may have chosen to make between arrangements for children below the age of 11 and those above it.

1994 guidance from the Department for Education encourages governing bodies to involve parents as fully as possible in the formulation and review of their sex education policies and programmes, not only as a matter of good practice but, because such involvement is likely to reduce the number of parents who have sufficiently strong reservations about the school's programme as to lead them to consider exercising their right of withdrawal.

The 2000 Guidance

This guidance was updated in the 2000 Department for Education and Sex and Relationships Guidance of the Department for Education and Skills. This stated that:

- Effective sex and relationship education is essential if young people are to make responsible and well-informed decisions about their lives. It should not be delivered in isolation and should be firmly rooted within the framework for PSHE and the National Curriculum.

- The objective of sex and relationship education is to help and support young people through their physical, emotional and moral development and would help young people learn to respect themselves and others and move with confidence from childhood through adolescence into adulthood.

- It would help pupils develop the skills and understanding they need to live confident, healthy and independent lives and deal with difficult moral and social questions.

- It states that "as part of sex and relationship education, pupils should be taught about the nature and importance of marriage for family life and bringing up children," but that the Government recognised "that there are strong and mutually supportive relationships outside marriage," and that "care needs to be taken to ensure that there is no stigmatisation of children based on their home circumstances."

- Secondary pupils should learn to understand human sexuality, learn the reasons for delaying sexual activity and the benefits to be gained from such delay, and learn about obtaining appropriate advice on sexual health.

- Effective sex and relationship education does not encourage early sexual experimentation. It should teach young people to understand human sexuality and to respect themselves and others. It enables young people to mature, to build up their confidence and self-esteem and understand the reasons for delaying sexual activity.

The 2002 OFSTED Report

The 2002 Report from Her Majesty's Chief Inspector of Schools followed from a recommendation that OFSTED, the Office for Standards in Education, should conduct a survey on sex and relationships education in schools and produce a guide to good practice.

The report it produced was based on evidence from inspection of 140 primary, secondary and special schools; discussions with 650 young people during these inspections; analysis of OFSTED inspections of primary, secondary and special schools carried out during 2000/01; and a postal survey of about 1,000 primary, secondary and special schools in20 local education authorities.

Main findings

The OFSTED report found that:

- Most of the primary and secondary schools taught about sex and relationships conscientiously and, for the most part, effectively.

- Pupils' **knowledge and understanding** of factual aspects of SRE were good, but school programmes needed to do more to develop **values and attitudes** and the **personal skills** needed to make sensible choices. OFSTED comment: "At all key stages, too many schools tend to judge achievement in SRE only in terms of factual knowledge."

- Over nine out of ten schools had SRE policies. Their quality was good in over half the primary schools and in three fifths of secondary schools. In one in ten of all schools, their quality was poor.

- The 2000 guidance from the DfES had had a positive effect, but too many schools had not reviewed their policies in the light of the guidance.

- Education about HIV/AIDS was receiving less attention than in the past, despite the fact that it remains a significant health problem. The rport found that the percentage of girls aged 14-15 "worrying quite a lot" about HIV/AIDS had gone down from 35% in 1995 to 12% in 1999, and boys from 27% to 10%.

- Education about parenthood did not feature in all secondary schools' programmes, even though most schools recognised its importance.

- Few schools engaged pupils in discussions when planning or evaluating their SRE programmes. Where such discussions had taken place, pupils valued them and the school gained fresh insights.

- In secondary schools, at both key stages, teaching about sexual health, including sexually transmitted infections, and the law in relation to sex, was poor in one in five lessons.

- Schools had been effective in addressing the concerns of parents, communities and religious groups about the SRE they provide. About four in every 10,000 pupils (0.04%) were currently being withdrawn from the nonstatutory aspects of SRE.

- Many parents were reluctant to play a greater role in discussing sex and relationships with their children because they felt they lacked the necessary knowledge and skills.

- The media, especially magazines for teenagers, were an increasingly important source of information and had a significant bearing on pupils' attitudes.

- Schools provided support and advice for individual pupils, but boys felt that this support and advice was often aimed only at girls. While not necessarily true, the perception discouraged them from seeking help.

- Access to advisory services depended in part on where pupils lived. Whatever the location of the services, many pupils were concerned about confidentiality.

- Support for pregnant schoolgirls varied in quality. School-age fathers did not receive enough guidance.

To improve the quality of education about sex and relationships in schools, it was important that:

- schools broadened their coverage and clarified their definition of achievement.

- SRE was taught by teachers with specialist knowledge and expertise.

- further guidance was given on teaching about sexuality and about parenthood.

- the coverage of HIV/AIDS was enhanced.

- assessment, monitoring and evaluation processes were improved.

- more advice was provided for parents, especially fathers, to help them to talk more fully about sex and relationships with their children.

- pupils were given better access to individual advice from specialist professionals.

Organisation of sex education

Sex education can be taught anywhere in the curriculum: in science; as a separately timetabled subject; within tutor groups; across the curriculum or ideally through a combination of the above approaches. Where there have been requests for the withdrawal of pupils from all or part of the sex education programme, schools should ensure that those aspects of sex education other than the requirements of the National Curriculum, are structured in the curriculum in such a way as to enable a pupil to be withdrawn. The right of withdrawal does not affect spontaneous discussion or the honest answering of questions that arise naturally in other curriculum areas. The DfE guidance notes state: 'Provided that such discussion is relatively limited and set within the context of the other subject concerned, it will not necessarily constitute part of a programme of sex education' (para 30 Circular 5/94).

Parental withdrawal

Pupils can be withdrawn by their parents from all or part of sex education that does not form part of the statutory National Curriculum. HIV, AIDS, sexually transmitted infections and non-biological aspects of sexual behaviour were removed from the

National Curriculum and now form part of compulsory 'sex education'. Defining the division between biological and non-biological aspects of sexual behaviour is left to the discretion of teachers. Teachers also have to consider where aspects of parenting, relationships and the ethical and moral dimensions of sex education will be placed within the curriculum. Parents are not able to withdraw pupils from sex education which continues to form part of National Curriculum (Science), nor from sex education comprised within other National Curriculum subjects, such as geography.

If a parent has withdrawn a pupil from sex education a teacher cannot give advice to that pupil on sexual matters without parental consent. However, a teacher who suggested that the child seek confidential information from, for example, their GP or Brook Advisory Centre, or any other medical or advisory service, would not be providing sex education, but merely giving information as to where advice, counselling (and treatment) could lawfully be obtained.

What should schools do if a request for withdrawal is made by a parent?

Schools should first discuss with the parents or carers the nature of their concerns and see whether they can be reassured. The DfE guidance notes that parents do not have to give reasons for withdrawal, but that schools may invite parents voluntarily to indicate their reasons for withdrawal, so that any misunderstandings about the nature of sex education provided by the school, can be resolved (para 37 Circular 5/94).

Where aspects of sex education arise naturally in other subject lessons within which there is a child or children who have been withdrawn from sex education teachers will need to balance the need to give proper attention to relevant issues with the need to respect pupils' and parents' views and sensitivities (para 30 Circular 5/94).

The right of withdrawal extends to all pupils attending maintained schools including those over compulsory school age. It does not apply to sixth form colleges or colleges of further education.

Once a request that a child be excused has been made, that request must be complied with until the parent changes or revokes it (para 36 Circular 5/94).

Content of sex education

Although sex education is compulsory in secondary schools, the content of this programme has not been clearly defined, other than including the study of HIV and AIDS and sexually transmitted diseases (Section 352-(3) Education Act 1996). Department for Education Guidance Circular 5/94 and Welsh Office 45/94 state:

"The Government believes that all pupils should be offered the opportunity of receiving a comprehensive, well planned programme of sex education during their school careers."

At the primary stage, the aim [of sex education] should be to prepare pupils to cope with the physical and emotional challenges of growing up, and to give them an elementary understanding of human reproduction.

In secondary schools sex education should, in the Secretary of State's view, encompass, in addition to the facts about human reproductive processes and behaviour, consideration of the broader emotional and ethical dimensions of sexual attitudes. It must include, at a point appropriate to the age and maturity of the pupils, education about HIV, AIDS and other sexually transmitted infections.

The Welsh guidance differs slightly in wording although not in substance.

The National Curriculum

Significant aspects of sex education remain part of the National Curriculum (Science). This must be taught to all pupils and parents cannot withdraw pupils from such lessons.

Curriculum guidance

Sex education and education for family life also form part of the cross curricular themes of the National Curriculum (NCC 1990a, 1990b). *Curriculum Guidance 5: Health Education* provides an excellent, developmentally appropriate curriculum for sex education, but this curriculum, itself, only has the status of guidance.

The National Curriculum for science contains the areas of study that must be taught and from which pupils cannot be withdrawn.

Specific learning objectives

The 2000 guidance states that for **Primary Schools:**

All primary schools should have a sex and relationship education programme tailored to the age and the physical and emotional maturity of the children. It should ensure that both boys and girls know about puberty and how a baby is born.

All children, including those who develop earlier than the average, need to know about puberty before they experience the onset of physical changes. In the early primary school years, education about relationships needs to focus on friendship, bullying and the building of self-esteem.

During the transition year before moving to secondary schools children should be taught about

- changes in the body related to puberty, such as periods and voice breaking;

- when these changes are likely to happen and what issues may cause young people anxiety and how they can deal with these; and

- how a baby is conceived and born.

And for **Secondary schools:**

Schools should set sex education within a broader base of self-esteem and responsibility for the consequences of one's actions.

Schools should set a framework for establishing what is appropriate and inappropriate in a whole-class setting and how to deal with individual questions.

Secondary schools should:

- teach about relationships, love and care and the responsibilities of parenthood as well as sex;

- focus on boys as much as girls;

- build self-esteem;

- the taking on of responsibility and the consequences of one's actions in relation to sexual activity and parenthood;

- provide young people with information about different types of contraception, safer sex and how they can access local sources of further advice and treatment;

- use young people as peer educators, e.g. teenage mothers and fathers;

- give young people a clear understanding of the arguments for delaying sexual activity and resisting pressure;

- link sex and relationship education with issues of peer pressure and other risk-taking behaviour, such as drugs, smoking and alcohol; and

- ensure young people understand how the law applies to sexual relationships.

Ethnicity

The guidelines state that research with families shows that "a range of children from black and other minority ethnic communities are less likely to talk to their parents about sex and relationships. Some young women and young men from some minority ethnic communities may rely on schools as their main, and sometimes only, source of sex education."

It is important for policies to be both culturally appropriate and inclusive of all children. Primary and secondary schools should consult parents and pupils both on what is included, and on how it is delivered. For example, for some children it is not culturally appropriate to address particular issues in a mixed group. Consulting pupils and their families will help to establish what is appropriate and acceptable for them. Generally, parents appreciate support from the school, if they are consulted and involved.

Relationships

Young people report that the emphasis of SRE is too biological and they want more opportunity to talk about feelings and relationships. This feedback from young people fits neatly into the PSHE framework with its emphasis on building self-esteem, and respect for self and others. The diversity of different relationships can be usefully discussed within this context.

Focus on boys and young men as well as girls and young women

Traditionally the focus has been on girls. Boys may have felt that sex education is not relevant to them and are unable or too embarrassed to ask questions about relationships or sex. Boys are also less likely to talk to their parents about sex and relationships. For these reasons, programmes should focus on boys as much as girls at primary level as well as secondary.

Teachers will need to plan a variety of activities which will help to engage boys as well as girls, matching their different learning styles. Single sex groups may be particularly important for pupils who come from cultures where it is only acceptable to speak about the body in single gender groups.

Special educational needs and learning difficulties

The SRE guidance states that mainstream schools and special schools have a duty to ensure that children with special educational needs and learning difficulties are properly included in SRE. The content and delivery may need to be adapted to meet individual needs. Some parents may have difficulty understanding their child's developing sexuality and it is important that they are consulted and involved in the development of the SRE curriculum.

Sexual identity and sexual orientation

The SRE guidance states that schools need to ensure SRE meets the needs of all pupils, regardless of sexual orientation. It says that young people, whatever their developing sexuality, need to feel that SRE is relevant to them and sensitive to their needs. The guidance states that there should be no direct promotion of sexual orientation. The role of SRE in framing sexuality, sexual identity and sexual orientation in a positive light is crucial. It is important to build tolerance as well as self-esteem and respect for self.

The National Curriculum for health education (NCC 1990) suggests that pupils at Key Stage 3 'be aware of the range of sexual attitudes and behaviours in present day society.'

The DfES 2000 guidelines state:

"It is up to schools to make sure that the needs of all pupils are met in their programmes. Young people, whatever their developing sexuality, need to feel that sex and relationship education is relevant to them and sensitive to their needs.

"Teachers should be able to deal honestly and sensitively with sexual orientation, answer appropriate questions and offer support. There should be no direct promotion of sexual orientation.

"Sexual orientation and what is taught in schools is an area of concern for some parents. Schools that liaise closely with parents when developing their sex and relationship education policy and programme should be able to reassure parents of the content of the programme and the context in which it will be presented.

"Schools need to be able to deal with homophobic bullying. Guidance issued by the Department (Social Inclusion: Pupil Support Circular 10/99) dealt with the unacceptability of and emotional distress and harm caused by bullying in whatever form - be it racial, as a result of a pupil's appearance, related to sexual orientation or for any other reason."

The 2002 OFSTED Report comments:

"Different interpretations of aims and values can produce confusion about what is deemed to be acceptable. For example, in too many secondary schools homophobic attitudes among pupils often go unchallenged. The problem is compounded when derogatory terms about homosexuality are used in everyday language in school and their use passes unchallenged by staff. Where problems arise, staff have often had insufficient guidance on the interpretation of school values and what constitutes unacceptable language or behaviour.

HMI Health Education From 516 states:

"Given the openness with which homosexuality is treated in society now it is almost bound to arise in one area or another of a school's curriculum. Information about and discussion of homosexuality, whether it involves the whole class, or an individual, needs to acknowledge that experiencing strong feelings of attraction for members of the same sex is a phase passed through by many young people, but for a significant number of people these feelings persist into adult life. Therefore it needs to be dealt with objectively and seriously, bearing in mind that while there has been a marked shift away from the general condemnation of homosexuality, many individuals and groups within society hold sincerely to the view that it is morally objectionable. This is difficult territory for teachers to traverse and for some schools accepting homosexuality as a normal feature of relationships would be a breach of the religious faith on which they are founded. Therefore Local Education Authorities, voluntary bodies, governors, heads and senior staff in schools have important responsibilities in devising guidance and supporting teachers dealing with this sensitive issue".

Overall there is a consensus that an effective sex education programme would and should include honest and objective discussions of a variety of sexual identities and behaviours. This would inevitably include discussions of homosexuality as well as heterosexuality, bisexuality, celibacy and the concept of sexual identity itself. The Sex Education Forum has issued guidance on teaching about homosexuality in Forum Factsheet 6. (See *References*).

Safer sex, HIV and STIs

Teaching about safer sex remains one of the Government's key strategies for reducing the incidence of HIV/AIDS and STIs.

Strategies for teaching about HIV/AIDS and STIs should include:

- helping pupils clarify their knowledge of HIV/AIDS and STIs;

- teaching them assertiveness skills for negotiating relationships; and

- enabling them to become effective users of services that help prevent/treat STIs and HIV.

The key messages for all sex educators, including schools, are:

- information and knowledge about HIV/AIDS is vital;

- young people need to understand what is risky behaviour and what is not;

- sex and relationship education should inform young people about condom use and safer sex in general;

- young people need skills to enable them to avoid being pressured into unwanted or unprotected sex (this should link with issues of peer pressure and other risk-taking behaviour such as drugs and alcohol); and

- young people need factual information about safer sex and skills to enable them to negotiate safer sex.

- young people need to be aware of the risks of contracting a STI and how to prevent it. A Health Education Authority study found that one in four young people believed that the pill would protect them from STIs.

- although the emphasis in sex and relationship education should be on prevention of infection, through delaying sexual activity and teaching the reasons for safe sex, pupils also need to know about diagnosis and treatment.

Teaching about HIV and AIDS

Schools will address education about HIV and AIDS within the curriculum - at secondary schools it is to be a compulsory part of the sex education curriculum. Primary school aged pupils are likely to have heard of AIDS and may have questions and misconceptions that need addressing. It is also important that schools consider wider issues for the support of staff, pupils and parents who may be infected or affected by HIV and AIDS. This could include the consideration of confidentiality and health and safety and bereavement amongst other issues.

A statutory order was issued to all schools in June 1994 removing HIV and AIDS from the programmes of study for National Curriculum (Science). However, maintained secondary schools and middle schools deemed secondary must provide a programme of sex education which includes education about HIV and AIDS and other sexually transmitted diseases.

Aspects of sex education can appear anywhere in the curriculum. The responsibility to educate young people about HIV and AIDS can and should be shared out across the curriculum and should utilise resources and services available from the wider community. Teaching about HIV and AIDS as with all health education is most effectively done by the use of active learning methods. The Sex Education Forum has produced detailed guidance on effective approaches to teaching sex in Forum Factsheet 12 (see *References*).

The requirement to teach about HIV and AIDS can be met in a variety of different ways, for example:

- The use of case studies. Case studies can provide students with the chance to explore different options open to fictional characters and examine factors which influence decision-making in a way which protects their confidentiality

- The use of role play. There are a number of resources and games developed specifically to enable teachers to engage pupils in role play around the issues of HIV and AIDS

- The use of peer education. Peer education is a method of health education which uses young people themselves as health educators. A small group of young people are given intensive training and this group then goes on to educate their peers. This method is gaining increasing popularity, especially among secondary school pupils and in the youth and community sector

- The use of theatre in education. There are a number of theatre in education companies which provide performances

and workshops around the issues of HIV/AIDS to schools. It is important that these performances are previewed to ensure that they are appropriate for the pupils' age and level of development and that they involve pupils actively, for instance by providing time and space for an active discussion after the play

- The use of outside visitors. It is often difficult for young people personally to identify with the issue of HIV/AIDS. One of the most popular methods of HIV education with young people is a visit from someone outside the school who has personal experience of the virus. This can have an enormous impact on young people, not only by giving a human face to the disease, but also by helping them to understand the pressures and stigmas experienced by people living with or affected by the virus. It is important that the young people themselves are able to set the agenda for the visit, and prepare questions in advance. The use of suitably qualified and experienced outside visitors can greatly enhance a school sex education programme. However schools should be careful that visitors are used in addition to, not instead of a planned programme of sex education. They must also ensure that any visitor is given a copy of the school's sex education policy and is aware of the ethos of the school and the way in which it has been decided to deliver sex education. Sex Education Forum Factsheet 8 provides guidance on the use of visitors (See *References*).

It is important that schools consider the use of outside visitors in their sex education policy, noting when or whether they will be accompanied in the classroom, how they will be prepared for and how their visit will be followed up.

Health professionals, for example school nurses, family planning or sexual health workers, are able to offer confidentiality and contraceptive advice. The Department for Education guidance 5/94 states:

"Teachers should take account of the range of expertise and other resources available to them, including the contribution which health authorities, other health service bodies, and health professionals - particularly doctors (including GPs) and school nurses - may be able to make (para 32)."

Health professionals are able to offer young people confidentiality and can provide a link between the school and relevant local services.

Schools should also be aware of other possible visitors such as theatre in education companies, peer educators, members of relevant voluntary organisations such as RELATE, Brook, or Terrence Higgins Trust.

Contraceptive advice to under-16s

Information and advice concerning contraception forms part of sex education, whether given on a one to one basis or in a group. If a pupil has been withdrawn from sex education they cannot be given such advice. However information regarding sources of confidential advice and treatment would not count as sex education and can be made freely available to all students.

Advice does not require consent, unlike the giving of medical treatment, and the decision as to whether to give such advice to a child, in confidence, is a matter of professional judgement for a teacher, having regard to any specific direction by the head. There are no restrictions on giving information concerning sources of confidential advice and treatment.

Many people are confused and anxious about the guidance contained in Circular 5/94 on confidentiality and contraceptive advice to under 16s. There have been no changes to the law in this area. It is only the language of the guidance that has changed. Advice contained in paragraphs 38-42 of Circular 5/94 suggests that teachers should at some point report disclosure or suspicions of unlawful activity to the head teacher who in turn should inform the pupil's parents. However, this is only guidance and is not legally binding. The following suggests how schools could deal with issues of confidentiality and contraceptive advice.

[Based on Beloff, M. QC (1994) Sex education in schools: joint opinion]

It is important to remember what teachers can do:

- They can provide all pupils with information about where and from whom they can receive confidential advice and treatment. They can provide education about types of contraception and where they can be obtained to all pupils as part of the National Curriculum

- Teachers should not promise confidentiality, but neither are they obliged to break it (see below)

- Unless instructed by the head teacher a teacher does not have a duty to inform a pupil's parents of evidence or suspicions of unlawful sexual activity.

Confidentiality

Teachers should not promise confidentiality. A child does not have a right to expect that incidents in the class room will not be reported to his or her parents, and may not, in the absence of an express promise, assume that information conveyed outside that context is private. No teacher could or should give such a promise.

However they are not obliged to break confidentiality.

It is a matter of professional judgement for a teacher whether he or she should indicate to a child that information could be offered confidentially and whether such confidence could then be maintained having heard the information.

The advice in the Circular does not seek to impose an absolute duty to break confidences, nor indeed is the Circular binding in law. A teacher is not bound to follow the Circular's advice, if, in the teacher's professional judgement, the child's best interests are better served by not doing so - subject to the parents power to excuse and the heads power to direct (that is unless parents have chosen to exercise their right to withdrawal, or the head teacher has instructed that he or she should be informed).

Teachers and others involved in SRE are often unclear about confidentiality. The Department for Education (as it was then called) (DfE, 1994) and Welsh Office Circulars (Welsh Office Education Department, 1994) offer advice on confidentiality but are not binding in law. The DfES's Child Protection Circular 10/95 Protecting Children from Abuse: The Role of the Education Service clarifies the position for schools regarding child protection issues.

The new SRE guidance aims to help schools in drawing up their own confidentiality policy and recommends that it includes the following components:

- An explanation as to how pupils and parents will be made aware of the school's confidentiality policy and how it works in practice.

- Reassurance for pupils that their best interests will be maintained at all times.

- Encouragement for pupils to talk to their parents or carers where possible, and sources of support for them to do so.

- Clarity for pupils so that they know that teachers will not always be able to maintain confidentiality.

- Reassurance for pupils that if confidentiality is to be broken, they will be told beforehand of the reason, and offered support as appropriate.

- Clear links between the school's child protection policy, in the event of a disclosure of abuse.

- Teachers are required to break confidentiality where they believe a young person is at risk of physical or sexual abuse. In which case, the school protection procedures should be followed.

- A guarantee that pupils will be told where they can access sources of confidential support and information.

- Using ground rules in lessons.

All schools should ensure that students are able to get support in school as well in the wider community. Some schools have set up general health clinics, and offer explicit advice and telephone numbers for sexual health services, Child Line and other helplines and youth advisory services. Young people are also able to access the information without embarrassment or delay if information is displayed publicly. It can also be available in leaflet form for individuals to take away.

If a teacher learns from an under 16 year-old that they are engaged in sexual activity, they should wherever possible encourage the young person to talk with a parent or carer, ensure that any child protection issue is addressed and that the person is adequately informed about contraception and safer sex. It is important that the policy on confidentiality is clear, meets the best interests of young people and is workable by staff.

Must parents be informed?
There is no basis in principle or authority for suggesting that there is any legal duty on a teacher, or a head teacher, to inform parents of matters which a child has confided to them. However if the head teacher instructs staff to follow the advice in paragraph 40 of the circular, failure to do so might be grounds for disciplinary action.

Must teachers inform heads?
A teacher does not have a general duty to inform the head of disclosures by a pupil. The decision as to whether to do so must be a matter for a teacher's discretion, unless the head issues an instruction that they should be informed, in which case the teacher must comply.

Could a teacher be committing a criminal offence?
The Sexual Offences (Amendment) Act 2003 created a new offence to protect those under 18 years of age in particular areas from abuse of trust in the form of inappropriate sexual relationships. The new offence applies to teachers and others in a position of trust. It will be an offence for a teacher to have a sexual relationship with a full-time pupil in the same school, residential school, or further education establishment who is under 18.

However the offences in the Act were developed to enable the prosecution of abusive and exploitative sexual activity. Guidance to the act states that that provisions about engaging children in discussion about sex "is not intended to cover health professionals, or anyone else providing sex education, advice or contraception to children."

The Act does not intend to limit children's right to SRE and sexual health support and advice. A person does not commit an offence if s/he acts for the purpose of:

- Protecting the child from sexually transmitted infections.

- Protecting the physical safety of the child.

- Preventing the child from becoming pregnant.

- Promoting the child's emotional well being by the giving of advice.

A teacher who gave a child under 16 advice relating to contraception, and who acted in what she or he honestly believed to be the child's best interests, would not be likely to incur criminal liability.

It is vital that these issues are considered by the governing body and that they make a statement in the school sex education policy that is understood by the head teachers, the staff, pupils and parents as regards how confidentiality will be dealt with in the school.

A training pack *Confidentiality In Schools* has been developed by Brook to help schools consider and develop practical codes of confidentiality.

Department of Health

Our Healthier Nation is a consultative green paper published in February 1998. It addresses social inequalities, targets the workplace and schools, and aims to ensure that all schools are 'healthy schools' through collaboration with the DFES.

The National Healthy Schools Awards Scheme was launched by the DfES in alliance with the Department of Health. Its aim is to ensure that all schools are healthy schools in accordance with *Our Healthier Nation*. It is based at the Health Development Agency.

A reduction in unintended teenage conceptions is one of the main aims of the UK's Sexual Health and HIV strategy.

Positive guidance on sex and relationships education

This section has been adapted with kind permission from Sex Education Forum, Factsheet 23 *Taking the initiative: Positive guidance on sex and relationships education.*

The sex and relationships education (SRE) guidance published by the DfES in July 2000. This had been highlighted as a priority in the *Teenage Pregnancy Action Plan* launched by the Prime Minister in 1999. It was published by the DfES in July 2000. The guidance (DfES 0116/2000) emphasises the need for effective SRE which is firmly rooted within the Personal, Social and Health Education (PHSE) and Citizenship Frameworks and is supported by the National Healthy School Standard (NHSS).

Why is it necessary to provide SRE in schools?

- Children and young people say that they want to learn more about sex and relationships.

- Parents say that although they want to talk to their children about sex and relationships, they want schools to help them.

- It is a legal requirement for schools to provide SRE.

Evidence shows that SRE can:

- make a positive contribution to children and young people's personal and social development; and

- help to prevent negative health outcomes such as unintended pregnancies and sexually transmitted infections.

SRE in schools is a legal requirement

The Sex and Relationship Education Guidance (2000) is supported in legislation by the *Learning and Skills Act* (2000). This requires that young people:

- learn about the nature of marriage and its importance for family life and the bringing up of children; and

- are protected from teaching and materials which are inappropriate having regard to the age and the religious and cultural background of the pupils concerned.

The evidence-base for SRE

- High quality SRE, when linked to confidential sex advice services, is shown to delay the start of sexual activity.

- School-based SRE contributes to meeting government public health priorities, such as achieving a reduction in teenage pregnancy rates and prevalence of sexually transmitted infections (STIs) including HIV.

- SRE that aims to prevent unwanted pregnancy or sexually transmitted infections should be initiated early, before patterns of sexual behaviour are established.

- Effective SRE offers an open and accepting attitude towards sex and sexuality.

- Young people need to be involved in their own learning. Therefore the use of active and participatory learning is important in SRE.

Implementing the SRE guidance

The guidance states that SRE should be firmly rooted within the framework for PSHE and Citizenship. Working towards becoming a healthy school through a Local Healthy Schools Programme will help schools develop a whole school approach that sets a positive and supportive ethos for SRE as part of PSHE. The following section looks at the links between SRE, the framework for PSHE and Citizenship and the National Healthy School Standard (NHSS) and the opportunities provided by these links.

The National Healthy School Standard - NHSS

The White Paper on Excellence in Schools (1997) set out the Government's intention to help all schools become healthy schools. This was driven by a belief in the role that education plays in promoting better health and emotional well being for all children and young people. The National Healthy School Standard is jointly funded by the (now) Department for Education and Skills and the Department of Health. The NHSS offers an accreditation scheme for local health and education partnership programmes. Local Healthy Schools Programmes support schools in developing as healthy schools.

The NHSS provides minimum criteria on a range of themes.

The minimum NHSS criteria for SRE

- The school has a policy which is owned and implemented by all members of the school including pupils and parents and which is delivered in partnership with local health and support services.

- The school has a planned SRE programme (including information, social skills development and values clarification) which identifies learning outcomes, appropriate to pupils' age, ability, gender and level of maturity and which is based on pupils' needs assessment and a knowledge of vulnerable pupils.

- Staff have sound, basic knowledge of SRE issues and are confident in their skills to teach sex education and discuss sex and relationships.

- Staff have an understanding of the role of schools in contributing to the reduction of unwanted teenage conceptions and the promotion of sexual health.

Healthy schools must work towards meeting legal requirements and take account of non-statutory guidance. You can find out more about the National Healthy School Standard by contacting the National Team based at the Health Development Agency on

020 7413 1865. They will be able to give you the contact details of your Local Healthy School Programme Coordinator.

For more about NHSS see
http://www.publichealth.nice.org.uk/indexsearch.aspx?ss=NHSS

PSHE and Citizenship Framework

A Personal, Social and Health Education and Citizenship Framework was published in 1999. From September 2000 it has been taught alongside the revised National Curriculum. It has four broad themes and aims to support the personal and social development of children and young people:

- Develop confidence and make the most of their abilities.

- Prepare to play an active role as citizens.

- Develop a healthy, safer lifestyle.

- Develop good relationships and respect differences between people.

To be effective, SRE needs to incorporate the three main elements of:

- Attitudes and values.

- Personal and social skills.

- Knowledge and understanding.

Developing a policy for SRE

The SRE guidance states that all schools must have an up-to-date SRE policy which is reviewed regularly. It is recommended that this forms part of an overall policy on PSHE and Citizenship. In accordance with the NHSS whole school approach, the policy should be developed in consultation with parents, young people, teachers, governors and the wider community. The following checklist uses the new guidance and the minimum criteria set by the NHSS as its starting point and will be helpful in developing and reviewing your policy:

- How have parents, pupils, staff and the wider community been involved in the policy development/review process?

- Does the policy set out the SRE provided within the PSHE framework as distinct from the National Curriculum Science Order?

- Does the policy include a moral and values statement which reflects the school's ethos and values, as well as being in line with the SRE Guidance which states, 'as part of sex and relationship education, pupils should be taught about the nature and importance of marriage for family life and bringing up children.'

- Does the policy address the need to build self-esteem and develop a sense of responsibility as well as information giving and social skills development?

- Does the policy include a statement on the school's position on specific issues such as confidentiality, accessing confidential support and sexual health advice, abortion, contraception and sexuality?

- Does the policy take into account the needs of ALL pupils at the school and national, local and in-school policies, such as equal opportunities?

- Does the policy identify partners in the wider community, particularly local health and social support services, who will be involved in the delivery of SRE? Is the policy explicit on the use of visitors?

- Does the policy address pupil-identified needs and evaluation outcomes as well as local and national priorities?

- Are resources, including human resources, relevant and up-to-date?

- Is there a commitment to in-service training for those involved in the delivery of SRE?

- Does the policy identify the date when it will next be reviewed?

Developing schemes of work

- Schemes of Work will need to be developed from the policy and should:

- specify aims and intended learning outcomes.

- ensure continuity and progression.

- consider differentiation for gender, faith and ability.

- provide opportunities for self-assessment.

- meet statutory requirements where appropriate.

- ensure a range of teaching strategies to meet different learning styles.

- offer advice on how to choose resources.

Organisation, planning and teaching strategies

Guidance from the Qualifications and Curriculum Authority (QCA) on PSHE and Citizenship suggests that, when planning a programme of PSHE and Citizenship (which will include SRE), schools should include opportunities in three curriculum locations to ensure a whole school approach:

- Designated curriculum time. Where there is sufficient support for specialist teams of PSHE tutors, designated courses have status with pupils who enjoy and benefit from structured and safe discussions.

- Teaching PSHE in and through other subjects/curriculum areas. Some subjects, such as science or RE, can provide a focus for discussing some elements of SRE.

- Occasional off-timetable experiences, such as 'health days'. These can provide a useful focus for an intensive study of SRE, but should be part of a carefully planned, ongoing SRE curriculum.

Curriculum planning for SRE should be part of the whole school planning process for PSHE and Citizenship.

Differentiated teaching is important in meeting the needs of all pupils. Pupils will have different abilities based upon their emotional and physical development, life-experiences, literacy levels and learning difficulties. Differentiated learning can be in terms of:

- Outcome - a task for all which the group can achieve at their own level.

- Extension of activities - a group which has finished first can be given a further activity to increase their understanding.

- Support on the task - an extra adult such as a school nurse can work alongside the teacher.

- Different resources - active learning techniques allow the teacher to manage more than one activity at a time.

- Grouping by ability - this may be by same level of ability or by mixed ability.

Both policy and practice need to identify how the needs of more vulnerable or excluded young people should be addressed. This approach is also advocated by the NHSS. The SRE guidance highlights the following, which will need to be covered:

Teaching strategies

Research shows that to be effective in meeting public health objectives and to ensure young people's interest and involvement, SRE needs to be taught using active and experiential learning. Use of such teaching methods allow young people to practise skills, use their knowledge and understanding, explore and exchange views.

The following teaching strategies support active learning:

- Sharing ideas

- Discussion

- Listening exercises

- Case studies and scenarios

- Trigger drawings, story boards, photographs as a basis for problem solving, role play and discussion

- Videos and films

- Using puppets

- Questionnaires and quizzes

- Story-telling

- Values continuums

- Role play

Teachers may need training and support in developing confidence in active learning methods.

Choosing and using resources

The guidance stresses the importance of choosing and using appropriate resources. The checklist below will help in clarifying what is appropriate.

Checklist for selecting a resource for health/sex education;

- Is it consistent with your agreed policy, course aims and objectives and values framework?

- Does it conform to the legal requirements for SRE?

- Is it appropriate to the needs of your pupils in terms of language, images, attitude, maturity and understanding and the knowledge required?

- Does it avoid racism, sexism, gender and homophobic stereotyping? Does it exclude any young people on the basis of home circumstance, gender, race, literacy, culture, faith and religion?

- Does it include positive images of a range of young people?

- Can it be used as trigger material for discussions of difference or exclusiveness?

- Can the resource be adapted for use with all of your pupils?

- Is it factually correct and up-to-date?

- Are there instructions on how to use the resource? Are they clear? Is the information for pupils distinguishable from that for teachers? Are there any handouts which can be photocopied and used to reinforce the learning?

- Is the resource well designed? Is it durable, easy to use and easy to store?

- Will it contribute to a broad and balanced curriculum that can be delivered within the PSHE and Citizenship Framework?

- Does it encourage active and participatory learning methods?

- If you have used this resource before what formal or informal feedback did you receive from young people about it?

(Adapted with permission from Health Development Agency, *Criteria for Choosing a Resource*.)

Visit the Sex Education Forum website www.ncb.org.uk for details of resources currently available.

Using outside visitors to support your programme

Using outside visitors can help support your SRE programme. They should be an integral part of the programme and not replace other input. The NHSS requires schools to have a code of practice for use of external agencies. In planning your programme, it is important that:

- the purpose and role of the outside visitor within SRE is clear.

- outside visitors are clear about the boundaries of their input.

- outside visitors are aware of the planned curriculum and relevant school policies, including confidentiality, and will abide by them.

- the aims and objectives of any session using outside visitors is clear, as well as the values framework within which they will work.

- the way they will work with the classroom teacher is planned and agreed.

- lines of accountability between the visitor and the school have been made explicit.

- learning outcomes are identified.

Monitoring, evaluation and assessment

Both young people and teachers should be fully involved in evaluation of SRE. The following checklist offers questions to consider when reviewing the programme:

- Skills - what have they learnt to do?

- Information - what new information have they learnt?

- Attitudes and values - what do they think, feel, believe?

- Did girls and boys engage equally with the activity?

- What do they need to learn next?

Feedback can be gathered in several ways. It should be attached to the lesson plan for future work, and fed back to other staff members involved in planning and delivering future SRE.

Support and training

Research shows that training is central to the success of SRE. Teachers need to feel confident to deliver young people's entitlement to SRE. The Institute of Education (University of London), for example, found that teachers who lacked experience avoided the issue of homosexuality altogether, or might simply touch on it within the context of HIV/AIDS.

Training opportunities via INSET, or national and local agencies will help increase confidence and skills to deliver high quality

SRE. There are also mechanisms for gaining support in both formal and informal ways. Advisory Teachers in the LEA, Health Promotion staff, local Teenage Pregnancy Co-ordinators and Healthy School Coordinators can all provide support in delivering SRE. The Government are committed to developing specialist SRE training for teachers.

Some areas have set up Local Sex Education Fora where workers from a range of settings come together once a term to share good practice and ideas and gain support.

Key government documents and resources

- *Sex and Relationship Education Guidance* (DfES 2000). Download from: www.dfes.gov.uk/sreguidance/sexeducation.pdf

- OFSTED Report of Sex and Relationship Education 2000. Download from: www.ofsted.gov.uk/publications/index.cfm?fuseaction=pubs.displayfile&id=67&type=pdf

- *The National Curriculum Handbook for Secondary School Teachers in England* (1999) DfES and QCA

- *National Healthy School Standard Guidance and Getting Started*. Guidance is forthcoming from the NHSS on meeting the sex and relationships education criteria of the National Healthy School Standard

- *Personal, social and health education at Key Stages 3 and 4. Initial Guidance for Schools* (2000) QCA, PSHE

- *Wired for Health Website* (www.wiredforhealth.co.uk)

- *Teenage Pregnancy*: Report by the Social Exclusion Unit (1999).

The Sex Education Forum produces a range of four and eight-page factsheets offering guidance and resources on a range of topics (currently 22 factsheets available). Topics include:

- Supporting the needs of boys and young men

- Supporting the needs of girls and young women

- Partnership with parents

- Contraception

- Sexual orientation, sexual identities and homophobia in schools

For details, phone 020 7843 1901 or go to www.ncb.org.uk

Useful addresses

For information, advice and support on HIV/AIDS and sex education first contact your Local Education Authority adviser, school nurse or local health promotion unit. The Sex Education Forum, an umbrella body bringing together 38 national organisations involved in supporting and providing sex education can offer advice on developing and reviewing your school sex education policy and provide details of resources and approaches to sex education.

AVERT

11-13 Denne Parade, Horsham, West Sussex, RH12 1JD.
Tel: 01403 210202
www.avert.org

MEDFASH

BMA House, Tavistock Square, London WC1H 9JP
Tel: 020 7383 6345
www.medfash.org.uk

Brook

421 Highgate Studios, 53-57 Highgate Road, London NW5 1TL
Tel: 020 7284 6040.
www.brook.org.uk

Provide resources for young people and professionals.

Consent Consultancy

Sexuality education and training for those working around sexuality and disability.
Tel: 01923 670796.

FPA

2-12 Pentonville Road, London N7 9FP.
Tel: 020 7837 5432.
www.fpa.org.uk

Provides training, consultancy and resources for professionals, as well as leaflets for young people.

Health Development Agency see NICE

The HDA has now merged with the National Institute for Clinical Excellence to become the National Institute for Health and Clinical Excellence.

IBIS Trust

Woodcote House, 178 Botley Road, Chesham, Bucks HP5 3FA
Tel: 01494778137

Information and advice concerning peer education.

NICE (National Institute for Health and Clinical Excellence)

MidCity Place, 71 High Holborn, London WC1V 6NA.
Tel: 020 7067 5800.
www.nice.org.uk

Relate (Relationship Education and Training Dept.),

National Education Officer, Herbert Gray College, Little Church Street, Rugby CV21 3AP.
Tel: 0845 456 1310.
www.relate.org.uk

Provides training for professionals in SRE.

Sex Education Forum

c/o National Children's Bureau, 8 Wakley Street, London, EC1V 7QE.
Tel: 020 7843 1901
www.ncb.org.uk

Information, advice and referral on sex education. As well as Factsheets (see above) the Forum publishes a termly newsletter *Sex Education Matters,* which brings together news of developments in sex education, new resources, research, conferences and details of practice issues.

Sheffield Centre for HIV and Sexual Health

22 Collegiate Crescent, Sheffield, S10 2BA.
Tel: 0114 226 1900
www.sexualhealthsheffield.co.uk

Training and consultancy.

Working With Men

320 Commercial Way, London SE15 1QN
Tel: 020 7732 9409.
www.workingwithmen.org

Provide resources and training for working with boys and young men.

References

Allen I (1987) Education in Sex and Personal Relationships. Policy Studies Institute

Wellings K and others (1994) Sexual Behaviour in Britain: The national survey of attitudes and lifestyles. Penguin

Parents, School and Sex Education (1994) HEA/NFER

NHS Centre for Reviews and Dissemination (CRD) University of York, 1997.

'Preventing and reducing the adverse effects of unintended teenage pregnancies', Effective Health Care Bulletin 3: 1-12

Oakley A and others (1994) Reviews of effectiveness No 2: sexual health interventions for young people. SSRU

Kane R and Wellings K (1999) An International Review of the Evidence: data from Europe. HEA

Frankham J and others (1995), Young Gay Men Talking. AVERT

Mellanby A and others. School Sex Education: An experimental programme with educational and medical benefit. BMJ 311, 7002, 414-417, 1995.

Douglas N and others (1997) Playing it Safe: Responses of secondary school teachers to lesbian, gay and bisexual pupils, bullying, HIV and AIDS education and Education Act 1996, HMSO, 1996.

Beloff QC: Sex Education in Schools: Joint Opinion. Association of Teachers and Lecturers and others, 1994.

White S: Confidentiality in Schools. Brook Advisory Centres, 1995.

Curriculum Council of Wales: Advisory Paper II Community Understanding: A Framework for Development of a Cross-curricular Theme in Wales, 1991.

DfES Circular 5/94 Education Act 1993: Sex Education in Schools, 1994.

DfES Sex and Relationship Education Guidance 2000. Download from www.dfes.gov.uk/sreguidance/sexeducation.pdf

DoH The Health of the Nation Key Area Handbook: HIV/AIDS and Sexual Health, 1993.

National Curriculum Council Curriculum Guidance 5: Health Education, 1990a.

National Curriculum Council   Curriculum Guidance 8: Education For Citizenship, 1990b.

OFSTED Report of Sex and Relationship Education 2002. Download from: www.ofsted.gov.uk/publications/index.cfm?fuseaction=pubs.displayfile&id=67&type=pdf

Welsh Office Circular 45/94: Sex Education in Schools, 1994.

Sex Education Forum Forum Factsheet 3: Positive guidance on sex and relationships education, 1994.

Sex Education Forum Forum Factsheet 8: Guidelines on the effective use of outside visitors in school sex education, 1996.

Sex Education Forum Forum Factsheet 6: Teaching about sexuality, 1995.

Sex Education Forum Forum Factsheet 12: Effective learning: approaches to sex education, 1997.

Sex Education Forum Forum Factsheet 23: Taking the initiative: Positive guidance on sex and relationships education, 2000.

Immigration and asylum and HIV

Getting specialist advice

Immigration is a complex and specialist topic where the law can change very quickly with little or no warning. This section highlights some HIV specific aspects. It is not a comprehensive summary of the law nor a substitute for individual legal advice. In every case, specialist advice should be taken as early as possible from a competent lawyer or advice agency. Suitable sources of help can be contacted at or through the organisations listed at the end of this section.

UK immigration law

There is one body of immigration law for the whole of the U.K. There are no regional or national variations. The immigration laws are implemented by the Home Office through its Border and Immigration Agency and the Immigration Service. The current immigration system finds most of its roots in the Immigration Act 1971 which has repeatedly been modified in many respects by subsequent legislation.

The Home Secretary has been given the power to draw up what are known as the Immigration Rules. These set out the different categories of persons who will be allowed to enter or remain in the UK and the requirements to be met. The Rules are being regularly updated and changed. The most recent consolidated version is called HC395 which has itself been amended many times, most recently by HC 398..

The Rules allow people to enter or remain in the UK for a myriad of reasons including as visitors, students, workers, business people, retired persons, innovators, highly skilled migrants, refugees and many more. There are detailed rules allowing family members of people already here to join them. These include provision for spouses and for unmarried partners where a relationship has subsisted for over two years (including same-sex relationships). The Rules contain nothing specific on persons with HIV.

In addition to the Rules there are policies and concessions that are referred to as being outside the Rules. Most of these are contained in the Immigration Agencys' Instructions.

The Rules and policies are published on the Border and Immigration Agency's website found at www.ind.homeoffice.gov.uk. From this site you can down load applicable forms and guidance notes.

Entering the UK

British citizens have an unconditional right to enter the United Kingdom. Nationals of other member states of the European Economic Area (EEA) (Austria, Belgium, the Czech Republic, Cyprus, Denmark, Estonia, Finland, France, Germany, Greece, Hungary, Iceland, Irish Republic, Italy, Latvia, Liechtenstein, Lithuania, Luxembourg, Malta, Netherlands, Norway, Poland, Portugal, Slovakia, Slovenia, Spain, Switzerland and Sweden) and their dependants, whether EEA nationals or not, are entitled to enter the UK in order to work, study or retire.

All other persons, with a few narrow exceptions, require leave (i.e. permission) to enter. These people are said to be subject to immigration control. On arrival in the UK they must present themselves to an immigration officer who will decide whether to grant them entry.

People from certain specified countries, as well as all applicants for certain forms of leave, require entry clearance (commonly known as a visa) in order to enter the UK. Entry clearance is a form of prior permission to enter and has to be obtained in advance from a British consular post abroad. Forms have to be completed and fees paid. Forms and guidance notes can be downloaded from the web site of the section in the Foreign and Commonwealth Office that runs the entry clearance system. This is found at www.ukvisas.gov.uk

Applications for entry clearance and leave to enter are dealt with strictly in accordance with the Immigration Rules which set out general grounds for refusal (Rule 320) as well as the specific requirements for each category.

Entering the UK: relevance of HIV status

Current government policy is that a diagnosis of infection with HIV or related symptoms is not a ground, in itself, for refusing entry into the UK. HIV infection has not been classified as an infectious disease justifying exclusion.

An individual can, however, be refused entry on medical grounds if in the opinion of the Medical Inspector that person, at the point of entry, is too sick to enter regardless of the fact that in theory he or she could satisfy the conditions of his or her leave to enter. Immigration Officers have power to require a person to submit to a medical examination and a person can be refused entry if he or she refuses to undergo a medical examination when asked to do so (Rule 320(17)).

Paragraphs 36 - 38 specify certain categories of passengers who should normally be referred to the medical inspector and the action that should be taken;

"36. A person who intends to remain in the United Kingdom for more than 6 months should normally be referred to the Medical Inspector for examination. If he produces a medical certificate he should be advised to hand it to the Medical Inspector. Any person seeking entry who mentions health or medical treatment as a reason for his visit, or who appears not to be in good mental or physical health, should also be referred to the Medical Inspector; and the Immigration Officer has discretion, which should be exercised sparingly, to refer for examination in any other case."

"37. Where the Medical Inspector advises that a person seeking entry is suffering from a specified disease or condition which may interfere with his ability to support himself or his dependants, the Immigration Officer should take account of this, in conjunction with other factors, in deciding whether to admit that person. The Immigration Officer should also take account of the Medical Inspector's assessment of the likely course of treatment in deciding whether a person seeking entry for private medical treatment has sufficient means at his disposal."

"38. A returning resident should not be refused leave to enter.on medical grounds. But where a person would be refused leave to enter on medical grounds if he were not a returning resident, or in any case where it is decided on compassionate grounds not to exercise the power to refuse leave to enter, or in any other case where the Medical Inspector so recommends, the Immigration Officer should give the person concerned a notice requiring him to report to the Medical Officer of Environmental Health designated by the Medical Inspector with a view to further examination and any necessary treatment."

These rules are likely to be adhered to in the usual way in cases of HIV. If there is evidence that an applicant is currently in need of regular medication or treatment, evidence of his or her ability to meet the costs involved is likely to be required. Paragraph 2.5 of Chapter 1, Section 8 of the Immigration Agencys Instructions (IDIs) on medical cases states;

"If a passenger is diagnosed as suffering from AIDS, HIV or any other serious illness this will not, in itself, be sufficient to justify refusal on public health grounds alone. However, port medical inspectors will continue to provide estimates of the cost of any treatment which may be required and thereafter it will be for the immigration officer to consider applications under the appropriate paragraphs of the rules."

When applying from abroad for entry clearance, there is no duty on a person to disclose their HIV status. If it is voluntarily disclosed it may lead to the application being referred to the UK for a decision and cause delay. Paragraph 3.2 of Chapter 1 Section 8 of the IDIs states;

"Applications made at a post abroad for entry clearance for persons who are suffering from a serious illness should normally be referred by the entry clearance officer to the Home Office . if the applicant meets the requirements of the Immigration Rules for the category specified. Evidence should also be forthcoming of the applicant's ability to meet the costs of any medical treatment that may be required during their stay. This is in addition to the usual requirements as regards maintenance, accommodation and intention to return..the fact that a person suffers from a serious illness is not in itself grounds for refusing entry clearance. However, where in any case it appears that public health may be risk because of the infectious nature of the disease (e.g. TB or hepatitis B or C), advice should be sought from the Department of Health."

An entry clearance or leave to enter is usually for a limited period and subject to various conditions, but in some circumstances may be for an indefinite period. The most common conditions are a prohibition on claiming welfare benefits and restrictions on employment. It is essential never to overstay a period of limited leave, even by a day, and to take advice in good time if for illness or any other reason an extension or variation of leave is sought.

European Economic Area law does accept that certain restrictions can be placed on the freedom of movement of persons within its jurisdiction on the grounds of public policy and public health (Directive 64/221, ANNEX). Infection with HIV has not been included in the list of diseases which might endanger public health and therefore justify exclusion. Although the directive does allow a discretion, it is extremely improbable that any country or region within the EEA could successfully deny freedom of movement of an EEA national on the grounds of HIV from exercising his/her rights within that country's borders.

Entering the UK for medical treatment

Rules 51-56 make provision for a person to enter the UK specifically to receive *private* medical treatment. Individuals have to meet the normal visitor requirements, such as not to take employment, and to be able to support and accommodate themselves (and any dependants) without recourse to public funds. They also have to prove that the treatment is of a finite duration and that they intend to leave at the end of it, and have the resources available to meet the costs of the treatment. It may be necessary to produce evidence of the arrangements that have been made for consultation or treatment. People are admitted for up to six months initially but may be granted extensions if they continue to fulfill the conditions. See also the IAI Chapter 2 Section 3.

Coming to the UK as a medical visitor is only really an option for people who have substantial financial resources.

There is no general right to come to the UK in order to obtain free NHS treatment. Nationals of the EEA, or their family members, and refugees and stateless persons living within the EEA have the right to NHS treatment without charge where the need arises during their stay. EEA nationals who wish to enter the UK for treatment (or who are referred to the UK for treatment) should obtain prior authorisation from their national social security institution which in principle should bear the cost.

Most NHS treatment is not automatically free of charge to other people from abroad. Access to the NHS depends on a combination of one or more of immigration status, length of residence, nature of the treatment required, and whether the need for it arose during the visit. The position is regulated by the National Health Service (Charges to Overseas Visitors) Regulations 1989 (SI 1989/306), as amended by the National

Health Services (Charges to Overseas Visitors) (Amendment) Regulations, (SI 1994/1535).

Certain NHS treatment is free to anyone at all. This includes testing and counselling for HIV or STIs at a GUM clinic (but not any subsequent treatment for HIV), family planning services, treatment for mental disorder, hospital accident and emergency treatment (but not in-patient care), and treatment for notifiable diseases and other conditions to which public health laws apply (not including HIV and AIDS).

Certain categories of people are exempt from any NHS charges. The main categories are:

- anyone in the UK for the purposes of employment.

- anyone taking up permanent residence.

- anyone who has resided in the UK for twelve months.

- refugees and asylum seekers.

- prisoners and immigration detainees.

- individuals where the services are provided in circumstances covered by a reciprocal agreement the individual's country.

Other categories of people are exempt from charges for treatment the need for which arose during the visit. This provision is intended to exclude travel to the UK specifically for treatment on the NHS of a pre-existing condition.

The NHS regulations refer only to hospital treatment, but GPs, dentists and opticians are advised to apply corresponding criteria in deciding whether or not to accept patients for treatment.

Remaining in the UK

Once a person has entered the UK they can remain for the duration of their leave as stamped in their passport or set out in their entry clearance. Prior to the expiry of their leave they can apply to the Border and Immigration Agency for an extension of stay in accordance with the requirements of the Immigration Rules. So long as the application is made before current leave expires the applicant will be lawfully in the UK until a decision is made. The Immigration Rules set out the circumstances in which extensions of stay may be granted. It is possible in certain circumstances to switch categories but certain nationalities are not allowed to switch. If the Rules do not allow such a switch, the individual concerned has to leave and apply for an entry clearance from abroad to return.

Applications for an extension of stay have to be made on the correct form and be supported by original documents. There are special forms for a variety of categories, including students, married and unmarried partners, family members, and EEA nationals.

Some categories of the Immigration Rules may eventually lead to permanent residence (e.g. marriage and some work permits) but others have an expectation that the applicant will eventually return home (e.g. visitors, short-term students). Ten years of lawful continuous residence can lead to permanent stay and 14 years of continuous residence may lead to permanent stay even if some of the time has been unlawful.

Remaining in the UK on grounds of HIV status

The Immigration Rules do not have a category that permits a person to remain in the UK simply because they are HIV-positive or have AIDS. There are a number of people who, whilst in the UK on a temporary basis, were diagnosed as HIV-positive and may have started treatment. When their current leave to remain comes to an end , and there are no grounds for extending it, they may not wish to return home because of their poor health and the lack of adequate medical treatment in their home country.

In the past it has been possible for such an individual to apply to remain in the United Kingdom on an exceptional basis by showing that "compelling and compassionate circumstances" prevail. Around 2000 and subsequently, the Home Office was relatively generous in its willingness to exercise such discretion with respect to those individuals seriously affected by HIV and AIDS, and prepared to grant permission to remain to individuals who had commenced life prolonging combination therapy in this country and who would, if forced to leave, be required to return to a country where such therapy was unobtainable or unaffordable. In those early years, families who were here as students or visitors and learnt whilst here of an HIV diagnosis were granted indefinite leave to remain. Later this became a four year period, with the ability to make a further application thereafter, then as numbers of applications grew, a one year period of further leave was given, prior to further application, followed ultimately by outright refusal; as in so many areas of immigration law, Home Office policy was swayed by the "numbers game."

The coming into effect of the Human Rights Act on 2 October 2000 imposed an obligation on public authorities not to act in a way that is in breach of human rights including Article 3 of the ECHR which provides that "no one shall be subjected to torture or to inhuman or degrading treatment or punishment". Whether it would breach human rights to remove a person who had AIDS from the UK was considered in 1997 by the European Court of Human Rights in the case of D -v- United Kingdom, (1997) 24 EHRR 423. That case related to a citizen of St Kitts whom the United Kingdom was proposing to return to his home country after serving a prison sentence for a drug-related offence. During the course of that sentence it was discovered that he had AIDS and that his life expectancy was very short. The UK persisted with its plan to remove him so he appealed to the European Court. The court found that his removal to St Kitts would constitute a breach of Article 3 of the European Convention on Human Rights. The court found that it would constitute "inhuman or degrading treatment or punishment" to withdraw from the individual concerned the medical treatment he was receiving in the United Kingdom and then force him to return to a country where no effective treatment or palliative care could be guaranteed, given that he was on the point of death.

Matters were to worsen with the House of Lords decision in the case of N (FC) and the Secretary of State for the Home Department, [2005] UKHL 31, on 5th May 2005.

"N" was a Ugandan woman who arrived in the UK in March 1998 and very soon thereafter was found to be seriously ill with Kaposi's sarcoma and a CD4 count of 10. The treatment which she received in the United Kingdom greatly improved her health to the point where doctors provided the opinion that, if the treatment continued, she would remain well for "decades". It was accepted by the court that, if she were returned to Uganda, "The cruel reality is that.her ability to obtain the necessary medication is problematic.and...her position will be similar to having a life-support machine switched off".

While repeatedly asserting how moved they were by N's plight, the Law Lords found that this plight was not "exceptional" enough to bring her within the scope of Article 3. They sought to distinguish it from the case of D:

"The essential distinction is not to be found in humanitarian differences. Rather it lies in recognising that article 3 does not require contracting states to undertake the obligation of providing aliens indefinitely with medical treatment lacking in their home countries. In the case of D and in later cases the Strasbourg court has constantly reiterated that in principle aliens subjected to expulsion cannot claim any entitlement to remain in the territory of a contracting state in order to continue to benefit from medical, social and other forms of assistance provided by the expelling state. Article 3 imposes no such 'medical care' obligation on contracting states. This is so even where, in the absence of medical treatment, the life of the would-be immigrant will be significantly shortened. But in the case of D, unlike the later cases, there was no question of imposing any such obligation on the United Kingdom. D was dying, and beyond the reach of medical treatment then available."

Basically, therefore, the House of Lords declared that there is a human rights obligation to permit to remain only those actually on their deathbed and not those who would face imminent death if returned home and deprived of their current treatment.

As a result of the Judgement in N, the IAI were altered, and can now be found at Para 3.3, stating in essence that leave to remain cannot be granted under the medical visitor provisions if treatment is to be on the NHS; that where UK obligations under the Human Rights Act are engaged Discretionary leave may be granted, by a specialist caseworker, subject to paragraph 3.4, which, following N, has been withdrawn for updating.

The Preface to the 2005 edition of Macdonald and Webber's Immigration Law and Practice had this to say:

" The House's decision in N reflects political preoccupations with the danger of the health service being swamped by health tourism rather than humanitarian ones. Having accepted the illogicality of distinguishing (for the purpose of expulsion) between terminally ill people and those saved from death by anti-retroviral treatment who will assuredly revert to a state of terminal illness shortly after expulsion, for want of suitable treatment in the country of return, their Lordships followed this doleful distinction, in delimiting the UK's obligation to refrain from expulsion, in a decision which faithfully follows a line of less than satisfactory Strasbourg cases and thereby risks condemning many hundreds of AIDS patients currently receiving treatment in the UK to despair and death in their countries of origin. "

However, all may not be completely gloomy on the horizon, as the case of N has been appealed to the European Court and pending a full decision the Court has ordered a stay of N's removal.

As a separate issue, there remains the possibility of an argument for those from Zimbabwe for example as to actual unavailability of ART (as opposed to the impossibility of accessing such treatment on grounds of cost) which could make such cases exceptional even as compared with "N" , and in cases such as ZT (2005) EWCA Civ 1421 the Secretary of State was advised to be sure that current conditions in Zimbabwe would not threaten the appellant's Article 3 rights on return. It is possible that a country guidance case specifically addressing HIV/Aids and Zimbabwe will follow.

Asylum applications on the basis of HIV status

Individuals may sometimes be able to lodge successful applications for asylum on the basis that they have a "well-founded fear of persecution" on being returned to their home country because of their HIV status. This may be appropriate where you can demonstrate that people who are HIV-positive or have AIDS are at risk of serious harm on account of this. The key legal issue relevant to this question is whether HIV status can be interpreted to define a "social group" for purposes of the 1951 Convention Relating to the Status of Refugees. It seems likely that people who are HIV-positive can be deemed to constitute a "social group" in light of the extremely important decision by the House of Lords in Shah and Islam [1999] 2 WLR 1015. That case related specifically to the issue of whether "women in Pakistan" constitute a social group but also separately addressed the issue of whether gay men and lesbians could do so (in both cases deciding affirmatively). It was held that the key factor in defining a "social group" should be an "unchangeable characteristic" and, in particular, stated that

there should be no additional requirement of "cohesiveness, co-operation or inter dependence".

To make a successful application on such a basis, asylum seekers would need to demonstrate the fact that individuals affected by HIV in their home country would indeed face persecution because of their status, either at the hands of their government directly or at the hands of other forces without the government providing adequate protection. A key to making such a successful application would be the collection of credible information confirming the existence of such persecution.

Other categories

Two other categories of immigration applications may be particularly affected by issues relating to HIV and AIDS:

- Carers

- Unmarried partners

Carers

A new policy was announced in August 1998 outside of the immigration Rules, relating to "carers". This policy permits "applications from persons here in a temporary capacity seeking leave to remain to care for a sick relative or friend who is suffering from a terminal illness such as cancer or AIDS" (Immigration Agency's instructions, Chapter 17, S2).

The "carer" category is meant to be a temporary arrangement but, in practice, it is often extended. Applications made to remain as a carer of a "relative" as opposed to a "friend" are treated differently. Applications to care for a "friend" are meant, in principle,   to be refused except in emergencies.

Such applications should be supported by a letter from a registered medical practitioner, a letter from the local social services department, if involved, evidence that alternative arrangements are being explored and full details of the patient's family in the United Kingdom and previous care arrangements, as well as evidence of the applicant's circumstances, both in his or her home country and in the United Kingdom. Where compelling and compassionate circumstances exist, the Home Office is often prepared to exhibit flexibility, but initial leave is limited to three months, with the possibility of a further twelve months thereafter, but any further concessionary leave highly unlikely.

Unmarried partners and civil partnerships

Since 2 October 2000, provisions have existed in the Immigration Rules (rule 295) relating to the admission of a foreign common law or gay/lesbian partner of a UK based person, where the couple concerned can demonstrate a relationship "akin to marriage" which has subsisted for at least two years. The Rule applies to both same sex couples and to heterosexual unmarried partners . The foreign partner may be seeking to join or remain with the British Citizen, an EEA National residing in the United Kingdom or any other person who has indefinite leave to remain in the United Kingdom or who falls into one of a number of categories of limited leave to remain which lead to indefinite leave. The couple should be able to demonstrate an ability to support and accommodate themselves without relying on public funds.

The Home Office has in the past been prepared to exhibit flexibility in applying the requirements of these arrangements in those cases where one or both members of the couple are affected by HIV. If, for example, recourse to public funds is necessary because of HIV-related illness, the Home Office may be prepared to exercise discretion outside the letter of the Rules.

From 5 December 2005, gay men and lesbians have been able to register their civil partnerships under the provisions of the Civil Partnership Act. The Home Office has said that it will amend the Immigration Rules to afford foreign civil partners the same rights as foreign spouses. This will afford another possibility for a foreign national in such a partnership to seek leave to enter or remain in the United Kingdom. While, again, the couple should be able to demonstrate an ability to support and accommodate themselves without relying on public funds, it is hoped that discretion will be exercised in compassionate cases.

Advice on other aspects of immigration and asylum law

As set out at the beginning of this section, it is essential that anyone seeking information on this subject go to the most up-to-date sources of advice and information. The following organisations can provide appropriate guidance.

Specific Immigration Advice Organisations

Joint Council for the Welfare of Immigrants (JCWI)
115 Old St, London EC1V 9JR
020 7434 3690 (advice line)

Refugee Legal Centre
Nelson House 153-157 Commercial Road, London, E1 2EB
020 7780 3200

Immigration Law Practitioners Association (ILPA)
Lindsey House, 40/42 Charterhouse Street, London EC1 6JN
020 7251 8383

ILPA is a consortium of immigration law specialists who can advise as to the whereabouts of specialist lawyers by region.

The Terrence Higgins Trust Advice Centre offers specialist immigration advice to people affected by HIV or AIDS.
020 7816 4605

Powers to regulate people with HIV and AIDS

Public Health (Infectious Diseases) Regulations 1988

Despite accepting that non-discrimination is the only effective approach to the epidemic and that attempts to regulate people with HIV are both unlikely to control the spread of the virus or benefit the individuals concerned, the Government has introduced discriminatory Regulations which can be used to detain people with AIDS.

The Public Health (Infectious Diseases) Regulations 1988 (SI 1988 No 1546) apply certain provisions of the Public Health Act 1984 to HIV and AIDS, but do not make either a notifiable condition (such as tuberculosis).

The following sections of the Public Health Act apply:

Section 35 states that a magistrate may order a medical examination if he or she receives a written certificate from a registered medical practitioner who has been nominated by the local authority stating that:

"(a) that there is reason to believe that some person in the district"

"(i) is or has been suffering from AIDS, or"

"(ii) though not suffering from such a disease, is carrying an organism capable of causing it, and"

"(b) that in his own interest, or in the interest of his family, or in the public interest, it is expedient that he should be medically examined, and"

"(c) that he is not under the treatment of a registered medical practitioner, or that the registered medical practitioner who is treating him consents to the making of an order."

This section therefore also applies to people suspected of being HIV-positive. The medical examination may include bacteriological and radiological tests and similar investigations.

Section 37 allows a magistrate to order the compulsory removal of a person with AIDS to a hospital. The magistrate must be satisfied, after an application by a local authority, that a person has AIDS and that proper precautions to prevent the spread of infection cannot be or have not been taken and that the person is a serious risk of infecting others. Space in a hospital must be available and the District Health Authority must consent.

Section 38, as amended by the Regulations, permits a magistrate, at the request of a local authority, to detain a person with AIDS in hospital for as long as is necessary in his or her opinion, if the person involved would on leaving hospital not take proper precautions to prevent the spread of the disease:

"(a) in his lodging or accommodation, or"

"(b) in other places to which he may be expected to go if not detained in hospital"

If a person with AIDS detained under section 38 discharged themselves they would be committing a criminal offence. Magistrates have the power to make these decisions in the absence of the affected person.

Section 43 authorises a local authority or doctor to prevent the removal of the body of a person who has died with AIDS from hospital, except direct to a mortuary or for burial or cremation.

Section 44 imposes a duty on anyone in whose premises a person has died with AIDS to take "such steps as are reasonably practicable" to prevent persons coming unnecessarily into contact with the body.

Both provisions carry criminal penalties.

Similar powers to compulsorily examine and detain persons with AIDS in Scotland exist under sections 45-59 of the Public Health (Scotland) Act 1897, which allow for people with any infectious disease to be so detained.

It is accepted that the regulations providing for detention are unlikely to be used in relation to AIDS. An earlier version of the 1988 regulations was controversially used in 1985 to detain a man in Manchester in hospital. A successful appeal was brought by the Terrence Higgins Trust on his behalf, but at that point he elected to stay in hospital voluntarily. The present writer is not aware of the detention power having been used since then.

Civil procedure: anonymity and non-disclosure

Introduction

It may be the case that a person with HIV is involved in some aspect of civil litigation and they do not wish their HIV status to be disclosed either to the other party or to the general public. This can be done either if a court case is heard in camera, i.e. in private, where the press and general public are excluded, or if reporting restrictions are imposed. It is in practice also possible to take practical steps to minimise the public disclosure of medical evidence.

In camera proceedings

Any court has the power to sit in camera where a public hearing would defeat the ends of justice (Scott v Scott [1913] AC 417 and R v Chief Registrar of Building Societies ex parte New Cross Building Society [1984] 1 QB 227). Other than cases involving children and mental patients, it is extremely unlikely that a court would sit in camera to prevent publicity in a case involving HIV. Two identifiable grounds exist which tend to indicate that a public hearing would defeat the ends of justice. These are:

(a) The subject matter of the litigation would be destroyed by a hearing in open court. Thus if the object of the proceedings is to keep certain information secret those proceedings need to be held in camera.

(b) Where a witness or a party is reasonably deterred from proceeding in public, a court is justified in sitting in camera. This point is more difficult to prove, but as a proposition it exists in law.

Reporting restrictions

As stated above, a Court would be most unlikely to be prepared to sit in private in an HIV-related case. There is a power for a court to order that a name or other information be withheld from publicity where a case is heard in public (section 11 Contempt of Court Act 1981). This power was considered in the case of R v Westminster City Council ex parte Castelli and Tristran-Garcia (1995) 7 Admin LR 840). The applicants were two men diagnosed with HIV who had earlier commenced judicial review proceedings against the Council for failure to house them and as a result of the publicity their case generated they sought to prohibit any further publication of their names, addresses or other means of identifying them.

The judge stated that the test to be satisfied before an order under s.11 would be granted was whether the applicant would reasonably be deterred from seeking justice at the hands of the court if not protected by a s.11 order. In the event the judge held that there was not sufficient material before him to establish the need for anonymity, especially since the proceedings raised questions of public interest, i.e. entitlement of EU nationals to public housing. However he also laid great emphasis on the fact that a further and insurmountable problem was that substantial publicity had already occurred as a result of one of the applicant's leave application. As he was unable to make a retrospective order, any order that was made at this stage in the hearing would be ineffectual. The applicants' names were already in the public domain and they had therefore lost their anonymity.

The judgment does however give helpful guidance on making applications for anonymity. It is stated that in cases where the applicant's name alone will not provoke publicity, then at the leave stage an application for anonymity and for a s.11 order can be made. This application would be dealt with ex parte and if necessary, in camera. If the court decides in favour of making the order, it will be granted for a short time to enable notice to be given to the press and the Attorney-General and there can then be a full hearing.

In cases where listing the matter by name will of itself give rise to publicity, the application for anonymity will have to be made as soon as the papers are lodged. The papers should not be lodged until the Crown Office has confirmed that the application for anonymity can be heard by a judge immediately.

Disability discrimination

The Disability Discrimination Act 1995 (DDA)

People with settled immigration status with HIV and AIDS are among the groups covered by the Disability Discrimination Act 1995 (DDA), which came into force on 2 December 1996. The DDA is the controversial product of a long and hard-fought struggle for civil rights for people with disabilities, and many campaigners are clearly dissatisfied with it. The Act is limited in scope, both in terms of how it defines disability, and in the restrictive nature of the rights and remedies it affords. In its first years the Act also lacked any strategic enforcement body, equivalent to the powers of the Equal Opportunities Commission or the Commission for Racial Equality in the fields of sex and race discrimination, however, it was remedied in 2000 with the creation of the Disability Rights Commission, and the 1995 Act has recently been updated and amended by the Disability Discrimination Act 2005.

There has been considerable criticism of the DDA's definition of disability for being narrow, functional, and ignoring the social experience of disability. There are particular problems from the point of view of HIV. Firstly, the 1995 Act did not automatically apply to everyone who is diagnosed HIV-positive. This has, however, changed as a result of the 2005 Act, which explicitly provides (section 18) that a person with HIV is to be "deemed" a disabled person for the purposes of the legislation. Secondly, it does not apply to anyone who is wrongly diagnosed or thought to be positive, or who is tested for HIV, and is discriminated against as a result. A functional test of disability is particularly inadequate as the basis for protection against discrimination which in the case of HIV is based upon stigma and fear, and where the level of symptoms (if any) is not the prime indicator of the degree of discrimination experienced.

Following is summary of the provisions of the DDA. Readers should be aware that caselaw has broadened the scope of the Act in some areas and in some instances has shed more light on previously grey areas.

What does the DDA do?

The DDA applies to people it defines as disabled (see below)in relation to discrimination in:

- Employment

- Insurance

- Access to other goods and services (see below).

Who is a disabled person?

A disabled person is someone who has a disability, or who has had a disability in the past (section 2). A disability is defined as *a physical or mental impairment which has a substantial and long-term adverse effect on [a person's] ability to carry out normal day-to-day activities* (section 1(1)).

Physical impairment is not defined.

Mental impairment includes the symptoms of mental illness if it is *a clinically well defined illness*, and learning difficulties (schedule 1 (1).

Substantial means more than minor or trivial.

Long-term means that the impairment has lasted or is likely to last at least 12 months, or for the rest of the person's life (which may be less than 12 months) (schedule 1(2)).

Normal day-to-day activities are exclusively defined as the following:

(a) mobility

(b) manual dexterity

(c) physical coordination

(d) continence

(e) ability to lift, carry or otherwise move everyday objects

(f) speech, hearing or eyesight

(g) memory or ability to concentrate, learn or understand

(h) perception of the risk of physical danger.

A person who has an *impairment which would be likely to have a substantial adverse effect* on their ability to carry out normal day-to-day activities, if it were not controlled by medication or other treatment (for example a person with epilepsy), will qualify as *disabled* (schedule 1(6)).

A person who has a *progressive condition* which results in an impairment which has *an effect* on their ability to carry out normal day-to-day activities, will qualify as disabled from that point onwards if the condition is likely eventually to result in an impairment which has a *substantial adverse effect* on their ability to carry out normal day-to-day activities. The Act includes HIV infection in a list of progressive conditions (Schedule 1 (8). The effect of this is to ensure that people with HIV are protected by the Act from the time when symptoms of illness are first experienced, even if at that stage these could not be described as having a *substantial adverse effect*, and even if the symptoms go away for a time.

What rights do disabled people have?

The DDA provides new rights in several distinct areas. The rights especially relevant to people with HIV or AIDS are in relation to employment, insurance, and the sale or rental of property. These rights are described within the relevant chapters.

Access to goods and services

The DDA provides a general right not to be discriminated against in the provision of goods, facilities and services. These are broad categories. A non-exhaustive list of examples is set out in section 19 (3) as follows:

(a) access to and use of any place which members of the public are permitted to enter

(b) access to and use of means of communication

(c) access to and use of information services

(d) accommodation in a hotel, boarding house or similar establishment

(e) facilities by way of banking or insurance or for grants, loans, credit or finance

(f) facilities for entertainment, recreation or refreshment

(g) facilities provided by employment agencies or under section 2 of the Employment and Training Act 1973

(h) the services of any profession or trade, or any local or other public authority (section 19(3)).

The DDA therefore includes pubs, cafes, restaurants, shops, banks, doctors, dentists, hospitals, courts, solicitors, train and bus stations, and the provision of utilities and telephone services. It makes no difference whether the service is one which is free of charge or paid for. Education and transport vehicles were not originally included in these provisions. This has now changed as a result of the 2005 Act and the Special Educational Needs and Disability Act 2001, although there are special provisions relating to transport: see section 21ZA of the 1995 Act, as inserted by section 5 of the 2005 Act.

What is discrimination?

It is unlawful for a service provider to discriminate against a disabled person by:

- refusing service.

- refusing to make a "reasonable adjustment" where required to do so under the Act.

- providing a lower standard of service, or providing it in an inferior manner.

- providing the service on less favourable terms (section 19 (1)).

Discrimination is defined as treating a disabled person less favourably than someone who is not disabled for a reason which relates to their disability, where the treatment is not *justified* under the Act (section 20 (1)), or failing to make *reasonable adjustments* when required to do so. A wide range of circumstances will justify treatment which would otherwise be discriminatory. These are if in the opinion of the service provider:

- the treatment is necessary not to endanger health or safety.

- the disabled person is incapable of giving informed consent.

- in the case of a refusal of service, or the provision of an inferior service, this is necessary because the service provider would otherwise be unable to provide the service to the public.

In each case, the opinion of the provider of services that one of the justifications applies must be reasonably held.

Duty to make reasonable adjustments

These provisions, which may require financial investment by a service provider, are being phased in over several years. Service providers are required to take *such steps as are reasonable in all the circumstances of the case* to:

- amend any policies, practices or procedures which make it impossible or unreasonably difficult for a disabled person to use the service (for example, a ban on dogs including guide dogs, or on wheelchairs in a cinema or restaurant).

- remove or alter a physical feature of premises, or provide a reasonable means of avoiding it, or a reasonable alternative way of accessing the service, if the physical feature makes it impossible or unreasonably difficult for a disabled person to use the service (for example, a self service petrol station could be altered for better use by people with disabilities, or else provide a free attendant service).

- provide auxiliary aids or services where they would facilitate use of the service by disabled people (for example, sign language interpreters) (section 21).

There will be limits on the amount of expenditure which can be required. Service providers are not required to take steps *which would fundamentally alter the nature* of the trade, profession or business (section 22 (6)).

Enforcement

In cases of discrimination relating to services, a legal claim of discrimination has to be made in the county court within six months of the incident complained of. It is expected that most cases will be dealt with in the small claims court, for which legal aid is not available. If a discrimination claim is relating to an employment issue, it would need to be lodged in an Employment Tribunal within three months. Compensation, including an element for injury to feelings, can be awarded.

Further information

Disability (official government website)
www.disability.gov.uk

RADAR (Royal Association for Disability and Rehabilitation)
www.radar.org.uk
250 City Road, London EC1V 8AF
020 7250 3222

Disability Rights Commission
www.drc-gb.org

DRC Information
Freepost, MIDO 02164, Stratford upon Avon CV37 9BR
Telephone 08457 622 633
Textphone 08457 622 644

Alternatively, a local Citizen's Advice Bureau may be able to help.

Employment and HIV

HIV in the workplace

Risks and discrimination

Largely because of combination therapy, more and more HIV-positive people are remaining well and living longer lives. Unfortunately, the discrimination against people living with HIV has not gone away. The workplace remains a major area where this discrimination takes place.

HIV is only transmitted by blood, certain sexual activities, and from mother-to- baby. Clearly therefore, HIV cannot be transmitted through ordinary social contact. In the vast majority of workplaces there is no risk of HIV transmission. Except for a tiny number of cases among healthcare and laboratory workers, nobody has ever been shown to have contracted HIV in the course of their duties at work.

Nevertheless, from time to time, AIDS panics have broken out in certain work places, where employees have refused to work with people who were or were thought to be HIV-positive, or have discriminated against them in other harmful ways.

There are a number of reports which document the type of discrimination experienced by people who are affected by HIV. In 2004, the Positive Futures partnership (see notes below) published a report "Can People with HIV Work?" that highlighted the attitudes of employers and employees in the UK towards PLHV. The report shows that problems related to HIV and the workplace are widespread and highlights the fact that people with HIV and AIDS are still very vulnerable to employment discrimination.

Also the many HIV organisations, still deal with many cases of blatant discrimination against people who are HIV-positive. Discrimination is particularly prevalent amongst employers who do not have HIV policies and amongst organisations outside of London and other major cities.

The key consequences of a failure to plan for HIV in the workplace are likely to be:

- Failure to follow infection procedures in situations where a risk of infection exists

- Unnecessary disruption in the workplace due to unfounded fears about the risks of HIV infection - 'AIDS panics'

- Mistreatment of employees, including discrimination and avoidable breaches of employment law, possibly leading to employment tribunal action

- Loss of skilled and highly trained staff through discriminatory practices or failure to plan for periods of ill health.

Most of the mistakes that employers have made in relation to HIV and AIDS have been the result of too little forethought and pre-planning. No organisation can legitimately argue that they are not affected by HIV/AIDS in any way.

It is essential that employers and trade unions prepare in advance for problems associated with HIV: strategies to avoid discrimination should be integral to this preparation.

Models of good practice

Although there are clearly many examples of HIV discrimination in employment, it is also important to stress that there are now many employers who have committed themselves by policy to provide good employment practice in relation to HIV and AIDS.

In 2004 NAT and the Positive Futures Partnership launched a new resource pack, HIV@Work to help employers deal with HIV issues in the workplace. The pack takes employers through the facts about HIV transmission and helps Human Resources Managers develop a fair policy on the issue as part of good practice on equal opportunities. There is also an additional pack aimed at workers in health and social care. Both packs are available for free download from the NAT website www.nat.org.uk

During 2005 - 2007 work is being undertaken by the Ensuring Positive Futures project to help break down the barriers to employment for PLWH in the UK. The partnership includes representatives from the HIV sector, but also trade unions, employer groups and others who will be working together trialling a number of initiatives. UKC is the leading member of this group and supporters include ACAS, Disability Rights Commission, General Federation of Trade Unions and Summittskills.

Although Ensuring Positive Futures was a three-year pilot project and is due to end in September 2006, its resources will remain available on the UKC website. For further information visit the Ensuring Positive futures website at www.e-pf.org.uk/

Government advice

Government advice to employers is that policy should be developed in order to plan in advance. *AIDS and the Workplace: a Guide for Employers*, published by the Department of Employment and the Health and Safety Executive, states that: (check latest version)

You need to think through in advance how to deal with any AIDS cases among your staff and how to handle any fears and prejudices that may arise. The most effective way to do this is to have an AIDS policy.

For any policy to work well it must have, and be seen to have, the support of management at all levels and of employees' representatives. Your policy should follow these principles:

- Since the risk of infection through normal workplace contact is negligible, there is no justification for discrimination against anyone with - or at risk of acquiring - HIV

- Individuals who know they are infected with HIV are not obliged to tell anyone in the company of their condition, but if the employer does know, confidentiality is assured

- People living with HIV will be treated no differently from anyone else suffering from life-threatening, non-contagious illness.

- Employers can avoid AIDS panics altogether or deal successfully with them through appropriate planning. A key element for success is the development of a consistent, formal policy on HIV in the workplace.

Ideally this should be:

- Developed in consultation with appropriate agencies such as trade unions, local and health authorities, and concerned voluntary agencies

- Developed before any problems and issues arise

- Communicated clearly and formally to all employees

- Accompanied by appropriate HIV/AIDS awareness education (which not only deals with basic facts about transmission, but also attitudes about sexual orientation and race)

- Accompanied by the availability of counselling for people's genuine concerns

- Monitored for successful implementation

- Evaluated and reviewed from time to time in the light of developing information.

The policy should not only exist in principle, but should also take the following form:

- Guidelines for appropriate and consistent implementation of the policy should exist at every level in the organisation

- Clear lines of responsibility for information and implementation need to be established

- Appropriate education involving participatory workshops and discussions rather than simply leaflets or videos.

This should be part of an overall profile of health and safety at work, including procedures to deal with other more infectious diseases.

Key policy guidelines for employers

Day-to-day issues

Policy details which relate to the day-to-day running of the organisation can be modelled on the following points:

- There will be no discrimination in recruitment against applicants externally or internally on the grounds that the applicant has HIV or AIDS

- No one will be dismissed on the grounds of HIV or AIDS

- Employees (and applicants for employment) should not be required to reveal their antibody status to their employer nor should they be required to undergo any kind of HIV test

- Any harassment or discrimination by a member of staff (including management) will be regarded as a matter for disciplinary action

- An employee with HIV infection should receive the same occupational benefits as any other employee

- Those who have responsibility for caring for people with HIV-related illness will be considered for special leave

- There is no medical, ethical or legal reason to treat an employee (or applicant) with HIV infection any differently than any other employee. If they are well they should be treated as employees who are well; if they are ill they should be treated as other employees with long-term or intermittent illness. Employees with HIV should be allowed to continue working as long as they are fit to do so

- There is no reason to redeploy an employee with HIV who is fit to work without their consent. In the rare cases where there is a genuine risk of occupational infection (such as in a job involving invasive medical techniques), retraining and redeployment at an equivalent level should be offered and confidentiality should be preserved

- If ability to work is impaired by HIV-related illness, the same kinds of changes in working arrangements should be made as for any other ill employee or an employee with a disability

- Users or clients of the organisation will not be denied services because they are HIV-positive or they have AIDS.

Policy on confidentiality and HIV

- Confidentiality should be ensured for all personal and medical information, including an employee's HIV status

- Only those people with a genuine reason to know that a person has HIV will be informed. No one will be informed without the written consent of the person affected by HIV

- An employee with HIV whose status is known should be protected from discrimination. This is most likely to be achieved through participatory education in the workplace

- Deliberate breaches of confidentiality will be considered a disciplinary offence.

Health and safety

There has never been a case recorded of HIV transmission during first AID but it is important employers consider the health and safety of all employees

- Protection against HIV infection for employees of the organisation should be a consistent part of general health and safety good practice, and in particular, part of standard infection control precautions against blood-borne viral infections such as hepatitis B. Good practice in infection control is more appropriate and effective than knowledge of the HIV status of individuals.

- Standard infection control guidelines should exist and be followed in first aid and other situations where there is a risk of blood contact

- Appropriate infection control equipment should be available, such as disposable gloves and aprons, paper towels, bleach and other disinfectants.

- Blood-borne viruses in the workplace, guidance for employers and employees   HSE ISBN 07176 2062X
www.hsebooks.co.uk

Employment law and HIV

Existing protection

From December 2006 people who are living with HIV are protected by the Disability Discrimination Act (1996). Before this date only those who have or have had symptoms or illnesses related to their condition were protected.

Employment rights

Employment law can be confusing and it is essential to get up to date information, and advice. ACAS have advisors trained in issues relating to HIV and can offer nationwide, impartial   free advice on all employment matters, both to employers and employees. The helpline is available from 9:00am to 4:30pm every week day and calls are charged at local rates.

Tel: 08457 47 47 47
www.acas.org.uk

Information and training

Laws relating to health and safety are another area which the employer should be aware of. Under Section 2 of the Health and Safety at Work Act, employers have a duty to provide adequate information, instruction and training to their workforce. This is also part of their common law duty of care. Under these laws employers may well have a duty to provide information about HIV and its modes of transmission.

Tribunal cases

There are very few cases related to HIV which have reached an employment tribunal. In those that have, the responsibility of the employers to follow proper investigation and procedures have been stressed:

- In 1987 a projectionist was sacked because fellow workers knew he was gay and were worried that he might have AIDS. The tribunal upheld the decision as fair. The case went to the Employment Appeals Tribunal (EAT) who advised that the employer should pay compensation. The EAT decision was based on the fact that the company had not held a proper inquiry

- In 1987 two solicitors at North Lambeth Law Centre refused to work with another solicitor because he was gay and they thought he would therefore have AIDS. After an internal inquiry both were sacked and an tribunal found their dismissal fair.

Although there are few related tribunal cases, many people affected by HIV have had problems in employment. One of the reasons why there have been so few cases reported is that many were settled out of court, or an employer offered a sum of money on termination of employment which was more than the tribunal was likely to award as compensation. The Disability Discrimination Act and the Human Rights Act now give much greater scope for people to challenge HIV-related discrimination.

It is worth noting that in 2000 one of the highest sums awarded under disability discrimination was an out of court settlement to a Mr Mark Hedley. Mr Hedley sued the supermarket Aldi, alleging disability and sex discrimination, after the firm made disputed claims that staff did not want to work with him and profits would suffer. The supermarket settled for an estimated £300,000.

Reasons for not requiring testing

The British Government, the World Health Organisation, the International Labour Organisation and the Council of Europe are amongst many who have stated clearly that there are no grounds for testing people for HIV either pre-employment or in employment. However, it would seem that until a law is passed to forbid such discriminatory practices then certain companies will continue to ignore advice

Confidentiality

The contract of employment has within it an implied duty of trust and confidence for both employer and employee. The duty of trust and confidence includes a duty for both employer and employee not to disclose confidential information obtained in the course of employment.

Employers are not legally entitled to disclose that an employee is HIV-positive unless the employee consents. The only exception to this rule is if it could be claimed that it was in the public interest for others to know - this is a standard defence to breach of confidence claims.

Even when disclosure without consent is justified, it should only be to those who have a real need to know the information. Disclosure should be on the basis that the information is strictly confidential and should not be further disclosed. Because

disclosure of a person's HIV status may have serious consequences, the employer would probably be justified in treating such a disclosure as a serious disciplinary offence.

The Data Protection Act 1998 (DPA) gives extra weight to confidentiality There are two sections of the DPA that are specifically relevant in relation to HIV: the first section is *Sensitive Personal Data*; the second section is *Rights in Relation to Health Records*.

The DPA gives strict rules to ensure that information about an individual is only used for the specific purposes for which it is intended. This has strong implications for maintaining confidentiality. The devastating effect that breach of confidentiality can have in relation to HIV means that employers should act scrupulously to ensure that they do comply with the Act.

Laws on confidentiality and HIV are further strengthened in Health Authorities by the National Health Service (Venereal Diseases) Regulations 1974. Section 1 1974.9 places Health Authorities, and by DHSS guidance, Local Authorities too, under an obligation to maintain confidentiality in relation to sexually transmitted infections.

The Human Rights Act 1998 came into force on 2nd October 2000. The right to privacy is one of the provisions of the Act, and this again gives extra strength to laws on confidentiality.

Disability and HIV-related illness

The Disability Discrimination Act 1995

The Disability Discrimination Act 1995 gives disabled people rights in the areas of employment, obtaining goods and services and buying or renting land or property.

It is within the category of progressive conditions that people who are HIV-positive and symptomatic are explicitly covered by the Act. People with progressive conditions are regarded as disabled under the Act providing that, as a result of the condition, the person has an impairment which has or has had an effect on their ability to carry out normal day-to-day activities. However, the effect on day-to-day activities does not have to be a substantial effect.

The employment provisions of the Act came into force in December 1996. In April 2000, the Disability Rights Commission was launched. The commission has the power to enforce the DDA. and further information on the act can be found on their web site. www.drc-gb.org

Complaints about discrimination

Disabled people who feel that their employer has discriminated against them can complain to an employment tribunal. There is no qualifying period of employment needed to take a case of discrimination to an employment tribunal. Claims must usually be made within three months of the discrimination taking place.

The Act explicitly outlaws victimisation of disabled people. Any victimisation of or discrimination against a disabled person is the employer's responsibility - regardless of whether or not it

occurred with the employer's knowledge or approval. www.acas.org.uk

Recruitment

An employer will have a defence against a discrimination claim only if they can justify that the less favourable treatment of a disabled person was for a reason which is material to the circumstances of the particular case and substantial. That is, the employer must show that the reason for treating a disabled person differently was genuinely relevant in a given situation. For example, an employer who rejects outrightly a job applicant because they disclose on their application form that they have had an HIV-related illness would not usually have a defence to their actions.

Always seek sympathetic legal advice before disclosing your HIV status to an employer or potential employer.

Victimisation and harassment

Under the DDA, people who are HIV-positive can now take claims of discrimination to an employment tribunal if they are being discriminated against or have been sacked because of their status.

It is the employer's duty to ensure that discrimination does not occur. It is therefore in the employer's interest to ensure that other employees do not victimise or discriminate in any way against colleagues who are HIV-positive.

Ill health retirement and dismissals

If a person is genuinely not able to continue to work for an employer, the most beneficial option for the employee is for the employer to offer some package of early retirement on ill health grounds. The package the employer is able to offer will, of course, depend on the size and resources of the organisation.

If dismissal is the only option, then legally the dismissal must come under one of two headings: either on health grounds after proper medical enquiry or for poor attendance.

If a person is dismissed because they are unable to do the job the employer must have sufficient evidence upon which to base the decision. This involves, preferably, both a report from the employee's doctor and an examination by a doctor on behalf of the employer.

If the employer makes a decision to dismiss on the grounds of poor attendance due to a succession of minor illnesses, this is a reason related to conduct. Therefore, the employee should be given warnings as appropriate, and an opportunity to improve. After that, if there is no improvement or explanation then the employer is eventually entitled to decide that enough is enough. However, no employer should consider dismissal without full consideration of the DDA Section 6 adjustments and modifications. If the employer is considering a dismissal on the grounds of poor attendance (reason related to conduct) then it is very important that flexible working arrangements have been fully considered. In the examples of adjustments that could be made under section 6, "allowing him to be absent during working hours for rehabilitation, assessment or treatment" is explicitly stated in the DDA.

Employer's duty to make a reasonable adjustment

Section 6 of the DDA states that an employer must take reasonable steps to prevent any physical feature of the premises, or any working arrangements that are made, from causing a substantial disadvantage to a disabled person.

The duty to make adjustments arises when a disabled person is placed at a substantial disadvantage as either a job applicant or as an employee. The duty to make adjustments would only arise at recruitment if the employer knew or could be reasonably expected to know that a disabled person was applying for a job.

Rights for carers

The Employment Relations Act 1999 gives a right to employees to take reasonable time of during working hours to attend to a *dependent*. The definition of *dependent* in the Act includes: a spouse, a child, a parent and:

- a person who lives in the same household as the employee, otherwise than by reason of being his employee, tenant, lodger or border" (Schedule 4, Part II, Section (3))

An employee is entitled to time off during working hours in order to take action which is necessary:

- (a) to provide assistance on an occasion when a dependant falls ill, gives birth or is injured or assaulted,

- (b) to make arrangements for the provision of care for a dependant who is ill or injured,

- (c) in consequence of the death of a dependant,

- (d) because of the unexpected disruption or termination of arrangements for the care of a dependant, or

- (e) to deal with an incident which involves a child of the employee and which occurs unexpectedly in a period during

which an educational establishment which the child attends is responsible for him.

In order to take time off, the employee must tell the employer, as soon as is reasonably practical, why she or he is going to be absent and how long they expect to be absent. It is recognised, however, that the employee may not be able to say how long they are going to be absent until they have returned to work.

The Act does not specify that time off for dependents should be paid leave, neither is there an attempt to quantify *reasonable* time off. The law does not state that the employee has to tell their employer the cause of an illness or injury merely the reason that time is needed in a specific circumstance.

Can an employer sack you because you have an HIV-related illness?

Government guidelines, *AIDS and the Workplace*, state that:

"HIV infection alone does not affect people's ability to do their job until they develop illnesses that make them unfit ... If they later become ill, they should be treated like anyone else with a life-threatening illness. Only if their illness affects their ability to do the job should their employer seek medical advice."

If you are dismissed because you are unable to do the job, the employer must have sufficient evidence upon which to base the decision. This involves, preferably, both a report from the employee's doctor and an examination by a doctor on behalf of the employer.

Or, if you are physically unable to carry out your contractual job, then the employer should consider the possibility of a move to different duties. The likelihood of there being suitable alternative employment will depend largely on the size of the firm involved. Furthermore, there is no duty for the employer to create alternative employment.

Seek legal advice if your employer is causing you difficulties in relation to time off for sickness.

Dismissal

If your employer sacks you, call ACAS or seek other sympathetic legal advice immediately. Time can be a very important factor in legal proceedings.

If you are in a trade union, contact your shop steward or representative.

If your employer asks you to resign, seek legal advice first before you make a decision.

Remember, if you resign from your job (even under pressure) you will most likely lose social security benefits for a period of time and you might not be allowed to bring a claim for unfair dismissal.

Contact ACAS 08457 47 47 47.for detailed information about employment rights or call one of the HIV organisations.

HIV testing and employment

Can an employer insist that you take an HIV test?

At recruitment?

There is no law to stop employers asking for an HIV antibody test as part of a company medical for all new recruits. But employers and/or company doctors must obtain your consent to be tested for HIV antibodies.

Does the employer have the right to know the test results?

No. Not without your permission. But, an employer can refuse an offer of employment if you refuse to give permission for the test or disclosure of the results. In addition, employers can also refuse employment if a test has been taken and showed positive. As with dismissal, there is a potential case for male job applicants to claim indirect sex discrimination if they are refused employment because they are HIV-positive. To date, this has not been tested in law.

Once employed?

The only way that an employer can insist on existing employees being tested for HIV antibodies is if the initial terms and conditions of service stated that this would be the case for the employee. Otherwise the employer is liable to claims of constructive dismissal, a claim for damages, breach of contract or wrongful dismissal.

Confidentiality

Employers are not legally entitled to disclose that an employee is infected with HIV unless the employee consents. The only exception to this rule is if it could be claimed that it was in the public interest for others to know.

The Data Protection Act (1998)

The *Data Protection Act* 1998 (DPA) gives extra weight to confidentiality. The new Act is much stricter than the previous 1984 Act. There are two sections of the DPA that are specifically relevant in relation to HIV: the first section is *Sensitive Personal Data*; the second section is *Rights in Relation to Health Records*.

The DPA gives strict rules to ensure that information about an individual is only used for the specific purposes for which it is intended. This further strengthens the need for employers to maintain confidentiality. The devastating effect that breach of confidentiality can have in relation to HIV means that employees could well have cases against their employer if a breach occurs.

The right to privacy under the Human Rights Act could also be cited in a tribunal case to challenge any breaches of confidentiality.

Trade unions

If there is a trade union where you work, think about joining it. A number of motions passed at TUC conferences have made it clear that all affiliated unions should adhere to equal opportunities for lesbians, gay men, bisexual people and for anyone affected by HIV. Some unions have produced specific information and guidelines on HIV. If there is more than one union recognised by your employer, check to see which union is the most progressive on HIV.

The employment of HIV-positive healthcare staff

In July 1990 a Florida dentist infected six patients during invasive dental procedures. A French orthopaedic surgeon, doing a long orthopaedic operation, has also transmitted HIV to a patient..

There may have been specific circumstances in the dental practice which led to the infections. Investigators are uncertain as to how exactly transmission occurred. Some researchers are uncertain as to whether the dentist really was the source of infection for his five patients, although the US Centers for Disease Control conducted an extensive investigation.

In spite of the risk of transmission of HIV from a health care worker to a patient being considered remote, the Department of Health has issued guidance on the management of HIV-positive health care workers and on the notification of patients treated by HIV-positive health care workers. The Department of Health's position is reflected in the statements of health care workers' professional bodies (i.e. the General Medical Council, the General Dental Council and the UKCC).

Health care workers are expected to:

- Seek medical advice and HIV antibody testing if they believe themselves to have been at risk of HIV infection

- If they are HIV-positive they are to seek medical and occupational advice from a physician

- If they perform 'exposure-prone procedures' (see below for definition), they must cease any further such work immediately and seek advice from an occupational health physician

- If exposure prone procedures have been performed, the health care worker must inform the local Director of Public Health or arrange for the physician acting on his/her behalf to do it. This information will be treated on a strictly confidential basis

- If they have not performed exposure-prone procedures, they must remain under regular medical and occupational health supervision and receive appropriate occupational health advice if their circumstances change.

Physicians/Occupational Health Practitioners treating health care workers with HIV are expected to:

- Inform the appropriate regulatory body and the Director of Public Health if they are aware that an infected health care worker has not sought or followed advice to modify their practice and/or are continuing to perform exposure prone procedures.

Employers are expected to:

- Ensure that all staff, including students, are aware of the professional regulatory bodies' statements of ethical responsibilities and occupational guidance for HIV-positive health care workers

- Ensure that medical information and records and the identity of the health care worker is kept confidential. (However, the duty of confidentiality is not absolute and there may be rare circumstances where disclosure of information is in the public interest. Disclosure of information without consent is acceptable only in exceptional circumstances, although the guidance specifies no mechanism by which the employer can be held accountable for any such disclosure)

- Arrange suitable alternative work or training for HIV-positive staff or, where appropriate, early retirement.

The Director of Public Health is expected to:

- Adhere to the same duties of confidentiality as described above

- Decide whether patients should be notified that they have undergone an exposure prone procedure at the hands of an HIV-positive health care worker. The guidance recommends that a notification exercise should be undertaken where the infected worker was the sole or main person performing the exposure prone procedure. However, the individual circumstances of each case must be considered before a public notification exercise is decided upon and the Director of Public Health should discuss their decision with the UK Advisory Panel before proceeding.

How far back Directors of Public Health should go in notifying former patients of the health care worker is likely to depend on how confidently the date of infection can be established. Where a clinical history cannot be obtained or if the health care worker has AIDS or has died, the Department of Health recommends notifying all patients who have undergone exposure-prone procedures in the past ten years.

What are exposure-prone procedures and who do the guidelines affect?

Exposure-prone procedures are those where:

"There is a risk that injury to the worker may result in the exposure of the patient's open tissues to the blood of the worker. These procedures include those where the worker's gloved hands may be in contact with sharp instruments, needle tips or sharp tissues (spicules of bone or teeth) inside a patient's open body cavity, wound or confined anatomical space where the hands or fingertips may not be completely visible at all times".

Although a normal vaginal delivery is not an exposure prone procedure,

"When undertaking a vaginal delivery an infected health care worker must not perform procedures involving the use of sharp instruments such as infiltrating local anaesthetic, or suturing of a tear or episiotomy, since fingertips may not be visible at all times and the risk of injury to the worker is greater. Neither can they perform an instrumental delivery requiring forceps or suction if infiltration of local anaesthetic or internal suturing is required. In practice, this means that an infected health care worker may only undertake a vaginal delivery if it is certain that a second midwife or doctor will also be present who is able to undertake all such operative interventions as might arise during the course of delivery".

The following procedures would not be considered exposure-prone as long as routine infection control procedures are adhered to at all times:

"Procedures where the hands or fingertips of the worker are visible and outside the patient's body at all times, and internal examinations or procedures that do not require the use of sharp instruments... Examples of such procedures include the taking of blood, setting up and maintaining IV lines, minor surface suturing, the incision of abscesses or uncomplicated endoscopies".

Patient notification of healthcare worker's HIV status-policy update

In December 2001 the Department of Health announced a new policy on the action to be taken whenever a healthcare worker is found to be HIV-positive. The new policy is based on advice from the Expert Advisory Group on AIDS and the UK Advisory Panel on Health Care Workers Infected with Blood Borne Viruses.

This new policy states that the risk of HIV transmission to patients will be assessed on a case by case basis using a criteria based framework. The extent of the patient notification exercise will depend on the level of risk of exposure. This may mean that in some instances there will no patient notification exercise, or it is limited in scope.

The decision to change the policy was reached in the light of the fact that there has never been a case of transmission of HIV from an infected health care worker to a patient in the UK detected, even though 22 extensive look back exercises involving tens of thousands of patients have been undertaken. This step has been taken in an effort to avoid unnecessary anxiety to patients and means that the policy is now more in line with that of the rest of the world.

Until this policy came into force all patients have been notified regardless of their level of risk. Under the new guidance, all patients that are notified will be offered pre-test discussion and an HIV antibody test.

HIV testing new NHS recruits

On the 2nd January 2003, the Department of Health announced that all new recruits to the NHS who will be involved in exposure-prone procedures will be tested for HIV and hepatitis C. The draft guidance is now available at the Department of Health website at www.doh.gov.uk.

If you think you may be HIV-positive and are a health care worker

If you think you might be HIV-positive the guidance states that you must seek medical advice and, if appropriate, an HIV test. Failure to do this is regarded as a potential breach in the duty of care to patients. If you are already aware of your HIV status, the chances are that you will also have taken some steps towards evaluating your professional practice and judging what risk is posed to patients. If you have not already informed a designated occupational health physician, you need to consider the consequences of this breach of guidelines on your future employment. Think what might happen if your confidentiality is subsequently breached, or you become symptomatic and unable to work. The most serious consequence of a failure to disclose is that you may be liable to disciplinary action from your employer.

Needlestick injuries, HIV infection and employment

Needlestick injuries raise a number of troubling issues for health care workers and managers, despite the rarity with which workers are actually infected through this route. Refer to the Department of Health's guidelines for the latest information. www.doh.gov.uk.

Guidelines for employers

- The UKC provides advice, training, information and support for all employers, trade union members or employees who may be infected or affected by HIV and AIDS. They also offer a wide range of services for people living with HIV from career guidance to skills training. (etc - whatever you want to write). See www.www.ukcoalition.org

- The National AIDS Trust is the leading independent policy and campaigning voice on HIV and AIDS. They produce materials aimed at both employers and employees. See www.nat.org.uk

- Employers Forum on Disability provide general advice and guidance on disability in the workplace. Publications include Employers Briefing Paper 13 - A practical guide to employment adjustments for people with HIV. See www.employers-forum.co.uk

- Health Development Agency (HDA) produces a range of publications on HIV and AIDS. *HIV and AIDS at Work: How to set up an HIV/AIDS policy* is aimed at employers, trade unions and health professionals. Some HDA publications are aimed at specific occupations, for example, seafarers. Some information in relation to HIV is available on their website http://www.hda-online.org.uk/

- The Disability Rights Commission (DRC) is an independent body, established by Act of Parliament to eliminate discrimination against disabled people and promote equality of opportunity. The DDA take on individual disability discrimination cases, including HIV related cases; provides information about the law, rights, information and publications for businesses and services, policy and campaigns. The can be contacted by post: DRC Helpline, FREEPOST, MID02164 Stratford upon Avon, CV37 9BR. Helpline: 08457 622 633. Textphone: 08457 622 644. Fax: 08457 778 878 or Website: http://www.drc-gb.org

Health & safety/first aid at work

The Health & Safety Executive and the Department of Health AIDS Unit provide written guidelines for various occupations, especially in the National Health Service.

Advice on first aid at work is available from The British Red Cross Society, the St. John's Ambulance Brigade or in Scotland, the St. Andrew's Association.

HIV employment and other issues abroad

The UK NGO AIDS Consortium is a networking organisation for charities sending employees to developing countries. The Consortium has published two booklets called *HIV/AIDS & Overseas Employment*. One booklet is for employers, the other for employees. The booklets are published and available from the Health Development Agency (HDA). For more enquires about working abroad contact at UK NGO AIDS Consortium for the Third World, Fenner Brockway House, 37-39 Great Guildford Street, London SE1 0ES. Tel: 020 7401 8231.

The CBI produce a booklet called *AIDS & Overseas Business Travel* available from the CBI, Centre Point, New Oxford Street, London WC1.

Trade unions and professional associations

The TUC offers a training pack and a joint statement on AIDS (with the CBI and ACAS). Available from: TUC Publications, Congress House, Great Russell Street, London WC1B.

Some unions have issued their own guidelines and codes of good practice. UNISON, for example, has produced several comprehensive publications on HIV and AIDS.

Many unions, however, have produced guidelines which address issues specifically to do with the industry or sectors they represent: some of the guidelines, therefore, do not necessarily carry information on the broader issues on HIV and AIDS or about safer sex.

Information for legal advisors

The publishers Butterworths have just produced two books which give guidance to legal advises about HIV and about sexual orientation:

Advising Clients with HIV/AIDS - A Guide for Lawyers edited by Avrom Sherr and Isabel Manley, concentrates on the legal implications of a client being HIV-positive or of developing AIDS. The book covers all issues which a client will need advice on, including disclosing one's status, criminal and civil liability, access to medical records and right to treatment, discrimination and employment issues, arranging financial affairs and living wills, family issues such as custody and guardianship of children, the rights and education of HIV-infected children and access to social services such as housing and welfare benefits. Published by Butterworths. ISBN 0 406 92931 9.

Advising Gay and Lesbian Clients - A guide for Lawyers, various contributors. The book provides detailed and practical coverage of issues of specific concern to lesbian and gay clients including in and outside employment, immigration issues, arranging financial affairs, inheritance tax planning and making wills, cohabitation, the family home, custody disputes, adopting and fostering children, donor insemination and the criminal law as it affects gay men. Published by Butterworths. ISBN 0 406 90303 4

Disability Discrimination Claims - An Adviser's Handbook by Catherine Casserley and Bela Gor. The book concentrate on the practicalities of bringing disability discrimination cases before the employment tribunal. Published by Jordans. ISBN 0 85308 642 7.

Referral for clients

National organisations giving legal advice to individuals who have employment problems, including discrimination, related to their HIV status are:

Terence Higgins Trust,
54 Grays Inn Road, London, WC1X 8JU, Tel: 020 7831 0330, info@tht.org.uk
www.tht.org.uk

UK Coalition of people Living with HIV and AIDS
020 7564 2180
www.ukcoalition.org
See also Ensuring Positive Futures: www.e-pf.org.uk

ACAS
www.acas.org.uk
08457 47 47 47

Specialist advice and consultancy for employers

The National AIDS Trust (NAT). NAT publishes materials to assist with the development of workplace policy and practices as well as its implementation. The *HIV@Work* pack draws together the information needed by employers seeking to develop or review their response to HIV/AIDS; Other workplace materials are currently being developed as part of the Ensuring Positive Futures project .
Tel: 020 7814 6767
www.nat.org.uk

The **UKCoalition of people living with HIV and AIDS** can provide consultancy, training, support and advice for employers, often free of charge or at a nominal rate.
020 7564 2180
www.ukcoaltion.org

The **ILO Code of Practice on HIV/AIDS and the world of work** is a blueprint for workplace action. It provides practical guidance for governments, employers and workers covering the key areas of prevention, behaviour change, non-discrimination and care.
www.ilo.org/aids

The Global Business Coalition on HIV/AIDS (GBC).
The GBC promotes the international business response to HIV/AIDS. Its membership includes many UK headquartered companies that have developed global policies on HIV/AIDS. Its website gives direct access to GBC materials on workplace and community responses to the epidemic and provides details of other resources and organisations that would help a multinational company determine their approach to HIV/AIDS, especially in countries of high prevalence
www.businessfightsaids.org
Tel: 001 212 846 5893.

Returning to work or study?

Introduction

Since the news of advances in treatments at the World AIDS Conference in Vancouver in 1996, dramatic changes have occurred in the lives of many people with HIV. The introduction of highly-active-anti-retroviral therapy (HAART) to delay progression of HIV disease and of viral-load testing to better monitor disease progression has created new optimism among people living with HIV and their treatment providers alike.

Up until that time services for people with HIV were geared towards benefit maximisation and determining when to retire from work. The first and most important point to make is that not everyone is capable of returning to work and not everyone wants to. There are those however who, upon realising that their new found level of health is lasting and that there is a prospect of a 'future', are starting to think more long term and consequently re-engaging with life. This includes the possibility of returning to work.

Why go back to work?

One of the very important decisions people have to make when thinking about going 'back to work' is what they actually want to 'go back' to. Some may choose to try and pick up where they left off. Others choose to use this as an opportunity to try something completely different. Many people in this situation view work from a very different perspective. They may be much more aware of what it is they want to achieve from working, rather than simply wanting to be 'employed'. It is a good time for people to assess what they value and what they want from work other than an income.

Working can provide many benefits to an individual; this includes companionship, stimulation, challenge, and a sense of fulfilment and increase in self-esteem and confidence.

The reality for others may be that due to the lapse in time since previous employment, they are unable to simply pick up where they left off. Many will require some form of training to equip them to return to the workforce either for returning their old line of work or if they wish to try something completely different.

Training and studying

The main options for people wishing to gain new skills would be to undertake some voluntary work, attend a course at a local college, enrol on a work experience placement, or avail themselves of various government training schemes.

Adult education is available at Community Colleges and Universities in a wide variety of subjects. The costs of these courses vary, but some may offer reduced fees to people on reduced incomes.

For information about other government training schemes, contact the local Jobcentre Plus. Further contact details can be found at the end of this chapter.

Volunteering

The main advantage of undertaking volunteer work is that it provides an opportunity for gaining new skills, as well as starting the process of introducing some structure into daily activities. It also provides an opportunity of experiencing working conditions, as well as offering an opportunity to check whether the person is ready to consider seriously returning to work.

Volunteering also provides an opportunity to relearn how to interact with colleagues in a working environment. One of the main outcomes of volunteering is that it can increase levels of self-confidence. Many people have found that volunteering has led them into paid work as a direct result.

What help exists for people who want to brush up their CV, or interview skills?

Assistance and advice with updating CV's is available through EPF; Contact the Case Manager at any one of the partner organisations for details. Local Jobcentre Plus can also assist with CVs and interview skills. Ask for an appointment with a Disability Employment Advisor. Similarly local Adult Education Services often run day sessions on CV writing. There are also many websites that offer free advice and guidance.

Disclosure

The decision to disclose or not at work is not a simple one. Some people choose to disclose because they feel more comfortable with their employer knowing so that they can assess whether they will be working in a supportive environment. Others however prefer to keep the information confidential to avoid possibly being discriminated against or having to deal with work colleagues' attitude towards HIV and AIDS. Not disclosing HIV status at work may lead to difficult situations if the person needs time off work because of illness or hospital appointments.

Setting up your own business

Many people with HIV have thought of setting up their own business as a way of taking control over their working hours and a way of dealing with not having to disclose their status to an employer. As with anyone setting up a business this should be approached with prudence and caution. The demands and responsibilities of running your own business should not be underestimated.

There are many Business Start-up courses around that offer basic advice on how to go about setting up your own business. It would also be advisable to contact the Small Business Advice Centre nearest you who can advise on all the various aspects and steps necessary for successfully setting up your own business, and New Deal at Jobcentre plus also offers advice and guidance.

Ensuring Positive Futures

Ensuring Positive Futures (EPF) is an innovative employability programme for people living with HIV and AIDS, delivered by a partnership of 24 organisations throughout Great Britain. This partnership includes HIV charities, trades unions, employers and government bodies all working together to support plwha in the workplace.

The five core partners are major HIV and AIDS charities: National AIDS Trust (NAT), Positive East (PE), Positively Women (PW), Terrence Higgins Trust (THT) and the lead partner, UK Coalition of People Living with HIV and AIDS (UKC). Collectively this partnership aimed to test new ways of working together to assist and support people with HIV enter, return to and remain in employment.

The project was always intended to be a pilot, funded on a three-year basis as an innovative equality project by the EU. It will be wound down by the end of 2007 but its materials will continue to be available on the EPF website at http://www.e-pf.org.uk/. Many EPF style services will continue to be run by organisations engaged in this programme.

EPF, through its Employer and Trades Unions Diversity Development (ETUDD) project also targeted trades unions and employers together to explore and develop increasingly effective ways of ensuring introduction and implementation of HIV friendly employment related policies and practices within the workplace.

EPF has been hugely successful in raising awareness of HIV in the workplace with the general population, employers, trades unions, community organisations, government bodies and the media. This was recognised in 2006 when Ensuring Positive Futures was the winner of the Guardian Public Service awards.

Benefits

How welfare benefits may be affected by work or study

Editor's note: This section is taken from the THT booklet Positive About Work and is reproduced by kind permission of The Terrence Higgins Trust.

The rules covering issues such as changes in circumstances, re-claiming benefit after a break in your claim, and whether or not the Department of Work and Pensions (DWP) can review your benefit can be a complex area of benefits law. There are some areas where this section can only highlight potential problems rather than provide definitive answers. Wherever possible you should seek advice from a welfare rights specialist before making a decision to start work or studying. In particular, if you have come from abroad, for example if you are an overseas student or an asylum seeker, you should always seek advice before breaking a benefits claim.

Employment - benefit implications

What will happen to the benefits that I am currently getting if I start work? Each benefit has different rules about working, and these are outlined below.

Can I work for just a few hours a week?

One of the limitations with the benefits system is that people are treated as being either incapable of all work, or else fully fit for work. There is no structure to support people who may be able to work occasionally, or who can work for part of a week, or those who can work full time but with limited capacity. If you are well enough to do some work, then the DWP will usually treat you as fit for work and you will then lose your entitlement to sickness benefits. There are a few exceptions to this, such as rules on Permitted Work, which are discussed below.

If the work is low paid, can I get any benefits to top-up the wages?

It is worth remembering that the disincentives to take up employment because a future salary would be lower than your current benefit entitlement, *the benefits trap*, is now largely a thing of the past. There are many benefits you can claim if you work part-time or your wages are low, and details of those are given below, and you are likely to find yourself financially better off than if you just stayed on benefits.

What happens if I have to stop work because of illness - will I be able to go back onto benefits at the same rate I currently get?

There are linking rules, which allow you to go straight back onto some benefits at the same rate, and under the same conditions, after a break in claim of up to 52 weeks. These linking rules only apply however if you have been claiming benefit on the basis of your incapacity for 28 weeks and stop claiming because you have gone into work. Over recent years there have been changes to many benefits. If you have been continuously in receipt of benefits, you may have been shielded from these changes. However, if you break your benefit claim without being able to take advantage of the linking rules described above, you will usually have to reclaim under the new (often-harsher) rules. Some of the main changes that you need to be aware of are included below.

Disability Living Allowance

Can I still get DLA if I am working?

DLA is not means tested, and entitlement to DLA is based on disability rather than incapacity for work: therefore there are no specific rules regarding working. It is possible to work full-time and receive DLA - even at the higher rates. Indeed, there are many people with HIV who qualify for DLA whilst in full-time work. In theory going back to work may not affect your DLA payments. However, if you are considering returning to work, this is likely to be because there is a change in your circumstances, for example an improvement in your health. This change may mean that the DSS can look again at your DLA to see whether you are still entitled to receive it.

Can the DWP stop my DLA?

The DWP can review your DLA at any time, if there has been *a relevant change in circumstances*. It may be possible to argue that starting work is not in itself a relevant change - as there are no specific rules regarding working and DLA. However, an improvement in your health that leads to better mobility or a change in the amount of care you need certainly is a relevant change of circumstances.

If the DWP decide there has been a relevant change in your circumstances, this does not mean your DLA will automatically be stopped. The DWP will look at your case again and will assess whether you still have care needs and/or mobility problems. The DWP may decide that you are still entitled to DLA, but possibly at a lower rate.

Do I have to tell the DWP if I start working?

If you are receiving DLA, you are obliged to tell the DWP if your circumstances change. If you are paid too much benefit because you *fail to disclose a material fact*, then you may have to repay the overpayment. There are no rules that prevent you working and claiming DLA, so it could be argued that starting work is not a material fact. However, if you feel able to work because your health has improved to a point where you no longer have care needs and/or mobility problems the clearly this would be a material fact that you have a duty to report to the DWP.

What can I do if my DLA is stopped?

If your DLA is stopped following a return to work, you should always get advice. It may be possible for you to appeal and argue that the DWP had no grounds to review your DLA because there had not been a relevant change in your circumstances. If the DWP did establish correct grounds for the review, then you may be able to argue that even though your circumstances have changed, you still have mobility problems and/or care needs which entitle you to DLA.

Can I claim DLA again?

If your DLA has been stopped, then you can make a fresh claim at any time if your health deteriorates. If you make this claim within two years of a previous award then you may be entitled to DLA immediately. Otherwise you will usually need to show that you have had care needs and/or mobility problems for at least three months before the DLA can be paid again.

Incapacity Benefit (IB)

It is not usually possible to do any work whilst claiming IB. This is because IB is paid on the condition that you are incapable of work. If you actually do any work, even if it is just a few hours a week, then the DWP will treat you as fit for work and your IB will stop. There are some limited exceptions made for voluntary work and work which is undertaken as part of the permitted work scheme.

How much voluntary work can I do?

In theory there is no limit to the number of hours of voluntary work that you can do for someone other than a 'close relative', whilst still being able to satisfy the Benefits Agency that you continue to be incapable of work. However, you should note that the DWP could take into account the amount of voluntary work you do as part of any personal capability assessment to determine your incapacity for work. It maybe advisable therefore, to restrict any voluntary work to less than 16 hours per week.

What is permitted work?

This is a scheme that allows you to do a limited amount of work whilst retaining your right to benefits. There are two levels of permitted work called the higher and lower limits.

The permitted work lower limit allows you:

- To work for less than 16 hours per week

- To earn no more than £20 per week

- To work for an indefinite period.

The permitted work higher limit allows you:

- To work for less than 16 hours per week

- To earn no more than £78 per week

- To work for a period of up to 26 weeks in the first instance with a possible extension of up to 52 weeks.

There are slightly different rules for people undertaking permitted work as part of a treatment programme or a supported employment programme.

You must inform the DWP before undertaking any permitted work. It is important to bear in mind that if you are getting Income Support on the basis of incapacity, and you undertake higher limit permitted work, your IS will be reduced pound for pound after the first £20 of your earnings. If you receive Incapacity Benefit no reduction will be made.

If I stop claiming IB, will there be any problems if I have to reclaim in the future?

There is a 52-week linking rule for IB, called the Welfare to Work Beneficiary scheme, for those who have been claiming benefit on the basis of incapacity for 28 weeks and who stop claiming because of starting work. This means that if you try to go back to work, but find your health is too poor, you can go straight back on to your previous rate of IB provided you give up work within the 52 week linking period and you provide a sick note form your doctor. If you successfully claim the disability element of the Working Tax Credit when you return to work, the linking period is extended further from 52 weeks to two years. In order to qualify for this protection you have to specifically request it within four weeks of starting work. Do not assume that you have the protection until you receive written confirmation from the DWP.

In April 1995, Incapacity Benefits was brought in to replace Invalidity Benefit. If you have been in receipt of Incapacity/Invalidity Benefit since before April 1995 then you may be getting transitional protection. This means your current benefit will be non-taxable and may include an earnings related addition (SERPS) based on your previous wages. If a fresh claim is made under the new rules, IB will be taxable and may be paid at a lower rate, as it will not include this addition. Seek advice if you think this may apply to you.

Income Support (IS)

Can I do any work whilst I am getting IS?

Most people with HIV will be claiming IS on the basis that they are incapable of work. Usually if you do any work at all, the DWP will class you as fit for work which means you can no longer claim IS.

There are some exceptions to this rule:

- If you are a single parent or a carer, then provided that you work for less than 16 hours a week, you can claim IS to top up your earnings

- If you undertake employment under the permitted work scheme.

- If the amount of work you can do is restricted because of ill health or disability, then it may be possible to qualify for IS under the disabled worker rule (sometimes known as the 75% rule).

You will probably need a letter from your doctor confirming that the number of hours you can work, or the amount you can earn, is only 75% or less than that of someone without your health problems. This rule is rarely used, and you may want to get advice from a welfare rights worker before contacting the DWP.

How will my wages affect my IS?

If you fall into one of the three groups described above, then you can continue to claim IS while you do some part-time work. However, your IS will be reduced by your wages. The DWP will usually ignore the first £20 a week that you earn (although sometimes only £5 is ignored). After this, your IS will be reduced pound for pound by your wages.

If I stop work, could I go straight back onto IS?

If in the future you find that you have to stop work because of ill-health, then you can claim IS again straight away.

If you had been claiming benefit on the basis of your incapacity for more than 28 weeks when you began work, and become incapable of work again within 52 weeks, you can reclaim benefit at the same rate as before under the 52 week linking rule.

This will be important, for example, if you had previously been paid Income Support at a higher rate, including, for example, a disability premium on the basis of long term incapacity for work, or help towards mortgage repayments.

If however, you are not covered by the52-week linking rule, then when reclaiming Income Support you may find that you are entitled to benefit at a lower rate than before. You may then have to wait for up to a year to regain the Disability Premium or up to 39 weeks for help with mortgage payments.

NB: if you get any rate of DLA, this means you can qualify for the disability premium straight away.

Housing Benefit/Council Tax Benefit (HB/CTB)

Can I get help with my rent and council tax if I start work?

It is possible to claim HB and CTB even if you work full-time, provided your wages are low enough. You will need to make a new claim as soon as you start work. The amount of benefit you get will depend on the level of your wages.

It may also be possible to get an extra 4 weeks of HB and CTB paid when you return to work, this is regardless of the level of your earnings. This scheme may apply to you; if for at least 26 weeks, you have been claiming Income Support, Income Based Job Seekers Allowance, Incapacity Benefit, or Severe Disablement Allowance. The payment should be automatic, but you have to inform the DWP or local authority within 4 weeks of starting work or increasing your hours.

Working Tax Credit

The Working Tax Credit (WTC) is a payment to people in work to top up their wages. It is slightly different from a benefit as it is administered by HM Revenue and Customs (formerly Inland Revenue) and not by the DWP. It is means tested but is not based on your current income but on your income from the previous tax year. It does not affect the amount of tax you pay, but if you qualify you will get a set amount of money each week or month from the government in addition to your salary.

The amount of WTC that you get depends on your circumstances and your income. The amount is made up of various elements, depending on whether you:

- are single

- in a couple

- have dependent children

- are a lone parent

- are over 50

- are disabled or severely disabled.

- work more than 30 hours per week

You will qualify for the disability element if you have been getting a qualifying disability benefit for at least 6 months prior to making a claim for WTC or you are currently getting DLA. If you are a disabled person you can only get WTC if you work more than 16 hours per week.

If you require child care because you are working or returning to work, WTC can pay 70% of any approved relevant childcare costs in addition to your WTC.

Please note if you are under 25 you will not normally be eligible for WTC unless you are responsible for dependent children, are disabled, or are over 50. If you are over 25 and not in these categories you will only qualify for WTC if you work over 30hrs per week.

Child Tax Credit (CTC)

You can claim Child Tax Credit if you are responsible for a child or children up until their 16th birthday or up until their 19th birthday if they're in full time education, whether you are in work or not, and your income is sufficiently low. CTC can be paid in addition to Working Tax Credit.

Job Seekers Allowance (JSA)

If you work part-time, i.e. less than 16 hours a week, you may be able to claim JSA to top up your wages. To qualify for JSA you will have to sign-on as unemployed at the local Job Centre. You will also have to show that you are available for work and are actively seeking work. You will usually be expected to show that you are looking for a full time job. However, you can place restrictions on the type of job you will take, provided these restrictions are reasonable because of your health problems. The amount of JSA you receive will depend on the level of your wages. Payment of JSA can be reduced if the Employment Service is not satisfied with your efforts to find full-time work, or if they believe you are setting unreasonable restrictions. It is a good idea to get advice before claiming JSA.

Job Grant

You may be eligible for a job grant if you start employment that is expected to last more than 5 weeks, and is at least 16 hours per week, and you have received either, Income Support, Incapacity Benefit, Job Seekers Allowance, or Severe Disablement Allowance for the previous 26 weeks. It is paid at two rates of £100 or £250 depending on your circumstances, and is paid automatically if you notify the DWP within 21 days of commencing employment.

If you are under 25 and the benefit you have been getting is JSA, you would not qualify for a job grant unless you are a loan parent.

Studying - benefit implications

If you are thinking about studying, you should contact your local education authority (LEA) to see if you qualify for a grant or for any help with course fees.

Each of the benefits has different rules on studying and these are outlined below. Contact a Welfare Rights worker for further advice on how your benefits will be affected if you go to college.

Disability Living Allowance

There are no specific rules regarding studying and claiming DLA. Generally, your entitlement to DLA will not be affected by studying.

Remember though that you do have an obligation to tell the DSS when your circumstances change. If your health has improved so that your mobility and care needs have changed, you have a duty to notify the DSS. There are more details under the section on DLA. in *Employment - benefit implications*.

Incapacity Benefit

There are no specific rules which prevent you studying whilst claiming IB. However, if you are studying full-time, this may lead the DSS to query whether you are genuinely too ill to work. For most people who have symptomatic HIV, this should not pose a problem, as the DSS will usually accept that you are unfit for work. In other cases it may be possible to argue that the nature of the course and the hours you are studying are very different from employment, and that although you are well enough to study it does not follow that you are well enough to work. You may be asked by the DSS to complete a form asking for details of the course and, whether the college offers you extra support because of your health problems.

Income Support

Full-time students generally cannot claim IS for the duration of their course - including holidays. IS can be claimed though if you are a full-time student and you are either a lone parent or a disabled student. The DSS will treat you as a disabled student if:

- You qualify for the disabled premium; or

- You have been too ill to work for at least 28 weeks; or

- You are deaf and qualify for a disabled student's allowance.

The amount of IS paid will be affected by any grant that you receive. In practice this usually means that your total income will remain almost the same as before you became a student. If you are getting IS, then you will also be entitled to full housing benefit and council tax benefit.

Housing Benefit

Full-time students usually cannot claim HB. However, you can get HB if you are a student and you fall into one of the following categories:

- You get Income Support

- You are a lone parent

- You are a disabled student.

Council Tax

If you are studying full-time, you should let the council know. If you are alone, or live with other students, then your home will be exempt from the council tax so you will not have to pay anything. If you live with other people who are not students, then seek advice, as there may be several ways of reducing your council tax bill.

Conclusions

This section provides only a brief summary of how welfare benefits will be affected by undertaking employment or studying. For more detailed advice people should contact a welfare benefits adviser.

The possibility of having a future is both exciting and anxiety provoking. There are many options available to people who find that treatments have either directly or indirectly improved their quality of life, and extended their life expectancy. Each individual needs to make their own informed choice based on what they want to do and what their state of health is. There are risks involved, but the potential benefits gained from opting for any of these choices are many. No one should feel coerced into any particular course of action. All of the options discussed above can be seen as goals in themselves, as each can contribute to increased quality of life. Going back to work is one of these options and one that an increasing number of people are undertaking.

Resources

Publications

UKC's into work guide: see www.e-pf.org.uk
tel: 020 7564 2180

HIV@Work - addressing stigma & discrimination, a resource pack for employers:
www.nat.org.uk

Can people with HIV work? - An employment perspective from the UK
e-mail: info@ukcoalition.org
tel: 020 7564 2180

Positive Nation - The UK's HIV & Sexual health magazine
www.positivenation.co.uk

Websites - Education

www.ucas.ac.uk

www.dfee.gov.uk

www.floodlight.co.uk

www.hero.ac.uk

www.prospects.ac.uk

www.learndirect.co.uk

Websites - Vacancies

www.job-opps.co.uk

www.charityjob.co.uk

www.jobsgopublic.com

www.jobhunter.co.uk

www.opportunities.org.uk

www.jobsunlimited.co.uk (The Guardian)

www.prospects.csu.ac.uk

www.jobcentreplus.gov.uk

Websites - Government

www.dfes.gov.uk

www.drc-gb.org

www.disability.gov.uk

Organisations

UKCoalition of People Living with HIV and AIDS
250 Kennington Lane
London SE11 5RD
020 7564 2180
www.ukcoalition.org

Positive East
159 Mile End Road London E1
020 7791 2855
www.theglobecentre.co.uk

Positively Women
347-349 City Road
London EC1V 1LR
020 7713 0222
www.positivelywomen.org.uk

Oasis North London
Unit 2000, Regis Road
Kentish Town
London NW5 3EW
020 7485 2466
www.oasisnorthlondon.org.uk

TerrenceHigginsTrust
52-54 Grays Inn Road
London WC1X 8JU
020 7831 0330
www.tht.org.uk

GeorgeHouseTrust
77 Ardwick Green North
Manchester M12 6FX
www.ght.org.uk

Legal Advice

Disability Rights Commission
08457 622633 (Mincom: 020 7211 4037

Disability Law Service
020 7791 9800 (Mincom 020 7791 9801)

DuncanLewisSolicitors - solicitors with experience in HIV legal matters
www.duncanlewis.co.uk (Freephone 0800 740 8081)

Small Business Advice Centres

Business Link 0345 567 765 (England)

Business Connect 0345 969 798 (Wales)

Business Shop 0345 787 878 (Scotland)

Northern Ireland Development Agency 0800 731 4741

EnterpriseCareers Services 020 7275 0346

New Deal - self-employment 0845 606 2626

Funding for Courses

The Department for Education and Skills produce a booklet called *Financial Support in Higher Education,* they also produce a booklet on disabled students' allowances (DSA) and how to apply for them, called '*Bridging the gap'* which you can obtain by calling their Freephone information line on 0800 731 9133.

Career Development Loans
www.lifelonglearning.dfes.gov.uk/cdl/
Freephone 0800 585 505

The Educational Grants Advisory Service
www.egas-online.org/fwa/index.html
020 7254 6251

The Student Loan Company Ltd
www.slc.co.uk/noframe/contacts/index.html
Freephone: 0800 40 50 10

Overseas students

Students from other European Union member countries can only apply for help with course fees from:

The Department for Education and Skills
www.dfes.gov.uk/studentsupport/index.shtml
Freephone: 0800 731 9133.

Disabled students

SKILL (National Bureau for Students with Disabilities)
Freephone: 0800 328 5050
www.skill.org.uk

Mental health and quality of life

Mental health

Introduction: We're well but were not happy

A survey that came out shortly before this chapter was written shed a revealing insight into the needs of people with HIV in Europe.

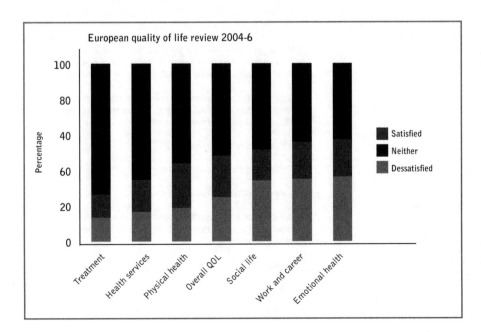

The European HIV Quality of Life Review (European Men's Health Forum) interviewed 534 people with HIV (24% of them women) from six European countries, plus African immigrants in those countries, about their health and HIV treatment, their satisfaction with their medical services, and their levels of satisfaction with work, relationships and general well-being.

With some simplification (merging 'very dissatisfied' with 'dissatisfied' and 'very satisfied' with 'satisfied'), the results look like this (see chart)

People were considerably more satisfied than not with their HIV treatment, their physical well-being, and their experience of health services. But only a minority were truly satisfied with their social life, their work and career, and their emotional well-being.

In other words HIV treatment and their physical health had a net positive effect on their overall quality of life. But their mental health, and their ability to fit in with normal life outside being a patient had a net negative effect.

Because surveys ask different questions it is difficult to say what the responses of another group of people or of patients with a different chronic condition would have been.

However it is at least superficially surprising that a group of people who suffer from one of the most feared and intractable illnesses in the world should, of all areas of life that may cause unhappiness, be least bothered about their health.

Or is it? In the developed world, through an extraordinary scientific effort, AIDS has been turned from a lethal affliction into a chronic manageable condition. This has involved people with HIV having hundreds of millions of pounds and years of health workers' and scientists' time being spent on them.

When the tide of deaths recedes, people with HIV may feel stranded and left to cope alone:

- They may be left to deal with personal issues like depression or addictions that contributed to their becoming HIV-positive in the first place (see **'mental health and sexual health' and 'long term mental health issues')**

- If they are newly diagnosed, they may feel shame for 'not having known better' (see **'adjustment disorders: reactions to diagnosis')**

- They find themselves living with a stigmatised and isolating condition and may be afraid to disclose what feels like the most significant fact in their lives to anyone

- They may miss a sense of being special, as 'plague victims' and objects of the compassion of celebrities (**see the Lazarus effect: reactions to recovery')**

- They may find themselves having to restart a career prematurely terminated by AIDS

- If they are long-term survivors, they may have lost partners and/or an entire supportive generation of friends to AIDS

- They are faced with having to negotiate a sex and love life in the face not only of possible rejection but of internalised shame about their condition and concern with body image (**see 'social issues: isolation and stigma')**

- Body changes may be imagined, but may be a real consequence of HIV treatment, and some treatments themselves cause psychological side-effects

But before we can explore these issues, we have to answer three fundamental questions first.

- What exactly is 'mental illness'?

- To what extent is it an **illness** (a disorder of the mind), and to what extent is it **unhappiness** (a disorder of the life)?

- Is it true that people with HIV suffer higher rates of it?

Quality of Life

Sigmund Freud said that the task of psychoanalysis was "To replace hysterical misery with common unhappiness." The best-selling self-help book *The Road Less Travelled* (Peck) opens with the statement that "Life is Difficult." The American Declaration of Independence enshrines a right to "the pursuit of happiness" but not to happiness itself.

These are reminders that anxiety, unhappiness, stress, loneliness, conflict and loss are part of any normal life and that we should be careful not to label as "mental illness" something that is in fact a normal reaction to a sudden change, poor resources, oppression or bad situation in life.

Over the last couple of decades, psychologists have become increasingly interested not only in disorders of the mind but in 'positive psychology' - the definition and measurement of happiness and what can influence it for good or ill. In doing so they have developed measuring tools which are not designed to diagnose mental illness but to measure broad satisfaction in life amongst entire populations - in some cases, between countries.

The definition and measurement of Quality of Life

Quality of life is the degree to which "life is good" for the individual. This is a partly subjective, situationally-specific synthesis of measurements of different aspects of the person's physical, psychological, spiritual and social 'health'.

Quality of life (QoL) studies started off in the field of palliative care, where they were used as a way of measuring the degree of

pain, discomfort and mental anguish patients were feeling in situations where these might need to be offset against quantity of life, in order to make treatment and care decisions in terminally-ill people. However Quality of Life indicators are now used to measure everything from the desirability of living in specific countries or cities to the degree to which medical and social services meet patients' and clients' actual needs. There is at least as much concentration on psychological indicators like stress and social ones like isolation as there is on physical ones. A key set of scales used are the ones developed by the World Health Organization in line with its definition of health as "A state of complete physical mental and social well-being."

QoL can be measured along a variety of different axes. In the Calvert-Henderson approach, which mainly measures physical health, QoL is measured in terms of:

- **Who** gets to live (mortality)

- **How long** that life will be (longevity)

- **How healthy** that life is (morbidity)

In a second and more sophisticated approach, the SF-36 questionnaire, QoL is divided into physical and mental health and further subdivided into:

- **Ability**

- **Role**

- **Pain**

- Mood

- Productivity and vitality

- Social role

In an approach used in the population sciences such as sociology, economics, as well as in human rights and policy, QoL may be measured in a three-step hierarchy:

- Provision of **basic needs**

- Provision of **opportunities** for growth

- Provision of **choice and control** over those opportunities

Because of the implicit hierarchy in this approach, there is a danger that more complex needs may be neglected if they are perceived as being secondary to the meeting of basic ones; or that the neglect of basic ones may mean that people have no realistic way of achieving more complex ones. This tripartite division of the Quality of Life has, in the University of Toronto's model, been reframed as

- **Being: who** one is: basic physical heal, emotional mood, moral outlook

- **Belonging: where** one is: physical environment, social support, friendship

- **Becoming: what** one can do: basic self-care, leisure, ambitions and goals

A truly holistic model of quality of life for people with HIV therefore needs to measure multiple indicators, of which the provision of effective treatment is only one.

The impact of treatments on Quality of Life, and of QoL on treatment

Even though people with HIV may be relatively well-informed about treatments compared with other unmet needs, HIV treatments may impact significantly on quality of life especially:

- When contemplating or undertaking the life changes necessary to start therapy

- When people are badly affected by drug side-effects

In turn, multiple factors affecting quality of life may impact upon patients' wish or ability to start therapy and their ability to adhere to regimens.

For instance, one French study (Vincent), injecting drug users with HIV were more likely to report having unsafe sex if they experienced more than three HIV-related side-effects. In another (Collins), drug-related lipodystrophy and body shape changes had multiple negative effects on quality of life. In a third (Duran), patients with lipodystrophy symptoms were 80% more likely to report difficulties with adherence.

However quality of life issues may also affect patients' ability to take HIV medication and therefore stay healthy. In one meta-analysis(Mehta), risk factors that affected adherence included side-effects; beliefs about the effectiveness of the treatment; beliefs about the severity of disease; youth; poor housing; low income; lack of childcare; mental illness; and illicit drug use. In one recent study (Horne), 25% of patients who had a clinical need for HIV therapy turned it down when offered: not taking therapy was associated both with the perceived need for the therapy and with a more-than-average concern about possible side-effects.

Doctors underestimate the impact of side-effects, especially those which may be stigmatising in general (such as lipodystrophy), or for specific populations (such as pigmentary changes). They may also perceive a patient dallying starting medication or deciding to take a treatment break as due to lack of understanding about treatments or to self-destructiveness. Doctors should respect patients' decisions even when they do not necessarily go with what is clinically indicated.

The oft-repeated assertion that HIV these days is a 'manageable condition' or that treatments enable people to 'live normally', while correct in terms of its impact on mortality compared with the days before HAART, may clash with a patient's feeling that their life is anything but manageable or normal. Deciding to start treatment is itself a significant change, and as research into stress has shown(Martin), positive changes in life can be as stressful as negative ones.

The measurement of Quality of Life

There is an increasing interest in QoL in health, education and disability studies, where the study of QoL has been defined as "An examination of influences upon the goodness and meaning in life, as well as people's happiness and well being."

It is about how we make life *both* meaningful and enjoyed.

The World Health Organization has developed a QoL scale based on a 100-question assessment instrument (**WHOQOL-100**)[1], which can be shortened to a 30-question version (WHOQOL-BREF). It has also developed a specific one for PLHAs.

Using as its basis the WHO definition of health as "A state of complete physical mental and social well-being", the HIV QoL assessment measures intensities of:

- Pain and discomfort

- Symptoms of HIV

- Positive feelings

- Body image and appearance

- Negative feelings

- Personal relationships

- Sexual activity

- Sense of forgiveness of self and others (self-acceptance)

- Spiritual connection

Another example is the **Calvert-Henderson QoL Indicator**.

This aims to answer three basic questions of a population:

- Who gets a chance at life (who gets to survive)?

- How long will that life last?

- How healthy will that life be?

In QoL studies there is much more emphasis on stress reduction and lifestyle choices these days as well as physical health, pain and discomfort. They look at the interrelationship between the health of the individual and the health of society. They consider, both on an individual and a society level:

- Education

- Employment

- Income
- Energy supply
- Quality of the environment
- Health
- Food
- Shelter
- Human Rights
- Income
- Social Infrastructure
- National security and policing
- Public safety
- Recreation

A third QoL measuring tool, much used in trials of the psychology of living with HIV, is the SF-36 Questionnaire.

SF stands for Short Form and as its name indicates uses just 36 questions. It divides QoL into two domains each containing four subdomains thus:

Physical health

Physical functioning - degree of ability in actions such as walking, keeling, bathing and dressing, stairs etc

Physical role - degree of difficulty and time spent on tasks

Physical Pain - magnitude, and degree to which it interferes with ability

General Health scale, and the degree to which it is improving or declining

Mental health

Vitality - degree of energy or 'go' versus fatigue or lethargy

Social functioning - extent of and time spent on social relations

Mood - degree to which sad, nervous, content

Emotional role - degree to which mood affects ability and productivity

The Centre for Health Promotion at the University of Toronto has developed probably the most sophisticated QoL assessment instrument. This measures QoL along three interacting domains, each with six subdomains.

It defines QoL as "The degree to which a person enjoys the important possibilities of their life".

It's about what you have.and whether what you have makes you happy.

Domain 1 - BEING
(Who one is - health and self-concept)

Physical Being
- Being physically able to get around
- My nutrition and the food I eat

Psychological being
- Being free of worry and stress
- The mood I am usually in

Spiritual being
- Having hope for the future

- My own ideas of right and wrong

Domain 2 - BELONGING
(Social relationships and integration)

Physical belonging
- My home and housing
- The neighbourhood I live in

Social belonging
- Being close to people - social circle
- Having a spouse or special person - primary relationship

Community belonging
- Being able to get professional services (medical, social etc)
- Having enough money

Domain 3 - BECOMING
(Achieving personal goals)

Practical becoming - domestic activities and paid work
- Doing things around my house
- Doing something creative/productive in my life

Leisure becoming - activities that promote relaxation and stress reduction
- Outdoor activities
- Indoor activities

Growth becoming
- Improving my health and physical fitness
- Being able to cope with changes in my life

Being, belonging and becoming are determined by both *importance* and *enjoyment*: what do I want in life? Do I have it? And does it make me happy?

The answers will be unique for each individual.

Control and opportunities are important for QoL: it's affected by the degree of control we have over our environment and what opportunities are available to us. A decent QoL should

1 Provide for basic needs

2 Provide for range of opportunities

3 Provide for control and choice of those opportunities

Of course, if someone is struggling with very basic needs such as health or housing at the first level, it may be overwhelming to ask them how they could make a change in their circumstances. But change is relative rather than absolute, and stress and unhappiness seem to be due not so much to life circumstances as to lack of control over them; this is the reason why in QoL surveys, inhabitants of prosperous countries do not in all cases report a better QoL than people in poorer countries (though prosperity s an important positive factor to QoL, as prosperity general equals the power to make changes.

Introduction and Quality of Life - References and reading

Calvert-Henderson Quality of Life indicators are at http://www.calvert-henderson.com

Collins E. Psychosocial Impact of the Lipodystrophy Syndrome in HIV Infection. AIDS Reader 10(9):546-551, 2000.

Duran S et al. Failure to maintain long-term adherence to highly active antiretroviral therapy: the role of lipodystrophy. AIDS 15(18), 2441-2444. 2001.

European Men's Health Forum. European HIV Quality of Life Review. Full Report, July 2005. Available from http://www.emhf.org/resource_images/HIVsurveyfinalresults.pdf

Horne R et al. Identifying the key beliefs influencing uptake and adherence to HAART: final results of a 12-month prospective, follow-up study. Eleventh BHIVA/BASHH Conference, Dublin, abstract 031, 2005.

Martin: For a very good overview of the relationship between stress and health, see Paul Martin: *The Sickening Mind: Brain, Behaviour, Immunity and Disease.* HarperCollins, 1997. ISBN 0 00 655022 3.

Mehta S et al. Potential factors affecting adherence with HIV therapy.AIDS 11(14), 1665-1670. 1997.

Peck, M Scott. *The Road Less Travelled.* First published 1978. Published by Arrow, 1990. ISBN 978-0099727408.

SF-36 - the SF-36 Questionnaire and literature can be found at www.sf-36.org

University of Toronto: The 2. 3. The adult QoL profile of the Quality of Life Research Unit can be seen at www.utoronto.ca/qol/profile/adultVersion.html

Vincent E at al. Impact of HAART-related side-effects on unsafe sexual behaviours in HIV-infected injecting drug users: 7-year follow-up. AIDS 18(9), 1321-1325. 2004.

WHOQOL-100 can be found at www.who.int/evidence/assessment-instruments/qol/documents/WHOQOL-100.pdf

WHOQOL-HIV can be found at www.who.int/mental_health/media/en/557.pdf

Mental illness

One problem with mental illness, then, is that in its milder forms it may be difficult to distinguish from normal reactions to life. Its definition and diagnosis is also notoriously subject to the influence of social and cultural norms: one reason advanced for the fact that black people and black men in particular are more likely to receive psychiatric diagnoses.

Broadly, however, mental illness is distinguishable from normal reactions to events because it is

- **Severe:** notably more severe in its subjective intensity and objective signs and symptoms than normal mental states

- **Persistent:** characterised by a quality of 'stuckness' and persistence: the person cannot 'snap out of it' and seems entangled in their condition

- **Disabling:** it prevents the person carrying out normal functions and in particular social functions: to some extent what lies at the core of most mental illness is a profound loss of the ability to relate to others.

To return to Sigmund Freud: he defined mental health as the abilities "to work and to love"; mental illness, then, implies a profound disability in a person's social and interpersonal roles and capacities.

The second problem with mental illness is that one is by definition talking about a condition that, until recently at least, did not display symptoms and physical changes that could be scientifically verified. There is no blood test for depression. If you hook up someone with dementia or epilepsy to a brain scanner or an EEG machine, atypical brain anatomy and electrical activity will be observed. But there is no equivalent set of diagnostic signs for something as clearly different from normal thought processes as active schizophrenia, let alone gradations in the severity of conditions most of us have had at some time, like depression.

This does not mean that subtle brain changes (in the activity of certain neurotransmitters, for instance) cannot be picked up; it means that there is not a gross pathology of the central nervous system process which has a clear cause, whether or not it is amenable to treatment.

There is also a philosophical dimension to the diagnosis of mental illness which is summed up in the saying that "if the human brain was simple enough to understand, we would be too simple to understand it". Mental ill-health affects not only our physical bodies but our social abilities and emotional being. This means that a pure 'medical model' where a physician - presumed not be affected or being part of the condition in question - diagnoses a condition and then applies expertise and treatments to effect a physical cure or relief.

Mental illness is both a physical condition in which very powerful changes can happen in the brain and body chemistry (as anyone who has had a panic attack or major depressive episode well knows), but is also a social illness; a disorder of the person's ability to relate to others. Loneliness is the strongest single predictor of mental illness: up to three-quarters of people with depression feel lonely, and vice versa. It is also strongly associated with physical ill-health (House), and, of relevance to the present chapter, with unprotected sex with casual partners in gay men (Martin)

Perhaps because of this two very different treatment modalities have arisen for mental illness:

- **psychopharmacology,** or the prescription of drugs to alter mind states

- **psychotherapy,** 'talking therapy' in which a cure is effected by discussing one's problems with a skilled practitioner. May be called counselling if of a short-term or less intensive nature.

These two modalities exist in uneasy relationship and it is not uncommon to encounter doctors who dismiss the effectiveness of psychotherapy for anything other than mild mental illness or psychotherapists who regard resorting to antidepressants as a defeat. In reality they are complementary; psychopharmacology deals with mental illness from the 'bottom up' by blunting or calming extreme emotions or mental states so that the person may begin to deal with their problems, while psychotherapy deals with the situation from the 'top down' by helping the individual to regain their lost sense of self-confidence and self-efficacy.

Different psychotherapies work in different ways according to how much stress they place on the patient-therapist relationship. For short-course therapies such as Cognitive-Behavioural Therapy (CBT), the therapist acts more like an instructor who prescribes different methods by which the patient can control negative thought patterns and behaviours. However for long-term and lifestyle problems where self-image may interfere with the patient's motivation to get better, more stress is played on using the therapeutic encounter as a 'model relationship' in which patients may experience attention and understanding they may have lacked and work out experientially how to alter maladaptive ways of being with others.

A meta-review (Gill 2005) of studies of the effectiveness of antidepressants found that patients given antidepressants were 63% more likely to recover from depression than patients given a placebo. However it also found that patients given a placebo were 3.45 times more likely to recover than patients given no treatment. This nicely quantifies the extent to which drugs can alter mental states above and beyond what the patient may be able to do for themselves in ideal situations where the belief that they can get better is itself the thing that cures.

Psychotherapy is sometimes criticised as being a treatment only those already motivated to change can benefit from, and furthermore that it is a 'western' or 'middle class' approach that depends on the ability to talk about mental experience in terms that are culturally similar to the therapist. In fact there is a huge evidence base as the effectiveness of psychotherapy in all sorts of settings. To give one example of relevance to this chapter (Bolton 2003), 341 men and women from 30 villages in rural Uganda diagnosed with major depression were randomised to receive group interpersonal therapy or no treatment. After 16 weekly sessions, the proportion of subjects meeting the criteria for major depressive disorder fell from 86 to 6% in the psychotherapy group as compared with a fall from 94 to 55% in the control group, or in other words psychotherapy worked 5-6 times better than doing nothing.

The investigators comment that they decided on group psychotherapy because they could not afford to prescribe antidepressants in the African context. This is ironic, as in the UK NHS-provided psychotherapy has long waiting lists and patients are more likely to be given a prescription for psychotherapeutic drugs and left to cope with issues than provided with what is seen as a costly and time-intensive resource.

Cost-effectiveness is a difficult thing to measure in a situation where outcomes are so subjective, both on the part of patient and therapist. However several studies (Browne, Burnand, Scott) have calculated that different kinds of psychotherapy for depression saved anything from £275 over two years to £4500 over doing nothing. Miller (2003) calculated that the depression-associated cost per patient of counselling for mild to moderate depression was £302 for counselling as against £342 for antidepressant prescription, which was statistically equivalent. However this is still an area where the evidence is weak, though qualitative surveys almost universally report that patients value therapy.

Diagnosis and categories

Because gross pathology is not usually present, diagnosis of mental health problems, except for organic impairment, has to rely on a skilled professional like a psychiatrist or psychologist (see **services** below) who forms an opinion of the patient's internal state of mind by means of an interaction or interview with the patient called the **mental state examination**. Like any doctor before the battery of lab tests that are now used became available, they will be looking out for unusual features in the person's quality of appearance, behaviour and relationship.

To be more precise, they are looking for unusual features in the person's:

- **Appearance and behaviour:** eg an unkempt appearance may indicate depression: unusual, bright clothes and makeup may indicate mania.

- **Rapport:** the degree to which the person is able to relate to the interviewer, and how this changes through the interview.

- **Speech:** whether it is slow, fast, easy, reluctant, comprehensible.

- **Mood:** elevated and euphoric, depressed, anxious, angry or irritable, labile (shifting rapidly), blunted (apparently emotionless), or incongruent (inappropriate to the situation).

- **Thought:** disorders of the stream of consciousness: sudden thoughts or blockages of thought which the person feels they have no control over: delusions: incoherency and unpredictability: repetitive and obsessive thoughts.

- **Cognition:** the general ability to form coherent thoughts and to comprehend.

- **Perception:** hallucinations, dizziness, distortions of time and space, 'out of body' feelings etc.

- **Insight:** self-awareness, including the awareness that something is wrong (if it is).

Reference is made to one of several diagnostic 'bibles' of psychology, of which the most often used is the Diagnostic and Statistical Manual (fourth edition) of the American Psychiatric Association.

This categorises mental illness and lists defining and distinguishing symptoms. Without attempting a comprehensive list, these are some of the more familiar and/or common conditions:

Adjustment disorder

Adjustment disorders are common and may happen to anyone. They are a period of mental turbulence the individual may go through after experiencing a sudden change or loss, such as bereavement, divorce, diagnosis with a serious illness (such as HIV), unemployment and so on. An adjustment disorder is diagnosed only if the person's reaction to the change interferes markedly with their ability to lead their normal life. People may react with anxiety, depression, avoidant behaviour (social isolation) or a mix of all three.

Anxiety disorders

In anxiety disorders the normal emotion of fear has run out of control and disrupts the person's life in some way. Anxiety disorders include agoraphobia and social phobia; the other specific phobias; stress disorder; panic attacks; and generalised anxiety disorder (a generalised state of jumpiness and fear about most situations). Anxiety has a large somatic component - as anyone who has had 'nerves' before an exam or presentation knows - and drug therapy often acts to calm down the physical symptoms of adrenaline overload such as pounding heart, cold sweats and hyperventilation so the person can function.

Two rather different and specific types of anxiety disorder are:

- **Obsessive-compulsive disorder.** In this the person finds themselves constantly 'having to' think or try not to think specific thoughts, or to perform specific actions. Compulsive handwashing or having to check that the gas is not left on many times are examples, but probably more disabling are the internal circling thoughts or 'ruminations' that people with OCD force themselves to think. Sufferers may have the conviction that they will do something terrible like murder someone or blurt out obscenities unless they perform specific actions or think specific things. OCD can be quite disabling. What looks like agoraphobia can sometimes be OCD, as the person is unable to leave the house because the rituals required to do so are too elaborate. The millionaire Howard Hughes was a famous sufferer from the condition. OCD is not a particular risk factor for HIV as OCD sufferers tend to be hyper-careful about sexual health, though there are case reports of OCD being set off by HIV diagnosis. However one way OCD very commonly presents is as fear of disease and, in particular fear of AIDS. Many of the 'worried well' who consistently plague helplines and agencies with unlikely scenarios for having caught HIV in fact have OCD.

- **Post-Traumatic Stress disorder.** A unique diagnosis in that there has to be a specific precipitating event before it can be called PTSD. This is a particular state of anxiety brought on by having participated in or witnessed a traumatic event such as a natural disaster, accident, war and so on. It is characterised by the 'Vietnam Vet' picture of hair-trigger nerves, nightmares and flashbacks to the traumatic event. May also be produced by prolonged and repeated traumas such as childhood abuse, in which case it is often more difficult to treat. Traumatic events unsurprisingly are very stressful and may cause post-traumatic stress (PTS) in themselves; for PTS to be considered a disorder the stressed behaviour has to persist more than six months after the event and/or be brought on later by additional stressors that reawaken memories of the event. The core cause of PTSD is **dissociation** (see below under **fight, flight or freeze**).

Cognitive disorders

These are organic, neurological damage to the ability to think; drug-induced amnesia, fever-induced delirium and dementia are examples.

Dissociative disorders

In these the person avoids specific events or the stress of life by mentally or even physically absenting themselves. They include depersonalisation, where nothing feels real to the person or they don't feel they are real (often part of a normal adjustment process such as grief or shock), fugue, where the person literally flees from their normal life, often with loss of memory, and dissociative identity disorder (DID), so-called 'multiple personality disorder', a rare but much-publicised condition in which the person compartmentalises their experience into different 'sub personalities' who may not be aware of each other's experiences.

Eating disorders

Bulimia and anorexia. Among the most difficult of common disorders to treat.

Factitious disorders

In these the person makes up a physical or mental illness in order to gain attention or contact, usually repeatedly. Although the actual illness complained of is not present, the pattern of behaviour may disrupt life enough to be a mental illness in itself. Sometimes called Munchausen's Syndrome when it applies to physical illnesses. Needless to say factitious disorders can be very difficult to distinguish from the real thing.

Impulsive disorders

An inability to control impulsive and often antisocial behaviour such as gambling addiction, kleptomania (compulsive stealing) or pyromania.

Mood disorders

The most common kind of mental illness, they may range in severity from mild depression ('the blues') to completely disabling mania or lifelong depression with **psychotic** (see below) delusions.

Divided into:

- **Bipolar affective disorder** ('manic depression') in which the person oscillates between mania (a heightened state of 'speediness' and euphoria which is distinguished from normal elevated mood by being socially maladaptive and out of touch with reality) to major depression.

- **Unipolar illness** in which the person relapses periodically from relative normality into sudden sharp periods of major depression.

- **Dysthymia** or minor depression. Has to last more than two years to be diagnosed. A general state of low mood, pessimism, and poor self esteem. Has been associated with sexual risk-taking; in one Australian study (Rogers) gay men with dysthymia were 2.36 times more likely than others to report unprotected sex with casual partners.

Major depressive disorder (MDD). This is distinguished from dysthymia by including more physical characteristics, and from unipolar depression by not being episodic. The person may feel and indeed be quite unable to get out of bed, care for themselves, etc, as well as suffering from crushing feelings of unworthiness, guilt and inadequacy. There is marked slowing of speech, concentration and memory without any obvious organic cause. Very high risk of suicide. Not associated with sexual risk because libido is also blunted.

Schizophrenia

About 1.1% of the world population has this condition. If there is a central characteristic of schizophrenia, it is **boundary loss**. A person with schizophrenia is unable to distinguish between their own thoughts and other people's. They may attribute their own thoughts to alien messages or perceive that slogans on advertising hoardings are intended specifically for them. They may experience a general inability to keep thoughts under control, with streams of thought sliding rapidly into each other, and may adopt incomprehensible (to the outsider) rituals to attempt to assert some control over disordered thought processes. This may or may not be accompanied by hallucinations and organised delusions.

Schizophrenia is an example of a mental illness that used to be thought of as caused purely by upbringing and psychological factors and is now thought to be largely genetic and physiological in origin, with subtle changes apparent in the brain, especially of long-term sufferers. Schizophrenics are rarely a danger to others (more often themselves) and the condition is treatable. Over a 30-year period, 25% of people who have had at least one episode completely recover, 35% will be much improved and relatively independent, 15% will be improved, but require extensive support, 10% will be hospitalised and unimproved and 15% will be dead (mostly from suicide). There is no evidence that people with HIV are more likely to have schizophrenia than average, but schizophrenics are more likely to have risk factors for HIV such as homelessness, survival sex and multiple partners, and 22% of men with schizophrenia in one survey (Cournos) had had sex with other men.

Sexual disorders

Divided into sexual dysfunction, sexual and gender identity disorders (transsexuality etc, or difficulty adjusting to it) and paraphilias or antisocial sexual behaviours such as exhibitionism, paedophilia, voyeurism, sexual sadism etc. Notoriously, homosexuality used to be included in this list until the APA removed it from DSM in 1973, ratifying this removal in 1975. However a person who is obsessed by fear of homosexuality or is deeply unhappy that they are gay may have a sexual identity disorder.

Somatoform disorders

Hypochondria or other preoccupation with illness, which may or may not actually produce physical symptoms. Differs from factitious illness in that the intention is not to deceive.

One very important point to note from DSM-IV is that as well as homosexuality, alcohol dependency and drug abuse are not in themselves seen as psychiatric disorders. Their use may indicate 'self-medication' for short-term crises or long-term personality disorders; people with narcissistic, antisocial or borderline disorders are particularly prone to addictions of this type. Equally, conditions ranging from schizophrenia (associated with cannabis and LSD), paranoia and anxiety (cocaine, methamphetamine and alcohol) depression (ecstasy and methamphetamine) and memory loss (alcohol) may be caused by prolonged drug use or even occasional use if the person is already unstable. However substance use in itself is not a diagnosis.

Another spectrum

Another way of classifying mental illness is to use a rather older classification which rates the disorder roughly in terms of the degree of control and insight the person has into their condition and its amenability to treatment. This breaks down mental and neurological conditions into four types.

Organic (neurological) disorders

Organic disorders are those in which there is a clear and physically testable pathological process going on in the brain. Examples include Alzheimer's disease, Parkinson's disease, Tourette's syndrome, epilepsy, stroke-associated brain injury, delirium and certain AIDS-defining illnesses such as toxoplasmosis and PML, not to mention HIV-associated dementia (see below). Depending on the part of the brain affected, the person may be quite 'sane' with their cognitive functions unaffected, as in Parkinson's disease, or may suffer complete loss of personality, as in Alzheimer's.

Certain conditions such as autism and schizophrenia used to be thought of as psychological in origin, but are now as likely to be seen as organic brain disorders (often made worse by the psychological and social impact of the illness).

Autism, for instance, may be related to a greater or lesser disturbance in development of a group of brain cells called 'mirror neurones'. In experiments on monkey, these were observed to fire when, and only when, another monkey was observed to do something. These neurones mirror the activity of a group of cells called 'canonical neurones' that fire when the person performs the task themselves. What this leads to is a condition in which the person, in a very profound way, lacks empathy. They do not have a 'theory of mind', which means an instinctive understanding that other people have minds similar to their own and may be presumed to be having the same thoughts and feelings when they do similar things. To an autistic person, therefore, all people are, to a greater or lesser degree, objects, and objects are not classified into things with more or less personal significance. This leads to symptoms such as fixations typical of autism, in which the person may obsess on particular repetitive activities in order to make sense of what is otherwise a meaningless (and painful) flux of experience (see Grèzes).

In the case of schizophrenia, research is still seeking a definitive cause. But what appears to happen is that genetic defects lead to a situation in which the neurotransmitters (messenger chemicals) dopamine and glutamate are synthesised in the wrong amounts - too much or too little - in different parts of the brain. Since neurotransmitters actually change brain architecture by creating and destroying synapses (the connections or 'routing switches' between cells), the result is a state in which the brain is wired up wrongly. Antipsychotic drugs effect a partial cure by changing dopamine levels in the brain, though in a global and unsubtle way (see Owen).

Psychoses

Psychoses are psychological disorders which are typical of what the lay person thinks of as 'madness'. The key characteristic is that the person has **lost insight** - they are no longer aware that their mind is functioning abnormally and will attribute symptoms and feelings to influences outside themselves or not think anything is wrong at all. In other words, they are delusory. Florid (unmedicated or uncontrolled) schizophrenia is still seen as a psychosis, but mood disorders such as bipolar illness and major depressive disorder become psychotic in nature when delusions are present. A manic person may believe themselves to be a great ruler or prophet, for instance, while a depressive may become convinced they have committed some dreadful crime and actually hand themselves into the police. Delusory elements may be present in other conditions such as hypochondria or anorexia (where the person is convinced they are fat despite being skeletal). Not all situations in which insight is lost are psychoses: total organic disorder, as in delirium, is not psychotic. A psychosis is something in which there is some structure of thought and cognition, but one which feels 'alien' and is at variance with reality. To quote the saying: "neurotics build castles in the air: psychotics live in them."

Neuroses

Neuroses form the overwhelming majority of mental ill-health. It is unfortunate that 'neurotic' has become a pejorative terms as it is still clinically useful.

A neurotic has not lost insight into their condition; on the contrary, they are only too aware, and sometimes exaggeratedly so, that there is something wrong with them. However they feel to a greater or lesser degree helpless to change this. They have not lost insight, but they have lost **self-efficacy**, a fundamental belief in their own mental balance and ability to deal with life.

In this there is hope, as people with neuroses are often highly motivated to change, though they may at the same time resist change.

Personality disorders

These form a category of mental illness or condition invented to cover the fact that there are a lot of people around who are not delusory, and do not generally feel that they are in an 'abnormal' state of mind, but whose lives seem to be shaped by significant defects in their ability to function socially. Personality disorder is something that is **global** - it is a way of being rather than a specific deficit or excess of some feeling or trait - and **enduring**, i.e. it is lifelong, or at least intractable to treatment.

Probably about 10% of the population has some degree of personality disorder, though this does not mean that they will all seek or need treatment.

DSM-IV defines personality disorder as "an enduring pattern of inner experience that deviates markedly from the expectations of the individual's culture.which is inflexible and pervasive across a broad range of personal and social situations." Essentially, people with personality disorders are misfits - and the causes are often thought to lie in inadequate parenting during childhood, or a 'misfit' between a child's needs and what their parents (and extended family and peers) were able to provide them. It organises personality disorders into three broad categories. We will look at a few of them in more depth.

Cluster A are the **paranoid, schizoid and schizotypal** disorders. People with these disorders may seem suspicious, cold or eccentric to others. They will tend not to relate easily to others because they are genuinely not very interested in socialising or because they are distrustful of others. They may be litigious or have odd beliefs.

Cluster B are the **antisocial, borderline, histrionic and narcissistic** disorders. These people may appear overly emotional, selfish, self-absorbed, dependent on or manipulative towards others. They appear driven by odd but very strong and inflexible emotional needs.

- **Antisocial personality disorder** is also known as psychopathy or sociopathy. The person essentially acts as if they have no conscience or regard for the feelings of others. It is estimated that 3% of men and 1% of women have a degree of antisocial disorder.

- **Narcissistic personality disorder** may appear on the outside like anti-social disorder, but unlike true sociopaths, the narcissist is driven by strong feelings of low-self worth which he (75% are male) dare not show to others. The person is someone who constantly shows off, has to be the centre of attention, and has a need to be praised and flattered; they will often be quite high achievers if work serves their purposes, but their personal relationships will tend to be shallow and brief as they cannot bear criticism. About 1% of the population may have this disorder.

- **Histrionic personality disorder** is typified by the 'drama queen'; the person depends on provoking strong emotional and usually sexual reactions in others (positive or negative). Traditionally more common in women, though this may be governed by social disapproval against sexually flamboyant women.

- **Borderline personality disorder** is typified by an alternately clinging and hostile style of relationship; the person desperately seeks love and approval but it is of such an all-or-nothing character that they inevitably become hostile and jealous. The Glenn Close character in 'Fatal Attraction' is often held up as an archetype of the borderline personality, though most people with this condition are more dangerous to themselves than others, as they are often prone to suicidality, self-harm and risk-taking behaviour, including substance and sexual addiction. The inner dilemma of the borderline person is that they feel empty or non-existent as a personality in their own right and are so both utterly dependent on others and yet hate that dependence. Borderline disorder is an increasingly common diagnosis, leading some psychologists to theorise about the role of weak family relationships and especially extended family in its cause. About 75% of those diagnosed are women, and there is a strong association with sexual or other abuse in childhood.

Cluster C are people whose lives seem governed by anxiety rather than suspicion (cluster A) or need (cluster B). They include **obsessive-compulsive disorder,** in which while not necessarily suffering from OCD to a disabling degree, the person is ruled by perfectionism and may be very 'stiff' and formal. People with **avoidant personality disorder** are governed by shyness and social inadequacy (as opposed to suspicion). Lastly, people with **dependent personality disorder** are afraid of being on their own and typically develop submissive or compliant behaviours in order to avoid displeasing people.

References - mental illness

Bolton P, Bass J, Neugebauer R, et al. Group interpersonal psychotherapy for depression in rural Uganda: a randomized controlled trial. JAMA 289: 3117-3124, 2003.

Browne G, Steiner M, Roberts J, et al. Sertraline and/or interpersonal psychotherapy for patients with dysthymic disorder in primary care: six month comparison with longitudinal two year follow-up of effectiveness and costs. J Affect Disord 68: 317-330, 2002.

Burnand Y, Andreoli A, Kolatte E, et al. Psychodynamic psychotherapy and clomipramine in the treatment of major depression. Psychiatr Serv 53: 585-590, 2002.

Cournos F. Sexual activity and risk of HIV infection among patients with schizophrenia. Am J Psychiatry 151: 228-232, 1994.

Diagnostic and Statistical Manual of Mental Disorders (DSM-IV). American Psychiatric Association, 2000. ISBN No. 0-89042-025-4.

Gill D. Antidepressants for depression in medical illness. Cochrane Rev Abstract. 2005. See http://www.cochrane.org/reviews/en/pk111999091612245715.html

Grèzes J. Activations related to "mirror" and "canonical" neurons in the human brain: an fMRI study. NeuroImage 18: 928-937, 2003.

House JS. Social relationships and health. Science 241(4865): 540-545, 1988.

Martin JI (http://www.ncbi.nlm.nih.gov/entrez/query.fcgi?db=pubmed&cmd=search&term=%22martin+ji%22%5bauthor%5d). Loneliness and sexual risk behavior in gay men. Psychol Rep. 81(3 Pt 1): 815-825. 1997.

Miller P, Chilvers C, Dewey M, et al. Counseling versus antidepressant therapy for the treatment of mild to moderate depression in primary care: economic analysis. Int J Technol Assess Health Care 19: 80-90. 2003.

Owen MJ. Schizophrenia: a genetic disorder of the synapse? BMJ. 330(7484): 158-159, 2005.

Rogers G. Depressive disorders and unprotected casual anal sex among Australian homosexually active men in primary care. HIV Medicine 4: 271-275, 2003.

Scott J, Palmer S, Paykel E, et al. Use of cognitive therapy for relapse prevention in chronic depression. Cost-effectiveness study. Br J Psychiatry 182: 221-227, 2003.

How common is mental illness in people with HIV?

Because diagnosis and definition is more subjective and interpersonal in mental than in physical illness, the estimates of the proportion of people with HIV vary according to how strictly disorders are defined. But nearly all surveys find higher rates of certain disorders than in the general population, particularly mood, substance abuse and anxiety disorders, as well as adjustment disorder after diagnosis or if treatment failure happens.

One 2002 study from the University of North Carolina, (Hooshyar) looked at 726 people with HIV and 215 co-infected with HIV and Hepatitis C receiving HIV primary care from the university's clinic, which serves a rural population. It found a 57.3% prevalence of depression among HIV-infected patients and a 69.8% prevalence of depression among patients co-infected with HIV and hepatitis C (HCV), compared with an estimated 5-10% in the general adult population of primary care patients.

Substance abuse, which affects an estimated 8.3% of the US population ages 12 and up, affected 28.8% of HIV-infected patients in the study, and 47.9% of HIV/HCV-infected patients.

The 2002 "What do you Need?" survey (Anderson) of 1,821 HIV-positive people in the UK found similar figures. Only a quarter of respondents were happy with their current quality of life across all needs. Forty per cent each complained of anxiety and/or depression and sexual problems. Thirty-three per cent reported sleep problems, 32% problems with self-confidence, 15% with relationships and 14% with drugs and alcohol, among other more social needs such as housing and childcare. Two-thirds related they had experienced at least one depressive episode over the past year.

The survey asked about three areas of need in 18 areas of people's lives:

3 areas of need:

1. Dissatisfaction with current state

2. Experience of problems in last twelve months

3. Whether they felt they needed more support

In detail, notable findings include:

In **housing:** 18% were currently unhappy: 21% had been in the last year: and 16% would like more support

In **eating:** 17% had current problems finding the right nutrition: 42% said they had at some point in the last year: 24% would like more support.

Sleeping patterns were a problem area - 32% currently had problems sleeping, 59% had experienced them over the last year, and 36% would like more help to get better sleep

Household chores - 18% felt unhappy about how to look after themselves

Mobility 15% felt unhappy about their ability to get around locally

Money: 28% felt unhappy about the money they were getting to live on: 31% had experienced problems in the previous 12 months: and 25% had ongoing problems getting enough money to live on and felt that further help or support would be useful

Drugs and alcohol: these were problematic to a lesser degree than might have been expected, with 9% unhappy about their ability to cope with drug or alcohol related problems, 14% with problems in the previous twelve months and 10% needing further help or support

Anxiety and depression on the other hand were widespread with 33% unhappy about their ability to cope with anxiety or depression, 67% with problems in the previous 12 months and 45% wanting further help or support. 19% felt they had not been given support when they had asked for it.

Friendship and **looking after children** were also problematic areas

Sex and relationships: sex was more problematic than relationships. 51% had a current relationship. 9% were unhappy about it, and 29% had experienced problems within a relationship in the previous 12 months: whereas 40% felt unhappy about their sex lives, 51% had experienced problems with sex in the previous 12 months, and 34% wanted further help.

Treatment and relationships with **health professionals** were the least problematic areas.

These are exceptionally high figures, even for HIV patients, and not all studies have shown such high rates. The US study did not control for depression caused by drug use as opposed to endogenous depression in this relatively poor and rural population, many of whom has intravenous drug use as their HIV acquisition factor. The UK survey was a social rather than psychiatric one and may have encouraged people to report general states of dissatisfaction rather than diagnosable mental ill-health.

Not all studies have found such high rates. A pre-HAART study of patients referred to the psychiatric liaison service at the Royal Free Hospital in London and compared 70 HIV patients with 70 from the general; population. It found that five times as many people in the HIV patient population were referred as in the hospital's general patient population. However it found that the prevalence of each group of psychiatric diagnoses was not significantly different between the HIV and control groups, except in the case of alcohol dependence, which was more common in the control group (21%) than the HIV group (4%), and drug use where, conversely, 44% of the HIV group and 30% of the control group fulfilled DSM criteria for a diagnosis of non-alcohol psychoactive substance abuse. A diagnosis of borderline personality disorder was made more often in the HIV group.

A study from San Diego (Chan) caught a positive change in people's mental health during the introduction of HAART. 2466 patients from the HIV Cost and Services Utilization Study were interviewed first in December 1996 and January 1997 and then again eight months later, after a number had started on HAART. It graded their severity of psychiatric disturbance on four scales rating major depression, dysthymia, generalised anxiety and panic tendencies. It did not find such high levels of alcohol and substance dependence as the North Carolina study, with 6% reporting heavy drinking and 11% substance abuse. And it found that the average number of psychiatric symptoms in patients declined by 20% during the eight-month follow-up period of the study.

Nonetheless it found that although the proportion of patients reporting any psychiatric problems declined by 10% during the study, it did so from 47% to 37% - indicating a prevalence of psychiatric disturbance of any kind of about double that in the general population, where one in six are estimated to suffer from at least one of the four conditions measured at any one time.

One particularly interesting study which teased out the contributions of age and drug taking to poor mental health among men with HIV was performed by the US Veteran's Administration (Justice 2004). It enrolled 1,803 patients, 1,047 of them with HIV and 756 without. Nearly all (97.65) were men, with 15 women apiece who were HIV-positive and negative. The majority (51.55%) were African American, with 10% more in the HIV-positive group. The HIV-positive group also had a lower level of educational attainment and were slightly younger.

They asked the patients' physicians to provide reports of mental health problems (major depression, dysthymia, generalised anxiety disorder and panic attacks) and drink and drug use using a standardised brief interview called the Composite International Diagnostic Interview (CIDI). They then took a select group of 28 HIV-positive and 22 HIV-negative patients from the larger group and subjected them to a battery of neurocognitive and psychiatric tests (NCP) and calibrated these against the results reported from their physicians.

This gave an interesting insight into the imprecision of mental health diagnoses. The psychometric tests gave very reliable results but were impractical to perform in most clinical settings, taking on average three hours and as much as six hours to perform. For depression the researchers found the CIDI interview

to have good negative predictive value - it agreed with the NCP diagnosis of *no* depression in 89% of those who did not have it. However although it was reasonably sensitive, correctly diagnosing depression in more than three-quarters of patients who according to the NCP tests had it, it was less specific, incorrectly diagnosing depression in more than a third of patients who according to the NCP test did not have it.

For heavy alcohol use the CIDI interviews were specific, misdiagnosing only 11% of patients as having drink problems when they in fact did not, it was poorly sensitive, missing fully two-thirds of those actually did.

For drug problems the results were similar with CIDI and NCP diagnoses of people who actually did have problem agreeing 90% of the time but missing 50% of those who did use recreational drugs.

And for organic cognitive impairment, the CIDI interviews picked up on memory problems very poorly with only a half of patients reporting problems who in fact had them, though they were better at diagnosing those who did not have problems.

In the NCP testing the sample sizes were too small for differences between HIV-positive and negative patients to reach statistical significance. However there was a trend for positive patients to have more current major depression (20% vs 7%, p=0.2).

By calibrating results from the larger group of patients it was found that although the raw data suggested that HIV-positive patients had higher rates both of mental problems and drink and drug use these statistics confounded each other. Positive patients did not have higher rates of mental problems independently of drink and drug use; it appeared that they had more mental problems *because* of drugs and alcohol and vice versa, not in so far as they had HIV. The statistical significance also disappeared when in multivariate analysis rates were corrected for ethnicity and educational attainment.

In multivariate analysis after weeding out these confounders it was found that HIV-positive patients in general were still found to have higher rates of drug use. However the most significant finding was that the reason positive patients had higher overall levels of mental poor health and drink and drug use was because, unlike the HIV-negative patients, these rates did not tail off with age.

Not unexpectedly, drink and drug abuse tends to tail off as people get older, Contrary to some popular stereotypes, so do rates of anxiety and depression. But they tailed off much *less* in the positive patients. For every ten years older, the positive patients were 30% more likely than negative patients of the same age to be currently depressed; 24% more likely to report lifetime depression; 18% more likely to be heavy drinkers; and 46% more likely to continue using recreational drugs. Only cognitive and memory performance, though it got poorer with age, got no poorer than it did in negative patients.

This study has one major limitation; although it controlled for ethnicity, it did not control for sexual orientation. Other studies have shown that gay men have higher rates of drink and drug use than the general population (Cochran 2004) and that whereas as heterosexual's drug using 'careers' tend to be over by their late 20s, gay men continue using drugs into middle age.

The question thus remains: were the researchers seeing a greater level of mental distress and drink and drug use in older patients because they had HIV - or because they were gay?

Is it HIV or sexuality?

Gay men (and lesbians) are known to have higher rates of depression, drinking and suicide than heterosexuals. One study (Cochran and Mays 2000) found that 19.3% of US gay men under 35 had at some point attempted suicide compared with 3.6% of exclusively heterosexual men (the 'exclusively' is important, as we will see in the next study).

Several studies indicate that gay men and lesbians are at greater risk for psychiatric morbidity than heterosexuals. Remafedi and colleagues found a higher risk for suicide attempts in lesbian, gay, and bisexual-identified youth, with 28.1% of young bisexual/homosexual boys, 20.5% of young bisexual/homosexual women, 14.5% of young heterosexual women, and 4.2% of young heterosexual men reporting suicide attempts.

The same pattern has been found among adults. Using data from the National Comorbidity Survey, Gilman and his associates found that people reporting same-sex sexual partners have consistently greater odds of experiencing psychiatric and suicidal symptoms compared with their heterosexual counterparts. Among men reporting same-sex sexual partners, the odds of experiencing an anxiety disorder were 1.3 times higher, the odds of experiencing a mood disorder were 1.7 times higher, and the odds of experiencing a substance abuse disorder were 1.5 times higher than odds for their heterosexual counterparts. Among women reporting same-sex sexual partners, the odds of experiencing an anxiety disorder were 1.8 times higher, the odds of experiencing a mood disorder were 2 times higher, and the odds of experiencing a substance abuse disorder were 2.4 times higher than odds for their heterosexual counterparts.

Participants also had higher odds of reporting suicide symptoms. Among men reporting same-sex sexual partners, the odds of having thought about suicide in their lifetimes were 2.2 times higher, the odds of having made a plan for committing suicide were 1.6 times higher, and the odds of having attempted suicide were 2.4 times higher than odds for their heterosexual counterparts. Among women reporting same-sex sexual partners, the odds of having thought about suicide in their lifetimes were 2 times higher; the odds of having made a plan for committing suicide were 2.6 times higher; and the odds of having attempted suicide were 1.5 times higher than odds for their heterosexual counterparts.

However, research on this population and the prevalence of psychiatric conditions is in its early phases, and some studies have found similar rates of psychiatric hospitalizations, and even somewhat lower rates of psychotic disorders among LGBT people compared with the general population (Hellman). Some LGBT people may have greater resilience because of the stresses and challenges that they experience. Although these possibilities are certainly worthy of further study, pursuing them is beyond the scope of this article.

One fascinating study (Paul) of suicide in gay men (which has been strongly linked to both depression and alcohol use) not only found much higher rates of suicidal thoughts and attempted suicide in gay men but also suggested some psychosocial reasons, rooted in society's views of homosexuality, why they might feel suicidal.

The study was part of the Urban Men's Health Study, a household probability-based sample of MSM (defined as either having had sex with a male since age 14 or self-identifying as gay or bisexual) in 4 US cities (Chicago, Los Angeles, San Francisco and New York).

It used demographics to identify areas with larger gay populations and then used random-digit dialing, weighted more towards areas with higher gay populations but not excluding areas with low ones, to call up gay male households. 2,881 men were interviewed using this sampling method, which while it may still exclude 'closeted' gay men who do not wish to identify as such to a researcher, at list avoids the pitfall of sampling only gay men who use the commercial gay scene or the internet, as many other studies do.

It found very high levels for both having at some point thought about suicide and having actually attempted it. Twenty-one per cent of the men interviewed had at some point made plans to kill themselves. This contrasts with figures of 8.87% and 14.66% derived from two studies of the general male population (the National Institute of Mental Health Epidemiologic Catchment Area study and the National Comorbidity Survey, both reported in Weissman).

There was an even bigger difference in actual suicide attempts. Twelve per cent of the men interviewed had attempted suicide at some point, of whom 45% (5.4% of the whole sample) had attempted it more than once. This compares with rates of 1.52%

and 3.19% in the two studies quoted by Weissman. Two-thirds of suicide attempts (8.3%) had taken place before the person's 25th birthday - this question was asked because suicide rates are higher among male teenagers than men in general.

HIV-positive gay men had somewhat higher suicide rates than HIV-negative men; 29% had had suicidal thoughts and 16% had attempted suicide (five to ten times the rate of men in general). However the rate of attempts before 25 was not higher, which may confirm that the higher rates among men with HIV were caused by the knowledge of and problems attendant on HIV rather than HIV infection being caused by suicidality/depression.

Men who identified as bisexual also had higher rates - 30% had planned suicide, 16% attempted it and 11% had attempted it before they were 25, possibly indicating higher rates of sexual confusion.

However the most fascinating (and discouraging) finding of the study was that suicide rates in gay men had increased in the last 25-30 years and that this increase was almost exclusively among gay youth. Those who had been 25 or under in 1971 (i.e. at least 44 by the time the survey was done, in 1998) were 33% less likely to have attempted suicide at some point than men who were 25 in the 1970s; 42% less likely than those who were 25 in the 1980s; and 69% less likely than those who had been 25 in 1991 or later or were under 25 now. When it looked specifically at suicide attempt when the respondent was under 25, an even stronger relationship with current youth was found.

"This evidence seems to run counter to expectations regarding the effect of an emergent gay culture and the prospect of earlier self-identification as gay or bisexual," say the researchers.

"Identifying as gay, lesbian, or bisexual at an earlier age simultaneously places youths at risk of victimisation while potentially cutting them off from social supports available to 'mainstream' adolescents and young adults (their communities or families). Other studies show that the risk of suicide is greatest at the developmental point when youths come to identify as gay or bisexual but have not yet told anyone. Similarly, it was recently reported that if one controls for stress, social support, and coping resources, no differences are found between gay, lesbian, and bisexual youths and heterosexual youths in terms of current suicidality. The increased suicidal risk in this age range appears to be not simply a mental health concern but rather a broader issue of the effect of societal discrimination and harassment."

So some of the lifetime history of depression and suicidality in gay men may come from being a troubled gay teenager. However when it comes specifically to HIV, older gay men with HIV show higher rates of depression and other mental health problems than HIV-negative men. One study of patients aged over 54 (not just gay men) attending St Mary's Hospital HIV Clinic and referred to the Imperial College psychiatry service found that the older adults were more socially isolated, had more employment worries and more sexual problems (primarily sexual dysfunction).

Africans with HIV and mental health

However we have to be careful not to make the assumption that higher rates of mental ill-health reported in gay men with HIV actually correlate with a higher real prevalence. Because mental ill-health is subjective, it is also dependent on cultural assumptions and taboos about mental distress and talking to strangers about it, and also about professionals' assumptions about presentation.

A study from West Middlesex Hospital (Malanda) found that sub-Saharan African patients with HIV were almost three times less likely to be referred for specialist mental health care than other patients. A case control investigation of those referred to mental health services showed that those Africans who were referred were more likely to be referred for assessment of possible organic brain disease, and more likely to be found to be suffering from major depression or organic brain disease. In other words, only the most gross and obvious levels of dysfunction resulted in referral.

The researchers considered reasons for the lesser likelihood of referral to the mental health service, including the possible failure of staff to recognise psychological morbidity in Black Africans, or reluctance and fear on the part of patients to be referred to services that may be perceived as threatening.

A 2003 study of African living with HIV in the UK (Project Nasah - Weatherburn) is an interesting contrast with the *What Do You Need?* survey. Also conducted by Sigma Research, it investigated the needs of Africans with HIV living in the UK. This used a similar question structure and methodology. Some areas of dissatisfaction and need were considerably higher than for the HIV-positive population in general.

Getting enough money was ten times more likely to be a problem for positive Africans than for people with HIV in general; housing seven times more likely; discrimination three times more likely; and relationships and mobility twice as likely. Eight times as many Africans complained of feeling unhappy about their knowledge of treatments.

Project Nasah was designed to look at the treatment information needs of the community. Ironically it found that treatment information was the one need they felt was provided for best, with it coming second to the bottom of a list of suggested issues that had caused problems in the previous twelve months - only 27% felt they had problems accessing treatment information. In contrast the top seven concerns were mentioned by over half of all respondents. They were money worries, depression and anxiety, sleeping problems, self-confidence, immigration status, housing problems and relationships. Four of these may be fairly said to be mental health problems or at least ones to do with happiness and quality of life - depression and anxiety were mentioned by 71% as a problem, sleeping by 57%, self-confidence by 56% and relationship problems by 51%.

Here is a summary of the percentage of Africans with HIV who stated that they had problems with other specific needs:

- Skills, training & job opportunities
  48%

- household chores & self care
  42%

- Mobility
  41%

- Sex
  40%

- Discrimination
  38%

- Looking after children (those with children)
  38%

- Eating & drinking
  37%

- Taking treatments (those on treatments)
  37%

- Friendships
  35%

- Dealing with health professionals
  28%

- Knowledge of HIV treatments
  27%

- Drugs & alcohol
  7%

Of these, three (depression and anxiety, sleeping problems and self-confidence) were mentioned as often by Africans as by a representative sample of HIV-positive white people, while Africans mentioned relationships as a problem twice as much. In contrast some other areas like money - and also HIV treatment information - were very much more likely to be mentioned as problems by Africans (only 4% of the white HIV-positive people mentioned treatment info as a need compared with 68% who reported depression). This may say something about the 'medicalisation' of people with HIV and the fact that other needs may be neglected.

Anti-HIV therapy and mental health

The question of efavirenz

Efavirenz (*Sustiva*) has been particularly suspected of causing long-term depression and sleep disturbance in a minority of people taking it that persists beyond the well-documented central nervous system (CNS) side-effects commonly seen in the first month on therapy. Some studies, such as one in Australia (Kelly), found that up to 40% of patients on the drug continued to report CNS side-effects during long-term follow-up, and that these persisted beyond 18 months in 16% of patients.

Allin and colleagues from King's College Hospital in London reported on a small group of six patients who had been referred over a two-year period from a single London hospital with acute severe psychiatric symptoms including suicidal ideation out of a total of 200 patients who had started medication with efavirenz. Suicide was out of proportion to the depressed mood and inner feelings of tension that were also reported and was attempted in two cases, with homicidal ideation additionally present in one of the six. All symptoms resolved when efavirenz was withdrawn. Four of the six patients had a prior psychiatric history but two did not.

Other studies however, (e.g. Blanch) have found that CNS side-effects fade away to below the level of statistical significance in all but a small minority of patients. If you are virologically suppressed on efavirenz but suspect that it may be causing symptoms like depression, anxiety, bad dreams or sleep disturbance, it may be possible to switch to either nevirapine or PI-based therapy. Many HIV physicians avoid giving efavirenz to people with histories of psychiatric illness.

The stigma of lipodystrophy

One of the ironies of HAART was that as soon as combination therapy became really effective, it started producing facial and bodily fat redistribution and shape changes that made some people look sicker or more distinctive than they ever had before.

The first paper to examine the psychological effects of lipodystrophy was written in 2000 (Collins). Qualitative data were collected from 33 individuals, including 14 heterosexual women and 19 gay men. Average age was 39 years, with a range of 29 to 56 years.

Body image was generally poor, with some respondents describing themselves as "grotesque," "deformed," or "damaged goods." Responses included: "I've basically decided that I will be unattractive to a potential partner. I find myself concentrating on the outside and choosing to overlook what might be attractive on the inside."

Self-esteem was also affected, with individuals describing feeling "unloved and unlovable." One said: "Like all gay men, I relied (perhaps too heavily) on physical attractiveness to define me and bolster my self-esteem."

Many claimed that they had been able previously to cope with HIV and still feel good about themselves but that now, with the body changes, coping has become increasingly difficult.

Effects on social relations related mainly to social withdrawal. Responses here included: "I don't really go out in public much anymore unless it is to the market, or occasionally to the movies -- in the dark. Strangers stare. Children point." "I feel I should go to the gym to do something about this, but I am too embarrassed to be seen in my gym clothes."

Sexual relations were frequently affected by the general feeling of unattractiveness. One person described his body changes as being "cruise suicide." Another said: "I feel self-conscious in public, sexually unattractive, so don't try to stimulate an already reduced libido." From a woman whose husband is negative and who gained 22.5kg (50 lb) within months of starting HAART: "He now refuses to have sex with me... only as my body changed has the HIV become an issue in our love lives. Now, he is afraid of catching HIV. Perhaps he was in denial before."

There were other issues related to current relationships. A number of respondents said they were afraid their partners no longer found them attractive. One said: "My lover left me because, as he has no lipodystrophy and no viral load, my face was a constant reminder of the HIV he allowed himself to ignore."

Disclosure issues were a common theme, with comments including: "People in my community can tell I am HIV-positive from just looking at my face. It is like the old KS [Kaposi sarcoma] lesion on the nose." "It is no secret what this face means. I have been open about my [HIV] status, but I prefer to announce it myself. Not have it plastered across my face." "All my students and co-workers started to tell me 'how skinny I was.' In my thoughts, this meant 'how sick you are.'"

After an article was published in a local newspaper describing lipodystrophy, one man said it had likely "outed" him to his family after he had been able to hide his HIV from them for 15 years. While forced disclosure relates to a loss of control, other experiences threaten locus of control. Examples were "I feel my body changes are out of my control, and it is concurrent with feeling my life is out of control." "There seems so little I can do to prevent this or correct it. All my doctor tells me is to work out and is not even sure that can help."

Feelings of helplessness and of loss of control can lead to depression. Depression and demoralization were frequently expressed themes in the sample: "I feel constantly dejected." "I have thought about killing myself seriously. I guess what keeps me going is the hope of T20 [a new antiretroviral drug being developed]." "I used to be able to stay quite positive about the inconveniences, feeling that it was worth it to still be alive. Now, I am finding it hard to keep that attitude - I'm feeling really sick and tired of dealing with AIDS and sometimes wonder if it is worth it anymore. I used to keep up with all the research and developments, and now I just cannot muster the oomph to do it. How much this bad attitude re AIDS is connected to the poor body image and resulting poorer self-esteem I cannot say. I can say they are happening at the same time."

Not surprisingly, given this treatment-associated burden, when treatments were developed that ameliorated the appearance of lipodystrophy they were welcomed by patients and improved their mental health.

In one study (Moyle) 30 patients were randomised to two arms for immediate or deferred treatment with polylactic acid (New-Fill) to correct the appearance of facial wasting. Patients provided self-assessment of appearance on a visual analogue (VA) scale and a Hospital Anxiety and Depression assessment (HAD).

Patient VA assessments, anxiety and depression scores improved with treatment. At week 12, immediately-treated patients had significantly better VA scores (7 vs. 1, p<0.001) and 33% less anxiety (6 vs. 9 p=0.056) than Del patients. Benefits on VA and anxiety scores persisted through week 24. Depression scores fell in both groups by week 24, by two-thirds in the immediately treated group and by a half in the delayed treatment group.

References: frequency of mental illness

Allin M et al. Frequency of serious psychiatric adverse events with efavirenz. *Antiviral Therapy* 8:L85. 2003

Anderson WJ (http://www.ncbi.nlm.nih.gov/entrez/query.fcgi?db=pubmed&cmd=search&term=%22anderson+wj%22%5bauthor%5d), Weatherburn P (http://www.ncbi.nlm.nih.gov/entrez/query.fcgi?db=pubmed&cmd=search&term=%22weatherburn+p%22%5bauthor%5d). The needs of people with HIV in the UK: findings from a national survey. Int J STD AIDS 15(12): 793-796, 2004. "What do you Need?" survey can be downloaded from http://www.sigmaresearch.org

Blanch J et al. Preliminary data of a prospective study on neuropsychiatric side-effects after initiation of efavirenz. Journal of Acquired Immune Deficiency Syndromes 27(4): 336-343, 2001.

Cochran SD, Mays VM. Lifetime prevalence of suicide symptoms and affective disorders among men reporting same-sex sexual partners: results from NHANES III. Am J Public Health. 90: 573-578, 2000.

Cochran SD (http://www.ncbi.nlm.nih.gov/entrez/query.fcgi?db=pubmed&cmd=search&term=%22cochran+sd%22%5bauthor%5d) et al. Prevalence of non-medical drug use and dependence among homosexually active men and women in the US population. Addiction 99(8): 989-998, 2004.

Collins E. Psychosocial Impact of the Lipodystrophy Syndrome in HIV Infection. AIDS Reader 10(9): 546-551, 2000

Gilman SE, Cochran SD, Mays VM, et al. Risk of psychiatric disorders among individuals reporting same-gender sexual partners in the National Comorbidity Survey. Am J Pub Health. 91:933-939. 2001.

Hellman RE, Sudderth L, Avery AM. Major mental illness in a sexual minority psychiatric sample. J Gay Lesbian Med Assoc. 2004;6:95-104.

Hooshyar D. Depression High Among HIV-Positive Patients: Rates Are More than Five Times Greater. AIDS Alert 19(3): 34, 2004.

Justice AC et al. Psychiatric and neurocognitive disorders among HIV-positive and negative veterans in care: Veterans Aging Cohort Five-Site Study. AIDS 18: S49-S59, 2004.

Kelly M et al. Long-term follow-up of efavirenz usage in patients with HIV disease. 12th Annual Conference of the Australasian Society for HIV Medicine, Melbourne, abstract 88, 2000.

Malanda S. Are we meeting the psychological needs of Black African HIV-positive individuals in London? Controlled study of referrals to a psychological medicine unit. AIDS Care 13(4): 413-419. 2001.

Moyle G. Polylactate (NewFill) Injections Subjectively and Objectively Improve Appearance and Reduce Anxiety and Depression Scores in HIV-positive Persons with Facial Lipoatrophy: A Randomised, Open Label, Immediate vs. Delayed Therapy Study. 42nd ICAAC Conference, San Diego, abstract H-1934, September 27-30, 2002.

Paul JP et al. Suicide Attempts among Gay and Bisexual Men: Lifetime Prevalence and Antecedents. American Journal of Public Health 92(8), 2002.

Remafedi G, French S, Story M, Resnick MD, Blum R. The relationship between suicide risk and sexual orientation: Results of a population-based study. Am J Pub Health. 88:57-60. 1998.

Weatherburn P et al. Project Nasah: An investigation into the HIV treatment information and other needs of African people with HIV resident in England. Sigma Research, February 2003. Can be downloaded from http://www.nat.org.uk/documents/final.nasah.pdf

Weissman MM, Bland RC, Canino GJ, et al. Prevalence of suicide ideation and suicide attempts in nine countries. Psychol Med. 29: 9-17, 1999.

Resource

The Lesbian, Gay, Bisexual and Transgender Mental Health e-Network

A useful database and collection of research and policy material on LGBT mental health in the UK. You need to register by going to http://kc.csip.org.uk/ and then clicking on the following link: http://kc.csip.org.uk/groups.php?grp=134

Mental health and neurological disorders in more detail

Dementia and brain impairment

Dementia can be a frightening subject. Other mental health problems are at least seen as things people 'grow out of' or which can be cured by the right mix of appropriate medication, a sympathetic therapist and improvements in quality of life. We can imagine coping with many of the ills HIV might throw at us, but not if it robs us of the very thing that does the coping - our sense of self.

So when an Aidsmap headline in February 2005 declared: "Over-50s at increased risk of cognitive impairment, even with

HAART" (referencing Valcour, Becker and Cherner), many people were concerned.

These studies appeared in a special supplement in the journal *AIDS*, which documented recent research aimed at finding if there was an increase in dementia and/or mental illness among people over 50 with HIV. Most alarming was a study that found that more than one in five HIV-positive people over 50 had dementia, and that HIV-positive people in general were three times more likely to experience cognitive impairment than the general population.

This is particularly worrying as the HIV-positive population is aging: an estimated 11% of people with HIV in both the US and the UK are already over 50 years old and this proportion will only increase as people live longer on HAART.

The first associations between AIDS and brain disease were made back in 1986, when two New York neurologists (Navia) unveiled alarming findings in the *Annals of Neurology*. They concluded that up to a third of their patients with AIDS had a specific group of deficits in cognitive (thinking) and motor (movement) skills - disabilities they named AIDS Dementia Complex (ADC).

This was followed a year later by a report in the *Annals of Internal Medicine* (Grant), which found neuropsychological deficits in many people with asymptomatic HIV disease. These deficits took characteristic forms, such as poor concentration, poor memory and loss of fine motor co-ordination.

However, the findings of these early studies were criticised at the time by others working in the field, including Dr Pepe Catalan, Consultant Psychiatrist at London's Chelsea & Westminster Hospital, whose own studies suggested that although HIV might have subtle mental effects, frank dementia was quite rare.

Catalan comments: "The original *Annals of Neurology* paper was based on autopsies of people who had died, and weren't necessarily representative of all people with AIDS. They were patients who had been specifically referred for neurological observation. In addition, what they called AIDS Dementia Complex was a loose diagnosis."

In a 1993 paper, Catalan wrote: "It is clear that the original description included more than dementia in the usual sense of the word, and that patients who had a variety of neurological and, possibly, psychiatric disorders were grouped together under a novel label."

Catalan and colleagues found that the pre-1996 prevalence of classical dementia in people with AIDS was no more than 7% in the last year of their life. A new category of Minor Cognitive Impairment (MCI) or Minor Cognitive-Motor Disorder (MCMD) was instead devised. This not uncommonly seen in HIV, presents characteristically as a mix of mild difficulties with concentration and memory, often accompanied by slight motor impairment - difficulty in making fine movements such as those required for handwriting or delicate repairs. "This is like a slightly advanced aging. You behave as if you're ten years older than you are," Catalan comments.

When HAART came along, AIDS-related dementia became a rarity. Catalan told *AIDS Treatment Update* that he - the chief psychiatrist at the UK's largest HIV mental health unit - had only seen two or three cases in 2002-5, in people diagnosed very late or who had not started HAART till very late. He said he had also seen cases of people improved physically on HAART, but whose brain impairment had not improved and turned out to be caused by something else - in some cases, alcohol abuse.

Catalan did do a case notes study in 1998 of people over 50 referred to the psychological medicine service from the Chelsea & Westminster HIV clinic, and found some form of neurological impairment to be more common in people with HIV over 50 compared with younger people - the rates were 13% and 4%, respectively. However these were people taken from the one-third of HIV patients who were referred to the mental health unit because they had some sort of psychological complaint in the

first place. He told *ATU* he had not seen rates of impairment as high as those found in the studies in *AIDS*.

In one of those studies, Becker and colleagues recruited 289 HIV-positive and 124 HIV-negative people into a study that subjected them to a battery of psychological tests designed to see how well they performed at specific tasks. The basic findings certainly sound alarming. The HIV-positive individuals were three times more likely to be impaired either by dementia or by a milder degree of impairment that Becker termed 'CIND' - Cognitively Impaired, No Dementia.

Among the HIV-positive group, only 69% fitted the definition of having 'normal' functioning compared with 89% of the HIV-negative group. Across all ages, 22% of HIV-positive individuals were found to have CIND and 9% had dementia. And no fewer than 22% of the HIV-positive over-50s had dementia, compared with none of the HIV-negative over-50s.

However, when one looks into Becker's results more deeply, they are not quite what they seem. When the same tests were performed again a year later, the results were actually better. Of the original 289 HIV-positive people, 169 (58%) returned for more testing, as did 83 of the 124 HIV-negative people (67%) returned- the rest were lost to follow-up. This time the rates of CIND and dementia in the HIV-positive people were 'only' 15% and 4.7% respectively.

Additionally, Becker defined both CIND and dementia very broadly. To have dementia, a person was only required to have quite low scores on two or more individual tests, which did not have to include memory-specific tests. To have CIND, a person needed only to have quite low scores in just one test area. For example, you could be fine at doing everything else but, say, be bad at naming animals starting with 's' - which is a standard verbal fluency test. Forty per cent of the people in Becker's study did not even notice they were impaired.

Catalan comments: "I can tell you that when patients start developing dementia, they definitely notice and are frustrated by their impairments. Again, a very loose definition of 'dementia' is being used."

Another concern is that Becker's sub-category of people over 50 was really very small. Only 22 HIV-positive people were over 50 and a scant three people were HIV-negative. With groups this small, it is highly likely that some of the results could be due to chance.

Most importantly, however, only 17% of Becker's HIV-positive participants were on HAART, so this study does not measure dementia in a population where the majority are on HAART, as is the case with people with HIV in the UK. Becker's study does however suggest that there may be increased incidence of cognitive impairment in the over-50s, possibly of a mild to moderate nature.

In another study in *AIDS*, Igor Grant, one of the original researchers into AIDS Dementia Complex and colleagues (Cherner) compared neuro-psychological abilities in 67 HIV-positive individuals aged at least 50 with those in 52 HIV-positive people aged 35 or less. He found that 64% of the over-50s had at least one deficit in one of seven cognitive or motor 'domains', compared with 54% of those under 35. Grant specifically excluded individuals who were current alcohol or substance abusers. However, the numbers in his study were so small that the differences between the over-50s and the under-35s did not achieve statistical significance.

Additionally, the study participants had quite advanced HIV infection: 69% of those under 35 had an AIDS diagnosis, as did 76% of the over-50s. Despite this, only 55% were on HAART, and, of these, 51% of the older group and 28% of the younger group had undetectable viral loads.

The third study was the study of veterans already quoted above (Justice) as showing that rates of depression and substance abuse do not decline with age in HIV-positive people.

In the Justice study people with HIV had a higher rate of memory problems than those who were HIV-negative, by between six and 14 percentage points according to age group. When people with depressive symptoms were excluded, the HIV-positive people had a higher rate of memory problems in their 60s than HIV-negative people did in their 70s.

But the 'big story' of this study was of the psychological factors that were not specifically to do with organic neurological impairment. Contrary to popular wisdom, it has been found that older people tend to have lower rates of depression than younger people. However, depression rates in the older HIV-positive people stayed quite high compared with similarly aged HIV-negative people. So did rates of drug abuse, with, for instance, 24% of HIV-positive people in their 60s reporting recreational drug use compared with 10% of HIV-negative people. This may, however, include phenomena such as 'medical marijuana' use for symptom control.

Pepe Catalan comments: "They didn't match the HIV-positive people with HIV-negative people who had other chronic medical conditions, like cancer or renal impairment. Essentially they were comparing healthy old people with less healthy ones. Nor were they controlling for risk factors like being gay, so we may just be seeing that older gay people are less happy than older heterosexuals."

Another study (Valcour) that specifically looked at dementia and organic cognitive impairment was of a group called the 'Hawaii Aging with HIV Cohort'. This was a prospective study of a group of older people specifically followed to see what problems they developed with age. Hawaii is a good location for a study like this, since 20% of the HIV-positive people in this state are over 50.

It found that whereas 88% of HIV-positive people aged 20-40 had normal or near-normal neuro-cognitive functioning, only 58% of those over 50 did. This looks like a conclusive result. However, Pepe Catalan stresses that this study did not use the very specific psychological tests used by the other studies, but only a doctor-evaluated estimation of how well a patient is coping, called the *Memorial Sloan Kettering Scale*. He says: "It's a very inaccurate measurement of functioning. It doesn't even require the doctor to ask the patient how they are, so it can be easily distorted by physician bias."

The final study (Ernst) in *AIDS* looked at organic brain impairment performed brain scans on people with HIV to see what changes were happening in the brain. It found that HIV infection was causing damage to cells in a part of the lower brain called the basal ganglia, and that this increased with length of infection. There was also less serious damage seen in higher cortical areas, which did not increase with length of infection.

Whereas the cortex controls higher functions like thinking, the basal ganglia control impulses towards movement. This is the same area that is damaged in Parkinson's disease, which may explain why a degree of mild motor impairment is the most common neurological symptom seen in people with AIDS. However, this study specifically excluded people on HAART - so what it really measures is the damage resulting from untreated HIV infection.

The *AIDS* studies do seem to show that as we get older we may expect to develop minor - and in a few cases major - motor, cognitive and memory problems sooner than HIV-negative people our age.

More on the causation of dementia

Three studies since the ones above were published in *AIDS* took a more precise look at exactly what is happening in the brains of HIV-positive people.

A genetic analysis of HIV taken from the brain of a patient who died with severe HIV-associated dementia (Salemi) has shown that dementia may be caused by rapid evolution of HIV in certain brain regions, leading to a cycle of infection of macrophages and inflammation.

HIV is known to enter the brain soon after infection and to spread through the brain by infecting macrophages, a type of white blood cell. To gain a better understanding of how HIV behaves in the brain, investigators extracted virus from various regions of the brain of a patient who had died with severe HIV-associated dementia. By comparing the genetic sequences in the virus particles in the different areas of the brain, they found evidence that HIV moved around the brain in distinct paths, and that it evolved at different rates depending on where it was in the brain.

The investigators found that migration of HIV occurred most commonly from the meninges - the membrane surrounding the brain - to the temporal lobes, as well as to other areas of the brain and spinal cord. The temporal lobes are a vital part of the system that encodes memory, particularly memories of auditory sensations such as speech, people's names and music.

They also found evidence that HIV in the meninges and temporal lobes evolved more rapidly than elsewhere. In the meninges, the patient's HIV had evolved 30 times more rapidly than other areas, while HIV in the temporal lobes had evolved 100 times more quickly. While the meninges are probably the site of initial brain infection with HIV, the temporal lobes are one area where damage to brain cells causes the symptoms of dementia.

The researchers found evidence that the regions of the virus's genetic material that enabled it to infect macrophages were expanded in the brain. They argue that these new HIV variants would normally be cleared by the immune system.

However, once HIV has damaged the immune system, the new HIV variants are no longer removed from the brain and they can go on to infect and activate macrophages. These then activate further macrophages, as well as release HIV particles, resulting in a large increase in the number of activated macrophages in the brain. These activated cells are responsible for the inflammation and brain cell damage that is thought to underlie dementia.

As this study only analysed HIV from one patient, these findings must be interpreted cautiously. However, they seem to confirm previous theories on how HIV-associated dementia develops and form a model that can be tested in future investigations.

Another study (Rempel) found another possible culprit for the brain damage caused by HIV - the viral toxin HIV produces called the tat protein. Tat is short for transactivator, and the viral protein's normal job as an upregulator of genes; it speeds up the molecular assembly line that produces new HIV viruses within an infected cell. HIV viruses lacking the tat gene are almost non-pathogenic.

HIV-infected cells continue to produce tat even when HIV treatment ensures they cannot produce whole viruses, and it circulates freely in the system.

Rempel and his team found that tat inhibits the action of an enzyme called neprilysin. This chemical has the vital job of getting rid of a protein called amyloid-beta. This is a kind of waste product that accumulates naturally in the brain unless it is cleared away. It obstructs signals flowing between nerves, and accumulations of it are the main cause of Alzheimer's disease. Biopsies of Alzheimer's sufferers' brains show them invaded by gritty "plaques" of amyloid-beta.

Rempel found that a very specific short length of the tat protein was responsible for inhibiting the action of neprilysin. This is potentially good news, as it may make it easier to develop an anti-tat pill. He also found that even youngish people with HIV who took treatment had some amyloid-beta in their brains. He took biopsies from 14 HIV-positive people who had died, six of whom had been diagnosed with AIDS dementia and whose average age was 44. He found accumulations of amyloid-beta in the brain of every patient. This was not in the hardened plaques seen in Alzheimer's sufferers, but in more diffuse clumps that would not cause dementia in themselves.

In *in vitro* experiments, the investigators observed that HIV-1 Tat inhibited neprilysin activity by 80%. Adding recombinant Tat directly to brain cultures resulted in a 125% increase in soluble amyloid beta levels.

"Surprisingly, said one of the investigators, "people who had been infected the longest had the most amyloid beta so there was not a correlation with age but rather length of infection. This, unfortunately, suggests that individuals infected with HIV-1 early may have an unusually high amyloid beta load at an early age, in their 40's or earlier. Clinically, we need to identify which individuals are harboring an increased amyloid beta load. Treatments will probably be similar to treatment of Alzheimer's, with antiretrovirals to keep viral load down. It would make sense that those with a high viral load may be at risk," she concluded.

Finally, a September 2005 study (Thompson) used brain-imaging techniques to reveal dramatic pictures that appeared to show a distinct pattern of thinning of the cerebral cortex (the brain surface, which controls the more sophisticated functions).

Thompson observed that patients with HIV infection had a reduction of up to 15% in the thickness of the cerebral cortex compared with 14 HIV-negative patients matched for age and HIV risk factor. This loss of brain tissue did not seem to be related to current viral load or whether the patients were taking HAART.

The loss was also concentrated in very specific areas, namely the parts of the brain dealing with movement and to a less extent touch and visual processing. This reinforces previous observations that often the only overt symptom of HIV brain impairment is mild clumsiness and movement problems.

Thompson told Gay.com: "The people in this study are not impaired at the level of neurological deficits that would interfere with their social functioning and work activities. The tests are basically tests of motor speed. These are generally subtle or fairly mild Minor Cognitive-Motor Disorder (MCMD) impairments. HAART does not appear to slow the damage. A protective barrier prevents drugs entering the brain, where HIV can multiply and attack cells unchecked."

Many questions remain unanswered by Thompson's study. His patients were given a battery of psychological tests and the HIV patients performed worse. However the brain scans revealed that the parts of the brain most reduced in the patients with the most functional impairment were not the ones most strongly affected by HIV infection.

Thompson told Gay.com that this was because the areas damaged by HIV were damaged in all patients: "The areas most affected by HIV are often so severely affected that the damage is "maxed out", and most patients have such severe loss that there is little correlation with variations in the levels of specific cognitive functions. Only in other areas do you see a range of thinning that links better with differences among the patients."

Secondly, current CD4 counts were strongly related to psychological performance. Only seven of the 22 patients studied had current counts under 200, with the majority between 200 and 600. A loose correlation between movement problems and low CD4 count was observed; three of the eight patients with moderate impairment had fewer than 200 CD4 cells, as did all three of those with more severe impairment. Thompson calculated that low CD4 count contributed about 35% of the loss in movement performance seen.

But again, the areas of the brain most reduced in people with low CD4 counts are not those most reduced in people with HIV infection per se, suggesting that two processes or a sequence of processes is involved. Those most strongly affected by CD4 loss were the frontal lobes, responsible for decision-making, and some parts responsible for memory.

What can be done about dementia?

Even though grim predictions in the early days of AIDS that we would end up with large numbers of demented HIV patients in wards have not come to pass, HIV dementia is still an alarming

subject as it is seen as a condition nothing can be done about. Luckily, this is not entirely true.

It is still unclear whether the functional brain impairments seen are mainly caused by HIV infection or other factors to which people with HIV are prone. Co-factors such as depression, lower testosterone levels, and alcohol and drug use can all affect mental functioning at least as much as HIV itself and these factors can, at least, be dealt with by specific therapies or interventions.

Another unknown factor is the effect of HAART's increased cardiovascular risks. Having high cholesterol levels is another predictor of brain impairment. This is because cardiovascular problems may cause tiny strokes in small areas of the brain, which could build up into a picture of dementia in the long run. Smoking is also a very significant factor here, and giving up cigarettes may be one of the best ways someone with HIV can protect themselves against the risks of dementia and cardiovascular problems as they age.

Although the last study cited found that antiretroviral treatment did not affect brain cell loss, other studies have shown the benefit of including in HIV drug regimens the drugs that best cross into the brain. The ones that do best are the nucleosides AZT and 3TC and the non-nucleosides nevirapine and efavirenz. Protease inhibitors cross very poorly, with the exception of indinavir. Taking these drugs before CD4 counts fall too low may provide some protection.

The study of drugs that can halt or reverse brain damage are in their early stages, though there have been promising results with the investigatory drugs memantine and seligiline, and a recent study found that taking omega-3 fish oils - and, indeed doing anything that preserves a good blood supply to the brain - helped guard against dementia in later life.

Lastly, it's important to remember that the brain is a very adaptive organ and that not all brain cell loss translates into performance loss. All but end-stage dementia is at least partially preventable by pursuing a life with a high level of intellectual stimulation and social interaction. This is sometimes called 'use it, don't lose it'.

A study published in the *British Medical Journal* (Richards) recently followed 2058 people who were born in 1946. One of the findings was that people with good reading scores either in their youth or in their late 40s were much less likely to be showing signs of dementia in their late 50s.

The brain is a very adaptable mechanism and, given the right environment, can often compensate for the gradual loss of nerve cells that comes with age. Leading a healthier and stimulating life can do much to prevent us getting slower as we get older.

References

Becker JT et al. Prevalence of cognitive disorders differs as a function of age in HIV virus infection. AIDS 18 (suppl. 1): S11 - S18, 2004.

Catalan J, Thornton S. Whatever happened to HIV dementia? International Journal of STD and AIDS. 4: 1-4, 1993.

Cherner M et al. Effects of HIV-1 infection and aging on neurobehavioral functioning: preliminary findings AIDS 18 (suppl. 1): S27 - S34, 2004.

Ernst T, Chang L. Effect of aging on brain metabolism in antiretroviral-naive HIV patients. AIDS 18 (Suppl. 1): S61-S67, 2004.

Grant, I., et al. Evidence for early central nervous system involvement in the acquired immunodeficiency syndrome (AIDS) and other human immunodeficiency virus (HIV) infections: Studies with neuropsychologic testing and magnetic resonance imaging. Annals of Internal Medicine, 107(6), 828-836, 1987.

Navia BA et al. The AIDS dementia complex. Annals of Neurology 19(6): 517-535, 1986.

Rempel HC. HIV-1 Tat inhibits neprilysin and elevates amyloid beta. AIDS 19(2): 127-135, 2005.

Richards M et al. Cognitive ability in childhood and cognitive decline in mid-life: longitudinal birth cohort study. BMJ 328 (7439): 552, 2004.

Salemi M et al. Phylodynamic analysis of human immunodeficiency virus type 1 in distinct brain compartments provides a model for the neuropathogenesis of AIDS. J Virol 79: 11343-11352, 2005.

Thompson PM et al. Thinning of the cerebral cortex visualized in HIV/AIDS reflects CD4+ T lymphocyte decline. Proc Natl Acad Sci U S A, online edition, 2005.

Valcour VG at al. Cognitive impairment in older HIV-1-seropositive individuals: prevalence and potential mechanisms. AIDS 18 (suppl. 1): S79 - 86, 2004.

Stress

Stress is not a mental illness in itself. Some degree of stress is an inevitable part of life and all significant changes may be stressful. It is how we handle stress that dictates whether the result is mental *dis*tress.

Stress is a two-part process: firstly, life throws an unusual challenge in our path (the **stressor**) and then our minds and bodies cope with it in a characteristic way (the **stress response**).

One of the best descriptions for exactly what stress does to the body and how it works is contained in Paul Martin's *The Sickening Mind*, which is an examination of how psychological stress and disease interact and reinforce each other. Martin defines stress as:

"The state arising when the individual perceives that the demands placed on him exceed (or threaten to exceed) their capacity to cope, and therefore threaten their wellbeing."

Stressors can be physical or psychological; physical ones include injury, disease, surgery, undernourishment and extremes of pain, heat or cold. However one of the reasons stress in modern-day society often results in distress is because most of the stresses of modern life are psychological; we are more likely to encounter an unreasonable boss than an enemy in battle.

Stress elicits a characteristic response in the body, called the startle response. Within a few seconds the **autonomic nervous system** fires and causes the hormone epinephrine (adrenaline) to flood the system. This increases blood flow to the muscles and away from the skin and digestive system. It dulls pain and dilates the pupils of the eyes (hence the pale skin, wide eyes and 'butterflies in the stomach' of fear).

Prolonged stress - lasting longer than a few minutes - causes a different part of the nervous system to send a second hormone, cortisol, to course through the body. Cortisol does two things: it turns the body's energy reserves into glucose for immediate use, and it dampens down the immune system.

The reason it acts on the immune system is in order to delay the inflammatory response that the body uses to direct the immune system to the site of injuries; cortisol enables us to 'keep going' when otherwise we would be sick from the effect of immune system chemicals (cytokines), which cause the characteristic symptoms of infection such as fever and aches. This is the reason why many people soldier on through stressful work then get sick as soon as they go on holiday. Artificial versions of cortisol - corticosteroids - are used medically to damp down inflammation in the same way.

The problem with long-term stress is that the immune suppression can make us sick eventually anyway.

By correlating stressful events in people's lives with subsequent sickness, psycho-immunologists have been able to devise a **stress scale** which predicts the amount of stress specific events may cause an average individual. See table for Top Ten.

Note that positive events are stressors too. And note how many events (death of partners, separation, serious illness, job loss) may be events typical of a life lived with HIV.

Fight, flight or freeze

The autonomic nervous system has two arms - the **sympathetic** and **parasympathetic** nervous systems. The job of the first is to produce the startle response and get the adrenaline going. The second is to do the opposite: by direct nerve signals and by releasing the hormone acetylcholine (alongside others) it causes the blood to flow back into the skin and away from muscles, gets digestion going again, and brings down the body's energy level. These two systems are complementary, like paired muscles that extend and flex joints. However they are not a zero-sum game: they may both be firing at once. An example is during sex, when the parasympathetic system causes erection by releasing blood to

Stress	Event value
Death of spouse	100
Divorce	60
Menopause	60
Separation from living partner	60
Jail term or probation	60
Death of close family member other than spouse	60
Serious personal injury or illness	45
Marriage or establishing life partnership	45
Fired at work	45
Marital or relationship reconciliation	40

the penis or clitoris and the sympathetic causes orgasm by contracting the genital muscles.

The purpose of adrenaline is to cause the individual to either **fight** the stressor or to **flee** from it. However, if the stressor can neither be defeated or run away from, a third way of handling stress comes into play - the **freeze** response, characterised by animals that 'play dead' when confronted by an attacker. What happens is that even while the sympathetic nervous is still firing the parasympathetic overrules it and paralyses the muscles.

Simplistically speaking, if the freeze response happens in response to a stressor, and particularly to long-term stress, mental distress is much more likely to result. Studies have shown that people who respond to an attack or a disaster by fighting the aggressor or running away are much less likely to suffer depressive or anxiety symptoms than people who freeze in terror. One of the reasons child abuse is so damaging is because children are not in a position to fight or flee.

When the 'freeze' response takes over, the result is **dissociation** - a feeling of unreality and detachment. The person, deprived of the ability to run away in reality, 'runs away' from the event internally. "It seemed so unreal," or "It was like it was happening to someone else," people will say. Unfortunately this also means that clear memories of the event fail to be laid down. It is believed that deprivation of a 'narrative' - a sequential memory of a traumatic event - is the cause of post-traumatic stress disorder, as it means the event is not placed by the brain where it belongs in time and therefore the unconscious mind still reacts as if the event were happening now.

Some stress is good for the system; the result otherwise is boredom, which is stressful in itself. This is the reason people go to roller-coaster rides and horror movies. The key difference between helpful and harmful stress is **control.** A work assignment may be daunting but if the individual believes they can accomplish it, they will do. Complementary therapies may help people suffering from chronic illnesses because they help the individual feel in control of the disease.

The freeze reaction, if long-term stress keeps it going, may result in two types of mental illness - the two most common types. If the parasympathetic response predominates, the result is depression (which is why depression is sometimes called 'learned helplessness'). If the sympathetic response does, the result is anxiety. Both may happen at the same time - and often do.

Further reading

Martin Paul. The Sickening mind - Brain, Behaviour, Immunity and Disease. Flamingo, 1997. ISBN 0 00 655022 3

The impact of mental illness on health

With the immune-suppressant effects of cortisol and other stress hormones, it is not surprising that there is an association directly between poor mental health and poor physical health. Numerous studies have found, for instance, that depression appears directly related to an increased risk of heart attack. However it is sometimes difficult to disentangle other health risks people with poor mental health may run (poor self-care, drink and drugs, etc) from the direct effects of stress.

One study (Cole) found that HIV replication rates in people on treatment who had been psychologically assessed as stressed and introverted were eight times higher than in patients with no mental health issues. Cole measured social inhibition by means of a psychological questionnaire and stress and direct measurements of autonomic nervous system (ANS) arousal in 54 gay men with HIV. Following baseline ANS assessment, HIV viral load and CD4 levels were monitored for 12-18 months to assess relationships between ANS activity and HIV pathogenesis. He found good correlation between elevated ANS activity and high scores for social inhibition. He also found that viral load set-point was elevated eight-fold in socially inhibited men, and that they showed poorer virologic and immunologic response to HAART. Effects were independent of duration of infection, Cole calculated that differences in ANS arousal could account for 64%-92% of way that social inhibition impacted on viral load.

A series of studies (Goodkin 1995) presented at a conference on psychoneuroimmunology (the science of how mental state impacts on the immune system) in 1995 found that natural killer cell activity and total lymphocyte count were related to the amount of stress gay men with HIV had experienced, and to their ability to cope with that stress, as measured by psychological tests.

A study (Cook) of 1716 HIV-positive women who paid 6-monthly visits between 1994 and 2001 to six HIV clinics found that after all other factors were controlled for, AIDS-related deaths were more likely among women with chronic depressive symptoms, and symptoms were more severe among women in the terminal phase of their illness. Mental health service use, on the other hand, was associated with reduced mortality.

Jeanette Ickovicz (2001) measured HIV-related mortality and CD4 decline over a maximum of seven years in 765 HIV-positive women aged16 to 55 years and compared mortality between women with no depressive symptoms, intermittent depressive symptoms, or chronic depressive symptoms. After controlling for clinical treatment, and other factors, women with chronic depressive symptoms were twice as likely to die as women with limited or no depressive symptoms. Among women with CD4 cell counts of less than 200, HIV-related mortality rates were 54%for those with chronic depressive symptoms, 48% for those with intermittent depressive symptoms and 21% for those with limited or no depressive symptoms. Chronic depressive symptoms were also associated with significantly greater decline in CD4cell counts.

Equally, psychotherapy can directly improve immune function by reducing stress. Another study by Goodkin and colleagues (1999) was a randomised controlled study of intensive group therapy for gay men who had lost partners between 1992 and 1995. A total of 166 men, 97 with HIV and 69 without, were randomly assigned to four groups; two therapy groups for men with and without HIV and two control groups. The men with HIV were largely not taking antiretrovirals, The HIV-positive men receiving group therapy maintained stable CD4 counts while those of the control group declined. When viral load testing became available, archived blood samples from 36 trial participants showed that the men receiving group therapy also had significant decreases in viral load.

A previous analysis of the study (Goodkin 1998) found that CD4 counts were also higher in the HIV-negative men who received therapy. It also found that plasma cortisol levels decreased significantly among men who received therapy compared to controls. There were a significantly reduced number of health care visits over the 6-month follow-up period among the men who had therapy.

In another study, Petrie and colleagues conducted a randomised controlled trial of 37 patients. They were randomly assigned to one of two groups and were asked to write for 30 minutes each day for just four days in a row. Half of them were encouraged to write (in private) a daily piece exploring their deepest feelings about HIV or other traumatic and emotional experiences in their lives, particularly topics they hadn't discussed with anyone before. The other half wrote about unemotional topics including what they had done the day before, and what they had planned for the next day, the next week, and the next year. In those patients who wrote about emotional experiences, HIV viral load dropped immediately after the writing period, and then increased gradually over the next 6 months, while T cell counts gradually and continuously increased during the next six months.

Depression and adherence

Lastly, depression and other mental health problems may have a very specific effect on people with HIV by making it difficult to adhere to HAART. In one study (Yun) of patients seen at a city HIV clinic between 1997 and 2001 adherence levels were related to depression scores. Out of 1713 HIV-infected patients, 57% were diagnosed as depressed; of those, 46% and 52% were taking antidepressants and antiretroviral treatment, respectively. Antiretroviral adherence was lower among depressed patients not on antidepressants than those taking antidepressants (p = 0.012). Adherence to antiretroviral treatment was higher among patients adherent to antidepressants vs. those non-adherent to antidepressant treatment. Antiretroviral adherence improved over a six-month period for all groups of patients, whether they were prescribed antidepressants or not and whether they actually took their antidepressants or not; however the largest positive change in adherence was seen in people prescribed antidepressants.

References

Cole SW. Psychological risk factors for HIV pathogenesis: mediation by the autonomic nervous system. Biol Psychiatry 15(12): 1444-1456, 2003.

Cook JA. Depressive symptoms and AIDS-related mortality among a multisite cohort of HIV-positive women. Am J Public Health 94(7): 1133-1140. 2004.

Goodkin K. Clinical aspects of psychoneuroimmunology. Lancet 21(8943): 183-184, 1995.

Goodkin K (1998)A Bereavement Support Group Intervention Is Longitudinally Associated with Salutary Effects on the CD4 Cell Count and Number of Physician Visits. Clin Diagn Lab Immunol. 5(3): 382-391, 1998.

Goodkin, K et al. A randomized controlled clinical trial of a bereavement support group intervention in human immunodeficiency virus type 1-seropositive and -seronegative homosexual men. Arch Gen Psychiatry 56: 52-59, 1999.

Ickovicz JR. Mortality, CD4 Cell Count Decline, and Depressive Symptoms among HIV-Seropositive Women. JAMA 285: 1466-1474, 2001.

Petrie KJ et al. Effect of written emotional expression on immune function in patients with human immunodeficiency virus infection: a randomized trial. Psychosomatic Medicine 66(2): 272-275, 2004.

Yun LW. Antidepressant treatment improves adherence to antiretroviral therapy among depressed HIV-infected patients. J Acquir Immune Defic Syndr. 38(4): 432-438, 2005.

Further reading

Karl Goodkin, Adriaan P Visser (eds.) Psychoneuroimmunology: Stress, Mental Disorders and Health. American Psychiatric Publications Inc, 2000. ISBN 0880481714

Depression

Depression, malignant sadness, melancholia, the blues, the black dog; by whatever name it has been called, depression has been a recognised part of the human condition throughout history.

Famous depressives range from King Saul in the Bible through to Samuel Johnson, Winston Churchill and Virginia Woolf.

Depression is very common; an estimated 121 million people worldwide are suffering from it at any one time. An estimated 5.8% of men and 9.5% of women will experience a depressive episode in any given year, and over a lifetime people have a 20% chance of having an episode of depression (statistics from WHO).

Depression is the leading cause of disability as measured by Years Lived with Disability (YLDs) and the fourth leading contributor to the global burden of disease (DALYs) in 2000. By the year 2020, depression is projected to reach 2nd place of the ranking of DALYs calculated for all ages and both sexes. Today, depression is already the 2nd cause of DALYs in the age category 15-44 years for both sexes combined.

Women are twice as likely to get depression as men, but men are more often casualties of it. Depression is responsible for about 60% of suicides (the other 40% being rational, as with people faced with a terminal illness, or impulsive ones, often under the influence of alcohol), and while women *attempt* suicide more often, men are between twice as likely (in Sweden) and 10 times as likely (in Ireland) to actually kill themselves than women. In the UK three times as many men kill themselves as women. Depression is the tenth biggest cause of death worldwide (worse than all varieties of viral hepatitis, for instance).

Gay men are three to six times as likely to commit suicide as heterosexuals (MYRBS)

Clinical depression is a medical condition, a serious illness that in no way has to be endured, 'put up with', or 'snapped out of'. Physically, it is caused by biochemical disorders that interfere with normal brain functioning. Although as with most mental conditions the biochemical causes are not completely clear, a major factor appears to be plunging levels of the neurotransmitter serotonin in the brain.

Serotonin has been mislabeled the 'happiness chemical'. It might be better labeled the 'confidence chemical'. Whereas dopamine, which is overproduced in the brains of people taking methamphetamine and cocaine, and underproduced in the brains of people with Parkinson's disease, gives people their basic biopsychological energy or 'go', serotonin appears to confer *social* energy and ease of discourse. It is found universally in animals that live in groups, and not just higher animals - ants have serotonin too.

Depression's persistence and universality made scientists think it must confer some evolutionary benefit - otherwise such an unbearable and disabling illness would long ago have disappeared via natural selection (people with major depression don't have sex). This lack of serotonin gives a clue as to what is going on. Studies of monkeys that live in social groups have shown that the dominant animal in the pack has far higher serotonin levels than subordinates and that if the dominant animal is defeated and loses status, his serotonin levels immediately plunge.

Moreover, artificially raising the serotonin levels in subordinate vervet monkeys with fluoxetine (*Prozac*) results in these individuals rising in status, in some cases to alpha rank (Raleigh). Dominant animals display an air of calm self-assurance, self-control, and self-directed behavior. Subordinates, on the other hand, appear fidgety, easily perturbed, and sometimes unpredictably aggressive; their behavior seems to be largely controlled by external stimuli rather than being self-directed.

Depression, in short, is all about status. Its evolutionary function is literally to 'shut down' the aggression of subordinates so that a society can function. It also serves to enforce a period of calm and recovery after suffering a loss or accident. Without depression people would be constantly disruptive, getting into fights and hurting themselves - as happens in people with depression's opposite, mania. That even great leaders like Churchill and Abraham Lincoln suffered depression shows that it may even be necessary to *reculer pour mieux sauter* - to withdraw so as to gather strength.

Unfortunately however depression also appears to have a strong hereditary component. Depressed parents have depressed kids, and may also bring up their children in a way that restrains their natural impulsivity so as not to create parental stress. Children brought up to be 'no bother' may end up as adult depressives.

So it is no wonder that people who belong to stigmatised groups (such as immigrants, drug users and - despite much social progress- gay men) should be more prone to depression, nor surprising that having a stigmatised disease should also lead to depression. An HIV diagnosis may in fact have a stronger impact on people who have *not* had previous experience of being stigmatised or losing status. For instance, a study of African-American men with HIV (Coleman) found that heterosexual men reacted to HIV diagnosis with worse depression than gay men - possibly because they were not so used to a perceived loss in status.

Clinical depression is distinct from reactive depression - the short-lived, unhappy feelings that may be linked to a particular event. Even grieving, although an intense emotional experience, is not in itself depression if it follows the expected course of eventually fading away. The defining psychological characteristics of depression are that it is *isolating* (the person does not express their unhappiness in a way that produces support) and *self-reinforcing* (the thought patterns that happen in depression serve to entrench the depression more deeply).

Symptoms of depression include:

- Persistent sad, anxious, or "empty" mood

- Feelings of hopelessness, pessimism

- Feelings of guilt, worthlessness, helplessness

- Loss of interest or pleasure in hobbies and activities that were once enjoyed, including sex

- Decreased energy, fatigue, being "slowed down"

- Difficulty concentrating, remembering, making decisions

- Insomnia, early-morning awakening, or oversleeping

- Appetite and/or weight loss or overeating and weight gain

- Thoughts of death or suicide; suicide attempts

- Restlessness, irritability

- Persistent physical symptoms that do not respond to treatment, such as headaches, digestive disorders, and chronic pain.

There is a high link between HIV and depression. HIV-positive people have an estimated prevalence rate of 22% to 45%, compared with 15% for the general population. In one study, depression, anxiety and problems sleeping were frequently reported by people with HIV. 72% said they experienced depression, 65% experienced anxiety, 48% had insomnia. In addition, 43% had symptoms of lethargy and 40% reported impaired concentration and mood swings (Carter, 2002).

Depression and anxiety are experienced by the overwhelming majority of people living with HIV, according to research conducted by the International Association of Physicians in AIDS Care (Horwath). More than 84% of doctors polled said that their HIV-positive patients "frequently or very frequently" had symptoms of depression, and 81% of doctors said their patients exhibited symptoms of anxiety. According to physicians, more than 71% of their patients experience headaches, lethargy and/or insomnia. Doctors overwhelmingly attributed their patients' psychiatric problems to the effects of their treatment, with 84% saying they believed HAART had a role in depression, anxiety or other mental health problems.

The patients seem to agree that *if* they have emotional or mental health problems, depression is by far the most common symptom - indeed it is nearly universal.

A survey of gay men attending the mental health service at a clinic in Massachusetts (Berg) over a 12-month period found that depression was the most common presenting problem, cited by 58.1% of clients, followed by anxiety at 38.2%. But when patients were asked to tick off their psychological symptoms in a checklist, nearly all (96.3%) described symptoms of depression and another 78.2% described 'low energy' - which is often a symptom of depression. Sixty-nine per cent described symptoms of anxiety too - which shows that the two mental states may often co-exist (as it did in the subordinate vervet monkeys).

What you can do about depression - a checklist

For specifics on treatment for depression, see **treatments** below. But a checklist may help readers currently depressed, especially as depression impairs concentration.

- Depression is **global -** it makes you think that a temporary setback ("I've lost a friend") says something about your entire personality ("I can't make friends"). Think about other occasions when what has just happened did not happen.

- Depression is **timeless** - it deceives you into believing you have always felt this way and always will. Remember that you have had happier times and that this will not last.

- Depression **reinforces itself** - it makes you think in chains of thought that make the depression worse ("I'm so depressed and helpless I'll end up in the gutter, which makes me more depressed"). Try to distract yourself from depressive chains of thought by attempting an activity that does not involve reflection and analysis.

- Depression makes you **inactive -** it cannot be 'thought out of', but exercise or physical activity can raise serotonin levels sufficiently for the depression to lift.

Depression makes you **antisocial** ("I'm such a drag, my friends all hate me"). Forcing yourself in a very structured way to talk to a friend or relative ("I'll do one five-minute phone call") can remind you that you form part of a social nexus and that others care about you. Pick with care though - 'misery loves company' and phoning a depressed friend may have the opposite effect.

References

Berg MB
(http://www.ncbi.nlm.nih.gov/entrez/query.fcgi?db=pubmed&cmd=search&term=%22berg+mb%22%5bauthor%5d). Mental health concerns of HIV-infected gay and bisexual men seeking mental health services: an observational study. AIDS Patient Care STDS.18(11): 635-643, 2004.

Coleman CL
(http://www.ncbi.nlm.nih.gov/entrez/query.fcgi?db=pubmed&cmd=search&term=%22coleman+cl%22%5bauthor%5d). Sexual Orientation a Predictor of Depressive Symptoms Among HIV-Infected African American Men: A Descriptive Correlational Study. Arch Psychiatr Nurs. 19(5): 236-241, 2005.

Horwath E. Psychiatric and Neuropsychiatric Manifestations of HIV Infection. J Int Ass Physi AIDS Care 1(Suppl 1) S1-S16. October 2002.

MYRBS - Massachusetts Youth Risk Behaviour Survey 1999. See http://www.doe.mass.edu/hssss/yrbs99/chapter8.html

Raleigh MJ, Brammer GL, McGuire MT: Male dominance, serotonergic systems, and the behavioral and physiological effects of drugs in vervet monkeys (*Cercopithecus aethiops sabaeus*). Prog Clin Biol Res 131: 185-197, 1983.

World Health Organisation: Mental Health: Depression. See http://www.who.int/mental_health/management/depression/definition/en/

Stress and anxiety

While anxiety may co-exist with depression, it may also manifest by itself. The most common development of what might be called 'malignant anxiety' is generalised anxiety disorder on GAD. Here the anxiety is not pinned on to a particular fear or object as in obsessive-compulsive disorder or phobias, but exists as a free-floating part of the person's experience. They worry about everything. They know they have got things out of proportion but there is nothing they can do about it. People who are well off agonise over money. Healthy people torture themselves with thoughts of fatal illnesses. Then they worry about the fact that they can't stop worrying. Then finally they worry because the anxiety gives them physical symptoms. GAD is second only to depression as a mental health problem. About two million people in the UK (3.3%) are thought to suffer from it and probably only about half are diagnosed. GAD is about twice as common in women as men.

Different cultures may manifest different rates of anxiety and depression. For instance, a survey of 51 recently-diagnosed HIV patients in India found that anxiety symptoms were nearly as common as ones of depression (36% and 40% respectively) whereas most of the studies above suggest that depression is 30 to 50% more common than anxiety.

Anxiety is a very physical condition and most people with GAD take themselves to the doctor because they have physical symptoms. In the case of HIV patients these may be blamed on HIV therapy (though some drugs can indeed cause anxiety, see below).

As well as worrying unreasonably about everything, the following symptoms may be present:

- Trembling

- muscular tension

- sweating

- lightheadedness or dizziness

- heart palpitations

- irregular breathing or hyperventilation

- heartburn/acid indigestion

- being easily fatigued

- difficulty concentrating or mind going blank

- irritability

- sleep disturbance (difficulty falling or staying asleep, or restless unsatisfying sleep)

Some people with GAD refer themselves because they fear they are having a heart attack, not only because of heart palpitations but because acid indigestion can cause nerve pain down one arm very similar to that stereotypical of a heart attack.

GAD can manifest itself as outright panic attacks, where the above symptoms intensify into a terrifying experience of fear and loss of control.

One study (Elliott) assessed the prevalence of GAD in people with HIV as high as 38%. Interestingly, significant associations were found with particular antiretrovirals and other drugs used in HIV, including d4T, ddI, AZT, fluconazole, foscarnet, and isoniazid (this study dates from 1998, before the widespread introduction of efavirenz).

Fatigue can be as much a symptom of GAD as of depression. In one study at King's College Hospital in South London (Henderson) 148 patients were assessed for fatigue and were also assessed for anxiety, depression, state of health and perception of state of health. Two-thirds of patients displayed some degree of fatigue. It was found that fatigue was not related to HAART or HIV disease stage. On the contrary, the more fatigued people had higher CD4 counts. Fatigue was also associated with high scores for depression and especially for anxiety, and for the functional impairment caused by these symptoms.

Another early (1992) study by Perdices found no relationship between HIV disease stage or CD4 count and anxiety. The study compared 207 HIV-positive gay men and 36 negative controls and stratified the HIV+ men into asymptomatic (101), ARC (72) and AIDS (34). The only predictors f mental anxiety were physical symptoms consistent with anxiety and psychosocial factors such as isolation.

In a study at the University of Pennsylvania Morrison compared anxiety and depression scores between 93 HIV-positive and 62 HIV-negative women. The women with HIV were far more likely to have major depression (19.4% vs 4.8%). They did not have higher rates of diagnosis of GAD; but when individual symptoms likely to be caused by anxiety were assessed, HIV-positive women scored 8.8 out of a possible 11 on an anxiety-symptom scale compared with 3.6 by the HIV-negative women. This shows how subtly anxiety may be masquerading as physical symptoms.

GAD may be caused by a general overload of stress, a constitutional tendency to overstimulation or - intriguingly - by a real anxiety. People may be worrying about crashing every time they drive a car or of catching HIV because, in the words of the British psychoanalyst Donald Winnicott, "the breakdown feared is the one that has already happened". Typically the person has suffered a life change or stressor of the type listed on the stress scale above and the hypervigilant state of anxiety is caused by failure to come to terms with it. Very often existential fears like ageing are involved too.

The classic case of hypervigilance caused by an event that is over is **PTSD - post-traumatic stress disorder.**

Post-traumatic stress disorder

We have already described PTSD above, but it may be particularly common in certain people with HIV, especially post-diagnosis. PTSD may be specifically caused by HIV diagnosis, especially if this happens in a traumatic fashion; it may be caused by circumstances leading up to the diagnosis such as partner abuse and rape, but triggered by the diagnosis; or it may be a causative factor in poor sexual health skills and risk behaviour. It is estimated that 3.6% of people in the USA meet diagnostic criteria for PTSD.

One non-HIV study (Marshall) shows how the trauma of war, danger and exile can cause PTSD in refugees. The researchers interviewed 450 Cambodians in the Long Beach area of California, the largest Cambodian community in the USA, two decades after the Khmer Rouge regime had forced them to flee Cambodia. It found that 62% met PTSD criteria (remember the US general prevalence is estimated as 3.6%), 51% criteria for depression and 42% criteria for both.

In one South African study (Olley) 149 recently diagnosed HIV-positive people, 105 of them women, were assessed for PTSD. The mean time since diagnosis was 5.8 months. Twenty-two patients (14.8%) met diagnostic criteria for PTSD. Twenty-nine per cent of patients with PTSD also had major depression compared with 7% without PTSD. No less than 54% of patients with PTSD felt suicidal compared with 11% of patients without it. Eight out of the 22 patients with PTSD were thought to have it directly as a result of their HIV diagnosis. The researchers commented that "female gender and a history of sexual violation in the past year were significantly associated with a diagnosis of PTSD.In some cases, PTSD is secondary to the diagnosis of HIV/AIDS but in most cases it is seen after other traumas, with sexual violation and intimate partner violence in women being particularly important."

In a US study (Leserman) 611 patients at rural clinics in southern states were assessed for PTSD. The researchers do not give the prevalence found in their abstract, but report that patients with more lifetime trauma, stressful events, and PTSD symptoms reported more bodily pain, and poorer physical, role, and cognitive functioning.

They continue: "Trauma, recent stressful events, and PTSD explained from 12% to 27% of the variance in health-related functioning, over and above that explained by demographic variables. In addition, patients with more trauma, including

sexual and physical abuse, and PTSD symptoms were at greater risk for having bed disability, an overnight hospitalization, an emergency room visit, and four or more HIV outpatient clinic visits in the previous 9 months. Patients with a history of abuse had about twice the risk of spending 5 or more days in bed, having an overnight hospital stay, and visiting the emergency room, compared with those without abuse. The effects of trauma and stress were not explained by CD4 lymphocyte count or HIV viral load; however, these effects appear to be largely accounted for by increases in current PTSD symptoms."

Another study (Smith) interviewed 145 non-hospitalised patients with diagnosed AIDS. It found that over half of them (53.8%) merited a PTSD diagnosis. Those with PTSD reported having significantly higher pain intensity and greater pain-related interference in performance of daily activities like working, sleeping, walking ability and general activity and mood, relations with other people and enjoyment of life. On average, participants reported being exposed to 6.3 different types of trauma over the course of their lifetime - and said that receiving an HIV diagnosis was rated as being among the most stressful.

What can be done about anxiety and PTSD

Drugs such as beta-blockers can control anxiety symptoms, and anti-depressants any attendant depression, and complementary therapies involving relaxing movement like t'ai chi or yoga can help. Relaxation therapies involving being still such as Reiki can make anxiety and PTSD worse, as they give the mind a chance to wander and can exacerbate feelings of helplessness and paralysis; people with histories of sexual and physical abuse will also often be unwilling to be touched.

Ultimately taking therapies seem to work best for anxiety and PTSD. In PTSD great care needs to be taken as simply to 'debrief' the traumatic event(s) will tend simply to reawaken the unprocessed (implicit) memories that cause symptoms. Various novel techniques such as EMDR (eye-movement desensitization and reprogramming) can be used to educate people out of psyching themselves up into anxiety states, and then a very careful and gradual re-remembering of the traumatic events may be possible, placing them into a narrative order and enabling the individual to make sense of what was terror and chaos. Highly skilled therapy is required and people should be referred specifically to a therapist skilled in working with PTSD.

References

Chandra PS et al. Anxiety and depression among HIV-infected heterosexuals--a report from India. J Psychosom Res 45(5): 401-409, 1998.

Elliott A (http://www.ncbi.nlm.nih.gov/entrez/query.fcgi?db=pubmed&cmd=search&term=%22elliott+a%22%5bauthor%5d). Anxiety and HIV infection. STEP Perspect. 98(1): 11-14, 1998.

Henderson M et al. Fatigue among HIV-infected patients in the era of highly active antiretroviral therapy. HIV Med 6(5): 347-352, 2005.

Leserman J (http://www.ncbi.nlm.nih.gov/entrez/query.fcgi?db=pubmed&cmd=search&term=%22leserman+j%22%5bauthor%5d). How trauma, recent stressful events, and PTSD affect functional health status and health utilization in HIV-infected patients in the south. Psychosomatic Medicine 67: 500-507, 2005.

Marshall GN, Schell TL, Elliott MN, Berthold SM, Chun CA. Mental health of Cambodian refugees 2 decades after resettlement in the United States. JAMA. 294(5): 571-579, 2005.

Morrison MF (http://www.ncbi.nlm.nih.gov/entrez/query.fcgi?db=pubmed&cmd=search&term=%22morrison+mf%22%5bauthor%5d) et al. Depressive and anxiety disorders in women with HIV infection. Am J Psychiatry 159: 789-796, 2002.

Olley BO et al. Post-traumatic stress disorder among recently diagnosed patients with HIV/AIDS in South Africa. AIDS Care 17(5): 550-557, 2005.

Perdices M et al. Anxiety, depression and HIV related symptomatology across the spectrum of HIV disease. Aust NZ J Psychiatry. 26(4): 560-566, 1992.

Smith MY (http://www.ncbi.nlm.nih.gov/entrez/query.fcgi?db=pubmed&cmd=search&term=%22smith+my%22%5bauthor%5d). The impact of PTSD on pain experience in persons with HIV/AIDS. Pain 98(1-2): 9-17, 2002.

Mental health and sexual health

Poor mental health may be a factor in becoming HIV-positive and after diagnosis it may be a factor in both the risk of contracting other STIs and of transmitting HIV. The decision to engage in risky sex may not always be a consciously made decision, but an attempt to satisfy some other need.

Firstly, anxiety and depression may be risk factors in themselves. One Australian study already cited (Rogers) found that gay men with dysthymia (but not major depression) were 2.36 times more likely to have unprotected sex.

A study from Connecticut (Kozal) found an even stronger association between mental distress and unsafe sex. The researchers interviewed 333 HIV-positive people (of all genders and sexualities) about their risk behaviour over the previous three months. Of these, 23% (75 people) had had unprotected sex with 191 separate partners, only 36 of whom (19%) were known to be HIV-positive themselves. About 5% of the clinic attendees were responsible for most of the unprotected sex with casual partners. There was no relationship between unprotected sex and any physical measurement such as viral load, CD4 count or HIV symptoms, nor with demographic variables such as race. Gay men had more unsafe sex because they had more partners. Once the influence of number of partners was factored out, so that the choice of whether or not to have protected sex was the only variable left, the *only* predictor of whether people chose to have unsafe sex was a higher mental distress score of a scale that measured depression and anxiety. People in the highest quartile of poor mental health scores were *ten times* more likely to choose to have unprotected sex than others.

In another study among gay men (Martin) social isolation was associated with sexual risk taking. A sample of 470 urban gay men completed a self-administered questionnaire. Participants scored high on loneliness in comparison to matched group of non-gay men and men who had unprotected anal intercourse with casual partners during the previous six months scored higher on Loneliness than other participants, but those who did so with primary partners scored the lowest. The researchers comment that "Episodes of unprotected anal intercourse with nonprimary partners might have been avoidance strategies to help participants cope with loneliness or other negative affect." In other words, loneliness may not just lead gay men to go out and have casual sex, it may also be a driver behind unsafe sex, as this comes to symbolise contact and satisfies a craving for it.

For many gay men, low self-esteem and internalised homophobia can impact HIV risk-taking. One study (Ross) linked internalised homophobia directly with increased risk of having HIV. Two hundred and two gay men attending sexual health seminars in Houston, Texas filled in questionnaires assessing how much they were out as gay, whether they enjoyed the company of other gay men, whether they had religious and moral views about the acceptability of being gay, and the degree to which they felt stigmatised. People with higher degrees of internalised homophobia were more likely to have HIV.

In one particularly interesting study of gay men (Imrie) 408 gay men with HIV attending the HIV clinic at the Royal Free Hospital in north London were surveyed to see if they had had an STI over the last 12 months and were then asked about four types of experience that other studies have shown are associated with high levels of sexual risk taking and poor mental health. They were asked if they'd started having sex below the legal age of consent (16 in the UK); whether they'd even been forced to have sex; whether they'd ever been paid for sex; and whether they had ever injected drugs, including performance steroids.

The researchers found that 125 or nearly one in four of the HIV patients (23.5%) had been diagnosed with an STI during the previous year.

Out of the whole patient group, whether they had had an STI or not, they found that 63% had first had sex before they were 16;

over a third (36%) had been paid for sex at some time; over a quarter (27%) had had an experience of non-consensual sex; and 12% had injected drugs (including performance steroids) during the last five years.

But the proportions of people with these risk factors were all much higher in the men who had had STIs. Of these men, 77% had had first sex before 16; 45% had ever been paid for sex; a third had had non-consensual sex; and one in six had injected drugs.

Putting it another way, men diagnosed with STIs were a third more likely to report first sex before 16 than those without STIs; 62% more likely to have ever been paid for sex; 42% more likely to have had non-consensual sex; and 80% more likely to have injected drugs. Of patients who reporting injecting drugs in the last five years, more than half had had an STI in the previous year.

The researchers comment that "receiving an HIV-positive diagnosis is not the end of the story" when it comes to addressing gay men's prevention needs. "An individual diagnosed with HIV comes complete with a life history in which the receipt of an HIV-positive diagnosis is often simply the climax to a list of negative sexual health experiences, and in which there may also be concurrent psychosocial health problems.

"Factors that may have initially predisposed men to becoming HIV infected are likely to continue to infect their sexual health beyond this point and for many years to come. More effective sexual health promotion for those with HIV infection requires innovative interventions which address individuals' historical antecedents for their current poor sexual health and risk practices."

Another study from the Royal London Hospital (Beck) found that gay men (HIV-positive and negative) attending a sexual health clinic reported high levels of both unprotected sex with serodiscordant partners (36%) and having had non-consensual sex (26%). Although this study did not find an association between a history of non-consensual sex and current unprotected sex, it did find that unprotected sex was associated both with depression and with "cognitions assessing the controllability or predictability of HIV risk". In other words if gay men had depression, that depression made them feel fatalistic about whether they caught HIV.

Gay men are not the only group among whom child sexual abuse and premature sexual experience have been associated both with depression and with sexual risk taking.

In a second study from the Royal London Hospital (Petrak) 137 out of 303 women attending the GUM clinic there (45%) reported experiences of child abuse, 26% of them child sexual abuse (CSA). Women who had experienced CSA were more likely to have previous STIs (p=0.0007) and more than one concurrent STI (p=0.004). "Women with a history of CSA reported significantly higher frequency of thought reflecting anticipated negative reaction from partners to suggesting condom use," say the researchers.

PTSD may be a consequence of CSA or a risk factor for HIV in its own right. In one early study of US army veterans (Hoff - published 1997, but data from 1992), the results indicated that the combination of PTSD and substance abuse increased the risk of HIV infection by almost 12 times over those without either.

Several studies have used qualitative interviewing to model why premature or non-consensual sexual experiences may lead to greater HIV and STI risk. In another early study of gay men (Bartholow - 1994 but data collected 1989-90), 1,001 gay men attending urban STI clinics were interviewed regarding abusive sexual contacts during childhood and adolescence. Sexual abuse was found to be significantly associated with mental health counselling and hospitalisation, recreational drug use, depression, suicidal thought or actions, social support, sexual identity development, HIV risk behaviour including unprotected anal intercourse and injecting drug use, and risk of sexually transmitted diseases including HIV infection. "Data suggest that sexual abuse may have a wide-ranging influence on the quality of life and health risk behaviour of homosexual men," comment the researchers.

Maureen Miller (1999) developed a model to account for the many ways CSA may lead to increasing sexual risk behaviour among women. She said that CSA could lead directly to sexual risk due to difficulty negotiating sex in adulthood; it could lead to sexual risk due to depression; it could lead to " initiation of and/or increasing reliance on drug use as a method of coping with the sexual abuse experience", and lastly that social factors such as social support, and social isolation could also influence risk taking.

Drink and drugs

The mention in several of these papers of drug use as a coping mechanism underlines how early experiences, mental problems and drug use may all combine to create sexual risk.

Remember however that drink and drug use *in themselves* are not defined as mental illnesses by DSM-IV. There has been an extensive literature in recent years particularly dealing with how drug use in gay men is related to HIV risk and acquisition. The Miller paper reminds us that people may take drugs for all sorts of reasons. They may use them to disinhibit themselves socially in order to meet partners; to heighten sensuality and sexual excitement; or simply because everyone else in their social circle uses them. None of these indicate mental distress, need be problematic or lead to addiction in themselves, or create a greater degree of risk to sexual health. A reminder that high-risk behaviour and drug use do not *always* go together in gay men came from a widely-publicised study (Clatts) of HIV-positive men who arranged HIV-only sex parties ('poz parties') in order to have unprotected sex. The researchers found that although the men involved had high lifetime levels of recreational drug use, there was very little use of drugs at the parties themselves.

Problematic drug use and/or HIV acquisition as a result of drug use is more likely when patients are either using drugs to escape mental distress or because drug use has *created* mental distress. People may use drugs:

- To disinhibit themselves sexually because sex creates anxiety when they are sober.

- To 'self-medicate' against anxiety and depression.

- Because drug use itself has led to poor mental health (e.g. ecstasy use leading to depression, methamphetamine to anxiety and paranoia) and the person is caught in a spiral of self-medicating for symptoms cause by their 'medication'.

This is not the place specifically to look at the interaction between drug use and HIV transmission/acquisition. There is an extensive literature, some of which is covered in sections on **drug use** and on **HIV transmission** in this manual.

References

Bartholow BN (http://www.ncbi.nlm.nih.gov/entrez/query.fcgi?db=pubmed&cmd=search&term=%22bartholow+bn%22%5bauthor%5d) et al. Emotional, behavioral, and HIV risks associated with sexual abuse among adult homosexual and bisexual men. Child Abuse Negl. 18(9): 747-761, 1994.

Beck A (http://www.ncbi.nlm.nih.gov/entrez/query.fcgi?db=pubmed&cmd=search&term=%22beck+a%22%5bauthor%5d) et al. Psychosocial predictors of HIV/STI risk behaviours in a sample of homosexual men. Sex Transm Infect. 79(2): 142-146, 2003.

Clatts MC et al. An emerging HIV risk environment: a preliminary epidemiological profile of an MSM POZ Party in New York City. Sexually Transmitted Infections 81: 373-376, 2005.

Hoff RA (http://www.ncbi.nlm.nih.gov/entrez/query.fcgi?db=pubmed&cmd=search&term=%22hoff+ra%22%5bauthor%5d) et al. Mental disorder as a risk factor for human immunodeficiency virus infection in a sample of veterans. J Nerv Ment Dis. 185(9): 556-560, 1997.

Imrie J et al. More to positive prevention than sexually transmitted infection screening. AIDS 19(15), 1708-1709, 2005.

Kozal MJ (http://www.ncbi.nlm.nih.gov/entrez/query.fcgi?db=pubmed&cmd=search&term=%22kozal+mj%22%5bauthor%5d) et al. Antiretroviral resistance and high-risk transmission behavior among HIV-positive patients in clinical care. AIDS 18(16): 2185-2189, 2004.

Martin JI (http://www.ncbi.nlm.nih.gov/entrez/query.fcgi?db=pubmed&cmd=search&term=%22martin+ji%22%5bauthor%5d). Loneliness and sexual risk behavior in gay men. Psychol Rep. 81(3 Pt 1): 815-825, 1997.

Miller M (http://www.ncbi.nlm.nih.gov/entrez/query.fcgi?db=pubmed&cmd=search&term=%22miller+m%22%5bauthor%5d). A model to explain the relationship between sexual abuse and HIV risk among women. AIDS Care. 11(1): 3-20, 1999.

Petrak J (http://www.ncbi.nlm.nih.gov/entrez/query.fcgi?db=pubmed&cmd=search&term=%22petrak+j%22%5bauthor%5d) et al. The association between abuse in childhood and STD/HIV risk behaviours in female genitourinary (GU) clinic attendees. Sex Transm Infect. 76(6): 457-461, 2000.

Rogers G. Depressive disorders and unprotected casual anal sex among Australian homosexually active men in primary care. HIV Medicine 4, 271-275, 2003.

Ross MW (http://www.ncbi.nlm.nih.gov/entrez/query.fcgi?db=pubmed&cmd=search&term=%22ross+mw%22%5bauthor%5d). Measurement and correlates of internalized homophobia: a factor analytic study. J Clin Psychol. 52(1): 15-21, 1996.

Sexual addiction and compulsivity

One form of addiction that is clearly an HIV and STI risk and which may impact on the individual in many other ways including broken relationships is addiction to sex itself.

The concept of sex addiction is still controversial in some circles. Gay men are wary of people who do not understand the gay lifestyle judging as pathological behaviours that are reasonably 'normal' in gay society such as sex in bathhouses, open relationships, the leather scene and so on. Other specialists say you can only apply the term 'addiction' to substance use, in which case sexual compulsivity might be a better term. It is not helped by media stories of Hollywood stars whose marriages break up, or pastors who are caught with prostitutes, blaming it on their 'sex addiction' and seeking 12-step programmes to cure it. But it has long been a recognised syndrome among psychiatrists. And, because of the ease of obtaining commitment-free sex on the gay scene, it is one gay men are particularly vulnerable to.

The classic work on sex addiction is *Out of the Shadows*, written by Patrick Carnes in 1992. It needs to be read critically because it is exclusively heterosexual in its case studies, and wedded to the 12-step model of recovery, which does not suit everyone.

However it describes a world many sex addicts get caught up in - a desperate quest for sex as a 'fix' that compensates for deep feelings of insecurity and loneliness, but which only serves to make them more lonely. People with sex addiction have no problem with sex: the thing they can't do is relationships. The sex becomes a substitute for, not part of, contact with other people and the testosterone rush of orgasm becomes a physical craving which remains unsatisfied. It is no coincidence, perhaps, that 'scoring' is used to mean both buying drugs and finding a sex partner.

In a recent issue of *Positive Nation* magazine (116, October 2005) one interviewee put it thus: "It was important I had a feeling of sexual power; that people found me attractive and that I could exercise that sexual power over them. I find I just can't switch off the cruise instinct. I have to do it, even when it pisses other people off. Like when I'm taking to friends but cruising over their shoulder at the same time. I've lost friends because of it."

Another interviewee found his addiction to anonymous sex only made sense when he was diagnosed with Borderline Personality Disorder. His experience of relationships had been typical of BPD: he would always become clinging and unbearably jealous with partners and suffer huge feelings of abandonment when they were not physically present. He realised he used sex as a way of avoiding relationships, not having them.

Sexual compulsivity is by no means an exclusively gay issue and many heterosexuals have similar issues. Because free sex is less available in the heterosexual world they may be more likely to get involved in the sex industry, either as clients or workers.

There are a number of 12-step and other groups around the UK where people who think they may have sexual compulsion problems can seek support.

Further Reading

Patrick Carnes. Out of the Shadows: Understanding Sexual Addiction. Hazelden, new edition 2001. ISBN 1568386214

Life stages: how HIV may impact upon mental health

Adjustment disorder: reaction to diagnosis

HIV diagnosis or (even more so) falling sick with an HIV-related illness are classic 'stressors' and virtually everyone will react with some degree of mental turmoil as they accommodate their new status - indeed if they don't, they may still be in the stage of denial (see below).

Any severe difficulty in dealing with a profound change of circumstances in life is known as an adjustment disorder. .A shattering event leaves the person scared, shocked, and uncertain. Everything one thought was safe and predictable turns out not to be, explains Professor Maurice Lipsedge, one of the pioneers of mental health services for people with HIV in the UK, who set up the first HIV mental health service at Guy's Hospital in London in the late 1980s. The times when people with HIV are most likely to experience an adjustment disorder are when they first test HIV-positive and, even more likely, when treatment fails and they start becoming ill (of course, for late testers, both of these may happen at once). Bereavement is another trigger, and rejection by a partner due to HIV status can also induce an adjustment disorder.

The particular 'flavour' of adjustment-shock people experience to HIV diagnosis may have changed in the post-HAART era. People are no longer faced with the stark news that they have a terminal illness that may kill them unpleasantly, and there may be fewer anxiety disorders or overt suicidal thoughts during this period. Instead there may be stronger feelings of shame, social isolation and stigma - people may feel they 'should have known better', have let themselves down, or have become ostracised from society (even if the ostracism is only in their own minds - see **stigma** below)

A classic theory of how human beings come to terms with bad news about their health was initially developed by the psychiatrist Elisabeth Kübler-Ross when she worked with cancer patients in the 1960s and was published in her seminal book *On Death and Dying* in 1970.

She was working with terminally-ill patients and indeed in the early days of AIDS was active in working with AIDS patients too. She developed a theory that people react to changed health status and the threat of death in five well-defined stages of accommodation which she labelled Denial, Anger, Bargaining, Depression and Acceptance.

Kübler-Ross's work has been criticised as being overly rigid and because it was initially applied to patients who were terminally ill and therefore geared towards acceptance of death rather than determination to survive. However she was at pains to stress herself that the stages overlap and may happen in a different order or that people may revert to earlier stages at different times. She also - and this is often ignored - wrote another chapter pointing out that human beings faced with illness face it with a sixth characteristic, hope, which is not lost till the person is near death.

Since then her work has been extended to apply to any situation of change which the person regards as a *loss*. This may be loss of a partner as in bereavement or divorce; loss of possessions and material status; loss of home or family; or loss of perceived health and sexual eligibility.

Stages only become psychopathological if the person becomes 'stuck; in them and is afraid to move on to, or lacks the capacity to develop, a different response.

Denial

At first faced with a loss the person may simply refuse to face it. There is nothing pathological in this itself. People who grieve often speak of an initial period of emotional numbness that enables them to carry on with normal life. During this period people often **isolate** themselves too, often because they lack the experience and language to talk about the new situation in which they find themselves. Denial may feel like a positive numbness or inability to react; it may feel like nothing is wrong and the person attempts to ignore their changed situation; or it may be more apparent than real, with the person experiencing shame or fear inside but acting externally as if all was well.

One way denial may become pathological is if the person reacts to their diagnosis by developing what is called a **manic defence**. Although bipolar illness ('manic depression') is not more common in people with HIV than it is in the general population, case reports (see Hutchinson, Yang) continue to appear in the literature of patients who had manic episodes, particularly around the time of progression from HIV to AIDS. Mania is a form of hysterical denial in which the person avoids feelings of despair or loss by 'hyping themselves up' into a state in which they feel super-confident, invulnerable and full of energy. Manic episodes have also been reported when patients start HAART, and it is unclear whether the drugs are having an organic effect or whether the change in status is to blame (see Wise).

People may persist in denial for years and it may be the reason people fail either to seek HIV testing despite illness and knowledge of risk factors or to seek treatment.

References

Hutchinson G. HIV mania as a marker for clinical deterioration in AIDS. West Indian Med J. 54(2): 149-151, 2005.

Wise MEJ. Neuropsychiatric complications of nevirapine treatment. *BMJ* 324: 879, 2002.

Yang CY (http://www.ncbi.nlm.nih.gov/entrez/query.fcgi?db=pubmed&cmd=search&term=%22yang+cy%22%5bauthor%5d) et al. Association of AIDS and bipolar mania with rapid progression to dementia and death. J Chin Med Assoc. 68(2): 92-95, 2005.

Anger

The person may go through a period of seeking 'someone to blame' for their status (and may seek legal advice) or may become very angry about other issues in their lives. Again, anger need not be pathological or impact negatively on the person's life; on the contrary, it may be the spur to get involved in AIDS activism or campaigning on other issues. It only becomes pathological if the person harms themselves or others or seeks refuge in drink or drugs to deal with feelings of rage.

Bargaining

In bargaining, the person attempts to guard against perceived negative changes or deterioration by performing specific activities. They may pursue an intensive fitness regimen or a programme of complementary therapies; they may pray to God in a methodical or intense way or devote themselves to good works. The underlying thinking is "If I do this perfectly enough, I will not get sick". Again bargaining is healthy if the activities turned to have a positive impact on health. It may become harmful if the person sticks rigidly to their chosen programme in the face of deteriorating health and regards other choices (such as taking HIV therapy) as 'failure'. Bargaining may also become pathological if it runs out of control and develops OCD-like characteristics, such as taking up an unreasonable amount of the individual's time and thinking.

Depression

Probably pretty sufficiently covered before - but this depression is specifically *reactive* depression dealing with loss or change, and far from being indicative of mental illness, may be a necessary stage the individual needs to go through to face the reality of their changed condition head-on without the illusions of the previous stages. They are taking a final farewell of whatever they feel they have lost - their life, a deceased partner, their HIV-negative status, a treasured job - whatever.

Acceptance

In the original Kübler-Ross model, this meant finally relinquishing hope and preparing to die. But it can equally well apply to an acceptance of one's changed (and possibly reduced) circumstances and a renewed capacity to embark on the next stage of life.

Further reading

Elisabeth Kübler-Ross. On Death and Dying. Routledge, 1989 (originally published Tavistock, 1970). ISBN 0 415 04015 9.

The Lazarus effect: reactions to recovery

Remember that positive events can be stressors too. One paradoxical result of the extraordinary medical achievement that was the development of HAART, with the resultant recovery, in some cases virtually from their deathbed, of a generation of people with HIV is that depression and anxiety may strike with particular force at the point they get better, not worse.

There aren't many scientific papers that document this phenomenon, usually called "The Lazarus Effect" or "Lazarus Syndrome" after the man raised from the dead by Jesus. But there have been several accounts of it in the gay press.

One correspondent calling himself "The Living Dead" emailed online agony uncle Angelo Pezzote at Westhollywood.com:

"I have been living with HIV for nearly 20 years. Like many, I thought I would be dead by now. Instead, the new drug protocols have kept me very healthy. However, I don't feel joy about my "second chance" at life. I am more depressed, anxious and scared than before there was any real hope for long-term survival."

Pezzote replied:

"You may be shell shocked and lonely, perhaps having seen your partner, young friends and cohort groups die from AIDS. Now older, you may find it difficult to reengage socially to build new support systems. You may face financial difficulties. Your disability benefits can be shut off. You may lack work because no one will hire you after having been out of the workforce for several years. You may face paying off huge debt that piled up while you were waiting to get sick and die. How's all this for your self esteem?"

There are a number of different components to the Lazarus syndrome, some universal to survivors of disaster, others specific to HIV.

- **Survivor guilt.** This was first noticed in Holocaust survivors after World War II. It may seem irrational that people feel bad for having survived while others died. But it can be an extremely potent feeling. The Italian writer Primo Levi was one such holocaust survivor. He was never able to completely 'forgive' himself for surviving Auschwitz and eventually committed suicide in 1987. He said of the holocaust: "The worst survived, that is, the fittest; the best all died." He himself only survived because his knowledge as a chemist was useful to the Nazis and he observed the death of countless friends and contemporaries. People who survive AIDS may blame themselves for the death of a loved one who did not. There are accounts of people offered HAART turning it down because they could not live with the guilt of seeing other family members die for lack of it.

Zinhale Tabethe, a member of the Durban-based Sinikithemba Choir of HIV-positive patients, spoke movingly about the issue at the opening of the 10th Retrovirus Conference in Boston in

2003. On a pilot programme of HAART herself, she spoke in front of other choir members not receiving HAART and visibly ill. She said:

"I am done asking myself, why me? Why did I have to be infected with HIV? Now I ask myself, why me? Why do I get to live when others next to me are dying without treatment?"

This leads on to an allied topic,

- **Multiple bereavement.** Communities such as gay men from 1980-95 and Africans to the present day may have entire families and circles of friends removed by AIDS and find themselves in middle age with none of the relatives and childhood friends others keep with them. In Africa this has reached tragic proportions as some people are facing survival after the death of every other family member, at least of their own generation.

- **Broken careers.** Many people took 'early retirement' assuming they would die and then found themselves having to re-learn to work in middle age at a time when they had lost skills and were less employable. In addition, many people piled up debts because they did not expect they would have to repay them. They may also face returning to the job market having spent a long time unused to the rigors of a nine-to-five job at a time when their health may still be uncertain, whether because of HIV or because of HAART side-effects.

- **Changed relationships.** Partners in a serodiscordant relationship where the positive partner was expected to die may have ignored tensions and disagreements. Given a new lease of life, the positive partner may seek a new partner who they are not tied to simply because they depend on them to care - or the negative partner may realise that the person they were expecting to live a few years with is not the one they want to live with till old age. Related to this is:

- **Renewed interest in sex.** People with AIDS may have gone through a period of not desiring sex or feeling ineligible at a potential partner. Feeling well again, their libido returns - but they are faced possibly with the challenge of learning to disclose their HIV status to prospective partners and certainly with seeking new partners at a time when they are older.

- **Loss of 'specialness'.** AIDS, for all its terror, was a newsworthy and 'glamorous' affliction, with sufferers celebrated in films and plays like *Philadelphia* and *Angels in America* and visited at their bedside by princesses. People may feel a perverse loss of special status now they are no longer 'dying' and may become depressed at realising they are just another ordinary person.

- **Prevention paradoxes.** This is a community rather than an individual concern, but some people with HIV feel at a loss how to present their condition. People determined to show that it is possible to live a full life, including a sex life, with HIV may also feel - or be accused of - underplaying the continued seriousness of HIV infection and encouraging others to rationalise about having unsafe sex. It becomes extremely difficult to know whether to present oneself as a 'victor' or a 'victim'.

- **Long-term mental health issues.** Finally, of course, mental health problems may have pre-existed HIV infection and may indeed have contributed to the individual having HIV in the first place. The need to deal with sex and substance addictions, difficulties with relationships, long-term depression or bipolar illness may become more urgent now that everything is not secondary to facing death. Worries about ageing and even possible neurological problems may be superimposed on these.

Social issues: isolation and stigma

Things like depression and anxiety are not just individual processes, they are social processes. As we said above part of the root cause of depression is the loss of social status, and the perception of that loss.

The Microsoft Word Dictionary defines stigma as the shame or disgrace attached to something regarded as socially unacceptable, but it has been more succinctly described as the process of 'othering' people: treating them as not full members of society, or people who do not deserve to be.

It has a strong moral component, especially as people with HIV tend to come from groups already stigmatised, but the roots of stigma go deeper than any particular religious or moral framework, probably as far back as evolutionary imperatives to avoid disease.

This does not mean stigma cannot be combated and resisted. It has been a problem to address because it is so pervasive and is a matter of half-conscious assumptions people make in their minds rather than a series of actions as such. Stigma in action is **discrimination**, which can at least be addressed legally within a human rights framework. But stigma operates more often on an individual and family level.

Furthermore, it is a two-part process. As the saying says, "It takes a victim to make a bully," and stigma is only complete as an operation when first, a person or group of people regard someone as a 'bad person,' and, secondly the person (sometimes reluctantly or unconsciously) *agrees with them*. The stigma becomes internalised, and depression can be seen as a way of acting out that internalised feeling of being unworthy. A recent USAID paper notes that: "the stigmatised often accept the norms and values that label them as having negative differences. As a result, stigmatised individuals or groups may accept that they "deserve" to be treated poorly and unequally, making resistance to stigma and resulting discrimination even more difficult."

Dr Virginia Bond took part in a four-country study on HIV related stigma and resulting discrimination in Zambia Tanzania & Ethiopia (2001-2003), and, Vietnam (2002-2004). The study was led by International Center for Research on Women (ICRW), Washington (see Resources), which has recently published a report synthesising the findings online (Ogden and Nyblade).

Some of the commonly observed forms of internalised stigma in the ICRW research included loss of hope, feelings of worthlessness (even suicidal feelings) and inferiority, and belief that they no longer had a future. Many people with HIV drop out of school or give up on long term plans. People internalising stigma also isolate themselves from society, friends and family.

Stigma mitigates the effect of HIV treatment and prevention programmes. Although there are waiting lists for testing and treatment services in some settings, in others, available testing services go underutilised and after an initial flurry of activity, enrolment at HIV treatment sites levels off. The demand for HIV services falls short of projections and clinic staff must engage in active case finding within the local communities.

Stigma often manifests as exaggerated fear of contact with and infection by a person with HIV, often despite the person having full knowledge of HIV risk factors. This is particularly troubling when medical personnel adopt these attitudes.

This fear of HIV transmission is amplified when public health campaigns focus primarily on negative images of sick and dying people with HIV and AIDS, as well as by sensationalised media reports about risk-taking behaviour or infected persons purposefully exposing others.

In the ICRW report, a nurse in Ethiopia explained:

"The wards don't have gloves, so how would you expect a nurse to go and attend to a HIV/AIDS patient? That's why you can find a patient lying in a pool of diarrhoea for many hours."

And a health worker in Vietnam admitted:

"We absolutely never inject [HIV] infected persons. We just give them medicines.... We also treat small children here, so we give [HIV] infected people no injections at all."

In addition, there was a tendency across contexts to create a continuum between guilt and innocence related to "how" someone got infected. On the innocent side of the continuum are children, followed by health workers infected by treating their patients; while on the guilty end are the drug users and sex workers. Given that sex work and drug use are already socially unacceptable, the "guilty" infected are doubly stigmatised.

An HIV-infected woman could be near either end of the continuum, depending upon whether she is believed to have become infected while faithful to her husband (innocent) or otherwise (guilty). The role of gender was another key similarity across all contexts. "Women generally bear the strongest brunt of this type of stigma," write Ogden and Nyblade. "The reason underlying this seems to be that women in all of these settings are expected to uphold the moral traditions of their societies. HIV is regarded as evidence that they have failed to fulfil this important social function."

Ogden and Nyblade divide stigma into four loosely defined groups: physical, social, verbal and institutional.

Social stigma

Isolated from community

Voyeurism: any interest may be morbid curiosity or mockery rather than genuine concern

Loss of social role/identity: social 'death', loss of standing and respect

Physical stigma

Isolated, shunned, abandoned

Separate living space, eating utensils

Violence

Verbal stigma

Gossip, taunting, scolding

Labelling: in Africa: "moving skeleton," "walking corpse," and "keys to the mortuary."

In Vietnam: "social evils," and "scum of society."

Institutionalised stigma

Barred from jobs, scholarships, visas

Denial of health services

Police harassment (eg of sex workers, HIV-positive activists in China, outreach workers in India)

One of the interesting things about this research is that though it shows some aspects of stigma are universal, they take different forms in different societies. Thus in an Asian country with a relatively new HIV epidemic, people with HIV are condemned morally; in African countries where the physical devastation of AIDS is more evident, fear of the stigmatised person is more prominent. This fear does not just take place on the levels of exaggerated fears of infection; these fears would not be so powerful if they were not founded in something much deeper; a fear that to associate with the (presumed) dying is somehow to catch not just their disease but their status as outsiders.

Stigma can impact on treatment and testing because it inhibits people from coming forward and it impacts on prevention because, for instance, insisting on condom use is tantamount either to admitting HIV seropositivity or that one has been unfaithful or, to give another example that to bottle-feed one's baby reveals one's status.

But most of all, it impacts on disclosure. It is perhaps fortunate that, if AIDS had to happen at all, the first community it impacted (as far as the world was concerned) were gay men, a group whose entire politics is about refusing to accept stigma. The process of 'coming out' as gay involves a process of refusing to agree to be ashamed of one's sexuality. People who aren't articulate gay men in developed countries - that is, virtually everyone else with HIV - have not had the same experience and groups of stigmatised people who try to self-organise, like sex workers, injecting drug users or indeed gay men in the developing world, may face fierce opposition.

Another difficulty of stigma is that it is not *entirely* irrational. It is rational for an HIV-negative gay man to think twice about having sex with a positive man. It is rational for a poor African family to regard a relative with AIDS as an economic burden.

The impact on mental health should be obvious. People who are stigmatised are *isolated*, and many surveys have shown that social isolation is the strongest predictor of any kind of mental illness. They are also *silenced*, and thus deprived (or deprive themselves) of the process that all psychotherapies try to facilitate.

Information and educational programmes addressing stigma in the individual have had only limited success in the past, so the ICRW report recommends a more in depth and interactive approach, "moderated by a knowledgeable and trusted facilitator. [and] ensuring that people have a deep enough understanding of what HIV is and how it is transmitted so that they are equipped to make correct assessments of actual HIV risk in any given life situation they encounter."

Another approach that incorporates many of these principles is palliative care. Although often associated with end-of-life care or home-based, palliative care is actually a "continuum of care" that begins from the time a person is diagnosed as HIV-positive. Palliative care includes psychosocial and spiritual support to help people with HIV/AIDS and their families cope with stigma and illness. It also includes more emphasis on comfort for people living with HIV/AIDS, relieving or lessening symptoms for people suffering from AIDS.

A well-designed and implemented palliative care programme can include a complete package of services adapted to deal with each social context of stigma, and lessen the burden of caring for a person with HIV in the community.

For more, see **palliative care** below.

In the UK, the report **Outsider Status** (Dodds) interviewed a mixed selection of Africans and gay men with HIV about their experiences of stigma. For the Africans, one of the most painful aspects of HIV stigma was that they had been used to turning to their own communities and families as their one source of support in a world that already stigmatised them as asylum seekers. Becoming HIV-positive made them feel outsiders in their own communities. One African man said:

'I have lost a brother in 1998, but we cannot talk about what killed him. If a person dies, you ask them, what is the problem. "Ah, so and so is bewitching him, so and so is bewitching him." You can't say because of the stigma. If I say, "My brother died of HIV", it takes the courage to talk about it in that manner. As it is now, I have failed. I say, "Today I want to tell my sister and my brother". Each time I leave a support group I say, "Today I want to tell them". But I have failed to tell them that I am positive. It is a stigma that I don't know how to deal with.'

And, as one African woman says, stigma means that HIV is always something that happens to 'other' people:

'They [African cultural organisations] do organise things and they will discuss HIV, but individuals talk about it as if it is happening to someone else and not them. When we go to African groups, they talk about educating people about HIV and nothing else.'

The results is that people with HIV become 'medicalised'; as one African man said,

'It [his family's reaction] kind of isolated me more, because I felt that the only person I could talk to was maybe my doctor, the counsellors, or other people at the clinic.'

One answer to this 'medicalisation' is to refuse to accept the passive role of patient ('patient' and 'passive' as words come from the same root) and join support groups and patients' rights organisations, not just as support members within HIV charities, but within the wider NHS.

This process goes far beyond a mere interest in one's own rights or in institutional structures; indeed one needs to gather confidence and knowledge before one can stand up for oneself. The way an individual can move from being 'acted upon' to being in charge of their own condition and life may be termed self actualisation or self management and is discussed under self-management of life with HIV below.

The gay men in the **Outsider Status** report felt, on the whole, a less keen sense of ostracism but one interesting finding was that rejection by their biological family was just as important to them as to the Africans. One man said:

'It is soul destroying to put them through that pain. Sometimes I so want to tell my mother or my sister, so that they understand me a lot better, but realistically I don't think they could tell me the things I need. So instead of feeling less isolated, it would probably isolate me more. I would have to handle that on top of everything else.'

The sense that one is a **burden to others** - or would be, if they knew the truth - is a central part of the experience of depression.

Gay men also felt a complex mix of shame at their own sexual behaviour and anger at the perceived irresponsibility of other gay men with HIV. One said:

'Isn't it part of the prejudice of HIV and part of the guilt that is attached to it, is that you already feel responsible? Or feel that you lack responsibility for allowing yourself to be infected in the first place?'

But another commented:

'I know people who do that on the Gay scene, shagging around to infect as many people as possible to make it easier for themselves.'

This illustrates the point that one of the things stigma does is to isolate stigmatised people from each other, not just from their own communities.

Stigma is a highly complex subject and not something that can be legislated away. Information and education programmes have only had limited success in the past in combating it, though continuing to help people explore, via facilitated groups, rational and irrational fears about HIV transmission and what it is like living with HIV will continue to form a valuable and necessary part of HIV education and social support. There are some online resources available designed to suggest interventions and measure their effectiveness.

Resources, toolkits and tools to measure the effectiveness of interventions

Understanding and challenging HIV stigma: toolkit for action

Growing out of ICRW's four-country study, this Toolkit provides "evidence-based guidance for launching stigma-reduction activities with key groups, including religious and political leaders, people living with HIV and AIDS, and community members."

The toolkit contains more than 125 exercises and was developed through interactive, participatory workshops in all three African countries, with a total of 75 participants from 50 NGOs. The toolkit since has also been adapted for use in Vietnam. The first edition was developed in Africa and is available in English and Kiswahili. An adaptation of the first edition for the Asian context is available in both English and Vietnamese.

http://www.changeproject.org/technical/hivaids/stigma.html

Reducing stigma and discrimination related to HIV and AIDS: training for health care workers

The training course guides health workers through an investigation of the root causes of stigma and discrimination while helping them to understand their own attitudes about HIV, AIDS, and individuals affected by these conditions and how these attitudes might affect the care they offer. The training also provides a review of clients' rights in receiving health care services, information about the use of standard precautions and proper infection prevention techniques to help minimise the risk of occupational exposure to HIV, and guidance in developing action plans to help the participants put what they have learned into practice at their service settings. The training employs participatory education techniques such as role-plays, small- and large-group discussions, and brainstorming.

http://www.engenderhealth.org/res/offc/hiv/stigma/

The Siyam'kela Project: measuring HIV/AIDS related stigma

Siyam'kela (SI-YUH-MU-GE-LAR) is an African word from the Nguni language. Translated it means "We Are Accepting" expressing a collective embracing, understanding and acceptance of a challenge at a particular time. The word has thus been interpreted as "Together We Stand" for this project.

Siyam'kela has been designed to explore HIV-related stigma and is a joint project of the POLICY Project, South Africa; The Centre for the Study of AIDS, University of Pretoria; The United States Agency for International Development (USAID); and The Chief Directorate: HIV/AIDS & TB, Department of Health.

The project is an excellent resource with research papers, stigma mitigation guidelines for faith-based organisations and the workplace, best practices, as well as a tool programmes can use to measure the progress of HIV/AIDS stigma mitigation.

http://www.csa.za.org/article/articleview/228/1/6/

References

Bond V et al. Kanayaka-"The Light is On": Understanding HIV and AIDS- related Stigma in Urban and Rural Zambia. Lusaka: Zambart Project and KCTT, 2003

Dodds C et al. Outsider status: Stigma and discrimination experienced by gay men and African people with HIV. Sigma Research, 2004. Available online from http://www.sigmaresearch.org

Ogden J and Nyblade L. Common at its Core: HIV-Related Stigma Across Contexts. International Center for Research on Women, 2005.

(see online http://www.icrw.org/docs/2005_report_stigma_synthesis.pdf)

Self-management of life with HIV

Introduction

Everybody 'self-manages' all the time. In terms of health self-management might include: eating well, taking exercise or taking steps to manage stress. This 'self-management' can be almost unconscious, particularly when we are otherwise healthy.

Most people will also seek to self-manage minor illness. Sales of non-prescription remedies bear this out and it is clear that the majority of responses to illness are some form of self-management behaviour.

Not surprisingly self-management is even more important to people living with complex, serious long-term conditions. This is as true of HIV as it is of Diabetes, MS or heart disease.

Historically self-management has been important to people living with HIV. In pre-HAART days many of the health strategies and much of the activism around HIV were a form of self-management. As early as 1987 the Frontliners book "Living With HIV" advocated an approach strongly rooted in self-management. This continues, the recent NAM book also called

"Living with HIV" is very much about "taking control" for yourself and self-managing the consequences of living with HIV.

For a person living with HIV today self-management will be about the social and emotional consequences of living with the condition as much as the medical consequences. It will be as much about dealing with the fears and frustrations of living with HIV as it will be about dealing with side-effects or planning meals around medications.

Medical management and self-management compliment each other and there is no conflict between them. A person who self-manages their condition well will make the very best use of the resources offered by the health care system. Health is often described as a "co-productive process" and self-management is part of this.

Everybody has self-management skills but their level, and how we use them, will vary from person to person and at different times during our lives. In addition at times we may lose confidence in our ability to self-manage - people often express this as a "loss of control." Fortunately it is possible to learn, or relearn, self-management skills and there are many interventions that seek to achieve this.

What is self-management?

One definition is:

"Self-management is the means by which people can develop confidence and skills to take control of the daily management of their illness. The aim is to achieve the greatest possible quality of life by working with professionals to make the best use of all resources."

LMCA, Supporting Expert Patients

There are many interventions designed to improve self-management skills. Most of them work by some combination of information provision, learning skills and changing attitudes. The balance between these elements varies but each plays a part:

1. Information

In order to manage life with HIV it is essential to have reliable, relevant and understandable information sources. Given the speed of change in treatments these information sources need to be regularly updated. The information needs of people living with HIV in the UK are well served by organisations such as NAM and THT. Much of this information focuses on things we can do for ourselves or on improving our understanding HIV and its treatment. Both reinforce attitudes supportive of self-management.

2. Skills

Life requires many management skills. These are analogous to those required in the workplace. Skills such as planning, problem solving and time management are all the more important when living with HIV. Juggling hospital appointments and medication regimes make these skills essential. Good communication skills are valuable to anyone but doubly useful if one has to deal with an issue like disclosure. Many of these skills can be taught.

3. Attitudes

Dealing with the emotional, physical and social consequences of living with HIV requires confidence that one can deal with them. This confidence is often lost as a result of the effect of living with HIV but it is possible to regain it.

Developing skills and changing attitudes can be more difficult than providing information. And information will not be used, to best effect, if users lack the skills to use it or the confidence that it will "work for them." For this reason self-management programmes that concentrate on skills and attitudes are particulary valuable. The **Positive Self-Management Programme** (PSMP), which originated in work undertaken at Stanford University in the USA, is an example of this type of programme.

Given that the PSMP has strong links to the approach widely used within the **Expert Patients Programme** (EPP) in Britain the rest of this section will focus on it, however much of what is said about the PSMP will be true for other "self-management" interventions.

Self-management in context

Self-management is very much of the moment. The government strategy for dealing with the effects of long-term (or chronic) illness has self-management and self-care at its centre. There has been recognition that the development of self-management skills

can make a significant impact on health outcomes and quality of life. This is reflected in government funding of the Expert Patient Programme, which has brought self-management programmes to every Primary Care Trust area in England and to most Local Health Boards in Wales.

The process which lead to this situation began with work carried out by Professor Kate Lorig (then a graduate student) at Stanford University in the 1970s. Initially her work focussed on the creation of a programme for people with arthritis. Its aim was to introduce them to a range of techniques which would allow them to feel more in control of their arthritis on a day to day basis. Crucially a second aim was to produce a programme, which could be delivered by people living with arthritis themselves - the courses were to be "lay led."

The research results for the initial arthritis programme were so successful that further work was undertaken to develop a generic approach applicable to any chronic disease. This course now known as the Chronic Disease Self-Management Course has been used successfully throughout the world. Today Professor Lorig heads a dedicated team at Stanford's Centre for Patient Education Research. They develop, promote and research the programme as well as providing training to course leaders.

Lay led self-management was introduced to the UK in 1994 by Arthritis Care who continue to run their "Challenging Arthritis" programmes to the present day. By 1998 the Chronic Disease Self-Management Course (CDSMC) was introduced to Britain with the British Liver Trust being one of the first organisations to be involved.

At about the same time a research project led by the Long Term Medical Conditions Alliance (LMCA) began. In partnership with eight of its member organisations LMCA sought to develop knowledge about self-management in a UK context and increase the number of self-management programmes being used. This project (the Living With a Long Term Illness or LILL project) ran for over two years, was highly successful and may be credited with "kick starting" the development of lay led self-management in the UK. It was also, given the involvement of the Haemophilia Society and British Liver Trust, the first time that people living with HIV experienced this form of self-management programme in Britain.

The statutory sector first began to show interest in the possibilities of lay led self-management soon after the successful completion of the LILL project. Government intent was first signalled by the publication of "The Expert Patient: A New Approach to Chronic Disease Management for the 21st Century" in September 2001.

This document included the following commitments:

- To appoint Expert Patients Programme trainers in each Strategic Health Authority area.

- To create central co-ordinating and training resources to promote self-management in both public and voluntary sectors.

- To run a nationwide programme of CDSMC.

- To scientifically evaluate the effectiveness of the program.

Much of this work has been carried out in partnerships with voluntary sector providers though it is fair to say that the sheer scale of the Expert Patients Programme has overshadowed voluntary sector delivery.

The Expert Patients Programme has been a great success. To date there have been more than 1400 CDSMC courses run by 600 volunteer lay tutors. Structures for training course leaders cover the whole of England and Wales and the programme is now being introduced in Northern Ireland. Quality standards have been agreed which ensure that programmes operate to the same standards nationally. Evaluation results to date have clearly demonstrated the potential benefits of lay lead self-management training and the CDSMC is increasingly seen as part of mainstream NHS activity.

Lay led self-management and HIV

Small numbers of people living with HIV have attended CDSMP courses since the beginning of the LILL project in 1999. A number have become more deeply involved in the programme and have trained in leading courses.

However it has always been unlikely that large numbers of people living with HIV would be attracted to EPP courses as the generic nature of the courses means that they are usually for mixed groups in local community settings. This, of itself, would make attendance difficult for anyone with concerns over disclosure.

A number of CDSMP courses have been run specifically for people living with HIV, notably at Positively Women in London and at THT in Bristol and Cardiff, but development was slow. Participants in at least one of the courses felt that the "action oriented" nature of the course was perfect for people living with HIV but that the course failed to address specific issues around sex and intimacy, disclosure and medication.

The real spur to lay led self-management of HIV in the UK has been the availability of a "condition specific course" - the Positive Self-Management Programme (PSMP).

The PSMP was developed at Stanford University in the mid 1990s by a team lead by Allen Gifford. The course is directly derived from the CDSMC retaining its advantages while addressing specific concerns related to living with HIV.

The PSMP was first offered as a pilot in San Francisco in 1994. Further pilots were conducted by Kaiser Permanente at their Medical Centres in Oakland and San Francisco during 1995.

British interest in the PSMP followed publication of initial research results from the American pilots. It came from a number of sources: people working in HIV services (some of whom were able to go to Stanford and receive training), senior trainers working in the EPP and people living with HIV who were already involved with the CDSMP.

At the outset it was very much a case of interested individuals working independently however all parties involved collaborated to ensure that the American programme was revised to be appropriate for UK circumstances. All have agreed to work with standard material and within agreed quality standards. These standards, also adopted by the EPP and voluntary sector providers of the CDSMC, have been published (Stepping Stones to Success - NHS Expert Patients Programme, 2005).

To date the majority of PSMP courses have been held in London (where they are offered by voluntary organisations and NHS "Living Well" programmes) and Manchester (where they are offered by Body Positive North West). As capacity to deliver courses grows, and more organisations become interested, a gradual spread to other areas is now beginning.

To date there have been approximately 30 programmes in the UK. There is a strong core of trainers who continue to develop the programme and British trainers are active in attempting to develop programmes in Europe and Africa.

The Positive Self-Management Programme

Several important assumptions underlie the PSMP:

- People with long-term (chronic) conditions, such as HIV/AIDS have similar concerns and problems.

- People with HIV/AIDS must deal not only with their disease but also with the impact it has on their lives and emotions.

- Peers with HIV/AIDS, when given training and a detailed leaders manual, can teach the PSMP as effectively as health professionals.

The process, or way the PSMP is taught, is as important, if not more important, than the subject matter that is taught.

PSMP Leaders Manual, Stanford University 2002.

These principles are exactly the same as those that underlie the CDSMC.

The PSMP consists of seven sessions each of which is 2 ½ hours in duration. They are generally completed over seven successive weeks. Groups of 8 -16 participants work together with two leader/facilitators in a highly participative process. Throughout the emphasis is on the group identifying problems and finding solutions for themselves.

At least one of the two leaders is a person living with HIV. The other leader may be a health professional or a person living with another long-term condition but the course is specifically designed to be delivered by lay volunteers with real experience of living with conditions. The "role-modelling" aspect of having a leader living with the condition is fundamental to the success of the approach. Many people involved with self-management believe that the best results can be achieved where both leaders live with a condition themselves

All course leaders will have attended a standard training programme and will have passed a process of accreditation. They are monitored regularly by trained assessors in order to ensure that quality standards are maintained.

PSMP Content

During the programme the following subjects are covered:

Overview of self-management and chronic conditions (figures indicate the weeks when covered):

- Medication issues: 1,2,3

- Goal setting: 1,2,3,4,5,6,7

- Problem solving: 2,3,4,5,6,7

- Dealing with difficult emotions: 2

- Cognitive symptom management: 2,4,5,6

- Working with your health care team: 3,4

- Evaluating common symptoms: 3

- Depression management: 4

- Changing negative thinking: 4

- Understanding laboratory tests: 4

- Making treatment decisions: 4

- Advance directives/ Living Wills: 5

- Sex, intimacy and disclosure: 5

- Communication skills: 5

- Fatigue management: 6

- Healthy eating: 6

- Exercise: 7

- Building support systems and finding resources: 7

- Future plans: 7

These activities can conveniently be divided into two types:

- learning skills, and

- using skills/information to deal with commonly experienced problems.

For example participants learn problem-solving skills then apply them to commonly experienced problems with medication such as poor adherence. They learn simple relaxation and distraction techniques and to use them to ameliorate common problems such as fatigue, anxiety or the side-effects of medications.

Learning skills

1. Action planning:

Action planning is simple step-by-step process to encourage participants to make successful changes in their behaviour. Goals are broken down into manageable units and worked on week by week. Success breeds success and growing confidence.

2. Problem solving:

Standard problem solving techniques are used to identify the real problems facing participants and to find workable solutions. The technique is practised in every element of the programme particularly when dealing with barriers people experience in achieving their action plans.

3. Cognitive techniques:

Participants are taught to use techniques such as breath control, distraction and guided imagery. Their use in symptom control is of value in itself but practice also encourages participants in becoming confident that they can "do something" for themselves.

4. Communication skills:

Participants learn listening skills, paraphrasing, the use of non-accusatory language and other communication techniques. Practising the use of these techniques is part of the basic course process.

Using skills to address common problems

The PSMP addresses the most commonly reported problems of people living with HIV. Many of these (for example dealing with depression, exercise or healthy eating) relate to anybody with a long-term condition and are covered in the CDSMC in much the same way. Others are more specific to HIV (for example much of the medication content and sex, intimacy and disclosure).

Each issue is dealt with in three ways:

1. Problem solving:

The group identify their problems and identify solutions together.

2. By provision of basic information:

The PSMP concentrates on the "essentials," key messages about which there is little possibility of argument. Thus the section on healthy eating concentrates on messages such as "5 a day," regular meals with all food groups and "drink more fluids."

3. By signposting other resources:

Throughout there is an emphasis on helping participants to identify sources of information and other resources for themselves. Each activity covered includes references to more detailed sources of information and there are specific activities that consider other community resources. In addition great care is taken to refer participants to health care professionals, as their most important resource, whenever appropriate.

Finding resources and information

The ability to find resources, particularly information, is an important part of building participants' confidence that they can increase their control over the situation. In this, signposting to outside sources can be more effective than providing the information in lecture form. In the US all programme participants receive a workbook ("Living Well with HIV and AIDS" Gifford, Lorig, Laurent and Gonzalez). This contains a mixture of generic self-management advice and more detailed advice on HIV related topics.

While this is an excellent book it had disadvantages in a UK context as it reflected US experience of living with HIV and treatment protocols which differ from British ones. In addition it was felt that any workbook would rapidly become out of date given the pace of change in HIV treatment.

In order to overcome these problems the references in the UK version of the PSMP are to NAM factsheets, Information Series booklets and the Treatments manual. Participants have indicated that they particularly value being introduced to this source of authoritative, readily available and multi-level information, which is continually updated. In addition participants are provided with a workbook developed by the EPP ("Self-Management of Long-term Health Conditions - A Handbook for People with Chronic Disease"- NHS Expert Patients Programme) which EPP use this alongside the generic CDSMC. This covers and reinforces the principles and techniques of self-management from the course and deals with issues common to anybody living with a long-term condition.

Building self-efficacy

The PSMP, like the other Stanford programmes, works by building participants Self-Efficacy in relation to their health. Self-Efficacy is the confidence or belief that you can make changes that will help you to manage aspects of life better. Participants often refer to this effect of the programme as feeling "more in control" or being "more confident."

Given that the programmes encourage changes in health behaviours, and that participants do in fact make changes it was initially assumed that reported improvements in health status resulted from changed behaviour. However further investigation showed little correlation between changes in behaviours and changes in health status and that the main factor was participants' beliefs about what they could achieve.

Work by Albert Bandura, Professor of Social Psychology at Stanford had demonstrated that:

- Belief in one's ability is a good predictor of motivation and behaviour.

- Self-Efficacy beliefs can be enhanced.

- Enhanced self-efficacy leads to improved motivation, thinking patterns and emotional well-being.

Thus someone who is confident that they can exert some control over the emotional distress resulting from their condition is likely to experience less distress. When new scales to measure these effects were developed it became clear that the principle effect of the programmes was in enhancing Self-Efficacy.

During the PSMP Self-Efficacy is enhanced in a number of ways:

1. Skills mastery:

Skills such as Action Planning, Problem Solving and relaxation techniques are learnt and practiced - the main skills are used repeatedly in different contexts during the course to ensure that they are internalised. The programme encourages success by keeping the skills simple and by encouraging participants in making small achievable steps. Participants are able to build on these successes and grow in confidence.

2. Modelling:

The techniques learnt in the course are modelled by the leaders when they are introduced. The fact that they are people living with HIV themselves is key to participants' belief that they too can achieve change. Confidence is also derived from observing and participating in the success of others within the group.

3. Reinterpreting symptoms:

The course challenges the belief that everything negative experienced by the participant is a direct result of HIV. It encourages problem solving behaviours, which build confidence that "something can be done" to break out of negative cycles.

4. Persuasion:

By setting goals, making action plans and learning skills in a safe environment people are persuaded to try new activities and make changes. The group support each other in successfully achieving against goals and in problem solving any barriers experienced and the effect seems to be cumulative.

It is clear that Self-Efficacy is a transferable attitude. Many participants make changes in areas of life, such as returning to work, which may not be directly connected to health. It is also apparent that for many participants regaining Self-Efficacy is a catalyst for longer-term changes which continue well after the programme.

Research - the CDSMC

To date there has been considerably more research relating to the CDSMC than the PSMP. Given that people living with HIV/AIDS experience many of the same problems as other people living with other severe long-term conditions, and that the core of the two courses is the same, one would expect similar gains.

The CDSMC has been subjected to research in a wide number of countries and contexts. Even when different research methods are used the results seem to be remarkably consistent with general improvements in both the medical and social effects of conditions:

"The accumulated research is impressive and sufficient to be able to describe the Chronic Disease Self-Management Course (CDSMC) and the Arthritis Self-Management Course (ASMC) as evidence based self-management courses."

Supporting Expert Patients, LMCA

Typical outcomes of attending a self-management course which are supported by most studies include:

1. Slowing of physical deterioration: Participants' physical status deteriorates slower than would have been expected following attendance.

2. Improved Self-Efficacy: Scores developed to measure Self-Efficacy show a marked improvement. People take active steps in respect of their health and re-engage with activities they wish to pursue

3. Improvements to psychological state: There is a decrease in levels of depression and anxiety.

4. Increased use of health promoting techniques: Not only do people adopt techniques such as exercise or relaxation they persevere with them. Long-term studies show a good proportion of participants still using techniques 12 months, and even four years, after their course.

5. Reduction in visits to doctors: While in some instances there was an increase in visits as participants sought to deal with issues raised, twelve months after participation a pattern of reducing visits is apparent.

6. Improved communication with doctors: This improvement occurs whether measured by course participant or clinician report.

To date published evidence related to UK experience is confined to that published in "From Patient to Person: The Living Well Report" - Jane Cooper, LMCA. This fully supports the typical results outlined above and suggests that self-management programmes can be effective in a UK context.

The much larger study being conducted by the EPP has yet to be published however some interim results have been reported at conferences. These suggest that for participants in EPP courses:

- 10% more take medicine as prescribed.

- 30% feel better prepared for consultations with health professionals.

- 30% show significant reductions in feelings of depression.

- 30% feel they have more energy.

- 20-30% felt pain, breathlessness and tiredness less intense.

- 30-50% were more confident they would not let pain, breathlessness, tiredness or depression interfere with life.

- 9% fewer visits to GPs.

- 6% fewer visit to A&E.

- 9% fewer visits to outpatients.

- 15% increase in visits to pharmacists.

Research - the PSMP

To date no UK research into the PSMP has been published. The main evidence relates to the initial pilot study in San Francisco. This study was a randomised control trial of 74 men living with symptomatic HIV/AIDS and looked at symptom severity, Self-Efficacy and health behaviours.

The results of the study for the group who had participated in the PSMP include:

- A reduction in the severity of symptoms reported.

- An increase in measures of Self-Efficacy for controlling symptoms.

- A trend towards greater physical activity.

Changes in use of anti-stress and relaxation techniques were not significant and there was no difference in knowledge about HIV/AIDS.

Although this study was relatively small it does support the idea that self-management will work for people living with HIV/AIDS in much the same way as for other conditions. Further research results, as yet unpublished but reported at conferences, suggest that people who have attended PSMP courses have significantly better medication adherence and higher CD4 counts when followed up over time.

Evaluations of British programmes are underway however to date results have not been published. Unfortunately there is no nationwide process of evaluation of the PSMP at present.

Self-management of HIV/AIDS: the future

There will always be a need for self-management skills for people living with HIV/AIDS. This need does not diminish with improving treatments though the skills and knowledge required may change. Self-management reflects and supports the opportunities offered by better treatment.

Self-management may play a role in developing a new activism among people living with HIV/AIDS. Active involvement in ones own health is often a significant step towards a desire for involvement in the health care system as a whole. There has been an increasing emphasis on public and patient involvement in the management of health services in recent years and many people who have been involved with the CDSMC and PSMP have gone on to roles in formal involvement structures.

The introduction of the PSMP to the UK is an opportunity to build on other approaches to self-management which have always been available to people with HIV/AIDS. The links between the PSMP and the CDSMC can contribute to this opportunity particularly given the importance of the EPP in future arrangements for the management of long-term conditions.

Many course leaders who live with HIV/AIDS now deliver CDSMC programmes. This can assist in breaking down barriers between people living with HIV/AIDS and people with other conditions.

Opportunities exist to use the approach to help other groups affected by HIV including young people living with HIV and partners and families of people living with HIV. It will be possible to integrate the PSMP with wider service packages. Already the NHS Living Well Programmes in London use the PSMP as part of an overall approach to supporting people.

At present the development of the PSMP on a national basis is held back by the lack of a central co-ordinating body. While there have been developments in parts of London and in Manchester it is difficult to see rapid national progress without the support of a national HIV organisation or possibly the EPP. At the very

least this central co-ordinating function is necessary to ensure that consistency and quality standards are maintained and that research and development into the approach continues.

Further reading

From Patient to Person: The Living Well Report - Jane Cooper, LMCA, 2004

Living Well with HIV and AIDS - Allen L. Gifford, Kate Lorig, Diana Laurent, Virginia Gonzalez - Bull Publishing 2000

Partnerships for Successful Self-Management - The Living With a Long Term Illness (LILL) Project Report - Jane Cooper, LMCA, 2001.

Patient Education: A Practical Approach- Thousand Oaks Publications 2001

Self-Management of Long-term Health Conditions A Handbook for People with Chronic Disease - NHS Expert Patients Programme - Bull Publishing, 2002

Stepping Stones to Success - An Implementation, Training and Support Framework for Lay led Self-Management Programmes - Department of Health, 2005

Supporting Expert Patients - How to develop lay led self-management programmes for people with long-term medical conditions, LMCA/NHS 2003

The Expert Patient: A new approach to Chronic Disease Management for the 21st Century - Department of Health, 2001

References

Lorig KR, Sobel DS, Stewart AL, Brown BW, Ritter PL, Gonzalez VM, Laurent DD, Holman HR. Evidence suggesting that a chronic disease self-management group intervention will improve health status while reducing utilisation and costs. Medical Care 37(1): 5-14, 1988.

Gifford AL, Laurent DD, Gonzalez VM, Chesney MA, Lorig KR. Pilot randomised trial of education to improve self-management skills of men with symptomatic HIV/AIDS. Journal of Acquired Immune Deficiency Syndrome and human Retrovirology 18(2): 136-144, 1988

Gifford et al. Effects of Group HIV Patient Education on Adherence to Antiretrovirals: A randomised control trial. Paper presented to the 8th Conference on Retroviruses and Opportunistic Infections 2001.

Websites:

Stanford University Centre for Patient Education Research: *www.stanford.edu* (http://www.stanford.edu)

Long Term Medical Conditions Alliance: *www.lmca.org.uk* (http://www.lmca.org.uk/)

Expert Patients Programme: *www.expertpatients.nhs.uk* (http://www.expertpatients.nhs.uk/)

Treatment for mental health problems

Mental health services have been characterised as the 'Cinderella service' of the NHS. Although it is true that compared with some of the high technology and advanced drug research conducted in other areas of medicine - including HIV - mental health has lagged behind, this is as much to do with the nature of mental illness as it is to tack of resources. The social nature of much mental distress means that there will never be a perfect pharmacological or surgical intervention to 'cure' or treat it. Mental health is as much a matter of learning to live as productively and successfully in society as one can it is of correcting some inner imbalance in the brain. This especially applies to the neurotic conditions like depression, anxiety and adjustment problems that form the vast majority of mental illness.

Because of this as well as NHS services a whole profession - counselling and psychotherapy - has emerged over the last century. While some therapists work within the NHS, others can only be seen privately or offer some of their time to voluntary organisations. This inevitably and unfortunately means that social inequality is built into mental health services: those that can pay for it tend to get the best help.

However, while there are not as many resources as there used to be in the provision of counselling and support within HIV organisations, it is still possible for people with HIV to get dedicated counselling or psychotherapy - usually of a time-limited nature - for free or at subsidised cost.

Emphasising counselling or psychotherapy does not imply that pharmacological interventions are not of value. In the case of people with severe problems like schizophrenia or bipolar illness they may be absolutely necessary for the person to live a life with any degree of quality. Even with more common conditions, the impact of severe depression or acute anxiety is often so intense - and intensely physical - that drug treatment is often necessary to help the person get into a state where they can think and respond clearly enough to benefit from psychotherapy.

However antidepressants and other drugs, though they may offer symptom relief, do not in themselves help the person resolve personal crises or address deep-seated life patterns that may have caused the mental distress in the first place. A number of studies (see, for instance, de Jonghe) have found that antidepressant treatments work better if combined with psychotherapy than they do alone, and cognitive therapy (see below) may have particular value in preventing the recurrence of depression (see, for instance, Bockting).

When it comes to anxiety, several studies (e.g. Antoni) have not only shown that cognitive psychotherapy helps to reduce anxiety symptoms but also improves the immune function of people with anxiety.

Seeking treatment

There are two barriers to accessing mental health help. One is waiting lists; while it may be possible to get a prescription for antidepressants from your GP as fast as for any other illness, psychiatry services as well as counselling offered by voluntary agencies may have long waiting lists of weeks to months. This particularly applies to psychotherapy accessed through the NHS.

The other barrier is to do with the nature of mental illness itself and the stigma against it. People may feel ashamed of having depression, anxiety or other conditions; they may even lack terms to adequately describe what they feel like inside. Depression, in particular, may 'creep up' on people so that what starts as a low mood may become an incapacitating illness step by step. It is also in the nature of depression for the person to feel that they 'should' be able to help themselves and that they do not 'deserve'

professional help. In many cases it is the patient's friends or family who make an initial referral for this reason, though it is important that the person acknowledges they have a problem for the more psychotherapeutic interventions to be successful.

A few definitions

There are a confusing (and rather similar-sounding) number of professional labels attached to people who work in mental health.

- **Psychiatrist**

This is a medically-qualified doctor who had undergone additional training to become a specialist in mental health. He or she may not have undergone training in psychotherapy, though many psychiatrists will have done. They will be the Responsible Medical Officer under the Mental Health Act if you are detained and authorise prescription of medication.

- **Psychologist**

This essentially means anyone who has completed a degree (usually at least a Masters) in psychology. A **clinical psychologist** is someone who works in a medical setting and who "aims to reduce psychological distress and enhance and promote psychological wellbeing". While not being in charge of patients' medication, they may be in charge of therapy programmes and case-management.

- **Psychiatric nurse**

This is someone qualified as a nurse who has taken additional mental health training. Some work in hospital settings and may be the first mental health professional you see if you refer yourself to A&E; others work within the community to help and monitor people with mental health problems.

- **Occupational therapist**

This is not a mental health specialist, but a therapist who works with people with any disability to help them improve their capacity to live a relatively normal life within their disability. May become involved with someone with mental health issues if their condition involves physical incapacity, e.g. dementia.

- **Psychotherapist/counsellor**

At present these terms have no legal definition as such: see **private counselling and psychotherapy** for the current regulatory and training framework. Anyone can in theory call themselves a counsellor or psychotherapist. However any worth consulting should have undergone a fairly rigorous process of training and accreditation.

- **The difference between counselling and psychotherapy**

The difference is in the main one of degree rather than kind; they are essentially the same activity. **Counselling** will more often tend to be of a time-limited nature and will try to help the client address specific presenting problems in their lives; **psychotherapy** will more often tend to be open-ended, with termination of treatment decided between practitioner and client, and will tend to address deeper, more unconscious and longer-term patterns of behaviour. There is a tendency for psychotherapy training to be longer and more theory-based than counselling training. However none of these are hard and fast rules; there is, for instance, an established school of brief psychotherapy and counselling may be open ended. Neither label implies more or less expertise or experience on the part of the practitioner.

- **Psychoanalyst**

This means a psychotherapist trained in a particular tradition. The strict definition is someone trained specifically in the teachings and tradition of Sigmund Freud. A broader definition includes the tradition of certain other pioneering figures in psychotherapy such as Carl Jung, Melanie Klein and Donald Winnicott. Psychoanalysis is in general a particularly intensive (and expensive) form of psychotherapy. It is more likely to involve several treatment sessions a week and most psychoanalysts (except some Jungians) use the traditional technique of the client lying on a couch rather than sitting on a chair.

Primary Care

General practitioners are often the first port of call for patients seeking help. GPs can prescribe drugs for the milder conditions, and many general practices have counsellors either attached to the practice or a register of counsellors they can refer people to. If either patient of doctor feels, however, that the condition is severe or in danger of becoming so, there should be no hesitation in recommending or seeking referral to a psychiatrist.

HIV care

The first port of call for many patients will be their HIV physician. Most of the larger HIV clinics have specialist teams of counsellors and mental health professionals attached to the clinic or who have short-cut referral arrangements with the clinic. Your HIV doctor him/herself may be able to prescribe antidepressants and other medication but for cost reasons this is becoming increasingly more restricted and they may want you to see the psychiatrist for assessment if you need any drugs for mental conditions. Practice varies by clinic.

Psychiatric care

Mental health services in the NHS, perhaps in acknowledgment of the atypical nature of mental illness, are organised and administered separately from primary care or hospital trusts. However in practice this makes little difference to referral pathways, as most large teaching hospitals will have a mental health unit attached.

The important thing for a patient to know is that referral to a psychiatrist does not mean that they are considered 'mad'; many people need psychiatric help to see them through a crisis.

Emergency referral

A person in severe crisis is a severely ill person, and episodes of severe mental illness, especially with life-threatening characteristics such as suicidality, violent behaviour, disabling panic attacks or drink or drug intoxication should be treated as medical emergencies. All hospitals with Accident and Emergency departments have a psychiatric liaison service with psychiatric nurses in attendance during the day and on call at other times.

For emergency situations where the person has to be detained for safety reasons, the **Mental Health Act** 1983 comes into play.

The Mental Health Act

This Act is currently undergoing revision in Parliament, and some revisions have caused controversy, dealing as they do with a small fraction of the population who have severe personality disorder that may *predispose* them to be a danger to the public but who do not have a diagnosed mental illness presently. However these changes are unlikely to affect the vast majority of people who come into contact with mental health services.

The Mental Health Act (MHA), in a nutshell, attempts to define 'mental impairment' or 'psychopathic disorder' in a legal rather than medical way as an illness which "is associated with abnormally aggressive or seriously irresponsible conduct on the part of the person concerned". However it does *not* define 'mental illness' per se, even though people do not have to have legally-defined 'mental impairment' to be detained under the MHA.

The Department of Health has attempted a definition of 'mental illness' that is not as such enshrined in law but may be used by

practitioners working under the Mental Health Act. It must include one or more of the following features:

- More than temporary impairment of intellectual functions shown by a failure of memory, orientation, comprehension or learning capacity.

- More than temporary alteration of mood of such degree as to give rise to the patient having a delusional appraisal of his situation, his past or his future, or that of others or to the lack of any appraisal.

- Delusional beliefs, persecutory, jealous or grandiose.

- Abnormal perceptions associated with delusional misinterpretation of events.

- Thinking so disordered as to prevent the patient making a reasonable appraisal of his situation or having reasonable communication with others.

Importantly, the MHA states very clearly that people must *not* be deemed to have a form of Mental Disorder "by reason only of promiscuity or other immoral conduct, sexual deviancy or dependence on alcohol or drugs".

The MHA empowers certain professionals to detain people who are considered to be a danger to themselves or the public and fit one of the above definitions. This is known familiarly as being 'sectioned'.

Sections 2 and 3 require two professionals (usually a psychiatrist and a social worker qualified under the Act) to authorise detention for, respectively, up to 28 days (non-renewable) for assessment and six months (renewable) for treatment.

Section 4, which is quite rarely used, allows a single medical professional to detain a person in an emergency situation for up to 72 hours.

Section 5 allows a doctor or nurse to prevent someone who is already in hospital on a voluntary basis from discharging themselves for up to 72 hours.

Sections 135 and 136 allow a police officer to take someone from a public place or from their home to a 'place of safety' (usually meaning a hospital) where they can be assessed. This is not a 'section' as such.

Other sections allow for particular types of detention ordered by courts in criminal cases.

Sectioning is not a course of action undertaken lightly by professionals and every effort will be made to get the person to agree to a voluntary admission unless they are incapable of doing so. A person's discharge from detention is usually ordered by the responsible professional (usually the psychiatrist) or, in the case of dispute, by a mental health tribunal, but can be requested with 72 hours' notice by the next of kin - though this can be blocked by the responsible medical officer.

Other sections of the Act specifically cover consent to treatment, and a whole different set of legislation - the law on **Capacity** - also comes into play to cover situations where the person may or may not have a diagnosed mental illness but may be incapable of understanding why they need treatment or giving informed consent to it. Capacity applies to situations where people are both physically and/or mentally incapacitated.

Voluntary organisations

Many organisations that offer HIV services or who work with groups vulnerable to HIV offer counselling on a free or (more often) low-cost basis. They may also offer support groups, therapy groups and workshops. Counselling is usually restricted to short-contract work (six to 24 weeks is typical), but onward referral to private therapists or (if appropriate) psychiatric services is usually possible.

Drug treatments for mental illness

This Manual does not seek to give specific recommendations for treatments. With mental illnesses - as with other conditions, but maybe even more so - a drug that suits one person may not work for another or produce unacceptable side-effects, and psychopharmacology is often a matter of judgement, experience and working with the patient to achieve better stability. However certain medications have interactions with HIV drugs that not all GPs, for instance, will know by heart so it is important that if you are prescribed drugs by someone who is not your HIV clinician you make them aware of what anti-retrovirals and/or other medication you are on. This includes complementary practitioners - see below.

This list only covers drugs used to treat diagnosed mental illnesses; there are a range of other drugs used for organic neurological disorders like epilepsy.

Antidepressants

- Tricyclic antidepressants (TCAs) were developed in the 1950s, including amitriptyline, nortriptyline (*Allegron*) and desipramine. Side-effects include confusion, drowsiness, dry mouth, weight gain, blurred vision and sexual problems.

- Monoamine oxidase inhibitors (MAOIs) include phenelzine (*Nardil*), isocarboxazid and tranylcypromine. These drugs can cause side-effects, including tremors, insomnia, weight gain and liver toxicity, and may interact with some foods to cause a sudden, life-threatening increase in blood pressure. As a consequence, these drugs are rarely prescribed.

- Selective serotonin re-uptake inhibitors (SSRIs) are the most recent type of anti-depressant to be developed. The group includes fluoxetine (*Prozac*), citalopram (*Cipramil*), escitalopram (*Cipralex*), fluvoxamine (*Faverin*), paroxetine (*Seroxat*) and sertraline (*Lustral*). Due to their better side-effect profile, these drugs are more frequently prescribed than the other drug classes. Nevertheless, a significant proportion of people experience early side-effects such as diarrhoea, insomnia, giddiness and nausea. These usually resolve after one to two months of treatment. Fluoxetine tends to be prescribed more frequently than other SSRIs because of a larger body of experience in its use and fewer concerns about potential for withdrawal symptoms. Citalopram is also often used because it has the least interaction with antiretrovirals. SSRIs also have fewer interactions with other drugs and do not usually cause weight gain, although they can affect sexual function. Impotence or delayed ejaculation are side-effects which may affect 10-20% of people taking fluoxetine, for example.

- Other drugs sometimes used as antidepressants include mirtazepine (which often causes weight gain) and venlafaxine (*Efexor*).

- Antidepressants of all classes have the potential for interaction with the protease inhibitors, especially ritonavir.

Drugs for anxiety

- Beta-blockers do not reduce anxiety as such but inhibit the effect of adrenaline on the sympathetic nervous system. They reduce the physical symptoms of anxiety such as racing heart, sweating, hyperventilation and so on, which may in themselves give rise to more anxiety. They also have many other uses such as correcting heart arrhythmias. Commonly-used ones include propanolol, atenolol, carvetidol and metoprolol. The potential exists for overdose if combined with protease inhibitors; side-effects include irregular heartbeat and kidney problems.

- Anxiolytics directly reduce anxiety and are perhaps better known as tranquillisers. The only class generally used these days are the benzodiazepines, which include diazepam, alprazolam and oxazepam. Lorazepam has a more strongly sedating effect and chlodiazepoxide is often used for alcohol withdrawal in people with dependency.

- Temazepam, loprazolam, nitrazepam and flurazepam are used solely as sleeping pills as their sedative effect is more pronounced; the latter two drugs can produce a 'hangover effect' of drowsiness the following day, as can zopiclone, a non-benzodiazepine. Doctors are reluctant to prescribe the benzodiazepines, especially for anxiety, as they all have the potential to cause addiction even after quite short-term use; however they are still sometimes prescribed on a short-term basis for acute anxiety and insomnia. When patients are taking protease inhibitors, especially ritonavir, indinavir and especially ritonavir, *extreme caution* should be taken when prescribing diazepam, flurazepam and alprazolam, and European agencies recommend that diazepam and flurazepam should not be co-administered with ritonavir, though US guidelines, which are more recent, just urge caution.

- The benzodiazepines midazolam and triazolam must not be co-administered with protease inhibitors.

- The old-fashioned barbiturates are now no longer prescribed as the window between an effective dose and a toxic dose is very narrow and becomes more so as the body develops tolerance to them.

Anti-psychotics

- These drugs are often mislabelled 'major tranquilisers'. While they do have sedative effects they do a lot more than this, calming down disordered thought processes and controlling other psychotic symptoms such as hallucinations. You don't have to have a diagnosed psychosis to be given an anti-psychotic; anyone has the capacity for entering a state of temporary psychosis, for instance during an extreme reaction to a recreational drug or during fever-induced delirium. No doctor would prescribe an anti-psychotic for sedation alone; these are strong drugs with a wide range of side-effects, the chief one of which is a Parkinson's disease-like syndrome in long-term users. Nonetheless they enable some people with illnesses like schizophrenia to lead relatively normal lives. The ones most commonly used are chlorpromazine, haloperidol, olanzapine and risperidone. This is not a complete list; these are just the most common 'first line' drugs. The antipsychotic pimozide must not be co-administered with protease inhibitors or efavirenz; data is incomplete on some of the others.

Bipolar illness and mania

- Salts of the metallic element lithium have a special place in psychopharmacology as they were until recently the only drug that seemed to work to prevent the mood swings of bipolar affective disorder ('manic depression') and particularly manic episodes. Lithium has a narrow therapeutic window between efficacy and toxicity; it needs to be taken strictly every 12 hours and drug levels in the patient's body need regular monitoring.

- The anti-convulsant (anti-epilepsy) drugs carbamazepine and valproic acid however are also now used in bipolar illness, especially when lithium has proved ineffective. Carbamazepine can cause liver toxicity.

Complementary remedies

- The herbal remedy St John's wort (Hypericum) has proven anti-depressant properties, and one recent study found it produced a 25% greater reduction in depression symptoms than the antidepressant paroxetine (*Seroxat*)(Szegedi). However, two different studies have found that St John's wort reduces the concentration of the protease inhibitor (PI) indinavir (Piscitelli) and the non-nucleoside (NNRTI) nevirapine (de Maat) in the body, in the case of indinavir by 80%. It also reduces oral contraceptive pill levels, potentially resulting in unwanted pregnancy, and interacts with anticonvulsants, potentially resulting in someone having a seizure or epileptic fit.

- A number of herbal remedies are used to calm anxiety. One of the few for which some evidence of efficacy exists is valerian; one study (Andreatini) found it had similar efficacy to diazepam in calming the psychological aspects of generalised anxiety disorder. However others have found no difference from placebo. No studies have as yet been conducted on the interactions of valerian with anti-HIV medications.

Many other complementary therapies may be useful in calming anxiety and relieving depression; for more details see the NAM **Directory of Complementary Therapies.**

References

Andreatini R Effect of valepotriates (valerian extract) in generalized anxiety disorder: a randomized placebo-controlled pilot study. Phytother Res. 16(7): 650-654, 2002.

de Maat MM et al. Drug interaction between St John's wort and nevirapine. AIDS 15(3): 420-421, 2001.

Piscitelli SC et al. Indinavir concentrations and St John's wort. Lancet 355(9203): 547-548, 2000.

Szegedi A et al. Acute treatment of moderate to severe depression with hypericum extract WS 5570 (St John's wort): randomised controlled double blind non-inferiority trial versus paroxetine. BMJ 330: 503, 2005.

Counselling and psychotherapy

Counselling and psychotherapy is a huge and growing profession and one which in the UK so far has no regulatory legal framework. In theory anyone can call themselves a counsellor or psychotherapist, though moves are afoot to institute an EU-wide regulatory framework to cover qualifications, training and standards. In the USA psychotherapy is a regulated profession and all people advertising as counsellors or therapists should be qualified psychologists.

In the UK there are two professional bodies, the **British Association for Counselling and Psychotherapy (BACP)** and the **United KingdomCouncil for Psychotherapy (UKCP)** which run voluntary training and accreditation schemes and regulate training standards and institutes. Both have directories of registered therapists on their websites and any therapist on their register will have undergone a rigorous professional training.

This does not necessarily mean they will automatically be the right therapist for you, however. Studies have shown that even in general medical practice, patients who have a good relationship with their doctor do better, and because psychotherapy is such an interpersonal activity, it is crucial to find a therapist who you trust and who understands your lifestyle, background and concerns. Indeed, the building of trust is often an essential part of what makes the therapy work.

It is therefore important when seeking a therapist to:

- If possible, seek therapists personally recommended by people you trust.

- If not, investigate one of the registers of therapists run by organisations that specialise in people with HIV or groups vulnerable to HIV such as Africans or gay men.

- 'Shop around'; this means that it is perfectly in order to arrange to see a number of therapists for an initial consultation before making a decision about who you want to work with.

A (very) brief guide to types of therapy

Psychotherapy is a very complex field. The sheer number of different theoretical approaches to the human mind and to the practice of therapy may seem to the person nervously stepping into the therapy world for the first time like a confusing array of choices all jostling for competition. It's important to keep in mind that most of the relatively meagre amount of research that has been done into counselling and psychotherapy shows that all theoretical approaches have roughly the same effectiveness (in the order of a 60 to 66% 'cure rate'). Certain techniques like cognitive-behavioural therapy are better researched because their short-term nature and slightly more structured method makes them easier to research, and CBT may be especially useful for anxiety disorders. In general the strongest predictor of success is a successful therapeutic relationship rather than the type of therapy, though of course your view of your therapist may be influenced by their theoretical and philosophical outlook.

Reference

Durham RC. Cognitive therapy, analytic psychotherapy and anxiety management training for generalised anxiety disorder. *British Journal of Psychiatry* 165: 315-323. 1994.

Psychoanalysis

We start with this because it was the original technique devised by the father of psychotherapy, Sigmund Freud (1856-1939).

Freud's most significant contribution to the history of thought was his assertion - pretty much accepted these days, but revolutionary in its time - that man was not, in essence, a rational animal. This overturned over two thousand years of thinking, ever since the Greek philosopher Aristotle asserted precisely the opposite. Freud did not 'invent' the unconscious mind - it had been known for centuries that many thoughts people had were half-conscious or half-expressed. But he was the first to advance the theory that the mainsprings of human behaviour were a series of entirely unconscious drives. He believed that mental illness symptoms were caused by the efforts of the conscious person to reconcile the demands of society with these animalistic drives and to balance them against each other while still retaining some conception of a coherent self.

Freud couched his theory in entirely psychological terms and many of his concepts these days seem old-fashioned, unscientific or even a bit 'mad' themselves, so it is worth keeping in mind that a lot of what he theorised turned out to be true in the subsequent century, as neurologists discovered the neural and endocrine pathways that drive much of our behaviour.

Psychoanalysis is an outwardly simple endeavour: the patient lies on a couch and is invited to 'free-associate' or say whatever comes into their head. However during his work with patients Freud discovered that patients had great difficulty simply 'coming out with it'. He devised a second theory, called **transference**, which said that the reason patients can't say what is on their mind is because the therapist comes to represent parental figures from the past. In this way Freud also devised the idea of therapy as a kind of 'test-tube relationship' - a venue in which the patient (or, to use the term more commonly used today, client) practices new ways of relating to people in the safe space of the consulting room by using the therapist as an 'object' against whom to bounce the desire, hatred, distrust, need and so on that the person may feel for other people and which may get in the way of them achieving satisfactory relationships.

Pure Freudian psychoanalysis is these days a rare commodity. Psychoanalytic training is lengthy and arduous, and a course of psychoanalytic treatment - which usually requires attendance at least three times a week - is exacting and expensive, a major personal commitment. However it is available, especially in London.

Contact

The British Psychoanalytic Society - www.psychoanalysis.org.uk - 0207 563 5002

Carl Jung and transpersonal therapy

The first split in the orthodoxy of psychoanalysis came when Freud's colleague and disciple, Carl Gustav Jung (1875-1961), split from Freud to form his own school after the First World War. Where Freud was a secular Jew, Jung was the son of a protestant pastor, and the flavour of his theories is explicitly spiritual, if not exactly religious. Jung was fascinated by mythology in non-European philosophy and devised a theory which in many ways turned Freud's ideas upside down. Instead of being driven by animalistic drives from below, said Jung, man was driven 'from above' by spiritual demands and ambitions and by the drive to become a more whole and complete person than he was now.

Jung called this process 'individuation' and said the spiritual desires were embodied in a series of cultural associations or collections of symbols he called 'archetypes' which tended to appear again and again in mythology, stories and dreams. He was so fascinated by the way human minds from many different cultures had similar 'stories' to explain themselves that he devised a theory of a 'collective unconscious'. This has been misunderstood to say that human beings were telepathically connected; in fact what Jung was saying was that the similarity in our myths and stories about ourselves is evidence of our common genetic and cultural legacy - another idea later borne out by scientific discoveries.

Jungian therapy is very interested in the client's creativity and in their dreams. It is in some ways one of the few therapeutic traditions which looks to making sense of the **future** rather than the past and in maximising the person's potential rather than helping them understand the legacy of past traumas as something that holds that potential back. For this reason it often seems to be particularly effective for fairly well-established people in the second half of life who are trying to 'make sense of' their lives.

Contact

www.jungian-analysis.org

The post-Freudians

Freud died in London, and the psychoanalytic tradition in the UK was carried on after his death by figures such as his daughter Anna Freud, Ernest Jones, Melanie Klein and in particular Donald Winnicott (1896-1971). The latter two took psychoanalysis in the direction of the analysis of children, and child therapists to this day are influenced by this tradition. Strict psychoanalysis has branched out into a large section of the general therapeutic industry usually called the 'psychodynamic' approach which still retains Freud's basic tenets but may offer a huge range of different techniques and settings.

One of the world's largest and most respected organisations offering psychodynamic treatment is the Tavistock Clinic, which is located just round the corner from both Freud's old house and the Jungian institute. It is an NHS Trust and is the largest single provider of psychotherapy to the NHS. Generally you would have to be referred by a GP though self-referral is possible. It offers psychodynamic psychotherapy to a wide range of targeted groups including Somalis, Bangladeshis, couples experiencing relationship and sexual difficulties, and people who have committed sexual offences or are worried they might.

Contact

The Tavistock and Portman NHS Trust: www.tavi-port.org - 020 7447 3862

Wilhelm Reich and body psychotherapy

A younger disciple of Freud's, Wilhelm Reich (1897-1957), took a side-step away from the psychoanalytic tradition by insisting on the importance of physical and bodily processes in the development of the mind. He developed a holistic theory of human nature, saying that there were not two separate entities called 'mind' and 'body' which had to be treated in different ways, but that mental liberation and bodily liberation were one and the same thing. Reich asserted that Freud's **libido**, the mental energy that lies behind and sustains our unconscious drives and desires, was in fact a physical and real energy he called 'orgone energy' and he devoted the latter half of his career to attempting to measure and use it.

Reich was a prickly and paranoid character, and also one of the inspirations behind the countercultural revolution of the 1960s, which prevented his ideas being taken seriously for a long time, at least in the UK (he has always been more influential in Europe). However many of his ideas have been borne out by later discoveries about the sympathetic nervous system and the effect of long-term stress on the body.

There is no such thing now as 'Reichian therapy' but his ideas were developed and elaborated by people like Alexander Lowen, Gerda Boyesen and Jack Lee Rosenberg and now form a distinct school of Body Psychotherapy. Body psychotherapists work with the body as much as the mind; many use techniques like massage and physical exercises as well as traditional talking therapy, not as complementary therapies in their own right, but to help the client experience the way stress, anxiety and depression have impacted on, and are perpetuated by, physical attributes such as muscle tone and posture. Body psychotherapy may be particularly valuable for people who experience difficulty expressing or acting on emotions or who suffer from psychosomatic illness.

Contact

The Chiron Centre for Body Psychotherapy - www.chiron.org - 020 8997 5219.

Group psychotherapy

Another development of psychodynamic therapy was to apply the theories of Freud to human relationships in families and groups. The work of the British psychoanalyst Wilfred Bion (1897-1979) was seminal in this area, and he devised a method of group analysis which looked at the way groups tend to replicate, for each member, the particular family conditions they grew up in.

Group therapy may be a particularly valuable kind of therapy for people whose problems are largely to do with being in groups such as social phobics, agoraphobics, or people who suffer from anger, envy or feelings of exclusion when they find themselves in social and work situations.

Contact

The Institute of Group Analysis - www.igalondon.org.uk - 020 7431 4431

Person-centred therapy and counselling

A radical departure from Freud happened in the USA around the time of the Second World War with the development of the theories of Carl Rogers (1902-1987). Rogers had more in common with Jung and Reich than Freud in his insistence that people basically strived towards goodness rather than away from animal desires. But his approach was quite different. Rogers developed a radically 'stripped down' theory of therapy (or rather, counselling; he was the first therapist to prefer this term). He based this not just on his own theories and personal convictions but on actual research he had done into what conditions seemed to be necessary for patients to improve in therapy. In this way, although his research was crude and small-scale, he was a pioneer in insisting that the effect of psychotherapy could be measured, and indeed should be.

Rogers developed a theory that three, and only three, simple conditions were necessary for therapy to be a success; the therapist must have 'congruence' which means they must be honest and genuine with the client; they must have empathy, or the ability to feel what the client feels; and they must have

respect for the client, which Rogers called an attitude of 'unconditional positive regard' towards the client. He said if therapists could observe these conditions perfectly, they were necessary and sufficient for any client to improve. The crucial word is 'if', of course; Rogerian therapy, while being very simple theoretically, imposes a doctrine of near-saintly consistency and warmth of behaviour on the therapist.

Because it is so accepting, what is now usually called 'person-centred therapy' may be especially suitable for clients with habitually poor self-image, and has been demonstrated to work successfully with clients with major depression.

Most organisations that offer counselling are influenced by Rogers' ideas, so there is no specific clinic or school of person-centred therapy to refer to.

Behavioural and cognitive-behavioural therapy

Another radical departure from Freudian theory was behavioural Therapy, the work of B F Skinner (1904-1990). Skinner was inspired by the work of earlier scientists like Ivan Pavlov (1849-1936) whose experiments on animals laid the foundations for 'operant conditioning'. This is the theory that animals and humans learn to associate specific behaviours with specific stimuli - which may be nothing to do with the original stimulus that the behaviour was at first a response to.

Skinner's ideas were diametrically opposed to Freud's. In essence he said that what went on in the mind was irrelevant; people were essentially 'black boxes' and that all that mattered was finding the right rewards and disincentives to change behaviour. His theories were immensely influential in the earlier half of the 20th century and he has been criticised for taking an essentially inhumane and controlling attitude towards changing human behaviour.

Much of what Skinner said has since been scientifically disproved, as more subtle ways of measuring the activity of the human mind proved that internal thought processes and emotional states were just as important in modifying and controlling behaviour as external stimuli.

However a modified version of behaviourism, **Cognitive Behavioural Therapy (CBT),** which treated thought patterns also as 'behaviours' that could be modified by therapists, was developed and now forms one of the strongest traditions of therapy in the UK.

Although relationship skills between therapist and client are as important for CBT therapists to have as any therapist, CBT therapists' relationship to clients is more like that of a teacher or instructor who helps them develop more positive thought patterns and less self-destructive behaviours. CBT therapists will both work directly with suggesting alternatives to the negative and repetitive thought patterns that characterise so much anxiety and depression (e.g. "If I receive a rejection it means no one likes me"), and will also give clients 'homework' so that they can expose themselves to stimuli (e.g. the object of a phobia) in measured 'doses' and can try out different ways of reacting to them.

CBT is especially useful for anxiety states, phobias and so on, but also has a proven track record of helping people with depression. Because (see above) it is one of the most widely-researched types of psychotherapy, it is also one of the types most easily accessible via NHS referral. It may not be so useful for people who have had therapy before or who have issues to do with their relationships with others that may need longer-term work.

CBT is quite a specialised form of therapy and you should only go to a therapist who is qualified to practise it.

Contact

British Association for Behavioural and Cognitive Psychotherapies - http://www.babcp.com - 01254 875277 - babcp@babcp.com . Website has a directory of CBT therapists in the UK.

Resources

Some organisations offering help for mental health problems

General

MIND (National Association for Mental Health) - www.mind.org.uk - 0845 766 0163. National Charity for people with mental health problems, has numerous local centres offering therapy and support throughout the UK, with 21 in London alone.

The Mental Health Foundation - www.mentalhealth.org.uk/ - comprehensive website offering information and contacts for all types of mental disorders.

Stress

Stress Management Society - www.stress.org.uk - 0870 199 3260. Company offering stress management training to companies and individuals.

Anxiety disorders

No Panic - www.nopanic.org.uk. Helpline 0808 808 0545. Charity helping sufferers from Panic Attacks, Phobias, Obsessive Compulsive Disorders, other related Anxiety Disorders, including Tranquilliser Withdrawal

National Phobics Society - www.phobics-society.org.uk - 0870 7700 456

Obsessive-compulsive disorder

Obsessive Action - www.obsessive-action.demon.co.uk - 020 7226 4000

Post-traumatic stress disorder

(From child sexual abuse): Survivors UK: info@survivorsuk.org.uk - 0845 122 120

(From torture and war crimes): Medical Foundation for the Care of Victims of Torture: www.torturecare.org.uk - 020 **7697 7777**

Depression

Samaritans - www.samaritans.org.uk - 08457 90 90 90 - jo@samaritans.org . 24-hour help for the depressed and suicidal.

Depression Alliance - www.depressionalliance.org - 0845 123 2320. Charity offering advice and support, runs local groups

Addictions: Drink, drugs and sex
Alcohol:

Alcoholics Anonymous: www.alcoholics-anonymous.org.uk - 0845 769 7555

Alcohol Concern: www.alcoholconcern.org.uk/ - 0800 917 8282

Drugs:

Narcotics Anonymous: www.ukna.org - 020 7730 0009

Release: www.release.org.uk - 0845 4500 215

(Gay-specific): Antidote: www.thehungerford.org

Sexual Compulsion:

Sexaholics Anonymous: www.sauk.org - 07000 725463- newcomers@sauk.org

Schizophrenia

SANE (Schizophrenia A National Emergency): www.sane.org.uk - 0845 767 8000

Bipolar affective disorder (Manic-depression):

MDF The BiPolar Organisation: www.mdf.org.uk . 08456 340 540

Borderline personality disorder

www.bpdworld.org

UK HIV organisations offering counselling (there are also many local ones)

The range of organisations offering counselling has changed as funding for this kind of support work has decreased for the voluntary sector. HIV-related counselling is now often easier to access through HIV clinics than through voluntary agencies. Nonetheless many voluntary organisations still offer counselling, often in liaison with local counselling organisations or clinics.

Other voluntary organisations offer a package of support which includes peer support, information and complementary therapies, and can also include one-to-one counselling at the organisation or accessed by them. Just because an HIV organisation doesn't explicitly offer 'counselling' as one of its services doesn't mean you won't be able to get counselling by asking them.

Terrence Higgins Trust

The Terrence Higgins Trust offers counselling at a number of centres in London. Some are attached to HIV clinics and some in the THT's own offices. It also offers counselling at every one of its regional offices. For a referral, phone THT Direct on 0845 1221 200.

THT regional offices are in:

Birmingham and Coventry (THT Midlands) - 01902 711 818 - info.birmingham@tht.org.uk . Also run MESMEN, gay men's counselling and support group - 024 7622 9292 or mesmen@tht.org.uk

Brighton (THT South) - 01273 764 200 - info.south@tht.org.uk

Bristol (THT West) - 0117 955 1000 (Bristol) or info.west@tht.org.uk. Also run services from Swindon.

Cardiff (THT Cymru) 029 2066 6465 - info.cymru@tht.org.uk

Leeds - 0113 236 4720 - info.leeds@tht.org.uk

Oxford - 01865 243 389 - info.oxford@tht.org.uk

Southend and Colchester (THT East) - 01702 340 791(Southend) or 01206 798 595 (Colchester) - info.southend@tht.org.uk

Other London organisations offering councelling

The majority of other London HIV organisations that offer counselling are now ones that offer counselling to affected groups.

- **CASCAID** - 020 3228 5121. Although this is an NHS-operated service it is mentioned specifically because it also offers counselling services in several HIV organisations in south London.

- **Positive East** - 020 8509 3440. Formed recently by a merger between the Globe Centre and London East AIDS Network, this organisation offers HIV counselling as well as their Gay Men's Wellbeing service

Gay and bisexual men, transgender etc.

- **Healthy Gay Living Centre** - 020 7835 1495. Counselling for gay men. This organisation has now merged with the Terrence Higgins Trust.

- **PACE** - 020 7700 1323.info@pacehealth.org.uk .Islington-based LGBT counselling and therapy centre that offers subsidised counselling and workshops to gay men, lesbians, bisexuals and transgendered people throughout London. PACE also has a register of private gay-affirmative psychotherapists.

- **Pink Therapy** - 020 7291 4480. info@pinktherapy.com . This is a private partnership and register of gay-affirmative psychotherapists, based in central London. Standard psychotherapy rates.

- **KAIROS in Soho** - 020 7437 6063. Promotes the health and well-being of the Lesbian, Gay, Bisexual and Transgender Community in central London. Low-cost therapy.

Africans and Afro-Caribbeans

- **Shaka Services** - 020 7735 6744. Counselling and emotional support for Africans and Caribbeans; based in Kennington, south London

- **Nafsiyat** - 020 7686 8666. An intercultural therapy centre in north London. Provides private therapy for and by people of colour and can offer free places to residents of Islington, Camden and Enfield.

Many African support organisations in London can provide or access one-to-one and group support for clients. 'Counselling' and 'psychotherapy' are not always culturally familiar terms to people of African origin, so many organisations use terms like 'emotional support', 'peer support' and 'confidential advice' instead. They include:

- **Uganda AIDS Action Fund** - 020 7394 8866. Provide emotional support, outreach and support groups for African people in London.

- **IVO (Innovative Vision Organisation)** - 0208 365 0349. Based in Tottenham, north London

- **HAAZ (HIV and AIDS Association of Zambia)** - 020 8214 1475. Based in Neasden, north-west London.

Other ethnic minorities

- **Naz Project** - 020 8741 1879 - npl@naz.org.uk . HIV and sexual health support for south Asians, Latin Americans, and Africans from the Horn of Africa region and Spanish and Portuguese-speaking countries.

Women, families and children

- **Positively Women** - 020 7713 0444. Provide an integrated programme of support for HIV-positive women.

- **Body & Soul** - 020 7383 7678 - info@bodyandsoulcharity.org . A UK charity supporting children, teenagers, women, heterosexual men and their families who are living with or closely affected by HIV and AIDS.

Non-THT organisations outside London

This is not an exhaustive list; it has been restricted to organisations specifically mentioning 'counselling' on their websites and which represent services for most UK regions, especially those not covered by the Terrence Higgins Trust.

- **East Anglia**/King's Lynn - E.A.S.T (Eastern AIDS Support Services) - 01553 776655 - mail@aids-east.org.uk

- **East Midlands**/Leicester - Leicester AIDS Support Services - 0116 255 9995 - reception@lass.org.uk

- **North-east**/Middlesbrough - Cleveland AIDS Support - 01642 254598 - vdm@clevelandaidssupport.org.uk

- **North-west**/Liverpool - Sahir House: 0151 708 9080 - info@sahir.uk.com

- **North-west**/Manchester: Body Positive North West - 0161 873 8103 - **info@bpnw.org.uk** (mailto:info@bpnw.org.uk)

- **Scotland**/Edinburgh: Waverley Care Solas - 0131 661 0982

- **Scotland**/Glasgow - PHACE Scotland - 0141 332 3838 - contact@phacescotland.org. Support and advocacy for people with HIV, also run a counselling service for lesbians, bisexuals, gay men and people questioning their sexuality. Have an office (PHACE Grampian) in Aberdeen.

- **South**/Brighton: Brighton Body Positive: 01273 693266

- **South**/Southampton: Ribbons Centre - 023 8022 5511. info@ribbons-centre.co.uk

Services for specific affected groups outside London

Gay and bisexual men, transgender etc

- **PHACE Scotland -** see above

- **MESMAC northeast** - HIV and sexual health services for gay men in northeast England. - 0191 233 1333

- **MESMAC Yorkshire** - 0113 244 4209. Based in Leeds, with other offices in Bradford, Wakefield and York.

- **Lesbian and Gay Foundation -** Based in Manchester. Counselling via 0845 330 3030 or via George House Trust on 0161 274 4499

Africans

- **Black Health Agency -** 0800 0967 500. Based in Manchester, offers support and advice to African people living throughout England.

Helping people live with HIV

This section is a condensed version of the 'Services for people with HIV' section in the last AIDS Reference Manual. Since then the 'living with HIV' section in the previous edition of the manual has been turned into a separate book, *Living with HIV*. Nonetheless there are still services and issues particular to living with HIV that people with the virus and professionals who work with them need to know, many of which impact directly on quality of life and the stress of living with HIV.

Many of these 'living with.' areas are covered in other chapters, especially the chapter on **The Law and HIV** and the chapter on **Employment and HIV.**

The range of services available

This section describes the types of services that are available to those living with HIV across the UK. What is available will depend very much on how developed services are in your local area, and you should check with your local Social Services Department, local primary care trust (PCT), or a local voluntary agency for exact details of what is available in your area.

These are listed in the *UK AIDS Directory*.

Local authority responsibilities

The NHS and Community Care Act (1993) split the responsibility for health and social care services between health authorities and local authority social services departments.

In 2002 the National Health Service underwent extensive re-organisation. England now has four Directorates of Health and Social Service (North, Midlands & Eastern, South and London), which together cover 28 Strategic Health Authorities (SHAs), which themselves contain 301 Primary Care Trusts (PCTs). Wales now has its own NHS Directorate as part of the National Assembly for Wales. By April 2003, it will have re-organised its existing five Health Authorities into three regional ones (South, Mid & West, North).

The division between health and social care sounds fine in theory, and there are many services which are clearly the responsibility of one or the other, e.g. hospital in-patient services are always funded by the NHS. In practice there are many community services, for example HIV drop-ins, which provide both health and social care. Different arrangements exist in different areas for the funding of HIV community services - in some areas the NHS takes the lead, whilst in others local authorities do. Sometimes, HIV services are jointly funded by both agencies.

Due to the way services are provided and funded it is difficult for those of us living with HIV to keep track of what is available and how it is best accessed. We suggest that whether your initial or primary contact with services is through a clinic, your GP, social services, or a voluntary organisation, you should ask for advice and information about services available to you.   Many health and local authorities publish leaflets containing details of all the HIV services available locally. However leaflets do go out of date, services change, and even the most skilled worker might not be able to keep up with everything that is on offer - so keep asking if you have needs that you think ought to be met.

If you are unwell, you may be eligible for a social services care manager who will be able to help you decide what services you might want, and help you make choices about your care (see *Social Services* below).

Hospital HIV services

Hospital HIV services play an important part in HIV care. In particular, regular health checks with an experienced HIV doctor are very important as a means of monitoring overall health, checking the strength of your immune system, and can be an important way of recognising infections early and even preventing some disabling illnesses. Avoiding or delaying visits to hospitals or clinics may lead to some problems getting worse and may cause unnecessary worry or distress.

This is particularly important if you are receiving treatment with anti HIV drugs. Regular tests to check that the drugs are working properly are an essential part of taking them.

Hospital services usually offer a lot more than tests and medical treatment. Most hospital HIV or GUM services have health advisers. They can offer regular support, answer questions about HIV and AIDS, about treatment and medical conditions, and can help you make the most of other services.

Many hospital clinics also have nutritionists to advise and help you with issues of diet, specialist counsellors and psychotherapists, social workers and occupational therapists who can assist and advise you on how to live as independently as possible. Some clinics may also arrange group meetings for patients to learn about developments in HIV treatment and care.

In response to the general consensus that for treatments to be effective, they need to be taken in the right doses at the right time on an ongoing basis, many clinics now offer specialist adherence or treatment support clinics which provide access to specially trained staff such as clinical nurse specialists, pharmacists and psychologists.

Dentists

All dentists can and should be able to offer dental care for people living with HIV. But, notoriously, not all are willing to do so. Telling your dentist about your HIV status could enable them to consider alternative treatments to protect you from unnecessary infections. If your dentist is unwilling to provide you with dental care, there are a number of specialist dental clinics who may either give you the treatment you need or give you details of local dentists who are willing to provide treatment for people with HIV. Your local PCT will be able to give you details of specialist clinics.

If you are unsure of how to find a dentist who is not going to discriminate against you because of your HIV status use your local voluntary organisation or health adviser to help you.

Involving your GP

Some hospitals are now attempting to work closely with local GPs to develop 'shared care' for people with HIV (and for other care groups). This means that many of us with HIV may (or already are) able to receive treatment and care through a partnership of a GP and a hospital clinic. For some of us this may be more convenient, especially if the hospital clinic is a long way from home and will certainly be of help with matters such as non-HIV, routine and out-of-hours care.

There is another reason for HIV clinics involving GPs - the cost of HIV therapy. Just before this article was written, the consortium of HIV clinicians and commissioners that provide HIV care in London announced that because there was a projected overspend of at least 4% on the HIV drugs budget for 2005/6, they were planning to severely restrict the list of drugs that could be prescribed by HIV clinics and would be referring patients to GPs for non-HIV related medication such as anti-depressants, sleeping pills, skin preparations, asthma drugs and various others.

HIV patients are often reluctant to get their GPs more involved in their care for three reasons:

- They have had problems registering with a GP anyway.

- They are not convinced that GPs have the expertise to help with HIV care.

- They are concerned with their GP knowing their HIV status due to worries about confidentiality.

Regarding the first point, many GP practices, especially in inner-city areas, are over-subscribed and for financial reasons practices are sometimes reluctant to take on patients with chronic conditions like HIV or hepatitis B/C. Anyone who has residency status in the UK is entitled to register with a GP and is also entitled to have a choice of GPs from within their PCT. In general you are required to register with a GP whose 'catchment area' includes your address, but you are entitled to a wider choice if you have special needs such as not having English as a first language.   If you are having difficulty registering with a GP, you can log on to http://www.nhsdirect.com or phone **NHS Direct** on **0845 46 47** and explain that you are having problems. In cases where you feel you have been discriminated against, phone up your local PCT and ask for **PALS - The Patient Advocacy and Liaison Service.**

At the end of this section is a list of the PCTs in London, including contact details for PALS, and information on how to take a complaint further.

Regarding the second point, the Sexual Health and HIV Strategy for England and Wales is clear that it is not government policy to get GPs involved in specialist HIV care such as deciding on anti-retroviral treatment regimens. The problem is partly a question of GPs themselves receiving better training in HIV and of GP practices taking on board the Strategy's suggestion that certain practices should specialise in sexual health. In the meantime it is vital that your GP is aware what HIV treatments you are on (and what complementary treatments, too) so they can prescribe with confidence that you will not experience drug interactions.

This leads on to the third point, which unfortunately is still an unresolved area. GPs cannot ethically lie to employers or providers of insurance when questioned directly about patients' HIV status. Some GPs however are happy not to record your HIV status in your files if requested. It is important to have a frank talk with your GP about this area - you are entitled to ask for information to be removed from your records if you don't want it there, though it is still important to make sure doctors are aware of your status.

If you were to decide that you feel happy to involve your GP more actively, you should discuss this with your hospital doctor or health advisor the next time you visit your clinic. Get them to tell you- or find out if they do not know- the level of knowledge, interest and expertise any prospective GP has about HIV. If you are unhappy with your GP you will be able to change to another one in your local area. Some GP surgeries also have practice nurses now and these may be able to offer you additional advice and support.

Most GPs are now classified as 'fund holders'. This means that they have budgets to buy some community services, e.g. district nursing.

What to do if you are unsatisfied

If you are unhappy with the health services in your local area there are mechanisms in place to deal with suggestions and complaints. It may be just a matter of seeking advice from an advocacy worker at a local HIV charity about how best to deal with your doctor or access the treatments or advice that you want.

All health services have formal and informal ways that we can express dissatisfaction with the service that we are receiving- or

trying to access. If you are dissatisfied with any of the health services you are receiving, you should raise this in the first instance with the person providing the service or their line manager. You do not need to put anything in writing at this stage. If you are still unhappy, you should contact the Chief Executive of the Hospital or Community Health NHS Trust, or the Chief Executive of the PCT. They are required to fully investigate your complaint and reply to you within a few weeks. This process can seem very daunting however- even at the informal stage of raising the issue with the person concerned or their manager. However, unless we tell the people who are paid to provide the services to us when we think they are getting it wrong, how can we expect things to get better?

IF ALL ELSE FAILS there are two further levels of complaint. The first is the Independent Complaints Advocacy Service (ICAS) which is an independent body set up by the Department of Health to assist people who want to take out serious complaints against the NHS. Its phone number is 0845 120 3784.

The last is the Parliamentary and Health Services Ombudsman which has the power to compel even the Department of Health to make changes. Phone 0845 015 4033 or email phso.enquiries@ombudsman.org.uk

Social services and community care

Social services departments provide a range of services designed to promote independent living for people with HIV and AIDS. These services can include:

- advice and information about the kinds of support and assistance available from the council, the NHS or voluntary organisations.

- help in the home.

- meals on wheels.

- help with transport or mobility.

- respite and convalescent care, "holiday" grants for you and/or someone who cares for you.

- loans of domestic electrical equipment.

- practical adaptations in the home.

- help with telephone installation and rental.

- emotional support for people with HIV and AIDS and their carers.

- social workers and occupational therapists.

- day centres and drop in services.

Not all of these services may be available in every local authority, and where they are, eligibility for them will often be dependent on residence, health status and financial need. Many services set eligibility criteria to ensure that these services are only given to people in greatest need.   Most Councils expect you to make a contribution toward the hourly cost of providing you with some social care services - e.g. home helps. This is especially true if you receive benefits such as the care component of Disabled Living Allowance, or have other income that can be reasonably expected to defray some of the costs of the help provided.

Remember that in the main the services provided to us via Social services are those that we have a legal right to - depending upon our needs. They are not "charity". Denial of any service that we believe we need can be challenged.

How to access social care services

In order to access these services you should be offered an 'Assessment' of your needs from your local Social Services Department. This is an opportunity for you to talk in detail about your needs and find out as much as possible about the services available to you. This assessment is then written up and should then be made available to you to comment upon and correct if necessary. Depending upon your assessed (and agreed) level of need, services will be offered to you

If you are ill

If you are ill and have complex needs a care manager should be allocated to you. This person is usually a Social Worker with a budget, who can arrange access to a number of different social care services, e.g. home helps, respite care etc. Their role is to ensure that you can have the social care services which you need. The full range of services is made available to you if and when you need them. Most services are only given to people in greatest need.

If you are well

If you are well, or have fairly 'low level' needs, you will be offered basic advice and support, as well as information about services available locally. These are often called 'open access' services because they are open to anybody who feels that they need them. Most of the services provided by voluntary organisations are open acce

If your health changes

Most people with HIV or AIDS have fluctuations in their health, and therefore in the level of services they may require at any time. As such, care managers should flexibly re-assess the levels of care and support provided.

You are entitled to request a new assessment if you feel your care needs have changed.

Do you need a carer?

Many people living with HIV, particularly those entitled to Disability Living Allowance will be entitled to some funding for a carer. Government grants have recently increased and your carer may well be entitled to extra financial help. If you have a carer they will also be eligible for an assessment of their care needs by social services (see *Caring for Someone With AIDS*).

If you are unhappy with social services

In some areas, the quality of services available is very good with well trained workers and extensive consultation with people using services. Unfortunately this is not always true and there have been cases where confidentiality has been abused or services have been of a poor standard.   Such instances are increasingly rare as local authorities become more experienced in working with people with HIV or AIDS.

However, if at any time you are dissatisfied with the services you have received, you should raise the issue with the member of staff who is supposed to be helping you, or with their manager. Where this does not resolve the problem, you should make a formal complaint - local authorities are now obliged to have a formal complaints procedure for people using services, and this procedure should be made known to all people using services.

It is important to make sure you know how to complain and local authorities should have leaflets explaining how their complaints procedure works. You may also find the advice and support of voluntary AIDS service organisations and self-help organisations very helpful should you wish to pursue a complaint, and in some cases they will pursue the complaint on your behalf. Non-AIDS specific disability organisations or agencies such as the Citizens' Advice Bureau may also be able to help.

If your complaint is not resolved through the complaints procedure you may wish to contact the local Government

Ombudsman. If the Local Authority refuses to assess your needs there are unreasonable delays, or if they do not provide you with the services you need you may wish to consult a solicitor who specialises in Community Care Law.

Managing community care budgets

New legislation was introduced in 1996 which allows local authorities to make direct payments to individuals so that they can purchase the community care services they require, rather than having such services provided by their local authority.

The Government is encouraging all local authorites to offer direct payments as an alternative to local authority services. By June 2001, 98% of local authorities were either running direct payments or are in the process of setting them up. Direct payments for community care were introduced following lobbying by people with disabilities, who wanted to see a system which would allow the disabled person to manage his or her own care independently.

Who is eligible for direct payments?

Anyone eligible to receive community care services who is disabled by physical illness (or a range of other disabilities) is eligible to receive direct payments. Recipients must be aged above 16 and must be willing and able to manage direct payments for themselves, and cannot have direct payments managed on their behalf by a carer or by another agency. People with dementia or other HIV-related brain impairment will not be judged eligible.

What can direct payments be used to purchase?

Direct payments can be used to pay for services such as cleaning, shopping, cooking, night sitting, basic nursing care and other forms of personal assistance which aid independent life in the community. The scheme allows the employment of a live-in 'personal assistant' who may take on all of these duties if a community care assessment deems this necessary, or it may simply meet the cost of occasional 'home help' type services provided by an individual chosen by the recipient, depending on the degree of need.

You should be told about the option of direct payments whenever you undergo a community care assessment - either an initial assessment or a re-assessment - if your needs change. You may have to lobby your local authority, or get an advocacy organisation such as your local self-help group for people with HIV, to advocate on your behalf as not every local authority offers direct payments to every group of disabled people.

Who can be employed to provide services?

The scheme allows recipients to choose their own paid carers, but payments cannot be used to pay close relations, spouses, partners or friends already living with you. However the current guidelines do not prevent you from employing a same-sex partner who does not live with you to provide care services if you wish to do so.

The scheme allows you to employ a personal care assistant who lives in your home, but this person must not be a relative or partner. However, exceptions may be made in rare circumstances where it is not possible to find a suitable care assistant in the locality. These regulations are designed to promote the independence of people with disabilities from their families, and to relieve the burden of unpaid care which frequently falls upon the families and partners of sick or disabled people.

Direct payments cannot be used to pay for local authority services. In other words, you cannot pay for services from your own local authority, or from local authority services in another district if you think those are better.

The scheme is likely to be particularly attractive to people with HIV who come from stigmatised social groups, since it will allow them to identify care assistance which is appropriate for them. For example, people from ethnic minorities may be able to identify someone from their own community who can provide the care they require far more easily than a local authority could do, and gay men may benefit similarly.

Recipients of direct payments will be expected to fulfil all the normal obligations of an employer, such as PAYE and National Insurance contributions, and will be required to manage their direct payments budget (for example, if they are receiving payments for care provided by two different individuals or agencies). Local authorities are expected to provide support to direct payment recipients in managing PAYE and national insurance, and in budgeting, as part of community care support.

How much money will be available to employ carers?

Personal assistance funded by direct payments will be charged at the same rates as local authority home care. The scheme is not intended to provide privatised home care 'on the cheap', but no extra resources will be available to local authorities to manage the scheme. Some local authorities are likely to find it difficult to introduce direct payments in the short term because they can't calculate unit costs for all the services they provide, or because they have concerns about the effect which direct payments might have on the standard of care available to those unwilling or unable to take up direct payments.

It has been suggested that direct payments may reduce the cost of home care by 30-40%, but it is very difficult to assess how true this will be for all local authorities given the difficulties they face in establishing accurate unit costs for delivering home care services.

Recruiting a personal carer

Some disability organisations have already opened personal assistance agencies through which disabled people can recruit personal carers. If large numbers of people with HIV chose to take advantage of direct payments, AIDS voluntary organisations might be called upon to provide similar services, but it is likely that direct payments will be most attractive to people with HIV in areas with social services departments which have less experience in dealing with the needs of HIV-positive clients.

The recruitment and training of personal assistants are likely to raise a host of issues which some voluntary organisations may be well adapted to cope with, due to their previous experience of developing voluntary and care services for people with HIV. However, the direct payments system is not designed to sub-contract the community care case management of people with HIV to the voluntary sector or to private agencies.

People with disabilities have already found that peer support is essential in the management of direct payments and in the recruitment, management and training of personal assistants. Whilst there is scope for AIDS voluntary organisations and self-help groups to develop such support, there is not always scope for this in areas where only one or two people with HIV might be taking advantage of direct payments. This raises issues of confidentiality, and of the need for a national or regional network of people with HIV receiving direct payments.

Recruiting a personal carer even if you do not satisfy the criteria for direct payments.

There is already the capacity for you to have an existing carer to provide you with your home care if your local authorities are providing or intending to provide home care services through an agency. This arrangement is known as an "informal carer arrangement" where the agency employs the person you want to provide you with your care and they then work for you. For tax and national insurance purposes your carer is employed by the agency - however they will not be asked to care for anyone else as an employee of the agency.

Resource
The National Centre for Independent Living

www.ncil.org.uk

Phone: 0207 587 1663

Text phone: 0207 587 1177

Email: info@ncil.org.uk

A national charity set up to advise disabled people and people who work with them on independent living and Direct Payments for disabled people.

Housing services

Your local authority housing department can offer you support, advice and information on all aspects of housing, whether you are a council tenant, private sector tenant, rent from a Housing Association, or own your home.

People with HIV or AIDS often encounter different problems with housing, such as homelessness, financial difficulties with rent or mortgages, harassment, possession proceedings or disrepair or unsuitable accommodation. If you are homeless or are threatened with homelessness, you may qualify for housing through your local authority although rules for eligibility can be particularly complex and restrictive. Remember that you do not have to be a council tenant to obtain advice or assistance from the council's housing department.

You should also seriously consider taking legal advice. Housing law is extremely complex and too many people seek legal advice too late.

You may also be able to get housing advice and information from local housing associations, from advice agencies such as Citizens' Advice Bureaux, or from voluntary organisations in your area (see *UK AIDS Directory* for details).

AIDS service organisations

There are a large number of voluntary AIDS service organisations providing a wide range of care, support, advice and education services (although there are considerable regional variations in the type and number of organisations available to you at a local level).

These organisations vary in size, the kinds of services they provide, whether they operate on national or local levels, and to whom they offer services. Most however have established themselves as a result of community-led initiatives to fight HIV and promote independent living for people with HIV or AIDS. Some organisations are partly or wholly led by people living with HIV, and some services are provided by people with HIV. Some of these organisations are therefore very aware of the needs of people with HIV or AIDS and are much more responsive to the communities they serve than is often the case with statutory services.

The services that voluntary organisations often provide include :

- social care, inc. help at home, and 'buddying' (where trained volunteers can offer long term emotional and practical support for people living with HIV or AIDS)

- telephone helplines

- support groups

- one-to-one counselling (see **counselling and psychotherapy** above for a list)

- 'drop-in' facilities where food is available as well as different kinds of therapeutic help such as massage, acupuncture or aromatherapy

- advice and information, by phone, in publications and from trained advice workers on benefits, employment, housing and legal problems.

A number of organisations also provide access to health and medical care and information about medical treatment, and a small number provide self help advocacy.

Finally, there are organisations concentrating on health promotion, sexual health education, equity for people with HIV and AIDS, and training for people providing services for people with HIV and AIDS.

For more information about these organisations and the services they provide, please see the *UK AIDS Directory*, or look at the *A to Z of services* later in this chapter to find details of some of the key organisations providing specific types of services.

Regional variations

It is unfortunately still the case that the level of services for people with HIV will vary according to where you live. Some local authorities will be providing a much better level of service than others. It is common for people to move in order to take full advantage of the services in a particular area - due to the concentration of services in London many move here from elsewhere in the country. However, there are considerable variations in both medical and social care even across London.

Furthermore, funding and resources do not always keep abreast with demand for services, so some services may therefore be difficult to get. It is therefore important to discuss your needs with whichever HIV service you are using.

Building a support network

It could be extremely useful to find out about what services are available and who provides them whilst you are HIV-positive and well or asymptomatic. Even if you don't think you need anything, familiarising yourself with local and health authority services, hospital clinics, voluntary AIDS service organisations, and GP surgeries (including whether your GP is a fund-holder) whilst you are well could cut down on the worry or stress of trying to get the help you need if you become unwell.

Making yourself known to local social services, or telephoning a voluntary AIDS service organisation to find out more about what services they provide can mean building up a list of named professionals, volunteers and telephone numbers before you need them, for when you need them.

Some people also find that using social care services whilst they are well is a good way of meeting other people with HIV. Sometimes such friendships can be an important form of peer support.

A to Z of services

Advice and advocacy

Knowing how to get advice about anything concerning being HIV-positive may seem a bewildering prospect, but there are many organisations which can either provide you with the information or help that you need, or point you in the right direction. You may also be able to obtain direct assistance in getting what you need from advocates, who will obtain services or information on your behalf. There are many people out there who are willing to help you - doctors, social workers and other professionals, volunteers or other people living with HIV.

Many local health and social services have key workers who act as points of contact for all other services you may need. Advocacy may also be available from local voluntary organisations, and there's help available to try to get you the best possible deal from the Department of Social Security and officials generally, whether it relates to your welfare or civil rights.

Some voluntary organisations provide Peer Advocacy - advice and help from someone of the same HIV status, gender and or ethnic background as yourself working alongside you to get your needs met.

Such organisations also lobby policy makers, government, providers and commissioners of services, with the concerns of those of us living with HIV.

UK Coalition of People Living with HIV and AIDS
250 Kennington Lane, London SE11 5RD
Phone: 020 7564 2180
Fax: 020 7564 2140

Terrence Higgins Trust
52-54 Grays Inn Road
London WC1X 8JU
Helpline: THT Direct 0845 1221200
Website: www.tht.org.uk

Bereavement and death

When someone dies there are many practical issues to deal with. With HIV infection there can be additional issues such as infection control or dealing with ignorance or prejudice.

The Department of Social Security publishes a free booklet entitled *What to do after a death*, which contains useful information about what must be done and what help is available. Many social and health care professionals can provide further information or assistance where a death has occurred, including how to register deaths and obtain medical certificates, who to contact about arranging funerals, and how to apply for financial assistance from the DSS Social Fund.

Most organisations which provide counselling for people living with HIV also provide emotional support for people who have been bereaved. Two specialist voluntary organisations offering bereavement counselling are:

Cruse Bereavement Project
Cruse House, 126 Sheen Road, Richmond TW9 1UR
020 8332 7227

Lesbian and Gay Bereavement Project
020 7403 5969

Children

Children with HIV infection will have special needs and concerns and there are agencies that have been established to deal with these. They can give advice on many issues including risks of HIV transmission, who to tell and how to deal with schools. Many local authorities have specific social care professionals who work with children and can provide you with particular help and advice. See *Children, adolescents and families* later in this volume for more detailed information about services available.

Cleaning

You can get help with cleaning if you need it, from voluntary organisations and from social services, either on a regular basis or for a short period if you are unwell. Contact your local voluntary organisation or social services department.

Clinical waste disposal

Local authorities or councils have a duty to provide free collection services for clinical waste e.g. needles, syringes, soiled dressings etc, and can collect waste from home. The service should be confidential - speak to a health or social care professional about referral, or contact your local authority's Environmental Health department - and you don't have to tell the service you have HIV.

Community care

The services you receive from you local authority will be provided under the heading of 'Community Care'. The Government's Community Care legislation aims to enable local authorities to help people live in their own homes 'in the community', rather than separating them from society in closed hospitals or other institutions. For more information, see *Services for people with HIV & AIDS*, above, or speak to a social care professional in your local social services department.

Community nursing

You can receive nursing care at home from district or community nurses, or from Clinical Nurse Specialists (HIV/AIDS). Community nurses can provide support, help and advice about changing dressings, help with IV drips, give injections, give you equipment to help with physical problems, give advice on health, or teaching other carers. Clinical Nurse Specialists (HIV/AIDS) have particular experience in providing advice, support and care for people living with HIV or AIDS and can provide intravenous therapy, symptom or pain control, advice about anti HIV drugs, and advice and care should you wish to die at home. Speak to your doctor or a social care professional about how to contact community nurses.

Complaining about services

Most voluntary AIDS service organisations and all hospitals, health and local authorities have formal complaints procedures should you feel you have been inappropriately treated or served. If you do experience problems or are unhappy with a service, give that person a chance to sort out any misunderstanding, keep a record of events, and know your facts. If you are still dissatisfied, ask the person you are dealing with to provide you with details of how to complain.

Complementary therapies

There are many different kinds of therapies available which may complement the medical treatment, health or social care you receive. Therapies such as massage, acupuncture, aromatherapy, relaxation, yoga and creative therapies are offered by many voluntary AIDS service organisations. To find out more, see NAM's *Directory of Complementary Therapies in HIV & AIDS*.

Dental services

All dentists should be able to treat people with HIV. If you tell your dentist you have HIV and they are unwilling to treat you, you may be able to get referred for specialist dental treatment by your GP or clinic doctor. Many hospitals have special dental clinics and your health authority may have a district dental officer who can direct you to community dentists experienced in treating people with HIV.

Family services

Many local authorities have specialist social care providers who work with children and families. Furthermore there are a number of organisations who provide service to families affected by HIV and AIDS, such as:

Positive Partners and Positively Children
Unit F7, Shakespeare Commercial Centre, 245 Coldharbour Lane, London SW9 8RR
020 7738 7333

See also *Positively Women* and *Body & Soul* above, under **counselling and psychotherapy: London organisations**

Food and nutrition

A number of services are available depending on where you live. Some local authorities provide 'meals-on-wheels' services. Many AIDS service organisations offer cheap meals at their centres and in some cases specialist meal deliveries to your home.

You may also be able to seek nutritional advice from dieticians who are often attached to hospital clinics.

The Food Chain
www.foodchain.org.uk
020 7272 7272
info@foodchain.org.uk

Provides meals free of charge to HIV-positive people in London who cannot cook for themselves.

Gay men

There are a number of organisations which focus on advice, support, sexual health education and information for gay and other men who have sex with men. See **counselling and psychotherapy** above for some that offer emotional support.

Some health authorities have dedicated gay men's workers who specialise in sexual health issues for gay men. There are also a growing number of hospital clinics in London who offer specific sexual health clinics for gay men, including gay men living with HIV or AIDS. A useful organisation to contact if you are a gay man living with HIV and want advice, support or information:

GMFA
Unit 42, Eurolink Centre, 49 Effra Road, London SW2 1BZ
020 7738 6872

Relies on gay male volunteers to develop and carry out sexual health education and information access initiatives.

Haemophilia

If you have HIV and haemophilia, you can get advice, support and help from:

The Haemophilia Society
Chesterfield House, 385 Euston Road, London NW1 3AU
020 7380 0600

They will be able to give you information about local groups offering help and information.

See also the chapter on *Haemophilia* later in this volume.

Health advisers and visitors

Clinic-based health advisers and community-based health visitors can provide you with a range of advice, support and information about living with HIV. They may also be able to refer you to other useful services.

Building a relationship with a health adviser in a clinic can be invaluable as they generally have more time to talk to you (and offer a broader perspective) than doctors.

Home care

There is help provided by both local authority social services and voluntary organisations for support with day-to-day household chores such as cleaning, shopping and cooking.

Nursing care at home is also available (see *Community nursing* above), and social services departments can be a source of help with home adaptations like stair-lifts, hand rails, bathing aids, telephone installation and washing machine/cooker/microwave loans.

Hospices and terminal care

A number of organisations provide care for people who are dying. Hospices provide hospital-style terminal care where medical staff can provide pain or symptom control. If you are terminally ill and wish to die at home, you can receive ongoing nursing care.

Housing and utilities

There are a number of potential problems related to HIV. You may have the threat of eviction or other harassment hanging over you. You may have difficulties in meeting rent or mortgage payments. You may be homeless or living in sub-standard accommodation. You may find you need certain home adaptations and special equipment. If you are experiencing any housing problems, it's important to seek advice or help as soon as possible. Local authority housing and social care professionals can be an invaluable source of help, as can organisations experienced in giving housing advice.

Languages, interpretation and translation

Many hospital trusts, health and local authorities have interpretation and translation services for people who do not have English as their first language. A number of helplines also have times when their phones are staffed by people speaking specific languages, including:

National AIDS Helpline
0800 917 2227
Call for details of language services offered.

Naz Project
Palingswick House, 241 King Street, London W6 9LP
020 8741 1879
Call for details of language services offered.

AFAS
6 Osnaburgh Street, London NW1 3DH
020 7383 0489
Support for French speakers.

Language Link
www.languageline.co.uk
020 7520 1430

Learning difficulties

There are a number of organisations who work with people with learning difficulties and many local authorities have specialist professionals who work with people with learning difficulties in need of specific social care.

Legal advice and services

See *Advice and advocacy*.

Leisure activities

Leisure passes are available from many local authorities for people who are unemployed, on income support or who are registered disabled - these can be used in various centres, swimming pools, gyms etc. Speak to a social care professional in your local social services department for more information.

Compass Support Group
c/o 36C Nevern Square, London SW5 9PE
020 7373 9091

Medical care

For information about medical care, see *Services for people with HIV and AIDS* above or the *HIV & AIDS Treatments Directory*. The following organisations can help you choose your treatments and decide how and if you can have these at home or at a local clinic or in hospital and give advice about up-to-date treatments and drug trials.

NAM
Lincoln House, 1 Brixton Road, London, SW9 6DE
020 7840 0050
www.aidsmap.com

AIDS Treatment Update, published monthly; free to people with HIV.

HIV i-Base
HIV treatment information for healthcare professionals and HIV-positive people.
Treatment phoneline: 0808 800 6013 - Mon, Tues, Wed 12-4pm.
www.i-base.org.uk

HIV Treatment Bulletin published monthly.

Terrence Higgins Trust
52-54 Grays Inn Road, London WC1X 8JU
Helpline THT Direct 0845 122 1200
www.tht.org.uk

Information centre, individual advice sessions, support groups.

Positively Women
347-349 City Road, London EC1V 1LR
020 7713 0444

Treatment information sessions and individual advice sessions.

Waverley Care Solas
2/4 Abbeymount, Edinburgh EH4 8EJ, Scotland
0131 661 0982
info@waverleycare.org

Treatment advice and information in Scotland. Phoneline open Mon-Fri 11-4.

Mobility

A number of taxi card and discount travel schemes are available. Social services workers should be able to advise about eligibility for local taxicard schemes, disabled driver 'orange badges', community transport schemes or travel permits.

Some AIDS service organisations can offer assistance with transport, and help with mobility around the house is likely to be available from home care providers (see *Home care* above).

Money and financial help

Contact the Terrence Higgins Trust for up-to-date advice on this subject. Benefits regulations change too rapidly and are too complicated to be included in the *AIDS Reference Manual*, and claimants require individual advice on how to claim successfully.

Occupational therapy

Occupational therapists or OTs are trained to help people who are ill or disabled live at home as independently as possible. If you are in hospital you can ask to see an NHS occupational therapist who will either help you prepare for when you go home, or will refer you to a local authority occupational therapist. Some local authorities have specialist HIV/AIDS occupational therapists, but all should have 'generic' OTs who will be trained and experienced in working with people with HIV or AIDS.

OTs can advice people with HIV and their carers on special equipment and adaptations to their home, advise and assist with rehousing, provide re-training and learning new skills following periods of illness, and provide advice, information and emotional support for problems which might affect your day to day routine.

Physiotherapy

A physiotherapist can help you deal with some of the special physical problems that illness can lead to. They can help you maintain your strength through special exercise and muscle development, help keep you moving if you are weak, advise on breathing problems, help you cope with the physical effects of neurological problems, swollen limbs or back problems. Physiotherapists work in hospitals, in clinics and in the community. If you attend a clinic, ask to be referred, or ask your GP.

Prisoners

The HM Prison Service Directorate of Health Care now has a focus on HIV training, care, support and liaison, looking at the provision of care and support for prisoners with HIV, training for prison staff, and liaison with health authorities and other groups working around HIV issues in prisons. The HIV Training and Liaison Officer can be contacted on 020 7217 6602.

Many health authorities and some health care providers are working with prisons and prisoners with HIV. To find out further information, contact your district health authority HIV Prevention Co-ordinator.

For more information see the chapter on **HIV and prisoners**.

Refugees

There are a number of organisations which can provide services to political or economic refugees from other countries. Some voluntary AIDS service organisations which offer services to people from particular minority ethnic or cultural backgrounds will be able to provide specific advice, support and information to people who have come to this country as refugees. You can also contact the Refugee Council or the Refugee Legal Centre.

See also **The Law and HIV.**

Refugee Council
www.refugeecouncil.org.uk
020 7346 6700
info@refugeecouncil.org.uk

Refugee Legal Centre
www.refugee-legal-centre.org.uk
020 7780 3200
rlc@refugee-legal-centre.org.uk

Religious support

There is a wide range of religious support and counselling available to people living with HIV infection or who are affected by it in any way. This may be through the mainstream or 'established' religious communities, or various other 'spiritual' organisations. Religious groups can offer both religious support and practical help.

A 'religious' response to HIV and AIDS should be a caring response, though in practice religious responses have varied from the truly compassionate to the completely inappropriate and judgmental. In no religion is there such a thing as one single agreed response to all the issues that HIV raises. For every harsh and intolerant attitude in any of the world's religions, there will be other compassionate and caring ones as well.

Respite and residential care services

In some parts of the country there are special HIV residential centres which are designed to feel more like home than hospital, and offer convalescence, respite, relief, on-going and terminal care. You may be eligible for respite care under the local authority's community care service, so speak to a social care professional.

Sex workers

Sex workers have specific needs in relation to HIV and AIDS which can be met by a number of organisations and groups. Access to condoms, sexual health education and care for people working in the sex industry is available from some hospitals and clinics, as well as independent or voluntary organisations and projects. See the *UK AIDS Directory* for a list of services for sex workers.

Sexual health services

Information, advice and care around your sexual health can be obtained from different places, especially hospital genito-urinary medicine departments or sexual health clinics. Many voluntary AIDS service organisations also provide advice and information about sexual health, preventing sexual transmission of HIV, and access to safer sex materials. For more information on specific sexually transmitted infections and what to expect when you go for treatment, see *Sexually transmitted infections and sexual health* in *Safer sex*.

Shared care

Many hospitals and clinics are beginning to devolve some of their medical treatment roles down to GP's, as part of the Government's NHS Community Care legislation. This may mean you will receive 'shared care and treatment' from both hospitals and a GP. It could be a good idea to find out as much information about shared care as possible, so speak to your clinic doctor or health adviser.

Shopping

You can get help with shopping if you need it, from voluntary organisations and from social services, either on a regular basis or for a short period if you are unwell.

Social workers

All local authorities and some hospitals have social workers, some of whom may be specialist in HIV/AIDS. However many social services have become less specialist and more 'generic'.

Social workers are there to help you live as independently as possible. A good social worker will give you advice and information about services you may be able to get from the local and health authority, the NHS and from voluntary and independent organisations. They can also help you get services organised, help you make grant and benefit applications, and provide emotional support. For more information about social services and community care, see *Services for people with HIV and AIDS* earlier in this chapter.

Telephones

Under the Chronically Sick and Disabled Persons Act, you may be eligible for assistance with telephone installation and rental. Speak to a social care professional in your local social services department.

Telephone helplines

There is a huge range of telephone helplines across the country, many specifically serving people with HIV and AIDS, others incorporating HIV issues into the services they provide for people such as those from different minority ethnic groups, lesbians and gay men or drug users. The National AIDS Helpline is a free and confidential service offering advice on HIV and AIDS and related issues.

National AIDS Helpline
0800 567123

Travel

Some countries restrict entry for people living with HIV or AIDS, so it's important to get as much information as possible before you travel abroad. It may also be a good idea to get information about treatments available in the country/countries you intend to visit. Information can be obtained from a number of sources. A list of travel restrictions for countries known to have policies on HIV and immigration can be found in *Travel* below.

Visual impairments

There are a number of sources of support, information and services for people who are visually impaired and living with HIV or AIDS. Occupational therapists can help with adaptations to your home (see Occupational Therapy above). The Royal National Institute For The Blind can provide information and a wide range of services to people who are visually impaired or blind, including Braille versions and audiotapes of leaflets.

Royal National Institute for the Blind (RNIB)

224 Great Portland Street, London W1N 6AA

Helpline: 0845 766 9999

Welfare benefits advice

Many voluntary AIDS service organisations can provide advice and information about welfare benefits and what you may be entitled to. It is a fact that many people do not claim the benefits they are eligible for, so it's important to know exactly what you may be able to claim for. Many drop-in or day care centres will have welfare rights advisers for you to see, or you can speak to a social care professional. You can also contact your local Citizens Advice Bureau.

Women

Women living with HIV or AIDS may have particular issues or problems, such as increased difficulties in accessing quality services, obtaining appropriate care, support and advice, or issues around child care. A number of organisations offer services, information, support and advice specifically for and by women, such as *Positively Women* and *Body & Soul*, which both run support groups for women who are HIV-positive. The *UK AIDS Directory* lists services specifically for women in all regions of the country, including women's support groups.

Books about women and HIV are listed in *Recommended resources*.

Many GP surgeries and hospital clinics have health and medical care designed specifically for women. Check to see if any of your local GP surgeries have 'well women' clinics.

Social services can offer support with child care and child minding. You can be referred to a social services department social worker through a specialist HIV social worker at the hospital you attend, or else through any voluntary organisation. See *Children, adolescents and families* for more on help with child care.

Positively Women
347-49 City Road, London EC1V 1LR
020 7713 0222

Travel

Advice on international travel

Entry restrictions

Find out about any entry restrictions in the countries you are planning to go to. You can do this by checking the list below, although for the most up to date advice you should contact the local embassies or consulates of each country you are intending to travel to. If you do this you should not reveal your HIV status or name to them. If you feel uncomfortable about calling an embassy or consulate directly, you can call one of the advice giving organisations like The Terrence Higgins Trust and have them call for you. Information about travel restrictions can change, so it is important to double check.

If entry restrictions exist in the country to which you want to travel, you will need to decide whether you want to take the risk of travelling. Few countries have restrictions on tourist travel for short stays, but any restrictions are evidence of an ill-informed policy, and this could translate into spot checks on people who are suspected of having AIDS. Anyone who is identifiably sick, a gay man, a drug user or a person from an African country where AIDS is endemic is likely to be more vulnerable to inspection.

You may want to contact an AIDS service organisation in the country to which you wish to travel (if one exists), and find out if they know what risks you run in entering that country. You may also want to ask whether particular airports have a reputation for particularly stringent vetting of incoming visitors.

You should ask the local organisation what you ought to do if you are denied entry or detained, and if they don't know, ask them to find out. You may feel more secure if someone - either a friend or someone in an AIDS organisation - knows you are coming.

Travelling with medication

It's often necessary for people with HIV/AIDS to carry medication with them when they travel - particularly medicine for preventing opportunistic infections (prophylaxis) and antiretrovirals.

Border entry points usually take an interest in medicines and pharmaceuticals. Drugs which are legal in one country may not be legal in others.

You have three options

- Sending your medicine ahead. If you have someone to send it to, this is an option, but make sure it has arrived before you leave for your destination.

- Purchasing the medicine in the country you have entered. You need to find out if this is possible, how it is done, how long this is likely to take and what costs are involved. In some countries like the United States this can be very expensive.

- Carrying the medication with you. You can choose to be open about what the medications are for. If you are not going to be open, then you need to be ready to answer the question 'what are these drugs for?'. Either way, a doctor's letter may be of help. It may be advisable to have your clinician write you a letter on generic hospital paper- which has no mention of HIV on it, and state that the drugs are for a chronic medical condition and are for personal use.

Whatever you decide to do, calculate how much medication you will need and then add on a few extra day's supply to be on the safe side. It may also be a good idea to take preventive medications for minor everyday problems such as insect bites or headaches which you are used to using. New medications can sometimes cause allergic reactions.

Travelling by air

If you are quite ill, or there is a high chance that you could become ill, then airlines will sometimes make special arrangements for you and ensure there is going to be a doctor on your flight. Airlines can refuse to carry people who are very sick or insist on special conditions such as being accompanied by an appropriate medical practitioner. While some airlines have very good records of being cooperative and helpful to people with HIV and AIDS, others do not. You can usually check out these issues before purchasing your ticket by contacting the airline's Medical Assistance department, anonymously if you prefer.

Long distance air travel can sometimes cause additional health problems for people who are experiencing respiratory problems or have damaged lungs.

Vaccinations

A full discussion of issues for HIV-positive people to consider when deciding which vaccinations to undergo can be found in the *HIV & AIDS Treatments Directory*.

If you are travelling to areas where malaria is present, it is essential that you take anti-malaria medication. If you are going to be in these areas for some time then investing in a mosquito net may be useful. You should discuss your travel itinerary with your doctor to ensure that the most appropriate anti-malaria drugs can be prescribed.

Travel insurance

Some travel insurance companies now provide cover for people living with HIV & AIDS. However, certain restrictions tend to apply and the premiums can often be greatly inflated. Coverage includes claims for medical expenses, for loss of deposit or cancellation owing to illness and for any additional expenses. It is worth shopping around to see who can offer you the best cover at the best price. NAM cannot recommend any particular company. It is most sensible to obtain a range of quotes and identify which company most meets your specific needs.

The Freedom Travel Insurance Scheme, which has been developed in partnership with the National AIDS Trust provides a comprehensive travel insurance product, which includes full medical cover (though this is subject to health screening, which can be completed on the internet or on the telephone).

Specialist providers

GoGay: www.gogay.com - 0870 458 3230 - enquiries@gogay.com

It's SoEasy: www.gaytravelinsurance.com - 0845 222 2226 - hello@hivtravelinsurance.com

Rothwell and Towler: www.travelfirst.co.uk - 01404 41234 - martin@rothwellandtowler.co.uk

Reciprocal medical care arrangements

Travellers to European Community countries should obtain an E111 certificate before they go. A form to apply for this is available from any Post Office. The form will tell you which countries are covered by reciprocal health care agreements with

UK, and what they consist of. You may not get all medical services for free in some countries. This is a special problem for the United States, and you should check with a US AIDS organisation before you go about what medical services will be available to you at your destination.

Support services at your destination

You may want to check with local AIDS organisations at your destination where to go for medical help if you need it.

Food and drink

Food and drink are often sources of infection when abroad, and this is especially important to bear in mind if you have a compromised immune system. Drink only water that has been boiled. This includes bottled water and milk. Avoid ice, unless you are sure it is made from boiled water. The same goes for ice-cream.

Food which has not been heated thoroughly is often a source of infection. However tempting they might be, meals bought from street vendors shouldn't be eaten unless you are confident they have been fully cooked in your presence. Avoid raw seafood and other raw foods, except fruit and vegetables which you have washed and peeled yourself.

For **Life insurance,** see under **Insurance and HIV testing** in HIV testing

International restrictions on people with HIV

How we collected this information

This record of entry restrictions was originally based on information provided to us by the London diplomatic representatives of each country in March 1997, and on entry restrictions summarised from a variety of sources by the US State Department in December 1998. Since that time we have updated the information annually.

The latest US State Department list is available at http://travel.state.gov/HIVtestingreqs.html The February 2001 version has been consulted in preparation for this edition.

In addition, further information was obtained from *The free movement of persons living with HIV/AIDS* edited by Dr Lieve Fransen, published in 1999.

In April 2001 the Deutsche AIDS Hilfe published its research into international entry and residence restrictions and access to treatments. In total information was received from 162 countries. The results were astounding, with over 60% of countries covered continuing to practice discrimination and exclusion against people with HIV/AIDS.

The document is available in full in both German and French online at http://www.aidsnet.ch/modules.php?name=Sections&sop=listarticles&secid=13 An English language version is planned.

The European AIDS Treatment Group is in the process of putting an English version of this document on its website - see www.eatg.org/hivtravel/ for progress.

The German survey asked about any entry or residency restrictions that would apply to HIV-positive German nationals. The research need to be carefully read in light of this. It may be that other European Union passport holders have the same rights of freedom of movement as German nationals, but the same cannot be said for passport holders from countries outside of the European Union.

Research of this kind is urgently needed.

When conducting our own research, we asked whether countries imposed restrictions on nationals of any other country, not merely the UK, it should not be assumed that the answers provided by London diplomatic representatives are automatically applicable to holders of other passports.

If you are in any doubt before you travel, check with the diplomatic representatives of the country you are planning to visit. Also check this against information from any local AIDS service organisations listed in *NAM's AIDS Organisations Worldwide* and *European AIDS Directory,* and tell them that you are coming. That way, if you are detained at a port of entry, at least someone will know, and may be able to provide help.

A to Z of countries

Albania
No restrictions.

Algeria
Citizens returning from work abroad and members of the armed forces will be required to take an HIV test.

Angola
All nationalities require a visa to enter Angola.

A negative HIV status certificate is required to obtain a residence visa to work. Ordinary, transit and residential visas do not require this.

Anguilla
For British nationals there are no restrictions although there are reports of entry being refused to other foreign nationals suspected of having, or known to have, AIDS.

Argentina
No restrictions on visits of less than three months. No distinction between applicants from different countries. The usual documentation is required for longer visits and residence applications. However, HIV screening is included in the health control of immigrants. Foreigners suffering from diseases that reduce their ability to work will not be admitted on a temporary or permanent residence permit.

Armenia
Entry prohibited for HIV-positive people. Also, people who fall ill during their stay in the country may be deported, although the actual legislation on this matter is still being prepared.

Aruba
HIV testing is required for intending immigrants.

Australia
Everyone except those with Australian or New Zealand passports must have a visa. For short business or tourism visits, travellers must sign a declaration of good health. Those who are unable to sign must provide details of any health problems. It is unlikely that those with HIV and AIDS will be denied entry for short visits, but each case is considered on its merits.

HIV tests are required for foreigners who want to immigrate permanently to Australia.

Anyone working in food handling, or in a classroom situation will be required to have a medical. This is largely to prevent the spread of TB.

For stays over one year in duration, a medical with chest X-ray and blood test is required. All cases are considered on their merits.

In general, HIV-positive status is not a problem unless there is a public health risk (i.e. TB) or considerable expense by the health service is involved, or access to limited treatment resources for Australians may be reduced.

Austria
There appear to be no entry restrictions as such although the city of Klagenfurt requires persons applying for a residence permit to be certified as HIV-negative. Health certificate is required with application for a residence permit for more and six months from non-EU citizens.

Azerbaijan
No known restrictions.

Bahamas
The Ministry of Health have recommended that HIV-positive people should not be allowed to enter the country.

Bahrain
No restrictions on stays of less than four weeks. No questions are asked - but if a person were to declare their HIV-positive status they would be refused entry. There are exceptions for diplomatic staff.

Individuals will not be permitted employment in food handling or patient/child care if they are HIV-positive.

Bangladesh
There are no specific entry regulations for people with HIV/AIDS, and this also applies to long-term residence. If is possible, however, that foreigners with HIV/AIDS are deported if the competent authorities find out about their condition.

Barbados
At present, no restrictions for holiday trips. A medical is required for a long-term stay, or for a work permit, and it is thought unlikely that an HIV-positive person would be allowed into the country on a long-term basis.

Belarus
All persons staying longer than three months must produce evidence of their HIV status.

Belgium
All non-European Community nationals intending to study or undertake work permit employment must undergo an HIV test by a Belgian-approved doctor in their country of origin. No visas are granted for people who test HIV-positive.

Belize
Foreign nationals applying for citizenship must produce a negative HIV test certificate on arrival issued not more than two months earlier.

Benin
No restrictions for short-time tourist stays. HIV testing required for longer-term stays.

Bolivia
No regulations for short tourism or business visits - but compulsory Yellow Fever Vaccine for all visitors. This live vaccine is not recommended for those with compromised immunity.

A medical with blood test is required for short- or long-term residency applications.

Anyone staying more than 90 days and applicants for work permits will be required to provide evidence of their HIV status.

Bosnia-Herzegovina

No entry restrictions for HIV-positive people, However foreigners applying for a permanent residence must present a negative HIV test result.

Botswana

HIV testing required from students beginning their studies.

Brazil

There are no entry restrictions for people living with HIV.

Brunei

No mandatory testing for short-term tourist stays. However, people known to be HIV-positive are prohibited from entering, and expulsed if HIV infection is detected. Doctors have a duty to immediately inform authorities.

Bulgaria

Foreign nationals intending to stay for 30 days or longer are tested within 72 hours of arrival. The test is also required from Bulgarian nationals who have been abroad for longer than 30 days.

Burkina Faso

There are no entry restrictions for HIV-positive persons. However, in order to obtain an entry visa, foreigners must be vaccinated against yellow fever, a live vaccine which is not recommended for those with compromised immunity.

Cambodia

Though a foreigner can be expelled if he/she poses a threat to national security, health is not mentioned as grounds for expulsion.

Cameroon

There are no restrictions on entry and residence entitlement relating to public health.

Canada

People entering Canada for short tourist stays or temporary residents for less than six months are nor required to disclose their HIV status or to be tested.

Mandatory HIV testing of all prospective immigrants occurs. However, a recent (June 2001) policy change means that the status of would-be immigrants who test HIV-positive will be decided on a case by case basis. People found to be HIV-positive will not be automatically excluded.

UK passport holders can travel to Canada without the need for a visa.

Chile

There are no specific restrictions for those wishing to travel to Chile. A medical certificate is needed for those applying for a work permit or residency. Foreign students are also tested for HIV. If a person is found to be HIV-positive he or she will be denied entry.

China

Foreign nationals applying for residence or intending to stay more than six months must have an HIV test certificate approved by a Chinese Embassy or consulate, or undergo a test in China within 20 days of arrival. It is reported that random testing at the point of entry is now unofficial Chinese policy. Entry is denied and deportation is likely for foreigners who are found to be HIV-positive. Testing is not required for entry or residency in Hong Kong.

Colombia

A medical certificate is required for those who are applying for a long stay visa, work permit or residency. Anyone who is suspected of being HIV-positive will not be admitted for short visits.

Costa Rica

People wishing to work or live in Costa Rica are requested to present a medical certificate. There is no specification regarding HIV status.

Cote d'Ivoire (Ivory Coast)

No restrictions for HIV-positive individuals.

Cuba

Foreign students, foreign workers and long-term foreign residents are screened for HIV; people found to be HIV-positive are reportedly repatriated.

Cyprus

All foreign workers and students are required to undergo medical examinations, including an AIDS test. Under immigration laws, any carriers of contagious and infectious diseases, including HIV/AIDS, are considered illegal immigrants and permission of entry is at the discretion of the Minister of the Interior.

Czech Republic

No restrictions.

Denmark

No restrictions.

Dominican Republic

A negative HIV test certificate is required for a work permit or application for permanent residency.

Ecuador

Those applying for a long-term residency are normally requested to test for HIV.

Egypt

All foreigners intending to stay in the country for three months or more must have an HIV test on arrival. Spouses of Egyptian nationals are exempt. Foreigners requiring work permits must be tested but their spouses are exempt. No residence or work permit will be granted if test result is positive.

Foreign defense contractors at Egyptian military establishments must produce an HIV test certificate.

El Salvador

No restrictions.

Estonia

No restrictions on entry for HIV-positive individuals unless applying for a work permit or residence.

Fiji

People with HIV/AIDS are not allowed to enter the Fiji Islands.

Finland

No restrictions. However, according to a clause in the Finnish law persons who "knowingly transmit" HIV may be deported.

Gabon

All travellers require a medical certificate to enter the country. No specific HIV restrictions apply.

Georgia

All foreigners staying longer than one month are required to provide evidence of their HIV status, provided that the test certification was issued at least 30 days before arrival.

Germany

Foreign nationals applying for residence in Bavaria and tourists staying more than four months must undergo an HIV test. Certain nationalities are exempt.

Ghana

No restrictions.

Greece

Non-EU foreign students and foreigners wishing to work in Greece are required to take an HIV test, as are women intending to work in 'entertainment centres'.

Guatemala

No restrictions but foreign residents who remain in the country for a prolonged period must undergo testing for HIV and AIDS.

Guyana

All foreigners staying longer than three months are required to provide evidence of their HIV status. However the restrictions may be lifted in the near future.

Haiti

No restrictions.

Honduras

No restrictions for tourist stays. Special regulations for people wishing to settle in Honduras.

Hong Kong

No HIV testing on entry. Intending immigrants must undergo HIV testing and AIDS examination.

Hungary

No restrictions for short-term tourist stays. No HIV testing on entry. An HIV test is required for anyone who wants to stay in the country for more than one year. Additionally, some employers may require their staff to undergo HIV testing.

All students over 18, anyone between the ages of 18 and 70 with a visa valid for at least one year and anyone extending a stay to a year or more must provide evidence of their HIV status.

Accredited journalists and diplomats are excluded from this requirement.

Iceland

In general, neither a medical certificate nor an HIV test result is required when entering Iceland.

India

No restrictions for short-term tourist stays. HIV testing required for anyone wishing to stay in India longer than one year. There are also specific regulations, which apply to all foreign students admitted to an Indian university. People with a known HIV infection are not granted visas.

Indonesia

There are no specific entry or residence regulations for people with HIV/AIDS. Neither a medical certificate nor an HIV test result is required when entering the country. Foreigners with a known HIV infection are not subject to specific residence regulations. There are no regulations regarding the control, deportation or expulsion of those concerned.

Iran

Foreign nationals intending to work in Iran or to stay for more than three months must produce an HIV test certificate.

Iraq

People with HIV/AIDS are not allowed to enter Iraq. A very recent test result has to be presented on entry, or else the test is performed on the spot. Those concerned are immediately expelled.

Exceptions: Holders of diplomatic passports or service passports while on official duty. People officially invited by the government and staying for 15 days or less. People older than 65. Children under the age of 12, who are in possession of a declaration from their parents, which states that they are not hemophiliacs and have never received a blood transfusion.

Ireland (The Republic of)

No specific entry or residence regulations for people with HIV/AIDS.

Israel

There are no specific entry regulations for people with HIV/AIDS travelling to Israel. The only condition is that they must have health insurance.

People intending to stay more than three months to work or study are required to show a medical certificate which includes information on HIV status.

Italy

No restrictions for people with HIV/AIDS.

Jamaica

No restrictions for people with HIV/AIDS.

Japan

No restrictions for people with HIV or AIDS who wish to travel or work in Japan.

Jordan

For a stay of more than 30 days, a medical examination by a Health Ministry laboratory is obligatory. In the case of positive test result, the applicant has to leave the country at very short notice.

Kazakhstan

A negative test result has to be provided when applying for a work or residence permit. It is recommended to carry a certified copy of a test result certificate in Russian language. This way it can be avoided to undergo an HIV test in Kazakhstan, a procedure that, in some cases, has to be repeated every three months.

Kenya

Foreigners may be excluded for refusing to undergo a medical examination. Though no entry restrictions have been specifically adopted relating to HIV.

Korea (Democratic People's Republic)

There is no legal provision regarding the entry of people with HIV/AIDS. Not everybody is requested to present a medical certificate or a specific document of an AIDS examination when entering the country. However, if a person's HIV-positive status becomes known, he/she is sent back to his/her country of origin. The reason given for this is the lack of experience with HIV/AIDS and the lack of treatment options.

Korea (South)

People with HIV are not permitted to enter the country. However, for a stay of up to 3 months, it is not mandatory to prove one's HIV status (for those visitors who do not require a visa). There are controls at the border regarding the HIV status. If a person's HIV-positive status becomes known, he/she is expelled.

Kuwait

No HIV testing is required for visitors or business travellers. The visa application for a long-term stay requires a doctor's certificate. In the case of an HIV infection, no visa is granted.

Kyrgyzstan

All foreigners excluding diplomats staying more than one month are required to provide evidence of their HIV status.

Laos

There are no specific entry or residence regulations for people with HIV/AIDS.

Latvia

No HIV testing on entry, but anyone seeking a residency permit has to present a test result.

Lebanon

Anyone planning to work in Lebanon must undergo an HIV test.

Lesotho

It is at the discretion of the border police as to whether or not a person may enter into Lesotho. However, no medical checks are carried out.

Libya

No restrictions for short stays, but HIV testing is obligatory for longer stays requiring a residence permit. In the case of a proven HIV infection, foreign nationals are required to leave the country immediately, or are not allowed to enter in the first place.

Lithuania

No restrictions.

Luxemburg

No specific regulations regarding the entry of people with HIV/AIDS, although Luxemburg law stipulates that entry can be denied on health grounds.

Madagascar

No restrictions.

Malawi

No entry restrictions. A health certificate is not required for longer stays and applications for residence permits either.

Malaysia

HIV testing for foreign nationals who apply for a work permit for unskilled labour.

Special provisions for domestic staff and construction workers from developing countries (Bangladesh, Pakistan, Indonesia, the Philippines); denial of permission to enter, or expulsion, if the HIV test result is positive.

Maldives

Long-term visitors are required to undergo an HIV test in the Maldive Islands.

Mali

There are no entry restrictions for HIV-positive persons. However, yellow fever vaccination is required. This is not recommended in immune compromised individuals.

Malta

No restrictions.

Marshall Islands

Temporary visitors staying more than thirty days and applicants for residence and work permits are required to produce evidence of HIV status.

Mauritius

HIV test required for foreign nationals who want to work in Mauritius or who apply for permanent residence.

Mexico

Foreigners with a known HIV infection are not subject to specific entry or residence regulations. The deportation of an HIV-positive person is only possible in the case of a very severe offence.

Micronesia

Anyone staying over 90 days and anyone holding a work permit is required to undergo an HIV test.

Moldavia

Foreign nationals who are HIV-positive are not allowed to enter Moldavia. A medical certificate is required on entry, although tourists are exempt. In addition, foreign tourists need to pass a health exam conducted by the Moldavian Health Authorities. Such a certificate is also necessary if a foreign national wishes to get married in Moldavia. HIV testing is required of anybody wishing to stay longer than three months.

Mongolia

A test result is requested on entry. However, this law is apparently not applied. Foreign students must have an HIV test on arrival, repeated several months later. Foreigners staying longer than 30 days may also be required to undergo testing, though this is not an official law and is only selectively applied.

Montserrat

Foreign nationals, including university students who are applying for or renewing work or residence must produce a negative HIV certificate.

Morocco

No restrictions.

Mozambique

No restrictions.

Namibia

No restrictions.

Nepal

No restrictions. However some foreign visitors with HIV have reportedly been deported.

Netherlands

No restrictions.

New Zealand

No restrictions for stays of up to twelve months.

From early 2005, New Zealand started undertaking HIV screening for migrants. The full set of changes, including screening for HIV, and a wider and updated set of tests for other expensive-to-treat conditions, was implemented for people seeking to be in New Zealand for longer than twelve months.

Nicaragua

No restrictions for short-term stays. For stays of more than three months, the residence permit has to be extended by the immigration authorities. In this case, the presentation of a medical certificate is requested.

Extended residency will only exceptionally be granted to HIV-positive people.

Nigeria

Immigration officers may refuse entry to any foreigners who are undesirable for medical reasons. Also, immigration officers may refuse entry to any foreigners living with HIV, whose home country would apply restrictions to Nigerian nationals.

Norway

Persons who stay in Norway for longer than three months are offered a voluntary tuberculosis test and an HIV test, in order to arrange for any necessary treatment as quickly as possible.

Myanmar (Burma)

No restrictions.

Oman

There is no clear information on whether or not HIV testing is required for tourists. Persons whose HIV-positive status becomes known are immediately deported.

Compulsory testing on entry for foreign nationals wishing to settle in Oman.

Pakistan

A medical examination is required of returning nationals, refugees and applicants for long-term stays.

Panama

An HIV test certificate is required of foreign nationals wishing to stay for more than 1 year, women wishing to work in "entertainment centres" and anyone wishing to extend an existing visa. HIV-positive people are refused entry.

Papua New Guinea

HIV testing required when applying for a work permit which is granted only if negative HIV test result can be presented.

Paraguay

Anyone applying for permanent residency in Paraguay is required to undergo HIV testing at the regional medical laboratory. No residence permit is granted if the test result is positive.

Peru

No specific entry restrictions. Those wishing to obtain a Peruvian marriage certificate are required to take an HIV test.

Philippines

No restrictions for short-term tourist stays lasting up to six months. Applicants for a permanent visa must undergo medical examination including an HIV test. This also applies to visitors who wish to extend an existing visa.

Poland

Applications for long-term stays require medical testing for HIV/AIDS.

Portugal

No restrictions.

Qatar

No HIV testing on entry. However, people whose HIV-status is known to the authorities are refused entry. Applicants for a work or residence permit must present a negative HIV test certificate (the date of the certificate must not be older than six months).

Romania

No restrictions.

Russian Federation

HIV-positive people are not permitted to enter the Russian Federation. No HIV testing is required on entry for short-term tourist stays (up to three months).

Rwanda

There are no restriction entries to people living with HIV. However in the case of serious illness, e.g. AIDS, residence permission can be refused.

Solomon Islands

Entry can be denied if it becomes known, that the person in question has an infectious disease.

St Kitts and Nevis

Foreign nationals seeking permanent residence, undertaking study and those applying for work permits may be asked to undertake an HIV test.

Saudi Arabia

HIV testing on entry. HIV-positive foreign nationals are expelled.

Senegal

There are no restrictions regarding entry for HIV-positive persons.

Seychelles

The law states that foreigners are undesirable if they are carrying infections they are capable of infecting other people with. Applications for residency must be accompanied by medical certification proving that the applicant is in good health. Visitors who are working for the government must produce a negative HIV result. This does not apply to those working in the private sector or who are only applying for a short stay.

Singapore

No restrictions for short-term tourist stays lasting up to six months. Compulsory HIV testing when applying for work permits. The main group targeted is foreign domestic staff employed in Singapore. Foreign nationals with AIDS or who are HIV-positive are expelled.

Slovakia

No restrictions for short-term tourist stays of up to three months.

South Africa

No restrictions for tourists with HIV/AIDS. HIV testing required of all mine workers (irrespective of their positions).

Spain

Anyone seeking residence, or a work or student permit, must submit to a medical exam, which may include an AIDS test.

Sri Lanka

No specific entry regulations for people with HIV/AIDS. No questions asked about HIV/AIDS on entry. However in cases in which an HIV infection is suspected, foreign nationals may be denied entry.

Sudan

Officially, people with HIV are not granted a visa and are not permitted to enter Sudan. A negative HIV test result must be presented at a Sudanese embassy or at Khartoum airport in order to obtain a visa. According to the embassy, this requirement is not enforced in practice.

Swaziland

There are no entry restrictions for people living with HIV.

Syria

Foreign nationals applying for work permits and foreign students must undergo an HIV test at one of three specified centres in Syria. A foreigner wishing to marry a Syrian national is required to take an HIV test.

Sweden

No restrictions for people with HIV/AIDS. In case of doubt, the health authorities may oblige a foreign national to undergo an HIV test. According to Swedish law, persons who come to Sweden and who have reason to believe they could be HIV-positive must consult a doctor and follow that doctor's advice.

Switzerland

No restrictions.

Tadjikistan

So far, it has been possible to enter the country without having to present an HIV test certificate. HIV testing is required for stays of more than 90 days.

Taiwan

An HIV test result must be presented by anyone wishing to stay longer than 90 days or applying for a residence or work permit. If the result is positive or if the person in question refuses to take the test, he/she is expelled.

Tanzania

No restrictions.

Thailand

According to the law, people with communicable diseases are not allowed to enter Thailand. However, no doctor's certificate is required at the border, so that an illness (as long as is not known) does not affect the granting of a visa.

Trinidad and Tobago

All foreign nationals applying for residence or to stay more than one year must undergo a medical examination. Those found to be HIV-positive or to have AIDS will be refused permission to stay.

Tunisia

There are no specific entry restrictions for HIV-positive people. Foreigners and students who intend to stay in the country for a long period are required to get tested on HIV/AIDS.

Turkey

There are no entry or residence restrictions applicable to HIV-positive persons.

Turks and Caicos

All foreign nationals applying for work and residence permits must have a medical examination on arrival, including an HIV test.

Uganda

As a rule, health certificates or HIV test results do not have to be presented on entry or when applying for a long-term stay.

Ukraine

No restrictions.

United Arab Emirates

Foreign nationals aged 18 or above, applying for or renewing work or residence permits must undergo an HIV test. Entry will be refused to those who test positive.

United States of America

In principle, the USA refuses entry to foreign nationals known to be HIV-positive. In exceptional cases, a stay of 30 days may be granted (for family visits, medical treatment, business travel or participation in a scientific, health-related conference).

HIV testing or a medical exam are not required. In the visa application form, the applicant has to say if he/she has a "communicable disease of public health significance". The visa will be denied if this is the case. An applicant who answers "no" despite better knowledge commits an immigration fraud, which leads to immigration prohibition.

HIV-positive foreign nationals lose their right to remain in the USA and are expelled if their status becomes known.

At present, as far as is known, this remains the US position. However on World AIDS Day, December 1 2006, President George W Bush announced that he was going to relax the travel restriction.

A White House press release said: "The President will direct the Secretary of State to request and the Secretary of Homeland Security to initiate a rulemaking that would propose a categorical waiver for HIV-positive people seeking to enter the United States on short-term visas.

"The President considers the participation of people living with HIV/AIDS a critical element in the global HIV/AIDS response."

A 1993 law prohibits HIV-positive people from receiving visas to visit the United States without a waiver. A categorical waiver would enable HIV-positive people to enter the United States for short visits through a streamlined process."

Exactly what this means is open to question. Currently most tourists entering the US from the UK sign an entry form you write on the plane before going through immigration instead of having to get a visa. However the form excludes admission to people "with a communicable disease" and under a 1987 bill the list of such diseases explicitly included HIV.

People with HIV are currently supposed to get individual Visa Waivers which involved queuing up at the embassy and having a stamp, usually in your passport that may identify you as HIV-positive to other countries and will certainly cause immigration to haul you aside for a few questions.

Unsurprisingly, a study published in early 2006 (Mahto) amongst HIV-positive patients in Brighton found that though two-thirds of travellers to the USA knew about the entry ban, only one in seven had sought a Visa Waiver: the majority simply lie on the entry form.

More worryingly, it found that in order to avoid detection as positive by immigration, one in nine patients stopped their HIV medication, half of them without consulting with their doctor.

The Los Angeles-based AIDS Healthcare Foundation welcomed the proposal.

"We applaud President Bush for his order rescinding this outright ban on HIV-positive foreigners entering the United States," said Michael Weinstein, AIDS Healthcare Foundation's President.

"Now, instead of more complicated 'special waivers,' HIV-positive people would obtain a 'categorical waiver' for business or tourist visas for visits up to 60 days. Although we would like to see an even more enlightened approach on this issue, this executive order is a vast improvement over current law, and we than the president for his leadership in this area of HIV/AIDS policy and law."

Friday's executive order may also begin to pave the way for the International AIDS Conference to once again be hosted by a city in the US - which, as the White House hints, is part of the intention. This has not occurred since the congressional legislation instituting the ban was first enacted in 1993.

Other AIDS activists were more skeptical "The devil will be in the detail," said Bob Munk of NAIDS InfoNet in New Mexico. "Will travellers have to disclose their HIV status to get the waiver?

This, at present, is unclear. The form you sign on the plane is marked "US Visa Waiver Program" but whether this means people with HIV can simply now sign the form as anyone else, or will still have to go through the process of applying for a visa is unclear.

The measures also only apply to visitors staying less than 60 days: a ban on long-stay visas and work permits is still in place.

At least a relaxation would mean removing the USA from the list of countries that impose a total entry ban on people with HIV.

An influential US think-tank, the Center for strategic and International Studies, has issued a report laying out the options for relaxing the ban. It can be accessed at www.csis.org/media/csis/pubs/movingbeyondinadmissibility.pdf

The two options open to the US government were laid out in the report as follows:

- **Legislation.** *The most comprehensive approach to address the current outdated policies would require congressional legislation. Congress could choose to strike the language contained in the Immigration and Nationality Act that specifically designates HIV as an inadmissible condition. This approach would provide a more expansive and permanent fix and address the inadmissibility policy for all categories of noncitizens. Such a change could also include returning authority to the secretary of health and human services to determine whether HIV should be considered a "communicable disease of public health significance," authority the secretary has for all other diseases. In parallel with that step, Congress could allow DHHS a reasonable but limited period in which to revisit the list of "communicable diseases of public health significance." This legislative approach would not preclude the administration from implementing a categorical waiver of the inadmissibility requirement for short-term visitors (and any other visa categories that are able to be included).*

- **Expanded waivers.** *For its part, the administration could choose to systematically expand the current HIV waiver options to include (1) additional categories of visa applicants, (2) additional flexibility in the duration of waiver periods, and (3) nondisclosure of HIV status for short-term visitors. This approach could first be applied to additional categories of nonimmigrants, but it might also be extended to additional categories of immigrants. It would provide one way of enabling at least some additional groups of noncitizens with HIV to enter the United States and would build on a process already underway. Some aspects of this expanded waiver approach may encounter obstacles based on limitations in the legal authority of the executive branch to modify waiver policies for specific groups of noncitizens. Further, it is largely an incremental approach; it may not be able to encompass all categories of noncitizens; it would not eliminate entirely the requirement for disclosure of HIV infection that some observers see as discriminatory; and it would not address the underlying differential treatment of HIV under U.S. public health law. In the meantime, however, the administration's current and laudable intention to streamline short-term nonimmigrant visa applications through a categorical waiver, as announced on December 1, 2006, could be expedited at relatively low cost. Although these two approaches are not mutually exclusive, each would undoubtedly raise complex questions about process and implementation. Policy deliberations could benefit from the establishment and input of a working group of relevant experts.*

As of the time of writing (April 2007) no decision has been made, so for now the US entry restrictions remain as they were before.

Reference
Mahto M et al. Knowledge, attitudes and health outcomes in HIV-infected travellers to the USA. HIV Medicine 7(4):201. 2006.

Uzbekistan

Anyone staying for more than 15 days is required to provide an HIV certificate and longer term visitors must renew their HIV certificate after the first three months in the country, and annually thereafter.

Venezuela

No regulations regarding the entry or residence of people with HIV/AIDS.

Vietnam

No specific entry or residence restrictions for people with HIV/AIDS. However the Vietnamese law requires HIV-positive people to report to the health control authorities on entry.

Yemen (South)

No restrictions for tourist stays of up to two months. A negative test result has to be presented for stays of more than two months and HIV-positive people are expelled immediately.

Zambia

No restrictions.

Zimbabwe

No restrictions.

Problems getting into the UK

Visitors 'suspected of having AIDS' have been refused entry by individual immigration officers on questionable legal grounds.

The Home Office claims that the policy is only to exclude people if it is suspected that the person needs extensive medical treatment without being able to pay for it. For further information on UK immigration law and HIV see *Immigration and asylum and HIV.*

The best advice and help for anyone encountering difficulties is available from:

Joint Council for the Welfare of Immigrants
www.jcwi.org.uk
020 7251 8708
info@jcwi.org.uk

United Kingdom Immigration Advisory Service
www.iasuk.org
020 7967 1200

Information and advice

- National HIV/AIDS services: are listed in NAM's *AIDS Organisations Worldwide* and the *European AIDS Directory.*

- Vaccination/immunisation: issues for people with HIV are discussed in the *HIV & AIDS Treatments Directory.*

- Help with travel for people with HIV may be available through the British Red Cross which has links in all other countries through the International Red Cross and Red Crescent. Help may also be available from organisations listed by country in NAM's *AIDS Organisations Worldwide* and the *European AIDS Directory* .

- The Foreign and Commonwealth Office Consular Department has a Travel Advice Section which is open 9.30am until 4.pm Monday to Friday (020 7008 0232 / 0233) may be able to give you information about travel restrictions and political problems abroad.

- Advice on other aspects of health abroad is also available from MASTA, the Medical Advisory Service for Travellers Abroad (0906 822 4100 - http://www.masta.org - enquiries@masta.org). This is not a free service.

- Advice (and a manual) for voluntary organisations sending volunteers or workers abroad is available from the UK NGO AIDS Consortium (020 7324 4780).

- General leaflets: The Traveller's Guide To Health produced by the Department of Health is available free from the Health Literature Line or your local library or Citizens Advice Bureau.

- You can also get general health information about travelling abroad by asking your doctor, who in turn can get guidance on health issues for travellers abroad from the Communicable Disease Surveillance Centre.

- First aid kits and clean needles etc. for travellers abroad can be bought from MASTA (see above).

Putting your affairs in order

Planning for all possibilities

HIV disease is not a death sentence and people who are newly diagnosed usually need reassurance about the quality of their future life, not how to prepare for their eventual death. However it is also the case that some at least of the fears about dying from diseases associated with HIV infection can be lessened by some basic long term preparation by the person with HIV (and their partner, if they have one) before illness makes this process much more difficult. These are important decisions and should not be left to the last minute.

Long term planning points to think about:

- Making a will and appointing an executor.
- Organising power of attorney.
- Organising property, money and papers in the best way.
- Settling disputes with family and friends.
- Making funeral arrangements.

Dying without a will

If anyone dies without making a will (sometimes called dying 'intestate'), strict rules govern who will inherit their property, including money and personal possessions. It is especially important to make a will if you are gay or unmarried or have a partner you wish to provide for.

If there is no will, the person is said to have died intestate, and the law decides who is to get what. Under the rules of intestacy, only a husband or wife, children and blood relatives are entitled to inherit under a complex formula.

Without a will, gay men and lesbians, unmarried partners, lovers and friends, however long the relationship and whatever the true wishes of the person dying might have been, have no automatic right to inherit anything. Although they might in limited circumstances be able to make a legal claim for financial provision out of the estate, this will be an expensive, slow and uncertain process. Only a husband or wife, children and blood relatives are entitled to inherit property and money.

You cannot choose who will make the funeral arrangements and take care of your affairs after death without making a will.

Making a will

You can decide what will happen to everything that belongs to you. You can make sure that your partner, friends or charities receive exactly what you wish, although you may not have a completely free hand if you have dependents, children, a spouse or a former spouse.

It is worth making a will even if you think have no property to speak of.

By making a will, you decide who will look after your affairs and take care of all the arrangements after your death - see *Executors* below.

If you have children under 18 you may be able to appoint someone to care for them after your death - see *Guardians* below.

You can express any particular wishes you may have about your funeral - for example, you might have a preference for cremation or burial, church service or informal wake.

A valid will can only be made by a person of at least 18 years of age and with the appropriate mental capacity both when giving instructions for the will and when executing it.

Mental capacity means that the person making the will must understand the nature of the act and its effects, the extent of the property which is being disposed of, and must be able to comprehend and appreciate any claims which ought to be considered, for instance by relatives. If there is any doubt at all then the advice of the person's doctor should be obtained.

Your will is something you need to think about calmly, while you are free of other pressures. Although a will can be prepared very quickly in an emergency, it is much better to take ample time to consider carefully what it should say and to make sure that you are happy with the arrangements you have made.

A valid will cannot be made by anyone suffering from mental incapacity. Because of the possibility that that might happen, it is very important to make it sooner rather than later. This will give you the comfort of knowing that your wishes have been recorded.

Making a will now does not mean that you can't change your mind later-see *Changing your will,* below.

Making a will is not a difficult process, but although standard do-it-yourself will forms are available from stationers it is better always to take professional advice from a solicitor or an advice centre dealing with wills. A will is a legal document and should be drawn up carefully and signed and witnessed in a particular way. If you write it yourself it may turn out to be invalid, or there may be legal ambiguities in what you thought were clear requests.

Executors

Your executor is the person you appoint in your will to look after your affairs after your death, and is responsible for carrying out the wishes in your will, including arranging your funeral. In some cases (for instance if children may inherit), you should choose two executors, not just one.

An executor should be someone you trust and who will be able to cope with any paperwork, with the help of a solicitor if need be. If at all possible, they should be on hand as it is very difficult to deal with someone's affairs from a long way away. If you must choose someone who lives abroad, there is a risk of uncertainty and additional legal expense unless they are able to spend time here. Many people appoint the person who is to receive most of their property and their money, but you may choose to appoint a close relative or friend whether or not they are to inherit anything, or sometimes their solicitor. It is sensible to check with your chosen executors that they are willing to undertake the task.

Work out roughly what you own and what debts you have. Remember to include money in the bank or building society, and your home if you own it. You do not need to list everything you own but it will help if you know what sorts of things you possess. Do you, for example, have any shares or National Savings Certificates, or any particularly valuable personal belongings, or life insurance? Make sure you leave this list somewhere obvious. You can only give away money and property after all your debts and liabilities have been paid and discharged.

Particularly if you are not well off, you should be aware that your funeral expenses are the first thing to be paid out of your property when you die, ahead of any debts or legacies. A funeral, especially one abroad, could use everything up. If there is not enough money to pay for it, friends or relatives may have to foot the bill, or depending on the situation, it could be paid for from social security.

If you own property in another country, it may be necessary to make a separate will in that country dealing with that property. You will need legal advice from a lawyer familiar with the law in that country.

If you have someone who is dependent on you and needs to be provided for, think of them first: if you don't plan to leave them everything, decide what they will need, and then consider what personal belongings, property, money or other assets you wish to leave to other people. You might also want to consider a gift to charity.

In some circumstances a spouse or former spouse, children or anyone you have maintained such as a partner may have a claim against your estate whether or not you have provided for them in your will. A lawyer will be able to advise you about this.

Some things that cannot be given away in a will

Your share in a jointly owned house or flat, joint account or any other jointly owned property may pass automatically to the other joint owner on your death, or may be subject to the terms of your will, or the intestacy rules. It depends on the exact legal basis of ownership, and you should seek legal advice about your particular circumstances, especially if a flat or house is involved. It is also possible to change the basis of ownership of joint property, but this must be done with legal advice.

Benefits such as 'death in service' benefits and discretionary payments from personal schemes payable by your employer cannot be left by will. If you have formally nominated someone to receive the benefit it will normally be given to that person, but the final decision will be at the discretion of the trustees of the scheme. You should check with your employer that you have made a nomination and that it is up-to-date.

Guardians

The law concerning the appointment of guardians to care for children is quite complicated, and you should always seek legal advice on your proposed arrangements. To summarise:

- If you are a single mother you can appoint a guardian in your will who will in most circumstances be entitled to care for your children on your death.

- However, if you are married to or divorced from the children's father, or if he has *parental responsibility*, the guardian you choose may not normally take over responsibility for the children until after the father's death.

- If you are a single father who has not been married to the mother, you have no automatic right to appoint a guardian, but should seek legal advice as you may be able to acquire *parental responsibility*.

See also *Children, adolescents and families*.

Changing your will

You can change your will at any time so long as you are fit to do so, so do not put off making one because you think you might change your mind.

Never try to change your will yourself. It can only be altered by a separate legal document called a 'codicil'. Do not try to prepare a codicil without professional advice. Alternatively you can have a new will drawn up and revoke the old one.

If you get married, any existing will is revoked unless it specifically refers to the proposed marriage. You should make a new will as soon as you marry. Divorce also affects your will and you should consider making a new will if you get divorced.

Enduring powers of attorney

A Power of Attorney is a document whereby the donor gives the power to act on his or her behalf to another person, the 'attorney'. This ensures that the person of the donor's choice is legally entitled to act for them should they become unable to handle their own affairs. A Power of Attorney can be 'ordinary' or 'enduring'. An ordinary power is usually employed for a specific purpose such as the sale of property or for a restricted period of time and it automatically lapses if the donor becomes 'mentally incapable'. An enduring power by contrast can have very wide powers and most importantly it continues after the donor is deemed incapable as long as it is clear that this is what the donor intended and the legal formalities have been followed.

For people who are concerned about the possibility of becoming seriously ill or mentally impaired the enduring power of attorney is more appropriate and it can be designed to take effect only when they become incapable of handling their own affairs.

Who can be an attorney?

The donor has almost complete freedom in their choice of attorney. The only restrictions are that the attorney(s) must be over 18 and cannot be a bankrupt. Most people choose their partner or spouse, a close friend or family member, or their solicitor.

Legal formalities

Enduring powers have strict rules to prevent any possibility of exploitation of the donor. They must take a specific legal form and they must be independently witnessed. Having said that, they are quick and easy to do in comparison with making a will. Standard forms for powers of attorney are available some local HIV agencies and from legal stationers.

Registration of enduring powers

If an attorney believes that the donor is or is becoming mentally incapable the enduring power must be registered at the Court of Protection for a fee. The attorney does not have to produce medical evidence to support the application but the donor and his or her family must be told in case they object. If there is an objection the Court will hear the objection before deciding to register the power.

Once registered the donor cannot revoke the enduring power of attorney without the intervention of the Court and neither can the donor change the scope of the powers. The attorney is also bound by the power of attorney and cannot stop acting as attorney until notice has been given to the Court.

Organising money, property and other affairs

Your home

It is especially important to consider what will happen if you die if you share a home with a partner to whom you are not married. In the case of joint ownership with a legal *joint tenancy* then on the death of one the property will automatically pass to the other regardless of any will. However if you are what is known as *tenants in common*, the share of a person who dies passes under the terms of a will, or to relatives under the rules of intestacy if there is no will. In this case, the surviving co-owner may have to sell the property. If you have a mortgage which is not covered by life insurance, and do not intend the house to be sold on your death, consider how it is to be paid. You may need to take legal advice to ensure your wishes will come into effect.

Bank and savings accounts

Once someone has died their bank and savings accounts will be frozen by the bank or building society, although they will usually release money to pay for the funeral. This does not apply to joint accounts which the surviving account holder can in most cases continue to use. It can take a long time for property to be sorted out after a death especially if the estate is complicated, or there are a lot of debts, or it is a large estate on which Inheritance Tax is payable. Where funds permit, and there is a surviving partner or dependent to provide for, it is worth considering how best to ensure their continuing access to funds during the administration period. The amount of the assets involved will influence the possibilities available and it is important to seek guidance from a solicitor or accountant.

Funeral arrangements

At first sight it may seem strange to suggest that funeral arrangements could be seen as long-term planning. But people often find reassurance in thinking about the kind of funeral they would like in the event of their death and in knowing that their wishes will be respected. It is also worth thinking about how it will be paid for. Cost is especially an issue if a funeral is planned to take place abroad.

People often do not realise the options that exist - there is certainly no need to have a religious service if they do not want one. People may also want to choose the music and readings they would like and to make dedications to those close to them. Many prefer to have a very simple funeral for close friends and families followed by a memorial event open to all those who wish to remember the deceased. After talking this over with their partner or family they should inform their executor who will have control over the funeral arrangements. Some people do not consider funerals or memorial services to be that important but they do mean a great deal to those who mourn. It is often the last chance for the rest of their lives.

Raising money from insurance policies

Alternatives to surrendering life insurance

Many people who take out life insurance policies find that within a few years their circumstances have changed to such an extent that the policy is no longer relevant to their needs. While financial advisers encourage people to take out life insurance policies, very few provide advice when their clients want to stop their premium payments. Financial advisers receive commission when policies are commenced, and they may be required to return some of this commission to the insurance company if the policy is terminated at an early stage.

The golden rule is to surrender life insurance policies only as a last resort. Life insurance policies can be quite valuable and a number are highly saleable, but only if the insurance policy is kept in force until a buyer can be found.

The people who surrender or abandon their endowment policies early fund the investment performance of those policyholders who hold out for the full term. Generally speaking, seven out of every eight policyholders surrender their policies before they mature.

Life insurance companies impose the vast bulk of their charges early on, so most, if not all, of what goes into the policy in the first two years will not actually be invested. Anyone surrendering a policy within three years will receive virtually nothing back. However, there are alternatives to surrendering insurance policies.

Making a policy paid up

This can often provide the best choice for people who need to cut down spending but are able to leave existing savings where they are. Making a policy paid up simply means ceasing to pay premiums with the agreement of the insurer.

This option is useful to people who would like some money to be paid out by the insurance company to their estate in the event of their death.

Borrowing against the policy

This option is available if the policy has been in force for some years, and can produce ready cash at better rates than bank loans. Normally you can borrow up to 85% of the policy surrender value, and you do not have to return any of the money borrowed until the policy is due to mature. Further details of this option are available from your insurance company.

Auctioning or selling the policy

This option will produce better returns than surrendering the policy. Typical sale or auction values are at least 25% above the surrender value, although they can be much greater. The policies are bought by people who will continue the payments until the policy matures or the life assured dies, at which time the insurance company will pay out the benefits to the person who has bought it.

Most buyers will never meet the 'life assured', nor will they know when that life assured dies.

Accordingly they generally value the policy on the assumption that they will only cash the policy in when it matures. However, if a life assured makes it known that his life is impaired i.e. that his life expectancy is shorter than usual, buyers may be prepared to pay more for the policy, as they would expect that the insurance company will be paying the death benefit sooner than would normally be the case.

Increasing numbers of people who have declared that their lives are impaired because of an HIV-related infection are finding that buyers are not prepared to pay as much for the policy as they might have paid a few years ago. As well as the current economic climate, this is also due to the general increases in life expectancy of people who are successfully receiving HAART.

Some firms buy policies with their own funds, which means that they can pay promptly rather than waiting for a buyer. Examples of such firms include Life Benefit Resources and International Viatical Settlements (UK). Both firms offer slightly different terms depending on the size of the policy, its remaining term and the policy holder's life expectancy. Eligible policies include Term Assurance, Whole of Life and Endowment policies, both unit linked and with-profits. Both firms will offer a free quote without obligation.

Other firms act as agents, and will need to find a buyer before the policy holder receives any cash. This can sometimes take time. Agents also take a commission from the transaction, usually between 10-12.5% of the price, which is deducted from the sellers proceeds.

Some firms act as auctioneers. The disadvantage of this process for someone with a terminal illness is the degree of disclosure of confidential information about your medical condition which may be required during the auction. Auctions also take place only occasionally, and policies may not attract a buyer, which entails a delay before any cash is received.

Reputable firms recommend that policy holders take independent advice, such as from a solicitor, before selling their policy. All firms in this field should be registered under the Financial Services Act. It is not advisable to deal with firms which are not registered. Firms buying policies from people who are diagnosed as having a terminal illness will seek medical confirmation of the prognosis which should be treated in absolute confidence.

Making a 'living will'

What is a living will?

A living will is a means of indicating your wishes about what sort of medical treatment you wish to receive in the event that you become unconscious or otherwise unable to communicate your wishes. Living wills are often also known as *Advance Directives*. Living wills are often, but not necessarily, associated with medical treatment at the end of life. They are also usually thought of in connection with requests to cease or refuse medical treatment, but a living will is really about expressing one's wishes about medical treatment, whatever they may be.

A living will is about medical treatment only. You cannot use it to say what is to happen to your property after your death, or to make funeral requests. To dispose of property you need to make an ordinary will (see above).

How to make a living will

There is no set legal format for a living will. Various organisations have produced their own forms for people to fill in, and some solicitors draw them up individually. Organisations producing forms include the Voluntary Euthanasia Society, the Patients Association, and the Terrence Higgins Trust (THT). The THT form was produced jointly with Kings College Centre of Medical Law and Ethics and is available free of charge from THT and other HIV organisations and care centres. It was produced in close collaboration with people with HIV, and specialist medical professionals, and is designed for people to fill in themselves without a lawyer.

You can use a living will to do either or both of the following:

- You can state in advance your wishes regarding medical treatment. These statements are called advance directives.

- You can appoint someone, called a health care proxy, to take part on your behalf in decisions about medical treatment.

The living will produced by THT sets out three possible scenarios:

- Physical illness from which there is no likelihood of recovery. In this case you can say what your wishes are if you develop an infection or other illness which cannot be cured and which has become so serious that your life is nearly at an end because of it.

- Permanent mental impairment in which an individual is suffering from an irreversible impairment to his/her mental functions which is so severe that the individual does not understand what is happening to him/her, and develops a physical illness from which there is no likelihood of recovery.

- Permanent unconsciousness from which there is no likelihood of regaining consciousness.

In each case, the document gives you the option of stating that you would wish to be kept alive by medical treatment, or of refusing treatment other than to keep you comfortable and free from pain.

It also gives you the opportunity to state your wishes about particular medical treatments or investigations about which you may have a preference. For instance, you may not wish to have certain sorts of painful tests, or to receive certain sorts of drugs. You might also have views about ventilation (artificial breathing), or the administration of food by tube.

It is best to discuss your wishes with your doctor partly to ensure that you have understood the options, and expressed your wishes in a way which makes medical sense, and partly so that if the time comes to put the Living Will into effect, there is evidence from your doctor on the points which have to be proved in order for it to be legally binding (see below)

Bear in mind that you can change or cancel a Living Will so long as you are fit to do so. What you decide now is not set in stone, and if your circumstances change you may wish to make a new Living Will, expressing slightly different views.

You can also use your living will to appoint someone, such as a partner, friend or family member, to take part in medical decisions on your behalf if you become unable to do so yourself. This person is known as your Health Care Proxy. You should discuss your intentions with the person you have in mind. You need to make sure that he or she is prepared to take on this role, knows your wishes about medical treatment, and is prepared to express them on your behalf. The role of the *next of kin* has some similarities, but the emphasis is on the administrative function of being someone for the hospital to contact in an emergency, rather than someone with whom issues might be discussed. *Next of kin* has no clear legal definition in this context, and you can name anybody. It is probably less confusing for the hospital if the same person is named as *next of kin* on your hospital notes and as health care proxy in your living will. You should also be aware that the law is unclear when it comes to disputes after a death. If there is any risk of arguments about who should arrange a funeral, it is worth remembering that the law gives this responsibility to the executor of a will, if there is one, but that hospitals will normally release a body to whoever they consider to be the *next of kin*.

As the law stands (see below) nobody at all, including your proxy has the right to express legally binding wishes about medical treatment on your behalf. If you are incapable of expressing a view, and have not made a valid advance directive, doctors are entitled to treat you in accordance with their assessment of your best interests. However, doctors often value knowing who it is that you have chosen to participate in decisions about your care, especially in a situation where there seem to be a number of people all claiming to know you best and all expressing different opinions.

Make sure that those close to you (especially your Health Care Proxy) know that you have made a Living Will and where to find it.

If you have to go into hospital, make sure your doctor there knows you have a Living Will and that a copy is in your medical notes. Ideally you should also discuss your wishes with a member of the medical team, both when you make the living will, and on admission to hospital.

What is the legal status of a living will?

Advance refusals of treatment

Most people who make a living will do so in order to refuse medical treatment. In principle, an adult of sound mind may refuse medical treatment.

An advance refusal of medical treatment will be legally binding if it is *clearly established and applicable to the circumstances*. Three conditions must be fulfilled:

- The maker must have had mental capacity (this in itself involves another complicated assessment, but in everyday terms implies that the person understood in broad terms the nature and effect of what they were doing, and possessed the ability to understand the available options and to make a choice).

- The maker must have been subject to no undue influence at the time of expressing the refusal

- The maker must have had in his or her contemplation the circumstances which have arisen. This means that they must have considered the likely future scenario, so that for example a refusal of treatment when facing a terminal illness would not necessarily apply after a road accident (re T (Adult: Refusal of Treatment) [1993] Fam 95).

The statement need not be in writing, but evidentially a clearly written, signed and witnessed document will be much easier to establish.

Artificial nutrition and hydration constitute medical treatment and may therefore be the subject of a valid advance directive (Airedale NHS Trust v Bland [1993] AC 789). It is likely that for public policy reasons a refusal of basic care (not defined but including warmth, comfort and hygiene - and arguably spoon feeding) will not be binding. Re C (Adult: Refusal of Medical Treatment) [1994] 1 WLR 290 confirmed that an individual may seek an injunction to enforce a refusal of treatment, and highlighted that a mental patient may have sufficient capacity to have his or her wishes concerning physical treatment respected.

Limitations

An Advance Directive cannot override statutory authority where this exists, for example provisions for compulsory treatment in the Public Health Act 1984 and the Mental Health Act 1983. A person who is lawfully detained under the provisions of the Mental Health Act may be treated for mental disorder regardless of their consent. A person with a disorder such as Anorexia Nervosa may be detained and receive treatment (including forcible feeding since in this instance the lack of eating is considered to be part of the mental condition).

There is also controversy the extent to which a pregnant woman may refuse medical treatment (notably a caesarian section) where medical opinion considers that the foetus's life may be at risk. It seems following a decision by the Court of Appeal on 26 March 1996 that a pregnant woman may continue to refuse treatment, even if that could risk the life of the foetus, so long as she has full mental capacity. However, capacity is likely to be strictly tested.

What is lawful is the refusal of medical treatment: a living will cannot be used to require treatment aimed solely at hastening death since that would amount to euthanasia which is illegal in the UK.

According to present law the refusal of medical treatment by children and young people under the age of eighteen is not legally binding, even though the consent to treatment of a young person of sufficient understanding is binding (Re R: (Minor, Refusal of Treatment) [1991] 3 WLR 592). A young person with a life threatening condition does not therefore have an absolute right to refuse medical treatment in the face of parental or medical opposition.

Advance requests for medical treatment

There is no right to insist on any particular treatment from the NHS, and the Courts have repeatedly stated that they will not interfere in questions of resource allocation or clinical judgement (R v Cambridge District Health Authority, ex p B (1995) 2 All ER 129)

Treatment from a private doctor is a matter of contract, but the doctor will be bound by professional ethics.

Healthcare proxies

Such an appointment is not at present legally binding, so it is up to the individual doctor how much weight to place on the views expressed by the proxy. This is in contrast with an attorney under a power of attorney, whose powers are legally binding, but only apply to dealing with property and financial affairs.

Further information

Advance statements about medical treatment, code of practice, British Medical Association, 1995.

Practical guidance to doctors on dealing with living wills

Mental Incapacity: Law Commission Report, 1995.

A major review of the law relating to incapacity and decision making. Proposals for reform include a statutory basis for advance directives and provision for health care proxies to be appointed along similar lines to the Enduring Power of Attorney.

Palliative care

What is palliative care, and why does it matter now?

The advent of antiretroviral therapy has brought greatly reduced morbidity and mortality among people living with HIV disease. Unfortunately, it has also meant that we often focus on the clinical aspects of therapy and viral suppression to the exclusion of the enduring principles of palliative care: attention to the physical, emotional and spiritual distress of those patients and families affected by life-threatening disease.

The WHO definition of palliative care is as relevant now as it was in the early days of the epidemic (*see* box 1). For people with advanced HIV in the 1980s and early 1990s, good terminal care was the best that could be hoped for when advanced stages of the disease were reached. During this time, a number of day centres, community services and specialist HIV hospices were developed. As the benefits of antiretroviral therapy were identified, the focus of care shifted to an emphasis on viral suppression. However, there are five important reasons why palliative care should be available from the point of diagnosis within the modern multiprofessional HIV care team.

Firstly, a significant proportion of HIV-infected individuals are unaware of their diagnosis, and present only with advanced disease. For these patients, palliative approaches to advanced disease management need to be incorporated with antiretroviral treatment options. For patients with advanced disease and severely compromised immune function, the challenges of immune reconstitution syndrome may further necessitate a joint approach between HIV medicine and palliative care teams. For these patients, antiretroviral therapy may be followed by a period of severe ill health as the immune system begins to increase its capacity to respond to infections within the body, infections that to date have been allowed to flourish unchecked.

Second, globally people with HIV continue to die at a higher rate than the uninfected (Sabin), and the virological failure rate with first- and second-line therapy remains a risk (Tamalet; Dragsted). Treatment failure or non-adherence can lead to progressive immunological failure and the development of life-threatening consequences. Therefore, the availability of antiretroviral therapy has not taken away the need for the historically defining feature of palliative care, i.e. high quality end-of-life care for those who need it, with the aim of providing a "good death". However, terminal care is less often required in resource-rich countries with universal access to antiretroviral therapy compared to resource poor countries.

Third, pain and other distressing symptoms may be experienced from relatively early in the disease trajectory, and antiretroviral drugs are associated with a significant rate of toxicities and side-effects (Heath) such as peripheral neuropathy and gastrointestinal problems. The availability of therapy has increased the need for specialist palliative care staff who can assess and treat the distressing symptoms associated with new therapies. The experience of symptom burden may compromise the ability to adhere to drug regimens as well as have a negative impact on the patient's quality of life. Such pain and symptom problems may be present from relatively early stages of infection, and involvement of palliative care is therefore appropriate for symptom control at any stage from the point of diagnosis.

Fourth, some HIV-related malignancies such as non-Hodgkin's Lymphoma, cervical carcinoma and colorectal and lung malignancies have not declined in incidence with HAART (Matheny; Yeguez; Powles). For patients whose cancers are not responsive to curative approaches, then the traditional terminal cancer care aspects of palliative care will be necessary. It is also required to support individuals through potentially curative cancer treatment, for cancers such as Non-Hodgkin's Lymphoma, anal squamous cell cancers, and Kaposi's Sarcoma.

Fifth, as a result of surviving longer, new co-morbidities have become apparent such as end-stage liver disease secondary to hepatitis C co-infection, myocardial infarction (Mary-Krause), and cerebrovascular disease (Rabinstein). Since its inception in the UK in the 1960s, the modern palliative care movement and the medical discipline of palliative medicine, have made significant contributions to patient care beyond malignant (i.e. cancer) care into other life-limiting diseases that are likely to be presented by patients. Patients may also require the spiritual and psycho-social support services of palliative care to help in coming to terms with their changing morbidity and mortality with respect to an uncertain prognosis.

For these reasons, the WHO has declared palliative care to be an essential component of the package of care for people living with HIV/AIDS in both resource-rich and resource-poor settings (SEE BOX2). However, the proportion of care that is symptom control, care for co-morbidities and terminal care will vary according to the country and availability of health care resources (e.g. diagnostic and curative cancer therapies, and antiretroviral therapy).

The World Health Organisation (WHO) definition of palliative care (2005a):"*an approach that improves the quality of life of patients and their families facing the problems associated with life-threatening illness, through the prevention and relief of suffering by means of early identification and impeccable assessment and treatment of pain and other problems, physical, psychosocial and spiritual.*"

The WHO statement on palliative care in HIV (2005b):"*Palliative care is an essential component of the package of care for people living with HIV/AIDSbecause of the variety of symptoms they can experience- such as pain, diarrhoea, cough, shortness of breath, nausea, weakness, fatigue, fever and confusion. At the community level, lack of palliative care places an unnecessary burden on hospital or clinic resources".*

The World Health Organisation (WHO) definition of palliative care (2005a):

"*an approach that improves the quality of life of patients and their families facing the problems associated with life-threatening illness, through the prevention and relief of suffering by means of early identification and impeccable assessment and treatment of pain and other problems, physical, psychosocial and spiritual.*"

The WHO statement on palliative care in HIV (2005b):

"*Palliative care is an essential component of the package of care for people living with HIV/AIDSbecause of the variety of symptoms they can experience - such as pain, diarrhoea, cough, shortness of breath, nausea, weakness, fatigue, fever and confusion. At the community level, lack of palliative care places an unnecessary burden on hospital or clinic resources".*

Holistic team care: the palliative total care approach

The philosophy of palliative care is that it aims to maximise the quality of life, and also aims to make death as comfortable as possible when it comes. Palliative care teams support the whole family unit, whoever they may be, and seeks to help those around the patient to come to terms with the diagnosis, to support them during the length of the disease, and to assist them into the bereavement phase. The palliative care team is multidisciplinary, and may consist of a doctor, nurse, social worker, dietician, occupational therapist, physiotherapist, psychologist, and spiritual professionals of many or no fixed denominations.

HIV care services have been progressive and multiprofessional in their care mix, but without the palliative care element these is a potentially significant loss to patient care. While not all patients will need palliative care, and palliative care may need to be introduced and withdrawn as different complex problems emerge and are resolved, it is crucial that links and referral systems operate to ensure that such care is available.

The addition of specialist input to address complex pain and symptom issues, and to support patients and families through challenging life changes, can make a large difference to clinical team services and assist in case loads. The evidence suggests that palliative care improves the health and wellbeing of people with HIV, particularly in the domains of pain and symptom control, anxiety, insight and spiritual well-being (Harding).

The challenges of HIV in the era of antiretroviral therapy have presented a new model of palliative care integration, necessitating a revised model from one of steadily increasingly palliative input as curative options lessen in cancer care (Figure 1). Figure 2 shows that in HIV care, palliative staff may increase their input and then withdraw according to need. The uncertain prognosis we currently face means that the palliative care team may not necessarily need to provide terminal care due to improved life expectancy with the new therapeutic regimes. However, they will be often be required to assist in the management of pain and symptoms, psychosocial and spiritual problems. The models show that palliative care has taken an increasing role in improving the quality of life and as well helping the patent and family to face its end.

The importance of joint care: HIV teams and specialist palliative care

The changing epidemiology of HIV disease in the era of HAART has resulted in new and evolving roles for palliative care. The shift has been from the more conventional (terminal) HIV palliative care of the 1980's and early 1990s to a greater focus on symptom-control in patients with a chronic disease like diabetes. These patients may continue to live for an extended period, and may need active treatment for one HIV-related condition and palliation for another simultaneously (Easterbrook).

The likelihood of active and palliative treatment, and the specialist skills that might be required of the two approaches, underline the importance of joint working. There are numerous examples of strong links and working systems of care between HIV medicine and palliative care, and these are the result of a sound understanding and respect for each other's roles, sound assessment of patient needs, and good communication. It is essential that HIV health professionals and palliative care teams work closely together. Both teams have specialist knowledge that may benefit the patient. The palliative care team need to be aware of signs of HIV disease progression, the implication of symptoms in the context of immune suppression, the importance of strict adherence to antiretroviral therapy and that drug interruptions must be supervised, the high level of drug interactions and adverse effects. Close liaison with the HIV team will enable the palliative care team to refer back for active treatment as appropriate. Also both teams' services may change and joint care ensures that individuals receive all available help and support.

What do palliative care teams do for people with HIV?

Palliative care teams will:

- Advise on control of treatment related symptoms.

- Palliate alongside active treatment in opportunistic infection and malignancy.

- Provide support around social needs.

- Help HIV teams to make appropriate treatment decisions.

- Help with psychological support.

- Be involved in terminal care (including supporting carers into bereavement).

Symptom control

Individuals with HIV can experience symptoms even in early infection but in advanced disease they experience a similar burden of symptoms as their fellow-sufferers with advanced malignancy. Anorexia, fatigue, pain, fever and cough are amongst the common symptoms in far advanced disease. Symptoms can arise from the direct effect of the HIV viraemia, as a result of drug therapy, opportunistic diseases, immune reconstitution or unrelated causes.

Pain is experienced by 50 -88% of individuals with advanced disease. Pain associated with infections (e.g. herpes simplex infection) is common even in early disease. Headache, arthralgia and myalgia are more common than in the non-infected population. Painful peripheral neuropathy occurs in up to 20% individuals receiving HIV medication although it

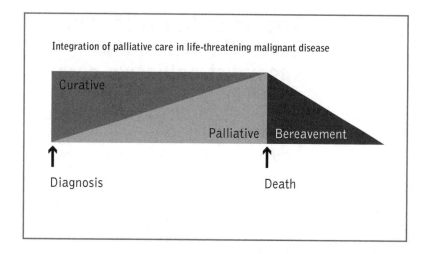

Integration of palliative care in life-threatening malignant disease

Curative

Palliative | Bereavement

↑ Diagnosis   ↑ Death

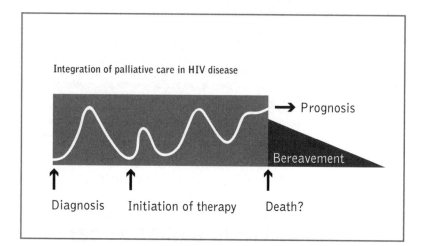

Integration of palliative care in HIV disease

→ Prognosis

Bereavement

↑ Diagnosis   ↑ Initiation of therapy   ↑ Death?

may be caused by drugs or HIV or both. It presents as a painful or numb feeling in both feet and sometimes the hands. Some individuals find benefit from non-drug therapies such as acupuncture or massage. Pain control may not be optimal in general HIV clinics and reasons given for this include the absence of advice about pain. The potential of antiretroviral medications for interactions must be considered when prescribing analgesics.

Nausea and vomiting occur commonly as a consequence of disease or medication including septrin and protease inhibitors which may have to be discontinued as a consequence. Tolerance to this adverse drug effect does develop in some individuals but antiemetic medication is often required. Diarrhoea is another common side-effect of antiretroviral treatment as well as being a consequence of the underlying HIV infection, and occurs with 32% of individuals on protease inhibitors.

Case Study

Charity is a 30 year-old woman from Zimbabwe who has been HIV-positive for ten years and taking antiretroviral therapy for the last four years. She was referred to the palliative care clinic with pain in her feet. She has felt tingling and sharp pains with numbness in both feet for two years. More recently the pain has increased and she has difficulty sleeping because of it. She has to wear "sensible" shoes and walking makes the pain worse. She has tried "over the counter" painkillers with little relief.

After assessment and investigations she is told that she has peripheral neuropathy. The cause may be her HIV or treatment or both. She has been stable on her current regime and both Charity and her HIV doctor are reluctant to change drugs. She is offered a range of treatment including complementary therapy, topical treatment and drug therapy. She starts on medication to treat the symptoms and finds that the tingling and sharp pains

reduce. She still has numbness and some pins and needles but she is content because she can sleep and wear shoes with heels.

Palliation alongside active treatment for opportunistic infections and malignancies

The HIV and palliative care teams complement each other in providing active and supportive care to individuals who may develop illness as a consequence of their immune suppression. This is outside the usual remit of palliative care teams who would normally restrict their involvement to those individuals with progressive, incurable disease. In practice, however, it makes sense to have teams placing priority on both aggressive treatment and quality of life issues.

Case Study

John is 40 and has been infected with HIV for fifteen years. He has been taking combination antiretroviral therapy for the last twelve years. He presented with pain and bleeding from his anus four months ago which was diagnosed as anal cancer. He was devastated by the news but was told that his scans showed localised disease only and that with treatment he could be cured. He agreed to have six weeks of chemotherapy and radiotherapy during which time he remained in hospital. He experienced increasing pain in his anus and rectum requiring regular morphine. He had diarrhoea and superficial painful ulcers of the skin at the site of his radiotherapy. During his treatment he felt out of control. He decided that he had to tell his family (including his rather frail elderly mother) about the cancer diagnosis although not all of them know about his HIV status.

The Palliative Care team were involved from his diagnosis of cancer to help him with information and support him emotionally come to terms with his new diagnosis. They also helped him to think about who he might want to share the information with and how. They saw him regularly during his treatment to address his symptoms and continue to provide psychological support. At his request they spoke with his mother to explain to her about his cancer diagnosis and the good prognosis. After his treatment finished his diarrhoea and pain slowly improved and the palliative care team continued to see John as an out patient to supervise the reduction in his analgesics.

Treatment decisions

There are some infections and malignancies that occur in HIV disease where it is not clear whether aggressive treatment is the right option. The views of the patient and their carers, the HIV team and the palliative care team may all help to make a balanced decision about what is appropriate treatment. There may come a point where the patient decides that although further life-prolonging treatment is possible they would rather pursue quality than quantity of life. These decisions require much discussion and appropriate information.

Terminal care

Palliative care teams are accustomed to providing holistic terminal care to patients with advanced progressive diseases of all types including HIV. Alongside symptom control, they will explore emotional and spiritual needs, try to address financial and practical issues including where the individual wishes to die and give support to carers and relatives. The patient's need for confidentiality must be respected although this sometimes leads to difficulties communicating with other health care professionals outside the immediate team and with the family. Funding for HIV community support and HIV specific inpatient hospice beds has reduced over the last decade which has made it more important for general palliative care teams to extend their services to the HIV population.

Social support

Case Study

Robert acquired HIV through intravenous drugs six years ago. He also has Hep C infection and despite treatment he remains Hep C positive. Over the last two years his liver function has been deteriorating and he has had repeated admissions with complications of his failing liver. He has found it impossible to tolerate taking antiretrovirals and he now has advanced immunosuppression with a CD4 count of 20. He has been seen by a liver transplant team but because he remains Hep C positive and has such poor immune function he has not been offered a liver transplant.

Robert is admitted again with jaundice and a distended abdomen because of ascites - a collection of fluid within the abdominal cavity. The palliative care team are asked to see him to help with pain and nausea. As they get to know him he tells them that he knows is very ill. He starts to talk about all the admissions he has had and how his quality of life has been poor for the past two years.

One night Robert suffers a large gastrointestinal bleed. He has a central line put in and an endoscopy. The bleeding settles but it is clear that he has terminal liver failure and time is limited. Robert tells the nurses and the palliative care team that he has had enough and wants the treatment stopped. His best friend comes in and agrees that Robert has told her that he would not want his life prolonged if he was terminally ill. The palliative care team represent Robert's view to the rest of the health care team looking after him and it is agreed that Robert is entitled to stop his treatment. He understands what he is saying and is mentally competent. He calls his family who he had been keeping at arms length and tells them what is happening. His family are understandably distraught and need a lot of explanation and support. Robert has his intravenous lines taken out and is able to go to his flat for the afternoon to arrange some paperwork. He realises that he will not feel comfortable at home and does not want to be a burden to his friend or his family. The palliative care team discuss the options, including transfer to a hospice, but Robert decides that he would rather stay in the hospital ward where he is well known and where he is familiar with all the nurses. He has his favourite photos brought in and his music and spends some days with his friends and family in a more cheerful mood. He dies on the ward and the hospital palliative care team are able to support him and his carers up to the end.

Who can provide palliative care?

Palliative care is not yet seen as a medical speciality in all countries. However, modern nursing and clinical training usually includes some introduction to palliative medicine and palliative care. Modern HIV care is a multiprofessional discipline, and members of the team should have the basic skills of holistic care required to meet basic palliative care needs. Intractable symptoms, anxiety and psychosocial/spiritual crises associated with incurable disease, and terminal care may all present challenges to the care team that require consultation with specialist palliative care staff. Clear referral guidelines are extremely helpful in identifying those patients who may benefit from specialist input. The availability of palliative care training to the HIV care team, as well as established named links to specialist palliative care, are important steps to ensuring that patients can access the care they need.

Palliative care may be provided in a number of settings:

- In patient hospital care
- Nursing homes
- Outpatient clinics
- Primary care settings
- In patients' homes
- Hospices

It may be provided by specialist voluntary-sector funded services such as Macmillan nurses, Marie Curie nurses or hospice staff, or by statutory sector hospital-based palliative care services and trained General Practitioners.

The palliative care model is strongly multiprofessional, and may include:

- Doctor
- Nurse
- Social worker
- Physiotherapist
- Welfare benefits adviser
- Occupational therapist
- Art therapist
- Music therapist
- Aromatherapist
- Dietician
- Counsellor
- Religious/spiritual advisor

When should we refer to palliative care?

People living with HIV disease may need a referral for palliative care input at any point though the disease trajectory, from the point of diagnosis into the advanced stages. However, not all patients will need to be seen by specialist palliative care. Modern, holistic health care services should be able to provide very basic palliative care by paying attention to the "total care" needs of the patent and their family, offering support when needed and applying basic knowledge of pain and symptom control.

More complex cases may require the specialist skills of a multiprofessional palliative care team. There are many appropriate reasons for referring to palliative care, and referrals should not be restricted to the terminal stages of the disease when the end-of-life seems imminent.

Some examples of when co-management between HIV and palliative care teams can improve the quality of overall care include:

- advising on and delivering expert pain and symptom control where distressing symptoms have persisted.

- managing the emotional and physical challenges experienced by patients and families facing advanced disease when the patient's health may deteriorate. Support may be needed to make treatment decisions and to come to terms with an uncertain prognosis.

- assisting in the adjustment to living with new and emerging co-morbidities such as cancers.

- assessing and managing complex health and social care needs for patient and families who are preparing for a discharge for the patient to be cared for at home.

In order to achieve best patient care and quality of life, and to ensure appropriate referrals are considered, HIV and palliative care teams should establish guidelines for referral criteria and patient co-management. These efforts can be very rewarding in understanding and respecting each other's specialties, and in establishing successful ways of harmonising active treatments and palliative care.

It should be remembered that the introduction of the palliative care team might raise some anxieties for patients and families due to its origins in terminal care. Patients may choose to refuse to see palliative care staff if they believe them to be solely responsible for end-of-life care, or may see their involvement as a sign that active treatment is to be withdrawn without discussion. Such misunderstandings can be avoided through ongoing integrated care systems where palliation is routinely introduced and withdrawn as appropriate. Some palliative care clinicians introduce themselves to patients as members of the "symptom control team" to allay such fears. It is important that HIV clinicians have a broad understanding of what palliative care offers to those *living* with HIV disease so that they may introduce the potential for referral to the patient without causing undue anxiety.

Further resources

Hospice Information Service
www.hospiceinformation.info

Palliative care in sub-Saharan African: a review
www.theworkcontinues.org/causes/pall_library.asp

Integrating palliative care into the continuum of HIV Care. An agenda for change. Workgroup on Palliative and End-of-Life Care in HIV/AIDS. Recommendations to the field. The Robert Wood Johnson Foundation. 2004.

References

Sabin CA. The changing clinical epidemiology of AIDS in the highly active antiretroviral therapy era. AIDS 16: S61-S68, 2002.

Tamalet C et al.. Resistance of HIV-1 to multiple antiretroviral drugs in France: a 6-year survey (1997-2002) based on an analysis of over 7000 genotypes. AIDS 17: 2383-2388, 2003.

Dragsted UB et al. Randomized trial to evaluate indinavir/ritonavir versus saquinavir/ritonavir in human immunodeficiency virus type 1-infected patients: the MaxCmin1 Trial. Journal of Infectious Diseases 188: 635-642, 2003.

Heath KV et al.. Emerging drug toxicities of highly active antiretroviral therapy for human immunodeficiency virus (HIV) infection. Current Drug Targets 4: 13-22, 2003.

Matheny SC. Clinical dilemmas in palliative care for HIV infection. Journal of the Royal Society of Medicine 94: 449-451, 2001.

Yeguez JF, Martinez SA, Sands DR, Sands LR, Hellinger MD. Colorectal malignancies in HIV-positive patients. American Surgeon 69: 981-987, 2003.

Powles T, Nelson M, Bower M. HIV-related lung cancer- a growing concern? Internatinal Journal of STD and AIDS 14: 647-651, 2003.

Mary-Krause M, Cotte L, Simon A, Partisani M, Costagliola D. Increased risk of myocardial infarction with duration of protease inhibitor therapy in HIV-infected men. AIDS 17: 2479-2486, 2003.

Rabinstein AA. Stroke in HIV-infected patients: a clinical perspective. Cerbrovascular Diseases 15: 37-44, 2003.

WHO 2005a. WHO definition of palliative care. http://www.who.int/cancer/palliative/definition/en/ 2005.

WHO 2005b. Palliative Care. http://www.who.int/hiv/topics/palliative/care/en/ , 2005.

Harding R, Karus D, Easterbrook P, Raveis V, Higginson I.J and Marconi K. Does palliative care improve outcomes for patients with HIV/AIDS? A systematic review of the evidence. Sexually Transmitted Infections 2004: in press.

Easterbrook P and Meadway J. The changing epidemiology of HIV infection: New challenges for HIV palliative care. Journal of the Royal Society of Medicine 94: 442-448, 2001.

Index

Index

Index

K

L

I

Index

S

T

U

V

W

Index

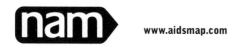 www.aidsmap.com

please make a
monthly
donation to nam today

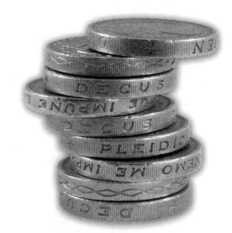

my details

name

address

telephone   email

signature   i would like to gift aid the donation* ☐

* Gift Aid Declaration
I confirm that I am a UK taxpayer and would like NAM to claim the Gift Aid on all donations that I have made since 6 April 2000 and all donations in the future until I notify you otherwise.
To qualify for Gift Aid, what you pay in income tax or capital gains tax must be at least equal to the amount that NAM will claim in the current tax year (currently 28p for every £1 donated).

☐ We publish a range of information resources on HIV & AIDS. Please tick this box if you would **not** like to be added to our mailing list.

☐ We occasionally undertake fundraising campaigns to help support our work. Please tick this box if you would **not** like to receive information about them.

---

i'd like to support NAM with a monthly gift of

☐ £25

☐ £10

☐ £5

☐ other   £ _____

DIRECT Debit

originator's identification number 679497

please return this form to

NAM, Freepost LON17995, London, SW9 6BR

tel   020 7840 0050
fax   020 7735 5351
email info@nam.org.uk
web   www.aidsmap.com

NAM is a UK registered charity number 1011220

Instruction to please pay NAM Publications Direct Debits from the account detailed in this instruction subject to the safeguards assured by the Direct Debit Guarantee. I understand that this instruction may remain with NAM Publications and if so, details will be passed electronically to my bank/building society. Banks and building societies may not accept direct debit instructions for some types of accounts.

instruction to your bank or building society to pay by direct debit

name of account holder(s)

account number   branch sortcode

bank name

bank address

bank postcode

please select a monthly payment date (if not selected the payment date will be the 1st)   ☐ 1st   ☐ 10th   ☐ 20th

date   signature   reference (for office use only)

The Direct Debit Guarantee
This guarantee should be retained by the payer. This guarantee is offered by all Banks and Building Societies that take part in the Direct Debit scheme. The efficiency and security of the scheme is monitored and protected by your own Bank or Building Society. If the amounts to be paid or the payment dates changes, NAM Publications will notify you 10 working days in advance of your account being debited or as otherwise agreed. If an error is made by NAM Publications or your Bank/ Building Society you are guaranteed a full and immediate refund from your branch of the amount paid. You can cancel a Direct Debit at any time, by writing to your Bank or Building Society. Please also send a copy of your letter to us.

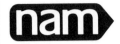

www.aidsmap.com

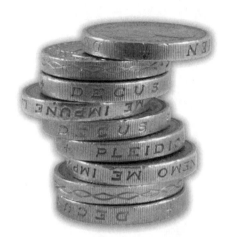

please make a
one-off
donation to nam today

my details

name

address

☐ We publish a range of information resources on HIV & AIDS. Please tick this box if you would **not** like to be added to our mailing list.

☐ We occasionally undertake fundraising campaigns to help support our work. Please tick this box if you would **not** like to receive information about them.

* Gift Aid Declaration
I confirm that I am a UK taxpayer and would like NAM to claim the Gift Aid on all donations that I have made since 6 April 2000 and all donations in the future until I notify you otherwise.
To qualify for Gift Aid, what you pay in income tax or capital gains tax must be at least equal to the amount that NAM will claim in the current tax year (currently 28p for every £1 donated).

i'd like to support NAM with a one-off gift of

☐ £10

☐ £50

☐ £100

☐ other £ _____

please return this form to

NAM, Freepost LON17995, London, SW9 6BR

tel   020 7840 0050
fax   020 7735 5351
email info@nam.org.uk
web   www.aidsmap.com

NAM is a UK registered charity number 1011220

payment method   ☐ cheque   ☐ charge my debit/credit card

card number

valid from   expiry date

name on card

issue number   3 digit security code

signature   date

card billing address

☐ as above

name

address